Medical Assisting
Administrative *and* Clinical Competencies

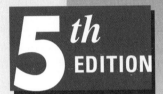

Lucille Keir, CMA-A
Barbara A. Wise, BSN, RN, MA(Ed)
Connie Krebs, CMA-C, BGS

THOMSON ™

DELMAR LEARNING   Australia   Canada   Mexico   Singapore   Spain   United Kingdom   United States

THOMSON

DELMAR LEARNING

Medical Assisting: Administrative and Clinical Competencies
Fifth Edition
by Lucille Keir, Barbara A. Wise, and Connie Krebs

Executive Director:
William Brottmiller
Executive Editor:
Cathy L. Esperti
Acquisitions Editor:
Rhonda Dearborn
Developmental Editor:
Deb Flis

Executive Marketing Manager:
Dawn F. Gerrain
Channel Manager—Career Education:
Mona Caron
Editorial Assistant:
Jill O'Brien
Technology Project Manager:
Laurie Davis
Technology Specialist:
Victoria Moore
Technology Production Coordinator:
Sherry McGaughan

Karen Leet
Art/Design Coordinator, Cover Design:
Robert Plante
Production Coordinator:
Nina Lontrato
Project Editor:
Shelley Esposito

Library of Congress Cataloging-in-Publication Data
Keir, Lucille.
  Medical Assisting: administrative and clinical competencies/ Lucille Keir, Barbara A. Wise, Connie Krebs—5th ed.
  p. ; cm.
  Includes bibliographical references and index.
  ISBN 0-7668-4146-4
  1. Medical Assistants   I. Wise, Barbara A.
  II. Krebs, Connie. III. Title. [DLNM: 1. Physician Assistants. 2. Clinical Competence. 3. Practice Management, Medical. 4. Vocational Guidance. W 21.5 K27m 2003]
  R728.8 K44 2003
  610.73'7—dc21
                    2002025907

International Divisions List

Asia (Including India):
Thomson Learning
60 Albert Street, #15-01
Albert Complex
Singapore 189969
Tel 65 336-6411
Fax 65 336-7411

Australia/New Zealand:
Nelson
102 Dodds Street
South Melbourne
Victoria 3205
Australia
Tel 61 (0)3 9685-4111
Fax 61 (0)3 9685-4199

Latin America:
Thomson Learning
Seneca 53
Colonia Polanco
11560 Mexico, D.F. Mexico
Tel (525) 281-2906
Fax (525) 281-2656

Canada:
Nelson
1120 Birchmount Road
Toronto, Ontario
Canada M1K 5G4
Tel (416) 752-9100
Fax (416) 752-8102

UK/Europe/Middle East/Africa:
Thomson Learning
Berkshire House
1680-173 High Holborn
London WC1V 7AA
United Kingdom
Tel 44 (0)20 497-1422
Fax 44 (0)20 497-1426

Spain (includes Portugal):
Paraninfo
Calle Magallanes 25
28015 Madrid
España
Tel 34 (0)91 446-3350
Fax 34 (0)91 445-6218

Notice to the Reader

TABLE OF CONTENTS

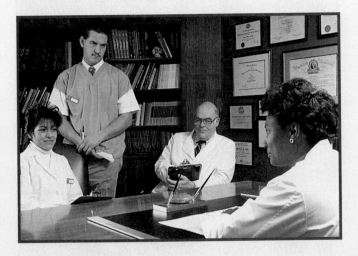

SECTION 1
MEDICAL HEALTH CARE ROLES AND RESPONSIBILITIES

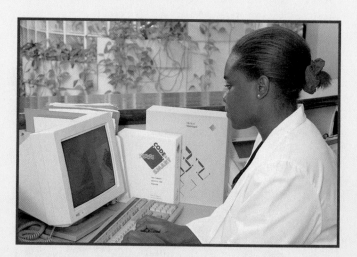

SECTION 2
THE ADMINISTRATIVE MEDICAL ASSISTANT 113

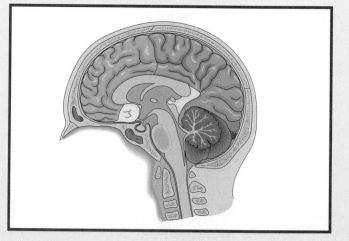

SECTION 3
STRUCTURE AND FUNCTION OF THE BODY   259

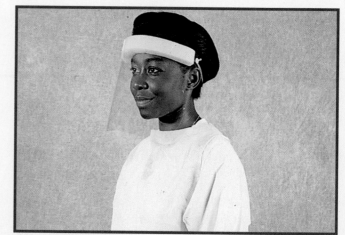

SECTION 4
THE CLINICAL MEDICAL ASSISTANT   525

CHAPTER 12
Preparing for Clinical Duties   526
Ⓒ Sterile Gloves and Gowns
Ⓒ Goves and Gown
Ⓒ Hand Washing
Ⓒ Infection Control
Ⓒ Removing Contaminated Items

CHAPTER 13
Beginning the Patient's Record   552
Ⓒ Weighing a Client
Ⓒ Taking a Temperature
Ⓒ Taking a Pulse
Ⓒ Counting Respirations
Ⓒ Taking Blood Pressure

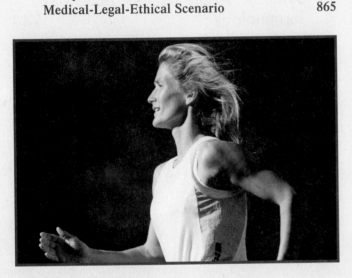

SECTION 5
BEHAVIORS AND HEALTH 865

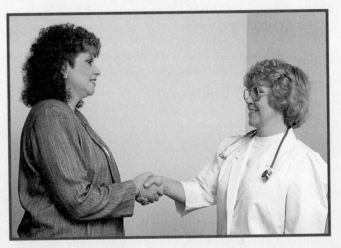

SECTION 6
EMPLOYABILITY SKILLS 909

■ MEDICAL ASSISTING SKILLS CD-ROMs QUICK LOCATOR

This is your link to Delmar's Medical Assisting Skills CD-ROMs, which are found on the inside back cover of this book.

Ⓐ = ADMINISTRATIVE SKILLS CD-ROM
Ⓒ = CLINICAL SKILLS CD-ROM

Text Chapter	Skills and Their Location on the CD-ROMs	Text Chapter	Skills and Their Location on the CD-ROMs
3	Ⓐ Legal Concepts	17	Ⓒ Hand Washing
5	Ⓐ Greeting Patients	17	Ⓒ Sterile Gloves and Gowns
6	Ⓐ Telephone Skills	17	Ⓒ Sutures and Staples
6	Ⓐ Telephone Messages	18	Ⓐ Prescriptions
6	Ⓐ Scheduling	18	Ⓒ Rectal Medications
6	Ⓐ Parts of a Letter	18	Ⓒ Oral Medications
6	Ⓐ Parts of the Envelope	18	Ⓒ Nebulized Medications
7	Ⓐ Medical Records	18	Ⓒ Skin/Topical Medications
7	Ⓐ Subject and Numeric Filing	18	Ⓒ Withdrawing from an Ampule
8	Ⓐ Billing and Collections	18	Ⓒ Medication from a Vial
8	Ⓐ Insurance and Coding	18	Ⓒ Mixing Medications from Vials
9	Ⓐ Insurance and Coding	18	Ⓒ Intradermal Medications
10	Ⓐ Banking	18	Ⓒ Subcutaneous Medications
10	Ⓐ Payroll Procedures	18	Ⓒ Intramuscular Medications
10	Ⓐ Purchase Orders	18	Ⓒ Z-tract Injection
10	Ⓐ Patient Receipts	19	Ⓒ Accidental Poisoning
11	Ⓐ Library (Anatomy & Physiology)	19	Ⓒ Heimlich Maneuver
12	Ⓒ Sterile Gloves and Gown	19	Ⓒ Administering CPR
12	Ⓒ Gloves and Gown	19	Ⓒ Applying a Splint
12	Ⓒ Hand Washing	19	Ⓒ Assisting with Casting
12	Ⓒ Infection Control	19	Ⓒ Cast Care and Comfort
12	Ⓒ Removing Contaminated Items	19	Ⓒ Applying Dry Heat
13	Ⓒ Weighing a Client	19	Ⓒ Applying a Cold Treatment
13	Ⓒ Taking a Temperature	19	Ⓒ Skin Puncture
13	Ⓒ Taking a Pulse	19	Ⓒ Bandaging
13	Ⓒ Counting Respirations	19	Ⓒ Dry Dressings
13	Ⓒ Taking Blood Pressure	19	Ⓒ Elastic Bandages
14	Ⓒ Weighing a Client	19	Ⓒ Safe Falling
15	Ⓒ Infection Control	19	Ⓒ ROM Exercises
15	Ⓒ Hand Washing	19	Ⓒ Applying an Arm Sling
15	Ⓒ Skin Puncture	19	Ⓒ Assisting with a Cane
15	Ⓒ Measuring Blood Glucose	19	Ⓒ Assisting with Crutches
15	Ⓒ Clean Catch Urine Sample	19	Ⓒ Assisting with a Walker
15	Ⓒ Testing Urine	19	Ⓒ Safe Lifting
15	Ⓒ Collecting Specimens	21	Ⓐ Writing a Resumé
15	Ⓒ Wound Specimens	21	Ⓐ Writing a Cover Letter
17	Ⓒ Infection Control	21	Ⓐ Writing a Thank You Letter

INDEX OF TABLES

INDEX OF PROCEDURES

■ INDEX OF PROCEDURES cont.

PREFACE

*M*edical Assisting: Administrative and Clinical Competencies, 5th Edition is a proven competency-based learning system with a 19-year history of success. The text is full-color throughout and written in an interesting, easy-to-understand format. The content covers the knowledge, skills, attitudes, and values necessary to prepare you to become a successful, multiskilled medical assistant. Information is presented in six major sections, which are divided into 21 chapters with a total of 80 units of instruction. There are hundreds of color photos, illustrations, charts, and tables to visually supplement and reinforce the written material. A student workbook, medical assisting skills CD-ROMs, instructor's manual, computerized testbank, and instructor's resource kit complete this learning system.

The text, workbook, and medical assisting skills CD-ROMs are comprehensive, covering the administrative, clinical, and general areas identified as necessary for entry level employment by the current Medical Assistant Role Delineation Study issued by the American Association of Medical Assistants (AAMA) and the National Board of Medical Examiners. The cognitive and performance competencies are identified by Learning Objectives, which are stated at the beginning of each unit of instruction or as Performance Objectives with each written administrative or clinical procedure.

A clear and concise presentation of human anatomy and physiology is included in the text. The structure and function of each system is followed by a discussion of the common diagnostic examinations and the diseases and disorders of that system. To facilitate learning, an expanded outline format organizes the description, signs and symptoms, etiology, and treatments for each disease.

The text, workbook, and medical assisting skills CD-ROMs are designed as instructive guides to learn the attitudes, behaviors, and skills necessary for a successful career as a multiskilled medical assistant in today's dynamic health care environment. They can be used in a variety of settings:

- a structured classroom setting, with the expertise of a qualified instructor
- for individualized instruction of learners in programs of diversified training because much of the content and format are appropriate for self study
- for on-the-job training in a physician's office, where the learning package serves as a supplement to employee instruction and as a resource manual

- for review by medical assistants who wish to prepare for the certification examination

Completion of the learning materials, including an understanding of the learning and performance objectives and application of the standard competencies during externship or employment, prepare the learner to successfully complete the CMA or RMA certification examination.

Two **Medical Assisting Clinical Skills CD-ROMs (Administrative and Clinical)** are found on the inside back cover of this book. This interactive software challenges you to apply content, think critically, develop competency in skills, and improve your knowledge base.

Together the authors have over 55 years of medical and academic educational preparation and employment experience. In addition, medical assistants, educators, nurses, physicians from general and specialty practices, a radiology technician, medical laboratory technicians, a medical engineer, and a bank manager have reviewed and contributed to this fifth edition.

WHAT'S NEW IN THE FIFTH EDITION?

Many changes were made to reflect the impact of technology, recent legislation, medical advances, and revised accreditation standards. Limitations on clinical laboratory procedures and the impact of this and other legislation on the operation of a medical office are explained. Other changes involve third-party payments, the shift to managed care, and the communication revolution. The anatomy and physiology content reflects advances in cellular biology applications, DNA sequencing, gene therapy, and the ever-changing diagnostic and treatment methods.

The major content changes are as follows:

General

- *New*—The appropriate areas of competence identified in the American Association of Medical Assistants (AAMA) Medical Assistant Role Delineation Study are identified at the beginning of each unit within the text. A chart of the study and a correlation to the text grid are included in Appendix A.
- *New*—An example of content in each unit of the book is identified, which addresses the standards for curriculum identified by the Commission on Accreditation of Allied Health Education Programs (CAAHEP). A listing of the required curriculum content is included in Appendix B and is accompanied with a correlation to the text grid.

- *New*—The program content requirements specified by the Accrediting Bureau of Health Education Schools (ABHES) are included in Appendix C along with a grid that correlates the standards to the text. At the end of each chapter, the program requirements are related to the content in a feature called "Relating to ABHES."

- *New*—The certification competencies for the registered medical assistant (RMA/AMT) credential are included in Appendix D.

- *New*—Content on the administrative and clinical skills CD-ROMs is identified in the book where it is appropriate to the subject matter being discussed.

- *New*—Web links that relate to the content were added to the end of chapters.

- *New*—A unit on complementary and alternative medical therapies is added to Chapter 20. This unit also includes discussion on the use of herbal supplements.

- *New*—Point-of-care and quality assurance are discussed.

- ***Revised and Expanded***—Medical-Legal-Ethical "Highlights" at the end each chapter is changed to "Scenario." These situations are followed by a feature called "Critical Thinking Challenge" that identifies areas to discuss and problems to be solved. Some challenges are related to the CAAHEP standards.

- ***Revised***—Information on career opportunities, career laddering, Bureau of Labor Statistics on employment forecasting, and professional credentials is included.

- ***Expanded***—Recent events in medicine are added to Chapter 1.

- ***Expanded***—Content on OSHA and safety in the work environment is included.

- ***Expanded***—Information on nutrition is included.

Administrative

- *New*—Content on the use of phone menus in physician's offices is added.

- *New*—Content on Internet use and downloading of information is added, and how to protect your system from a virus is also discussed.

- *New*—Cautions with accepting packages and opening mail as released by the U.S. Postal Service are discussed.

- *New*—Information is added to the management chapter regarding insurance and professional on-site reviews. A collection of topics usually evaluated is included in Appendix E.

- *New*—Content is included concerning the manager's responsibilities when moving an office.

- ***Expanded***—Information on filing and charting is included.

- ***Expanded***—Additional information on electronic communications and the use of computers is included.

- ***Revised***—Parts of speech and spelling rules are organized in a different format to make them easier to understand and use.

- ***Revised***—New mail classes and services of the U.S. Postal Service are included.

Insurance

- *New*—Information is included on the change of administration for Medicare to Centers for Medicare and Medigap Services. Also discussed is the effort to educate the public on services.

- *New*—The upcoming ICD-10 release is discussed.

- ***Expanded***—The types of HMOs are expanded to include point-of-service.

- ***Expanded***—Assurance of coverage is expanded to cover preauthorization, precertification, and predetermination. Also, content is added concerning identifying primary and secondary coverage responsibility.

Anatomy and Physiology

- *New*—Pediatric Perspectives are included in the content where appropriate to explain the differences or special considerations when the patient is a child.

- *New*—The most common medications or medication classification for treatment of the diseases are discussed.

- *New*—New guidelines for treatment of strokes are added.

- ***Revised and Expanded***—The diagnostic examinations with each system are included.

- ***Revised and Expanded***—The content on physiology includes recent research findings regarding the functions of the body.

- ***Revised and Expanded***—The content covering treatment of diseases and disorders includes current practices.

Clinical

- *New*—Examples of charting are included after each clinical procedure.

- *New*—Discussion and examples of log book entries are included.

- *New*—OSHA Guidelines including Standard Precautions are identified at the beginning of each procedure when appropriate.

- *New*—Content regarding Automated External Defibrillator (AED) is included.

- ***Expanded***—The medication discussion is expanded to include new medication and methods of administration.

- ***Expanded***—The discussion on progress notes is added.

- ***Revised***—The discussion of diagnostic procedures is updated.

- *Revised*—Burn classifications are changed to reflect new descriptions.
- *Revised*—CPR procedure is revised to reflect new terminology.
- *Deleted*—Because of recent CLIA regulations, laboratory tests that can only be performed by Clinical Lab Technicians are deleted from the text.

COMPREHENSIVE LEARNING PACKAGE

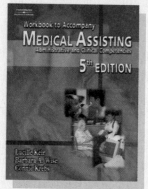

Student Workbook (0-7668-4150-2) contains unit-specific assignment sheets with a variety of review questions (including questions related to AAMA, CAAHEP, and ABHES), vocabulary and skill exercises, forms to complete, puzzles, and other activities that reinforce the text content. Continued in this edition, *the anatomy and physiology section is in full-color*. The workbook also includes Performance Evaluation Checklists for determining student competency of administrative, clinical, and general competencies of the text and *includes a point rating for each step*. The checklists correlate with the steps in the textbook procedures and reflect the performance objectives. The organization of the workbook places the assignment sheets in the same order as the text content. The Performance Evaluation Checklists are numbered as they are in the textbook and are in one complete section in the back of the workbook to make them easier to locate and use. Evaluation Checklists include a documentation section for students to practice charting the appropriate procedures.

A Certificate of Completion, to be completed and signed by the instructor, is included at the back of each workbook.

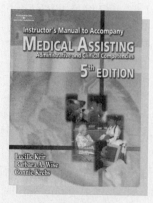

Instructor's Manual (0-7668-4147-2) has been improved to make it easier for instructors to identify answers to student workbook questions and exercises. The questions as well as the answers have now been included to facilitate evaluating the workbook assignment sheets. The Instructor's Manual includes:

- Correlation guide from the fourth to the fifth edition, identifying what features are new, expanded, or revised and where they can be found

- The AAMA Medical Assistant Role Delineation Study and an indepth correlation to the content in the text to help you identify skills taught in the program to a review committee
- The CAAHEP standards and an indepth correlation to the content in the text to help you identify the curriculum content for program approval
- The ABHES course content requirements for a medical assistant program and a correlation to the content of the text
- The complete Registered Medical Assistant (RMA/AMT) required certification competencies
- Instructional strategies and suggestions for presenting the course content, including integrating technology into the curriculum
- Instructional suggestions, organizational tips, and sample lesson plan format
- Section on establishing an externship program along with suggested tracking forms
- Chapter by chapter workbook questions with correct answers plus additional suggested activities for each chapter
- Documentation record of student scores for assignment sheets and performance evaluation sheets, which may be used in lieu of a gradebook, if so desired

Electronic Classroom Manager (0-7668-4148-0) includes the following:

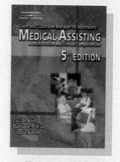

- **Computerized Testbank**—includes over 1,800 questions and answers. Question types include multiple choice, true and false, matching, completion, short answer, and art labeling. Instructors can also add their own questions or let the software create tests in just a few minutes.
- **Power Point® Presentation**—is a valuable resource for instructors that contains over 200 slides that outline a summary of key points from each chapter.
- **Electronic Lesson Plans**—include complete presentation outlines for each chapter in the text.

Instructor's Resource Kit (0-7668-4149-9) is a comprehensive 3-ring binder packed with instructional support for instructors at any level of educational program. It includes sections on:

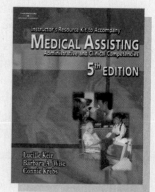

- **Concepts and Principles of Teaching and Learning**—discusses what teaching is, how students learn, basic learning principles, and steps in the learning process.

- **From Objectives to Evaluation**—discusses the purpose and benefits of identifying objectives, how to evaluate student competence, and how objectives and evaluation provide a solid framework for a competency-based education.
- **Instructional Strategies**—identifies ideas and methods of planning that make up the media of content presentation; describes a variety of methods for delivering instruction.
- **Lesson Plans**—discusses four-step lesson planning and design along with complete presentation outlines for each of the textbook units.
- **Class Activities**—provides additional ideas, activities, and materials to reinforce lessons, to make learning more relevant, and to help students apply concepts from theory to practice.
- **Transparency Masters**—includes individualized sheets that can be photocopied into overhead transparencies, aiding in the visual presentation of material.
- **Electronic Classroom Manager**—includes the computerized testbank, power point, and electronic lesson plans.

WebTUTOR™ on WebCT™ (1-4018-1400-X)
Text bundled with WebTUTOR™ on WebCT™ (1-4018-0398-9)
WebTUTOR™ on Blackboard™ (1-4018-1401-8)
Text bundled with Blackboard™ (1-4018-0397-0)
Designed to complement the text, WebTUTOR™ is a content-rich, web-based teaching and learning aid that reinforces and clarifies complex concepts. The WebCT™ and Blackboard™ platforms also provide rich communication tools to instructors and students, including a course calendar, chat, email, and threaded discussions.

Medical Assisting Administrative and Clinical Competencies, 5th edition Curriculum (1-4018-3991-6) is a great tool that enables instructors and administrators to create a Medical Assisting program while integrating content from this text and other Delmar Learning titles.

Delmar's Medical Assisting Video Series: Administrative and Clinical Procedures is a collection of 15 tapes with over nine hours of instruction to complement Delmar's medical assisting texts. They cover administrative, clinical,

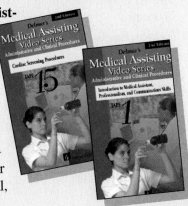

and laboratory procedures and interpersonal skills and characteristics.

Delmar's Medical Assisting CD-ROM (0-8273-8404-1) is a multimedia interactive program developed specifically for the field of medical assisting. The CD-ROM's menu structure is based on AAMA's new Role Delineation Study plus an add-on Managed Care Segment. The CD-ROM can be used as a stand-alone program or as an integrated enhancement to any medical assisting textbook.

Delmar's Medical Assisting Exam Review by J. P. Cody (0-8273-7183-7) is a comprehensive guide that prepares certification candidates to successfully pass either the CMA exam sponsored by the American Association of Medical Assistants or the RMA exam sponsored by the American Medical Technologists.

Value Package—the following innovative Delmar Learning product can be purchased separately, or you can package it with *Medical Assisting: Administrative and Clinical Competencies, 5th Edition* in a convenient and affordable value package.

- **Text and Delmar's Anatomy and Physiology CD-ROM Value Package** (1-4018-9528-X) is intended for any course where a brief review of anatomy and physiology is desired. This CD-ROM presents this important content in an accesssible and engaging manner. Organized by body system, the CD-ROM is perfect for self-guided learning or review. The software features separate quiz and tutorial modes to allow you to test your mastery of key content. Rich illustrations and activities make anatomy and physiology content interesting.

The use of the textbook, reinforced by the medical assisting skills CD-ROMs, Student Workbook, and the instructional assistance in the Instructor's Manual, Electronic Classroom Manager, and Instructor's Resource Kit, provides a complete, multiskilled competency-based learning system that is innovating, easy to comprehend, and provides the necessary competencies for a career in medical assisting.

ACKNOWLEDGMENTS

A textbook of this nature requires the input and assistance of many friends, professional colleagues and acquaintances, subject matter experts, the publishing team, and the group of reviewers. We owe them all a great deal of appreciation and recognition for their willingness to contribute their time and expertise to assist with this revision.

Special recognition is due to the following:

- **Anne Burns,** RPh, Clinical Assistant Professor and manager of the Proficiency Practice Laboratory, The Ohio State University College of Pharmacy, and **John Nance,** RMA, instructor, for assistance with Chapter 18 on medications.
- **Mary Mike Dunlevy,** RT(R)(M), radiology technician, for assistance with radiology procedures.
- **Michelle Heller,** CMA, RMA, prior instructor and now director of a medical assistant program, for her extensive review and revision of Chapter 7, Records Management, and Chapter 10, Medical Office Management.
- **Kim Knueven,** RN, BS previous office manager, now program director for Delmarva Foundation engaged in on-site reviews, for her contributions to Chapter 8, Collecting Fees, and Chapter 10, Insurance.
- **Holly Herron Meader,** RN, MS, Life Flight trauma nurse and critical care outreach manager, for reviewing and making recommendations for emergency care and first aid in Chapter 19.
- **Susan L. Newell,** Key Bank branch manager, for providing assistance related to cash, checks, and banking procedures in Chapter 10.
- **Sonia Papas,** MT, for her assistance with Chapter 15, Laboratory Procedures.
- **Lee A. Speck,** MT (AMT), LMLT (ASCP), Smith, Kline, Beecham Laboratories, for review and recommendations for Chapter 15, Laboratory Procedures.
- **James B. Soldano,** MD for reviewing the content regarding physical examination in Chapter 14.
- **Warner M. Thomas,** Jr. Attorney at Law, for his review and recommendations of Chapter 3, Medical Ethics and Liability.
- **Lynette Veach,** MA, MLT (ASCP), instructor in a medical assistant program, for assistance with Chapter 15, Laboratory Procedures.
- **Kent Vedder,** BSME, manager of manufacturing and engineer for a medical plastics company, for his assistance with electronic communications, data retreival, and prevention of computer viruses.

Invaluable contributions from physicians, nurses, and educators were truly outstanding. Their involvement took hours of reviewing, identifying and recommending content to be deleted, added, or technically updated in the 13 units of the anatomy and physiology chapter. Words are inadequate to express our appreciation.

Very special acknowledgment to the following:

- **Stephen D'Ambrosio,** PhD, Professor of Radiobiology and Pharmacology, The Ohio State University, College of Medicine, for resources and assistance with cellular structure and genetics in Unit 1.
- **William A. Barker,** MD, orthopedic surgeon, for his review and comments on Unit 5, The Skeletal System, and Unit 6, The Muscular System.
- **Cheryl Baxter,** RN, MS, pediatric nurse practitioner, for her insights related to children and the information for Pediatric Perspectives throughout Chapter 11.
- **Phil Diaz,** MD, The Ohio State University researcher and practicing physician specializing in pulmonary diseases, for review and assistance with The Respiratory System, Unit 7.
- **Christine Dombroski,** RNC, NP, nurse practitioner in OB, GYN, and Women's Health, for her review and extensive revision of Unit 13, The Reproductive System.
- **June Elek,** RN, MS, CAN, nurse manager, diabetes services for Riverside Methodist Hospital, for her assistance with Unit 11, The Urinary System, and Unit 12, The Endocrine System.
- **Lisa Smith,** RN, MS, AOCN, clinical nurse specialist (oncology) and pain management director, Riverside Methodist Hospital, for extensive revision of Unit 9, The Immune System.
- **Michelle Steed,** RN, BSN, clinical care manager, and **Luann Toth,** RNC, assistant nurse manager in urology services and dialysis with Riverside Methodist Hospital, for their assistance with Unit 11, The Urinary System.
- **Kelly J. Zyniewicz,** MD, dermatologist, for her review and recommendations for Unit 4, The Integumentary System.
- **James English,** MD, family practice physician and former anatomy and physiology instructor at The Ohio State University College of Medicine, for his contribution to this revision (his fourth time). His remarkable investment of time to review Units 2, 3, 8, 10, 12, and part of 13 is truly outstanding.
- **Elaine Glass,** RN, MS, OCN, clinical nurse specialist at the Arthur G. James Cancer Hospital and Research Institute, for sharing her materials on The Immune System, Unit 9.

■ **Henry A. Wise,** MD, urologist, who reviewed and provided extensive comments on The Urinary System, Unit 11, and male reproductive content in The Reproductive System, Unit 13.

REVIEWERS

The authors are particularly grateful to the reviewers who continue to be a valuable resource in guiding this book as it evolves. Their insights, comments, suggestions, and attention to detail are very important in guiding the development of this textbook.

■ **Jerri Adler,** CMA, CMT
Coordinator/Instructor
Lane Community College
Eugene, Oregon

■ **Jennifer Barr**
Chairperson, Medical Assisting Technology
Sinclair Community College
Dayton, Ohio

■ **Adrienne Lynne Carter-Ward,** BA, CMA, NRMA
Skadron College, Csi
San Bernardino, California

■ **Elizabeth L. Clark,** BA, CMA
Interim Program Director/Instructor
Everett Community College
Everett, Washington

■ **Lisa L. Cook,** CMA
Medical Assistant Program Director
Eton Technical Institute
Port Orchard, Washington

■ **Cindy Correa**
Healthcare Educational Consultant
Denver, Colorado

■ **Karen Hulse,** MT (ASCP)
Lenape Technical Institute
Ford City, PA

■ **Mary Marks,** MSN, RNC, PbT (ASCP)
Program Coordinator, Medical Assisting and Related Health Programs
Mitchell Community College
Mooresville, North Carolina

■ **Sharon McCaughrin,** CMA
Corporate Director of Education
Ross Medical Education Center
Warren, Michigan

■ **Susan R. Royce,** MS
Maria College
San Diego, California

■ **Janet Sesser,** RMA, CMA
Corporate Director of Education for Allied Health Programs
B.S. Education Administration
High-Tech Institute, Inc.
Phoenix, Arizona

■ **Melanie Schmidt,** RMA, MLT
Arizona College of Allied Health
Phoenix, Arizona

■ **Kathy Tozzi,** CLPN, RMA, AHI
Director of Education
Cleveland Institute of Dental-Medical Assistants, Inc.
Mentor, Ohio

DEDICATION

We gratefully acknowledge the support and encouragement of our families, loved ones, and friends throughout the preparation of this edition. We especially appreciate the wonderful friendship we share, which goes far beyond the pages of this book. Because of our experiences in employment and education, we felt a need for this text. We therefore wish to dedicate it to you, the reader, for you are the reason it was written.

APPRECIATION TO DELMAR LEARNING

The authors especially wish to acknowledge and commend the editors and staff of Delmar Learning for their guidance and expertise during the preparation of this edition. A special thanks goes to Deb Flis, who patiently encouraged and pleaded for manuscript until we finally got it finished. Her assistance and dedication to the development of the text was truly outstanding.

Acquisitions Editor—**Rhonda Dearborn**

Developmental Editor—**Deb Flis**

Editorial Assistant—**Jill O'Brien**

Art and Design Coordinator—**Robert Plante**

Project Editor—**Shelley Esposito**

Production Coordinator—**Nina Lontrato**

Technology Project Manager—**Laurie Davis**

Production Assistant—**Sherry McGaughan**

Marketing Manager—**Dawn F. Gerrain**

Marketing Coordinator—**Mona Caron**

HOW TO USE THIS BOOK

Medical Assisting: Administrative and Clinical Competencies, 5th Edition, is designed to help you acquire the knowledge and skills necessary to become a successful medical assistant. Several unique features will enhance your learning experience, including:

Chapter Openers

1 Each chapter begins with a brief overview of the content presented in the chapter. This two-page opener lists the *Units* of study and *Objectives* that can be used to self-test your understanding of the material. The *new* feature, *Areas of Competence (AAMA)*, identifies the administrative, clinical, or general area of competence discussed in each unit. *Words to Know* identifies the medical and general terminology used in the unit. These are listed alphabetically and appear in **red** the first time they are used. These terms are all defined in the glossary at the back of the book.

Anatomy and Physiology Section

2 This comprehensive anatomy and physiology chapter is organized into 13 general body system units. Each body system unit includes the structure and function of the system and the common diagnostic examinations and tests used to determine pathological conditions specific to that body system. Each body system unit also includes *Common Diseases and Disorders* that highlights the description, etiology, signs and symptoms, and treatment of the disease or condition. Phonetic pronunciations assist in building your vocabulary. The *new* feature, *A Pediatric Perspective*, explains the medications, treatments, and special considerations to take when the patient is a child.

Procedures

Administrative and clinical competencies are presented in complete, step-by-step procedures with distinct components. ***Title*** identifies the procedure competency. Icons indicate whether the procedure is administrative 📋 or clinical ✋. ***Purpose*** states the reason for performing the procedure. ***Equipment*** lists the materials and supplies needed to perform the task. The *new* procedure heading, ***OSHA Guidelines***, emphasizes safety and Standard Precautions pertaining to the procedure. ***Performance Objective*** states the competence (or task), the conditions for its performance, and the standard by which it will be evaluated. Throughout the steps, ***Notes*** identify specific instructions, and ***Rationales*** explain why a step in the procedure is required. *New* ***Charting Examples*** at the end of clinical procedures encourage correct documentation of a patient's chart.

Patient Education Boxes

These colored boxes alert you to issues and information that may be discussed with patients regarding tests and examinations, providing information to assist patients and their families in actively participating in their own health care.

Administrative and Clinical Skills CD-ROMs

Icons in each unit direct you to the ***Administrative and Clinical Skills CD-ROMs*** in the back of the book for interactive and engaging practice activities to help you better understand concepts you are learning in the book.

Medical-Legal-Ethical Scenarios

These situations at the end of each chapter have medical, legal, or ethical implications. *New* ***Critical Thinking Challenge*** questions expand the scenarios and help you focus on delineation competencies.

A CAAHEP Connection and Relating to ABHES— NEW Features

7 *A CAAHEP Connection* in each unit gives an example of content related to the CAAHEP standards. *Relating to ABHES* lists program requirements related to the content in each chapter. Both of these new features are designed to increase your understanding of knowledge and skills required of medical assistants.

Web Links

Web Links at the end of each chapter provide web site addresses that give you practice using the Internet to locate additional chapter-related information. **8**

Color Photographs and Illustrations

9 Throughout the book are visual images to aid in the explanation and understanding of the subject matter. Full-color *illustrations* help differentiate human structures and organs, and explain physiological processes. *Color photos* throughout provide realistic examples of the material described.

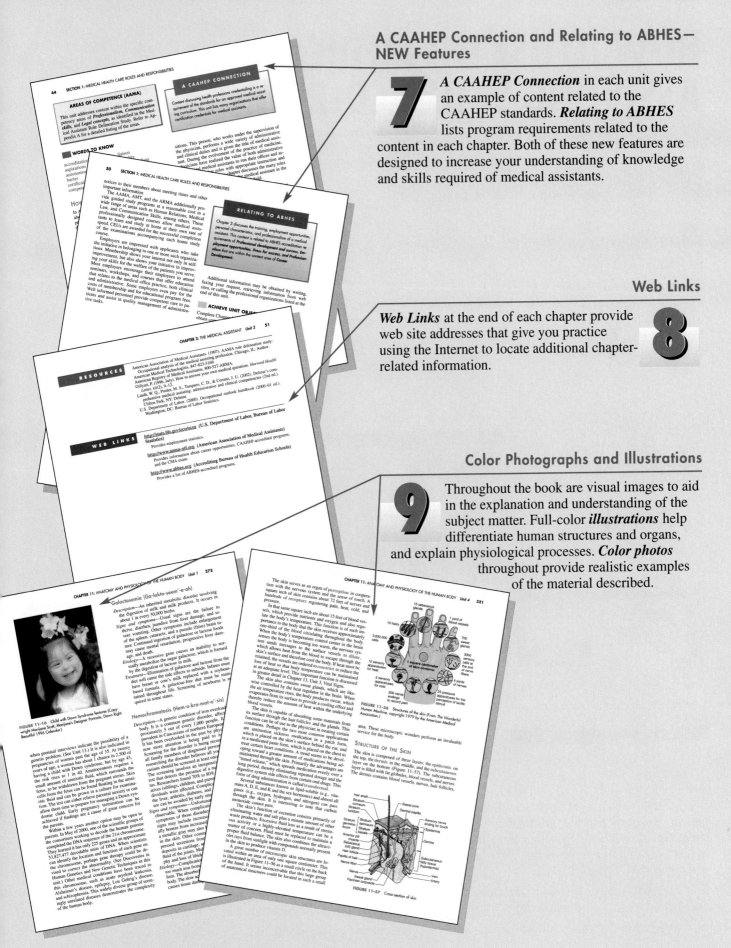

HOW TO USE THE MEDICAL ASSISTING SKILLS CD-ROMs

The Skills CD-ROMs are designed to accompany *Medical Assisting: Adminstrative and Clinical Competencies, 5th Edition,* so you can review and reinforce the important concepts you are learning in the textbook. By using these CDs, you'll challenge yourself and make your study of medical assisting concepts more effective and fun.

ADMINISTRATIVE SKILLS CD-ROM

The Administrative Skills CD-ROM is designed with you, the user, in mind. Several medical assistants lead you on a verbal guided tour through the medical office.

An introductory tour gives you an overview of the entire office. To navigate through the office, click on the area you wish to visit.

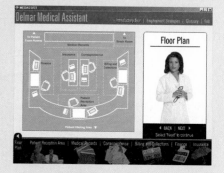

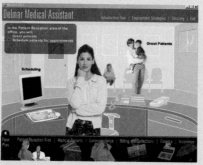

The medical assistant will give you an overview of the tasks and responsibilities associated with each area, and guide you through your many choices. In the patient reception area, for example, you may click on the active areas such as the computer, the phone, the answering machine, or the patient to brach into different content areas.

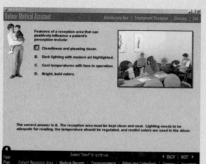

The medical assistant will give you instruction so that you understand the various aspects of each area. Activities include multiple choice questions with correct and incorrect responses noted, scheduling appointments by dragging and dropping the information into the appointment book, filling out a message pad, and maintaining a telephone log.

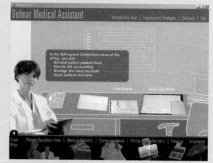

In other areas, such as billing and collections, you will be asked to complete a patient receipt by entering information into the correct area, fill out a daily log sheet, use the pegboard system, complete a super bill and ledger card by entering and highlighting information, complete a patient charge slip, write a check, and complete a deposit slip.

In the library, you can test your knowledge of legal and ethical principles by completing a crossword puzzle, or you can complete activities and games related to anatomy and physiology.

A comprehensive glossary allows you to check your understanding of important key words and phrases.

CLINICAL SKILLS CD-ROM

The Clinical Skills CD-ROM is designed to be easy to use. It includes basic clinical skills used in medical assisting, a glossary of words used in the office, important infection control information, a help feature, and a tutorial that will assist you in using the CD-ROM.

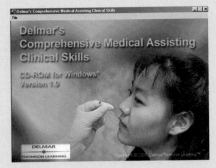

Clicking on the skills menu will take you to the main menu of skills you will be reviewing.

At any time you may return to this menu by clicking on the *Main Menu* button.

The skills menu lists each of the clinical skills contained on the CD-ROM. Click on the button of the skill you wish to study.

As you choose each skill, a menu will appear listing each of the sections included with the skill. By clicking on the buttons, you will navigate through the skill.

If you need to go back to the previous screen, just hit the *Previous* button.

The *Next* button takes you to the next step in the procedure.

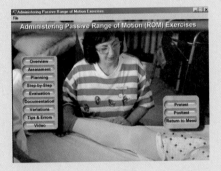

Each skill includes a pretest and a post-test section, so you may enhance your learning by checking your knowledge before and after viewing the skill.

Each question on the pretest and post-test gives you a chance to answer correctly. You will be asked if that is the answer you want to go with, and you are able to change your answer. The correct answer will be displayed, and your score will be tallied as you advance through the questions.

At the end, your final score with your percent rate for passing will be given. You are able to reset the questions and try again by simply clicking on the *Reset* button.

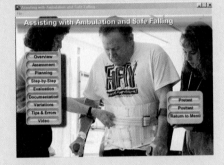

A glossary of terms is included to help you with your medical terminology. To find a term, just scroll down or use the buttons to advance you to the place in the alphabet where the word is found.

SECTION 1

Medical Health Care Roles and Responsibilities

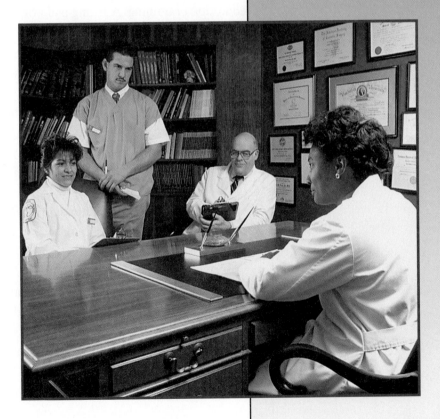

Health Care Providers

Health care providers have held prominent positions in society since the beginning of time. A look into the history of medicine reveals that for thousands of years, disease was thought to be the result of evil spirits and demons, brought on by disobedience to the gods. Therefore, early medical practitioners were primarily religious leaders. Eventually, scientific interest led to the discovery of microorganisms and understanding of the human body. Unit 1 of this chapter highlights ancient, medieval, and modern health care practitioners.

Because of the complexity of health care, many other health care practitioners and specialists are needed to provide complete patient care. These professionals are also members of the health care team. They work in a variety of settings providing specialized care or services related to their education or training. A listing and brief discussion of various team members is included in Unit 2.

Current medical practice has become very technical and is constantly undergoing change due to clinical research and development. Because of the vast amounts of accumulated knowledge and clinical procedures, it is impossible for a physician to provide competent care in all areas of medicine. In order to meet the needs of patients, some physicians become medical specialists, spending additional years in the study of one particular field of medicine. Unit 3 lists many specialties, practitioners' titles, areas of practice, and types of patients treated.

Because of the great technologic advances in health care which have controlled plagues, increased survival rates, and extended the years of life, another major problem has developed: overpopulation. Unless controlled very soon, the masses of people will outstrip the world's capacity to support their existence. The current presence of air, water, and land pollution and the destruction of vital resources are evidence of impending problems. Once again disease, famine, and epidemics of viruses yet unknown and uncontrolled, may affect the people of the world.

UNIT 1

A Brief History of Medicine

◼ OBJECTIVES

Upon completion of the unit, meet the following performance objectives by verifying knowledge of the facts and principles presented through oral and written communication at a level deemed competent.

1. Spell and define, using the glossary at the back of the text, all the **Words to Know** in this unit.
2. Explain how the caduceus may have been acquired as the medical symbol.
3. Explain the reason Hippocrates is known as the Father of Medicine.
4. State why many of Galen's findings were invalid.
5. Explain the differences in the role of the physician, the surgeon, and the barber-surgeon.
6. Identify the contributions of Jenner, Pasteur, Lister, Roentgen, Reed, Barton, Blackwell, Nightingale, Curie, Papanicolaou, Domagk, Banting, Fleming, Salk, Bernard, Sabin, and DeBakey.

AREAS OF COMPETENCE (AAMA)

This unit addresses content within the specific competency area of *Instruction* as identified in the Medical Assistant Role Delineation Study. Refer to Appendix A for a detailed listing of the area.

◼ WORDS TO KNOW

acupuncture
anesthesia
apothecaries
apprenticeship
asepsis
caduceus
cautery
chloroform
disease
epidemics
ether
exorcism
guilds

Hippocratic oath
infectious
pandemic
physicians
plague
practitioners
Roentgen
scientific
surgeons
surgery
trephining
vaccination

ANCIENT HISTORY

To fully understand the high technical level of current health care and the responsibilities of those who provide it, we must look back at its history and learn how it has developed. Ancient times were filled with **infectious dis-**

ease and **epidemics** as well as illnesses and injuries caused by dietary deficiencies and unhealthy or hostile environments. Eighty percent of primitive human beings died by the age of 30 as a result of a hunting accident or violence. Primitive individuals lived primarily alone, so there was little risk of widespread diseases or **plagues**. However, when they began settling in communities, farming, and domesticating animals, epidemic diseases were caused by overcrowding, filth, and the natural presence of microorganisms. Initially, tuberculosis, tetanus, malaria, smallpox, typhus, typhoid, and later leprosy ravaged early civilizations.

Because these ancient people did not understand the concept of microorganisms or the function of the human body, the presence of disease was credited to evil spirits and demons brought on as punishment for disobedience to the gods. Therefore, medical practice became the role of priests or medicine men. "Treatments" involved rituals to drive out demons. At times, a surgical procedure called **trephining** was performed. This remarkable operation involved cutting a hole in the skull with a flint knife presumably to treat migraines, epilepsy, paralysis, or insanity. Later, it was used to treat head injuries incurred in battle or from accidents. Archaeologists have examined hundreds of skulls and determined that some trephining ended in death, but surprisingly, the majority showed healing and several years of survival.

Evidence has been found in Egyptian tombs and on papyri which indicates that the people of the area around the Nile River had developed a level of medical practice as early as 3000 BC. Egyptian **physicians** were priests who studied medicine and **surgery** in the temple medical schools. They too tried to drive out evil spirits with spells. If this failed, they used concocted repellents to fight the demons. These were made from the excretions of the lion, panther, gazelle, and ostrich. Insects, either crushed or alive, were swallowed along with the backbones of ravens and fat from black snakes. In addition to the "black magic," they also used about one third of the medicinal plants still used in pharmacies today.

Egyptians believed that blood in the body flowed through canals like those constructed along the Nile for irrigation. When it was thought that the body's canals were "clogged," they were opened by bloodletting or the application of leeches. The leech not only removed blood and disease toxins but also produced hirudin in the process, which prevented coagulation. The use of leeches continued until the 19th century and is being reintroduced today in specific traumas where a large amount of blood is present within the tissues. Egyptian physicians (priests) were very conservative in treating patients. They adhered to rules of the Sacred Books so they would be free from blame if a patient died. If the physician tried a different treatment and the patient did not survive, the physician was executed; therefore, medical progress was impossible. The conservative physicians became famous and were in high demand. An Egyptian named Imhotep was considered outstanding and became the physician for the royal family. As a reward, he was given deity and named the Egyptian God of Medicine.

People from surrounding regions had medical problems similar to the Egyptians. The average person lived in squalor, drank filthy water, and had very poor personal hygiene. By the year 2000 BC, the ruler of Babylon established a legal code for medical practice that set fees for services and established rules of conduct. It provided that the physician's hands be cut off if the physician killed a patient or destroyed the patient's sight. It is worth noting that these stiff penalties applied only to patients from nobility—a slave just had to be replaced.

The Sacred Books tell of priest-doctors in India around 1500 BC and listed their deadly diseases as malaria, dysentery, typhoid, cholera, the plague, leprosy, and smallpox. The Hindus had the world's first nurses and hospitals. There was extensive use of drugs, including those for **anesthesia** that undoubtedly assisted with the main Hindu contribution to the art of healing: surgery. Their knowledge of anatomy was limited but their **surgeons** performed a fairly technical form of cataract and plastic surgery. Early writings reveal that they used approximately 120 surgical instruments in many different operations. The Hindu environment was greatly improved with walled sewer drains and underground water pipes. Their level of medical knowledge and drugs spread to other lands through trade, migration, and by conquerors.

The Chinese, India's neighbor, had a highly developed center of early medical learning. Their belief in evil spirits as the cause of illness gradually changed; they began searching for medical reasons for illness. About 3000 BC, the emperor, who was known as the Father of Chinese Medicine, had a document called *Great Herbal* (a translation) which contained over a thousand drugs; some are still in use today. The art of **acupuncture** was originally used as a means to drive out demons. Today, the ancient procedure has become a respected alternative form of treatment. Acupuncture consists of the insertion of needles of various metals, shapes, and sizes into one or several of the 365 specified spots on the head, trunk, and extremities. It is believed to relieve internal congestion and restore the equilibrium of the bodily functions.

The Greeks also played a large role in the development of medicine. Beginning about 2000 BC, they invaded many lands and established a remarkable civilization. They acquired knowledge from their conquered, but still practiced the religious/healing rituals. They believed Apollo, the Sun God, taught the art of medicine to a centaur who in turn taught others, including Asklepios, the Greek God of Healing, who lived around 1250 BC. The priests in the temples of Asklepios (also called Aesculapius) used massage, bathing, and exercise in treating patients. They also depended on the magical power of large, yellow, nonpoisonous snakes. After patients purified themselves by bathing and made offerings to the god, they were given tablets to read that described cures of former patients. Then they were put into a drug-induced sleep in the temple. During the night, the snakes licked the wounds and Asklepios applied salves. The god was usually depicted holding a staff with a serpent coiled around its shaft. This is probably the origin of the medical symbol known as a **caduceus** (Figure 1–1), even though it shows two instead of one coiled serpents, as did the staff of Aesculapius. Both are accepted as symbols of medical practice.

The Greeks absorbed ideas, drugs, and earlier methods of treatment from their predecessors. Their great interest in the unknown led them to question the accepted knowledge and seek information themselves. They began to investigate the causes of and reasons for illness in nature, which started the tradition of medical inquiry. About 500 BC, Alcmaeon dissected animals to study sight and hearing. Another Greek named Empedocles believed that blood gave life and the heart distributed it around the body. Medical schools began to observe what

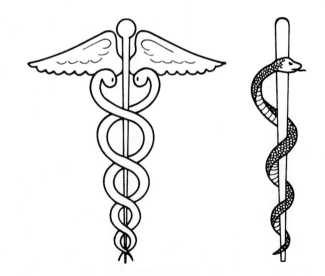

FIGURE 1–1 A caduceus (left) and the staff (right) of Aesculapius

happened in illness rather than accept the teachings of the past. Hippocrates, the founder of scientific medicine, was born in about 460 BC on the Island of Cos. During his 99 years of life, he took medicine out of the realm of priests and philosophers and produced an organized method of gaining knowledge through the means of observation. He taught that illness was the result of natural causes and not punishment for sin. He advocated examining a patient's environment, home, and place of work. He stressed the importance of diet and cleanliness. He felt medical knowledge could only be acquired through accurate clinical observation of the sick. He discovered that the course of certain diseases could be traced by listening to the chest of a patient. Over 2000 years passed before a French physician named Laennec invented the stethoscope to improve this method of observation (Figure 1–2).

Hippocrates studied with the most distinguished teachers of the day. He practiced in many parts of the Greek world and was admired for his cures. He wrote many detailed studies among which are ones on prognostics, fractures, and surgery. He is best known for his code of behavior known as the **Hippocratic oath**, which medical schools still teach and physicians repeat as they enter practice. For all his accomplishments, Hippocrates became known as the Father of Medicine.

Aristotle, a contemporary of Hippocrates, was a philosopher and scientific genius, and became the tutor of Alexander the Great. He brought together medicine, biology, botany, and anatomy. His findings were based upon animal dissection because human dissection was illegal where he lived. However, in Alexandria, Egypt, human dissection was legal. Students throughout the ancient world went there to study and use its library of 700,000 books. Alexandria became the center of learning and the home of a famous medical school. However, it declined with the rise of the Roman Empire, and medicine reverted to supernatural theories of disease.

Medicine was held in very low esteem in the Roman Empire. The Romans distrusted and despised the wandering Greek physicians who came to Italy about 200 BC, many as slaves. Roman men treated their own families with early, primitive methods. In 46 BC, Julius Caesar gave physicians citizenship rights and they began to achieve status. But the great demand for physicians opened medicine to anyone and little clinical teaching took place. The teachings of Hippocrates were largely ignored and rival schools of medicine argued about his ideas.

About this time Claudius Galen, a physician from Asia Minor, emerged, professing to following the teachings of Hippocrates. He was born in 129 AD and became a surgeon for a gladiatorial school after minimal medical training. He received much experience treating the severe wounds the gladiators received in the arenas. He later went to Rome and quickly became famous, but his arrogance caused hostility from other physicians and he was forced to return home. He was called back to Rome by Marcus Aurelius, the emperor. Galen successfully cured the emperors stomachache, and he remained in Rome until his death in 199 AD. Galen produced over 500 books during this time. His theories were accepted for the next 1300 years because he claimed they had the authority of Hippocrates (Figure 1–3). However, he had ignored observation and explained diseases as unbalanced "humors." The body was believed to be composed of and regulated by the four fluids (humors) of life, namely the blood, phlegm, black bile, and yellow bile. An imbalance or disturbance of the humors was thought to result in illness. He prescribed diets, massage, exercise, and drugs to cool, heat, dry, or moisten the body as needed. His beliefs regarding blood and circulation set back medical progress.

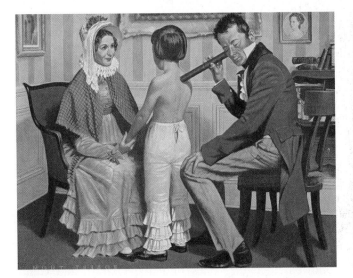

FIGURE 1–2 Laennec and the stethoscope (Courtesy of Parke-Davis and Company, copyright 1957.)

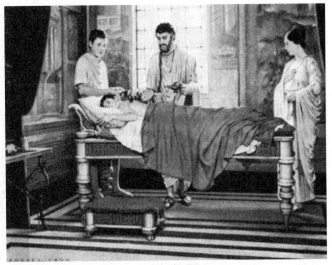

FIGURE 1–3 Galen: An influence for 45 generations (Courtesy of Parke-Davis and Company, copyright 1957.)

He did believe that knowledge of anatomy was necessary, so he dissected pigs and apes and related his findings because human dissection was still illegal. His viewpoints went unchallenged until the 16th century.

The Romans made almost no contribution to medicine but established superior methods of sanitation and water supply. They realized disease was connected to filth and overcrowding. They drained the marshes to reduce the incidence of malaria. There were laws to maintain public health and clean streets. They built an extensive underground sewer system and pure water aqueducts capable of bringing an estimated 300 million gallons of drinking water a day into the city. The emperor provided for teachers of medicine to maintain a supply. Medical officers and surgeons, usually Greek, served in the army. A private hospital system was also developed, first for the wealthy and slaves, then for the campaign armies. Later, public hospitals were founded and the hospital movement expanded with the growth of Christianity and its tradition of caring for the sick.

Despite Rome's advances, the empire began to fall as political, social, and economic factors collapsed. The real cause, however, was the spread of disease which resulted from the disuse of the drainage system and the return of the swamps which followed invasions by other empires. The resulting malaria and smallpox killed thousands. In 542 AD, the remnants of the eastern Roman Empire were destroyed by the first major historically known **pandemic** (a disease occurring at the same time in different places) of the bubonic plague. It had come from China and had spread through trade routes to Egypt along the coast of North Africa to Palestine, Syria, and into Europe. It affected all the known world.

MEDIEVAL HISTORY

The great Roman Empire was overrun by barbarians. Europe was controlled by Teutonic tribal groups. The people were agricultural and established health standards vanished. The centers of learning and medicine decayed. From the 5th to the 16th centuries, there was no progress in medical knowledge or practice. There was a blend of pagan magic, superstition, and herbalism. According to Hastings in *Medicine, An International History*, the Anglo-Saxon settlers in Britain believed illness was caused by "nine venoms, the nine diseases, or of 'worms', elves, and witches." It was treated with charms and incantations or with herbs, some of which were effective. However, the settlers lived in filth and had a total absence of sanitation and personal hygiene. Writings from the 6th to the 10th centuries tell of epidemics of smallpox, dysentery, typhus, and plague. In addition, there was widespread famine.

Eventually, medicine passed into the hands of the Christian Church and Arab scholars. The church did not foster medical science. They recommended prayer and fasting because they believed that illness was a punishment for sin. In 391 AD, a religious fanatic mob burned the great library at Alexandria. Christianity forbade human dissection, so anatomy and physiology died except for the erroneous pages of Galen. Priests again became healers, using **exorcism** and holy relics to cure the sick. Parts of the body were assigned a patron saint who could cure and inflict disease. The church did care for the sick and established religious orders that provided care. Most monasteries had rooms and herb gardens to care for their own sick and members of the general public. The monasteries also took on the task of translation and transcription of the ancient manuscripts of the classical physicians, a task which preserved and circulated information before the invention of the printing press.

A second storehouse of medical knowledge was in the Moslem Arab Empire which, by 1000 AD, extended from Spain to India. The Arabs were eager for knowledge and the classical learning was translated into Arabic. Medicine began a revival. Arab physicians learned much about epidemics, but their great knowledge of chemistry resulted in their major medical contribution in pharmacology. They also continued the Roman system of hospitals, including at least four major teaching centers. One had specialized wards for specific conditions. All patients were admitted regardless of race, creed, or social status. Upon departure, patients were given sufficient money to cover their convalescence.

One of the greatest physicians was known as Rhazes, the Arab Hippocrates. He was 40 before beginning medical study and was responsible for the construction of a hospital. He produced about 150 books including a medical encyclopedia weighing 22 pounds. He based his diagnosis upon observation of disease and his major contribution was distinguishing smallpox from measles. Anatomy was still based upon Galen. Because it was considered unclean to touch the human body with the hands, the Arabs were not good surgeons. This was left to inferior practitioners; however, Rhazes is credited with the use of animal gut sutures to sew wounds. The major surgical instrument was the **cautery** (a red-hot iron) applied to wounds and infected ulcers to "burn out the poison," always very painful and disfiguring and often fatal.

The union of medical knowledge from both the East and West produced an outstanding medical school at Salerno, Italy, around 850 AD. It was believed to be founded by a Jew, a Roman, a Greek, and an Arab and was open to both men and women of all nationalities. Because it was not a church school, it could teach medicine using a sound basis. It became the convalescent center for wounded Crusaders. By the 12th century it had a highly organized curriculum upon which students were examined and issued degrees to become the first "true" doctors. Both anatomy and surgery were taught, but it was still based upon animal dissection. Other medical centers followed, including ones in Paris, Oxford, and Cambridge. Despite earlier beliefs, however, religious and scholarly factions prohibited advancement. Hippocrates and Galen remained the unquestioned authorities. Medical teaching was predominately oral since books were scarce (for example, the medical school in Paris had only twelve books at the end of the 14th century). Dissection was rare. One university did secure the right to dissect one executed criminal every three years, but it allowed only a superficial examination of the chest and abdomen.

Medieval European surgeons' practice was limited to nobility, the high clergy, and wealthy merchants. Other patients and minor surgeries were treated by ignorant barber-surgeons. They cut hair, practiced bloodletting, opened abscesses, and occasionally did amputations—all with the same razor. Their trademark became the white poles around which they wrapped their blood-stained bandages. The red and white pole has descended to barbers today.

The Roman tradition of hospitals continued but public health and personal hygiene was gone. The environment was overrun with disease. Famine and population movement due to wars increased the problems. Typhus was flourishing due to the custom of wearing the same underclothing, which was often infested with fleas. Tuberculosis was endemic due to poverty and food shortage. Tuberculosis of the neck was common and its principal remedy was "the king's touch." In one month in 1277 AD, Edward I touched 543 persons attempting to affect a cure. Smallpox was returned to Europe by the Crusaders in the 13th century causing at least 20 epidemics. Danish ships even spread the disease to Iceland.

Two of the greatest medieval diseases, however, were leprosy and the bubonic plague. Leprosy was present in the early centuries, brought perhaps by the Roman soldiers. It was one of the few diseases recognized as being contagious, but was believed to be a result of sins against God. The afflicted were herded into leper houses outside the towns, forbidden to marry, proclaimed dead citizens, and ordered to wear a black cloak with white patches. In 1313, King Philip the Fair wanted to burn them all, but was forbidden by the church. Incidences of leprosy decreased with the coming of the "Black Death" (or, the bubonic plague) which killed many lepers. Black Death was a term used to describe the dark, mottled appearance of the corpse due to hemorrhages beneath the skin. (In 1905, it was determined that this disease was caused by a bacillus which grew in fleas of infected black rats.) The disease was devastating. Symptoms included sudden shivering, headache, vomiting, and pains in the abdomen and limbs, followed by delirium. Large, painful boils appeared at the body joints and unless treated, proved fatal in five days. Other variations included the pneumonic plague, which affected the lungs and caused death in three days, and the septicemic plague, caused by direct bacillus injection into the blood by the flea, which caused death within 24 hours.

The plagues probably began after flooding drove rodents inflicted with fleas from their habitats. China reported 13 million deaths. The plague traveled to India, Asia Minor, Egypt, and North Africa. One army fighting for a trading port realized they were becoming infected, catapulted their infested corpses into the port, and fled homeward to Sicily. This same sequence occurred in other areas, thereby carrying the plague into other ports. By 1352, all of Europe, Iceland, Greenland, and Russia were infected. The plague was blamed on a corrupt atmosphere: foul vapors created by Jupiter, infection from decomposing bodies of a plague of locusts, and, the most favored, invisible arrows shot by Christ. All were attributed to the wrath of God. Finally, the Jews were blamed. All Jews living in Switzerland and Germany, approximately 28,000 people, were put in wooden buildings and burned alive. Before it subsided, it is estimated that 30% of the total European population died. There were four additional outbreaks before the end of the 14th century. In *Medicine, An International History,* Hastings states, "infectious disease has been a more deadly enemy to man than war—hence the ghastliness of the modern concept of bacteriological warfare." The Black Death was not forgotten, and fear of the plague was an important motivation to stimulate a return to medical learning.

EARLY MEDICAL PIONEERS

Beginning in Italy in the 14th century, there was a revival of culture and concern for life. Gradually, people began to escape the limitations of the church. There was a new attitude toward the human body. The classical artists, Michelangelo, Dürer, and da Vinci, began to practice dissection in order to draw the human body—especially the bones, muscles, and internal organs—accurately.

An anatomist named Vesalius was from a medical family in Brussels. He was the student of a strong believer in Galen. The teacher thought the new anatomical discoveries were merely changes that had occurred naturally since Galen's time. Vesalius was not convinced and did his own dissections on corpses that he took from the gallows or bought from grave robbers. He determined that the structures he dissected were all the same and not as Galen had described. In 1537 he became a professor of surgery and anatomy, and four years later, while dissecting a monkey, he discovered that Galen's descriptions had been the result of animal dissection, not human. He published a book on the human body which contained over 300 illustrations proving Galen's errors; however, he made little attempt to discuss physiology or the function of organisms.

It was in 1578 when an Englishman named William Harvey observed that blood in the arteries always flowed away from the heart while blood in the veins flowed toward it, with valves that prevented it from changing direction. He also calculated that two ounces of blood passed with each heartbeat; therefore, with 72 beats per minute, the body would require 270 pounds of blood for just half an hour. He also realized that the same blood had to be pumped repeatedly. He knew blood passed through the lungs to be purified, but he died without discovering the capillaries between the arteries and veins.

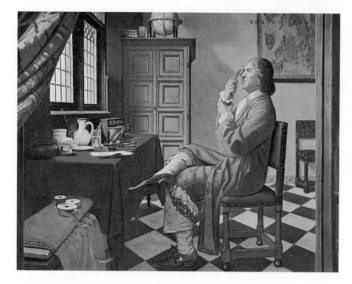

FIGURE 1–4   van Leeuwenhoek and his microscope (Courtesy of Parke-Davis and Company, copyright 1957.)

The microscope was the invention of an Italian named Malpighi and a Dutchman named van Leeuwenhoek (Figure 1–4). Malpighi first saw capillaries in 1661. van Leeuwenhoek was a wealthy merchant and in his leisure built over 200 microscopes (some which magnified up to 270 times), allowing him to see, for the first time, red blood cells.

An outstanding surgeon of this era was a Frenchman named Pare. He studied four years at the Paris hospital and earned his Diploma of Barber-Surgeon. For the next 30 years, he accompanied the army in its many battles, making discoveries first-hand. He accidentally discovered a wound dressing of egg yolk, oil of roses, and turpentine; this was the only thing he had left after his traditional boiling oil used to cauterize wounds ran out. He also discovered it was possible and much more successful to tie bleeding vessels with a ligature, rather than to burn them. He invented special forceps to grasp arteries and developed new techniques for treating fractures and dislocations. He was not well recognized by his peers because he could not use the Latin or Greek language of the formally educated physicians; however, he became Europe's greatest surgeon and served four French kings.

Intensive intellectual activity toward the end of the 17th century resulted in the development of scientific societies in different countries. The most famous was the Royal Society of London, established by Charles II in 1662. It was there that the mystery of circulation was solved and the recognition was made that oxygen was responsible for the change in the color of blood in the lungs. Soon after, pipes were inserted into veins and arteries of animals to measure blood pressure and attempts at transfusions were made.

The practice of medicine in the beginning of the 17th century was divided among the members of three **guilds** (an association of persons engaged in a common trade or calling for mutual advantage and protection): the physi-

cians, the surgeons, and the **apothecaries**. The physicians were the most prestigious because they usually possessed a university degree. They preferred studying, teaching, and debating the theories of disease to actually dealing directly with the sick. They limited their practice to the upper classes. The surgeons were considered inferior to the physicians. They were divided into two classifications: Surgeons of the Long Robe or, the more humble, barbersurgeons. Only a few surgeons held university degrees. They were trained largely in hospitals or through **apprenticeships** (a period of time when one is bound by agreement to learn some trade or craft). Barber-surgeons used their razors for opening veins as well as barbering. The apothecaries were tradesmen and were permitted to treat people with the drugs they made, prescribed, and sold. They were the general **practitioners** for the masses and also learned through apprenticeships.

MODERN MEDICAL PIONEERS

The discovery and conquest of the Americas had far-reaching medical impact. Colonists from Spain, Portugal, Holland, and France who landed in Southern, North, and Central America brought the diseases from the Old World and infected the Native Indians who had no built-up resistance. Entire native tribes were destroyed, making it easy to occupy their lands. However, the Indians were infected with syphilis and "sent" it back to Europe with sailors. Syphilis flourished and spread throughout Europe. Reportedly, one third of all the people in Paris alone were infected.

In the first settlement at Jamestown in 1607 there were only six medical men among the 208 settlers. Within three years, the population was reduced by half. This state of health continued for the next century, caused mainly by the fear of eating unknown fruits and vegetables. In addition, some settlers returned to Europe and there was a shortage of female settlers. There were only three or four trained physicians in all of Virginia before 1700. The Virginia Company offered free passage to apothecaries and their families to increase medical immigration. It was necessary for the settlers to practice self-medication using herbs and old practices. Bleeding was still practiced for fevers, infections, and even toothaches. One French surgeon reportedly bled his patient 64 times in eight months. To aid in digestion, some physicians recommended swallowing grit. Queen Anne's physician, the President of the Royal Society, prescribed drinking 50 live millipedes in water twice daily. The preparations in the medicines still contained ingredients recommended in ancient Egypt.

Humans had been "practicing" medicine for thousands of years, but only in the last 250 years, since the development of the microscope and the discovery of microbes, has it progressed. In the 18th century, medical science developed rapidly because of advances in the modern sciences of physics and chemistry, which gave the physicians new tools and new methods. Brothers William and John Hunter were born in Scotland and they both studied medicine. William became a surgeon in London and John became a surgeon in the army. After leaving the service, John devoted himself to practicing surgery and to the teaching and studying of anatomy. He was especially interested in comparing the bodies of animals with one another and with humans. John Hunter has been called the Founder of Scientific Surgery because his surgical procedures were based on sound pathologic findings. In 1778, he introduced artificial feeding by inserting a flexible tube into the stomach of a patient. His great collection of anatomic and animal specimens is in the museum of the Royal College of Surgeons in London, England.

With the emphasis on scientific inquiry, medicine changed rapidly. Many people made contributions that changed medical practice. Following is a list of the more familiar men and their contributions.

Edward Jenner (1749–1823) was an Englishman who studied under John Hunter. In May 1796, he gave the first **vaccination** to an eight-year-old boy using the pus from a cowpox lesion on the hand of a dairymaid. After two months, he injected the child with smallpox but the disease did not develop. The Royal Society rejected his discovery so he published it himself.

Gabriel Fahrenheit (1688–1736) was a German physicist devoted to the study of physics. He improved the construction of the thermometer, introduced the thermometric scale which is known by his name, and developed the first mercury thermometer. It became available in England in the 1740s.

Rene Laennec (1781–1826), a Frenchman, invented the stethoscope in 1816 out of necessity. He had an obese patient and could not hear the heart and lungs with just his ear. Originally, the stethoscope was a piece of rolled paper but was later refined into a wooden tube that fit the doctor's ear. Nineteenth century physicians carried it in their top hats.

Dr. Phillipe Pinel (1755–1826), a Frenchman, was the first physician to call for the humanitary treatment of mental patients. He thought mental illness should be treated as a disease and not a crime. In medieval and early modern times, mentally ill persons were burned as witches or kept in chains. Some had been manacled for 40 years. It was a popular 18th century pasttime to watch the antics of the chained inmates of Bedlam, the Bethlehem Hospital in London.

Dr. W.T.G. Morton (1819–1868) was practicing medicine in Massachusetts in the mid-1800s when he introduced the use of an anesthetic in the form of **ether** to make his patients more comfortable during surgery. After he died, the city of Boston erected a monument in recognition of his contribution. The use of ether stimulated research into other safer methods of relieving pain.

Dr. James Simpson (1811–1870) of Edinburgh University in Scotland began to use **chloroform** as an anesthetic. It was sprinkled on a towel held over the patient's face. Oliver Wendell Holmes, a writer and physician, suggested the word anesthesia to describe ether and chloroform. The word comes from two Greek words meaning "not feeling."

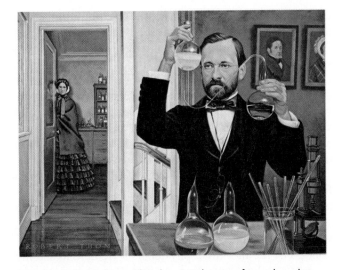

FIGURE 1-5 Pasteur: The chemist who transformed medicine (Courtesy of Parke-Davis and Company, copyright 1957.)

Louis Pasteur (1822–1895) was born in a small town in France and studied to become a chemist (Figure 1–5). He was working for some wineries trying to discover why their wine often became sour. With the aid of a microscope, he discovered that microorganisms were the cause and that they could be destroyed by heating and sealing the wine. His name is well known because it has been used to name the process that eliminates dangerous microbes from milk: pasteurization. Almost as important was his discovery of a vaccine for the treatment and prevention of deadly rabies. It was first given to a bitten, critically ill child in 1885. The child recovered and the occurrence of death from rabies, which was common, dropped to below 1% worldwide with the vaccine's extended use.

Joseph Lister (1827–1912) was born near London, England (Figure 1–6). He was respected as a surgeon, but despite his skill, many patients died of wound infections.

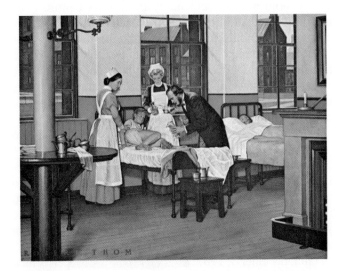

FIGURE 1-6 Lister introduces antisepsis (Courtesy of Parke-Davis and Company, copyright 1957.)

In 1865, he was reading Pasteur's research articles and thought infections might be caused by microbes in the air. At first, he used carbolic acid as a skin disinfectant, but it was too strong and he severely burned the patient's skin. By adjusting the strength of the solution used on wounds, his hands, the instruments, and the surgical dressings, the wounds healed without becoming infected. He also devised a carbolic spray to pump into the air in the operating room to kill organisms in the air. He laid the foundation for later techniques of medical **asepsis**.

Wilhelm von Roentgen (1845–1923), a German professor of physics, discovered x-rays, perhaps the greatest technical aid to the field of medicine. The name was chosen because he was uncertain about the nature of the invisible rays. Later, they were called **Roentgen** rays in his honor. For the first time, physicians were able to see into the body without operating. At first, Roentgen rays were used to diagnose fractures and the presence of foreign bodies. Later, it was learned that instillation of opaque liquids, either by mouth or injection, allowed viewing of the stomach, brain, kidneys, and bronchial tubes.

Dr. Elias Metchnikoff (1845–1916) was a Russian Jew who devoted much of his life to studying ways to prolong life. Louis Pasteur invited him to work at the Pasteur Institute. He became the director after Pasteur's death. In 1908, Metchnikoff was awarded the Nobel Prize in medicine for his study of the way white blood cells protect us from disease.

Frederick Banting (1891–1941), a young Canadian surgeon, discovered and isolated insulin in 1921. This breakthrough enabled people with diabetes to lead near-normal lives.

Gerhard Domagk (1895–1964), a German bacteriologist, began experimenting with a red dye called prontosil in 1932. By experimenting on mice, he discovered it killed or weakened many germs among the coccus family. This discovery led to the development of sulfa drugs, which cured 9 out of 10 patients with coccal infections.

Sir Alexander Fleming (1881–1955), in 1932, noticed that a mold which accidentally got on his culture plate had prevented the growth of the bacteria around it. He cultured the mold but did not realize its potential. This was the beginning of the development of penicillin. Nothing further was done until 1939 when doctors Howard Florey and Ernst Chain reinvestigated its properties. After months, Florey isolated the chemical substance and proved it effective as a germ killer in humans.

After World War II, surgeons were looking for ways to transfer tissues and organs from one person to another. Heart surgery was performed in the 1940s to repair defects. By 1960, surgeons had successfully placed artificial heart valves, plastic arteries, and pacemakers in the heart. In 1954 kidneys were transplanted. Even though the surgery was successful, the body often rejected the organ and the kidney failed after a year or two.

On December 3, 1967, Dr. Christian Barnard performed the first successful heart transplant in South Africa. His first attempt failed, but in his second attempt the patient survived for 19 months.

EARLY LEADERS IN AMERICAN MEDICINE

Thomas Bond was born in Maryland. Because there were no domestic schools or hospitals in which to serve an internship, he studied in France, England, and Scotland at medical schools affiliated with hospitals. These experiences taught him the value of hospital care for the sick. When he returned to Philadelphia to practice, he tried to secure money from friends to support building a hospital. He made no real progress until he enlisted the help of Benjamin Franklin. Franklin believed in his project and wrote about the proposal in the newspapers. When it was clear the money offerings would not be sufficient, Franklin proposed a bill before the Assembly; the bill passed in May 1751, and the first patients were admitted to The Pennsylvania Hospital in Philadelphia in 1756. A distinguished Frenchman, M. deWarville, visited the hospital around 1788 and reported it superior to most hospitals he had visited in France. The hospital was clean, and both black and white patients were being cared for in the same wards. It was not the first hospital in the American colonies, but it is recognized as the oldest surviving institution for the care of the sick in the United States.

In 1762, William Shippen, Jr., returned to Philadelphia from his study of anatomy under John Hunter in England. He placed an announcement in the *Pennsylvania Gazette* offering a course of anatomical lectures. He had only 10 students for the first course, but following years enrollment climbed as high as 200. Because of the interest in anatomy during this period, it was not unusual for bodies to be stolen from graves so that they could be dissected and studied.

William Beaumont (1785–1853) was a surgeon in the U.S. Army during the War of 1812. In 1822, he treated a young man who was in serious condition because of a bullet wound in his stomach. The treatment was successful and the man regained his health, but the flesh never healed completely. As a result, Dr. Beaumont was able to use the open area as a laboratory to study the action of the stomach. These studies added to our understanding of the digestive process.

Ephraim McDowell (1771–1830) was an American physician who studied at the then most famous medical school in the world, the University of Edinburgh. He practiced medicine in Kentucky and was a skilled surgeon. In the early 1800s Dr. McDowell performed an operation never before recorded. He removed a large ovarian tumor that would otherwise have killed his patient. When neighbors and friends found out he was going to perform the operation they called him a murderer. However, the surgery was successful and the patient lived many more years. McDowell was not recognized for his achievement until years later after he had performed other similar operations. Present day surgeons still use many of his techniques for this surgery.

At the time Beaumont and McDowell were practicing medicine, the causes of infection were not understood. Many patients developed blood poisoning or gangrene and died from these complications.

Walter Reed (1851–1902) was a major serving in the U.S. Army in Cuba when he realized the need to find the cause of yellow fever. He was forced to seek out volunteers who were willing to be given the disease. Certainly these people, some of whom died, also made a great contribution to medicine, although their names are not remembered. Dr. Reed's work in stamping out yellow fever made it possible to build the Panama Canal.

Theobald Smith (1859–1934), born in Albany, New York, was a professor of bacteriology. He was responsible for the establishment of a department of animal pathology in 1916 near Princeton University. His research laid the foundation for the prevention of diseases like typhoid, diphtheria, and meningitis, which are now prevented by use of vaccines.

Alexis Carrel was born in 1872 in France. He came to the United States after he received his medical degree and became a staff member of the Rockefeller Institute. He discovered in his study of body tissues that severed arteries could be joined and again carry on their function. His research work, which was carried out on animals, showed that it is possible to transplant bones and blood vessels and various organs of the body. He was awarded the Nobel Prize in medicine in 1912 for his work in joining blood vessels.

In 1949 there were 43,000 cases of polio in the United States alone. Dr. Jonas Salk and a group of researchers at the Harvard Medical School successfully isolated the polio virus after discovering that it grew in human intestines and was carried in water and food to other contacts. In April of 1954, Dr. Salk began massive trials of a vaccine. By the end of that summer, 1,830,000 children in America had been successfully protected.

Following vaccination, some of the children developed polio, and there was a lot of discussion regarding the use of the vaccine. In 1953, after a time of trial and testing, Dr. A. B. Sabin developed an attenuated oral vaccine composed of dead viruses. It stimulated production of antibodies in the human body and was 90% effective in preventing polio. The vaccine has been called one of the miracles of modern medicine. In 1961 the U.S. Public Health Department licensed Sabin's vaccine saying it produced immunity quicker, involved no injection, and lasted longer.

On December 24, 1954, a group of doctors at Peter Bent Brigham Hospital in Boston, MA, performed the first successful kidney transplant. In prior attempts, the patient had always died because the doctors did not understand that organs had to be compatible. This time, acting on a hunch that twins might be genetically alike, the kidney transplant to a patient from his twin was successful.

Also in Boston in 1962, the first severed limb was successfully reattached. A 12-year-old boy had leaped off the ladder on a slow train and then crashed into a tunnel entrance, severing his right arm at the shoulder. He was rushed to Massachusetts General Hospital along with his severed arm still in the sleeve of his coat. A team of surgeons worked for three and half hours to reattach his arm. The boy eventually regained use of the extremity.

In Holland in 1938, William J. Kolff tried to develop an artificial kidney device after helplessly watching his young patient die from kidney failure. A short time later, a colleague introduced him to a new product called cellophane, and he was able to use it to perfect his machine. After World War II, he brought it to the United States and joined the staff at the Cleveland Clinic in Ohio. The early treatments required long periods of time, three to four days each week, being attached to the machine. In 1966, with the help of colleagues at The Engineering Science Group, Kolff developed a dialyzing unit that encircled one arm and a fluid reservoir with activated charcoal that could be worn around the waist. This mechanism provided continuous dialysis and allowed for freedom from the machine.

A gigantic leap in diagnostic capabilities came about during the 1950s, with the use of radioisotopes. Before then, only x-rays could see inside the body, and that image was a still, flat picture. Doctors had to rely on palpation and tests for additional information. With the use of isotopes, however, organs could be visualized clearly with a scanner and observed for function as they absorbed, retained, or disposed of the isotope. Isotopes can be composed of iodine, fluorine, mercury, gold, copper, arsenic, or technetium. The type used depends on the organ being studied.

About midway through the 20th century, a breed of "medical supermen" came into being. They performed risky brain surgery, transplanted organs, and installed artificial parts. Cataracts were "popped out" and plastic lenses inserted in their place. And with prosperity came the explosion of plastic surgery to respond to the whims of clients. Heart surgery became an everyday occurrence.

REPLACEMENT PARTS

Many things have been developed to take place of the body's natural parts such as sea coral for bone, artificial metallic joints, plastic eye lenses, and lifelike limb prostheses. However, some artificial parts have truly been lifesavers. Late in 1950, Dr. Michael DeBakey of Baylor University in Waco, Texas, successfully replaced arteries with Dacron tubing and patients did not experience immune reactions. Later Teflon tubing was also used. Dr. Charles Hufnagel of Georgetown University Medical Center in Washington, D.C. replaced a heart valve with the first artificial one in 1953. In 1957, Dr. C. Walton Lillehei and two electronic engineers perfected a pacemaker with silverplated wires going through the chest and attaching to the surface of the heart.

A Swedish doctor, Ake Senning, was the first to implant a pacemaker, but the short battery life made it impractical. In May of 1970, the first pacemaker with a 10-year battery was implanted in a French woman. By July 1972, two U.S. surgeons had implanted the first nuclear-powered pacemaker, which had an extended period of use.

By 1960, Dr. DeBakey and his team developed the first auxiliary heart pump and attached it to a patient experiencing heart failure. The patient died three days later from pneumonia. In April 1966, an improved model was used; however, the patient died after five days, even though the pump was still working. Research has continued on the perfection of artificial organs but it has not been particularly successful. In July 2001, the first totally implantable artificial heart, developed by the AbioCor company was placed in a patient who had only a few days to live. The heart battery is powered externally through the skin. The expectation was that the patient would only live for about 60 days. He survived twice as long, dying on November 30, 2001, because of a stroke and internal bleeding. As of this date, at least two additional patients have received artificial hearts and are apparently doing well. Because this is an experimental device, little information is being released about the procedure or the progress of the patients.

A newly developed device allows continuous monitoring of a person by sensors imbedded into a self-contained, vestlike garment that only weighs 10 ounces. It is called SmartShirt, Life Shirt, or Health Buddy Appliance, depending on the manufacturer. The vest is capable of measuring 30 physiologic signs such as cardiac and respiratory function, measuring oxygen levels through an attached finger clip, identifying the location of a bullet hole in the chest, and measuring vital signs. The data is stored on a memory card of a handheld computer that clips on a belt. The device has applications for hospitalized patients, law enforcement, race car drivers, and the chronically ill, whose data can be assessed over the web with the proper connections.

A huge step in modern medicine is the ability to use stem cells to correct many problems within the body. Stem cells are extracted from an embryo when it has developed about 150 cells. They are grown in a culture and can develop into all of the body's tissues. Many researchers see stem cells as a way to treat many diseases. Healthy stem cells can replace diseased ones to cure patients with incurable diseases. To date the most promising early research is in diabetes. Stem cells can develop into pancreatic tissue to replace that which is nonfunctioning. The use of stem cells is a highly controversial process that is filled with ethical, moral, and legal implications. Reportedly, stem cells will be able to:

- repair brain cells damaged by Alzheimer disease
- replace corneas
- provide muscle or bone for any body part
- replace heart valves
- repair/replace damaged liver cells
- repair spinal nerves
- repair/replace skin after burns
- repair bone cartilage in joints

The cells themselves will be capable of multiplying indefinitely to make more stem cells. This scientific discovery may be one of the most significant of the century if scientists can "grow" new body parts on demand, and insert healthy cells where damaged ones are developing.

Another very significant scientific discovery will also change the practice of medicine. An international effort has resulted in the defining of the human genome, the identification of the genes in the DNA of cells. The ability to know which gene certain characteristics come from or which gene is responsible for certain diseases and disorders, opens the possibility for scientific intervention into an unknown number of areas. As with stem cell technology, manipulating genes is also filled with ethical, legal, and moral issues. On the positive side, DNA determination is an asset in identifying risk of disease, criminal activity, and identification of casualties. Chapter 11, Unit 1, discusses the Genome Project and its applications.

Presently many body parts can be replaced with artificial substitutes and in some cases, such as heart valves, with matching parts from animals. But replacing the vital functioning organs, like the heart, lungs, kidney, or pancreas, can be relatively successful only with transplants from a compatible donor. Efforts are being focused on the importance of designating oneself as a donor to meet the needs of thousands who are enrolled on waiting lists, anticipating their lifesaving gift.

Many modern-day miracles of medicine are being performed nearly every day, but only after time is it possible to determine which ones will truly make a difference. Innovations are apparently limited only by the imagination and perseverance of scientists and researchers.

THE IMPACT OF GOVERNMENT ON HEALTH CARE

In 1946, Congress passed the Hill Burton Act that provided for the improvement and construction of hospitals. Big cities renovated existing buildings and established ICU units, trauma centers, and outpatient services. Small towns and rural areas were provided with regional health centers. Professional administrators began to manage hospital operations.

Private clinics sprung up to care for specific diseases. Hospitals that once cared for tuberculosis (TB) patients are now closed because of the success of antibiotics. Large mental institutions are also gone as a result of the efforts to assimilate these persons into society. Custodial nursing homes and the hospice movement were developed to meet society's needs.

Following World War II, big medical centers with schools of medicine, nursing, pharmacy, dentistry, and allied and public health began accelerating research. Research was also being carried out by pharmaceutical firms, independent institutes, the armed forces, and health departments. New equipment (such as the electron microscope), new techniques using nuclear and molecular biology, biophysics, and the recent breaking of the genetic code have revolutionized research.

The federal government has provided much impetus and influence in the growth of medicine through funding, grants, and regulations. Legislation gave status to Public Health Services and the Food and Drug Administration. In 1953, the two became part of the Department of Health, Education, and Welfare, which has since become the Department of Health and Human Services.

Building on the successful organizations of the National Cancer Institute (1937) and the old Hygenic Lab of the Public Health Services, Congress passed acts that ultimately led to the creation of the National Institutes of Health (NIH), which are clusters of research institutes that focus on major diseases.

Congress also enacted legislation in 1965 in an effort to establish an effective and comprehensive federal health care program in the form of national health insurance with Medicare for the aged and Medicaid for the poor. Now there is an effort to try to control the massive costs of these programs.

THE IMPACT OF CONSUMERS ON HEALTH CARE

In the 1960s, many critics of mainline medicine became organized. There were organized efforts to stop vaccinations programs, the fluoridation of water, and the use of animals in research. A more subtle criticism was voiced against modern therapeutic practices. There were complaints about unnecessary surgery, excessive use of drugs, over-medicalization of childbirth, intimidating and painful procedures, and the use of heroic measures for prolonging life.

A more informed society began to question the previously unquestioned medical authority. Grievances from organized consumers, senior citizens, churches, and feminists groups began opposing specific medical practices and demanded more humane environments and treatments. Because of the lack of confidence in the medical establishment and the authoritarian manner of practice, many people defected to alternative health therapies (refer to Chapter 20, Unit 4).

Recognizing problems, medical schools began addressing the issues of philosophy, social concerns, and ethics and incorporated these courses in their curriculum. Other forms of medical care such as osteopathy and optometry flourished and became accepted by mainline medicine. Chiropractic medicine was without orthodox approval but flourished. Other options to medicine were Christian Science and faith healing among fundamentalist churches.

There was a great search for humane treatment by literate lay people. There was a revival of homeopathy and consideration of the whole person in holistic medicine. There was a renewed interest in herbal medicine and folk remedies.

Contacts made overseas by military and traveling Americans exposed them to Asian medical and health concepts. It generated interest in Zen, yoga, and martial arts. Acupuncture gained a measure of official acceptance following President Nixon's visit to China, and it is prominent in Asian-American communities today.

The promotion of physical exercise, sports, and recreation is directed toward promoting and maintaining good health. This is evident in the popularity of activities such as body building, aerobics, and running, as well as the proliferation of gyms and health clubs.

A sizeable portion of the population is now vegetarian. Health food stores have proliferated. There is a growing feeling of nonestablishment: a "heal thyself" attitude. There are "fat farms," multiple fad diets, liposuction, television and video exercise enthusiasts, and a mountain of health-related books. Pressure from activists forced the development of food labels to identify the nutritional content of foods. The relationship between food and the major illnesses of heart disease, diabetes, and stroke are being studied.

The sexual revolution in the past four decades fostered the idea that more frequent, less inhibited sex was healthy. Accommodation to homosexuality occurred. The liberation of women and the freedom of sexual behavior brought a new role to the physician. Sexually transmitted diseases, antibiotic therapy, birth control, sex-change surgery, breast enhancement, sterilization, and abortion all created new areas of counseling and treatment.

A new era developed. Sexual hygiene and education and birth control devices became common topics of discussion. Studies of sexual habits were conducted by two famous teams; Alfred Kinsey and colleagues from 1948 through 1953 and William Masters and Virginia Johnson from the 1960s through 1980.

In 1980, rigorous campaigns were begun to encourage the use of condoms in an effort to control the spread of STDs, especially the newest one, acquired immunodeficiency syndrome (AIDS). There was a great deal of public exposure to sexual behavior.

On another front, fighting influenza became easier with the development of flu immunizations. At first, a monovalent vaccine was only partially effective because scientists were unaware there were multiple strains of the virus. In August 1972, scientists from the National Institute of Allergy and Infectious Diseases announced success with a polyvalent vaccine that had a combination of live viruses that could be produced fairly rapidly to meet an influenza threat. This was more effective. Today, vaccines are tailored to match the upcoming year's anticipated strain, so the response is much more effective.

Physicians are now faced with a new problem to solve. Because of people's lack of physical activity and the convenience of prepackaged food, fast food, junk food, and eating out, the population has become obese and is displaying a number of medical conditions relating to obesity. Not only is this a problem for the adult population, but also for children who are becoming obese at alarming rates. In addition to treating diseases, physicians now find themselves dealing with dietary problems and prescribing preventative and curative therapies in an attempt to get at the real cause of the health problems. Unfortunately no magic pill has yet been discovered, and human nature being what it is, the problem of obesity will not be an easy one to solve.

WOMEN IN MEDICINE

The earliest known women in the field of medicine were at the famous medical school in Salerno, Italy, from 1099 to 1179. The most famous was Trotula Platearius (1100 AD). Her specialty was obstetrics and gynecology. Her textbook, *Diseases of Women,* was a major publication for seven centuries. She married a physician and had two sons, both of whom were physicians.

In England in the 16th century, women were allowed to practice medicine. Then, attitudes changed and women were often persecuted as witches if they tried to cure sickness. In the mid-19th century, even though there was still much opposition, women once again won the right to be trained and qualified as doctors.

Dr. Elizabeth Garrett Anderson (1836–1917) was the first woman to qualify as a doctor in Britain. A hospital is named after her. In 1872 she opened the New Hospital for Women. It was staffed entirely by women.

Clara Barton (1821–1912) cared for the wounded in the Civil War. In the course of this work she not only nursed the wounded but recognized the need for support services to meet the emotional and spiritual needs of the soldiers. After the war she worked at locating missing soldiers. She learned of the Red Cross in 1869 when she visited friends in Geneva, Switzerland. In 1881 she formed the American Red Cross and served as its first president.

Elizabeth Blackwell (1821–1910) was the first woman in the United States to qualify as a doctor (Figure 1–7). She was rejected by 17 schools before being accepted by

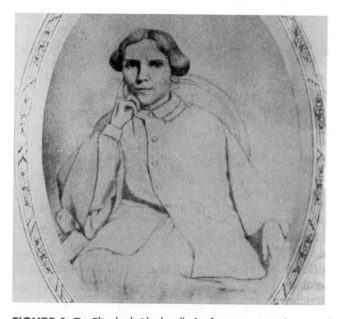

FIGURE 1–7 Elizabeth Blackwell, the first woman in the United States to qualify as a doctor (Courtesy of Hobart and William Smith Colleges.)

the medical school at Geneva, New York. She was granted her degree in 1849 from the college that is now called Hobart and William Smith Colleges. In 1853, Dr. Blackwell, with the help of two other women, who were also doctors, her sister Emily, and Dr. Marie Zackrzewska, opened a dispensary and medical college for women in New York. They opened a hospital exclusively for women in 1857 despite great opposition.

Florence Nightingale (1820–1910) was the founder of modern nursing. She was born into a wealthy family who were of the opinion that ladies found a suitable husband, were married, and raised children, period. She was greatly influenced by Elizabeth Blackwell, who was a close personal friend. Nightingale studied nursing in Europe and used her knowledge in the Crimean War to care for the wounded and sick. She established a school for nurses in 1860 at St. Thomas Hospital in London.

Dr. Aletta Jacobs (1854–1929) was Holland's first woman physician and opened the world's first birth control clinic in Amsterdam in 1882.

Marie Curie (1867–1934), born Mary A. Sklodowska in Warsaw, Poland, was the first world-famous woman scientist. She discovered the element radium. She won the Nobel Prize in physics with her husband, Pierre, and Henri Becquerel and later won the Nobel Prize herself in the field of chemistry. Her work led directly to the treatment of cancer with radium.

Elsie Strang L'Esperance (1878?–1959) was born in Yorktown, New York. She graduated from Woman's Medical College of the New York Infirmary for Women and Children established by Elizabeth Blackwell. Her concern for the early treatment of cancer led her to establish the Strang Clinic. Her effort represented the first organized attempt to detect cancer in its early stages. The clinic offered complete physical examinations to apparently healthy women to determine the presence of cancer. Major advances were made in the Strang Clinic, including the work of Dr. George Papanicolaou in the diagnosis of cervical cancer. His discovery, the Pap test (using a shortened version of his name) has become a routine screening examination and has saved the lives of thousands of women. Evaluations of the rectum were also studied through use of proctoscopy.

Gerty Theresa Radnitz Cori (1896–1957) was the first American woman to win the Nobel Prize for medicine and physiology. Dr. Cori worked with her husband on the overall process of carbohydrate metabolism in the body.

Dorothy Hansine Anderson (1901–1963) was born in Asheville, North Carolina. She was denied a residency in surgery and an appointment in pathology at the University of Rochester because she was a woman. She was accepted as an assistant in pathology at Columbia and in 1930 was appointed to the teaching staff. Her research into celiac disease of the pancreas led to the discovery of a previously unrecognized disease entity which she called cystic fibrosis. She ultimately developed a simple method of diagnosing this disease. She wrote major publications in the 1940s on chemotherapy for respiratory tract infections in cystic fibrosis.

Grace Arabell Goldsmith (1904–1975) was born in St. Paul, Minnesota, and received her medical training at Tulane University School of Medicine. Her main interest was nutrition. In the early 1940s she instituted (at Tulane) the first nutrition training for medical students anywhere in the world.

Dorothy Hodgkins was born in 1910 in Egypt of British parents. Her work in analyzing the structure of vitamin B_{12} as a vital substance in the fight against pernicious anemia won her the Nobel Prize for chemistry in 1964.

In 1983, *Ebony* magazine reported that only two black women in the United States, Drs. Alexa Canady and M. Deborah Hyde-Rowan, participated in the field of neurosurgery. They were excellent students and had experienced discouraging remarks from faculty members in medical school. Remarks such as "you don't fully understand all that is involved in neurosurgery" and it is "too difficult a field for a woman" did not stop them from realizing their goals. The women are proud of their accomplishments and say "it shows that black women have the determination, discipline, and dedication to succeed in an area such as neurosurgery."

Today, women continue to struggle with determination to achieve positions of leadership in the medical field. Many specialty areas are still dominated and controlled by men. Access to medical schools and opportunities to practice have improved, though. Extensive education and medical practice commitments can present a challenge to female physicians who also want to have and raise children. However, these challenges are being managed and women are making their mark as health care providers.

ACHIEVE UNIT OBJECTIVES

Complete Chapter 1, Unit 1 in the workbook to help you obtain competency of this subject matter.

UNIT 2

The Health Care Team

OBJECTIVES

Upon completion of the unit, meet the following performance objectives by verifying knowledge of the facts and principles presented through oral and written communication at a level deemed competent.

1. Spell and define, using the glossary at the back of the text, all of the **Words to Know** in this unit.
2. List and discuss the allied health care professionals described in this unit.
3. Explain why it is necessary to have a basic understanding of other health care team members.

AREAS OF COMPETENCE (AAMA)

This unit addresses content with the specific competency areas of *Patient care, Professionalism, Communication skills, Legal concepts,* and *Instruction* as identified in the Medical Assistant Role Delineation Study. Refer to Appendix A for a detailed listing of the areas.

WORDS TO KNOW

admissions clerk
certified medical
   assistant (CMA)
certified nurse assistant
   (CNA)
certified ophthalmic
   technician (COT)
chiropractor
cytologist
dental assistant
dental hygienist
dietitian
electrocardiogram
   technician (ECG tech)
emergency medical
   technician (EMT)
health unit coordinator
histologist
laboratory technician
licensed practical nurse
   (LPN)
multi-skilled health care
   assistants
nurse midwife
nurse practitioner
nutritionist

occupational therapist
occupational therapy
   assistant (OTA)
office manager/business
   office manager
paramedic
patient care technician
   (PCT)
pharmacist
pharmacy technician
phlebotomist
   (accessioning tech)
physical therapist
physician assistant (PA)
podiatrist/chiropodist
prophylaxis
psychologist
radiologic technologist
radiology technician
registered nurse (RN)
respiratory therapy
   technician
ultrasound
unit clerk
ventilatory
x-ray technician

ALLIED HEALTH PROFESSIONALS

In addition to the physicians you will work with, there are many other health care team professionals, and you should have a basic understanding and respect for their roles in patient care. Each one performs a specific set of duties for which they were trained. Defined hereafter are the many skilled areas, educational requirements, and primary duties of the most frequently encountered health professionals who cross paths in daily patient care. Many of these members you may not work with directly, but you may have contact with them by telephone or by written communication. Often patients can have several health problems at the same time, and cooperation with other members of the health care team to accommodate the patient is vital. Knowing the role each professional plays in the total health care of patients will enable you to speak more intelligently with others in the medical field and become more efficient in your role as the medical assistant.

Admissions Clerk

An **admissions clerk** in the hospital or medical center has basic medical terminology and administrative medical office skills. Obtaining a basic medical history and other important information from patients when they are admitted is the primary duty of this person. A college degree is desirable, but not essential.

Certified Ophthalmic Technician

Certified ophthalmic technicians (COTs) are valuable members in the field of ophthalmology. Often they are initially medical assistants with a versatile background in both administrative and clinical office procedures and a basic understanding of medical terminology. Additional training is necessary and certification is required to perform delicate ophthalmic tests and procedures for patients. All COTs must also keep current with the latest treatments, medications, and equipment in assisting patients and physicians.

Certified Nurse Assistant

The **certified nurse assistant (CNA)** provides basic nursing skills and patient care to those in nursing homes and retirement and adult day care facilities under the supervision of the registered or licensed nurse (Figure 1–8). CNAs are also referred to as nurse aides, nurse technicians, and orderlies.

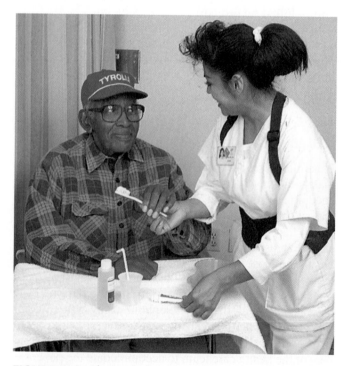

FIGURE 1–8 The nursing assistant assists with daily living skills.

Chiropractor

A **chiropractor** is highly trained and skilled in the mechanical manipulation of the spinal column. The degree of Doctor of Chiropractic, DC, is awarded after the individual completes two years of premedical studies followed by four years of training in an approved chiropractic school.

Certified Medical Assistant (CMA)

The **certified medical assistant (CMA)** is someone who has graduated from a Commission on Accreditation of Allied Health Educational Programs (CAAHEP)–approved medical assistant program and has successfully passed the certification examination of the American Association of Medical Assistants. The CMA assists the physician in both administrative and clinical duties in the health care field according to the state laws that govern medical practice. Medical assistants are versatile health care professionals.

Cytologist

A **cytologist** is a laboratory technician who specialized in the study of the formation, structure, and function of cells.

Dental Assistant

A **dental assistant** helps a dentist in the performance of generalized tasks, including chairside assistance, clerical work, reception, and some radiography and dental laboratory work. The person learns duties in school or on the job and becomes certified by taking the national certification examination to become a CDA, Certified Dental Assistant.

Dental Hygienist

A **dental hygienist** is a person with special training to provide dental services under the supervision of the dentist. Services supplied by a dental hygienist include dental **prophylaxis**, radiography, application of medications, and provision of dental education chairside and in the community.

Electrocardiogram Technician

Electrocardiogram (ECG) technicians are skilled in performing electrocardiograms and may be employed in medical clinics and hospitals.

Emergency Medical Technician

Emergency medical technicians (EMTs) are trained in and are responsible for the administration of specialized emergency care and the transportation to a medical facility of victims of acute illness or injury. All EMTs have ongoing training following certification and must be recertified every two years.

Histologist

A **histologist** is a medical scientist who specializes in histology, which is the science dealing with the microscopic identification of cells and tissues. Histologists are employed in private laboratories, clinics, and hospitals.

Laboratory Technician

A medical technologist or **laboratory technician** is one who, under the direction of a pathologist or other physician or medical scientist, performs specialized chemical, microscopic, and bacteriologic tests of blood, tissue, and bodily fluids. Those who have successfully completed the examination by the Board of Registry of the American Society of Clinical Pathologists, or a similar professional body, are designated as certified medical technologists (CMTs).

Multi-Skilled Health Care Assistants

Multi-skilled health care assistants are coming of age as a result of health care reform. In the efforts to hold down the cost of health care, many medical facilities have become more and more interested in the health care worker who offers a variety of skills in the area of patient care. There is a vast array of titles for this multi-skilled person that seem to vary from one facility to another, as do the expectations of the job. Some medical centers refer to this employee as a patient care technician (PCT). A background in medical assisting and/or nurse assisting is most helpful, and most often required. Additional training is provided by the nursing staff with certification exams that follow. Under the supervision of registered nurses, the duties of this position range from performing vital signs and ECGs, to turning patients, drawing blood, and changing dressings, as well as many other responsibilities.

Nurses

Nursing is the practice of those activities contributing to the health or recovery from illness. The following are specialized areas of nursing:

Nurse Midwife   A **nurse midwife** is a professional registered nurse who has had extensive training and experience in labor and delivery. Most states require a certification in addition to the state nurse license. The midwife assists the birthing mother throughout her pregnancy, the delivery of her infant at home or in a medical facility, and the postpartum period. Nurse midwives manage normal pregnancies and deliveries that potentially have no risks of developing complications.

Nurse Practitioner   A **nurse practitioner** is a **registered nurse (RN)** who, by advanced training and clinical experience in a branch of nursing (they usually hold a Master's degree), has acquired expert knowledge in that special branch of practice. Nurse practitioners are employed by physicians in private practice or in clinics.

Registered Nurse   In the United States an RN is defined as a professional nurse who has completed a course of study at a state-approved school of nursing and passed the National Council Licensure Examination (NCLEX-RN). RNs are licensed to practice by individual states. Employment settings for RNs include hospitals, convalescent homes, clinics, and home health care, to name a few.

Licensed Practical Nurse   Sometimes referred to as licensed vocational nurses, **licensed practical nurses (LPNs)** are trained in basic nursing techniques and direct patient care. They practice under the direct supervision of an RN or a physician and are employed in hospitals and convalescent centers.

Nutritionist

A **nutritionist** studies and applies the principles and science of nutrition (the study of food and drink as related to the growth and maintenance of living organisms).

Dietitian   A **dietitian** has specialized training in the nutritional care of groups and individuals and has successfully completed an examination and maintains continuing education requirements of the Commission on Dietetic Registration. This member of the health care team assists patients in regulating their diets. Dietitians are employed in hospitals and clinics. One of the duties of a nutritionist or dietitian is to instruct patients to select a daily well-balanced diet.

Occupational Therapist

An **occupational therapist** practices occupational therapy most often in the hospital setting. An occupational therapist may be licensed, registered, certified, or otherwise regulated by law. Occupational therapy is defined by American Occupational Therapy Association as: "the use of purposeful activity with individuals who are limited by physical injury or illness, psychosocial dysfunction, developmental or learning disabilities, poverty and cultural differences, or the aging process to maximize independence, prevent disability, and maintain health. The practice encompasses evaluation, treatment, and consultation."

Occupational Therapy Assistant

The **occupational therapy assistant (OTA)** is an important member of the health care team. The certified occupational therapy assistant, or COTA, generally has achieved an associate's degree in applied sciences, and works under the direction of a registered occupational therapist. The duties include assisting patients in learning (or relearning) self-care, functional duties of their employment, and recreational activities according to their individual needs.

Office Manager/Business Office Manager

An **office manager** or **business office manager** has managerial skills in the business operations of the medical office or clinic (or hospital). A degree in business administration is most desirable.

Paramedic

Paramedics are also called paramedical personnel and allied health personnel. They act as assistants to physicians or in place of a physician, especially in the military. They are trained in emergency medical procedures and supportive health care tasks.

Pharmacist

A **pharmacist** is a specialist in formulating and dispensing medications, licensed by individual states to practice pharmacy (the study of preparing and dispensing drugs). Pharmacists are employed in hospitals, medical centers, and pharmacies. Training consists of two years of postgraduate study in pharmacology.

Pharmacy Technician

Pharmacy technicians assist licensed pharmacists in preparing medications for patients and, in certain cases, administering the medicine. They also assist in clerical duties such as telephone communication, typing, and filing and often in patient education regarding medicines. Requirements and duties may vary in different states; however, professional certification can be obtained through individual state pharmacy boards.

Phlebotomist

In some areas, skilled **phlebotomists** are referred to as **accessioning technicians** because they are extensively trained in the art of drawing blood for diagnostic laboratory testing. Most often they are lab technicians. They must be nationally certified and are employed in medical clinics, hospitals, and laboratories. (Under the supervision of a physician, the medical assistant who has had instruction, practice on a training arm, and evaluation proving competency in this skill may perform this procedure to obtain blood specimens for analysis.)

Physical Therapist

A **physical therapist** is licensed to assist in the examination, testing, and treatment of physically disabled or handicapped people and those patients who are going through a physical rehabilitation program following accident, in-

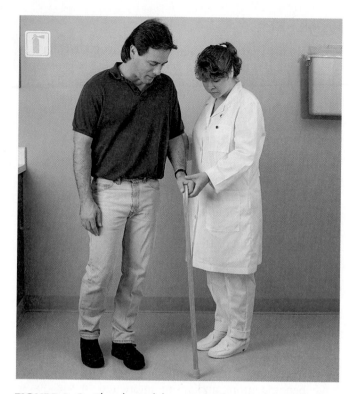

FIGURE 1–9 The physical therapist explains to the patient the correct way to use ambulatory equipment.

jury, or serious illness through the use of special exercise, application of heat or cold, and use of **ultrasound** therapy, and other techniques (Figure 1–9). They qualify by having a Bachelor's of Science degree in physical therapy or getting a special 12-month certificate course after obtaining a Bachelor's of Science degree in a related field.

Physician Assistant

A **physician assistant (PA)** is a person trained in certain aspects of the practice of medicine or osteopathy to provide assistance to the physician. These individuals are trained by physicians and practice under their direct supervision and within the legal license of a physician according to the laws of each state. Students who have successfully completed pre-med requirements can apply for the required two-year physician assistant program.

Podiatrist/Chiropodist

Podiatrists and **chiropodists** are trained to diagnose and treat diseases and disorders of the feet. They may be awarded these degrees: DSC—Doctor of Surgical Chiropody; PodD—Doctor of Podiatry; and with further training, DPM—Doctor of Podiatric Medicine.

Psychologist

Psychologists specialize in the study of the structure and function of the brain and related mental processes. They have a graduate degree in psychology and training in clinical psychology. They provide testing and counseling services to patients with mental and emotional disorders. Psychologists have private practices or may be a part of a group family practice.

Radiology Technician, Radiologic Technologist, X-Ray Technician

An **x-ray technician**, **radiology technician**, or **radiologic technologist**, Figure 1–10, is one who has had specialized training in the various techniques of visualization of the tissues and organs of the body and who, under the supervision of a physician radiologist, operates radiologic equipment and assists radiologists and other health professionals. Competence must be proved by the American Registry of Radiologic Technologists.

Respiratory Therapy Technician

Respiratory therapy technicians are graduates of an AMA-approved school designed to qualify persons for the technician certification examination of the National Board for Respiratory Care. These members of the health care team perform procedures of treatment that maintain or improve the **ventilatory** function of the respiratory tract in patients. The training period for this field is usually a one-year program in a hospital setting.

Unit Clerk

A **unit clerk** performs routine clerical and reception tasks in a patient care unit of a hospital. This position requires a self-motivated, mature individual to handle the stress of

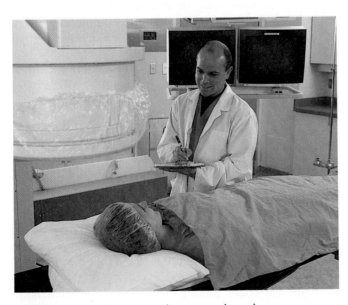

FIGURE 1–10 The x-ray technician explains the x-ray procedure to the patient.

A CAAHEP CONNECTION

Standards identify a professional component of allied health professions and credentialing as an essential area of instruction. This unit addresses a variety of professionals and briefly describes their training and roles in health care. It will help you understand how they fit into the total field of patient care.

---

the hectic pace of coordinating personnel and their duties at the nurses' station. Also called unit coordinator, unit secretary, **health unit coordinator**, administrative specialist, ward clerk, or ward secretary. Training is on the job or possibly included in a health care program such as medical assisting.

Because medical assistants are the most versatile of all health care workers, it is reasonable for them to seek employment in any of the previously mentioned areas of the medical field. Once these persons have gained basic entry-level skills in medical assisting, they are able to adapt easily to a specialty practice with additional training (the amount of which would obviously depend on the type of practice).

ACHIEVE UNIT OBJECTIVES

Complete Chapter 1, Unit 2 in the workbook to help you obtain competency of this subject matter.

UNIT 3
Medical Practice Specialties

OBJECTIVES

Upon completion of the unit, meet the following performance objectives by verifying knowledge of the facts and principles presented through oral and written communication at a level deemed competent.

1. Spell and define, using the glossary at the back of the text, all the **Words to Know** in this unit.
2. Identify the primary medical specialties and give the abbreviations for those that have them.
3. List eight health care professionals with doctoral degrees. Explain who should be called doctor.
4. Name employment possibilities for medical assistants other than with MDs and DOs.

5. Identify and spell correctly the title of each practitioner in each of the specialties.
6. Describe the educational process of becoming a physician.

AREAS OF COMPETENCE (AAMA)

This unit addresses content with the specific competency areas of *Patient care, Instruction, Legal concepts,* and *Instruction,* as identified in the Medical Assistant Role Delineation Study. Refer to Appendix A for a detailed listing of the areas.

■ WORDS TO KNOW

allergy	nuclear medicine
anesthesiologist	obstetrician
cardiologist	occupational medicine
chiropractic	oncology
competency	ophthalmologist
dentist	optometrist
deprivation	orthopedist
dermatologist	osteopathy
diplomate	otorhinolaryngologist
doctorates	pathologist
endocrinologist	pediatrician
gastroenterologist	perception
geriatrician	podiatrist
gerontologist	practitioner
gynecologist	preventive
hematologist	proprietorship
immunology	psychiatrist
infertility	psychologist
internist	psychotherapy
internship	pulmonary
licensure	radiologist
maintenance	radionuclides
manifestation	residency
manipulation therapy	surgeon
misalignment	traumatic
nephrologist	urology
neurologist	

HEALTH CARE PROFESSIONS

Ideally, all physicians dedicate their lives to acquiring skills in the art and science of diagnosing and treating disease and maintaining health. Each physician has this same goal. It is, however, impossible for a physician to study in detail every field of medicine. Because of this fact, some physicians become medical specialists. This means that they have chosen to gain expertise in one particular area of medicine. Some doctors additionally have a particular interest that is not a specialty, but is an area they feel worthy of their time and effort and effective in helping their patients toward better health. These areas are viewed as subspecialties or areas of special interest.

Because medical assistants generally are employed by physicians in their offices, they need a basic understanding of the various medical specialties and special interests. The medical assistant who works for a general practitioner may need to initiate contacts with specialists through referrals.

The medical assistant must then be knowledgeable about these areas to help reinforce or clarify the physician's directions to the patient. Moreover, knowing about these various practices will also help the medical assistant to decide in which area to seek employment. Most specialists maintain office practices and have a need for medical assistants just as general and family practitioners do. Adapting to these special areas after acquiring basic skills and knowledge should be relatively easy. A medical assistant interested in advancement must be willing to put forth the necessary effort.

To help you get familiar with these specialties, Table 1–1 contains basic information concerning each area. You should note that a few specialty practices are not listed in the table. One of those practices is the specialty practice of emergency medicine or traumatic medicine. In this case, the referral may be initiated by the family or general practitioner's office if, when the patient phones in for advice concerning a condition, the patient's symptoms suggest a true emergency or urgency, then referring the patient to an urgent or emergency care center is certainly the procedure. And too, physicians who practice in the specialties of anesthesiology and pathology are usually hospital-based; rarely do they have private practice offices where patients are seen. These specialists work as members of the health care team contributing their expert skills and knowledge in serving patients. More precise knowledge of all these practices will come with experience and further study.

The field of general practice covers perhaps the broadest spectrum. The general practitioner sees all kinds of patients with all kinds of problems. Most can be handled by the general practitioner. If, however, the symptoms of a case suggest a serious or perhaps unknown cause, the patient may be referred to a specialist for further diagnosis and/or treatment (Figure 1–11). When the patient's specific need or problem has been remedied or the recovery plan has been established, the patient returns to the "family doctor" for continued care.

The following pages will introduce you to many fields of medical practice and allied health professions. Because treating patients is a team effort, gaining a basic knowledge of the duties involved in each type of practice will help you better serve the patient. Better communication between colleagues who understand each other leads to more efficient patient care.

TABLE 1-1

MEDICAL SPECIALTIES

Specialty	Title of Practitioner	Area of Specialization	Types of Patients Seen
Allergy	Allergist	Diagnosing and treating conditions of altered immunologic reactivity (allergic reactions)	Adults of all ages, children, both sexes
Anesthesiology	Anesthesiologist	Administering anesthetic agents before and during surgery	Adults of all ages, children, both sexes
Cardiology	Cardiologist	Diagnosing and treating abnormalities, diseases, and disorders of the heart	Adults of all ages, children, both sexes
Chiropractic	Chiropractor (Chiropractors are not physicians, but they are licensed in their field of practice. They hold the degree of DC, or Doctor of Chiropractic.)	Manipulative treatment of disorders originating from misalignment of the spinal vertebrae	Adults of all ages, children, both sexes
Dentistry	Dentist (Dentists are not physicians, but they are licensed in their field of practice, which can range from general to highly specialized. They hold the degree of DDS, or Doctor of Dental Surgery.)	Diagnosing and treating diseases and disorders of the teeth and gums	Adults of all ages, children, both sexes
Dermatology	Dermatologist	Diagnosing and treating disorders of the skin	Adults of all ages, children, both sexes
Endocrinology	Endocrinologist	Diagnosing and treating diseases and malfunctions of the glands of internal secretion	Adults of all ages, children, both sexes
Family practice	Family practitioner	Similar to general practice in nature, but centering around the family unit	Adults of all ages, infants and children of all ages, both sexes
Gastroenterology	Gastroenterologist	Diagnosing and treating diseases and disorders of the stomach and intestines	Adults of all ages, children, both sexes
Geriatrics	Gerontologist or geriatrician	Diagnosing and treating diseases, disorders, and problems associated with aging	Older adults, both sexes
Gynecology	Gynecologist	Diagnosing and treating diseases and disorders of the female reproductive tract; strong emphasis on preventive measures	Female adolescents and adults
Hematology	Hematologist	Diagnosing and treating diseases and disorders of the blood and blood-forming tissues	Adults of all ages, infants and children, both sexes
Infertility	Infertility specialist	Diagnosing and treating problems in conceiving and maintaining pregnancy	Couples who desire to have children but cannot
Internal medicine	Internist	Diagnosing and treating diseases and disorders of the internal organs	Adults of all ages, children, both sexes
Nephrology	Nephrologist	Diagnosing and treating diseases and disorders of the kidney	Adults, children, both sexes
Neurology	Neurologist	Diagnosing and treating diseases and disorders of the central nervous system	Adults, children, both sexes
Nuclear medicine	Nuclear medicine specialist	Diagnosing and treating diseases with the use of radionuclides	Adults, both sexes

(continued)

TABLE 1–1

MEDICAL SPECIALTIES (Continued)

Specialty	Title of Practitioner	Area of Specialization	Types of Patients Seen
Obstetrics	Obstetrician	Providing direct care to females during pregnancy, childbirth, and immediately thereafter	Pregnant females
Occupational Medicine	Occupational medicine specialist	Diagnosing and treating diseases or conditions arising from occupational circumstances (e.g., chemicals, dust, or gases)	Adults of all ages, both sexes
Oncology	Oncologist	Diagnosing and treating tumors and cancer	Adults of all ages, children, both sexes
Ophthalmology	Ophthalmologist	Diagnosing and treating diseases and disorders of the eye	Adults of all ages, children, both sexes
Optometry	Optometrist (Optometrists are not physicians, but are licensed in their field of practice. They hold the degree of OD, or Doctor of Optometry.)	Measuring the accuracy of vision to determine if corrective lenses are needed	Adults of all ages, children, both sexes
Orthopedics	Orthopedist	Diagnosing and treating disorders and diseases of the bones, muscles, ligaments, and tendons, and fractures of the bones	Adults of all ages, children, both sexes
Otorhinolaryngology	Otorhinolaryngologist (Commonly referred to as an ENT [ear, nose, and throat] specialist.)	Diagnosing and treatment of disorders and diseases of the ear, nose, and throat	Adults of all ages, children, both sexes
Pathology	Pathologist	Analysis of tissue samples to confirm diagnosis	Usually has no direct contact with patients
Pediatrics	Pediatrician	Diagnosing and treating diseases and disorders of children; strong emphasis on preventive measures	Infants, children, and adolescents
Physical medicine	Physical medicine specialist	Diagnosing and treating diseases and disorders with physical agents (physical therapy)	Adults, children, both sexes
Podiatry	Podiatrist (Podiatrists are not physicians, but they are licensed in their field of practice. They hold the degree of DPM, or Doctor of Podiatric Medicine.)	Diagnosing and treating diseases and disorders of the feet	Adults, children, both sexes
Psychiatry	Psychiatrist	Diagnosing and treating pronounced manifestations of emotional problems or mental illness that may have an organic causative factor	Adults of all ages, children, both sexes. (Note: Child psychiatry is a further specialized field dealing exclusively with children and adolescents.)
Psychology	Psychologist (Psychologists are not physicians, but they are licensed in their field of practice. They hold the degree of PhD, or Doctor of Philosophy.)	Evaluating and treating emotional problems. These professionals give counseling to individuals, families, and groups	Adults, children, both sexes

(continued)

TABLE 1-1

		MEDICAL SPECIALTIES (Continued)	
Specialty	Title of Practitioner	Area of Specialization	Types of Patients Seen
Pulmonary specialties	Pulmonary/thoracic/cardiovascular specialist	Diagnosing and treating diseases and disorders of the chest, lungs, heart, and blood vessels	Adults, both sexes
Radiology	Radiologist	Diagnosing and treating diseases and disorders with roentgen rays (x-rays) and other forms of radiant energy	Adults of all ages, children, both sexes
Sports medicine	Sports medicine specialist	Diagnosing and treating injuries sustained in athletic events	Adults, especially young adults (athletes), both sexes
Surgery	Surgeon	Diagnosing and treating diseases, injuries, and deformities by manual or operative methods	Adults of all ages, infants, children, both sexes
Traumatic medicine	Emergency physician (Commonly referred to as ER or trauma physician since most work in hospital emergency rooms.)	Diagnosing and treating acute (traumatic) illnesses and injuries	Adults of all ages, infants, children, both sexes
Urology	Urologist	Diagnosing and treating diseases and disorders of the urinary system of females and genitourinary system of males	Adults of all ages, infants, children

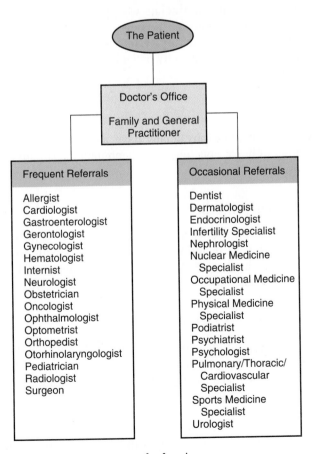

FIGURE 1-11 Frequency of referrals

A CAAHEP CONNECTION

The standards for curriculum indicate content be included that discusses health professions and credentialing. This unit contains information on the types of medical practice and the specialty areas within the field of medicine.

Physician Education

All physicians invest a minimum of nine years in learning how to practice medicine, which is the art and science of the diagnosis, treatment, and prevention of disease, and the **maintenance** of good health. Until recently, their training, education, and practical experience included a four-year college degree in pre-med, four years in medical school, and one year of **internship**. Following this and successful completion of the state board examination for **licensure**, the person was then considered a general **practitioner** and was ready to begin a private practice. This license to practice medicine is renewed periodically throughout the physician's life. Today the phrase "postgraduate year following medical school" (PGY-1) denotes the **internship** stage of training. Specialty areas require additional years of study in the particular area of choice. It is usually between two and six years and is commonly known as **residency** or PGY-2, 3, 4, and so on. After satisfactorily accomplishing all requirements, the physician is awarded a certificate of **competency** in the specialty area and is recognized as a **diplomate** of that specialty.

Types of Practices

The actual business of practicing medicine may be conducted in several ways. Many physicians prefer to have a solo practice, or sole **proprietorship**, meaning that the individual alone makes all decisions regarding the practice. Being employed as a medical assistant in this type of office requires that you have both administrative and clinical skills essential for the smooth operation of that practice, especially if you are the only employee.

In a partnership, two or more physicians have a legal agreement to share in the total business operation of the practice. In this case, usually two to several medical assistants (or other members of the health care team) are employed to care for patients and conduct business.

A group practice consists of three or more physicians who share a facility for the purpose of practicing medicine. In this legal contract the doctors share expenses, income, equipment, records, and personnel. Many times these practices are a health maintenance organization (HMO) or an independent practice association (IPA) type of practice. You will learn more about these in Chapter 9. Usually, several professionals make up the health care team in this setting. Medical assistants, lab technicians, radiology technicians, nurses, physician assistants, and the physicians work together in providing health care.

SUBSPECIALTY/SPECIAL INTEREST AREAS

In the following you will be introduced to the subspecialty (S) or special interest (SI) areas that branch off from a particular specialty practice. A brief description and definition of each area will give you a basic idea of the roles they play in the health care team. As you learn and study the duties and responsibilities of the medical assistant, you may realize a particular area of interest of your own. When the time comes for your internship and then later for you to begin the job search for gainful employment, you will have a basic understanding of the variety of practices so that you will be better prepared to make a decision of where to apply.

Acupuncture

This method of treatment originated in the Far East and has been gaining in popularity in western countries since the 1970s. This procedure involves the insertion of fine thin needles into specific sites of the body to alleviate pain or to treat a specific body system or area (its use is still controversial). (SI)

Adolescent Medicine

This area branches from pediatrics and specifically deals with youngsters aged 11 to 20 years, or the years of puberty to maturity. (S)

Aerospace Medicine

Physicians who extend their practice of medicine to this area do research in the effects of the environment in space on people. The areas of greatest concern are pathology, physiology, and psychology. (SI)

Alcoholism (Chemical Dependency)

These physicians treat patients who have addiction to alcohol and drugs. (SI)

Allergy and Immunology

An **allergy** is an acquired hypersensitivity a person exhibits to a substance that normally does not cause a reaction. Physicians interested in allergies sometimes combine these areas because they are closely related. **Immunology** is the study of how the body deals with immunity to disease (it is a subspecialty sometimes practiced alone). (S)

Cardiology (Cardiovascular Disease)

A **cardiologist** is a physician who specializes in treating diseases and disorders of the heart. Because the heart is the center of the circulatory system, a cardiovascular specialist is one who treats only patients with heart and blood vessel problems. (S)

Diabetes

As implied, these physicians have a special interest in treating only patients who have been diagnosed with diabetes. (SI)

Emergency Medicine

Physicians practicing this subspecialty are concerned with the diagnosis and treatment of patients with conditions that have resulted from injury or trauma or from sudden illness. (S)

Gynecologic Oncology

The subspecialty of gynecology that deals with the diagnosis and treatment of cancer of the reproductive tract of females of all ages is called gynecologic oncology. (S)

Hypertension

A physician who subspecializes in this area treats patients who have high blood pressure (hypertension). (SI)

Hypnosis

This method of treatment is becoming more popular with physicians. This procedure is used mainly in **psychotherapy** in which the patient is induced into a trancelike sleep to help change the memory or the **perception** of something in that person (such as weight control or an unwanted behavior like smoking). Its use in medicine is to help patients deal with pain and stress, which affect their overall health. (SI)

Nutrition

This area of special interest includes patients with disorders or diseases related to how the body uses food and drink for growth and maintenance. (SI)

Pediatric Allergists

These physicians deal only with treating children who have allergies. (S)

Preventive Medicine

This branch of medicine deals with the prevention of both mental and physical illness and disease. It is sometimes referred to as General Preventive Medicine (GPM). (S)

Rheumatology

Physicians in this subspecialty treat inflammatory disorders of the connective tissues and related structures. (S)

Sleep Disorder

As the name implies, physicians who deal with these patients are interested in the various stages of sleep and the effects of sleep **deprivation**. (SI)

Surgery

Most of the subspecialty areas of this branch of medicine and **osteopathy** are listed below:

- Cardiovascular
- Colon (and rectal)
- Cosmetic (plastic and reconstructive)
- Hand
- Head and neck
- Neurologic
- Orthopedic
- Pediatrics
- Spine
- Thoracic
- Urologic
- Vascular

With the great strides that medical science achieves, the field of medicine continues to evolve with remarkable new

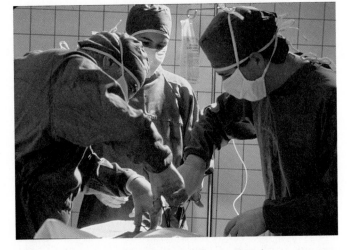

FIGURE 1–12 A successful operation requires the cooperation and expertise of the surgeon and the entire surgical team.

treatments, medications, and discoveries. Being an integral part of the health care team is exciting (Figure 1–12). New areas of special interest and subspecialties are ever-changing with the latest findings. Keeping abreast of these changes by attending ongoing educational programs to increase your knowledge will help you to become not only more confident in your work, but a most valuable medical assistant as well.

A NOTE REGARDING DOCTORS

As you progress in the field of medical assisting, a basic understanding of the frequently misused term *doctor* will be helpful. The term comes from Latin; it means *to teach.* Persons who hold doctoral degrees (**doctorates**) are entitled to be addressed as "Doctor" and to write the initials that stand for their doctorate after their name. The abbreviation "Dr." is the proper way to address a physician or any other type of doctor who has earned this title. In the medical field, the abbreviation "Dr." denotes that the person is qualified to practice medicine. In other fields, it means that the person has achieved the highest academic degree awarded by a college in the particular discipline. The doctors with whom you will be coming into contact include:

- Doctor of Chiropractic (DC)
- Doctor of Dental Medicine (DMD)
- Doctor of Dental Surgery (DDS)
- Doctor of Medicine (MD)
- Doctor of Optometry (OD)
- Doctor of Osteopathy (DO)
- Doctor of Philosophy (PhD)
- Doctor of Podiatric Medicine (DPM)

Doctor of Medicine and Doctor of Osteopathy

One of the areas of greatest confusion is the differentiation between MDs and DOs. Holders of either degree are licensed physicians. The degrees themselves originate from somewhat different schools of thought. (Interestingly enough, it was an MD who founded the osteopathic movement that now produces DOs.) Physicians of both schools must satisfactorily complete board examinations in the state where they wish to practice medicine.

The development of osteopathy has become an accepted medical treatment because of the efforts of a physician named Dr. Andrew T. Still. In 1874, Dr. Still began to practice the philosophy of osteopathy (the practice of being concerned with the patient as a whole person) and to use an alternative method to treat them. He was concerned with the overuse of drugs and medicines and feared that surgery was used too quickly to relieve patients' suffering. Because there was no college that taught the practices of osteopathy, Dr. Still traveled the country giving demonstrations to those who were interested about how to alleviate illness with **manipulation therapy**. His sons later joined him in giving instruction to students in the first school of osteopathy. The premise of osteopathy is that relieving structural stress increases the body's functional capabilities and allows the body to heal itself.

The charter for the American School of Osteopathy was obtained in 1892 in Kirksville, Missouri. This later became the Associated Colleges of Osteopathy and the degree of Doctor of Osteopathy (DO) was accepted. During World War II, osteopathic physicians became respected and appreciated for their services to both soldiers

---

RELATING TO ABHES

Chapter 1 discusses the history of medicine and the contributions of the many professionals, both past and present, involved in providing health care. This content is related to the ABHES accreditation requirement of *Professionalism* that is within the content area of **Career Development**.

---

and the general public. Today, there is a mutual respect among physicians of MD and DO degrees.

In the United States today, medical licensing boards permit DOs to perform the same duties as MDs. Should you find employment working for either a DO or MD, you will be able to apply the same administrative and clinical knowledge and skills.

Although you are training primarily to assist physicians, with a little adaptation you could also move into assisting chiropractors, psychologists, or podiatrists. To move into the dental or optometric field would require additional training.

ACHIEVE UNIT OBJECTIVES

Complete Chapter 1, Unit 3 in the workbook to help you obtain competency of this subject matter.

RESOURCES

American Medical Association (1999–2000). Health professions directory (27th ed.). Chicago: Author.

Clayman, C.B. (Ed.) (1989). Encyclopedia of medicine. New York: Random House.

Hastings, R.P. (1974). Medicine: An international history. New York: Praeger.

Johnson Publishing Company (1983, September). Neurosurgery. *Ebony.*

Jones, B.E. (1978). The difference a D.O. makes. Oklahoma City, OK: Times-Journal Publishing Company.

Lippincott's textbook for medical assistants. (1997). Philadelphia, PA: Lippincott-Raven Publishers.

Marks, G., and Beatty, W.K. (1973). The story of medicine in America. New York: Scribners.

Medical assisting: A patient centered approach. (1999). Princeton, NJ: Glencoe/McGraw-Hill.

Mosby (1998). Mosby's medical, nursing, and allied health dictionary (5th ed.). St. Louis, MO: Author.

Raven, S., and Weir, A. (1981). Women of achievement. New York: Harmony.

Sicherman, B., and Green, C.H. (1980). Notable American women: The modern period. Cambridge, MA: Belknap.

Thomas, C.L. (1997). Taber's cyclopedic medical dictionary (18th ed.). Philadelphia, PA: F.A. Davis.

Venes, T. (2001). Taber's cyclopedic medical dictionary (19th ed.). Philadelphia, PA: F.A. Davis.

WEB LINKS

http://www.abms.org **(American Board of Medical Specialties)**

This web site provides information on specialization and certification in medicine.

The Medical Assistant

The American Association of Medical Assistants (AAMA) describes the medical assistant profession as follows: "The medical assistant is a professional, multi-skilled person dedicated to assisting in patient care management. This practitioner performs administrative and clinical duties and may manage emergency situations, facilities, and/or personnel. Competence in the field also requires that a medical assistant display professionalism, communicate effectively, and provide instruction to patients."

During the evolvement of the practice of medicine, physicians have come to realize the value of medical assistants. Many years ago, physicians could treat patients alone. There was no need for appointments, filing of insurance forms, or extensive record keeping. There was rarely any thought of a lawsuit.

Times have changed dramatically. It is now necessary to document every transaction between the physician or the office staff and the patient to validate appropriate and responsible care. Accurate and comprehensive records are vital. Attention to every office management detail is essential as well.

This chapter discusses the training opportunities and job responsibilities of a medical assistant. It also describes highly desirable personal characteristics that will help make you a valuable asset to the physician. In addition, it identifies those attributes of professionalism which elevate your working experience to a higher level and provide you with personal satisfaction.

UNIT 1

Training, Job Responsibilities, and Employment Opportunities

■ OBJECTIVES

Upon completion of the unit, meet the following performance objectives by verifying knowledge of the facts and principles presented through oral and written communication at a level deemed competent.

1. Spell and define, using the glossary at the back of the text, all the **Words to Know** in this unit.
2. Name the two factors that are causing increased employment opportunities in the health care field.
3. Identify three types of schools that offer programs in medical assisting.
4. Explain the purpose of the *Developing a Curriculum* (DACUM) and the Role Delineation Study.
5. List the 10 areas of competence identified by the Role Delineation Study.
6. Explain the term "career laddering."
7. Identify the 14 fastest growing health occupations, according to the United States Department of Labor.

AREAS OF COMPETENCE (AAMA)

This unit addresses content within the specific competency areas of *Professionalism, Legal concepts,* and *Instruction* as identified in the Medical Assistant Role Delineation Study. Refer to Appendix A for a detailed listing of the areas.

■ WORDS TO KNOW

administrative
analysis
associate's degree
bookkeeper
certificate of completion
clinical
competency
compliance
confidential
curriculum
DACUM
hygienist
license
methodical

nuclear medicine
   technologist
professional
proprietary
radioactive agents
receptionist
rehabilitation centers
rehabilitative therapy
Role Delineation Study
secretary
therapeutic
therapist
ultrasound technologist

You have chosen to become a medical assistant. In a brochure published by the AAMA entitled "Plan Your Career as a Medical Assistant," a series of questions is listed to help the interested individual decide whether to pursue the career. The questions are:

- Do you like people?
- Do you want variety in your work?
- Can you "take hold" and get things done?
- Are you **methodical** and accurate in what you do?
- Can you be trusted with **confidential** information?

If you can answer yes to these questions, you may have the appropriate characteristics of a medical assistant. You will be pleased to learn that, according to the United States Department of Labor, this occupation is one of the health care areas identified to experience significant growth in the near future. Health occupations make up 47%, nearly half, of the total 30 identified fastest growing occupations. Specifically, medical assisting is expected to be one of the 10 fastest growing occupations through the year 2008.

In this unit, you will learn about the training and responsibilities of a medical assistant. You will also read about opportunities for employment in medical assisting as well as how experience, together with additional training, can qualify you for other health care jobs in the future.

Health care occupations have developed from the physician's need to enlist the help of other persons to provide technical and efficient care for greater numbers of patients. In addition to medical assistants who work directly with the physician, a large number of highly technical and **professional** people perform a great number of diagnostic and supporting functions. In the 1998–2008 Employment Occupational Outlook Bulletin, the United States Department of Labor data indicated that 14 health care related occupations would be growing faster than the average overall workforce through the year 2008. Opportunities would be plentiful in these broad occupational groups, with a predicted average growth rate of 29.6%.

Table 2–1 lists the projected percentages of growth in the fastest growing health occupations. Table 2–2 also lists data available from the United States Department of Labor. The first two columns show the 1998 and the 2008 projected employment figures of representative health care occupations. The third and fourth columns show the increase percentage of employment (except for ECG technicians) and the number of jobs anticipated within the 10-year period. Note: All data are listed in thousands, so three zeros need to be added to each number. The last two columns show the total number of new employees needed within the 10 years and indicate the most significant source of education for the job.

The health occupations boom is the result of two factors: the extended lifetimes of Americans and the rapidly evolving medical technology. Data has shown that the population over age 85 is growing at a rate of four times the total population. As people age, they develop more health problems and therefore require more services. With the development of new diagnostic tests and methods of treatment, someone must be trained to operate the equipment

TABLE 2-1

PROJECTED PERCENTAGES OF GROWTH IN THE 14 FASTEST GROWING HEALTH OCCUPATIONS

Occupation	Projected Growth (Percent Increase)
Medical assistants	58%
Personal care and home health aides	58%
Physician assistants	48%
Medical records and health information technicians	44%
Physical therapy assistants and aides	44%
Respiratory therapists	43%
Dental assistants	42%
Surgical technologists	42%
Dental hygienists	41%
Occupational therapy assistants and aides	40%
Cardiovascular technologists and technicians	39%
Speech-language pathologists and audiologists	38%
Ambulance drivers and attendants, except EMTs	35%
Occupational therapists	34%

and provide the service. Occasionally, it means that a completely new field of employment is needed, such as has occurred with **nuclear medicine technologists**.

Another shift has resulted from the changing nature of how health care services are being delivered. A good example of this is the explosion of home health care; see Table 2–2. Employment in this area is expected to increase 58%. This reflects the growing population of the elderly and the disabled who will need assistance, but the trend will be toward providing it in their homes instead of within a more expensive health care facility. Note: It may be speculative on the author's part, but it seems that the family physician may once again need to visit these persons at home if they are to be served. If a financial incentive from insurance companies were offered to physicians, home visits would probably occur.

TRAINING

Since you are reading this text, you are probably enrolled in a formal training program to acquire the knowledge and skills needed to become a medical assistant. Thirty years ago it was relatively easy to be hired and trained on the job.

This may still take place in some offices, usually where there are multiple employees so work can continue while a new person learns. But today, with the fast-paced, complex level of skills required to provide medical care and conduct the business affairs of the practice, the value of a trained employee is recognized as a real asset by the physician.

Training programs vary in length and design. In many states, vocational education offers medical assisting programs. It can be an educational option in public high schools, usually for junior and senior students. Vocational programs may also be offered at the adult level to meet the needs of post-high school individuals. Many technical and community colleges offer training as well. Programs leading to a **certificate of completion** or diploma are usually one year in length. An **associate's degree** program would require two years of course work and include subject areas which complement the **curriculum**. Another major source of training is available from private **proprietary** schools. This training may also vary in length and content depending upon the school's philosophy, affiliation, and educational goals.

Regardless of the type of school, the *basic* medical assistant curriculum should be similar. From 1979 through 1996 The AAMA maintained a document called the **DACUM** (*D*eveloping *a Cu*rriculu*m*). This publication identified the areas of practice and the **competencies** required for the occupation of medical assistant. This document was updated in 1984 and 1990. In 1997, the DACUM was replaced by the **Role Delineation Study**. Two groups of practicing certified medical assistants (CMAs) were surveyed by the National Board of Medical Examiners and AAMA. Based upon the groups' practical experiences, they listed all current competencies essential for medical assistants. The lists of competencies were combined with the 1990 DACUM to form a survey instrument which was sent to a random sample of CMAs who represent many areas of practice, geographic locations, and a variety of backgrounds. The responses were evaluated and became the content for the areas of competence for entry-level medical assistants found in the Role Delineation Study. The AAMA Curriculum Review Board finalized the list of competencies which became the *Standards and Guidelines of an Accredited Educational Program for the Medical Assistant* and replaced the previous *Essentials*.

The Role Delineation Study identifies three broad areas of practice: Administrative, Clinical, and General (Transdisciplinary). These are further divided into 10 areas of competence as listed in Table 2–3. The complete Medical Assistant Role Delineation Chart illustrating all skills (standard and advanced) within each area of competence is shown in detail in Appendix A. A grid which correlates the competencies to the text follows the Delineation Study Chart. These competencies are deemed necessary by the AAMA for the entry-level practice of medical assisting. In this text, the competency areas discussed within the content of each unit are identified at the beginning of the unit. You can increase your understanding and application of the study by referring to appendix A for more specific

TABLE 2-2

CURRENT AND PROJECTED EMPLOYMENT IN 18 HEALTH OCCUPATIONS (FROM U.S. DEPARTMENT OF LABOR, BUREAU OF LABOR STATISTICS BULLETIN 2522)

Occupation	Employment*		Employment Change, 1998–2008		Total Job Openings Due to Growth and Net Replacements* 1998–2008	Most Significant Source of Training
	1998	Projected 2008	Percent (increase)	Number* (increase)		
cardiovascular technologists	21	29	39.4%	8	13	associate's degree
clinical lab technologists and technicians	313	366	17.0%	53	93	bachelor's degree associate's degree
dental assistants	229	325	42.2%	97	131	OJT moderate-term
dental hygienists	143	201	40.5%	58	90	associate's degree
ECG technicians	12	10	−23.1%†	−3†	3	OJT moderate term
emergency medical technicians (EMTs)	150	197	31.6%	47	84	postsecondary-vocational training
home health aides	746	1,179	58%	433	502	OJT short-term
licensed practical nurses (LPNs)	692	828	19.7%	136	286	postsecondary-vocational training
medical assistants	252	398	57.8%	146	208	OJT moderate-term
medical records technicians	92	133	43.9%	41	63	associate's degree
medical secretaries	219	246	12%	26	62	postsecondary-vocational training
nurse aides, orderlies, attendants	1,367	1,692	23.8%	325	515	OJT short-term
occupational therapy assistant, aides	19	26	39.8%	7	12	associate's degree
pharmacy assistants	61	71	15.9%	10	25	OJT short-term
pharmacy technicians	109	126	15.7%	17	44	OJT moderate-term
physician assistants	66	98	48%	32	43	bachelor's degree
registered nurses (RNs)	2,079	2,530	21.7%	451	794	associate's degree
surgical technologists	54	77	41.8%	23	36	postsecondary-vocational training

Note: OJT = On-the-job training

*Numbers are listed in thousands

†Note surplus

identification of the knowledge and skills within each area that are covered in the unit content. Mastery of the competencies will prepare you to successfully complete the certification examination administered by the AAMA and acquire the CMA credential as evidence of your qualifications. (This is more fully discussed in Chapter 2, Unit 3.)

An organization that governs programs of educational preparation of medical assistants is the Commission on

TABLE 2-3

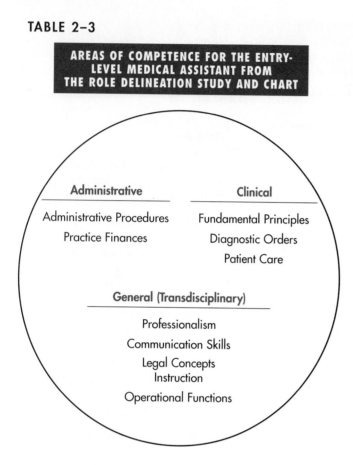

AREAS OF COMPETENCE FOR THE ENTRY-LEVEL MEDICAL ASSISTANT FROM THE ROLE DELINEATION STUDY AND CHART

Administrative

Administrative Procedures

Practice Finances

Clinical

Fundamental Principles

Diagnostic Orders

Patient Care

General (Transdisciplinary)

Professionalism

Communication Skills

Legal Concepts

Instruction

Operational Functions

Accreditation of Allied Health Education Programs (CAAHEP). General educational requirements cover the program length, the facility, the administration and faculty, library access, finances and other areas of operation. In addition, specific criteria are established in cooperation with the AAMA regarding the preparation of medical assistants. The curriculum must cover content in at least eight specific areas, plus provide an externship of a minimum 160 contact hours of practical experience. Educational programs desiring to acquire this accreditation standard participate in an on-site review process that measures their compliance to the established standards. If successful, the program is awarded approval by CAAHEP. This is a very desirable credential and qualifies graduates from CAAHEP-approved programs to take the AAMA test for certification as a medical assistant.

This text addresses all eight areas of the CAAHEP curriculum requirements. Throughout the text, content that reflects a specific requirement is identified by a feature known as "A CAAHEP Connection". This helps you to connect what you are reading to the curriculum standards. The total CAAHEP Curriculum Standards are located in Appendix B and are followed by a grid that correlates the standards to the text. In addition, the accompanying workbook provides for evaluation based on the objectives stated in the text. This feature means that the curriculum content is *competency-based*, which meets another requirement of the CAAHEP standards.

An externship component, the last curriculum requirement, is included in the Instructor's Guide that supplements this text.

Another accrediting agency of medical assistant programs is the Accrediting Bureau of Health Education Schools (ABHES). The course content required for an ABHES-accredited program is located in Appendix C and is followed by a grid that correlates, by chapter, the text with the requirements. At the end of each chapter, in a feature called "Association with ABHES", the content is compared to the ABHES course requirements. Graduates of ABHES-accredited programs are eligible to take the CMA examination after one year of work experience.

In 1999, there were about 450 programs accredited by CAAHEP and more than 140 accredited by ABHES. There are other options for acquiring a credential from educational programs, and they are discussed in Unit 3 of this chapter.

JOB RESPONSIBILITIES

The role of the medical assistant is to provide skillful execution of administrative, clinical, and general duties as an integral and supportive part of the physician's practice. Performing clinical skills are an extension of the physician's role of assessment, examination, diagnosis, and treatment. Performing administrative skills help manage the business affairs of the practice. The performance of general skills are concerned with legal, ethical, moral, and professional conduct in the execution of your duties.

The following lists are examples of the variety of skills to be acquired in administrative, clinical, and general areas.

ADMINISTRATIVE
Schedule appointments
Prepare correspondence
Handle telephone calls
Complete insurance forms
Obtain initial patient data

CLINICAL
Take medical histories
Take vital signs
Assist with medical procedures
Prepare patient for examination
Prepare medications

GENERAL (Transdisciplinary)
Demonstrate initiative and responsibility
Treat all patients with compassion and empathy
Use medical terminology appropriately
Teach methods of health promotion
Work as a team member
Maintain confidentiality
Document accurately
Follow federal, state, and local legal guidelines

Many other tasks are performed regularly. A particularly important one is patient teaching. It is a task that requires special attention to the patient's response to ensure there will be **compliance** with the instruction. The assistant must carefully explain and/or demonstrate the procedure or activity and follow up with questioning to confirm understanding. The assistant should not assume something has been learned until the patient can explain or perform it.

It is also important for medical assistants to have a basic understanding of the anatomy and physiology of the human body. This knowledge helps in the comprehension of the need for diagnostic and treatment procedures ordered by the physician. A working knowledge of medical terminology is also essential in order to communicate with other health care professionals and to assist patients in understanding information or instructions given to them.

Another major responsibility of a medical assistant is the legal, moral, and ethical issues which are confronted on a daily basis. The medical assistant must be constantly aware of these concerns in order to respect the values of others and to eliminate the chance for personal or employer liability. This subject matter is more fully discussed in Chapter 3. To get an overview of all the tasks a medical assistant will be expected to perform, look through the "Procedures" list in the front pages of this book (page xi). Job responsibility, however, goes beyond just the execution of procedures; it includes a personal commitment to assist the physician in every way possible in order to provide total quality patient care.

EMPLOYMENT OPPORTUNITIES

The practice of medicine has changed dramatically. In earlier times, physicians could treat patients without any assistance. Today, medical assistants work in physicians' offices, clinics, hospitals, and other facilities, performing both administrative and clinical duties, under the supervision of the physician. The efficient medical practice requires much attention to detail to provide the best care possible to patients. It is essential to keep thorough records. The need for a **receptionist, secretary, bookkeeper,** and technician, in addition to a medical assistant or nurse, may be required. Some small individual practices may still be able to operate with only one support person, who will handle all the administrative, clinical, and operational duties alone.

Some physicians like to manage their office operations themselves, but most prefer to concentrate on patient care and give office management responsibilities to a professional member of their staff. This person can discuss fees, arrange collection of accounts, order supplies, perform banking activities, schedule staff hours, pay office expenses, and do many other operational duties. Medical assistants who have office experience and administrative ability are often given the responsibility of performing the duties of the office manager.

Medical assistants who specialize in certain fields may have other responsibilities. A podiatry assistant may make castings of feet, take x-rays, and assist in surgery. Ophthalmic assistants administer diagnostic tests, measure eye muscle function, explain proper care and use of safety glasses and eye shields, and demonstrate the care and insertion of contact lenses.

You should be encouraged by the employment opportunities in not only medical assisting but also related medical careers. According to the latest statistics, 208,000 additional medical assistants will be needed by the year 2008 in order to meet replacement and additional needs. The position of medical secretary will need 62,000 additional people, whereas the related areas of nurse assistant and orderly will require 325,000 new people. It is interesting to note that 10,829,000 people were employed overall in the health service industry in 1998 (latest figures available). October 2000 data of a portion of that group shows the following number to be employed in offices and clinics:

Medical offices and clinics	1,948,700
Dental offices	682,100
Chiropractic/optometry offices	176,500
Other health practitioners	458,800

Physicians prefer to hire experienced workers or graduates of formal programs in medical assisting especially if they have passed a national examination. Salaries vary depending upon experience, skill level, and geographic location. The median annual earnings of a medical assistant in 1998 was $20,680 and varied among the following largest employing groups:

Offices and clinics of medical doctors	$20,800
Hospitals	$20,400
Offices of osteopathic physicians	$19,600
Health and allied services	$19,300
Offices of other practitioners	$18,500

CAREER LADDERING

You may be completely satisfied as a medical assistant and find great pleasure in your work. This is very admirable—you are providing a valuable service. But perhaps, after a period of time, you decide you would like to pursue another occupation for personal reasons, achievement needs, or financial gain. The term *career laddering* refers to other occupations in which you might be employed based upon your interest, training, and experience. The "ladder" can be lateral or vertical. In addition to the advancement to a medical office manager, there is hospital-based employment which medical assistants can fulfill. Examples of lateral jobs are ward clerks, admissions clerks, medical records clerks, medical secretaries, phlebotomists, and ECG technicians.

Other job opportunities may be possible with some additional instruction, and you may already possess a portion of the skills. Patient care technician, a developing job category, is seen as an alternative position for a medical assistant. It is also hospital based and incorporates skills from medical, nursing, and medical laboratory assisting. The job tends to be defined by the employing facility who also is currently providing the training. At this time, there is no recognized criteria or standards of practice.

The following brief descriptions of other health careers will provide you with some information about the type of employment, the training required, and an average salary amount. Each of these positions would require additional training but would also provide you with a personal challenge and reward your efforts. NOTE: The salary scales are based on 1998 data (the latest available) and may vary widely according to geographic area.

Additional information is available from the web sites of state and federal governments, educational organizations, and professional associations. Refer to suggested web links at the end of this chapter.

Licensed Practical Nurses (LPNs)

Where Employed LPNs work under the supervision of registered nurses and physicians. They work in hospitals, nursing homes, private home care, and physicians' offices and clinics. The growing elderly population will increase the need for LPNs in nursing homes, group homes, and residential care facilities (Figure 2–1).

Training Training is usually a one-year program of classroom and clinical practice. All LPNs must pass a state licensing examination to begin practice. Training is available at approved schools of practical nursing operated by vocational-technical schools and community colleges. A current **license** is required in order to work as an LPN. Renewal is subject to continuing education credits in most states.

Salary Average annual salary is approximately $26,940 for a 40-hour week, excluding shift differentials.

Emergency Medical Technicians (EMTs)

Where Employed EMTs work for private ambulance services or municipal fire, police, or rescue squads. EMTs provide immediate, on-site care in cases such as auto accidents, heart attacks, drownings, injuries, and shootings. EMTs transport patients to a medical facility (Figure 2–2). They work in teams under the direction of a dispatcher. There are three levels of practice: basic, advanced, and paramedic. The growing population and an increase in a total number of elderly people will increase the need. There is a high turnover rate for EMTs because of the stressful nature of the job.

Training The basic training course is from 100 to 120 hours of classroom instruction plus 10 internship hours in a hospital emergency room. Training is provided by vocation-technical schools and community colleges in conjunction with hospitals, police, fire, and health departments. There are certification exams for each level which must be passed to work in that capacity.

Salary Salaries vary according to the level of expertise and the employer. A basic EMT earns approximately $23,000 to $24,000 annually, on average. The average paramedic EMT earns $28,500 to $30,000.

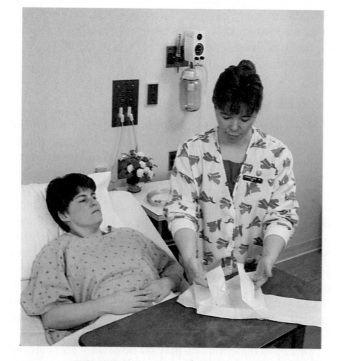

FIGURE 2–1 Licensed practical nurse

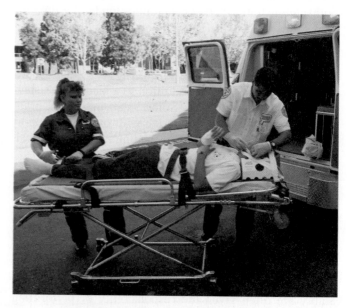

FIGURE 2–2 Emergency medical technicians

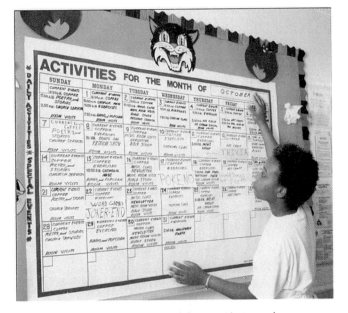

FIGURE 2-3   Recreational therapist/activity director

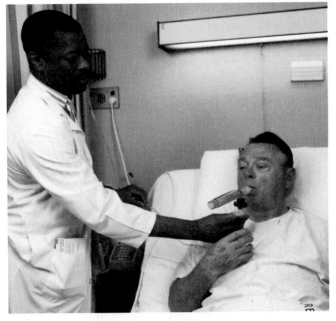

FIGURE 2-4   Respiratory therapist (RT) administering intermittent positive pressure breathing (IPPB) treatment

Recreational Therapists

Where Employed   Recreational **therapists** work in hospitals, **rehabilitation centers**, nursing homes, senior citizen facilities, and community recreational departments. They may assess a patient's condition by consulting medical records, the family, and the patient. A **therapeutic** program of individual or group activities can be developed by a recreational therapist, and may contain sports, arts, crafts, music, or outings. With advances in medical technology, more people survive illness and trauma and require **rehabilitative therapy**. Again, the increased number of elderly will require a larger amount of services.

Training   A bachelor's degree is the usual requirement, but an associate's degree program may be sufficient for some positions such as a nursing home director of activities (Figure 2–3). Certification by the National Council for Therapeutic Recreation requires a bachelor's degree.

Salary   A recreational therapist earns approximately $26,000 to $27,500 annually. Nursing home activity directors range from $16,500 to as much as $26,500 per year. Federal government employment of recreational therapists earn about $35,000 annually.

Respiratory Therapists

Where Employed   Respiratory therapists normally work 40 hours per week, but may work irregular night and weekend hours. Almost all work is in either respiratory care, anesthesiology, or pulmonary care departments of a hospital (Figure 2–4). Some may be employed by medical rental companies, home health care providers, and nursing homes. The increasing elderly population and the rapid rise in the number of acquired immune deficiency syndrome (AIDS) patients will increase the need for therapists.

Training   Most programs are two years in length. There are four-year and advanced two-year programs which are helpful for acquiring a supervisory position. In addition, there is a one-year technician program which permits employment in some settings. Most employers require all levels to obtain the Certified Respiratory Therapy Technician credential (CRRT). An advanced level certification is a Registered Respiratory Therapist (RRT).

Salary   The respiratory therapist's average annual salary is approximately $34,800.

Dental Hygienists

Where Employed   Almost all dental **hygienists** work in private dental offices. Some may work in public health agencies, schools, hospitals, or clinics. They regularly work 40 hours per week, but may often work part-time in more than one office. Dental hygienists provide preventive dental care by examining, cleaning, and taking x-rays of the teeth. They also remove sutures, teach oral hygiene, and provide restorative work. Population growth, higher incomes, and more elderly with natural teeth will increase the demand for dental services.

Training   Training is obtained at accredited dental hygiene programs of two or four years in length. All hygienists must pass the American Dental Association's

National Dental Examination in order to be licensed in their state of practice.

Salary   The average annual salary is approximately $44,000 but varies greatly in relation to the number of hours worked.

Nuclear Medicine Technologists

Where Employed   About 90% of nuclear medicine technologists work in hospitals, with the remaining 10% working in clinics and physicians' offices. Hospital employees usually work irregular hours and on-call rotations. Technologists locate and track **radioactive agents** that have been introduced into a patient's body as part of a diagnostic examination. The radioactive material, absorbed by a specific organ, produces images which are recorded on the photographic film of high-tech cameras. Technologic advances will increase nuclear medicine practice and the number of procedures, therefore requiring more technicians.

Training   There are different levels of training, varying from one to four years in length, that permit performance of various functions. **Ultrasound** and radiologic **technologists** complete one-year certificate programs (Figure 2–5). Advanced practice in nuclear medicine technology requires a two-year certificate or associate's degree. Many states require licensure. Federal standards covering administration and operation of radiation detection equipment must be met.

Salary   The average technologist salary for a 40-hour week, excluding shift differentials, is approximately $39,610 annually.

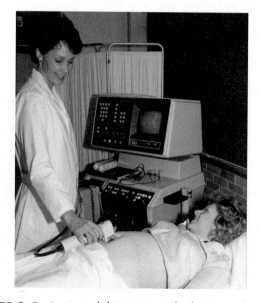

FIGURE 2–5   Registered diagnostic medical sonographer performing fetal ultrasound

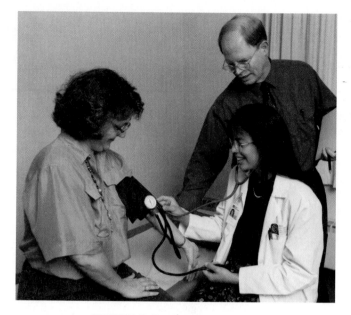

FIGURE 2–6   Physician assistant

Physician Assistants (PAs)

Where Employed   PAs are employed primarily in physicians' offices and clinics and work about 40 hours per week (Figure 2–6). Some hospitals employ PAs in their emergency department, on two 24-hour or three 12-hour shifts per week. Approximately 30% work in smaller communities where physicians are scarce. Depending on the state where they are licensed, PAs can treat injuries, suture wounds, apply splints and casts, examine patients, order and interpret lab and x-ray procedures, make diagnoses, treat, and prescribe most medications.

Training   The average PA program is two years in length and is offered by medical schools, vocational-technical schools, and four-year colleges. Graduates from accredited programs that become certified by an examination can use the letters PA-C following their name. Almost all states require certification. Recertification every six years, plus 100 hours of continuing education every two years, is required to maintain the certificate.

Salary   The average annual salary is approximately $47,090, with surgeons paying a slightly higher wage.

Pharmacy Technicians

Where Employed   Pharmacy technicians work in pharmacies in hospitals, grocery stores, and retail pharmacies. Opportunities also exist with pharmaceutical firms and wholesale pharmaceutical distributors. Duties include the preparation of prescriptions under the direct supervision of the pharmacist (Figure 2–7). Pharmacy technicians may also work in the retail side of the business. In some hospitals, pharmacy technicians dispense routine medica-

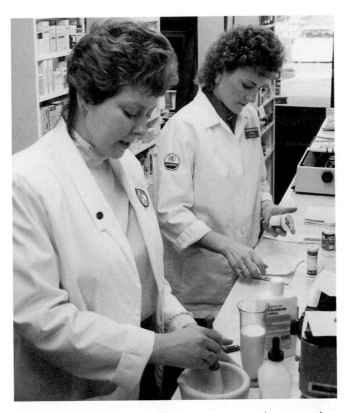

FIGURE 2–7 Pharmacy technicians prepare medications to be dispensed by pharmacists. (Courtesy of the Michigan Pharmacists Association and the Michigan Society of Pharmacy Technicians.)

tions to patients under the supervision of registered nurses (RNs).

Training The length of preparation varies and can occur during on-the-job training or by completing a certificate program or a two-year associate's degree college program. A National Pharmacy Technician Certification Examination is available through the Pharmacy Technician Certification Board. It offers the title of certified pharmacy technician (CPhT).

Salary The average pharmacy technician salary is $25,780 per year for a 40-hour week, but the job may require hours outside the regular 8-to-5 time frame.

Occupational Therapy Assistants

Where Employed Employment is under the supervision of a registered occupational therapist. Hospitals, rehabilitation facilities, retirement homes, psychiatric institutions, and nursing homes employ occupational therapist assistants (OTAs). Their duties involve helping individuals with mental or physical disabilities to learn or regain their highest level of functioning. This is achieved through activities that teach fine motor skills, day-to-day life skills, and the arts. OTAs prepare activity materials; maintain supplies, equipment, and tools; and document an individual's progress.

A CAAHEP CONNECTION

Knowledge of allied health careers, the training required, and the credentialing necessary for practice are important components of medical assisting curriculum. This brief discussion provides basic information regarding the training and duties of other members of the health care team so that you can make an informed career change, should you so choose.

Training OTAs must obtain an associate's degree and pass a national certification examination.

Salary The average OTA working a 40-hour week earns $28,690 annually.

Obviously, there is much opportunity within the health care field. Regardless of whether you remain a medical assistant or choose to practice in another field, you must be prepared to continue with life-long learning to maintain competency in your area of practice. At the present time, it appears that your efforts will be rewarded with the security of employment opportunities in the future. You are fortunate—this is not true in many fields of work.

ACHIEVE UNIT OBJECTIVES

Complete Chapter 2, Unit 1, in the workbook to help you obtain competency of this subject matter.

UNIT 2
Personal Characteristics

OBJECTIVES

Upon completion of the unit, meet the following performance objectives by verifying knowledge of the facts and principles presented through oral and written communication at a level deemed competent.

1. Spell and define, using the glossary at the back of the text, all the **Words to Know** in this unit.
2. List the 17 highly desired character traits of health care workers.
3. Identify five personality qualities desired.
4. Name the four voice characteristics desired.
5. Give two reasons why health care workers need to be concerned about their appearances.
6. List the nine things that contribute to a professional appearance.

WORDS TO KNOW

accurate	innate
adapt	intelligence
appearance	monotone
attitude	patience
confidential	perceive
cooperate	perseverance
courteous	personality
dependable	posture
discreet	punctuality
empathy	reliable
enthusiasm	respectful
flexible	self-control
honesty	tact
initiative	trait

HIGHLY DESIRABLE CHARACTERISTICS OF HEALTH CARE WORKERS

There are many personal character **traits** that are highly desirable for health care workers. Some characteristics seem to be almost **innate**, while others must be learned. All traits can be enhanced by consciously making an effort to improve them. Your ability to work well with your employer, supervisors, and coworkers and your effectiveness in dealing with patients is greatly influenced by your personal characteristics.

First, let us examine some character traits as they relate to the manner in which job responsibilities are performed. As you read and consider the content, try to *honestly* examine your own character traits. Then we'll look at a few **personality** qualities and consider the messages they send when there is either verbal or nonverbal interaction with others.

Character Traits

For each of the following character traits, rate yourself on a scale of 1, 2, or 3: 1 = not usually, 2 = usually, and 3 = always. Can you score at least 30?

Accuracy   (detailed correctness, exactness): Performing procedures in the correct manner is extremely important. Findings may be inaccurate or the process unsafe if you are careless. The **accurate** recording of patients' remarks and findings from vital signs or other assessments is ex-

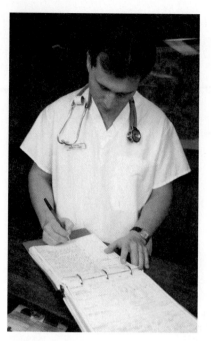

FIGURE 2–8 Accuracy is important when recording information.

tremely important, as is the preparation of medications and injections. Hopefully, you will always be conscious of accuracy (Figure 2–8).

Adaptable   (the ability to adjust, to make fit): In employment, it will often be necessary to **adapt** to a change in a situation to benefit the operation of the office, such as changing your schedule to work for someone or performing duties not usually your responsibility. Your willingness to be **flexible** and to **cooperate** will be noticed by your employer or supervisor and, in the future, if you should need someone to adapt to your situation, that individual will be more willing to work it out with you.

Conservative   (to be cautious, prudent; to handle with care; not wasteful): You will be handling equipment, materials, and supplies daily. It is important that you conserve office equipment usefulness and not carelessly waste products. Treat the things in the office as if they were your own. Waste is lost profit.

Courteous   (to be polite, well-mannered): You will be a representative of your employer and are expected to be **courteous** to coworkers, patients, and office visitors. This will not always be easy. It is never easy to be nice to someone who has been making it difficult for you. But, be courteous in spite of difficulties, and you will know you acted properly—it might even change the situation for the better.

Dependable   (can be relied upon, responsible): Can people depend on you to carry out your responsibilities without the need of constant supervision? When you agree to do something, do you always follow through? If you are **dependable**, you are at work, organized, and ready to start the day when the first patient arrives. When you are dependable, the physician and the office staff know you are reliable and can direct their attention to other matters.

Discreet (prudent, cautious—especially in speech): You must use good judgment in any discussion regarding a patient. You have access to **confidential** information that is not for discussion outside the office. The only exception is when there is a need to share information with other health professionals to whom you are making a referral for therapy or treatment (Figure 2–9). Always be **discreet**—never give out information about a patient over the phone or in writing without the patient's written permission. Even the completion of the patient's insurance claims requires the patient's authorization.

Empathy (trying to identify one's feelings with those of another): Empathy is not the same as sympathy. Most patients do not want you to feel sorry for them; they just want you to try to understand how they feel. **Empathy** is the ability to put yourself in another person's place. Imagine you are wheelchair-bound with a condition that requires you to depend upon others for all your needs (Figure 2–10). Everyone feeling sorry for you will not be of any benefit, but, if everyone could see the situation from your viewpoint, they would realize that you just need physical assistance and their support.

Enthusiasm (zeal, intense interest): **Enthusiasm** shows in your facial expressions and the general manner in which you carry out your responsibilities. Your **posture**, voice, and mannerisms should all indicate the fact that you like what you are doing. You usually will look your best and do your best when you are enthusiastic, and people will enjoy being around you. Enthusiasm must be

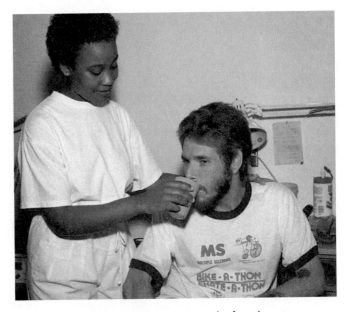

FIGURE 2–10 Have empathy for others.

genuine, however, or it becomes an effort for you and it won't convince anyone else.

Honesty (trustworthy; the quality of being truthful): You know the saying "Honesty is the best policy." In health care this is extremely important. You cannot lie about something you did or did not do for a patient because you are dealing with a living human being. You cannot use "white out" to correct a mistake but you can admit to the mistake so that it can be amended or counteracted. **Honesty** also refers to being trustworthy. You will have access to office equipment and supplies, coworkers' personal belongings, and perhaps money; you *must* be trustworthy. No business can tolerate or afford a thief or a liar.

Initiative (ambition; hustle; setting something in motion): A person with **initiative** is a self-starter and a valuable member of a health care team. This member recognizes work to be done—even though it may not be an assigned job—and will either do the work or offer assistance. A self-starter does not have to be told or reminded of routine tasks. A person with initiative will also volunteer to take on a task or project to learn something new.

Patience (calmness in waiting; tolerant): It is very hard to be "patient" with a patient when you have many tasks to do. The elderly, especially, require **patience** because they are often slow to move and need assistance (Figure 2–11). If they are also lonely, they may take advantage of having someone to talk to. You are sure to have a "chronic complainer" who goes on and on about symptoms or need for treatment until it begins to bother you. In your haste to stay on schedule and keep ahead of the physician, you will have to learn how to *politely* explain to patients that another person or

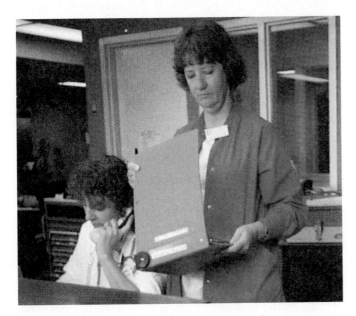

FIGURE 2–9 Be discreet in providing information.

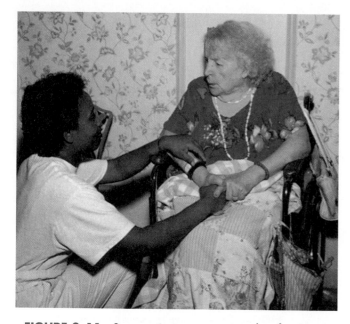

FIGURE 2-11 Some patients may require a lot of patience.

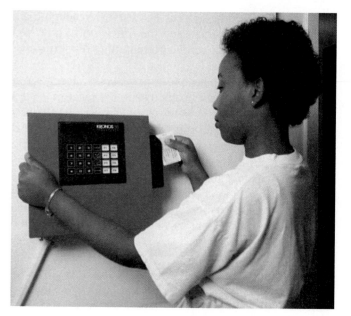

FIGURE 2-12 Being punctual is important.

duty needs your attention now and you must move on. The physician cannot afford for you to be impolite or impatient.

Perseverance (persistent, continued, or prolonged effort): **Perseverance** means to stick with a task until it is completed. Posting financial information, completing insurance forms, or filing may be postponed at times until it becomes a real task to accomplish and requires self-discipline to persevere until it is done. You may also need this quality when having difficulty getting a piece of equipment to function properly or when performing a certain procedure. In this manner, perseverance and patience go hand in hand.

Punctual (in exact agreement with appointed time): You are expected to be at work and on time every day (Figure 2–12). **Punctuality** is a part of being dependable. When you arrive at the established time and are ready to assume your responsibilities, the entire office will operate more smoothly. In contrast, when you are late, it often seems that you never get "caught up" and your whole day goes poorly. This is a trait you definitely can acquire with self-discipline.

Reliable (trustworthy, dependable, responsible): This trait is similar to being dependable. If you are **reliable**, the physician knows you can be expected to perform in the same consistent manner as you have in the past. In both your personal and professional life, you know how important it is to have someone who is reliable and who will always be there should you have the need.

Respectful (showing regard for; considerate; courteous): Being friends with everyone with whom you work will

probably not happen. You will have differences of opinion at work and at home about how people act or what they say. You don't have to agree with them, but realize they have a right to their actions and respect that right. Even if you do not care for someone personally, it is important to be courteous and **respectful**. That is the mark of a mature, civil person. There will be patients with whom you'll have difficulty, but you must always be tolerant and considerate. The trait of being respectful is necessary for good human relations.

Self Control (show restraint; in check): Being in control of your actions is very important. There will be times when you may be tempted to blurt out remarks or display some negative action, but it is not appropriate in the workplace. **Self control** is also very important when there is something trying that has to be done. Then, you must concentrate even harder on not losing your composure. Losing self-control usually makes matters worse because then you must apologize for your actions. Lack of self-control could also result in the termination of your employment.

Tact (delicate skill in saying or doing the right thing): **Tact** is a trait that may not be easy to acquire. Often, we respond to actions and statements *before* we think. Tact is being able to perceive a situation and knowing the right thing to say or do when dealing with people in a difficult situation. Tact is especially difficult and important when dealing with ill people. You must be very careful about what you say when responding to their questions.

This is the end of the discussion of highly desirable character traits. How do you rate?

PERSONALITY QUALITIES

In addition to the character traits discussed, there are other personality qualities that affect the way character traits are **perceived** by others. An individual could show initiative, dependability, honesty, and other traits, but if they are not likeable, they will not get along well with their coworkers. These qualities might be more difficult to acquire since they seem to be connected to one's personality. *New World Concise Webster's Dictionary,* 10th edition, defines personality as "existence as a person; the assemblage of qualities, physical, mental, and moral, that set one apart from others." Let's look at some of these qualities that we like in people.

Friendly Attitude and Genuine Liking of People (real, concerned, caring viewpoint): A friendly **attitude** will be recognized by the persons you deal with in the office. You should know and use the names of your patients while carrying on conversations with them. Be friendly, but at the same time maintain a professional relationship. You can show a true concern for their welfare without becoming personally involved. For example, if an elderly person needs assistance but has no family support, you cannot take this on personally but you can contact community resources to arrange for the assistance. Good interpersonal relations require dealing with people so that your self-image and theirs remain positive and intact. Courtesy is never out of style. A simple "please" and "thank you" is appropriate with all ages.

Intelligence (ability to apply the mind effectively to any situation; clear thinking plus good judgment): **Intelligence** is not just a high IQ or a college degree, for neither of these is of value if the owner can't appropriately apply knowledge to life situations. You can acquire knowledge from study and experience. There is no end to what you can learn; that information, effectively applied, is intelligence. Everything you learn affects you and, in turn, the people with whom you interact. Use every opportunity to expand your knowledge—not only of health care, but also of the world of information that is available (Figure 2–13). You will find that a willingness to learn advances your professional status. You will also find that your professional skills will improve with experience and new technology. Your knowledge can be expanded by observing, reading, and attending seminars. Physicians will often sponsor your attendance at workshops and educational seminars if you show an interest in learning.

Another good source of information is the Internet. Once you learn to "surf the net" you can bring up information on almost any topic. You should, however, be cautious of any information you read or download. There are no standards by which web sites are held or judged, and the person providing the information may be without qualifications. Remember also that any research, wonderful discovery, or cure may not be worth the time it takes

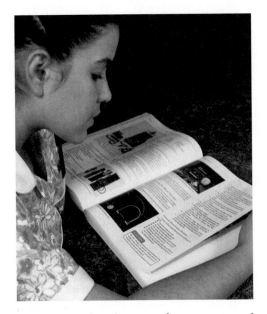

FIGURE 2–13 Take advantage of opportunities to learn.

to read it. Be very cautious. Consider the source of the information. If it is from a known educational institution, the national or state government, or a recognized organization, it is probably reliable.

Pleasant Personality (cheerful, agreeable personal qualities): A pleasant personality is tremendously important because of the continuous stream of persons with whom you will come into contact. Because of their illnesses, the situation will not always be the best, but if your contact with them is cheerful and pleasant, it will make their time in your office a little easier to bear. Your interaction with the physician and other team members will be much more enjoyable if you are pleasant. No one enjoys being around someone who is always complaining or is negative about everything. It has been said that success is 90% personality. Impressions about people are, at least initially, formed from the way we perceive their personality. A chance at success may not occur if the perception is negative.

Pleasant Voice (pleasing to hear): A voice has four characteristics: pitch, force, quality, and rate. The pitch of your voice refers to its highness or lowness. If you have a medium pitch, you are fortunate because it is considered the most pleasing to hear. If you are told your voice sounds high, consider exercises to lower its pitch. Record your voice and listen to it. You can also determine your pitch by using a piano. Sing "ah" to find the lowest note you can sing, then sing up the scale four whole notes. This will be your best speaking voice pitch. If you currently speak above it, practice reading aloud at the new note pitch. This will also allow you to develop variety in the range of your pitch. Without variation, your speech will be **monotone**, which is unpleasant to hear. The force of your voice makes it possible for you to be heard. You generally need little force in office communications; in fact, you must guard against being overheard by patients. If you do find it necessary to increase the intensity of your voice, be careful it does not become irritating. The quality of your voice is reflected in the manner in which you pronounce vowels. Relaxation exercises will improve vocal quality. A good exercise for the jaw muscles is a yawn. The rate of your speech is determined by how long you hold sounds and by the pauses between words and phrases. Most of us speak too rapidly. Communication requires understanding, and it is extremely hard to understand someone who runs their words together and does not enunciate clearly. Again, you can improve your rate of speech by listening to your recorded voice as you read aloud. With practice, you can adjust your rate and improve your communication skills. Practice is also needed to eliminate using "uh," "er," and "you know" when you speak. A simple pause, while you think of what to say, is much more pleasant for the listener.

Genuine Smile   (real expression): A genuine smile is a welcome sight to patients and visitors entering a physician's office. It conveys that you acknowledge them and are interested in being of service. You may be surprised by how many smiles you receive in return. Besides, it's hard to be unpleasant with someone who is smiling at you.

PERCEPTION AS A PROFESSIONAL

There are two other observations about you that speak very loudly, yet do not require a word to be spoken. Since you are a health care worker and consider yourself to be a professional, you are expected to "look the part."

Good Health   (state of wellness): The patients and visitors coming into a physician's office gain the first impression of the practice from the medical assistant or receptionist who greets them. A neat, attractive person has a good psychological effect on everyone. To look your best, you must be in good health. This requires a routine of rest, well-balanced meals, exercise, and recreation. As a health care professional, you are perceived as an example. What message are you sending? If you need medical attention, you should see your personal physician without delay. No patient wants to receive medical attention from someone who appears unhealthy. Patients may resent, and rightly so, any exposure to illness. Many people are in a rather fragile state of health. They come to the physician to get assistance with their own illness or injury; they do not need to be exposed to additional problems.

Personal Appearance   (individual image; a look; visible): Your **appearance** says volumes about you. Neat, well-groomed professionals look self-confident, display pride in themselves, and give an impression of being capable of performing whatever duties need to be done (Figure 2–14).

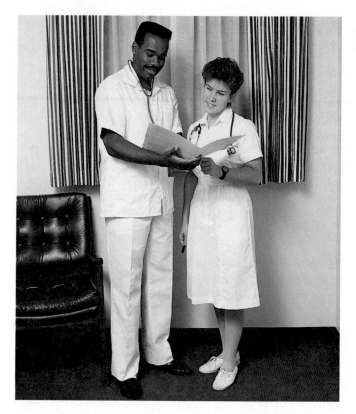

FIGURE 2–14   Present a professional appearance.

Not only does the patient feel the provider is competent, but the provider also feels good. We have all experienced days when we didn't feel good about the way we looked that, in turn, affected our performance. In order to present yourself in the best possible light, you must adhere to some general guidelines for a professional appearance:

1. *Cleanliness* is the first essential for good grooming. Take a daily bath or shower. Use a deodorant or antiperspirant. Shampoo your hair at least two to three times a week, depending upon its oiliness. Brush and floss your teeth daily.
2. *Hand care* is critical. Take special care of your hands. Keep hand cream or lotion in convenient places to use after washing your hands. Since this is done frequently, hands tend to chap and crack, which can allow organisms entry into your body—a risk you cannot afford. Also, keep your fingernails at a moderate length and manicured. If you work in a uniform and want to use nail polish, choose clear or light shades. Even in street clothes, bright or trendy colors are not appropriate for the office.
3. *Hair* must be clean and away from your face. Long hair should be worn up or at least fastened back. It is not a good idea to have to keep pushing your hair out of the way while working with patients. You only add their organisms to your environment, and perhaps take them home with you. Patients may also be susceptible to "receiving" something from your hair if you touch them after arranging your hair.

4. *Uniforms* must be clean, fit well, and be free from wrinkles. Uniform shoes should be kept clean with clean shoestrings. Hose are to be free of runners. It is a good idea to keep an extra clean uniform and pair of socks or hose at the office in case of accidents. Attention must also be given to undergarments worn beneath the uniform. Bright colors and patterns can usually be seen through the uniform's fabric. Underwear is best disguised if it closely matches your skin coloring because the contrast with your body will not be as visible. Test different shades to see which looks the best.

5. *Jewelry,* except for a watch or wedding ring, is not appropriate with a uniform. Small earrings may be worn but still may get in the way when you use the telephone. Not only does jewelry look out of place, it is a great collector of microorganisms. Novelty piercings, such as nose rings and tongue studs, are not appropriate for professional grooming. Save the wearing of these for after work hours.

6. *Fragrances,* such as perfume, cologne, and aftershave lotions, may be offensive to some patients, especially if they are suffering from nausea. If you feel it necessary to wear something, use one with a light, clean smelling fragrance. Leave the heavy aromas for after work.

7. *Cosmetics* should be tasteful and skillfully applied. All major department stores have sales people who can help you select and learn to apply products that will enhance your appearance. Save bright eye shadows, false eyelashes, and vivid lipsticks for leisure times.

8. *Gum* chewing can be very unprofessional. A large piece of gum interferes with speech, and cracking gum is totally unacceptable. If you feel you need gum for a breath concern, use a breath mint or mouthwash instead.

9. *Posture* affects not only your appearance but also the amount of fatigue you experience. The ease at which you move around reflects your poise and confidence. To check your posture, back up to a wall, place your feet apart (straight down from your hips) and try to insert your hand through the space between your lower back and the wall. If you can, you need to improve your posture. Pull your stomach in, tuck under your buttocks, and try to place your spine against the wall. Your shoulders should be relaxed with your head held erect. This will probably feel very unnatural, but practice keeping your body straight and head erect when you walk and you will see how much better you look and feel.

A lot of different elements make up our personal characteristics and have a definite effect upon how we feel about ourselves and how others perceive us. This discussion should help you to evaluate yourself and help identify things you can do to improve your effectiveness when interacting with people.

A CAAHEP CONNECTION

Personal attributes, whether character traits or personality qualities, are important to your success as a medical assistant. Instruction regarding these characteristics is therefore identified as an essential element in the curriculum for medical assistant.

ACHIEVE UNIT OBJECTIVES

Complete Chapter 2, Unit 2, in the workbook to help you obtain competency of this subject matter.

UNIT 3
Professionalism

OBJECTIVES

Upon completion of the unit, meet the following performance objectives by verifying knowledge of the facts and principles presented through oral and written communication at a level deemed competent.

1. Spell and define, using the glossary in the back of this text, all the **Words to Know** in this unit.
2. Describe the origin of the medical assistant profession.
3. Describe the history and purpose of the AAMA and the American Registry of Medical Assistants (ARMA).
4. Explain the definition of medical assisting according to the AAMA and the ARMA.
5. Describe and discuss the original and current AAMA logos.
6. Describe the three levels of membership with the AAMA and the value of each level.
7. Define and discuss the meaning of professionalism.
8. Explain the *Standards of Practice* set by the American Association of Medical Technologists (AAMT).
9. Explain the purpose of continuing education and how to acquire it.
10. Identify the qualifications for and methods of acquiring medical assistant certification from the AAMA, AAMT, and ARMA.
11. Describe methods for revalidation of medical assistant certification from the AAMA, AAMT, and ARMA.
12. Explain advantages of membership in one or more of the professional organizations contained in this unit.
13. List additional purposes of the AAMA and the ARMA besides membership.

AREAS OF COMPETENCE (AAMA)

This unit addresses content within the specific competency areas of *Professionalism, Communication skills,* and *Legal concepts,* as identified in the Medical Assistant Role Delineation Study. Refer to Appendix A for a detailed listing of the areas.

A CAAHEP CONNECTION

Content discussing health professions credentialing is a requirement of the standards for an approved medical assisting curriculum. This unit lists many organizations that offer certification credentials for medical assistants.

■ WORDS TO KNOW

accreditation
aspirations
autonomous
barter
certification
competent

liaison
morality
professionalism
pro tem
registry
revalidation

HOW MEDICAL ASSISTING BEGAN

In *A Brief History of Medicine* in Chapter 1, you learned about the many pioneers in this field. These leaders in the practice of medicine obviously had the best interest of their patients in mind as they treated them as efficiently as they could with what little was available. The sick went to be treated without an appointment and they waited as long as necessary to be seen by the physician. Payment for medical care was a **barter**-type, often with food or whatever the patient or the family had of value. If one had no means of payment, the doctor treated the person anyway. No medical records were kept because they were not even thought to be necessary in those days. Because the physician was considered to be a valuable close family friend whose knowledge and life-saving skills were well respected by the entire community, it was very rare for a lawsuit to be filed against the physician.

Since those days, the practice of medicine has changed dramatically. Accurate and comprehensive records are vital in the managed care of patients. Documentation of every transaction between physician and patient is a must. The efficiently-run medical practice requires absolute attention to every detail to protect the reputation of the physician and to make it possible to render the best care possible to the patient. Since medical school offers little or no background in managing the "business of medicine," the physician must entrust this responsibility to a competent individual. Even today, the common term "my office nurse" is often used by physicians in reference to a member of their office personnel. This can often be misleading as there may in actuality be no nurses employed in the facility. Using this term casually is not a wise practice because it is deceiving to the public. The art and skill of nursing is for the most part aimed toward the critically ill and those patients requiring bedside care. Obviously, in an ambulatory setting such as an office or clinic, and in some departments in medical centers and hospitals, medical assistants can be and are employed in a wide variety of po-

sitions. This person, who works under the supervision of the physician, performs a wide variety of administrative and clinical duties and is given the title of medical assistant. During the evolvement of the practice of medicine, physicians have realized the value of both administrative and clinical medical assistants to run their offices and assist in many other roles with appropriate instruction and evaluation. Unit 1 of this chapter discusses the many roles and responsibilities that await the medical assistant in the wealth of opportunities in the medical field.

HISTORY OF PROFESSIONAL ORGANIZATIONS

The American Association of Medical Assistants

In 1955, medical assistants from 15 states met in Kansas City, Kansas, and adopted the name American Association of Medical Assistants (AAMA). The representatives elected **pro tem** officers and made plans for an organizational meeting to be held the following year. In October of 1956, physicians and advisors of the American Medical Association (AMA) met with 250 members of medical assistant societies from 16 states. At this meeting, the AAMA was officially founded with advice, assistance, and moral support from the AMA. The founder and first national president of the AMA was Maxine Williams (Figure 2–15). The primary purpose of the AAMA was to raise the standards of the medical assistant to a profes-

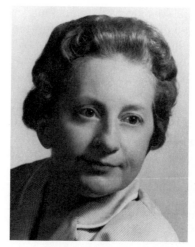

FIGURE 2–15 Maxine Williams, founder and first national president of the AAMA (Courtesy of the American Association of Medical Assistants.)

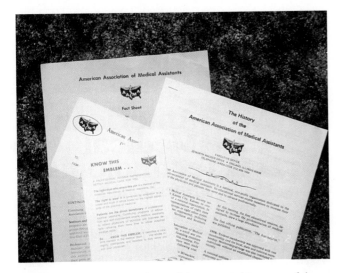

FIGURE 2-16 Original logo of the AAMA (Courtesy of the American Association of Medical Assistants.)

sional level. Physicians realized then, as they do now, that health care professionals were needed to assist them in a multitude of office duties for which nurses had not been trained. They also needed help in the physician/patient relationship. Another concern was that of instilling in young people a desire to carry the profession of medical assisting into the future. The *Maxine Williams Scholarship Fund* was established to award several $500 scholarships annually to students who were seriously interested in pursuing a career as a medical assistant. (NOTE: The scholarships are awarded on the basis of interest, need, and aptitude. Applications are available from the AAMA executive office. Applicants must have the completed form postmarked no later than May 1 of the year in which the scholarship will be used.)

In 1958, a national emblem was selected for use on AAMA stationery and official publications (Figure 2–16). The current logo for AAMA, introduced in 1978, is shown in Figure 2–17. The AMA received word from the United States Department of Health, Education, and Welfare that medical assisting had been formally recognized as an allied health profession and that its educational programs were eligible for federal funding by the Bureau of Health Manpower.

The AAMA Board of Trustees approved the current definition of medical assisting in February 1991: "Medical assisting is a multi-skilled allied health profession whose practitioners work primarily in ambulatory settings, such as medical offices or clinics. Medical assistants function as members of the health care delivery team and perform administrative and clinical procedures."

The American Academy of Professional Coders

The American Academy of Professional Coders (AAPC) was founded in 1988 to promote professionalism and encourage and support education, networking, and certification. Setting high ethical standards for its 22,000 members is a top priority. The AAPC offers training through their *Independent Study Program* and the *Professional Medical Coding Curriculum* and two distinct types of certification examinations. The Certified Professional Coder (CPC) is one who codes for professional services. The Certified Professional Coder-Hospital (CPC-H) is one who codes for the outpatient facility. *Specialty Proficiencies* provide further indication of a qualified professional in the coding field. In order to remain in good standing, credentialed members are required to submit continuing education units (CEUs) annually. The AAPC offers continuing education through its annual national conference, workshops, and the *AAPC Coding Edge,* the bimonthly news magazine that contains educational news for coding professionals. For further information, contact the AAPC at 800-626-2633 or at the web site http//:www.aapc.com. The current logo for AAPC is shown in Figure 2–18.

The American Registry of Medical Assistants

The American Registry of Medical Assistants (ARMA) is incorporated in Massachusetts and registered with the United States Federal Government. Their charter was obtained in 1950. One must be a graduate of an accredited medical assisting program to be eligible for ARMA certification. There is no national examination; the final examination of the medical assistant program is considered to be a sufficient screen of entry-level knowledge. Applicants with a minimum of three years on-the-job training

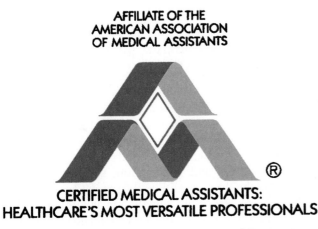

AFFILIATE OF THE
AMERICAN ASSOCIATION
OF MEDICAL ASSISTANTS

®

CERTIFIED MEDICAL ASSISTANTS:
HEALTHCARE'S MOST VERSATILE PROFESSIONALS

FIGURE 2-17 Logo of the AAMA (Courtesy of the American Association of Medical Assistants.)

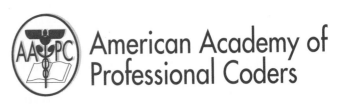

American Academy of Professional Coders

FIGURE 2-18 Logo of the AAPC (Courtesy of the American Academy of Professional Coders.)

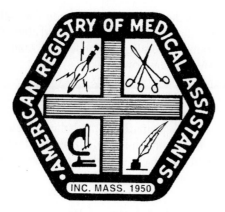

FIGURE 2–19 Logo of the ARMA (Courtesy of the American Registry of Medical Assistants.)

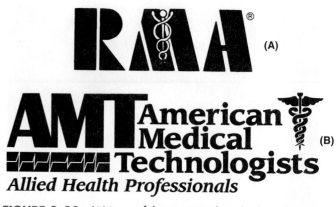

FIGURE 2–20 (A) Logo of the Registered Medical Assistant, representing a credential awarded by the American Medical Technologists Association; (B) logo of the American Medical Technologists (AMT) (Courtesy of the American Medical Technologists Association.)

and experience are eligible for ARMA certification with a letter of recommendation from their physician-employer. The letter must indicate the length of service, duties performed, and the doctor's determination that the applicant is qualified to be certified. There is a registration fee and annual dues as well as a five-hour requirement of continuing education per year to stay current in the field.

Since many medical facilities require medical assistants to have certification or registration to be considered for employment, this organization is helpful in offering members the immediate credentials of registered medical assistant (RMA). The current logo of the ARMA is shown in Figure 2–19. The RMA credential signifies that one is a registered medical assistant. The ARMA defines a medical assistant as one who is an integral member of the health care delivery team, qualified by education and experience, recommended to work in the administrative office, examining room, and physician's laboratory; who is also a liaison between the doctor and patient; and who is of vital importance to the success of the medical practice. The ARMA is not associated with the AMT or the AAMA.

American Medical Technologists Institute for Education

In 1976 the American Medical Technologists (AMT) association organized a nationally recognized body to address the needs of medical assistants and award the title of Registered Medical Assistant (RMA) following the successful completion of an Accrediting Bureau of Health Education School's (ABHES) accredited medical assisting program, and after passing the national registry examination. Other criteria for registry through the AMT are that one must have graduated from a nonspecific accredited medical assistant program and have been employed full-time in the medical field for one year or part-time for two years. The current logos of the RMA and AMT are shown in Figure 2–20. The RMA must complete continuing education credits to stay current in the field.

A national board of directors is elected to conduct the business of the organization such as educational programs, legal concerns, certification, and other national issues. The national board appoints state and local members to council positions. This leadership group works directly with the needs of the membership. Members receive a professional publication, *AMT Events*, which provides timely information regarding educational seminars, the annual meeting held in late June, test sites for certification, and home education programs. The AMT registers other health care professionals including phlebotomists, medical lab assistants, and medical lab technicians, which the medical assistant could become with additional study and training. Those who desire to become RMAs through the AMT must send the application form to the AMT Registry Office by the deadline date with the application fee, a copy of your high school diploma or GED certificate, a copy of the notarized cardiopulmonary resuscitation (CPR) current certification, and any other pertinent documentation. All information sent to this office must be in English.

Professional organizations for continuing education and membership are listed at the end of this chapter.

American Association for Medical Transcription (AAMT)

One who interprets and transcribes patient information from oral to printed form with the use of a typewriter or word processor is known as a medical transcriptionist. These professionals are medical language specialists who must possess excellent skills in the areas of listening, English grammar and punctuation, spelling, and transcription technology. Additionally, the medical transcriptionist must have a solid foundation in anatomy and physiology, disease processes, medical-legal and ethical areas, and professionalism.

The AAMT is the professional organization for the advancement of medical transcription and for the education and development of medical transcriptionists as medical language specialists. This organization was incorporated in 1978 in Modesto, California. The AAMT publishes a bimonthly journal to inform association leaders of important relevant information. State or regional component associations offer members delegate representation at the national convention, and local chapters offer educational opportunities. Voluntary certification by examination is offered by the AAMT. This certification is valid for three years. The certified medical transcriptionist must achieve 30 continuing education credits (CEU) in each three-year cycle for recertification or successful reexamination. The AAMT offers a national convention, continuing education programs, workshops, and seminars for members. This organization also publishes materials specifically for those in the medical transcription profession.

Professional Secretaries International® (PSI)®

This organization offers the administrative medical assistant many benefits. PSI® promotes competence and recognition of the professional and represents the interests and welfare of persons working in and preparing for secretarial and related positions. Certified Professional Secretary® (CPS)® is the registered service mark for the rating that has become the recognized standard of measurement of secretarial proficiency. To attain the CPS® rating, a secretary must meet certain education and work experience requirements and pass the two-day examination. The six-part examination is administered each May and November by the Institute for Certifying Secretaries, a department of PSI®. The CPS® examination has six parts: behavioral science in business, business law, economics and management, accounting, office administration and communication, and office technology.

PROFESSIONALISM

On your journey of study to become a medical assistant you must also become aware of just what a professional is and what that means to you. One who is trained and skilled in the methods of the profession is the coined definition which can apply to *any* profession regarding technical and ethical standards of the particular skill area. In an article in the January/February 1987 issue of AAMA's the *Professional Medical Assistant (PMA)* magazine, Barbara Smith defined **professionalism** as "a state of mind. It is a particular blend of self-esteem, self-confidence, enjoyment of life, respect for the feelings of others, as well as specific knowledge and skills."

The AMT outlines the requirements of professionalism in the *Standards of Practice* (Figure 2–21). All AMT members, RMAs, and every member of the health care delivery team are urged to follow these standards.

True professionalism goes well beyond a mere definition. Standards of conduct are certainly a noble consideration, especially in the revered field of medicine. The physician and the field of medicine, in general, have always been highly respected and admired by society. And, rightfully so, those who seek the services of professionals in the health care field have expectations of being treated with respect and dignity. It takes a certain type of person to work with the sick and injured day in and day out. You have been introduced to the personal characteristics that health care professionals should possess. Those necessary attributes are used perpetually in patient care. It is all part of being a professional. In the AAMA Role Delineation Study, there are nine areas of competency under Professionalism which are identified as follows:

- Project a professional manner and image
- Adhere to ethical principles
- Demonstrate initiative and responsibility
- Work as a team member
- Manage time effectively
- Prioritize and perform multiple tasks
- Adapt to change
- Promote the CMA credential
- Enhance skills through continuing education

Professionalism is a complex issue. It is your personal standard of conduct, morality, and ethics. It is having the will to excel in your vocational aspirations and to go above and beyond what is expected of you. Professionalism is seen in those who aspire to become certified and **revalidate** when the time comes. The professional is one who seeks out the ways and means to grow personally as well as professionally and encourages others to do the same. The leaders of these organizations, the pacesetters of the AAMA, the AMT, and the ARMA, have paved the way of the professional medical assistant. You are learning a fine tradition of the example they set for the future of the profession of medical assisting and in the establishment of continuing education programs. You have a great opportunity because of the efforts of a few medical assistants who saw the vision of the profession and had the desire to do something about it. That is what professionalism is all about. They did something above and beyond their 9-to-5 job. The seeds they planted have taken root and have bloomed into a formally recognized profession.

The AAMA, AMT, and ARMA Examinations

Furthermore, the AAMA, AMT, and the ARMA certification/recertification examinations cover content on professionalism. Areas from which questions may be derived are:

- professional organization
- accepting responsibility for own actions
- performing within ethical boundaries
- code of ethics
- patients' rights
- current issues in bioethics

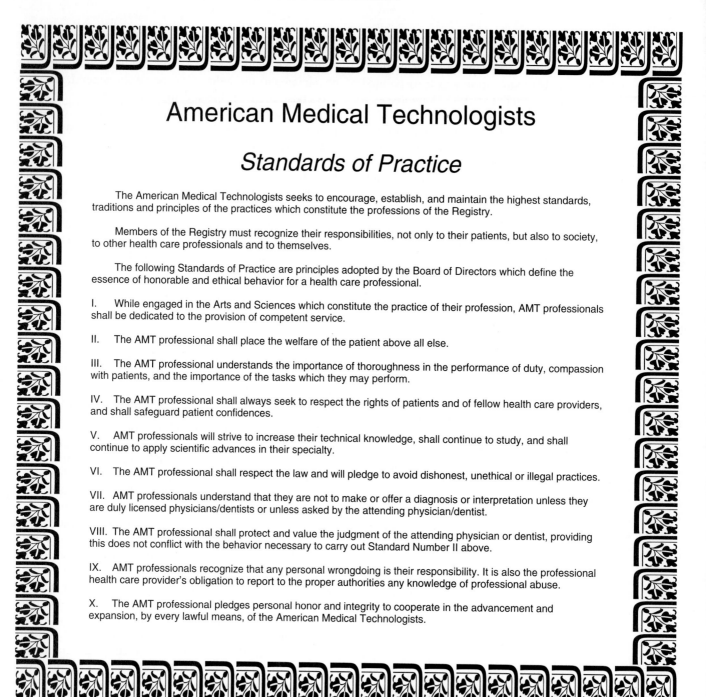

American Medical Technologists

Standards of Practice

The American Medical Technologists seeks to encourage, establish, and maintain the highest standards, traditions and principles of the practices which constitute the professions of the Registry.

Members of the Registry must recognize their responsibilities, not only to their patients, but also to society, to other health care professionals and to themselves.

The following Standards of Practice are principles adopted by the Board of Directors which define the essence of honorable and ethical behavior for a health care professional.

I.   While engaged in the Arts and Sciences which constitute the practice of their profession, AMT professionals shall be dedicated to the provision of competent service.

II.   The AMT professional shall place the welfare of the patient above all else.

III. The AMT professional understands the importance of thoroughness in the performance of duty, compassion with patients, and the importance of the tasks which they may perform.

IV.   The AMT professional shall always seek to respect the rights of patients and of fellow health care providers, and shall safeguard patient confidences.

V.   AMT professionals will strive to increase their technical knowledge, shall continue to study, and shall continue to apply scientific advances in their specialty.

VI.   The AMT professional shall respect the law and will pledge to avoid dishonest, unethical or illegal practices.

VII. AMT professionals understand that they are not to make or offer a diagnosis or interpretation unless they are duly licensed physicians/dentists or unless asked by the attending physician/dentist.

VIII. The AMT professional shall protect and value the judgment of the attending physician or dentist, providing this does not conflict with the behavior necessary to carry out Standard Number II above.

IX.   AMT professionals recognize that any personal wrongdoing is their responsibility. It is also the professional health care provider's obligation to report to the proper authorities any knowledge of professional abuse.

X.   The AMT professional pledges personal honor and integrity to cooperate in the advancement and expansion, by every lawful means, of the American Medical Technologists.

FIGURE 2-21   AMT *Standards of Practice* (Courtesy of the American Medical Technologists.)

- maintaining confidentiality
- releasing patient information
- intentional tort
- invasion of privacy
- slander and libel
- promote competent patient care
- working as a team member to achieve goals
- team member responsibility

Keeping all these points in mind as you learn and practice your skills will help you toward your goal of becoming a concerned and **competent** medical assistant.

COMPETENCY OF PROGRAMS

The AAMA has established an **accreditation** process for programs that prepare individuals to become medical assistants. Over 221 medical assisting programs at the postsecondary level in various schools and colleges nationwide have been accredited by the Committee on Allied Health Education and Accreditation (CAHEA), an **autonomous** committee of the AMA and an accrediting body sanctioned by the United States Department of Education.

All schools and colleges that offer accredited medical assisting programs must follow the AAMA's Occupational Analysis/Role Delineation Study outcomes in designing their curriculum. These statements of competence are an integral part of the document called *The Standards and Guidelines of an Accredited Educational Program for the Medical Assistant.* It is this document that specifies the requirements an educational facility must meet in order to be accredited by the AMA/AAMA review boards. *The Standards and Guidelines* are the minimum standards for accrediting educational programs that prepare individuals to enter into an allied health profession recognized by the AMA. It is this level of quality that qualifies medical assisting as a profession.

BECOMING CERTIFIED

At the 1995 AAMA convention in San Antonio, Texas, the certification board voted that as of February 1, 1998, only those individuals who have successfully completed an accredited medical assistant program may sit for the national certification examination. The AAMA certification exam is designed to evaluate entry-level competency in medical assisting. Administrative and clinical skills, anatomy and physiology, human relations, medical terminology, professionalism, communication, and medical-legal issues are included in this exam. It is offered twice each year at over 100 test centers nationwide. The National Board of Medical Examiners serves as an educational test consultant and works with the AAMA in preparing the examination. To be eligible for the certification exam you must be a graduate of a CAAHEP accredited medical assistant program or a graduate of an ABHES-accredited program with one year of documented work experience.

Since 1998 certified medical assistants (CMAs) must recertify every five years to demonstrate current knowledge of administrative, clinical, and general medical information. A CMA remains current through December 31 of the fifth year following certification or recertification. Recertification reinforces the validity of the CMA credentials and helps maintain continued acceptance by physicians, patients, and other health care professionals. This requirement may be met in one of two ways:

1. By earning 60 recertification points through continuing education courses or academic or other formal credit that has relevancy to medical assisting, with the points distributed equally among the three areas covered in the examination.
2. By retaking the certification examination.

Those who sit for the exam and are successful in achieving a passing score are entitled to the CMA designation following their names. Figure 2–22 shows a photo of the official CMA pin from AAMA. NOTE: There are also attractive pins sold in uniform shops around the country that say "medical assistant" or "certified medical assistant" as accessory items. Even though these pins inform the onlooker that one is a medical assistant, they are not authorized by the AAMA and

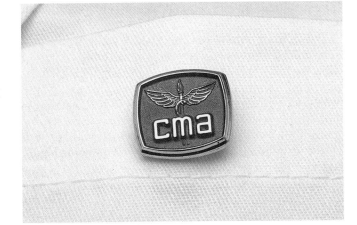

FIGURE 2–22 Certified medical assistant (CMA) pin (Courtesy of the American Association of Medical Assistants.)

do not reflect the wearer's credibility regarding AAMA certification.

In addition to sitting for the national certification exam after completing studies in medical assisting, you should carefully consider the many benefits of joining the AAMA. An *active member* must be a CMA or an individual who was an active member on December 31, 1987 and who maintains continuous active membership. An *associate member* is one who is not eligible for another category of membership but who is interested in the profession of medical assisting. Those enrolled in a medical assistant program may become student members at a reasonable cost. Student membership may be retained for dues one year after graduation if active or associate membership is not chosen.

One of the best and most appropriate ways for you to continue your education is through AAMA tri-level membership (local, state, and national levels). Hundreds of educational programs offering CEUs are conducted throughout the year. Physician advisors are among the professionals who speak at the monthly meetings and other educational activities. Many physician employers and/or office managers offer financial assistance to employees to encourage attendance and participation in seminars, workshops, and conventions where important current topics are shared. Members are entitled to special rates for all educational pursuits offered by the organization as well as many other financial advantages (such as group rates). Soon after joining, members automatically begin receiving AAMA's bimonthly magazine, *Professional Medical Assistant (PMA),* which is devoted to educational articles that are written by experts in allied health and related fields. This magazine contains current medical research reports, the latest state and federal health legislative news, education program announcements, and articles offering CEU credit. Most organizations at the state level keep members informed with a news publication containing educational articles as well as dates for programs, meetings, and other activities relevant to the medical assistant. Many local chapters send notices to their members about meeting times and other important information.

The AAMA, AMT, and the ARMA additionally provide guided study programs at a reasonable cost in a wide range of areas such as Human Relations, Medical Law, and Communication Skills, among others. These professionally designed courses allow medical assistants to learn and study at home at their own rate of speed. CEUs are awarded for the successful completion of the examinations accompanying each home study course.

Employers are impressed with applicants who take the initiative in belonging to one or more such organizations. Membership shows your interest not only in self-improvement, but also shows your initiative in improving your skills for the welfare of the patients you serve. Most employers encourage their employees to attend seminars, workshops, and courses that offer education that relates to the medical office practice, both clinical and administrative. Some employers even pay for the costs of membership and for educational program fees. Well informed personnel provide competent care to patients and assist in quality management of administrative tasks.

RELATING TO ABHES

Chapter 2 discusses the training, employment opportunities, personal characteristics, and professionalism of a medical assistant. This content is related to ABHES accreditation requirements of *Professional development and success, Employment opportunities, Dress for success, and Professionalism* that are within the content area of **Career Development**.

Additional information may be obtained by writing, faxing your request, retrieving information from web sites, or calling the professional organizations listed at the end of this unit.

ACHIEVE UNIT OBJECTIVES

Complete Chapter 2, Unit 3, in the workbook to help you obtain competency of this subject matter.

RESOURCES

American Association of Medical Assistants. (1997). AAMA role delineation study: Occupational analysis of the medical assisting profession. Chicago, IL: Author.

American Medical Technologists, 847-823-5169.

American Registry of Medical Assistants, 800-527-ARMA.

Gillyatt, P. (1996, July). How to answer your own medical questions. *Harvard Health Letter,* xii(2), 9–12.

Lindh, W. Q., Pooler, M. S., Tamparo, C. D., & Cerrato, J. U. (2002). Delmar's comprehensive medical assisting: administrative and clinical competencies (2nd ed.). Clifton Park, NY: Delmar.

U.S. Department of Labor. (2000). Occupational outlook handbook (2000–01 ed.). Washington, DC: Bureau of Labor Statistics.

WEB LINKS

http://stats.bls.gov/oco/ocos **(U.S. Department of Labor, Bureau of Labor Statistics)**

Provides employment statistics.

http://www.aama-ntl.org **(American Association of Medical Assistants)**

Provides information about career opportunities, CAAHEP-accredited programs, and the CMA exam.

http://www.abhes.org **(Accrediting Bureau of Health Education Schools)**

Provides a list of ABHES-accredited programs.

Medical Ethics and Liability

During the past 20 years the number of patients bringing lawsuits against physicians has increased dramatically. Medical liability insurance rates have increased so much that physicians in some areas are practicing without liability insurance (although not all states permit this). Laws may vary in different states, but ethical standards are the same in every state. **Ethics** deals with **moral** choices and rules of conduct. All members of professional organizations that deal with patient health care and have a high regard for morality and competence follow a code of ethics specific to their profession.

UNIT 1

Ethical and Legal Responsibilities

OBJECTIVES

Upon completion of the unit, meet the following performance objectives by verifying knowledge of the facts and principles presented through oral and written communication at a level deemed competent.

1. Spell and define, using the glossary at the back of the text, all the **Words to Know** in this unit.
2. List licensure requirements for physicians.
3. Describe methods of licensure.
4. List exceptions to the need for licensure.
5. Define the components of public and private law.
6. Recognize the differences between ethics and law.
7. Identify areas of medical ethics of particular concern to medical assistants.
8. List the five primary elements of the American Association of Medical Assistants Code of Ethics.
9. Describe the reason diagnostic related groups are causing an ethical issue for physicians.
10. Name one societal group being denied health insurance.
11. List ethical considerations surrounding the life of a fetus.
12. List and define the three categories of medical transplants.
13. Name the most common type of transplant.
14. Describe a living will.
15. Name four examples of tort law.
16. Define the term *emancipated minor* and give examples.
17. Describe the three parts of the physician-patient contract.
18. Define the terms *implied consent* and *express consent.*
19. Prepare common consent forms used in medical offices.
20. Define the term *privileged communication.*
21. List instances of legally required disclosure.
22. Explain the terms *defamation of character, libel,* and *slander.*
23. Describe the conditions for revocation or suspension of a medical license.

AREAS OF COMPETENCE (AAMA)

This unit addresses content within the specific competency areas of *Professionalism, Communication skills, and Legal concepts*, as identified in the Medical Assistant Role Delineation Study. Refer to Appendix A for a detailed listing of the areas.

WORDS TO KNOW

agent
artificial insemination
assault
battery
biennially
civil law
coercion
confidentiality
criminal law
defamation
emancipated minor
enact
endorsement
ethics
explicit
expressed
forged
fraudulent

genetic
implied
incompetent
intimidation
liability
moral
non compos mentis
peer review
proxy
prudent
quackery
rational
reciprocity
revoke
senility
statutes
surrogate
tort

Our founding fathers saw a need for regulation of the practice of medicine and in colonial days medical practice acts were in effect for the protection of citizens. These acts were gradually repealed because it was believed the Constitution gave everyone the right to practice medicine. This resulted in a period of time in the nineteenth century when **quackery** was common. After a Supreme Court decision in 1899 upheld a state's right to establish qualifications for people wishing to practice medicine, all states soon had once again established medical practice acts. Most state **statutes** define two basic elements that constitute the practice of medicine. One is diagnosis and the other is the prescribing of treatment. Only a licensed physician (and some mid-level practitioners) can engage in the diagnosis and prescribing of treatment for the physical condition of human beings. In general terms, medical practice acts define the practice of medicine and establish requirements for licensure and grounds for suspending or **revoking** a license.

LICENSURE REQUIREMENTS

Licensure requirements are established by each state. A physician is usually required to:

- be of legal age ⌊18⌋
- be of good moral character
- have graduated from an approved medical school
- have completed an approved residency program or its equivalent
- be a resident of the state where the physician is practicing
- have passed the oral and written examinations administered by the National Board of Medical Examiners and the state where the physician is practicing

Physicians who have all the necessary requirements for licensure may also be licensed by **reciprocity** or **endorsement**. A physician who has been licensed in one state and wishes to move to another state may be granted a license by reciprocity if it is determined that the original licensure requirements are equal to the requirements in the new state. Many physicians take the test administered by the National Board of Medical Examiners at the same time they take their first state test. The high standards of the national board make it possible to obtain a state license by endorsement when the national board examinations have been successfully passed.

Physicians are required to renew their license annually or **biennially**. You should be sure the physician has a record of all continuing medical education credits (CMEs) earned since the previous renewal as this is a requirement in many states. Physicians earn CMEs by attending seminars and scientific meetings as well as university courses. The renewal notice will notify the physician of the number of CMEs necessary to renew the license.

There are some exceptions to the rule requiring a current state license to practice medicine. Any physician is free to administer first aid outside the state of residence.

Physicians in military service must be licensed to practice medicine in their home states. They do not need to be licensed in the state where they are stationed as long as they practice only on the military base.

Each state's Board of Medical Examiners provides procedures for revocation or suspension of licensure. In some states the board has the power to revoke a license, and in other states a special review committee has this authority.

A physician may lose the license to practice medicine if convicted of a crime such as murder, rape, violation of narcotic laws, or income tax evasion. A medical license may also be revoked for unprofessional conduct. The most usual offenses in this category are betrayal of patient-physician confidence, excessive use of drugs and alcohol, and inappropriate sexual conduct with patients.

A license may be revoked because of proven fraud in the application for a license. In some cases **fraudulent** diplomas are used. Fraud in the filing of claims for services that were not rendered and fraud in the use of unproven treatments are also grounds for revocation of a license.

A CAAHEP CONNECTION

The curriculum standards specify the inclusion of **Medical law and ethics** as they relate to guidelines and requirements for health care. This unit discusses the AAMA's Codes of Ethics, professional licensure, and basic legal documents involved with health care.

Physicians who are found to be incompetent to practice because of **senility** or mental incapacity also may have their license revoked.

ETHICAL CONSIDERATIONS

Whereas laws concern matters enforced through the court system, ethics deals with what is morally right and wrong. The ethical standards established by a profession are administered by **peer review**, and violation of the standards may result in suspension of membership. The American Medical Association Principles of Medical Ethics was revised in 1980 and updated in 2001. It is reprinted here so that you can see what is expected of a physician.

Physician's Code

Preamble: The medical profession has long subscribed to a body of ethical statements developed primarily for the benefit of the patient. As a member of this profession, a physician must recognize responsibility to patients first and foremost, as well as to society, to other health professionals, and to self. The following Principles adopted by the American Medical Association are not laws, but standards of conduct which define the essentials of honorable behavior for the physician.

Principles of Medical Ethics

I. A physician shall be dedicated to providing competent medical care, with compassion and respect for human dignity and rights.

II. A physician shall uphold the standards of professionalism, be honest in all professional interactions, and strive to report physicians deficient in character or competence, or engaging in fraud or deception, to appropriate entities.

III. A physician shall respect the law and also recognize a responsibility to seek changes in those requirements which are contrary to the best interests of the patient.

IV. A physician shall respect the rights of patients, colleagues, and other health professionals, and shall safeguard patient confidences and privacy within the constraints of the law.

V. A physician shall continue to study, apply, and advance scientific knowledge, maintain a commitment to medical education, make relevant information available to patients, colleagues, and the public, obtain consultation, and use the talents of other health professionals when indicated.

VI. A physician shall, in the provision of appropriate patient care, except in emergencies, be free to choose whom to serve, with whom to associate, and the environment in which to provide medical care.

VII. A physician shall recognize a responsibility to participate in activities contributing to the improvement of the community and the betterment of public health.

VIII. A physician shall, while caring for a patient, regard responsibility to the patient as paramount.

IX. A physician shall support access to medical care for all people.

(Adopted by the AMA's House of Delegates June 17, 2001.)

Medical Assistant's Code

As an agent of the physician, you, the medical assistant, are also governed by ethical standards: The American Association of Medical Assistants (AAMA) Code of Ethics is, in many respects, similar to that of the American Medical Association (AMA).

A code of ethics is made up of statements regarding how individuals affiliated with an organization should conduct themselves. Refer to the AAMA's Code of Ethics and Medical Assistant's Creed in the shaded boxes of the text. The Code of Ethics indicates that medical assistants will abide by ethical and **moral** principles as they relate to the profession. It also states that medical assistants should strive to deserve the high regard of the medical profession and the general public. It continues with five specific pledge statements concerning how medical assistants will conduct themselves in the performance of their profession. In addition, the Medical Assistants' Creed contains eight statements that medical assistants agree to accept as evidence of their desire to practice their profession to the best of their ability. By adhering to these two ethical standards (Medical Assistant's Code of Ethics and Medical Assistant's Creed), you will uphold the professional quality of medical assisting.

The physician must release patient information when the patient authorizes the release or if the release is required by law. State laws vary regarding release of information. Information that must be reported includes:

- Births and deaths
- Cases of violence such as gunshot wounds, knifings, and poisonings
- Sexually transmitted diseases
- Suspected cases of child abuse, elder abuse
- Cases of contagious, infectious, or communicable diseases

Medical assistants should check with local authorities for the procedures to be followed in making these reports. They need to be aware also of other required local reports. When a physician moves or retires it is important that the original records be kept until the period for filing of liability suits has expired. A copy of the records is provided to a new physician if one takes over the practice.

You will often find it necessary to make decisions based on the professional nature of your employment. Patients can be extremely insistent at times, but you must be firm in carrying out the expectations of your employer and your profession. A patient may, for instance, demand that you call in a prescription for medication when the physician is not immediately available. You have to stand your ground and say that only the physician can give you the orders to do this. You then carefully record on the chart the request of the patient and how it was taken care of. *Never put yourself in the position of practicing medicine.*

The Federal Drug Administration has established five categories, or "schedules," which classify chemical substances with specific regulations as to their use. The states also have laws that further define the use of drugs. It is important for the medical assistant to understand that only the physician (and some midlevel providers) can legally prescribe medications. The medical assistant must understand that certain medications cannot be refilled and that restrictions limit the number of times some medications can be refilled. Some medication orders must be accompanied by a written prescription before they can be filled, while others can be called in by telephone. It is important to remember that all patients should be scheduled to see the physician at regular intervals to check all medications they are currently taking.

The United States Department of Justice Drug Enforcement Administration publishes a physician's manual that gives all the information necessary for office personnel to understand the provisions of the Controlled Substances Act. This booklet is free and is furnished on request.

The Drug Enforcement Administration also publishes a *Physician's Manual,* which includes 12 recommendations for physicians about the care and security of prescription pads to help reduce the number of **forged** prescription orders:

1. Prescription blanks should be stored in a safe place (locked cabinet) to discourage theft. There should be a minimum number of prescription blanks used.
2. Schedule II controlled substances are to be written in ink or typed and signed by the physician.
3. The prescription should contain the amount of the medication in Arabic or Roman numerals as well as the written number to deter changing the amount.
4. Unless absolutely necessary, the amount (number) of a controlled substance should be limited when writing prescriptions.
5. The amount of controlled substances carried in the doctor's medical bag should be kept at a minimum.
6. If the physician keeps a medical bag in the car, it must be locked in the trunk.
7. Use caution when prescribing controlled substances to a patient who has disclosed that another doctor has prescribed a controlled drug. Check with the doctor at the patient's medical facility, or examine the patient to make a decision regarding a prescription for a controlled drug.
8. Write only orders for medication on prescription blanks to discourage a forged prescription. Write memos or notes for patients on note pads.
9. Prescription blanks should never be signed in advance.
10. Controlled substances must be accurately recorded and maintained to comply with the regulations of the Controlled Substance Act.

11. Verify prescription orders with the pharmacist to assist her with the dispensing of the correct medication.
12. To report or obtain information regarding prescription medications, contact the nearest DEA field office.

CODE OF ETHICS
of the American Association of Medical Assistants

The Code of Ethics of AAMA shall set forth principles of ethical and moral conduct as they relate to the medical profession and the particular practice of medical assisting.

Members of AAMA dedicated to the conscientious pursuit of their profession, and thus desiring to merit the high regard of the entire medical profession and the respect of the general public which they do serve, do pledge themselves to strive always to:

A. render service with full respect for the dignity of humanity;
B. respect confidential information obtained through employment unless legally authorized or required by responsible performance of duty to divulge such information;
C. uphold the honor and high principles of the profession and accept its disciplines;
D. seek to continually improve the knowledge and skills of medical assistants for the benefit of patients and professional colleagues;
E. participate in additional service activities aimed toward improving the health and well-being of the community.

MEDICAL ASSISTANT'S CREED

The creed of the American Association of Medical Assistants reads as follows:

I believe in the principles and purposes of the profession of medical assisting.
I endeavor to be more effective.
I aspire to render greater service.
I protect the confidence entrusted to me.
I am dedicated to the care and well-being of all people.
I am loyal to my employer.
I am true to the ethics of my profession.
I am strengthened by compassion, courage, and faith.

(Copyright by the American Association of Medical Assistants, Inc. Used with permission.)

LEGAL AND ETHICAL ISSUES

A Library:
Legal Concepts

In the practice of medicine it can be difficult to distinguish between legal and ethical issues. The trend in the United States is to demand good health care as a right for everyone. However, not all citizens are willing to finance such a program. The use of diagnosis related groups (DRGs) in determining the payment hospitals will receive for Medicare patients raises both ethical and legal questions. The problem with the system arises when patients may be discharged too early simply because the hospital will not be paid for more than the DRG-allowed number of days. The physician knows the legal responsibility is to the well-being of the patient, but the hospital must have money to stay in business, and the physician wants to stay in good standing with the hospital. In a case in California *Wickline v. State of California, 1986,* a physician was held liable for releasing a patient too early. In fact, the physician had failed to protest the third party's decision to shorten the patient's recommended hospital stay. In this case, the third party payer was a California Medicare agency called MediCal.

Insurance companies are presenting more ethical questions to medical care providers when they refuse insurance to individuals who have acquired immunodeficiency syndrome (AIDS) and human immunodeficiency virus (HIV).

Many ethical considerations surround the life of a fetus, an infant's birth, and the newborn: New technologies allow us to have more control over birth by detecting *in utero* abnormalities. The improved techniques of **artificial insemination** bring before the court system the problems associated with **surrogate** motherhood and paternal responsibility. Many advances have been made in the use of fetal tissue in transplants. Our society must study the ethical and emotional considerations of ending a pregnancy if a serious **genetic** deficiency is found before birth or allowing the infant to be born handicapped. We seem to have more questions than answers at the present time.

The use of transplants has added another series of ethical problems. Medical transplants are divided into three categories:

- Autograft: transplantation of a person's own tissue from one body site to another (can also be used to describe transplant between identical twins)
- Homograft: transplantation of tissue from one person to another
- Heterograft: transplantation of animal tissue to a human being

The blood transfusion is the most common transplant. Nearly all the major organs of the body may be transplanted, and research continues to improve these possibilities.

THE UNIFORM ANATOMICAL GIFT ACT

The Uniform Anatomical Gift Act was passed in 1968. By 1978 it was reported that all 50 states had established some system of organ and tissue donor identification so that individuals can ensure that when they die they will be identified as a donor. Any person of sound mind and legal age may donate any body part after death for research or transplant. The family may make this decision for the donor if the donor has not done so while living. The time of death must be determined by a physician who will not be involved in the transplant in any way. No money can be exchanged for making an anatomical donation. Many states allow residents to mark and sign a donor card on the back of their driver's license.

Different ethical problems affect the use of organs from living donors. As the technology of transplantation becomes more readily available, the demand for organs will grow. Human organs should never be sold for profit, but our western ethics are not always followed worldwide. In a book titled *Law, Liability, and Ethics for Medical Office Personnel,* Myrtle Flight discusses the medical community's concern over the sale of human organs for transplant. One source estimated that since the year 2000, most of the poor in India are surviving with only one kidney as the result of the common practice of selling their kidneys to wealthy foreigners.

Another ethical issue of concern is the ability to *grow* tissue and organs from manipulated stem cells or cultivated *donor* tissue. This research is highly controversial yet highly motivated by the need for replacement organs to sustain life. The experimentation continues. We can only hope that the scientists making the decisions have high moral and ethical standards and value the dignity of human life.

Living Will

The health care team will provide a larger percentage of care to geriatric patients as the quality of care extends life expectancy. It is important that everyone in the office listen to older patients and allow them to make decisions regarding a living will (Figure 3–1). A majority of the states now have laws that define policies on withholding life-sustaining procedures from hopelessly ill patients. The living will is signed when the patient is competent and must be witnessed by two individuals. The effect of this living will is to protect the wishes of the patient who may become incompetent and thus unable to make **rational** decisions. The patient and all family members should discuss these issues while the patient is still rational and can fully comprehend the implications. A chosen family member should then be made aware of the responsibility of carrying out the patient's wishes as it becomes necessary. Copies of the living will should be filed with the family, the primary physician, and the family's attorney.

THE FOLLOWING IS AN EXAMPLE OF A LIVING WILL FOR THE STATE OF FLORIDA. PLEASE CONTACT CHOICE IN DYING AT (212) 366-5540 TO RECEIVE A COPY OF APPROPRIATE ADVANCE DIRECTIVES FOR YOUR STATE.

FLORIDA LIVING WILL

INSTRUCTIONS

PRINT THE DATE — Declaration made this ______ day of ______________, 19____.

PRINT YOUR NAME — I, ______________________, willfully and voluntarily make known my desire that my dying not be artificially prolonged under the circumstances set forth below, and I do hereby declare:

If at any time I have a terminal condition and if my attending or treating physician and another consulting physician have determined that there is no medical probability of my recovery from such condition, I direct that life-prolonging procedures be withheld or withdrawn when the application of such procedures would serve only to prolong artificially the process of dying, and that I be permitted to die naturally with only the administration of medication or the performance of any medical procedure deemed necessary to provide me with comfort care or to alleviate pain.

It is my intention that this declaration be honored by my family and physician as the final expression of my legal right to refuse medical or surgical treatment and to accept the consequences for such refusal.

In the event that I have been determined to be unable to provide express and informed consent regarding the withholding, withdrawal, or continuation of life-prolonging procedures, I wish to designate, as my surrogate to carry out the provisions of this declaration:

PRINT THE NAME, HOME ADDRESS AND TELEPHONE NUMBER OF YOUR SURROGATE —
Name: ______________________
Address: ______________________
______________________ Zip Code: __________
Phone: ______________________

SAMPLE

© 1995 CHOICE IN DYING, INC.

FLORIDA LIVING WILL — PAGE 2 OF 2

I wish to designate the following person as my alternate surrogate, to carry out the provisions of this declaration should my surrogate be unwilling or unable to act on my behalf:

PRINT NAME, HOME ADDRESS AND TELEPHONE NUMBER OF YOUR ALTERNATE SURROGATE —
Name: ______________________
Address: ______________________
______________________ Zip Code: __________
Phone: ______________________

ADD PERSONAL INSTRUCTIONS (IF ANY) — Additional instructions (optional):

I understand the full impo[illegible] is declaration, and I am emotionally and mentally competent to make t[illegible] declaration.

SIGN THE DOCUMENT — Signed: ______________________

WITNESSING PROCEDURE

TWO WITNESSES MUST SIGN AND PRINT THEIR ADDRESSES —
Witness 1:
Signed: ______________________
Address: ______________________

Witness 2:
Signed: ______________________
Address: ______________________

SAMPLE

Courtesy of Choice In Dying 9/95
200 Varick Street, New York, NY 10014 1-800-989-WILL

© 1995 CHOICE IN DYING, INC.

FIGURE 3–1 Sample living will form (Reprinted by permission of Partnership for Caring, Inc., 1620 Eye Street, NW, Suite 202, Washington, DC 20006, 800-989-9455.)

Choice in Dying, Inc., now stresses the importance of also completing a durable power of attorney for health care form, authorized by either your state's statute or some other legal authority. This allows you to appoint another person (known as your **agent**) to make health care decisions for you if at any time you become unable to make them yourself. It is strongly advised that you appoint an agent, assuming there is someone who can be trusted to make the decisions you would make if you could, and who is willing to act for you in this way. The appointed **proxy** (agent) must be aware of your wishes and understand the complete document before giving consent to carry out the agreement. It may be helpful to record the wishes of a living will and power of attorney on a videotape so there could be no doubt that you made the statements regarding care. It is also recommended that a copy of the video be kept by the appointed attorney. The video dialogue should state the date it is made, who has copies, and the living will/advanced directives of the patient.

A medical "Miranda warning" law approved by Congress and signed by President George Herbert Walker Bush gives patients legal options for refusing or accepting treatment if they are incapacitated. The law, which took effect in November 1991, applies to hospitals, hospices, nursing homes, health maintenance organizations (HMOs), and other health care facilities that receive money from Medicare and Medicaid programs. Under the law, patients must receive written information explaining their right-to-die options according to their state laws. The law stipulates that hospitals and other providers must note on medical records whether patients have legal directives on treatment. Providers also must have procedures to ensure that they comply with a patient's wishes.

Every member of the medical care team should be current in cardiopulmonary resuscitation (CPR) certification. An ethical question arises when the older or terminally ill patient does not wish to be resuscitated in the event of a cardiopulmonary arrest. The courts have held that individuals have the right to make decisions that affect their own deaths.

LEGAL MATTERS

In the United States the laws are divided into the categories of public law and private law. The various branches of public law include **criminal law**, constitutional law, administrative law, and international law. Criminal law deals with offenses against all citizens. The practice of medicine without a license is an offense under the criminal law. Constitutional law defines the powers of the government and the rights of its citizens. Each state has a constitution which defines its powers over matters not covered by the federal government, which are spelled out in the United States Constitution. Administrative law is concerned with the powers of government agencies. International law is concerned with agreements and treaties between countries.

The practice of medicine is primarily affected by private law or **civil law**, specifically by contract law and torts law. The patient-physician relationship is considered a contractual one. A **tort** is defined as any of a number of actions done by one person or group of persons that causes injury to another. Violations of tort law may be intentional or negligent. Negligence is an act or failure to act as a reasonably **prudent** physician under the same or similar circumstances that directly or proximately causes injury to a patient. The negligent causing of an injury, when committed by a physician in the course of professional duties, is commonly referred to as *malpractice*. Intentional torts also result in professional **liability** suits. Libel and slander are two forms of **defamation**. Libel refers to written statements; slander refers to oral remarks. **Assault** is defined as a deliberate attempt or threat to touch without consent. Another intentional wrong is **battery**, which is the unauthorized touching of another person. A patient has a right to refuse treatment. If any treatment is provided without consent, a charge of battery may be filed by the patient. Other civil laws govern property ownership, corporations, and inheritance.

The contract between a patient and a physician has three parts (Figure 3–2). They are the offer, the acceptance, and the consideration. The offer takes place when a competent individual indicates a desire to become a

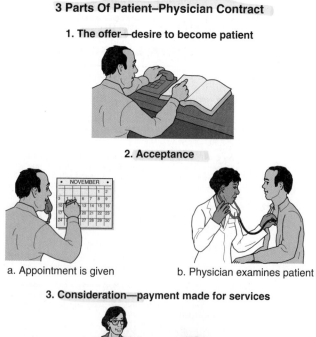

3 Parts Of Patient–Physician Contract

1. The offer—desire to become patient

2. Acceptance

a. Appointment is given

b. Physician examines patient

3. Consideration—payment made for services

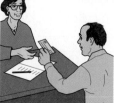

FIGURE 3–2 This cartoon illustrates the three parts of the patient–physician contract.

patient. The acceptance takes place when an appointment is given and the physician examines the patient. The consideration is the payment given in exchange for services. When a child is a patient, the parent is expected to pay. A young person is considered to be a minor until reaching full legal age, known as the age of majority. The statutes defining the age of majority vary from state to state. The medical assistant needs to be aware that the rights of minors in medical treatment are changing. More than half of the states allow minors the right to consent to treatment or consultation for pregnancy, contraception, venereal disease, drug abuse, or alcoholism.

An **emancipated minor** is an individual who is no longer under the care, custody, or supervision of parents. The emancipated minor may be married, in the armed forces, or self-supporting and living apart from parents. An emancipated minor can legally consent to medical care.

An individual who has been judged by the courts to be mentally **incompetent** must have an appointed guardian. The general legal term for all varieties of mental illness is *non compos mentis*. The guardian is responsible for both the payment of bills and the care of the patient. In this case the parents are not responsible for payment. When a patient-physician contract is entered into, the physician is responsible for the care of that patient until the physician officially withdraws from the case or the patient discharges the physician.

The contract between the patient and the physician may be either **implied** or **expressed**. An express, or written, contract must be entered into if a third party is to be responsible for payment. If this agreement is not in writing, it is not possible to press for payment. There are also implied consent and express consent agreements between patients and physicians. The fact that the patient has come to see the physician implies consent for treatment. The instances when express consent is required are:

■ proposed surgery or other invasive treatments such as lumbar punctures, sigmoidoscopies, and biopsies
■ use of experimental drugs
■ use of unusual procedures that may involve high risk

There are exceptions to the rule for surgery. Minor procedures generally involve only an explanation by the physician and oral consent of the patient. Notes regarding this conversation, however, need to be entered by the physician in the patient's medical record.

The American Medical Association has developed recommended standardized consent forms to be used by physicians (Figure 3–3). It will be your responsibility to know what consent forms your employer uses. The physician may wish to develop forms individualized for the practice. It is important that these be **explicit** as to what is to be done. Experiments have been conducted using a tape recorder to keep a record of the information given the patient before a consent form is signed. These were discussions with patients who had to be told they had cancer. The results showed that most of these patients had lit-

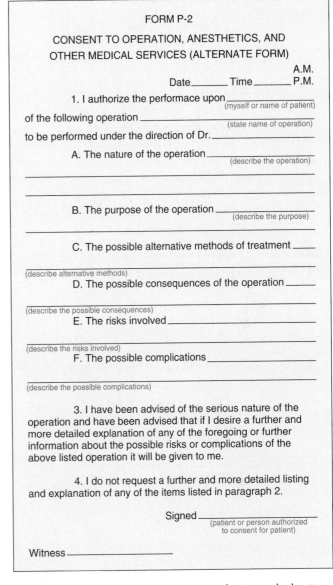

FIGURE 3–3 Consent to operation, anesthetics, and other invasive services (Courtesy of the American Medical Association.)

tle or no memory of what had been discussed because they were extremely upset by the diagnosis. In some of these cases the patients were certain they had not been fully informed, but replay of the tape proved they had been. The medical assistant should understand that the physician must be legally responsible for obtaining informed consent from a patient. You should not be given that responsibility. Informed consent is necessary to avoid a claim of assault and battery. The law describes this as a threat to make a physical attack on someone and carrying out the attack. You will be expected to prepare consent forms and ideally be present to listen so that you may help determine whether the patient understood before signing the consent form.

If an all-purpose form is used, it is important to cross out the paragraphs that do not apply. You may be asked to sign

Form P-22
CONSENT TO TREATMENT

Date ____________ Time ____________ A.M./P.M.

I have been informed by Dr. ________________________ of the nature, risks, possible alternative methods of treatment, possible consequences, and possible complications involved in the treatment by means of ________________________

____

____

for the relief of ________________________

____

Nevertheless, I authorize Dr. ________________________ to administer such treatment to me.

Signed ________________________
(Patient or person authorized to consent for patient)

Witness ________________________

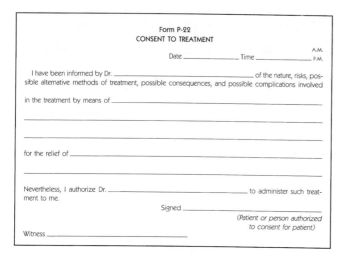

FIGURE 3–4 Consent to treatment (Courtesy of the American Medical Association.)

Form P-17
REQUEST FOR STERILIZATION

Date ____________ Time ____________ A.M./P.M.

We, the undersigned husband and wife, each being more than twenty-one years of age and of sound mind, request Dr. ________________________, and assistants of his choice, to perform upon ________________________ (name of patient), the following operation: ____________

____
(state nature and extent of operation)

It has been explained to us that this operation is intended to result in sterility although this result has not been guaranteed. We understand that a sterile person is NOT capable of becoming a parent.

We voluntarily request the operation and understand that if it proves successful the results will be permanent and it will thereafter be physically impossible for the patient to inseminate, or to conceive or bear children.

Signed ________________________
(Husband)

Signed ________________________
(Wife)

Witness ________________________

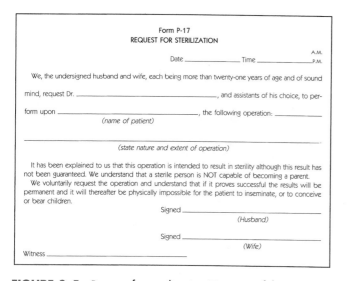

FIGURE 3–5 Request for sterilization (Courtesy of the American Medical Association.)

as a witness. What you say when you ask a patient to sign after the physician has explained the risks is important. A suggested statement is: "If you have no further questions for the doctor and you understand the consent form, will you please sign it?" You can help the patient by indicating the line where the signature is required, or ask the patient to sign on the line you have marked with an "X".

If a physician is to treat a patient with unusual or experimental medication, it is best to use a consent to treatment form (Figure 3–4). When a physician is to perform a sterilization procedure, it is preferable to have both husband and wife sign a request for sterilization form (Figure 3–5).

Patients have the right to privacy when they are being examined and treated. Even though many physicians have arrangements with medical facilities to offer training opportunities for medical students or residents, the patient always has the right to refuse to have observers present. Patients must first be asked if it is okay with them for observers to be present during the examination. If the patient refuses, no **intimidation** or **coercion** should be expressed to make the patient change the decision. Physicians may protect themselves by having an authority to admit observers form signed (Figure 3–6).

Form E-1
AUTHORITY TO ADMIT OBSERVERS

Patient ________________________ Place ________________________

Date ____________

I authorize Dr. ________________________ and the ________________________ Hospital to permit the presence of such observers as they may deem fit to admit in addition to physicians and hospital personnel, while I am undergoing (operative surgery) (childbirth), examination, and treatment.

Signed ________________________

Witness ________________________

FIGURE 3–6 Authority to admit observers (Courtesy of the American Medical Association.)

Information contained in a patient medical record and information exchanged between a physician and a patient are considered privileged communications. Every patient has a legal right to privacy and **confidentiality**. Information disclosed to the health care team must be kept in the strictest confidence, and you must be ever mindful of the legal implications of handling patients' records. Information concerning patients may be given to another member of the health care team, such as a laboratory technician or referring physician, only when it pertains directly to the course of treatment. For example, another medical office may telephone you to inquire about a patient's medical history for diagnostic purposes, to confirm symptoms, or to verify birth date. In complying with referral appointments or scheduled tests, patients will have given *implied consent* for necessary information to be transmitted concerning their condition. Implied consent means that the patient has expressed a desire to become a patient by making an appointment, being examined by the physician, and making payment for services rendered.

Medical information may be given to parties not concerned in the patient's treatment only when the patient has signed a release of information form.

A large number of states have privileged communication statutes that have been **enacted** to offer additional protection to the patient. You will find that curious and well-meaning friends and relatives will ask about patients, yet you must remember to give only information that has been authorized by the patient. Each time a patient authorizes release of information the form must state specifically who is to receive what information covering what time period. This authorization must be kept in the medical record.

All health care providers must be aware of any state regulations governing the reporting of HIV positive tests. At issue is the right of the patient to confidentiality and the rights of citizens to be protected from accidental exposure to the HIV virus. Such exposure might occur when police, fire, emergency medical service, or other medical personnel come into direct contact with the blood or body fluids of a patient.

In all fifty states, confirmed cases of HIV/AIDS constitute a reportable condition either by statute or administrative regulation.

ACHIEVE UNIT OBJECTIVES

Complete Chapter 3, Unit 1, in the workbook to help you obtain competency of this subject matter.

UNIT 2
Professional Liability

OBJECTIVES

Upon completion of the unit, meet the following performance objectives by verifying knowledge of the facts and principles presented through oral and written communication at a level deemed competent.

1. Spell and define, using the glossary at the back of the text, all the **Words to Know** in this unit.
2. List rights of the physician in providing medical care.
3. List rights of the patient in receiving medical care.
4. Describe the correct procedure for terminating the physician-patient contract.
5. Define and give examples of abandonment.
6. Define and give examples of professional negligence.
7. Give an example of an implied agreement.
8. Describe the precaution that should be observed in giving written instructions to a patient.
9. List the reasons for keeping medical records.
10. Describe who owns medical office records and who has a right to the information in them.
11. List the record keeping necessary to provide legally adequate records.
12. Describe the kinds of notes that are not appropriate in a patient chart.
13. Name the six basic principles for preventing unauthorized disclosure of patient information.
14. List six office procedures that can cause problems when the physician is involved in a lawsuit.
15. Describe the acceptable method for making changes in medical records.

AREAS OF COMPETENCE (AAMA)

This unit addresses content within the specific competency areas of **Administrative procedures, Professionalism**, and **Legal concepts**, as identified in the Medical Assistant Role Delineation Study. Refer to Appendix A for a detailed listing of the areas.

WORDS TO KNOW

abandonment	harmonious
breach	liability
chronologic	mores
competent	obligate
confrontation	procrastination
criterion	rapport
defamation	*res ipsa loquitur*
deposition	*respondeat superior*
doctrine	*subpoena duces tecum*
encompass	venereal

PHYSICIAN AND PATIENT RIGHTS

Physicians have the right to determine whom they will accept as patients. Physicians who have been in practice for a long period of time may also build up a patient load that is as large as one person can care for adequately. Because a physician must care for all patients accepted, it is not unusual for a physician to decide to see no new patients. A physician may not, on the other hand, refuse to provide emergency service if assigned to an emergency, and most physicians will provide emergency service whenever the need exists. Because they do not have to continue the patient's treatment once the emergency services have been provided, the patient is stabilized, and the patient's regular physician takes over the case.

Physicians have the right to decide what types of medicine they wish to practice and where. They have the right to establish their own working hours, to charge for their

A CAAHEP CONNECTION

It is important to know the legal guidelines regarding the practice of medicine, the rights of the patient, the physician, and the staff, and a basic understanding of laws applied to personal actions. It is essential that the medical assistant protect the patient's confidentiality and respect the legal status of the chart. This unit provides an introduction to these concepts.

services, and to take a vacation if they provide names of qualified substitutes to care for their patients while they are unavailable. Physicians have the right to change the location of their office but must notify patients in advance to give them adequate time to make alternate plans for medical care.

Patients have the right to receive care equal to the standards of care in the community as a whole. Patients have the right to choose the physician from whom they wish to receive treatment from the listing of physicians who are enrolled in their particular insurance plan. Of course, a patient may always see any physician desired as long as they take full responsibility for payment of services rendered; this means that the patient pays cash at the time of service if the patient's insurance plan will not cover the services of that particular physician. If a patient becomes a member of an HMO, the right to choose a physician may be restricted to physicians who are members of the chosen HMO. A patient has the right to accept or reject treatment, and to know whether the prescribed treatment has side effects, what the prognosis is, what effect the treatment will have on the body, and any treatment alternatives.

A physician may choose to withdraw from the care of a patient who does not follow instructions for treatment or keep follow-up appointments or who leaves a hospital against medical advice. Withdrawal must be by means of a letter sent by certified mail with return receipt requested as proof the letter was received. The return receipt should be filed in the patient record. The letter should state the reason for the withdrawal and needs to state the date the withdrawal will become effective (Figure 3–7). If the patient needs follow-up, the letter should recommend that the patient make an appointment with another physician. It is appropriate to indicate that a copy of the medical records will be sent to the new physician if the patient will send written authorization to do so. The letter should be signed by the physician.

A patient has a choice and a right to change physicians. The patient should notify the physician but if this does not take place in a written form the physician may send a letter confirming the dismissal. This letter should also be sent by certified mail, return receipt requested, and a copy of the letter and the receipt should be filed in the patient chart.

A physician who has begun care of a patient must carry through until the patient no longer needs treatment or decides to see a different physician, or the physician has withdrawn from care. A physician who has undertaken care of a patient and is then not available to continue that care may be sued for **abandonment** unless coverage for the patient by some equally qualified physician is provided. If a patient is admitted to the hospital and the physician does not see the patient right away to check on the patient's condition and order treatment, the physician may risk being accused of abandonment by the patient or by a family member of the patient. If a physician is ill, the office staff must refer patients who need care to other qualified physicians who will care for them.

Physicians are not **obligated** to provide follow-up care when they see a patient for preemployment or insurance examinations, or on other occasions when the request comes from someone other than the patient (e.g., when a school athletic department requests assessment of a potential athlete).

MEDICAL ASSISTANT RIGHTS

The medical assistant has the right to be free from sexual discrimination. This may involve a man or woman being refused employment because the job is usually filled by someone of the opposite sex. It can involve not receiving promotions, being paid less for the same work, or being treated as inferior in any way.

Title VII of the Civil Rights Act of 1964 defines sexual harassment as "Unwelcome sexual advances, requests for sexual favors, and other verbal or physical conduct of a sexual nature when submission or rejection of this conduct explicitly or implicitly affects an individual's employment, unreasonably interferes with an individual's work performance or creates an intimidating, hostile or offensive work environment." Sexual harassment can occur in a variety of circumstances.

- The victim as well as the harasser may be a woman or a man. The victim does not have to be of the opposite sex.
- The harasser can be the victim's supervisor, an agent of the employer, a supervisor in another area, a coworker, or a nonemployee.
- The victim does not have to be the person harassed but could be anyone affected by the offensive conduct.
- Unlawful sexual harassment may occur without economic injury to or discharge of the victim.
- The victim has a responsibility to establish that the harasser's conduct is unwelcome.
- A written account of each incident of sexual harassment should be documented with the names of witnesses, date, time, and place of occurrence.

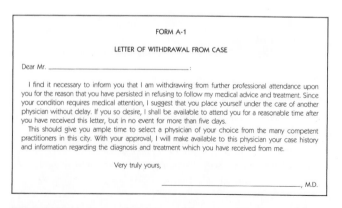

FORM A-1

LETTER OF WITHDRAWAL FROM CASE

Dear Mr. _____ :

I find it necessary to inform you that I am withdrawing from further professional attendance upon you for the reason that you have persisted in refusing to follow my medical advice and treatment. Since your condition requires medical attention, I suggest that you place yourself under the care of another physician without delay. If you so desire, I shall be available to attend you for a reasonable time after you have received this letter, but in no event for more than five days.

This should give you ample time to select a physician of your choice from the many competent practitioners in this city. With your approval, I will make available to this physician your case history and information regarding the diagnosis and treatment which you have received from me.

Very truly yours,

_____, M.D.

FIGURE 3–7 Letter of withdrawal from case (Courtesy of the American Medical Association.)

It is in the victim's best interest to directly inform the harasser that the conduct is unwelcome and must stop. Each instance reported to authorities is handled on a case-by-case basis and involves a thorough investigation.

NEGLIGENCE

Torts is the branch of private law that deals with **breach** of legal duty. Torts **encompass** such wrongs as invasion of privacy, personal injury, malpractice, and slander or libel. The tort of negligence is a primary cause of malpractice suits.

Physicians are expected to be as well trained and to exercise the same degree of skill with the same degree of judgment as other physicians in similar circumstances. These criteria are used in determining the standard of care. In lawsuits involving specialists, the standard of care is that practiced nationally rather than that in a given community.

In a case of negligence the patient must establish that he or she was examined by the physician, that the physician did or did not do something another physician under similar circumstances would or would not have done, whichever the case may be, and that the negligence injured the patient. Testimony of a physician as an expert medical witness is almost always necessary in a case of negligence. In some cases the testimony of an expert witness is not required. In these instances the **doctrine** is *res ipsa loquitur*, or *the thing speaks for itself*. These cases involve such situations as a sponge or instrument left in the patient during surgery, an injury done to the bladder while performing a hysterectomy, or an infection caused by the use of unsterilized instruments. The doctrine has different interpretations in different states.

Physicians are responsible for the actions of their employees. This **liability** is expressed in the doctrine of *respondeat superior (let the master answer)*. This is the law of agency, and you are an agent for the physician. Any individual entering the profession of medical assisting is considered to be accepting a position as a health care professional. If you violate the standard of care, you create the basis for a medical malpractice lawsuit. The physician is responsible for the acts of the medical assistant in the care of patients, and it is reasonable to expect the care to be as professional as the care given by the physician. A medical assistant is not licensed to practice medicine and cannot decide for a patient what care should be given.

After a Roche Laboratories medicolegal seminar, the Los Angeles County Medical Society sent the following directive to its doctors:

> When you ask your office assistant to instruct or refill a prescription, you are placing both the assistant and yourself in jeopardy. The physician's aide who directs a pharmacist to fill or refill a prescription becomes guilty of practice of medicine without a license. A physician who directs his assistant to do this places his license in jeopardy by assisting an unlicensed person to practice medicine. The conclusion of this directive is that when you want a pharmacist to fill or refill a prescription, let him or her hear the doctor's own telephone voice, or better, have written orders on a regular prescription blank.

Negligence is doing or not doing something that a *reasonable* person would do or not do in a given situation. Malpractice is a *professional's* negligence. Under ordinary circumstances, a medical assistant performing the administrative duties of a receptionist or secretary would be considered a person who could be charged with negligence. A medical assistant performing clinical procedures such as drawing blood or administering injections would be considered a professional and could be charged with malpractice.

Medical assistants who have had special training are expected to perform at a higher standard of care than those with no special knowledge or training. The medical assistant is not always covered by the physician's insurance, but insurance is available for the protection of medical assistants if they want to purchase their own coverage (or have the employer purchase it for them).

The Good Samaritan Act

The Good Samaritan Act originated in California in 1959 to protect the physician who gives emergency care from liability for any civil damages. The physician can help in an emergency without fear of being charged with neglect or abandonment for follow-up care. Now all states have Good Samaritan statutes. The statute requires that emergency care be given to the best ability of the person providing the care. In some states, the statute includes coverage for any health professional or citizen with first aid skills. The Good Samaritan law does not cover physicians if they receive compensation for the emergency care, however.

An implied agreement is considered to be a legal contract in a medical office. The medical assistant should never make a promise of a cure. You should be certain the patient understands that the instructions you give come directly from the physician or from written instruction sheets. When you hand a patient a written instruction sheet you need to be certain that the patient can read the instructions. Illiterate people are often reluctant to let anyone know that they cannot follow the directions for use of medications or preparation for a diagnostic test. One indicator of illiteracy might be the patient who becomes a "pest" by asking over and over for office staff to explain the instructions given by the physician. This patient might also ask you to explain a printed instruction sheet as a means of getting you to read it aloud. Informative videos that present detailed instructions regarding procedures, tests, and examinations for patient education are available from many pharmaceutical companies (or you can make them yourself) for patients to view while they are waiting to see the physician. Their questions and any further explanation can then follow at the end of their office visit.

The importance of doing everything possible to avoid a medical malpractice suit cannot be overemphasized. Simply being accused can have severe effects and repercussions on the physician, the physician's practice, and family. Those physicians who are wrongly accused of serious charges of neglect or malpractice can have ongoing problems with public mistrust and other issues depending on the extent of publicity. This misfortune can affect the livelihood of the physician and ruin the physician's medical practice. A physician can be ethical, honest, and **competent**, and still be sued for medical malpractice by a single patient who for some reason did not realize the expected result of treatment. This is another reason why the medical assistant is vital in providing patient education to supplement the physician's orders. The great increase in malpractice cases has caused physicians to order more tests and x-rays than are really necessary because they may feel the need to protect themselves from the possibility of missing a diagnosis and therefore being sued by the patient. The medical assistant is an extremely important person in the practice of preventive medicine in the medical office. When a friendly, **harmonious** interpersonal relationship is found in the office (known as **rapport**), the patient is much less likely to feel angry about anything associated with the care received. The well-trained medical assistant will understand the basic skills in good human relations and will then avoid **confrontations** that could lead to lawsuits against the office.

The following is the beginning of a chapter regarding medical office staff written by Melvin M. Belli, Sr., an internationally known attorney:

A woman once came to me with a complaint that she'd been incorrectly treated by a "dumb doctor."

"How do you know he's dumb?" I asked her.

"Because everybody who works for him is dumb."

It's common for patients to relate a doctor to his or her staff. Therefore, quite often, patient dissatisfaction with an office assistant will put the doctor on a malpractice spot.

(Reproduced with permission from Belli, M. M., Sr., & Carlova, J. [1986]. For your malpractice defense. Oradell, New Jersey: Medical Economics Company, Inc.)

The patient who suffers nerve damage as the result of a medical assistant giving an improperly administered injection may sue both medical assistant and physician under this doctrine. You should always inform the physician immediately of any mistakes you have made in the care of a patient so that corrective measures may be taken. You should never attempt to perform a procedure for which you have not been trained. Finally, you should be sure you understand your job responsibilities as outlined in a written procedures manual, which should be periodically updated.

You must be especially careful what you say about a patient within hearing distance of anyone but the physician or other office personnel. Statements regarding patients may be considered **defamation** of character and a breach of confidentiality. If you should make public the fact that a patient has a venereal disease, for example, this could be damaging to the patient.

You play an important role in preventing negligence by scheduling appointments for careful follow-up, knowing how and where to reach the physician at all times during the day, and making sure that the telephone is adequately covered at all times. The patient who feels well cared for will not be anxious to sue the physician. The patient who can never reach the physician for advice or who has difficulty obtaining an appointment will be much more apt to sue on the grounds of negligence.

The medical assistant should investigate the use of an arbitration agreement procedure by contacting the local or state medical society. Not all states have an arbitration statute at the present time, but it is well worth investigating as a possible way to settle legal problems without going to court.

Because the incidence of malpractice suits has increased, the medical assistant may need to be involved in preparing materials for court. This may include the professional training and experience of the physician as well as the patient medical record.

The attorney may agree to taking the testimony of the physician by **deposition**. A deposition is oral testimony and may be taken in the attorney's office or the physician's office in the presence of a court reporter. Some depositions are also videotaped.

A medical assistant may also receive a *subpoena duces tecum* to appear in court with patient records. This occurs when the physician is not available at the time needed in court.

Statute of Limitations

A statute of limitations is a law that designates a specific limit of time during which a claim may be filed in malpractice suits or in the collection of bills. Each state is obligated to protect individuals by establishing the statutes that regulate the time period. It is important to research the current law by contacting your state medical association.

MEDICAL RECORDS

The medical office staff must understand the importance of maintaining complete, accurate, up-to-date records on all patients. You must have complete records to give adequate care to patients. Your records may be used in research into certain illnesses or forms of treatment, and your records must be complete for protection in case of a lawsuit. A patient record that would meet this criterion would include: (1) personal information such as full name, address, occupation, marital status, and insurance carrier; (2) patient's personal family, sociocultural, and medical history; (3) all details of physical examinations, laboratory and x-ray findings, diagnoses, and treatments;

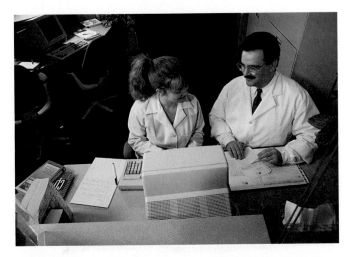

FIGURE 3-8 To help avoid an error, this medical assistant checks with her supervisor to clarify information regarding a patient's condition before recording it on the permanent record.

and (4) consent forms for procedures done and authorization forms for release of medical information. **Procrastination** cannot be tolerated in handling medical records. As legal documents, they are subject to critical inspection at any time (Figure 3–8).

You should always take a medical history in a private room or ask the patient to personally complete the information. Make entries on the patient medical record only as requested by the physician. All entries should be factual. All results of findings on a patient should be recorded even if they are normal or negative. Errors on a medical record must be corrected by drawing a single line through incorrect material and adding your initials, the date, and the reason for the change. All prescription refills should be recorded along with missed appointments, the reason for the missed appointment, and follow-up. Requests for medical information should be recorded along with the information given. Any failure to follow the treatment or advice of the physician should be noted. All notations should be in black ink, as pencil is too easily erased. Blue ink, as well as other colors, and pencil do not copy well. This is a concern for duplicating reports and records for referrals. Standard abbreviations should be used. Upon the death of a patient, a copy of the death certificate should be filed in case of subsequent requests for information. A quality medical record indicates quality medical care.

Medical records are considered the property of the physician who treats the patient. No record should be shown to a patient without the knowledge of the physician, as there may be some reason the patient should not see all of the record.

Each office should have a written policy regarding releasing information from a medical record. This policy must take into consideration local or state statutes. In some states, the legislature has given the patient, the physician, or an authorized agent the right to examine or copy the medical record. The requirement of confidentiality regarding the medical record is no longer recognized when the patient initiates a malpractice claim against a physician.

Physicians cannot agree on whether patients should be allowed to review their own records. The physician must be careful of personal opinion notes placed in the chart if there is a possibility the patient will be reading it. The following are two examples of patients reading medical records that were not recorded for their viewing:

A female patient was being professionally treated by a young physician when the doctor was suddenly called away from his office and left her medical record open on his desk. The patient read the first sentence: "This woman is a crock." Needless to say, she became very distraught and angry. (From Personal comments in medical records may cause trouble. [1976, January 12]. *Medical World News*, 128.)

While waiting to see a physician, a patient had been given her own record. Curious, she took out the notes and read them only to find that the doctor had written on the heading of the page, "Beware, hysterical and manipulative, determined to be unwell." She left immediately. (From Case conference: Fain would I change that note. [1978]. *Journal of Medical Ethics, 4,* 207–209.)

Any review of the chart by the patient should be done when the physician is present to interpret medical terms or abbreviations. Some physicians give patients a copy of their medical records and believe this reduces any anxiety regarding their health.

Prevention of unauthorized medical information regarding a patient requires that the following are practiced:

- Confidentiality applies to every patient regardless of their personal characteristics or lifestyle.
- Be aware of laws (federal, state and local), ordinances, regulations and rules, as well as public health programs.
- All requests from third parties require the patient's signature for medical information to be released. Keep a current "signature on file" form in the front of the patient's chart.
- Never give out medical information about a patient when you are not certain that a signed permission form exists.
- Patients should be provided with medical information regarding their diagnosis and treatment, and it is their decision to release or not to release that information. Documentation should be obtained with the patient's signature before disclosing medical information to anyone.
- If you are legally required to release medical information regarding a patient because of the seriousness or risk of the disease spreading to others, it should first be discussed with the patient.

For legal and practical purposes it is a wise choice to ask the patient at the initial office visit who in their family should receive medical information regarding the patient's health status; then have the patient sign the appropriate form and list all of the names provided. This directive protects the patient's confidentiality and will also protect the practice from potential problems if the staff pays attention to this important information.

The AMA has several forms for authorization for disclosure. It is a good policy to refuse to answer a telephone question as to whether an individual is a patient; a person coming to the office for information regarding a patient should produce an authorization to disclose information before any is given. It is important to check the specific details authorized to be released and to ask for photo identification of the individual or organization requesting the information. The signed authorization should be placed in the patient chart with a copy of the information released. According to Myrtle Flight, "when the information requested is disclosed, it must be accompanied by a note forbidding redisclosure" (*Law, Liability, and Ethics for Medical Office Personnel*, 134).

The complete, unaltered medical record is a legal document and is the best defense for a physician who is charged with malpractice. The first step a lawyer will take in a malpractice case against a physician is to obtain a copy of the patient's records and have them examined by an independent physician. The following office procedures have caused problems in malpractice suits:

1. Procrastination or delay in filing lab test results or reporting them to the physicians.
2. Incomplete medical records.
3. Illegible records.
4. Unexplained altered medical records.
5. Faking or forging a document or signature.
6. Loss of records.

There are acceptable methods of making changes in medical records. A single line should be drawn through an incorrect entry. The initials of the person making the correction should be written in the margin along with the date the error was discovered. The corrections should appear in the record in **chronologic** order.

In addition to having complete, up-to-date records you must be aware of the need for keeping these records even after care has ceased or the patient has expired. Records

---

RELATING TO ABHES

Chapter 3 discusses the ethical and legal responsibilities of both the physician and medical assistant as well as issues related to the application of laws related to patient care. The rights of the patient, physician, and medical assistant, as well as the liability of professional health care personnel, is covered. This content is related to the ABHES accreditation requirements of *Medical and ethical issues in today's society, Medical jurisprudence,* and *Legal terminology* that are within the content area of **Medical Law and Ethics.**

Medical-Legal-Ethical Scenario

Sharon Durbin, CMA, has been filing charts all morning. During a break, another medical assistant, Lisa Ford, was charting a prescription refill on a patient's chart. When she brought the chart back, it was wet with coffee she had spilled on it. Lisa gave the chart to Sharon, asked her to put it away for her, and walked away. Sharon called her back and told her she could not put a wet chart back in the cabinet. Lisa took back the chart and proceeded to replace several pages of progress notes, including the file cover. She hastily scribbled the information (making many errors) and threw the soiled pages in the trash. Then she gave the chart back to Sharon to file.

CRITICAL THINKING CHALLENGE

1. What should Lisa have done?
2. Who is responsible for the patient's record?
3. What would you have done?

4. Should the supervisor, physician, or office manager be called about this? If so, why?

should be kept as long as the statute of limitations is in effect on a case history. A few states designate the length of time records must be kept. Federal law dictates that you and your office have a responsibility to see that necessary records are kept for any narcotics used in the office. You also may be responsible for keeping accurate financial records. Within the following pages of this book, when-

ever appropriate, points will further remind you of the medical-legal importance of the subject matter.

ACHIEVE UNIT OBJECTIVES

Complete Chapter 3, Unit 2, in the workbook to help you obtain competency of this subject matter.

RESOURCES   Flight, M. (1998). Law, liability, and ethics for medical office professionals (3rd ed.). Clifton Park, NY: Delmar Learning.

WEB LINKS   http://www.aama-ntl.org (American Association of Medical Assistants)

Provides information for the medical assisting profession, including the bylaws of the organization.

Interpersonal Communications

One of the most important skills a medical assistant can possess is the art of communicating effectively with others. Both clinical and administrative duties require a constant exchange of written, oral, and nonverbal information.

You must be able to convey messages to many different people and receive vital information in the same manner. You will have daily contact with patients, colleagues, and other professionals, by phone, face to face, or by letter. Telephone and written communications and office mail will be discussed later in this text. This chapter deals with both verbal and nonverbal messages. Understanding how one gives and receives these is vital in the exchange of communication.

In dealing with patients and their families, learning to listen and to offer advice in a calm, professional manner will help to reduce unnecessary stress for all concerned. Times of sadness and pain can be extremely difficult for those closely involved. You can be instrumental in providing comfort and compassion to those in need.

Because the medical office is usually a very active place with many people coming and going, asking questions, and making payments or appointments, intraoffice communication can become hurried and ineffective. A harmonious team effort makes for an efficient and pleasant work environment. If an atmosphere of accord and cooperation exists among the staff, patients will sense this during their visits. If an uneasy situation exists, with friction evident, this may add to a patient's apprehensions and anxieties. Working together for the single purpose of providing quality health care to patients in a relaxed and friendly manner will help ease the daily pressures for the members of the medical office team and contribute greatly to their collective effectiveness.

UNIT 1

Verbal and Nonverbal Messages

OBJECTIVES

Upon completion of the unit, meet the following performance objectives by verifying knowledge of the facts and principles presented through oral and written communication at a level deemed competent.

1. Spell and define, using the glossary at the back of the text, all the **Words to Know** in this unit.
2. Describe the basic pattern of communication.
3. Give examples of nonverbal communication.
4. Explain how verbal and nonverbal communication can sometimes be misinterpreted.
5. Describe ways that tone and speed of speech can affect the message.
6. Discuss the importance of dress in nonverbal communication.
7. Explain *perception* and state its importance in communication.
8. List and explain the three types of listening and how they effect communication.

AREAS OF COMPETENCE (AAMA)

This unit addresses content within the specific competency areas of *Patient care, Professionalism,* and *Communication skills,* as identified in the Medical Assistant Role Delineation Study. Refer to Appendix A for a detailed listing of the areas.

WORDS TO KNOW

active listening	incongruous
articulate	intangible
conceptualize	interpret
contradict	intuition
convey	perception
distort	scrupulously
empirically	

To become effective in the art of communication, it may help to **conceptualize** the communication process (Figure 4–1). The message originates with the sender. The encoded message takes form based upon the sender's reference points (or frames of reference), and off it goes. The message is picked up by the intended receiver, who immediately begins to decode it based on reference points (or frames of reference). In responding (or providing feedback) the whole process is reversed: the original receiver becomes the sender, and the original sender becomes the receiver. In receiving this feedback, the origi-

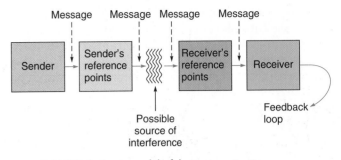

FIGURE 4–1 A model of the communication process

nal sender (now the receiver) can assess and evaluate how well the original message was received and **interpreted** and make any necessary adjustments or clarification.

The whole process seems simple enough, and generally it works well. However, many things can happen to affect the quality of the message or even **distort** it. You must be aware of these potential problems.

Foremost is the issue of reference points. For example, the spoken messages may include terminology familiar to you but unknown to the patient. Therefore, though the message will be heard, it may not be understood. Talking to patients on a level that they can easily understand is a skill requiring quick judgment. You will have to adapt to a vast number of different personalities in **conveying** information.

Some patients may be hearing- or sight-impaired, developmentally disabled, or non-English speaking, and will therefore require extra understanding. If a patient is in some way disabled, a family member or friend usually accompanies the person, thereby helping with your task of transmitting necessary information. It is important, however, that you speak to all patients directly and acknowledge their presence. It is rude and impolite to discuss their health care with another person and ignore the patients as if they were not even present.

There are many sources of interference or distractions, such as: others talking, phones ringing, phone conversations, coworkers, pagers, interruptions, music, and, more often in pediatrics and family/general practice, little ones crying. The patient could also be preoccupied with what the doctor has just told her, or she could have something personal bothering her. It is best to speak one-on-one with the patient in an area where there will not likely be any distractions or interference. The following gives an example of a conversation where the medical assistant is using active listening skills with the patient during triage:

Medical assistant: "Now Mrs. Owen, tell me what problems you have been having."

Mrs. Owen: "Well, I've been having a lot of indigestion lately, about a month or so, and I take antacids for it but it isn't going away. It bothers me a lot in the evening."

Medical assistant: "Okay, Mrs. Owen, you say that you've been having what you think might be indigestion for approximately a month and it seems worse at night, and you take antacids for this problem. Does it help?"

Mrs. Owen: "It seems to a little but this indigestion never goes away completely."

Medical assistant: "Could you tell me what other kinds of medication you are taking?"

Mrs. Owen: I only take aspirin sometimes for arthritis pain."

Medical assistant: "So you are taking aspirin. How much and how often?"

Mrs. Owen: Come to think of it, I have been taking aspirin about 3 or 4 times a day for the past 2 months."

Medical assistant: "I wrote all of this down for the doctor to talk to you about in just a little while. Is there anything else that you need to see Doctor Lang about today?"

Mrs. Owen: "No, thanks. I just want my stomach to feel better."

The spoken word must be delivered in an **articulate**, clear manner if the intended message is to be received. Correct pronunciation and proper grammar help to convey meaning. You must also be aware of the rate of the spoken word. Patients need to be spoken to in an unrushed manner so that the information has a chance to register and questions can be asked. Speaking in a pleasant tone of voice is necessary to keep the listener's interest in what you are saying. You must also remember to look the person in the eye while you are conversing. Eye contact makes people pay attention to the words you are saying because it gives them a feeling of importance and expresses a sincere interest in their well-being (Figure 4–2).

Listening involves giving attention to the persons who are trying to communicate with you. **Active listening** is

the participation in the conversation with another by means of repeating words and phrases, or in giving approving or disapproving nods. This signals to the message sender that you are hearing and following what is being said. This method of conversation is highly recommended for health care providers and patients in communicating needs, because it requires both parties to interact. The listener must make an effort to pay attention and follow the speaker. Distractions can create problems and interfere with what is being said; it takes concentration and self control to keep focused on a topic when there are many activities and interruptions going on, as often happens in a medical facility. Taking a patient into an exam room or to a quiet space away from noise is the most practical way to communicate important information.

Common courtesy is an art which seems to have been lost to some degree. In a professional setting it is essential to be **scrupulously** polite. *Please, Thank you, Excuse me,* and *May I help you?* should be words in frequent use. In this way the entire health care staff will show respect for others and a sense of caring.

PERCEPTION

Perception in the context of communication may be considered as being aware of one's own feelings and the feelings of others. The feelings you have about other people's moods and the way they act are perceptual, nonspoken communication between you. **Intuition** is another term for perception in this sense. While they cannot be measured **empirically**, these feelings may be strong indeed. Therefore, they must be recognized and reckoned with.

Being perceptive is a skill acquired with experience and practice. Keeping your eyes and ears open to the needs of others and what is going on will help you develop it. Developing the ability to perceive your own needs is a part of perception that will enhance your effectiveness. Planning and thinking ahead will help you develop in this area.

BODY LANGUAGE

The image you project is of utmost importance. Your overall appearance sends out messages to anyone who looks at you. Appropriate dress, uniform, or businesslike attire should be worn. Your professional appearance sends a nonverbal message that you have authority and confidence and are in charge.

Proper attire may vary with the medical specialty. For instance, many pediatric practices prefer medical assistants to dress in street clothes so as to make young patients feel more at ease. Children sometimes associate a white uniform with an unpleasant hospital visit, so wearing colorful prints with patterns of cartoon characters that children recognize is suggested. These scrub-type uniforms also come in a variety of colors, so the whole office team can be uniformed; furthermore, they are easily laun-

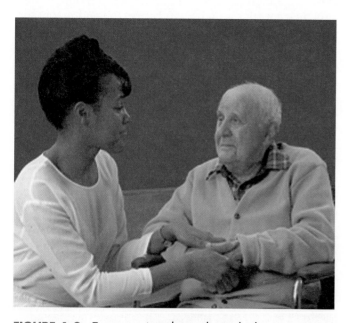

FIGURE 4–2 To communicate better, the medical assistant stoops down to speak with the patient in the wheelchair at eye level.

dered and are very comfortable. Psychiatry and psychology medical office assistants may also be more inclined to wear businesslike dress, for clinical duties are few, if any, and a uniform may not be necessary. However, casual wear is considered unprofessional, and jeans, sandals, and excessive jewelry are out of the question during working hours. Looking like a professional will not only encourage the respect of others for your profession, but it will help you to feel an integral part of the health care team.

Personal hygiene should be impeccable, because setting a good example for others is a part of your responsibility in the care of others. Daily showering, clean attractive hair, and neatly manicured nails shows others that you take pride in yourself and gives them a model to pattern themselves after.

Another part of your appearance, something **intangible** but very real, is your attitude. Your attitude shows *everyone* who sees you or speaks to you (by telephone or in person) how you feel about your work, others, and yourself. You display your attitude in the way you get along with others and interact with them. Body language is a complex communication process. It involves unconscious use of posture, gestures, and other forms of nonverbal communication. It is possible to **contradict** a verbal message by an inappropriate or **incongruous** facial expression. Even when a person says nothing and thinks that the message being sent is positive, body language will send the true message. When a person says for instance, "I'm OK," and you see the person grimacing with pain, the conflicting message shows through the true message. Many of us remember that our parents (or grandparents) could "read us like a book." It seems that body language is nothing new; it was the projection of attitude perceived by those who got to know us well. The importance of a positive attitude cannot be overemphasized. The many hassles and conflicts that can, and do, arise with patients and colleagues during everyday activity in the busy medical office can be handled much more effectively if you possess and project a positive attitude. Constant complaining only makes situations worse and breeds contempt. Having a good outlook on life carries over into every area and promotes well-being. Pleasant, agreeable working conditions increase productivity and efficiency besides giving one a sense of satisfaction on the job.

Facial Expression

Part of perception is being aware of how others think you feel, or see you. You create this impression partly by your facial expression. The most common example of a positive, happy facial expression is a smile (Figure 4–3). This nonverbal signal conveys a positive attitude. Frowning and looking glum only add to other people's troubles. It is especially important to be pleasant and friendly to those seeking medical attention, because their worries

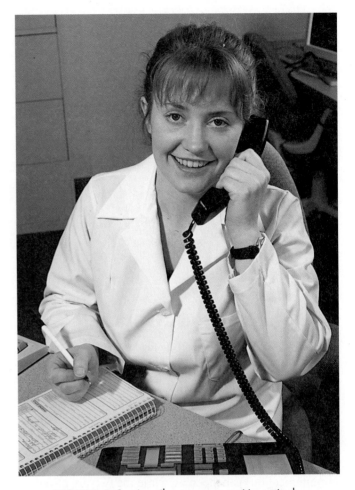

FIGURE 4–3 A smile conveys a positive attitude.

concerning their condition are already on their minds. Adding your troubles to theirs is highly inappropriate. A positive attitude and a receptive awareness will show in your facial expression.

Eye contact shows that you are interested in giving and receiving messages of mutual concern and interest. It has been said that the eyes are the windows of the soul. Looking into another's eyes while engaging in conversation permits an open, honest transmission of thoughts and ideas. Looking away while people are talking to you makes them feel that what they are saying is not important. Interest and attention soon disappear and the intent of your message may be distorted or lost.

Gestures

Still another way of transmitting nonverbal messages is by gesturing. Gestures are body movements that enhance what is being said. You may know people who seemingly could not talk if they had to sit on their hands. Try to follow their example. Using hand and body gestures to accentuate a point can help the receiver understand your meaning. To emphasize the subject matter in conversation, gestures help to convey the message. In Figure 4–4,

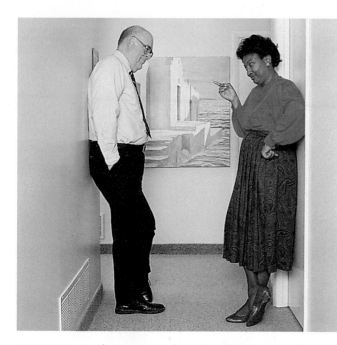

FIGURE 4–4 The woman is obviously telling the man about some frustrations she has, while he passively listens.

a woman's body language shows her feelings of frustration. She is facing her coworker and making eye contact with him. Her coworker has his hands in his pockets as he leans against the wall with his legs crossed, thereby looking rather passive. All of this body language (nonverbal communication) is happening while the two are also conversing verbally.

In your dealings with patients you will encounter many people who are from different cultures, countries, and social backgrounds. Some gestures, facial expressions, or remarks may be offensive to them. Use caution when you are not sure of a remark or gesture; it may be taken the wrong way. It is a good practice to have an interpreter for patients who do not speak the same language that you do. You can ask the interpreter to explain those things which you are not sure of and to alert you to those things you should be careful of in dealing with patients in the future.

There are many gestures that we use daily that have become such a part of our personalities that we do not even realize we do them anymore. Some of them are positive and some are not. Some that are positive and very popularly known are thumbs up, okay, high-five, applause, winking, and a handshake. These are all ways of showing signs of acceptance, encouragement, appreciation, and friendliness (Figure 4–5). If you pay attention, the intended message is clearly understood without saying anything at all. Some of the ways of telling if a person is upset or not interested (negative body language) are crossed arms, looking at one's watch, rolling of the eyes, tapping of the foot or fingers, sighing, and talking under one's breath. And there are still other gestures that are very rude and socially unacceptable. Usually it helps to ignore the patient who seeks attention by using this type of behavior. If this is not effective, it may be necessary to call for

assistance from a supervisor, security, or the police if nothing else works. It should not be a part of your job description to put up with verbal or physical abuse of any kind. If the patient is mentally ill or is under the influence of drugs or alcohol, a certain amount of understanding and tolerance must be employed by all. However, seeking assistance in these situations before a problem escalates is always recommended.

A handshake is a sign of friendship. Another meaningful body movement is a hug to convey feelings of warmth and affection. A comforting touch helps patients feel that you care and gives them a sense of security and acceptance. Studies have shown that patients who have been touched, by a hand on the shoulder or a hand held, respond significantly better in treatment than those not touched. Patting someone on the back and saying "Good for you" is a positive reinforcer. You might do that in praise of a patient who followed the prescribed treatment of the physician and lost 10 pounds and who needs positive recognition of these achievements to encourage continued compliance. There are, however, patients who may be offended by your touching them or whose religious beliefs, culture, or ethnic origin do not allow this. When touching patients in the office to offer comfort or praise, do so in the presence of other professionals for your protection against possible misunderstandings. This will safeguard you from being unfairly accused of touching someone inappropriately.

There is also a proper distance you should maintain when speaking to another. If you are engaged in a personal conversation, the accepted space between two peo-

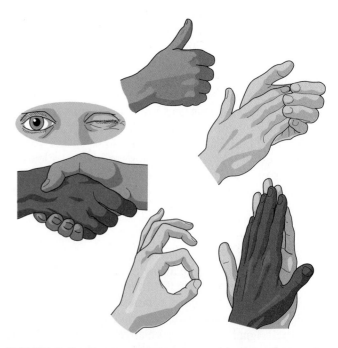

FIGURE 4–5 Common positive gestures (clockwise, from top): thumbs up, applause, high-five, okay, handshake, and winking. Note that some gestures may not be perceived as positive to persons from other cultures or backgrounds.

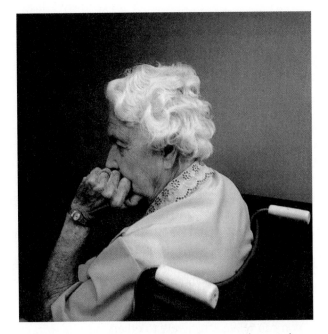

FIGURE 4–6 The patient is silent and seems to be avoiding eye contact with others. Her nonverbal language could indicate that there is an underlying problem that needs to be addressed.

ple is from 1.5 to 4 feet. For social conversation among people, the distance between people is from 4 to 12 feet, which is about the distance you and your patients will be communicating. In a public setting the space can be 12 to 25 feet. In addition to touch, gestures, language barriers, and talking to patients, you must remember to do the best you can, in general, and try to keep in mind these points while communicating with patients.

In reinforcing a patient's actions, you should display a positive attitude, facial expression, gestures, and eye contact—all the communication skills so far mentioned. In addition, your tone of voice should be happy and sincere. Patients who believe you are pleased with their progress are more willing to strive to follow future treatment because of the resulting positive feelings.

Another powerful nonverbal communication tool is silence. This method can indeed be most frustrating for the person to whom it is directed. In dealing with patients who exhibit this nonverbal way of communicating, it is best if the inexperienced medical assistant ask for help from a supervisor, a physician, or another staff member who has skill in dealing with this type of situation (Fig-ure 4–6). Patients who exhibit behavior such as this may have serious underlying problems.

ACHIEVE UNIT OBJECTIVES

Complete Chapter 4, Unit 1, in the workbook to help you obtain competency of this subject matter.

Medical-Legal-Ethical Scenario

Jackie has been working all morning and into her lunch hour to catch up on transcribing overdue reports and referral letters. Kelly and Sabrina just came back from lunch and are still laughing about a funny story they heard. Jackie hears them and instantly thinks that they are talking and laughing about her. She ignores them when they come into the area where she is. Kelly starts to bring the first afternoon patient in and is still smiling and occasionally chuckling about the funny story. The patient thinks he is being made fun of and sarcastically asks, "What's so funny?" Sabrina overhears the man, comes to Kelly's rescue by explaining the story, and they all have another laugh about it. Jackie was on the phone while this was going on and still thinks she is the reason for the laughter. This misunderstanding continues all afternoon.

CRITICAL THINKING CHALLENGE

1. What is going on here?
2. Does Jackie have a reason to be upset?

3. What should Kelly and Sabrina have done to alleviate the brewing situation?

UNIT 2

Behavioral Adjustments

■ OBJECTIVES

Upon completion of the unit, meet the following performance objectives by verifying knowledge of the facts and principles presented through oral and written communication at a level deemed competent.

1. Spell and define, using the glossary at the back of the text, all the Words to Know in this unit.
2. List the commonly used behavioral defense mechanisms and give an example of each.
3. Explain what could happen to a person who habitually uses one or more of the defense mechanisms listed in this unit.
4. Explain why it is necessary to know yourself before you can relate effectively to others.
5. List problem-solving steps, and apply them to a particular problem you may have.
6. Explain the importance of mental and emotional status in regard to overall health.

AREAS OF COMPETENCE (AAMA)

This unit addresses content within the specific competency areas of *Professionalism* and *Communication skills*, as identified in the Medical Assistant Role Delineation Study. Refer to Appendix A for a detailed listing of the areas.

■ WORDS TO KNOW

adjustment	projection
analytical	rationalization
ardently	regression
compensation	repression
denial	strategem
displacement	sublimation
intellectualization	suppression
malinger	unobtrusive

We discussed in Unit 1 of this chapter how keeping a positive attitude is of primary importance in our interactions with others. Even though we strive for a good rapport with coworkers, patients, family, and friends, we must realize that we are human beings. Perfection in any relationship, even the best one, is certainly a desirable goal, but rather unrealistic. Understanding ourselves and others is essential in meaningful communications. Often in our daily transactions of conveying and receiving messages, we use certain coping skills to keep ourselves

from getting hurt or to protect our image. These complex strategems are called defense mechanisms.

DEFENSE MECHANISMS

These defenses are largely unconscious acts we use to help us deal with unpleasant and socially unacceptable circumstances or behaviors. They help us make an emotional adjustment in everyday situations. Surely we all use various defense mechanisms from time to time. However, habitual use can cause one to become somewhat out of touch with reality.

Repression

The most commonly used defense mechanism is repression, which is the forcing of unacceptable or painful ideas, feelings, and impulses into the unconscious mind without being aware of it. Certainly, we have all wished something unpleasant would happen to another person when we have experienced feelings of hostility, jealousy, or intense anger from interacting with that person. These feelings do not vanish, but are placed in our unconscious and may surface in dreams or subtle unobtrusive behaviors.

Repression, like all of the defense mechanisms, tends to protect us from unwanted messages about ourselves that make us feel bad.

Suppression

Suppression is a term to describe a condition in which the person becomes purposely involved in a project, hobby, or work so that a painful situation can be avoided. There are those who, rather than face a difficult problem within a relationship, for instance, throw themselves into their work so much that there is little or no time for the relationship. This is a good way to avoid communication because the legitimate "work" has to be done. However, people only fool themselves until something has to be done to relieve the stress this kind of behavior causes.

Displacement

Displacement is the transfer of emotions about one to another. A typical example of displacement for the medical assistant might be as follows: In the course of the day, a medical assistant has many duties to perform for many others, and one patient in particular becomes overly demanding and rude. The medical assistant holds back the strong feelings that arise and deals with the situation professionally. Later in the evening at home, the medical assistant feels all the pent-up anger surface and explodes at a family member. Although this is done unconsciously, after the fact the medical assistant realizes that actions have been displaced from where they originated to an innocent, unsuspecting target.

Projection

In **projection**, you might unconsciously blame another person for your own inadequacies. An extreme form of projection can lead to hostile, even aggressive behavior if you perceive another person to be the cause of the painful feelings. For example, an obese patient who has gained a few pounds may blame the medical assistant by saying that the scales were set up or read incorrectly.

Rationalization

With **rationalization**, you justify behavior with socially acceptable reasons and tend to ignore the real reasons underlying the behavior. This self-disciplined, unconscious act is relatively harmless. However, habitual use of this defense mechanism, as well as all the others discussed in this unit, can become nonproductive or even destructive because they distort reality. A typical rationalization might be, "I dieted strictly all day; therefore, it's okay to eat a couple of candy bars later in the evening after supper."

Intellectualization

Intellectualization is still another means of denying socially unacceptable feelings or strong feelings that cannot be easily expressed. With this mechanism, you use reasoning to avoid confronting emotional conflicts and stressful situations. For example, you might discuss all the facts and provide endless information about how to begin caring for an elderly relative, elaborating on special diets and home health care to avoid dealing with the true feelings of sadness that may accompany the person's illness.

Sublimation

Sublimation is used unconsciously to express socially unacceptable instinctive drives or impulses in approved and acceptable ways. An example of sublimation might be a 30-year-old father who is a frustrated athlete forcing his child to excel in a sport. Or, an artist may unconsciously direct sexual impulses in the form of constructive writing, sculpture, painting, or photography.

Compensation

Compensation is somewhat similar to sublimation in that it is positive. When you use this defense mechanism, you use a talent or an attribute to the fullest to compensate for a realized personal shortcoming. For example, a person who can no longer participate in sports because of illness or injury may find satisfaction in writing about the game, helping with coaching, or becoming an ardent fan of a well-known team.

Temporary Withdrawal

Temporary withdrawal is a defense mechanism that is a retreat from facing a painful or difficult situation. This avoidance of something that is unpleasant is another way of protecting ourselves from disagreeable feelings. Watching TV or reading excessively to avoid dealing with an issue are common types of withdrawal.

Putting off issues only makes the situation worse. The longer the withdrawal goes on, it produces anxiety and makes the problem more difficult to face.

Daydreaming

A healthy type of temporary withdrawal that all of us do from time to time is daydreaming. This is a way to momentarily escape from reality and relax. At times, you can become very creative and return refreshed from daydreams. If, however, this form of escape is done too often and for too long of a time, it becomes unhealthy and should be of concern to you.

Malingering

Another common defense mechanism is **malingering**. When you malinger, you deliberately pretend to be sick to avoid dealing with situations that are unpleasant or cause anxiety. A malingering individual might stay home sick on a day when he or she was to give a presentation, when in fact, that person is not sick and is actually enjoying the time at home.

Denial

Denial seems to be a commonly used defense mechanism. It is the refusal to admit or acknowledge something so you do not have to deal with a problem or situation. When you are not accepting the phases of life that may produce anxiety, you sometimes use denial as an emotional defense. Denial is usually seen only in psychosis in adults who have reacted to a traumatic situation of extreme stress.

When one who has been given the diagnosis of a terminal illness does not accept the reality of it and believes that a recovery is certain, that person is going through the denial stage.

Regression

Regression is behaving in ways that are typically characteristic of an earlier developmental level. This usually happens in times of high stress.

For example, a college student consoles herself during final exam week with eating hot fudge sundaes as she did as a child with her mother whenever problems at school piled up. Occasionally we may see someone regress to sucking their thumbs or twirling their hair when they are stressed or very tired.

Indeed, we all use many and perhaps all of these defense mechanisms from time to time. Because they are mostly used without conscious awareness, they may be relatively harmless. However, habitual use of defense mechanisms can veil reality and interfere with facing personal issues and crises, as well as with open and honest communication with others.

Procrastination

This defense mechanism is a threat to us all. It robs us of time and energy if we let it become a habit. Procrastination is defined as "always putting off until tomorrow what you could do today." This is surely familiar to you. There is nothing wrong with doing as much as you can within reason and ability in a day and leaving some things to do the next day. The problem with procrastination is that it becomes easier to put off more tasks. This creates stress on the job for you and coworkers because there is so much to do the next day, and catching up is difficult. Occasional procrastination is understandable, but if it becomes a habit, it is detrimental to your character and your workload. Coworkers will not be pleased to always bail you out because you never complete your work on time. You must be aware of this and not give in to a habit of procrastinating so that you will be more productive.

PROBLEM SOLVING

In our complex daily lives, we use many coping skills to deal with our difficulties. Defense mechanisms have already been discussed. Another approach to handling interpersonal problems and concerns is to develop problem-solving skills. Taking a step-by-step approach helps one look realistically and logically at a problem. This method encourages **analytical** thinking and confident decision making. Here is an outline of the basic steps in problem solving:

1. Determine just what the problem is and write it down. Ask if there is a problem chain or a series of events that is a contributor.
2. Gather facts and ideas to help you decide what to do about it.
3. Use analytical and creative thinking. (List your decisions and what you think their outcome will be.)
4. Prioritize your decisions and begin testing them one by one until results are satisfactory to you and others concerned.

If results are not pleasing, begin again with step one. Often, step one alone triggers an answer to a problem. Sitting down and writing out what the problem actually is can be most therapeutic. Once you begin to use this skill to think logically about major problems, such as changing employment, relocating geographically, or locating a suitable day care facility, you will begin to think more logically in all matters. Making a habit of this skill will increase your peace of mind and reduce stress because you will deal with problems more efficiently and spend less time and energy worrying about what to do. This skill can be a great stride toward eliminating procrastination.

The medical assistant who concentrates on patient education may want to pass this helpful skill on to patients.

MENTAL AND EMOTIONAL STATUS INFLUENCING BEHAVIORS

Medical assistants, in both administrative and clinical capacities, have many opportunities daily to observe patients' mental and emotional states. These observations have a direct influence on the medical assistants' behaviors, which in turn directly influence their overall health. We must keep in mind that all medical personnel are patients too. Therefore, all of the information we learn about patients applies to us as well.

Stress in life can lead to ill health. A true understanding of one's self is the primary key to understanding others.

Learning about yourself requires you to take a good hard look at who and what you really are. When assessing your "self," your individual presence may come to mind first. This presence comprises both your physical self (your body) and your self-image (how you view yourself). Another aspect of self, as termed by psychologists, is the "self-as-process." This refers to the ongoing process inside each of us that deals with constant changes, or adjustments, in our lives.

Your response to others is dealt with by your social self. You have many different roles with which you identify **ardently**. Finally, you have an "ideal self." This is what you picture yourself to be—the perfect model you have of yourself.

We are, indeed, complex beings, capable of doing just about anything we choose. Unfortunately, many of us never come close to realizing our true potential. This may be due to never having to look at ourselves squarely. Sometimes it can be quite difficult and even unpleasant to be honest about ourselves.

A good way to begin a basic assessment of yourself is by making a list of all the strengths you have, as well as all your weaknesses. This technique can help point out your abilities and qualities and identify areas that need to be changed. Keeping a journal or a diary, even if only temporarily, is another way to vent feelings, look at problems, and realize and assess your behavior patterns to better know your true self.

An ideal time to reevaluate yourself and renew your goals and aspirations is annually on your birthday. Many people prefer the traditional New Year's resolution. Knowing yourself will help you become a more complete person and will help you relate to others more effectively.

COMMUNICATING EMOTIONAL STATES

In Unit 1 of this chapter, we discussed verbal and nonverbal messages. Communication is a complex process, and one must be aware of all of its facets so that complete information exchange may occur.

The perceptive medical assistant should be able to decide what "feeder questions" to ask a patient to determine whether the look on the patient's face matches the patient's emotional demeanor. The following are feeder questions the medical assistant may use to find out the emotional states of the patients they interview. After greeting the patient with a kind "hello," the medical assistant may want to ask "What seems to be the problem today?" or "What brings you here to see the doctor today?" or "Can you tell me about the problem you seem to be having?" or "Can we talk about what has been giving you concern that brings you in to see the doctor?"

For a follow-up visit, ask "Are you feeling any better since you were in to see the doctor last?" or "You don't seem to be feeling too well; do you feel any better?" or "Can you tell me how you've been doing since you were here last?"

Hearing patients' answers can provide a general idea of how they feel emotionally. Of course, one can only accomplish this by taking time to find out. That means giving the patients your undivided attention, if only for a few minutes. Unfortunately, many health care professionals lack the skills and perhaps even the concern to establish this rapport, and therefore fail to develop this skill. Remember that the manner in which you speak, your tone of voice, and your body language convey your attitude. Make sure that you show professionalism and compassion when you serve all patients. The medical assistant can be instrumental in pointing out factors that can interfere with a particular treatment approach planned by the physician (Figure 4–7). Patients will likely respond to and comply with the doctor's orders far more readily if the medical assistant imparts a genuine concern for their well-being with each contact.

1. Travel (business or pleasure)
2. Work schedule (irregular hours)
3. Relocating/moving
4. Lifestyle/cultural influences
5. Economic concerns
6. Comprehension of physician's orders
7. Disability/mental incompetence
8. Being unclear about the directions or the importance of the treatment plan

FIGURE 4–7 Factors that can interfere with patient compliance in treatment plans

If a patient seems quieter than usual, the medical assistant may determine after talking to the patient (with eye contact, of course) that the patient is preoccupied by some problem or matter that he or she will reveal if you show interest and take time to listen. Often a statement that begins with "I" can open up a conversation with another person. For instance, you may say to a patient, "I noticed as you were walking in today that you don't seem to be as lively as usual. Is anything in particular bothering you?" This gives patients a feeling that you really pay attention to them, that you care about how they are, and that you are showing it. This can make the patient feel more at ease and may gain better compliance with the physician's orders. If the patient is not allowed to express certain feelings, he or she may not be attentive enough to listen to the physician's orders, which need to be followed for optimal health benefits. The medical assistant plays an important role in assisting both physician and patient in providing quality health care.

Using the statements that begin with "I" can be of help to the health care team as well. You can also use an "I" statement with a coworker, such as, "I noticed that the filing is getting piled up; need some help?" This way of offering help is much easier to answer with a positive response because the person is not being accused of doing a poor job of filing. The blame falls on the volume of filing, not the coworker. When conversing with coworkers it is important to speak sincerely and to communicate your feelings as professionally as you do with patients. This can prevent a serious situation from happening because the habit of giving and expecting respect and courtesy has been established.

■ ACHIEVE UNIT OBJECTIVES

Complete Chapter 4, Unit 2, in the workbook to help you obtain competency of this subject matter.

UNIT 3

Patients and Their Families

■ OBJECTIVES

Upon completion of the unit, meet the following performance objectives by verifying knowledge of the facts and principles presented through oral and written communication at a level deemed competent.

1. Spell and define, using the glossary at the back of the text, all the **Words to Know** in this unit.
2. Explain why it is important to develop rapport with patients and their families.
3. Describe means of safeguarding the patient's right to confidentiality.

4. Describe the patient's options in relation to the physician's treatment plan.
5. Describe the stages that follow diagnosis of a terminal illness.
6. Describe your role in dealing with the terminally ill patient.
7. Explain the purpose of the living will.
8. State the purpose of the hospice movement.
9. List the services of the hospice movement.

AREAS OF COMPETENCE (AAMA)

This unit addresses content within the specific competency areas of *Professionalism, Communication skills, Legal concepts,* and *Instruction,* as identified in the Medical Assistant Role Delineation Study. Refer to Appendix A for a detailed listing of the areas.

▮ WORDS TO KNOW

absurd	incomprehensible
advance directives	living will
commiserate	inevitable
devastate	marginal
fortitude	nonchalant
holistic	solace
hospice movement	terminal
hostility	

The medical profession's first responsibility is to the patient. Thus you must be able to relate to people of all ages, from tiny infants to senior citizens. The development and growth of your own personality and interests will help you do so.

The ability to converse about a variety of subjects shows an interest in people and makes you interesting to be with. Conversation with patients helps to ease their anxieties and encourage a sense of friendship and trust. At times a patient needs to express pent-up feelings, and you will often be the one who provides this necessary listening service. Sincere empathy will often begin to relieve the inner fears and anxieties of a patient who is experiencing an illness for the first time.

Patients and family members may need to discuss again the treatment plan the physician has already discussed with them. Often patients do not hear all of what has been said by the physician because they have been preoccupied with worry about their illness. Their questions may sometimes seem trivial, but to the patient they are real and pressing issues that need immediate attention. Be mindful of those patients who are disabled, are from another culture, or speak another language. Offer compassion as best as possible when conversing with them about patient care. An interpreter should be scheduled to translate for the patient and family members if no family member speaks English. Provide translators with printed patient education materials that they can review with the patient.

This is the reason that giving printed instructions to patients is so important. If the patient is preoccupied when the instructions are given, printed material is also given to the patient, who can read the information later. Usually a phone call will be initiated by the patient at a later time to have questions answered or for clarification or reassurance about something.

Many patients have never before experienced sickness or injury. They may never have set foot in a health care facility. Having to face strange new surroundings, unfamiliar medical language, and possibly puzzling procedures will add to a patient's apprehensions. The way the patient is treated in these new situations will determine how the patient and members of the family accept the diagnosis and prognosis of the patient's condition. Tact and good communication skills will help to promote rapport with all patients and their family members.

RIGHT TO PRIVACY

As mentioned previously, every patient has a legal right to privacy and confidentiality. Information disclosed to the health care team must be kept in the strictest confidence, and you must be ever mindful of the legal implications in handling patients' records. Information concerning patients may be given to another member of the health care team, such as a laboratory technician or referring physician, only when it pertains directly to the course of treatment. Another medical office may telephone to inquire about a patient's medical history for diagnostic purposes, to confirm symptoms, or to verify a birthdate; patients, when they agree to a referral appointment or scheduled test, will have given implied consent for necessary information to be transmitted concerning their condition. In the daily routine, such procedures do not require consent forms to be signed by the patient. If this were not true, very little could be accomplished besides handling forms.

Medical information may be given to parties not concerned in the patient's treatment *only* when the patient has signed a release of information form. Medical insurance forms, for instance, have a section patients must sign to authorize the release of information to insurance companies (Figure 4–8). Only those persons specified in writing by the patient may receive information concerning the patient's condition. Usually the medical facility has a patient information release form, which is completed during the initial visit. Persons to contact in case of emergency are listed by the patient; this is when you should inquire about who may be informed about the patient's condition. This document should be filed in the patient's chart for future reference.

Many patients have answering machines and email. You must have a signed permission form on file to leave a message on an answering machine (or voice mail) or email concerning the patient. There may be others listen-

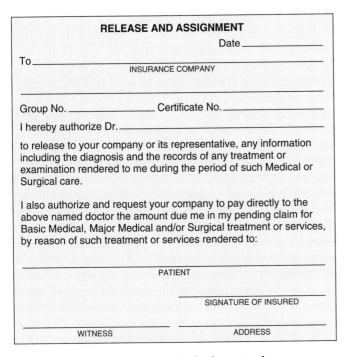

FIGURE 4–8 Release of information form

ing to or reading your message(s) before the patient retrieves the message(s), and the patient may not want the information known to others. Even a reminder of an appointment should have signed permission before a message is left. The privacy of each patient must always be protected. Those of legal age have the right to privacy in all matters of treatment, and even parents may not be given information about a family member's condition unless specific written permission accompanied by the patient's signature is secured.

In the normal course of conversation with a patient, you may be told personal information that should be kept to yourself, unless doing so would be harmful to the patient. The patient will usually tell you how far the information should go, or whom to tell or not to tell. Emotional stress and other critical data should be relayed to the physician, for it may have some bearing on the condition of the patient. You must use judgment in this important area. A patient who is experiencing domestic problems, for instance, may be asking for help by telling you about their situation.

There also will be patients who have no medical insurance to cover the cost of treatments or other diagnostic procedures; you should guide them to seek public assistance, if possible. Patients usually realize that professionals can put them in touch with assistance and sometimes expect that it will be forthcoming if they merely suggest that help is needed. Tact is required in handling delicate matters of this nature. Patients trust the medical profession to safeguard matters discussed in the privacy of the medical office. Directly asking each patient who may receive this confidential information and having appropriate release forms signed will ensure that the patient is

aware of what has been done and will also protect you from liability.

CHOICE OF TREATMENT

Advising patients of the choices they have in the treatment of their illnesses is often part of your responsibilities. A full explanation of the diagnosis, prognosis, and options in treating the condition are given to the patient by the physician. However, some patients have a difficult time making up their minds and may need additional information and further discussion before deciding to accept a treatment plan (especially when it involves a major event such as elective surgery). There are life-threatening situations in which patients must make these decisions quickly. Often family members must help patients with these difficult decisions.

You play an integral part in reinforcing the physician's orders. You should become proficient in identifying those patients who still seem confused after leaving their conference with the physician. Restating what the physician has already said may be all you need to say to some patients to initiate their compliance. Some patients may have had trouble with the wording used by the physician and look to you to interpret. It is difficult at times to make clear to patients all that is involved in the course of treatment. Great skill in perception is essential for all health care team members to ascertain if the treatment approach is fully understood by the patient. Perception is a valuable skill which takes time and experience to master.

It is prudent to advise patients to seek a second opinion if they harbor any doubts concerning their condition. It may be that patients disbelieve the diagnosis. Having a second, or even a third, opinion will help them to accept their illness. Many insurance companies encourage patients to seek other opinions before treatment is initiated. This is wise, especially if the patient is troubled about the possible outcome.

Patients still may have difficulty in complying with physicians' orders (e.g., regarding weight reduction, exercising, or taking prescribed medicine). Patients must be given sound reasons for following the advice of the physician even though they already know that it is for their own good. The prescribed treatment plan will most likely change the patient's lifestyle. The patient who has just been diagnosed as hypertensive may have to cope with several lifestyle changes, such as losing weight, following a special diet, and giving up cigarettes. If reinforcement and encouragement are not sufficiently provided to the patient by members of the health care team, cooperation may be **marginal**. The risks of not following the physician's advice should be outlined in the simplest terms. Acting **nonchalant** or showing no interest in the patient will not be much help in prompting a patient to follow orders.

The final choice is always the patient's, to accept and follow the outlined plan of treatment or not. Knowing what is best does not always dictate compliance. Motivation is the key. Giving patients realistic suggestions can help them accept a treatment plan that may initially have seemed impossible to follow. Changing behavior will probably be resisted. The patient who experiences setbacks, who does not remember to take medication, or who breaks away from the prescribed diet will need additional encouragement to get back on track. You can be of particular value in this type of situation. You must always be reinforcing with your remarks made to patients concerning the intended goals of treatment. Furthermore, by being a good role model, you subtly reinforce the physician's advice. An assistant who should be but is not following a weight-reduction plan will give a negative impression to a patient who has just been told to do so by the physician. A patient who has been instructed by the physician in personal hygiene will be less likely to follow advice if the medical assistant does not also heed the advice.

In conversing with patients you will find that their areas of interest will prompt ideas for encouraging compliance with treatment. One good motivator is the physician's fee for services. Many patients quickly realize that they should follow the physician's advice, for it will certainly be more costly in the long run if they do not.

Approach–Avoidance Conflict

Approach–avoidance behavior protects one from reaching a set goal that seems too difficult to complete. This is a personal conflict and can cause one considerable stress. The person wants to reach a goal, but keeps avoiding the final step of the plan. Think of the patient who makes an appointment for the removal of a mass in the colon. The patient schedules the appointment, yet when the time comes for it, the patient cancels because he or she fears that the results of the surgical biopsy will be cancerous tissue. Every time a person who has approach–avoidance conflict sets a goal or makes a plan of some magnitude, the outcome is that the person does not follow through because the person is afraid of the end result.

TERMINAL ILLNESS

Dealing with patients who have been diagnosed as having a terminal illness is a challenging and rewarding experience: challenging because of its difficulty and rewarding because of the knowledge that you are giving supportive care when patients and their families need it most.

Many patients have a hard time accepting the diagnosis. Their initial reaction is to deny it. Indeed, knowing that one's life is about to end is an almost incomprehensible fact. Patients wrestling with this new reality claim that the diagnosis is absurd, but ignoring the problem cannot provide solace.

As frustration mounts and anger becomes apparent, patients may feel isolated, for they see others as the picture of health. Feelings of hostility are natural and in-

evitable. Patients in this plight may lash out at anyone with whom they come in contact. Blaming themselves and others becomes a means of dealing with their anger for a time. Questioning becomes a way of venting anger for some. "Why does this have to be?" is the most troublesome question. Following this stage of anger is a period of depression. This is the reaction to the final realization of the course of their illness. Patients in this stage are usually ready to talk about their illness, hoping someone will understand. It is a difficult subject to talk about, but you may be influential in helping them to respond and talk about their fears. Eventually patients attempt to accept the terminal illness by bargaining, or seeking ways of "buying" more time. This sometimes gives them inner strength to live a while longer: they are holding on to see someone be married, wanting to hold the new grandchild, or waiting for someone to return from the service. In this stage of bargaining, patients may look for spiritual inspiration. The zest for life is strong and the fight is one not easily given up.

In the final stages of terminal disease, patients come closer to accepting the course of their disease. This is truly a sad time for patients and their families. To know that one may not see the next spring, or to know that one will no longer experience the joys and pleasures of loved ones, can be devastating to the patient. Empathy and genuine compassion may be offered to a patient who is reaching out for comfort. You will be touched deeply, and your fortitude will be challenged to the maximum in interacting with the patient and family members during this most stressful time (Figure 4–9).

Finally, patients resign themselves to impending death. An inner peace is often evident in patients in this final stage of their illness, and they are more willing to make plans for their final days.

Some patients prefer to spare family members the ordeal of prolonging treatment when their physicians reach the decision that death is likely to occur in the near future. Late in 1991 a law was passed in the United States that requires all health care providers to inform and advise patients and their families of advance directives. The living will is a legal document that allows patients to terminate medical procedures that would sustain their lives if they became unconscious or unable to make further deci-

---

The stages of terminal illness:

1. Denial
2. Anger
3. Bargaining
4. Depression
5. Acceptance

FIGURE 4–9   The stages of terminal illness

sions (see Figure 3–1, pg. 57). This document is not recognized in all states in the United States, but it is fast becoming a more acceptable way for patients to let others know when they want to have their life support discontinued. Advance directives also refers to the living will because it gives direction to those who will be following the wishes of the patient who prepared the legal document. With this legal form, the patient can state exactly how far lifesaving efforts should go or can establish a do not resuscitate (DNR) order. This documentation helps the patient and family avoid an agonizingly long period in waiting for the inevitable.

When the patient signs this document, a copy should be filed with the physician, the attorney, and the family. In assisting patients with this procedure, it is helpful if you remind them to make sure that all details have been worked out and that the family has been properly informed about who is responsible for honoring the document. Patients now know that they have a right to die with dignity and that they have a choice in making their last days of life more meaningful.

For many years a concerned group of individuals has recognized and **commiserated** with grief-stricken, terminally ill people. This concerned group has formed the **hospice movement** to provide some health care to those with terminal illness. In recent years the hospice movement has gained strength. Instead of the tiring and impersonal surroundings that are sometimes associated with hospital care, hospice helps the family provide care so that patients can remain in their comfortable, familiar home surroundings during the last days of their lives and be among their family members and friends more conveniently. Support and caring assistance is given to help the family learn to cope with the turbulence of the patients and their illness. Efforts are coordinated with physicians and hospital staffs when necessary to give patients the best possible care.

Patients and their families in this stage of the patient's illness may need more spiritual guidance. The counsel of a minister, priest, or rabbi, may also be found through hospice because **holistic** care is the purpose of the hospice movement. Once the patient has been informed by the physician that he or she has a terminal illness, you should refer patients to the local hospice movement for consultation.

Society is returning to the idea that there is a human need to share the experiences of birth and death with loved ones. These natural parts of life have been largely removed from our experience for some time now. We have even become uneasy in talking about them. The need for human love during significant times is evident in the return to the practice of entering and leaving this world at home.

ACHIEVE UNIT OBJECTIVES

Complete Chapter 4, Unit 3, in the workbook to help you obtain competency of this subject matter.

UNIT 4
Office Interpersonal Relationships

OBJECTIVES

Upon completion of the unit, meet the following performance objectives by verifying knowledge of the facts and principles presented through oral and written communication at a level deemed competent.

1. Spell and define, using the glossary at the end of the text, all the **Words to Know** in this unit.
2. Describe relationships between the medical assistant, the employer, and coworkers.
3. List positive methods for dealing with stress.
4. Describe the reasons for staff meetings.
5. Explain methods of intraoffice communication.
6. State the purpose of an employee evaluation.
7. Describe the obligations of the employer and the new employee in providing a smooth transition in the workplace.

AREAS OF COMPETENCE (AAMA)

This unit addresses content within the specific competency areas of *Professionalism* and *Communication skills*, as identified in the Medical Assistant Role Delineation Study. Refer to Appendix A for a detailed listing of the areas.

A CAAHEP CONNECTION

Knowledge of the basic principles of psychology, mental health, and applied psychology as discussed in this unit are curriculum requirements of the standards for an approved program in medical assisting. These components are essential for success in this field.

WORDS TO KNOW

description	perplexing
evaluation	petty
externship	transition
obligation	

The medical assistant employed in a medical office or clinic must learn to positively relate not only to patients but to other members of the health care team as well. Dealing with the needs of patients on a day-to-day basis can sometimes become an overwhelming task. Schedules in most medical practices can easily become overbooked; sometimes it seems everyone has an emergency and must be seen by the physician today! Health care employees should be able to shift gears and handle these situations gracefully and efficiently. The essential ingredient in running a medical office smoothly is cooperation. When each employee contributes, the result is a good team that works together for quality patient care.

The field of medicine is by its nature stress-filled. Patients are troubled by an abnormal state of health and are naturally anxious and on edge. They may exhibit their feelings by acting irritable and uncooperative at times. They not only expect but demand patience and understanding from medical personnel.

STAFF ARRANGEMENTS

Picture the ideal medical office where patients and medical staff are going about the business at hand in a pleasant, efficient manner. Everyone gets along well with everyone else, patients are smiling and friendly, and every interchange is courteous. The schedule is kept down to the minute, all the filing is caught up, the phone rings only when there is nothing else pressing at the moment, referral reports are all back, and everything runs like clockwork. This picture is unreal. This ideal situation is what every medical practice hopes to achieve, but to bring this model practice into existence would require the perfection of all persons involved. This is, of course, impossible. Nevertheless, each member of the staff has a unique set of values, principles, and standards, and each must respect the others to ensure compatible relationships.

The number of employees varies in each type of medical practice. Some physicians in private practice employ only one medical assistant to perform both administrative and clinical duties. This is a tremendous responsibility and requires a highly motivated and mature personality. There are offices where many health care professionals work together, as in group practices and clinics. A medical assistant's compensation may sometimes seem minimal when the job includes long hours and limited benefits. A good rapport with the employer is necessary to accomplish the objectives of daily patient care. Usually a good friendship develops between the physician and medical assistant over a period of time, and working together is an enjoyable learning experience for both. Interest in each patient is easy to cultivate since individual contact is made at each office visit. You may get to know patients even better than the physician because of frequent phone conversations with patients. You will soon become the physician's right hand by supplying important patient information obtained in this manner.

Communication lines must remain open with this one-to-one relationship, as in all employer-employee relationships. If misunderstandings occur, they must be rectified as soon as possible. More complex problems can mushroom if incidental misunderstandings are not cleared up. Solutions to these problems must be worked out together. You will have to be assertive in decisions concerning administrative, clinical, and personal employment matters. Being on one's own as a medical assistant in a private practice has its rewards as well as its disadvantages.

Many physicians in both private and group practices find it necessary to employ several medical assistants. Although this can be an enjoyable experience for all members of the staff, a great deal of cooperation and respect for one another is necessary for a harmonious relationship among the staff members to be maintained. Specific job **descriptions** encourage each employee to remain in a particular area to promote efficiency. Overstepping boundaries may cause friction and misunderstandings: at the same time, all staff members must be willing to pitch in where help is needed. Again, a positive attitude is needed to create a pleasant work environment.

The physician usually delegates responsibility for office management to one of the employees, most often the one with greatest seniority, qualifications, or both. This frees the physician to attend to patients and also relieves the physician of personnel management. This is a major area of importance, especially in large clinics with many employees, and, as a rule, it is an area physicians are not trained to handle. Often these supervisory or personnel management positions are filled by registered nurses, but they also have little or no specific training in medical office management. Their training centers primarily around the hospital model and direct patient care. Since a trained medical assistant can, in most states, perform most of the procedures that a nurse can, under the supervision of a physician, resentment may arise. You must come to grips with this reality before accepting a position where it may be a source of irritation and discontent.

Physicians and office managers appreciate the versatility of the medical assistant, respect their initiative and industriousness, and employ them with pride and satisfaction. However, each medical practice has its own unique office policy regarding employees. There are still some physicians who would rather take charge of their own office business affairs.

Working closely with others can have both positive and negative effects. In a large office practice or clinic, when there are many employees, a certain amount of give and take must prevail. Completing assigned tasks is expected so that the work is shared equitably. **Petty** differences should be settled with tact. Sharing enlightening experiences and significant events with other employees is a natural inclination. This is fine if it does not interfere with patient care. A certain amount of self-discipline and self-control is necessary in a professional setting. Remaining aware of the situation at hand will help you perceive what is appropriate.

INTRAOFFICE COMMUNICATION

Many physicians hold regular staff meetings that all employees are expected to attend. They are usually held in the medical office either before or after patients have been seen, and are announced far enough in advance so that arrangements can be made to attend. Many staff meetings are scheduled at regular times, (e.g., the second Friday of each month, a meet-and-eat meeting at noon every other Wednesday). At these meetings decisions concerning office policy changes are reached and problems are discussed. This is a time for new ideas to be expressed and exchanged. It also allows all members of the staff to get to know each other.

Some situations between employees may be impossible to iron out. These are usually personality conflicts, and the usual course of action, if the situation does not improve, is termination of one of the employees (usually the one who is more troublesome or less valuable to the practice). This kind of **perplexing** problem may be discussed during a staff meeting. Personnel managers are often aware of these problems before they are reported, and they are usually handled privately.

Employers sometimes use office meeting time for in-service programs, such as training in cardiopulmonary resuscitation. Some employers encourage holiday celebrations on occasion to promote better working relationships.

An intraoffice memo is a means of communicating important information to members of the staff, especially between regularly scheduled staff meetings. Each employee is instructed to read the memo and initial it, indicating that the information has been received, and then pass it on to another employee. This helps ensure that all employees are informed. Word of mouth is not a sure way to relay an important announcement, for it may get distorted en route.

Some offices and clinics use a bulletin board as a means of intraoffice communication (Figure 4–10). Notices of educational programs, seminars, or meetings are posted for all members of the staff to read, in an area such as the staff room or eating area.

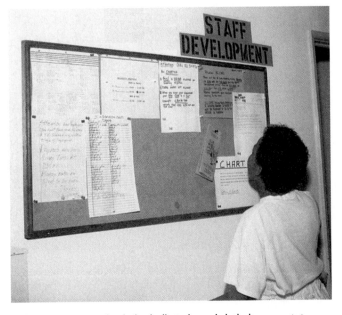

FIGURE 4–10 Check the bulletin board daily because it is a valuable resource for current information about professional meetings, educational seminars and workshops, staff activities, and in-service programs.

CAREER ENTRY

According to recent statistics, there is an increasing need for qualified medical assistants across the nation. Employers in the health care field are recognizing the benefits of employing medical assistants who have had specific training in this most versatile field. This, of course, eliminates the need for extensive and expensive additional training on the job. **Externship** plans are very successful in cooperative programs because they provide soon-to-graduate medical assistant students experience in different offices. The supervisor agrees to allow the instructor to periodically visit the facility and observe the student's performance. Other training programs not accredited by the AAMA require only that students observe for a certain number of hours to fulfill the program's standards. In either case, the trend is most welcomed following the past practice of hiring assistants without any training in the field, who sought either full-time or part-time employment in the physicians' offices or clinics.

The **transition** from student to medical assistant, at any age, poses certain adjustment considerations to all concerned in the health care setting. Employers have an **obligation** to assist the new employee in feeling accepted in the profession and to give helpful advice with patience. The new employee is obligated to strive to perform skills with both proficiency and efficiency. An effort to get along with others is required of each member of the health care team. A smooth transition with a new member of the team is possible if each employee recognizes the

A CAAHEP CONNECTION

Professionalism, getting along with and respect for others on the health care team, and communicating with patients and their families are all discussed in this chapter to prepare you for the field of medical assisting.

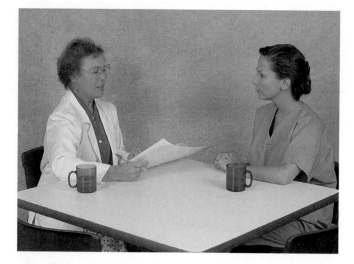

FIGURE 4–11 This supervisor and medical assistant have established a good rapport by maintaining open communication during the evaluation process.

individual worth of each person and the value of each position in fulfilling the health care needs of the patients.

EMPLOYEE EVALUATION

In most employment situations, an **evaluation** of work performance is made on an annual basis. This is filed in your record. The initial employment review is usually held after a probationary period of 30, 60, or 90 days. In this meeting, you and your employer will discuss your job performance. Evaluation forms outline the most important qualities and abilities needed for the job and include a section for strengths and weaknesses to be listed. An example of an employee evaluation form can be found in Chapter 21, Unit 2 with further discussion on securing employment. Employers are always aware of an employee's behavior. Little goes unnoticed when you share a daily routine. Your attitude shows at all times. Even though the word *attitude* may not be a part of the evaluation, the other categories cover it comprehensively.

Initiative is an important factor. Demonstrating resourcefulness will help you advance in your career. Following office policy is also important. Being on time and being dependable on the job are always pleasing to employers. Absences and tardiness are difficult to tolerate from employees who make it a habit. Another area of extreme importance to employers is the quality and quantity of your work. Performing assigned tasks in a reasonable amount of time, without needing to be reminded, is a valuable trait.

The employee evaluation need not be a threat to the conscientious medical assistant. It is a time when questions about advancement and salary may be openly discussed. If you have lived up to the standards of the job, your performance should receive a favorable review.

Some employers find that annual evaluations motivate employees and keep communication lines open (Figure 4–11). Others choose not to have official evaluations, but wish employees to discuss whatever is on their mind at any time. For some office personnel this works quite well. For the private practice physician with one or two medical assistants this is usually the case.

ACHIEVE UNIT OBJECTIVES

Complete Chapter 4, Unit 4, in the workbook to help you obtain competency of this subject matter.

RELATING TO ABHES

Chapter 4 discusses the power of both written and verbal communication and how relationships, environment, and culture affect our interactions with patients and coworkers. This content is related to the ABHES accreditation requirements of *Dealing with difficult patients with normal/abnormal behavior* and *Emotional crises/patients and/or family* within the content area of *Psychology of Human Relations.*

Medical-Legal-Ethical Scenario

Two medical assistants, Julie and Marcia, have been employed in the same family practice office for the past few months. It is a very hectic day and they have been working through the lunch hour because the schedule is so overbooked. Julie has been very short-tempered and rude with some of the patients who have complained about having to wait so long to see the doctor. The clinical supervisor is on jury duty this week and both assistants are handling everything in the office. Marcia is taking the phone calls and is pleasant and courteous to all the patients. She also rooms patients and does basic triage of their conditions. She is, however, running out of patience when she finds Julie sitting in the break room looking at a magazine. When Marcia asks Julie to come out on the floor to room patients and help answer the phone, Julie gets angry and states that she didn't get a lunch hour and needs a break and tells Marcia to leave her alone.

CRITICAL THINKING CHALLENGE

1. What should Marcia do about this situation?
2. Should Marcia tell the doctor about Julie's behavior?

3. Is there any way that Marcia can suggest Julie needs a refresher course on professionalism?
4. What would you do in this situation?

RESOURCES

Milliken, M. E. (1998). Understanding human behavior (6th ed.). Clifton Park, NY: Delmar Learning.

Physicians' desk reference. (Updated annually). Oradell, NJ: Medical Economics.

WEB LINKS

http://www.epic.org (Electronic Privacy Information Center)

This web site is a public interest research center in Washington, D.C., established in 1994 to focus public attention on emerging civil liberties issues and to protect privacy, the First Amendment, and constitutional values.

http://www.mentalhelp.net (Mental Help Net)

This web site, maintained by a psychologist, provides information on mental health, including defense mechanisms.

The Office Environment

A physician's office should be a safe, secure, and environmentally friendly workplace. The office staff must use constant vigilance to maintain that status. This chapter discusses the many aspects of the office environment as they relate to both patients and staff. Safety involves not only the use or condition of the physical equipment and furnishings in the office, but also the human activities of office personnel, visitors, and patients. The protection of staff, office equipment, and materials is very important. The working environment must allow for a focus on the provision of care rather than concern about personal safety.

The efficient design of the office is also a great asset to its ability to function effectively. **Provisions** for individuals who are physically challenged make the office environment a friendlier place for these people. Having the appropriate office management equipment available allows the office to operate more efficiently, and applying the principles of ergonomics assures that employees will be able to function more effectively and safely. This chapter discusses the preparation of the office to receive patients and considers the importance of the patients' and visitors' perception of the office.

UNIT 1

Safety, Security, and Emergency Provisions in the Medical Office

■ OBJECTIVES

Upon completion of the unit, meet the following performance objectives by verifying knowledge of the facts and principles presented through oral and written communication at a level deemed competent.

1. Spell and define, using the glossary at the back of the text, all the **Words to Know** in this unit.
2. Name four things to check to assure safety in a reception room.
3. List four hazards in a reception/business office area.
4. Name three things in an examination room that might be unsafe.
5. List nine items that are covered by OSHA or CDC regulations.
6. Name the three elements necessary for fire.
7. List four ways a fire might start.
8. Name six items that are considered to be protective barriers to prevent skin and mucous membrane exposure to pathogens.

■ WORDS TO KNOW

assault	precautions
barrier	prevention
biohazardous	provisions
emergency	reception
environment	safety
evacuated	security
extinguisher	universal precautions
hazard	ventilation
irrational	volatile

AREAS OF COMPETENCE (AAMA)

This unit addresses content within the specific competency areas of *Fundamental principles, Operational functions,* and *Patient care,* as identified in the Medical Assistant Role Delineation Study. Refer to Appendix A for a detailed listing of the areas.

A SAFE, HEALTHY ENVIRONMENT THROUGHOUT THE MEDICAL OFFICE

The medical office, like the home, is a place where you should feel safe and secure. But just like a home, it takes conscious effort to assure that the office has a protective, healthy **environment**. The medical assistant is part of the team responsible for recognizing any **safety**, security, or operational **hazard**, helping to eliminate it, and warning coworkers and patients of any dangers.

Safety in the Working Environment

The physician's office environment must ensure the health and safety of the physician and staff, and all persons being treated, as well as those accompanying them. This refers not only to the physical surroundings in the office but also the general maintenance of the facility, the mechanical condition of the equipment, and the procedures used to control the presence of harmful microorganisms. The effort to reduce or eliminate exposure to harmful organisms is known as *infection control.*

All types of health care settings must maintain procedures to control the transmission of organisms. By the very nature of the services provided, health care workers are constantly coming into contact with patients who are ill or who may have contagious diseases. The patients in this setting are also exposed to organisms from other patients. It is extremely important for the health and safety of all concerned that the spread of these organisms be prevented. Awareness has been heightened by the ever-present possibility of the spread of hepatitis and HIV viruses.

For the protection of employers and employees, federal and state agencies have established legislation dealing with policies, procedures, and guidelines to reduce disease transmission. The United States Department of Labor established regulations through the Occupational Safety and Health Administration (OSHA). These guidelines deal primarily with requirements of employers to provide employees with safe working conditions to protect them from harmful exposure and substances. An example of this regulation is the provision of latex and vinyl gloves to protect employees during patient contact.

The United States Public Health Department has the Centers for Disease Control and Prevention (CDC) in Atlanta, Georgia. It is the CDC's responsibility to collect data on pathogens and diseases and establish guidelines to prevent their spread. The CDC has developed a system of classifications or categories of infectious diseases related to their method of spread. It was this agency that established guidelines concerning contact with blood and body fluids referred to as **universal precautions**. These guidelines were developed to control the spread of hepatitis and AIDS. Universal precautions have since been incorporated into guidelines called Standard Precautions. These expanded precautions are set infection control guidelines to be used by all health care professionals for all patients. The new guidelines combine the basic principles of the universal precautions with the recommendations of personal protective equipment used to provide protection from all body fluids regardless of whether blood is present or not.

A third governmental agency also establishes regulations for the safety of patients and health care workers. The Clinical Laboratory Improvement Amendments (CLIA) legislation is governed by the United States Department of Health and Human Services. It is their responsibility to assure the public is safeguarded by regulating all testing of specimens coming from the human body. All clinical laboratories must adhere to the strict regulations set forth by the legislation. The original standards were strengthened in response to the public's complaints regarding misread Pap smears that resulted in unnecessary deaths. Laboratory tests are now categorized in relation to their complexity, and laboratories are only approved to perform testing in relation to their level of certification.

This discussion is only an introduction to the regulations. They are more thoroughly discussed in Chapter 12 and are specifically described as appropriate with each clinical procedure.

Safety in the Reception Room

A safe environment begins at the front door. The **reception** room requires a safety check every morning to assure it presents no hazards for patients and visitors. Observe the condition of the furniture carefully. Pay attention to chair and table legs—they must be stable and able to support appropriate weight. Lamps and electrical cords should be examined. Bulbs should not dim or flicker and cords should be in good condition with no evidence of fraying. Be sure lighting is adequate so that even people with impaired vision can see well. Check the floor to be certain there is neither carpet wrinkles nor anything lying on the floor that might cause someone to fall. Avoid the use of decorative or throw rugs.

Safety in the Receptionist/Business Office

In the receptionist/business office area, pay special attention to file drawers and cupboard doors. NEVER open more than one file drawer in a vertical file at a time because the unbalanced weight could cause the cabinet to tip forward. Many people have sustained back and extremity injuries from the automatic reaction to "catch" a cabinet. Also, be careful with opened bottom drawers. They can easily fall over. Wall cupboards pose another safety hazard. If the door is left open, you could strike your head quite forcefully when you stand up or raise up from underneath. All electrical cords must be kept behind desks and other office furnishings so that they will not be tripped over. All equipment should operate properly and show no evidence of electrical shorts or damage.

Safety in the Examination Room

The examination table must be cleaned after each patient. The table must operate properly and the medical assistant must be thoroughly competent in its use. Assist patients as necessary to sit or lie on the table. If the use of a stool is necessary, be exceptionally cautious to guard against the patient stepping on the edges, which could cause it to tip. Very ill patients, elderly patients, and children should not be left alone on an examination table where they could fall. Small children accompanying a parent are best left with another office staff member while the parent is in the examination room.

Children, and some adults, also have a natural curiosity about "things" on the examination room cabinets or counters. Anything which might be hazardous or could become contaminated should be kept out of sight. Prescription pads should not be left lying around where they could be stolen and possibly used to obtain controlled substances. In an examination room, there is a lot of equipment with electrical cords that must be positioned so that they will not interfere with movement or walking in the room.

Safety in the Laboratory Area

Chemicals kept in the office for laboratory work must be properly labeled and stored. Chemicals that could become **volatile** when kept beyond their expiration date must be monitored carefully. The testing of patients' urine, blood, and other specimens requires special procedures. Containers for the disposal of used equipment and **biohazardous** waste must be readily accessible. A strict adherence to standard precautions is essential to the maintenance of a safe and healthy office environment.

GENERAL OFFICE SAFETY

Fire

Fire **prevention** is very important to everyone's safety. Only three elements need to be present for a fire to start: heat, fuel, and oxygen (Figure 5–1). Today, there are rare exceptions to the "no smoking" regulations in medical and public facilities. Yet, there is still a possibility of a

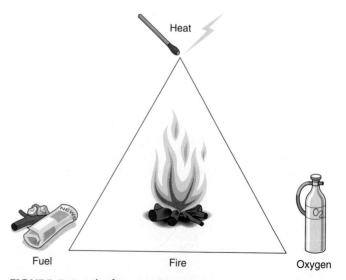

FIGURE 5–1 The fire triangle—elements needed for combustion (burning)

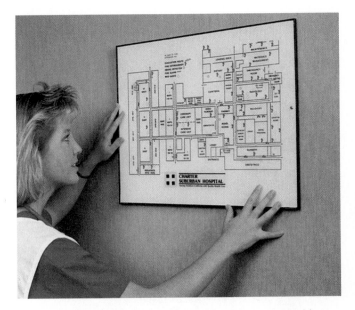

FIGURE 5–2 Know your quickest route to exit the building.

carelessly discarded match or cigarette ash dropping onto furniture or being discarded into a trash container. Some facilities provide floor model ashtrays just outside their entrance for disposal of smoking materials. If the ashtrays contain sand in which materials can be placed, they are relatively safe. However, types with metal tops that open

can be an ideal place for a fire to start because people tend to use the ashtray as a receptacle for their trash. Any regular ashtray may contain smoldering, smoking materials that are best emptied into a toilet and flushed rather than into a wastebasket, which could later burst into flame.

Fires can also be started by other causes. A defective outlet or frayed wires on any electrical appliance or office equipment could short out and start a fire. Coffee pots and water sterilizers can also boil dry and cause a fire. It is a good policy to unplug all electrical appliances whenever the office is closed.

The office should have an established policy regarding the procedure to follow in case of fire. There should be a planned route of escape prominently posted (Figure 5–2). All patients and office staff must be **evacuated** from the building, and the fire department must be notified. Exit signs should be clearly posted. All stairways and hallways should be free from clutter to allow quick, safe passage. When appropriate, knowing the location of the fire **extinguisher** and using it properly could prevent a fire from spreading. This knowledge should be everyone's responsibility (Figure 5–3).

Natural Disasters

A severe weather warning is another event that requires an established policy on what to do in case it comes up.

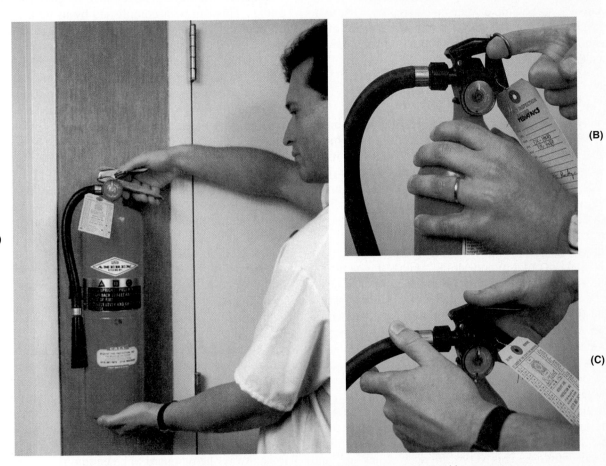

FIGURE 5–3 A, B, and C Know the location of the fire extinguisher and how to use it.

Natural disasters such as strong electrical storms and tornados are unpredictable and can claim lives if necessary steps are not taken. In these instances, people must remain inside and take shelter in the pre-determined safest area. In areas where there is danger from earthquakes, it is wise to stand in doorframes or beneath a sturdy structure. It may be dangerous to go outside where you could be struck by falling trees and buildings or come into contact with downed power lines. Yet, remaining in a multistory building may not be the safest policy, either. People living in high risk areas generally know the appropriate action to take.

Electrical power is sometimes disrupted during such an **emergency**. Never use an elevator during a threatening situation because the power could go off, trapping everyone inside until power is restored or they are rescued. Large medical facilities may have electrical generators to provide emergency lighting during emergency situations. Battery-powered lights should always be available and accessible.

Routine fire and weather drills prepare people psychologically to act in a safe and responsible manner. A practical time to review drill procedures is at a staff meeting or during new employee orientation. Those who are prepared have a greater chance of surviving a crisis than those who do not know what to do or how to act. Keeping calm and confident in times of emergency helps to reduce panic and **irrational** behavior in oneself and others. It is not practical to decide at the time of such an emergency what to do with the patients and the staff. Each member of the office team should be assigned specific duties and know how to carry them out safely and efficiently.

Spills and Dropped Objects

It is very important to clean up spilled liquids immediately. When the spill involves bodily fluids such as blood or urine, universal precautions must be observed by using gloves and placing materials in a **biohazardous** bag (Figure 5–4). The area must be thoroughly cleaned with an effective disinfectant or a 10% solution of household bleach. The used paper towels or cloths should also be discarded into the hazardous waste container.

Objects dropped on the floor must also be picked up immediately in order to prevent falls. Glass fragments are best picked up using a brush or broom and dust pan. Glass must be discarded in such a way that it will not puncture the plastic bag liner of the waste receptacle—this could accidentally cut someone's hands when it is removed. Fragments could be carefully wrapped in layers of newspaper or placed inside empty cardboard or plastic containers before being deposited into the receptacle.

Another substance that is present in a physician's office is mercury. This hazardous material is found in glass thermometers and blood pressure monitors. If either piece of equipment is broken, mercury will be released and require safe removal. It is very difficult to "pick up" and

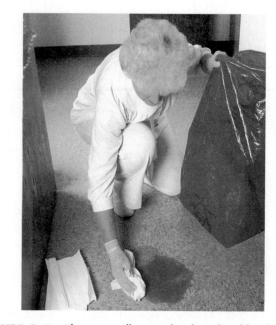

FIGURE 5–4   Clean up spills immediately. When blood or other body fluids are involved, universal precautions must be observed.

must not be touched with the bare hand. Mercury is a liquid metal, but it has unusual properties. When it is touched, it scatters into small individual "balls". These fragments of liquid can be rejoined by gathering them together. This can be accomplished by using a 3 × 5 card and pushing the segments together into a larger drop. By using two cards, the mercury can be "scooped" by one card onto the other one and dropped into the hazardous waste disposal bag along with the fragments of glass. Care must be taken to not drop the mercury from the card, for should it drop to the floor, it would scatter for several feet and make cleanup very difficult.

Emergency Phone Numbers

A list of emergency phone numbers should be posted by the phone for quick access. Such numbers may include but are not limited to: police, fire department, emergency service, poison control center, building security, utility companies, hospital emergency room, and a hospital admissions office. When an urgent situation arises, you don't want to have to search for phone numbers.

Safety Items

The installation of handrails in hallways and bathrooms within the office assists elderly patients and weak or motor impaired people in moving throughout the office with greater stability and less chance of falling. Be certain the floors are clear from any materials and that carpets are smooth and secured—loose rugs are very dangerous, especially over tile or vinyl flooring. The medical assistant must always be on guard to be certain no one falls.

Personal Safety

All health care workers must practice standard precautions to protect themselves against acquiring HIV, hepatitis B, or other infectious diseases. **CAUTION:** All patients should be considered infected because medical history and examination cannot reliably identify all patients infected with HIV or other blood-borne pathogens. Protection involves the use of appropriate **barrier** precautions to prevent skin and mucous membrane exposure when there is contact with blood or other body fluids of any patient. This means the appropriate use of gloves, face shields, masks, protective eyewear, and aprons and gowns as needed. Persons likely to be in an emergency situation also need to make use of mouthpieces, **ventilation** bags, and other ventilating devices in order to avoid direct contact with saliva or possible blood due to an injury. Precautions are identified later in this text as they become necessary within procedures. Look for the glove icon at the top of a procedure instruction.

SECURITY IN THE MEDICAL OFFICE

The increased incidences of crime makes security a prime concern. A criminal may think a physician's office has cash from daily receipts or from people in the office, such as employees or patients, and decide to commit a robbery. There is also the concept that large amounts of drugs are kept on site and could be easily attained. Unfortunately, sexual **assault** can also occur when the interior office is accessible from the reception area. In order to provide a degree of **security**, police recommend that doors between these areas be equipped with snap locks to prevent unwanted entry. Also, any opening between the two areas, such as a window, should be covered with a grill if it is possible to climb through it. (This author knows of an incident when an intruder crawled through the reception room window and assaulted a nurse who was working alone in an office.) If there are private entry doors, be certain they are kept locked at all times. If you must enter or leave the office after dark, be especially alert. The outside

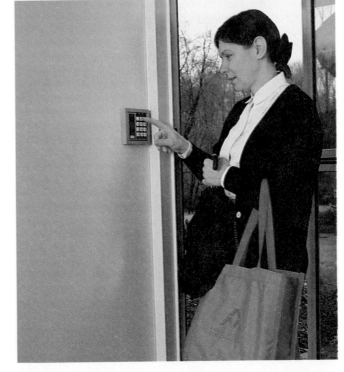

FIGURE 5-5   Enter the security code before opening the door.

area should be well lit. If building security people are available, ask for an escort.

Many offices today are equipped with electronic security systems. If you are the first staff member to arrive at work, it will be necessary to enter the code before opening the door or enter the code on an internal key pad before the entrance delay expires (Figure 5–5). Both these systems lend a feeling of safety and security, but be aware, it only takes a few seconds for someone to grab your purse or force you to hand over office money or drugs. Never enter the office if there is evidence of forced entry or if it appears that someone might either be inside or has been inside. Leave and call building security or the police at once.

▮ ACHIEVE UNIT OBJECTIVES

Complete Chapter 5, Unit 1, in the workbook to help you obtain competency of this subject matter.

UNIT 2

Efficient Office Design

▮ OBJECTIVES

Upon completion of the unit, meet the following performance objectives by verifying knowledge of the facts and

---

A CAAHEP CONNECTION

Asepsis and *Infection control* are important to your safety as well as that of your coworkers and patients. Knowledge of legal guidelines and requirements for health care providers are essential components in the curriculum for medical assistants. This unit discusses the government agencies involved in health care legislation and the day-to-day safety considerations in a medical office environment.

principles presented through oral and written communication at a level deemed competent.

1. Spell and define, using the glossary in the back of this text, all the **Words to Know** in this unit.
2. Explain what an efficient office design is and why it is important.
3. Describe the Americans with Disabilities Act of 1990 in regard to a public facility.
4. Design an office setting that includes provisions for those with physical disabilities.
5. In a facility that was not originally designed to provide for persons with a disability, describe the steps that should be taken to remedy this situation.
6. List ways for dealing with disabled persons effectively and considerately.
7. Explain where to obtain information for persons who have a disability.

AREAS OF COMPETENCE (AAMA)

This unit addresses content within the specific competency areas of *Professionalism* and *Communication skills*, as identified in the Medical Assistant Role Delineation Study. Refer to Appendix A for a detailed listing of the areas.

■ WORDS TO KNOW

anticipation	handicap
Braille system	implementation
communicable diseases	insomnia
contamination	mandate
cultivate	pantomime
design	protocol
disability	signer
feasible	triage area

In a medical facility where patients are treated for sickness, disorders, injuries, and a variety of illnesses, safety and well-being should always be the primary concern. In providing care for those who come in and out of the office daily, many things must be considered, including the design of the facility. Quality care begins long before patients come in for appointments to see the physician. Each medical facility is the result of long hours of planning and **anticipating** the needs of all who frequent the premises.

DESIGNING THE MEDICAL FACILITY TO ACCOMMODATE PEOPLE WITH DISABILITIES

The original blueprint of the facility contains the basic floor plan. Several considerations are necessary when designing a blueprint so that the basic floor plan is **feasible** and can accomodate people with disabilities.

The Americans with Disabilities Act

According to the Americans with Disabilities Act (ADA) of 1990, all public facilities must be accessible to all persons with physical **disabilities/handicaps**.

All offices, clinics, medical centers, and the like constructed before 1990, that were not already **designed** to accommodate persons with physical disabilities, had to be updated to comply with this federal **mandate**. The mandate stated that these public facilities must be adapted so that persons with disabilities and those in wheelchairs could easily and safely:

Enter and exit buildings.
Reach door handles to open and close doors.
Travel from floor to floor (elevators are a must for buildings that have more than one floor).
Proceed through hallways and doorways.
Use phones, drinking fountains, and restrooms.
Do all else that the general population is free to do in public places.

So that people with disabilities can enter any public facility, every facility must be altered, if not already designed to accommodate all persons. Ramps must be permanent so that those in wheelchairs can have access to buildings without assistance.

Provisions must be included for disabled persons regarding reception area, examination and treatment rooms, and all other areas including workstations and restrooms. Office equipment and furniture must be arranged with consideration for receiving people with disabilities. There should be a wide enough path through the reception area and in exam rooms for a wheelchair or walker so that a patient won't feel awkward. Those architectural barriers which prevent people with disabilities from entering public facilities must be eliminated according to many state and federal laws. It is wise to check the regulations governing this matter in your area.

Accommodating the Needs of Hearing- and Vision-Impaired Patients

For persons with hearing and vision impairment, accommodations must also be made. The **Braille system** must be provided for people who are blind to give them instructions and information for directions and identification of their whereabouts. If this is not possible, office staff must escort the person to and from the facility and give appropriate instructions verbally to assist them in getting around safely.

Those who are hearing-impaired need to have a **signer** (sign language interpreter) available to communicate their needs, or else they must face the person speaking so that they can read the speaker's lips. When speaking to a hearing-impaired patient, stand in the light so that the person reading your lips can see well enough without straining. There should not be anything in your mouth, such as gum or food, when speaking. Taking it a little slower than a normal conversation may also be helpful for the person. Using gestures and **pantomime** can be of great assistance, too. Remember that when you speak to a person who is hearing-impaired (deaf), speaking in a very loud voice will not help the person to hear you. Speak in a normal tone and face the person so that the person can see you as you talk as naturally as possible. Body language and appearance are additionally important. It should be noted that one should talk directly to the person who is deaf rather than to the interpreter, just as one should speak directly to *anyone* with a disability and not just to the person(s) accompanying them. It is appropriate to ask questions necessary for adequate health care, but personal questions are inappropriate. Employees with disabilities must also be considered with the same respect and attention.

NOTE: When talking to patients, regardless of the disability, it is important to be aware of your physical presence in relation to theirs. When talking to someone who is confined to a wheelchair for any length of time, it is considerate to sit so that your eye level is the same as the person in the wheelchair, so the person does not have to keep looking up to hold a conversation with you. (This position, as you can imagine, would be quite uncomfortable for a prolonged period of time.)

PLANNING THE LAYOUT OF A GENERAL PRACTICE

The reception area should have comfortable but supportive seating that is comfortably spaced for both individuals and groups. For a general practice, the area where patients are received should accommodate all ages and help them to feel at ease. Most offices supply children with safe plastic toys that should be washed after each use. Soft colors which are warm and simplistic are the most appealing decor. Proper ventilation and moderate temperature are necessary for comfort. Lighting should be varied for those who wish to sit quietly as well as for those who would like to read while they wait for their appointments. Background music that is instrumental is most appropriate. Soft music soothes the soul and helps one to relax. Reading material for all ages should be available in the reception area for patients waiting to see the physician.

Many offices have a television in the reception area that is turned to a learning/health channel or that is playing patient-educational videos. The sound should be clear and audible but not excessively loud. The television's position in the room should be elevated and in a corner area away from the traffic pattern. Figure 5–6 is an example of a layout for a general practice clinic. Notice the traffic flow from entrance to exit as a patient travels through the entire facility. Specific assistance should be provided for patients with particular needs (Figure 5–7).

Using this design as a reference, follow the traffic flow of office staff, patients, and others who visit the facility. Efficient office design allows for the traffic pattern to flow without retracing steps to eliminate unnecessary walking for the employees and others alike. It also yields to the patient a feeling of expediently advancing through the facility. A well-planned layout allows people to enter the facility and proceed with whatever may be necessary; therefore, time seems to pass more quickly. Often, patients feel as though they are in a medical facility for a lot longer than they really are—waiting to see the physician or for results of a test can seem like forever. When patients are detained in the facility either before or after their examination with the physician because of a temporary back-up in the schedule, they especially appreciate having their needs met in an orderly fashion: being called into the **triage area**, progressing to an exam room, having lab tests performed, having preliminary exam/health history information taken, receiving treatment/medication, receiving patient education provided, etc. If attention is given to the patient to make the time seem to go faster for them, then the patient is more likely to be satisfied.

Facility layout has a lot to do with how work patterns flow. If a medical facility has no available waiting area for very ill patients and everyone—sick and healthy—must stay together in the reception area, it makes for an uncomfortable situation. All patients waiting for appointments are placed at risk for possible **contamination** of **communicable diseases**. However, if the facility has an interior reception area for those who are very ill, the sick patient can be removed from the general reception area as soon as they arrive. The ideal design would have a central reception area with access through two doors: one for well and ambulatory patients, and another (wheelchair width) that opens automatically for those who are very ill. With this design, the contagious and more acutely ill patients would not come in contact with those who are not really ill (those for checkups, rechecks, etc.); the healthy patients could then avoid coming into contact with an illness during their well visit.

Of course, a medical facility does not have to be huge with many rooms to be efficient. Efficiency has to do with many points. The management of the schedule is a vital part of a practice. Scheduling will be discussed at length in Chapter 6. What is important to keep in mind is the relationship between office design layout and schedule and how they affect each other. Understanding the flow process is essential in efficient use of time and space. Once the staff realizes this fact and makes the proper adjustments, **implementation** of efficiency practices is possible.

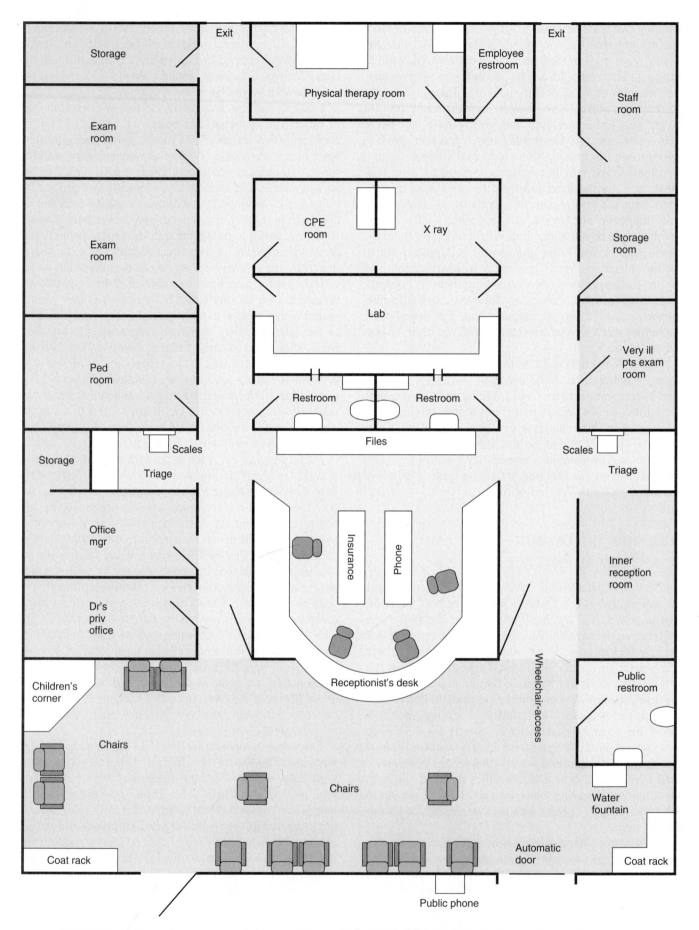

FIGURE 5–6 Trace the steps through this general practice facility to follow the efficient design of caring for patients.

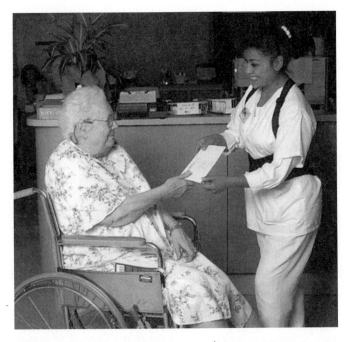

FIGURE 5-7 Many patients may need some assistance in getting around the facility carefully.

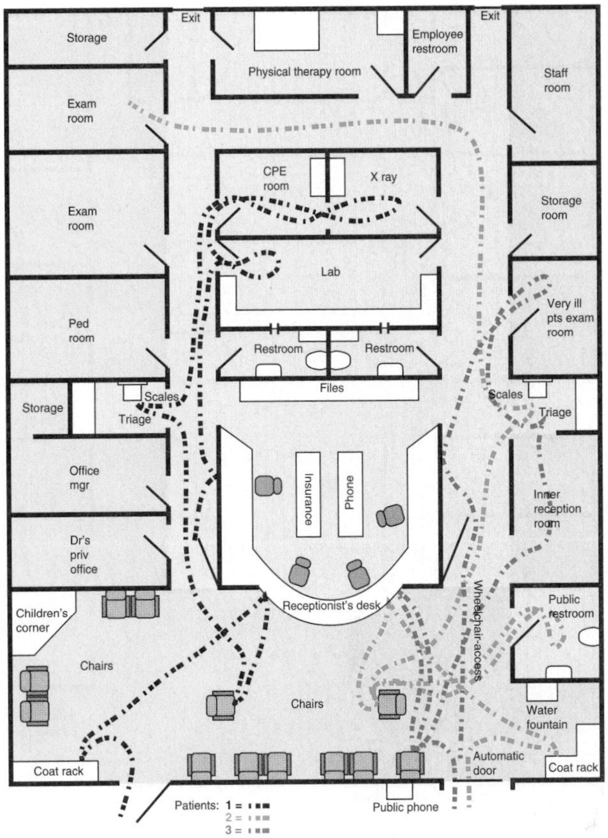

A General Practice Scenario

Follow Figures 5–8, 5–9, 5–10, and 5–11 as you read the following scenario to see how these factors can work together for optimum efficiency. This example shows small numbers, representing patients and office staff, from the point of entry throughout their completed office visit.

The physician and one part-time and three full-time staff members are beginning their day of providing health care to patients in a general practice facility. To prevent bumping into others when walking in the hallways, it is a standard practice to keep to the right just as you do in automobile traffic in the United States. If this is an understood policy among staff members, the patients will follow it also, and the traffic pattern will flow in an orderly fashion.

Patient #1, who is scheduled for a complete physical examination, enters the general reception area, places belongings on the coatrack, reports to the receptionist's desk, and takes a seat in the reception area (Figure 5-8).

Patient #2 enters shortly thereafter and does the same as patient #1. Patient #1 is called in to the clinical area and is escorted by a clinical medical assistant (A-1) to the triage area where a health history is taken. While this is taking place, patient #2 waits a few more minutes, uses the restroom, and returns to the reception area. Patient #1 is then shown to the complete physical exam (CPE) room and prepared to see the physician.

Patient #3 is a sick child with a high fever and rash who is brought into the reception area and placed in a chair near the door while the parent reports their arrival to the receptionist. The clinical medical assistant A-1 is alerted by the receptionist and calls patient #3 into the inner reception area. Triage and assessment are completed

FIGURE 5-8 Patients 1, 2, and 3 are taken to rooms for assessment and treatment as quickly as possible.

for the child and the physician is informed that the child is ready to be examined in the ill-patient exam room.

Patient #4 enters the general reception area. Patient #4 needs to have the medical assistant change a dressing on a burn. Patient #2 is taken to the clinical area for triage and assessment by clinical medical assistant A-2, where it is determined that he needs an ECG for follow-up care of a hospitalization for a heart attack that occurred a few weeks earlier. The physician reads the ECG and discusses the results with the patient. He makes an appointment for a re-check in four weeks and leaves the office.

The part-time medical assistant arrives at the rear entrance, clocks in, and puts her belongings in the staff room. She then proceeds to the receptionist's desk to assess the patient flow and begins her duties of preparing patients. She calls patient #4 into the second exam room on the left. The doctor checks the progress of the burn, the MA dresses it, and the patient leaves the office after making another appointment and a payment on the account.

Patient #5 enters the general reception area, reports to the receptionist that she is here for a re-check of her medications for diabetes and hypertension, and sits down in the reception area.

Patient #6 enters the general reception area coughing, sneezing, and feverish. The physician is called to see this sick patient. He is treated and leaves the office.

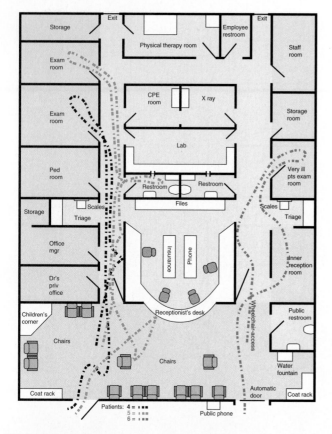

FIGURE 5–9   Patients 4, 5, and 6 are taken to rooms to be treated for their needs.

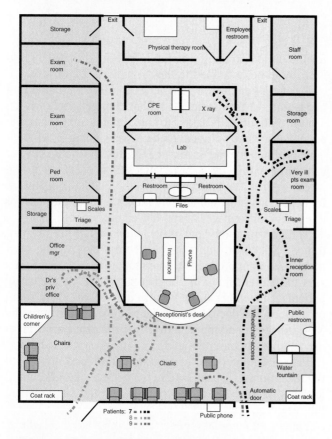

FIGURE 5–10   Patients 7, 8, and 9 are prepared for an examination by the physician.

Patient #4 is escorted back to the treatment room for a dressing change. (See Figure 5–9.) The physician examined and treated the sick child first, then examined patient #1 and ordered an ECG, chest x-ray and lab tests. Following these procedures, patient #1 stopped at the receptionist's desk and made a return visit appointment before leaving. The parent of the sick child took care of the charges incurred by the child's visit, made a re-check appointment for the following week, and exited through the same door they had entered. (The child was only in the far end of the general reception room and the inner reception room for a very brief period. The parent was able to leave the child in the exam room with one of the medical assistants for a short time while the business was handled and then the child was taken home.)

Then enters adolescent patient #7 with a knee injury. The receptionist sees her across the room and reports her arrival to clinical medical assistant A-2, who calls her in through the door near the water fountain. She helps patient #7 to the inner reception area to await the physician's exam for a possible x-ray of the knee. The doctor examines the patient, orders an x-ray, and the patient is treated and leaves the office, following a stop at the receptionist's desk for a return appointment in two weeks.

Patient #5 has a glucose test and is checked by the doctor after weight and blood pressure are measured. She stops at the desk to pay her bill, makes another appointment, and leaves the office.

Patient #8, who has had problems with stress and **insomnia**, enters and speaks to the receptionist. The MA takes her to the physician's office for a consultation appointment. Another appointment is made at the receptionist's desk before patient #8 leaves.

Patient #9 arrives, sits, and is silent. The receptionist greets the patient, calls him to the desk and asks quietly what he is to see the doctor for today. The receptionist is told that he has been having headaches and made the appointment with the physician over the phone the night before. (See Figure 5–10.) This patient is escorted to the last room on the left for an examination. The doctor refers him to a neurologist, and the patient stops at the desk for the appointment to be made by the receptionist.

Child patient #10 enters and reports at the reception desk that she is here for her allergy shot. The clinical medical assistant A-1 is notified. The child is brought in for the injection and requested to wait 20 minutes for observation. At the end of the time period, there are no problems noted and the patient leaves the office.

Patient #11 enters the waiting room and reports directly to the receptionist, complaining of nausea. Clinical medical assistant A-2 is notified immediately and calls the patient into the inner reception area through the door near the water fountain. The restroom is directly across from the reception area for the patients' convenience and comfort. The doctor sees this patient and then leaves.

Patient #12 enters the reception area and reports to the receptionist. The patient has a badly burned hand sustained at work the previous evening. The receptionist

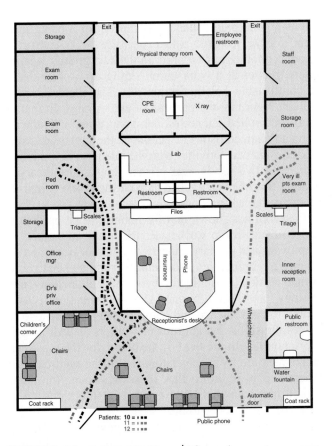

FIGURE 5–11 Patients 10, 11, and 12 are given necessary care.

calls the patient to the desk and begins obtaining information regarding the injury. Clinical medical assistant A-1 takes the patient to the exam/treatment room. (See Figure 5–11.)

This process continues daily, until all patients are examined and treated and the business is settled.

As you follow the number patterns on the floor of the layout of the facility, you can see that most of the steps taken by both the patients and the staff are minimal. This is, of course, the goal of the design for maximum efficiency. Infection control is more easily attained by keeping those who may be contagious in basically one area of the office. Necessary equipment and supplies should be within a few steps of where they will be used. Anticipation of needed supplies is an art and skill that needs to be **cultivated** by those who prepare patients to see the physician. This is most beneficial to the physician and the patient because it saves time and reduces stress for both parties. Knowing what is or might be necessary for a patient *before* the physician sees the patient is the most efficient way to handle traffic flow. Sometimes, of course, this is not possible. Also, the office policy and **protocol** of the facility will certainly be a factor in whether procedures are performed or not.

Additionally, financial coverage of medical care must be a consideration. Many procedures must be preauthorized for payment. Seeing as many patients as possible in a day will bring in the greatest amount of revenue. If the day's

patient flow of the schedule gets backed up too often, it can result in a decline in the return of patients to the medical facility. Even though it is not the most pleasant thought, the consideration that medical practice is a business is a reality. Time is money, and patients in volume bring financial success to the office. When the flow of traffic goes well, so does the workforce that contributes to this success. The old saying "in one door and out another brings more company" is a good thing in this arena. An efficient way to design patient/staff traffic flow follows: The patient is received in the reception area, enters an exam room for treatment, stops at the appointment desk, settles payment, and then exits.

As you continue to learn about medical assisting, you will be able to understand the effects of design layout in relation to patient care and how it personally affects your work. As you progress in your career, you will appreciate being efficient in the steps you walk through each day. In Unit 3 of this chapter, ergonomics will be discussed. This topic is important because it will help you to realize the importance of the work environment in relation to yourself.

ACHIEVE UNIT OBJECTIVES

Complete Chapter 5, Unit 2, in the workbook to help you obtain competency of this subject matter.

UNIT 3
Ergonomics in the Medical Office

OBJECTIVES

Upon completion of the unit, meet the following performance objectives by verifying knowledge of the facts and principles presented through oral and written communication at a level deemed competent.

1. Spell and define, using the glossary in the back of the text, all the **Words to Know** in this unit.
2. Explain ergonomics as it relates to the medical office.

3. Explain the reasons for and the importance of including ergonomics in planning for any facility.
4. List the main concerns for employment sites regarding ergonomics.
5. Describe the use of light and color in regard to the medical office.
6. List ways to prevent problems related to repeated use of computers and video display terminals (VDTs).
7. Explain the importance of adjustable components at a workstation.
8. Describe the relation between proper back support and posture.
9. Explain the importance of noise control.

WORDS TO KNOW

aesthetic
amenity
carpal tunnel syndrome (CTS)
controversial
cumulative trauma disorder (CTD)
discipline
emergency medical service (EMS)

ergonomics
evoke
glare screen
mandate
ocular accommodation
precise
renovate
video display terminal (VTD)

AREAS OF COMPETENCE (AAMA)

This unit addresses content within the specific competency areas of **Patient care, Legal concepts,** and **Operational functions**, as identified in the Medical Assistant Role Delineation Study. Refer to Appendix A for a detailed listing of the areas.

THE SCIENCE OF ERGONOMICS

During the 1990s, **ergonomics** came to the forefront of the workplace, even though this science has been around for over 50 years. Its origin was during World War II when attention to the success of pilots was vital to the outcome of the war. In order to make the duties of the pilots as effective as possible, a team of designers and planners were called upon to determine the detailed changes that had to be made to make the pilot's job easier and more **precise** and therefore improve performance.

This scientific **discipline** continues to advance and is becoming highly technical regarding the well-being, safety, and productivity of employees. A 1994 poster from the Division of Safety & Hygiene in cooperation with the Society of Ohio Safety Engineers states, **"Make Sure that Your Job Fits You . . . Ergonomics is the Answer."** The picture that goes along with this statement shows a male blue-collar worker in uniform being measured for the job with a tape measure by a seamstress. There is another male worker in the background wearing safety glasses at a workstation sitting on a chair that is of comfortable height for his job. The picture **evokes** thought regarding the purpose of ergonomics. Ergonomics is the applied science of being concerned with the nature and characteristics of people as they relate to workplace design and activities with the intention of producing more effective results and greater safety. In industry in general this science applies to both the workers and the products that are produced.

Research has shown that for humans to be productive and efficient in the workplace, the health and safety of employees is a primary concern. In another definition the science of ergonomics also includes study and analysis of human work as it is affected by individual anatomy, psychology, and other human factors. Attention is also geared to convenience and comfort. This science also includes the skills and abilities of workers as well as their shortcomings. In the field of medicine, for the most part, employees are by nature interested in the well-being of others. So it is fitting that those who care for others should first have their own health and safety ensured as they provide services to others.

All of us require the same basic physical needs: oxygen, food, water, and protection. As you will study, these basic needs must be met before other needs and desires can be realized. These basics satisfy our human needs and make it possible for us to share feelings and care for ourselves and others.

THE ERGONOMIC DESIGN OF A MEDICAL FACILITY

Often, the inefficiency of the staff lies in the design of the facility. If the planners were not aware of the nature of the business that was to take place there, the problem may never be completely solved. Some medical practices are moved into an office space where another type of business totally unrelated to medicine previously resided. Valiant attempts are made to **renovate** the facility to accommodate a productive practice. However, many spaces are just not easily adapted and do not accommodate the practice of medicine efficiently. Sometimes the answer may be to bring in an efficiency consultant who will observe for a day or longer (depending on how complex the problem seems to be) in order to determine what needs to be done. An outsider is always more objective and will see more readily any trouble areas that need attention. A medical facility that has a goal of treating ambulatory patients must have an efficient traffic pattern so that there is only a minimal waiting time for each patient. Another consideration is that the office must be easily accessible to all persons who may visit (Figure 5–12).

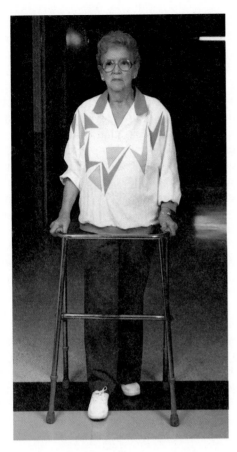

FIGURE 5–12 This photo shows a patient using a walker.

CONSIDERATIONS IN MEDICAL FACILITY LAYOUT AND DESIGN

Among the many considerations that need to be studied for an ergonomically sound workplace are:

- original floor plan or blueprint; layout
- connecting hallways/walkways
- actual room space
- environmental factors
- lighting
- acoustics
- decor
- children's area
- adaptability
- psychological/human factors

This includes a vast array of considerations, of which discussion follows.

Layout

Since the layout of a facility is the basis for the list of complex considerations, its importance cannot be overstated. The layout determines the available space and traffic pattern. Most people—medical personnel in this instance—seem to adapt to just about any situation. Even though space *does* limit work in some ways, there is flexibility with employees. They do the best they can with what they are given and establish a comfortable routine.

Hallways and Walkways

In any public facility, access for the physically challenged in entering and exiting the premises is a federal mandate. The walkways from the parking lot and hallways into the office must always be clear for safe passage. Ramps for wheelchairs are required wherever necessary. Within the office, aisles must be wide enough to allow a wheelchair to clear the passage without blocking the path of others. This applies to visitors and employees alike. If there are stairways connecting floors, an elevator must be available for those who are unable to climb stairs. This applies to all patients (and employees) who have various conditions (physical limitations or medical disabilities) that would prevent them from using the stairs. Assistance animals (usually well-trained dogs) must be permitted on the premises to attend to their dependent owners.

Actual Room Space

The actual space of each room should be proportionate to the purpose of the room. In existing buildings, adaptation for the ideal in efficiency is not always possible. The reception area needs to be large enough to accommodate several people at a time. Another consideration is that of having enough room for **emergency medical service (EMS)** ambulance service personnel to transport a patient to see the physician, especially if a stretcher is required. Also, many offices and clinics have many physicians on staff which yields to an increase in the number of people at any given time being present in the reception area. Overcrowded rooms, especially in the medical office setting, can be harmful to those who are not seriously ill when they are exposed unnecessarily to those who are. Having access to a public rest room is a convenience as well as a necessity for patients who are ill. A drinking fountain and a public telephone are also public service **amenities**.

Environmental Factors

The room temperature of a facility is one of the most critical of all environmental factors. If it is uncomfortably hot or cold, it can affect work performance and change one's attitude drastically. Proper ventilation is also necessary, but drafts should be avoided. The use of window coverings may be necessary to keep out direct sunlight that could also cause overheating.

Another consideration to the environment is the presence of foul odors. Keeping the office clear of trash and other messes will help to control this problem. Daily cleaning and routine "in-depth cleaning" will control odors and eliminate the possibility of potential pests. In the event of an unwanted odor, a room freshener spray may be used. A citrus scent is fresh smelling and will help diminish the offensive odor quickly (avoid spraying directly at persons who are seated in the reception area). Odors may also signal a problem with overheating of equipment, chemical leaks, or other serious potential health hazards. A quick response to any such odor is critical to the health and safety of all present.

Lighting

The ideal in making a room bright is accomplished with the use of both electrical and natural lighting. Because some facilities have no windows to allow for natural light, this presents a challenge in obtaining an adequate amount of light. Fluorescent lighting is usually the choice because it is the most cost-effective, even though natural lighting is the best. In offices where it is possible, skylights are popular. This can improve mood and behavior because it gives one a feeling of openness and light. Many facilities make use of indirect lighting, lamps, and overhead lights in a variety of ways to provide light for a particular need and/or to use as an aspect of the interior decorating. The avoidance of glare is advised with all lighting as it can impair one's vision and is uncomfortable as well. Mirrors and wall hangings, in addition to wall coverings, must be included in the assessment of lighting and glare capabilities for any room. Reflections from a metallic print wallpaper can be very annoying. NOTE: A safety factor that must have constant attention is the lighting of hallways, doorways, and stairways. The facility should also call attention to all exits. Accidents can be prevented by supplying proper lighting and by regularly checking to assure this is maintained.

Light and the Computer For those who work with computers on a routine basis, a **glare screen** should be used. The monitor or **video display terminal (VDT)** should be positioned to prevent excess glare entering from windows or reflecting from interior lighting (Figure 5–13). The operator must also have eye examinations and vision screening on a regular basis to stay on top of any difficulties that may develop. A frequent exercise for computer operators is to look into the distance away from the computer to prevent **ocular accommodation** which can cause headaches and blurring of vision. Looking away from the screen should be done for at least five minutes every hour of the workday. Lubricating eye drops may also be helpful to prevent dry, itchy eyes.

To prevent conditions of **cumulative trauma disorder (CTD)** and **carpal tunnel syndrome (CTS)**, ergonomists recommend that computer operators work with a special keyboard (Figure 5–14). A wrist support built into a standard keyboard can also prevent these problems (Figure 5–15). Using a vertical document holder that is either free-standing or attached to a flexible equipment arm helps to diminish eye strain and promotes good posture

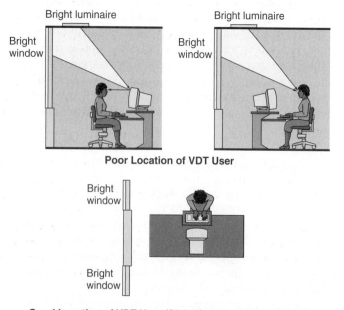

FIGURE 5-13 Proper positioning of the VDT will prevent glare from incoming light from windows and artificial lights in the room.

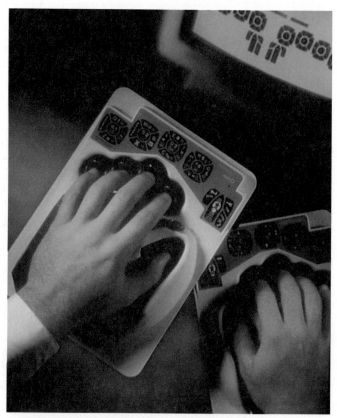

FIGURE 5-14 This keyboard is adapted to the hands for a natural position that is ergonomically correct. (Courtesy of Data Hand Systems, Inc.)

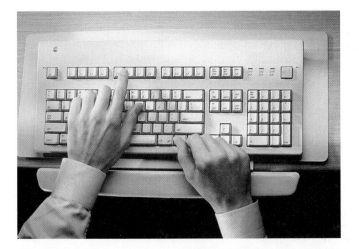

FIGURE 5–15 Keyboard with built-in wrist support (Courtesy of Steelcase, Inc.)

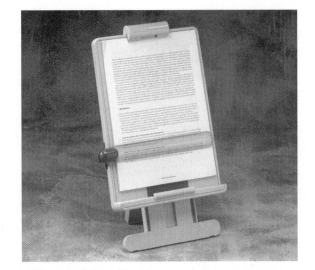

FIGURE 5–16 Vertical document holder (Courtesy of Eldon, a division of Newell Rubbermaid.)

(Figure 5–16). Those who must sit for long periods of time should stand, stretch, and move about periodically in order to relax muscles and increase circulation. Planning the workload so that there is a balance of keying, telephone communications, preparing documents, and filing will prevent slumps. This varied schedule of duties also helps to stay mentally alert.

Acoustics

Equally as important for the comfort and well-being of others is attention to the acoustics in a facility. Noise can be kept to a moderate level with the use of fabrics: furniture, carpet, drapes, and other items can absorb sound. A soft, general medley of instrumental-type music can be comforting and relaxing for employees and patients alike. Background music can help eliminate the silence that makes some people uncomfortable. It also can be a deterrent to keep patients in the reception room from listening to the receptionist's conversations on the phone and with patients or others at the window. The music selected can be varied but not too loud (under 50 to 60 decibels) because it could be offensive to some patients. Loud noise can be very stressful and can evoke a variety of emotions and possibly hearing loss if it is over 90 decibels for long periods (hours) of time. The same concerns apply to televisions in the reception area. A channel that is positive and uplifting is more acceptable to those waiting. There are some offices that use the television set in the reception area for patient education. Videos that inform patients about the latest in medical news, diet and exercise, or other valuable information can be very helpful in increasing the knowledge of those in the care of the physician. Educational videos can also be helpful in keeping those waiting from arguing over what to watch. Also, in very large medical centers, there are often decorative water fountains that produce a very favorable sound called "pink noise" from the water falling.

Decor

The decor of the facility is vitally important, as it is the first impression a person processes when entering the office. The environment should be bright and fresh to look at because this subconsciously begins to set the tone of one's attitude. Employees who are in the facility daily should have not only safe but pleasant surroundings for their well-being, too. The decor can have a psychological impact in keeping a positive outlook. In a facility where colors and lighting are dark and sparse, those employed and those who visit may experience a feeling of sadness or depression upon entering and also lose interest in activity. Where light colors are used with soft, but adequate lights, one gets a feeling of comfort and warmth from the surroundings. Everyone feels more positive and energetic in bright and colorful rooms. Use of greenery and plants (either live or artificial) give a nice touch, as do aquariums; remember, though, that they need regular care and/or replacement as necessary for **aesthetic** purposes.

Children's Area

Remember, if there is a special area for children in the reception room, it should have routine and sometimes immediate attention, especially when a sick child has been playing in the area. Particular attention needs to be given when there are little ones who tend to put everything in their mouths. You will need to pay special attention to this area to prevent disease transmission.

Adaptability

Adaptability of an office is also of critical concern. For employees to efficiently perform their duties, the facility should yield a pattern of fluid workability. This includes

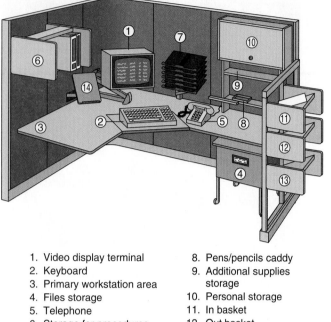

1. Video display terminal
2. Keyboard
3. Primary workstation area
4. Files storage
5. Telephone
6. Storage for procedures manuals and equipment
7. Forms caddy
8. Pens/pencils caddy
9. Additional supplies storage
10. Personal storage
11. In basket
12. Out basket
13. Additional basket
14. Document holder

FIGURE 5–17   In this workstation, all of the components can be adjusted to fit an individual's needs of safety and comfort to promote productivity.

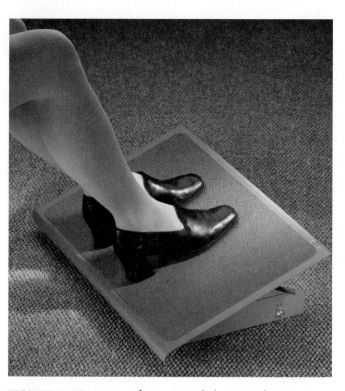

FIGURE 5–19   Using a footrest may help to avoid posture problems. (Courtesy of 3M Office Products.)

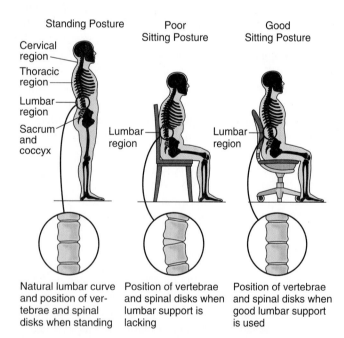

FIGURE 5–18   The illustration shows the effects of improper posture relating to back problems. Proper back support, as shown in the last picture with the back straight, will help to prevent this.

adequate space for performing all necessary functions in the most efficient way possible. Figure 5–17 provides an example of a workstation for an administrative medical assistant who has a variety of duties to perform daily.

Making each job as easy and efficient as possible for optimum use of time and space is the goal of ergonomics. For those who sit most of the day at work, proper seating is necessary in order to avoid back and other work-related conditions. Figure 5–18 shows the effects of one's posture while standing and sitting in two different types of chairs. An adjustable chair is desirable for comfort and support of the back. A footrest may also be helpful in promoting good posture (Figure 5–19).

Patients and other visitors will easily find their way around the facility if thought has been given to their needs regarding the most frequently used areas. This includes rest rooms, a drinking fountain, seating, reading materials, and so on. If those who are providing health care to patients can easily perform their duties, there is a feeling of confidence among those present. Employees who do not constantly have to backtrack and bump into others can become efficient and feel good about accomplishments. In a crowded facility where steps are repeated and someone is always in the way, levels of frustration mount quickly.

Psychological/Human Factors

With all considerations for an ergonomically sound workplace, the psychological aspect is by far the most critical. Getting along with others is the single most important factor in employability. Outlining the various areas of concern for the philosophy of ergonomics is the basis for

A CAAHEP CONNECTION

Protection of the office staff and those who come to the office is important. The use of appropriate equipment and environmental considerations makes a comfortable and safer work environment. It adds to the pleasure of the staff and therefore benefits not only them but the patients as well.

good working relationships. Having one of these areas altered can trigger a potential problem. Careful consideration to all areas is necessary for a smoothly run office and for good public relations to progress.

ACHIEVE UNIT OBJECTIVES

Complete Chapter 5, Unit 3, in the workbook to help you obtain competency of this subject matter.

UNIT 4

Preparing for the Day

OBJECTIVES

Upon completion of the unit, meet the following performance objectives by verifying knowledge of the facts and principles presented through oral and written communication at a level deemed competent, and demonstrate the specific behaviors as identified in the performance objectives of the procedures, observing safety precautions in accordance with health care standards.

1. Spell and define, using the glossary at the back of the text, all the **Words to Know** in this unit.
2. List five things to check in a reception room environment.
3. List four tasks to do before opening the office, in addition to the reception room check.
4. Explain why being the receptionist is an important position.
5. List at least five responsibilities of the receptionist.
6. Demonstrate "Open the Office" procedure.
7. Demonstrate "Obtain New Patient Information" procedure.
8. Identify five pieces of information found on a completed charge slip.
9. List four things you will find inside a new patient's chart folder.
10. List two reasons to use a "checklist."
11. Demonstrate "Close the Office" procedure.

AREAS OF COMPETENCE (AAMA)

This unit addresses content within the specific competency areas of *Administrative procedures, Practice finances, Communication skills,* and *Instruction*, as identified in the Medical Assistant Role Delineation Study. Refer to Appendix A for a detailed listing of the areas.

WORDS TO KNOW

atmosphere	environment
appointment	insurance
brochure	intervention
communication	preliminary form
confidentiality	receptionist
diversion	schedule

PREPARING FOR THE DAY

There is no set list of things to do in order to prepare for the day. Preparation procedures vary according to the type of practice, number of physicians, weekly schedules, and a lot of other variables. Some doctors may not see patients everyday. Surgeons frequently reserve a day or two a week for surgery and have office hours on the other days. Physicians who are affiliated with university schools of medicine will teach and work with medical students and may see personal patients only one or two days a week. The following content discusses general things that need to be considered when preparing to receive patients in the office.

Opening the Office

The staff should arrive at the office in time to make preparations for receiving patients. If adequate time is not available, it seems like you can never get organized or "caught up." There are several things that need attention before the first patient arrives. Procedure 5–1 "Open the Office" addresses many of these tasks.

1. *Unlock the reception room door.* This refers to the door to the outside hallway or building exterior. The door between the reception room and the interior of the office should probably be locked from the reception room side for safety reasons, as discussed in Chapter 5, Unit 1. Be certain that the lock is set on the outside door so that it does not relock itself when it is closed. Check any open/closed sign for proper reading.
2. *Observe the physical environment of the reception room.* Studies have shown that the reception room **atmosphere** can be an **intervention**, or, in other words, a "go between" or mediation to the outcome of the office visit. Atmosphere affects how people ex-

PROCEDURE

5-1 Open the Office

PURPOSE: To prepare the office to see patients.

MATERIALS: A simulated office, if available; otherwise, role-play explaining the procedure.

PERFORMANCE OBJECTIVE: Following all the steps in the procedure, role-play the actions necessary to prepare a medical office to see patients. Actions must be verbally described while performing.

1. Unlock the reception room door.

2. Adjust heat or air conditioning for the comfort of the patients.

3. Check for safety hazards in the office. **Note: Check for frayed electric wires, damaged furniture, objects on the carpet which might cause patients to fall.**

4. Check magazines for condition and date. **Note: Be sure magazines are current. Torn or damaged magazines should be removed from the waiting room.**

5. Check the telephone answering device or call the answering service for any messages.

6. Pull the charts of patients to be seen. **Note: Write or stamp with today's date. Check the patient's previous visit to see if any studies were ordered. Rationale: Results must be filed in the chart before the patient is seen.**

7. Check examination rooms to be sure they are clean and stocked with supplies. **Note: This is necessary in case the physician may see a patient after office hours and may not have put things away.**

8. Fill and turn on sterilizer.

9. Prepare hazardous waste disposal containers.

10. If it is the policy of the office, prepare a list of the patients to be seen and the times of their appointments and post and/or place copies in designated areas.

---

perience their environment and may have a relationship to their response to treatment:

- *Check the temperature.* The room temperature should ensure the patient's comfort.

- *Look at the room's appearance.* The room should appear pleasant and well maintained. The arrangement of chairs can "say" secluded or sociable, which affects **communication** in the room. The presence of large plants and attractive paintings soften the office **environment**. The choice of color and lighting affects behavior. Soft colors and subdued light tend to calm the hostile person. The use of relaxing background music has become commonplace in medical and dental offices. Aquariums can provide diversion and have an enjoyable bubbling sound. Try standing in the reception room and looking around. Be conscious of the sights, sounds, and even smells you perceive. Ask yourself, "What does this office 'say' to me?" Hopefully it is a favorable response.

- *Perform a safety check.* Review "Safety in the Reception Room" in Chapter 5, Unit 1. Remember to make a daily visual check of electrical devices, furniture, floors, and lighting before any patients arrive. Care should be taken to make the whole office "accident-proof." An incident in the office can result in a patient filing a suit for alleged pain and injury. If anyone should be injured, no matter how

insignificant it may seem, the medical assistant must have the individual examined by the physician. If the patient should claim they were not injured and refuse examination, the incident must still be carefully recorded on their chart and the refusal of care noted. Some physicians may require a signed release of responsibility in order to protect against a later claim of injury.

- *Check the reading material.* Neatly arrange magazines. Make them accessible in several seating areas. Remove torn and very outdated material. Encourage the physician(s) to subscribe to a variety of reading materials appropriate to both males and females of all ages. Many physicians have a prepared **brochure** which describes their practice, discusses the office policies, and provides information regarding appointments, office hours, and other useful details. Often there is a short biographical sketch of the physician(s). The brochure should be given to all new patients and a supply placed in the reception area for anyone who may be interested. An assortment of informative health-related pamphlets may also be found in a display rack (Figure 5–20). These should be attractively arranged and restocked as needed. Copies of professional medical journals or similar technical material is not appropriate for general display.

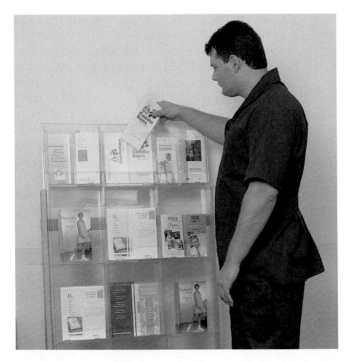

FIGURE 5-20 Office practice brochures and other handouts should be accessible to patients and visitors.

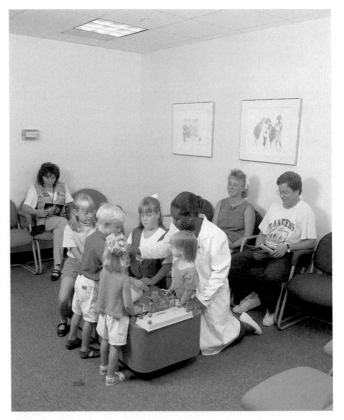

FIGURE 5-21 The medical assistant may need to entertain children while parents are in the examination room or physician's office.

■ *Check the toys and books.* If there are children's toys or books provided, they require constant monitoring. All toys should be washable and of a safe design and material with no sharp edges or parts small enough for a child to swallow. The toys should be cleaned regularly. During daily inspection, remove any broken or visibly soiled toys or books. If at all possible, the children's play area should be situated in a corner or within a half-walled space to contain things within a controlled area to reduce the possibility of adults falling over objects on the floor. In some offices, it may be necessary for the medical assistant to keep children entertained while adults are being examined (Figure 5-21). In pediatricians' offices, there are usually two reception rooms, or at least a room with a separate section, each with its own play area. One is considered the well area while the other is the "sick" area. This allows for the separation of children with fevers, coughs, nausea and vomiting, diarrhea and other disease conditions from the well children.

■ *Display the smoking policy.* In view of regulations against the use of smoking materials in a public area and the overwhelming evidence of the effects of secondhand smoke, a medical office probably does not permit smoking. Be certain the "No Smoking" sign is displayed and that it is enforced. There should be no ashtrays accessible.

3. *Retrieve telephone messages.* Retrieve and record all messages on the answering machine. If an outside service is used, call and obtain the messages.

4. *Pull charts.* Look at the appointment book or run a hard copy from the computer of all patients who have appointments that day. Pull the charts of previously seen patients. Be certain to attach reports of any previously ordered studies to the chart. Have materials ready for initiating charts for scheduled new patients. This process can often be done the night before to lessen morning preparation duties. Many offices like to post a copy of the day's **schedule** in a common area for reference. Some physicians want a list of patients and appointment times on their desk for their personal use.

5. *Inspect examination rooms.* Visually inspect all rooms for cleanliness. Even if they were cleaned when closed the previous office day, the physician may have seen a patient after–hours. Replace examining paper and be certain waste receptacles are emptied. Observe room temperature and plug in any disconnected electrical equipment. Be certain everything is in working condition. Restock supplies so that needed materials are available.

6. *Check common work areas.* Check for cleanliness and be certain everything is in order. Check the water level in the sterilizer and turn it on. Be sure hazardous waste disposal containers are available for use in all areas where needed.

THE RECEPTIONIST

A **Patient Reception Area:**
■ Greeting Patients

The medical assistant may fulfill the role of the **receptionist**, whose responsibility it is to greet and receive patients. This is a very significant role. The receptionist is usually the first person a patient encounters in the office. It is extremely important that this initial experience be very positive. Greet the patient promptly and courteously. Make an extra effort to make the patient feel at ease. (Studies have shown that a patient forms their initial impression of the office in the first four minutes of the office visit.)

The receptionist may be perceived as the doorway into the office. A pleasant tone of voice and the maintenance of eye contact is important when talking to patients. Attempt to call them by their full name (e.g., "Connie Krebs"). Listen intently to the patient's remarks and explain thoroughly any requests you make of them. Take opportunities to show that you care about their concerns and problems. Be especially careful NOT to ask questions or discuss matters that may be personal in a voice that can be heard by others in the reception room. Instead, bring the patient into the office to obtain this information. Respect your patient's right to **confidentiality**.

The receptionist must look and act professionally. Good grooming is essential. When you are neat and clean it conveys the impression of confidence and a business-like manner. Acting professionally is evident in the manner in which you deal with patients, both in the office and over the phone, with visitors, your coworkers, and your employer. It also shows when you perform your duties efficiently and effectively.

The receptionist is usually charged with answering the phone, making routine calls, and scheduling **appointments**. This responsibility requires an understanding of common diseases and disorders and the basic office operational procedures. It often demands tactful dealings with patients. The receptionist must determine when to enlist the assistance of other professionals in dealing with patients' concerns and requests.

The receptionist should be positioned within the office in such a way as to have a clear view of the reception room. If the space is within the office proper, behind a wall with a glass window partition, the reception room may not be easily seen. The area must be observed frequently to monitor the activity and to check for new arrivals who may fail to come to the window. This separated physical arrangement does have the advantage of providing privacy while engaging in a telephone conversation, talking with a patient, or performing duties.

It is important to monitor the social climate of the reception area. Be alert to any annoying behavior which may cause an unfavorable impression of the office. Some people may become involved in a conversation with another patient who eventually becomes overzealous and opinionated. The best solution to the problem is to take the offender into an examination room where he/she can wait to be seen by the physician. Children often become restless, noisy, and irritable while waiting. Occasionally, their parents do not notice the behavior or are unaware that others are being annoyed. They make no attempt to amuse the child. Unless you can tactfully suggest another toy or book as a **diversion**, it may be necessary to move this patient into an examination room as well. Remember: People are affected by their environment.

Be especially alert if a very ill patient enters the office. The ill patient should not have to sit and wait in a reception room. As soon as possible, assist the patient into an examination room where the patient can be made comfortable until the physician can see them. Remember to ensure the patient's safety. Warn the patient (and advise any companions) to be careful while lying on the narrow examination table.

Charge Slips

The receptionist may also be given the responsibility of preparing the charge slip which accompanies the patient's chart. This form is often called the routing slip or encounter form. Medical offices usually have a slip that lists the procedures, with the respective codes, which are performed in the office. The charge slip has a space for the patient's name and date and may request additional information. Some large clinics prepare "charge cards" which are used to stamp the patient's name and account number on the charge slip. When the physician completes the examination or treatment, the charges are entered on the slip and it is given to the patient with instructions to take it to a designated person on the way out of the office.

Forms will vary from one type of practice to another. Where computers are used, the form will be designed to be compatible with the software program being used. Figure 5–22 is an example of a computerized charge slip specially designed for a medical practice. This form will probably be preprinted with the patient identification information that is stored in the computer.

New Patients

The receptionist is usually responsible for the completion of the new-patient information form (Figure 5–23). If this is to be done in an interview format, be sure that others cannot overhear the questioning process. Usually, a new patient is given the form and a clipboard and requested to complete the information. A pen or pencil should be provided. It is important to give clear instructions and ask if there are any questions. Be observant. If the patient seems reluctant to accept the form, appears confused, or is not making progress, they may have a reading problem. Quickly offer to assist. Check to be sure this **preliminary form** is complete and signed by the responsible party.

At this time, it is normally routine to request **insurance** cards from the patient so that they may be copied, on both sides, for the necessary billing information. If necessary, verification of coverage can be obtained by phoning the in-

PATIENT INFORMATION							

PATIENT'S LAST NAME | **FIRST** | **INITIAL** | **BIRTHDATE** | **SEX** ☐ MALE ☐ FEMALE | **TODAY'S DATE**

ADDRESS | **CITY** | **STATE** | **ZIP** | **RELATIONSHIP TO SUBSCRIBER** | **INJURY DATE**

SUBSCRIBER OR POLICYHOLDER | **INSURANCE CARRIER**

ADDRESS | **CITY** | **STATE** | **ZIP** | **INS. I.D.** | **COVERAGE CODE** | **GROUP**

ASSIGNMENT AND RELEASE: I HEREBY AUTHORIZE MY INSURANCE BENEFITS TO BE PAID DIRECTLY TO THE UNDERSIGNED PHYSICIAN. I AM FINANCIALLY RESPONSIBLE FOR NON-COVERED SERVICES. I ALSO AUTHORIZE THE PHYSICIAN TO RELEASE ANY INFORMATION REQUIRED.

IDENTIFY
OTHER HEALTH COVERAGE ☐ YES ☐ NO
DISABILITY RELATED TO: ☐ ACCIDENT ☐ INDUSTRIAL ☐ ILLNESS ☐ OTHER
DATE SYMPTOMS APPEARED, INCEPTION OF PREGNANCY, OR ACCIDENT OCCURRED:

SIGNED _____ Date _____
(PATIENT, OR PARENT, IF MINOR)

✓	DESCRIPTION	CPT/MD	FEE	✓	DESCRIPTION	CPT/MD	FEE	✓	DESCRIPTION	CPT/MD	FEE
	OFFICE VISITS	NEW PT			LABORATORY (Cont'd.)				PROCEDURES		
	Moderate Complex	99203			Wet Mount	87210			EKG 93000	93005	
	Moderate/High Comp.	99204			Pap Smear	88150			Resp. Function Test	94010	
	High Complexity	99205			Handling	99000			Ear Lavage	69210	
	OFFICE VISITS	EST. PT			Hemoccult Stool	82270			Injection Inter. Jt.*	20605	
	Minimal	99211			Glucose	82948			Injection Major Jt.*	20610	
	Self Limited Comp.	99212			INJECTIONS				Anoscopy	46600	
	Low/Moderate Comp.	99213			Vitamin B12/B Complex	J3420			Sigmoidoscopy	45355	
	Moderate Complex	99214			ACTH	J0140			I & D*	10060	
	High Complexity	99215			Depo-Estradiol	J1000			Electrocautery*	17200	
	CONSULTATIONS	OFFICE			Depo Testosterone	J1070			Thromb Hemor.*	46320	
	Moderate Complexity	99243			Imferon	J1760			Inj. Tendon*	20550	
	Mod. to High Comp.	99244			Tetanus Toxoid	J3180					
	HOME	EST. PT			Influenza Vaccine - Flu	90724			MISCELLANEOUS		
	Moderate Complexity	99352			Pneumococcal Vaccine	90732			Drugs, Supplies, Materials	99070	
	ER				TB Tine Test	86585			Special Reports	99080	
	Moderate Severity	99283			Aminophyllin	J0280			Services After Hrs.	99050	
	High Severity	99284			Terbutaline Sulf.	J3105			Services 10pm - 8am	99052	
	LABORATORY				Demerol HCL	J0990			Services Sun. & Holidays	99054	
	Urinalysis - Complete	81000			Compazine	J0780			Counseling	99403	
	Hemoglobin	85018			Injection Therapeutic	90782					
	Culture, Strep/Monilia	87081			Estrone Susp.	J1410					

DIAGNOSIS:

☐ Allergic Rhinitis	477.9	☐ Chronic Fatigue Synd.	300.5	☐ Hemorrhoids	455.6
☐ Anemia	280.9	☐ COPD	496	☐ Hiatal Hernia	553.3
☐ Angina Pectoris	413	☐ Costochondritis	733.99	☐ Hiatal Hernia & Reflux	530.1
☐ Anxiety	300.00	☐ CVA	431	☐ HVD	402.10
☐ Aortic Stenosis	424.1	☐ Cystitis	595.9	☐ Hyperlipidemia	272.4
☐ ASCVD	429.2	☐ Deg. Disc. Disease, CX	722.4	☐ Hypoestrogenism	256.3
☐ ASHD	414.9	☐ Deg. Disc. Dis., Lumbar	722.52	☐ Hypothyroidism	244.9
☐ Asthma	493.9	☐ Depression, Endogenous	296.2	☐ Impacted Cerumen	380.4
☐ Atrial Fibrillation	427.31	☐ Dermatitis	692.9	☐ Influenza, Viral	487.1
☐ Bigeminy	427.89	☐ Diabetes Mellitus, Adult	250.0	☐ Irritable Bowel Syndrome	564.1
☐ BPH	600	☐ Diarrhea	558.9	☐ Laryngitis	464.0
☐ Bronchitis, Acute	466.1	☐ Diverticulitis	562.11	☐ Menopausal Syndrome	627.2
☐ Bronchitis, Chronic	491.9	☐ Esophagitis	530.1	☐ Mitral Insufficiency	396.2
☐ Bursitis	726	☐ Fibrocystic Breast Disease	610.11	☐ Moniliasis	112
☐ Cardiomyopathy	425.4	☐ Fissure in Ano	565.0	☐ Myocardial Infarction	410.9
☐ Carotid Artery Disease	433.1	☐ Gastroenteritis	558.9	☐ Neuritis	729.2
☐ Cerebral Vascular Disease	437.9	☐ Gout	274.9	☐ Osteoarthritis	715.9
☐ CHF	428.0	☐ HCVD	429.2	☐ Osteoporosis	733.0
☐ Cholecystitis	575.1	☐ Headache, Vascular	784.0	☐ Otitis Media	382.9
		☐ Headache, Migraine	346.9	☐ Parkinsonism	332

☐ Peripheral Vascular Dis	443.9
☐ Pharyngitis	462.0
☐ Pneumonia, Bacterial	482.9
☐ Pneumonia, Viral	480.9
☐ Prostatitis, Chronic/Acute	601
☐ Rectal Bleeding	569.3
☐ Renal Failure, Chronic	585
☐ Rheumatoid Arthritis	714.0
☐ Sinusitis	461.9
☐ Supraventr. Tachycardia	427.0
☐ T.I.A.	435.9
☐ Tachycardia	426.89
☐ Tendinitis	726.90
☐ Tonsillitis	463
☐ Ulcer Duodenal	532.9
☐ Ulcer Gastric	531.9
☐ URI	465.9
☐ UTI	599.0
☐ Vaginitis	616.10
☐ Vertigo	780.4

DIAGNOSIS: (IF NOT CHECKED ABOVE) | REF. DR. & #

DOCTOR'S SIGNATURE / DATE | **NO SERVICES PURCHASED** | SERVICE PERFORMED | ACCEPT ASSIGNMENT | TODAY'S FEE

INSTRUCTIONS TO PATIENT FOR FILING INSURANCE CLAIMS

1. MAIL THIS FORM DIRECTLY TO YOUR INSURANCE COMPANY. ATTACH YOUR OWN INSURANCE COMPANY'S FORM.

OFFICE ☐ | YES ☐ | AMT. REC'D TODAY

E.R. ☐ | NO ☐

PLEASE REMEMBER THAT PAYMENT IS YOUR OBLIGATION, REGARDLESS OF INSURANCE OR OTHER THIRD PARTY INVOLVEMENT.

HOME ☐ | TOTAL DUE

FIGURE 5–22 Charge form for a medical clinic (Courtesy of Bibbero Systems, Inc., Petaluma, CA, 800-242-2376, http://www.bibbero.com.)

PATIENT INFORMATION

DATE:

PATIENT'S NAME	MARITAL STATUS					DATE OF BIRTH	SOCIAL SECURITY NO.	
	S	M	W	DIV	SEP			

STREET ADDRESS ☐ PERMANENT ☐ TEMPORARY	CITY AND STATE		ZIP CODE	HOME PHONE NO.

PATIENT'S EMPLOYER	OCCUPATION (INDICATE IF STUDENT)	HOW LONG EMPLOYED?	BUSINESS PHONE NO.

EMPLOYER'S STREET ADDRESS	CITY AND STATE	ZIP CODE

IN CASE OF EMERGENCY CONTACT:	DRIVERS LIC. NO.

SPOUSE'S NAME

SPOUSE'S EMPLOYER	OCCUPATION (INDICATE IF STUDENT)	HOW LONG EMPLOYED?	BUSINESS PHONE NO.

EMPLOYER'S STREET ADDRESS	CITY AND STATE	ZIP CODE

WHO REFERRED YOU TO THIS PRACTICE?

IF THE PATIENT IS A MINOR OR STUDENT

MOTHER'S NAME	STREET ADDRESS, CITY, STATE AND ZIP CODE	HOME PHONE NO.

MOTHER'S EMPLOYER	OCCUPATION	HOW LONG EMPLOYED?	BUSINESS PHONE NO.

EMPLOYER'S STREET ADDRESS	CITY AND STATE	ZIP CODE

FATHER'S NAME	STREET ADDRESS, CITY, STATE AND ZIP CODE	HOME PHONE NO.

FATHER'S EMPLOYER	OCCUPATION	HOW LONG EMPLOYED?	BUSINESS PHONE NO.

EMPLOYER'S STREET ADDRESS	CITY AND STATE	ZIP CODE

INSURANCE INFORMATION

PERSON RESPONSIBLE FOR PAYMENT, IF NOT ABOVE	STREET ADDRESS, CITY, STATE AND ZIP CODE	HOME PHONE NO.

☐ COMPANY NAME & ADDRESS	NAME OF POLICYHOLDER	CERTIFICATE NO.	GROUP NO.

☐ COMPANY NAME & ADDRESS	NAME OF POLICYHOLDER	POLICY NO.

☐ COMPANY NAME & ADDRESS	NAME OF POLICYHOLDER	POLICY NO.

☐ MEDICARE	MEDICARE NO.	☐ MEDICAID	PROGRAM NO.	COUNTY NO.	ACCOUNT NO.

In order to control our cost of billing, we request that office visits be paid at the time service is rendered. We would rather control our billing costs than be forced to raise our fees.

AUTHORIZATION: I hereby authorize the physician indicated above to furnish information to insurance carriers concerning this illness/accident, and I hereby irrevocably assign to the doctor all payments for medical services rendered. I understand that I am financially responsible for all charges whether or not covered by insurance.

_____
Responsible Party Signature

FIGURE 5–23 New-patient information form (Courtesy of Bibbero Systems, Inc., Petaluma, CA, 800-242-2376, http://www.bibbero.com.)

PROCEDURE

5-2 Obtain New Patient Information

PURPOSE: To obtain initial information from a new patient.

MATERIALS: An assigned "patient," a patient initial information form, a clipboard, a pen, a mock insurance card, a charge slip, chart folder, tabs, and typewriter or computer.

PERFORMANCE OBJECTIVE: In a simulated situation, clearly communicate instructions and complete the steps in the procedure to obtain patient information and assemble all required materials.

1. Take new patient to private area to ask preliminary questions, or ask new patient to complete a data sheet. **NOTE: Give the patient a clipboard and pen and offer assistance, if needed. Ask the patient to return the form when it is completed. A medical history is a potential legal doc-**ument. Check to be sure the form is completed accurately and legibly, and signed where appropriate.

2. Prepare a patient folder by typing the patient's name on a label and attaching it to the tab of the folder.

3. Transfer information from the form to the chart sheet.

4. Copy the insurance card (both sides).

5. Insert the chart, sheets, information form, and insurance card copy in folder.

6. Prepare charge slip.

7. Place the folder in the area reserved for charts of patients to be seen. **NOTE: If you have received any referral material on a new patient, be sure to place it with the chart.**

surance company. The copy of the card and the preliminary form are placed in a folder along with chart sheets and any other referral materials received. If the filing method is numeric, the patient's name or number is typed onto a label which is attached to the tab of the folder. Before the patient is seen, the charge slip is completed and attached to the chart. The chart is then placed in a designated area until the patient is taken to an examination room. Then it is placed in a holder on the door outside the room, ready for the physician when the patient is seen. Procedure 5–2 discusses the steps in obtaining new patient information.

CLOSING THE OFFICE

At the end of the day, the examination rooms should be restocked and cleaned, and discarded material should be placed for pick-up. This saves time the next morning. Charts must be collected, checked for completeness, and filed in a locked cabinet. If there is not time to file, place charts in a separate folder of "charts to be filed" and place in the cabinet to be filed the next day. (Some doctors may dictate their notes, which must first be typed onto the chart before it can be filed.) All electrical appliances and the sterilizer must be turned off. Receipts collected during the day can be taken to the bank for deposit or locked in the office safe. If there is time, tidy the reception area and pull the next day's records. Always take a walk through the office to complete your checklist of things to do. Activate your answering system and turn off the lights. Activate the alarm system, if available, and securely lock the door. See Procedure 5–3.

ACHIEVE UNIT OBJECTIVES

Complete Chapter 5, Unit 4, in the workbook to help you achieve competency of this subject matter.

A CAAHEP CONNECTION

Entry level competency for medical assisting requires that you perform basic medical office functions to prepare the office for the day. It is also essential that you communicate effectively with new patients and make adaptations to their individualized needs as you initiate new patient records.

RELATING TO ABHES

Chapter 5 discusses safety and security in a medical office, the importance of ergonomics and an efficient design, and preparing the office for patient care. This content is related to the ABHES accreditation requirements of *Office safety and security* within the content area of **Medical Office Business Procedures/Management** and *Universal precautions in the medical office* within the content area of **Medical Laboratory Procedures.**

PROCEDURE

5-3   Close the Office

PURPOSE: To prepare the office to be closed.

MATERIALS: A simulated office, if available; otherwise, role-play explaining the procedure.

PERFORMANCE OBJECTIVE: Following all the steps in the procedure, role-play the actions required to close the office. Actions must be verbally described while performing the procedure.

1. Check to see that records are collected and filed in locked cabinets.
2. Place any money received in safe or take to the bank to be deposited.
3. Turn off all electrical appliances. **NOTE: Many offices ask that you unplug electrical appliances. Rationale: Eliminates the chance of electrical fire.**
4. Check that rooms are cleaned and supplied for the next day.
5. Straighten reception room if time allows.
6. Pull charts for the next day if time allows.
7. Activate answering device on phone or notify answering service and indicate when you will be back in the office.
8. Turn off lights.
9. **NOTE: Activate alarm system, if available.**
10. Set lock and close door.
11. Check to assure that it is locked.

Medical-Legal-Ethical Scenario

Consider the following situation: Mrs. Diaz is a young woman whose husband recently left her with two small children. Because she was married and began her family soon after graduating from high school, she has not acquired specific employable skills or gained much work experience. She is currently enrolled in a job training program but found it necessary to seek public assistance until she is able to get a good job. She is making her first visit to the physician's office and has just completed the new patient information form and given it to the receptionist.

Ms. Brown reviews the form for completeness and notices the patient is on welfare. Across the crowded reception room she calls to Mrs. Diaz, "I'll need a copy of your Medicaid card so I can bill welfare for this office visit." Mrs. Diaz feels embarrassed as she complies with the request. She wonders how many people in the room think she is just too lazy to work. Because the receptionist was so inconsiderate, she also wonders if the physician will treat her with indifference.

Fortunately, Ms. Brown was overheard by the office manager who warned her that her action was very inappropriate and that she was noting this on her performance record. She also told Ms. Brown that she should apologize to Mrs. Diaz for her thoughtlessness.

CRITICAL THINKING CHALLENGE

1. The Medical Assistant Role Delineation Study identifies behaviors that Ms. Brown has not mastered. Look in Appendix A and identify at least one statement in three different areas where she failed to meet the standard for behavior. Explain how they relate to this scenario.
2. Can you put yourself in Mrs. Diaz's place?
3. How would you feel?
4. Does a person's nationality or skin color affect how they are perceived?
5. Do you think the office manager or the patient should mention this situation to the physician so that other people are not treated the same?
6. What could be done in the office to assure that this type of situation does not occur again?

RESOURCES

American Medical Association (1995). The physician's current procedural terminology. Chicago, IL: Author.

Simmers, L. (2001). Diversified health occupations (5th ed.). Clifton Park, NY: Delmar Learning.

WEB LINKS

http://www.osha.gov **(Occupational Safety and Health Administration, United States Department of Labor)**

This web site provides information on safety and security in the workplace.

http://www.usdoj.gov/crt/ada/adahom1.htm **(ADA Home Page)**

This web site provides information on the Americans with Disabilities Act.

http://www.ctdnews.com **(CTD News)**

This web site has information on cumulative trauma disorder injuries and workplace repetitive stress injuries. It also has OSHA Ergonomics Standard Updates.

The Administrative Medical Assistant

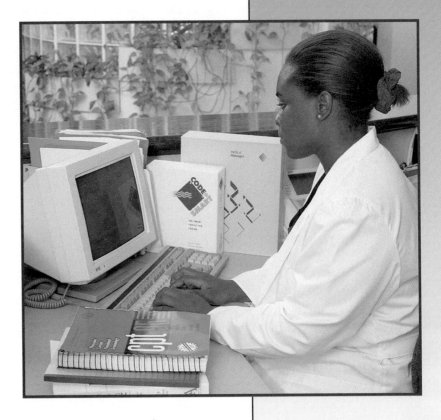

Oral and Written Communications

The office assistant must have sufficient knowledge of medical terminology to deal efficiently with the unending variety of telephone calls received daily. A pleasant voice and good listening skills are essential. Practicing patience and demonstrating compassion to those in need of such attention are important. The medical assistant needs to have legible handwriting for recording appointments and messages. Typing or keyboarding skills are necessary if appointments are to be made on a computer. The student who enjoys keyboarding or working on a computer has an opportunity to develop this skill as an administrative medical assistant. You will have an opportunity to demonstrate your knowledge of anatomy, medical terminology, spelling, grammar, and punctuation when you answer the office phone and as you complete progress notes on charts. You will use these skills also in the completion of correspondence. You may have the responsibility of processing incoming and outgoing mail. Written communication skills must be as flawless as possible. A number of people may view the letters or forms you send out and each will receive a mental picture of you and your office—good if the work is neat and correct, and definitely questionable if it is inaccurate or messy.

UNIT 1

Telephone Communications

■ OBJECTIVES

Upon completion of the unit, meet the following performance objectives by verifying knowledge of the facts and principles presented through oral and written communication at a level deemed competent, and demonstrate the specific behaviors as identified in the performance objectives of the procedures, observing safety precautions in accordance with health care standards.

1. Spell and define, using the glossary at the back of the text, all the **Words to Know** in this unit.
2. Organize desk space for efficient use of the telephone.
3. Demonstrate a professional method of holding and answering the phone.
4. Describe methods of screening incoming calls.
5. Locate information in a telephone directory.
6. Demonstrate a procedure for referring a patient to another health facility.
7. Describe the different types of phone calls that a medical assistant may have to answer in the medical office, and explain how they should be handled.

AREAS OF COMPETENCE (AAMA)

This unit addresses content within the specific competency areas of *Administrative procedures, Fundamental principles, Professionalism, Communication skills, Legal concepts, Instruction,* and *Operational functions* as identified in the Medical Assistant Role Delineation Chart. Refer to Appendix A for a detailed listing of the areas.

■ WORDS TO KNOW

bogus
colleague
confirmed
empathy
etiquette
expressed

personality
pertinent
rely
screening
verify

ANSWERING THE TELEPHONE

Ⓐ **Patient Reception Area:**
■ Telephone Skills

The telephone is the center of all activity in the medical office just as it is with any business. The professional attitude conveyed is critical to the success of the business of practicing medicine. The medical assistant who handles phone calls must be courteous, articulate, and a careful and active listener. The rapport established by the medical assistant will contribute to successful communication with patients. Most medical facilities have telephones with two or more phone lines. This means that someone should answer each line as soon as possible or at least by the third ring. It seems that on some days all lines ring continually and there is no letup. Because of this situation, an automatic answering device is available that will come on with a recording that asks the caller to please hold and explains that the call will be taken as soon as possible in order of the calls. The responsibility of responding to calls takes a great deal of maturity and patience. Over time, one develops the knowledge of what to ask and when to ask it to determine how serious a situation or condition is.

Phone Menus

Most business phone systems have a menu for the caller to be connected to the proper person or department. By pushing the correct number as directed by the recorded message (e.g., "Press one to reach the billing department, press two to speak to the scheduling department, press three for prescription refills,"), the caller can be connected to the desired party. The system is designed to be more efficient and not only keep the caller from being on hold for too long, but to help avoid being disconnected. The caller should be instructed at the beginning of the recorded message to hang up immediately and call EMS/911 (as applicable to the caller's geographic area) if there is a medical emergency. Each call should be answered as soon as possible no matter what the nature of the call is. Courteous and expedient return of a call is not only most efficient, but it promotes a positive atmosphere.

Telephone Triage

An established phone triage manual should be kept near the phone for reference so that each assistant who answers the phone will ask the same standard questions and give the same standard advice which the physician has pre-authorized. The assistant must learn how to logically proceed through a set of questions that will reveal the caller's condition and help to determine, if necessary, how soon the patient should be seen by a physician. This process is called telephone triage. If the assistant does not know how to handle a patient, or if the questions have not been addressed in the manual, referring the problem to one who is more experienced is necessary and appropriate. Never guess in response to a patient's questions and do not treat any question lightly. If there is a serious telephone emergency that cannot be handled in the facility, it is best to refer the patient to an emergency medical service (give the phone number to the person if they do not know it) and explain that they will send someone as soon as possible to help. It may be best to direct the person to an emergency room of the nearest hospital. It is a sensible practice to have all emergency phone numbers listed by each phone in the office. In stressful times, this will be helpful in giving the patient phone numbers they might need quickly or in calling an emergency service for the patient. The assistant must ask questions of coworkers and supervisors as they learn how to best deal with problems. If you are speaking to a patient face-to-face at the office and you must answer the phone, say to the patient, "Excuse me for a moment, please," answer the phone call, and then continue with what you were doing. Every emergency call must be handled immediately.

Non-emergency Calls

If the person on the phone needs additional information, or if the call is going to take a while, excuse yourself from the phone call by saying, "May I put you on hold for a moment?" However, if it will be more than one minute the caller should not be put on hold; in this case say, "May I call you back with that information?" Be sure to check the patient's phone number before hanging up because it may have changed since the patient's last appointment. Find out a good time to call back. There may be times when the patient has to wait to speak to the physician. In this case, you should check back each minute until the doctor answers to let the patient know that he has not been forgotten. During the time the caller waits, many medical facilities provide the caller with a pleasant recording with reminders of immunization updates, the services and procedures offered by the staff, when routine office hours are, what to do and whom to call in an emergency, and other relevant information. This gives the person who is waiting helpful information while the time passes. The assistant must beware of leaving callers on hold for too long. You can be sure that callers will let you know how long they had to wait and how many times they heard the entire recording.

If you need to transfer a patient's call to another department or office, first give the caller the phone number, extension number, and the person's name to whom you are transferring them in case there is a disconnection. You should signal (or page) the person and when the person answers, explain who is waiting to speak to her, and give a brief summary of what it is regarding. You may say, for example, "Excuse me, Ms. Winters. Mr. Robert James is on line three with a question about his insurance." Ms. Winters may respond with, "Yes, I can talk to him." You should then say, "Thank you, I'll transfer him now. Go ahead please, Mr. James." Then listen to make sure the call was transferred before you hang up. All of this needs to be done quickly and efficiently with a pleasant tone and a polite attitude. This process is much more polite and acceptable than yelling across the room or down the hall for another member of the staff to pick up the phone to speak to someone, or worse, asking the caller to hold while you "find" the person requested, regardless of whether the person is a patient or not. When a patient is calling for information, remember to pull the file and have it ready for the physician along with any test/lab reports that may be the reason for the call. If you have a public address system where everyone can hear the page, be very careful with confidentiality and merely say, for instance, "Dr. Smith, you have a call on line two." You may have to repeat the page if the call is not answered within one minute. Make sure you tell the caller that the person they wish to speak with has been paged and will be with them as soon as possible. If there is no way to announce a call over a loud speaker, simply use a small note to confidentially let the doctor know who is waiting to speak to him on the phone and which line the patient is on. There may be times when the physician is close to the phone; simply ask the doctor to take the call and tell him who is calling and what the call is regarding. Remember to say please, thank you, excuse me, and so on when appropriate. Establishing good communication, especially over the phone, is essential to building good rapport. It is important to make a list or a log of all phone calls and note who the person is that you should call back. You should also ask when it is best for a return call, repeat the number to ensure that you wrote the correct number down, and follow through with the request as close to the time as possible. This considerate practice should almost eliminate the frustration of playing "phone tag," which is repeatedly calling back and forth and never getting to speak to the intended party.

DOCUMENTING TELEPHONE MESSAGES

Ⓐ **Patient Reception Area:**
■ Telephone Messages

Documenting telephone messages is of vital importance and should be treated likewise. Of primary concern is the issue of confidentiality. Data regarding patients may not be given out over the telephone to anyone unless the patient has given written permission for the release of specific information with a signature. It is equally important that the date, time, a brief message regarding the call, and the initials of the person who responded to the call be recorded. Then any questions concerning a call may be further explained by the person whose initials are on the message. All calls, regardless of what you may think about their importance, should be documented in the same manner. All messages that are urgent should be given priority and handled as soon as possible to prevent further discomfort, pain, and anxiety for patients.

There are commercial answering services available that provide physicians with a practical way to handle all calls during lunch breaks, evenings, weekends, vacations, and any other time necessary. This can be a convenient service for the physician and office staff. There seems to be a greater acceptance of this type of answering assistance because the caller gets to speak to a live person instead of listening to a recording. In an emergency situation, people are more easily comforted by another human voice even if the doctor is not available. However, problems can arise with these systems because the business employing the service is unable to know all of the persons who answer the phone lines. There is the risk that someone who is not adequately trained may be too abrupt or possibly rude to a patient. Yet, keeping the human element integrated within professional boundaries is the most desirable way to build rapport when communicating with patients.

Voice mail, pagers, and other answering service devices make communications much more accessible than ever before. Answering machines are especially good to use for short time blocks such as during lunch time. If the standard in your medical office is an answering machine that records messages whenever the physician is not in the office, it should tell the caller how to contact the physician or how to leave a message. This must be done day and night, 365 days a year. Messages need to be played back and recorded as soon as possible. Then, all of the calls need to be returned in the order of their importance within an appropriate and reasonable time period. Remember to check the fax machine because messages and other patient-related information can be faxed to the office at any time. Returning phone or fax-requested patient information should also be done promptly. Confidentiality is a primary concern. All documents with information regarding patients should be kept out of reach of others who are not part of the medical office staff. Some physicians prefer to have patients call them at their home, while others employ an answering service to screen calls and take only urgent cases at home. In this instance, the one who screens the calls will contact the doctor at home (or wherever, usually by pager) and have the doctor return the patient's call.

A telephone message pad and pen should be placed by each office telephone. You cannot **rely** on memory in a busy office where there are constant interruptions. Individual offices have a variety of methods for recording telephone messages. You may use a preprinted duplicate message pad; the top sheet is removed and the carbon remains as a permanent record of calls received. The office may use a secretarial notebook that is dated each day; calls are recorded and checked off when returned. You need to develop a follow-up method to be sure calls have been returned. The call pad or messages should not be filed until the requests have been given a response. Some offices have a stamp made up to indicate in the patient chart a telephone communication and a brief note with the date the patient was contacted. It is not advisable to have loose slips of paper in the file as they are too easily lost. If it is desired to keep these in the chart, they should be filed shingle fashion on a sheet of bond paper with the latest call on top. The slips should be fastened with a piece of transparent tape horizontally across the top of the slip. A vertical piece of tape along the side prevents curling of the edges of the slip, ensuring that it is easy to read.

Self-stick telephone message forms are helpful in establishing effective control of patient calls. One form comes in a single looseleaf style with a stub (like that of a checkbook or loan payment book) which remains in a binder for future reference. Another style has a duplicate copy which remains in a spiral binder and provides a master reference for future review. When a call is received from a patient, the message form is completed. After completing the form, tear it at the perforation and attach the form to the patient's chart by removing the adhesive protection strips at each end on the back of the form. If a patient call requires a return call from the physician, the form is stuck to the front of the patient's chart and given to the physician. When the physician completes the call and records the message, the form is simply removed from the front of the chart and restuck in the proper location on the inside of the chart for future reference (Figure 6–1). Another telephone message form is a log sheet and message slip with carbon. The benefits of this system are that you do not have to rewrite the message in the patient's chart, use a telephone stamp, or be concerned about loose slips of paper falling out of the chart. The carbon copy is a permanent record of calls for reference. Examples of telephone message forms are shown in Figures 6–1 and 6–2A. Figure 6–2B illustrates the recording of a message from a patient on a chart.

The important items of a telephone message are:

- Caller's full name, spelled correctly
- Brief note indicating the nature of the call
- Action required
- Date, time of call, initials of person receiving call
- Phone number of caller; include the area code if this is a long distance call

If the telephone has a speaker phone or a headset, your hands will be free to use a pen to either write a message or use the keyboard to log in the patient's call, retrieve the

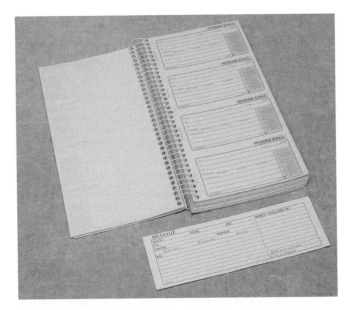

FIGURE 6–1 These telephone message forms have a carbon copy that stays intact for a permanent record of each call.

PHONE MESSAGE

For _____ Date _____ Time _____ AM/PM

Mr/Ms _____

Of _____

Phone _____ Page # _____ Fax _____

☐ Phoned   ☐ Please call—urgent
☐ Returned call   ☐ Stopped in
☐ Will call again   ☐ Wants appointment
☐ Personal   ☐ See me for message

Message

_____

_____

_____

_____

_____

_____

Call taken by _____ Date _____ Time _____

FIGURE 6–2(A)   Telephone message form

Date/time
Mr. Silvers called to let Dr. Lang know that his dentist, Dr. Edwin Blair, gave him an antibiotic, penicillin 500 mg, #32, 4x da, for 8 days, for an abscessed tooth.

FIGURE 6–2(B)   Example of recording a phone message on the patient's chart

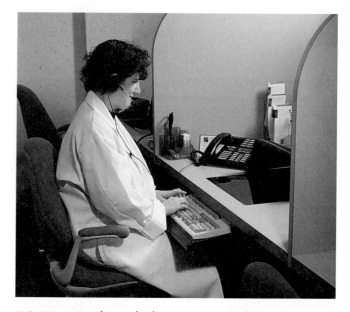

FIGURE 6–3   This medical assistant is using the headset to answer calls to free her hands to use the keyboard, take messages, open mail, and so on.

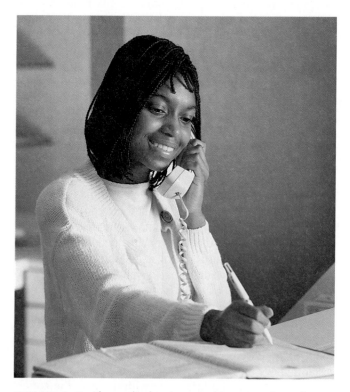

FIGURE 6–4   The medical assistant in this picture shows the proper distance in holding the phone receiver. Even though the caller cannot see this receptionist, her pleasant attitude is evident.

patient's file, or schedule an appointment. Figure 6–3 shows the medical assistant using the headset in phone conversation. The proper position of a phone with a receiver is shown in Figure 6–4. When you hold the receiver of the telephone, it should be 2 to 3 inches in front of your mouth so that the caller may clearly hear your voice. Many professional offices have cordless phones, speaker phones, or phones with long cords on the receiver part of the phone for ease in accessing files as needed. The hold button, transfer extension dialing, conference calling, and other various features may vary from office to office. You should be honest about your knowledge and experience with phone systems. You must ask to have a certain feature explained and demonstrated to you if you do not know how to use it. You must use proper technique with a telephone system or the caller may be rudely interrupted or accidentally disconnected during a call. Since you never know who is on the other end of the phone, always answer as promptly as possible in a professional manner. Emer-

gencies can happen at any time and your efficiency on the phone could affect the outcome.

The following example highlights the proper manner of a polite and efficient way to answer a call: "Good morning, Central Medical Center, Ellen speaking, how may I help you?" The caller usually is prompted to give you her name after saying hello to you and explains the reason for the call. Your response should be appropriate and spoken in a pleasant tone of voice to each caller. Make sure that you get the complete name and phone number of the patient in case your call is interrupted. This is a safe practice to follow in case the call is an emergency and you get cut off. If the information that the patient gives you is not clear, you must say, for example, "Could you please repeat that for me?" or, "Would you spell your name for me again, please?" It is better to ask someone to repeat what was said initially than to have to go back over the whole conversation and redo all of it—the patient may wonder if you paid attention to *anything* that was said. You should convey confidence rather than insecurity. If you cannot understand someone because their voice is too soft, ask them to speak a little louder. If the person talks too loud, ask if they could speak a little softer, faster, slower, and so on, as indicated by the way the caller sounds to you. It is also a good practice to ask patients each time you speak to them (over the phone or in person) if there is any change in their address, phone, and so on, to keep files current.

When you are finished with the conversation, it is best to allow the caller to hang up first. If you hang up first you might miss something the patient wanted to add. It is not considered professional to say "Bye-bye" when you finish the call. You should say "Goodbye."

When you have more than one telephone line coming in to the office, never answer the second line with "Hold the line, please," and then go back to your first call. You need to place the first call on hold properly and find out who is on the second line. Then you can determine whether or not it is an emergency and if it is not, ask the second caller to hold for you to finish the first call. Make all calls as brief as possible. You should keep any personal calls and personal business calls to a minimum.

Your voice is an important part of your **personality** at any time, but over the telephone, your voice *is* you. Callers form a picture of you as they listen to your voice. Does your telephone personality reveal a confident, courteous, friendly, and efficient medical assistant? It is equally easy to be heard as uncertain, irritated, abrupt, or inefficient.

Since the phone call is often the first contact a patient has with the office, your manner of speaking and the **empathy** you convey are critical to your success as a receptionist.

COMMON TYPES OF PHONE CALLS

The process of **screening** calls requires you to be aware of the most frequent types of phone calls that will be received in the medical office. They are:

- Referrals
- Patients who are calling for appointments, prescriptions, or the results of tests
- Emergency calls
- Other physicians, hospitals, or laboratories
- Personal calls and general business calls

A workbook and cassette titled *Handling Patients' Telephone Calls Effectively,* used in the Department of Practice Management as a guideline for workshops on this important aspect of the management of a medical office, is available from the American Medical Association.

Appointments, Prescriptions, and Test Results

Patients who phone for appointments should be given a choice of two appointment times. Usually one of the times will be satisfactory and this will eliminate the patient asking for multiple dates and times that are not available. Do not say "When would you like to come in?" It is better to say "Do you prefer mornings or afternoons?" Do not say "Are you a patient here?" It is better to say "When did we last see you?" Do not say "What's the problem?" It is better to say "Can you tell me what seems to be the problem, so that we can schedule you properly?" The appointment should be **confirmed** by reading the scheduled time back to the patient after it has been recorded in the appointment book.

You will find that patients will frequently ask to speak with the physician. Never say "The doctor is busy," as this may give the impression that the doctor does not want to be bothered by the caller. Be aware of the statements you make in reporting why the physician cannot speak on the telephone. It would be much better to state "The doctor is with a patient now. May I take a message and we will return the call as soon as possible?" The caller will usually respect the right of others to have the full attention of the physician and will not expect to interrupt the doctor except for an emergency.

Prescriptions

Each office will have its own rules for giving information to patients regarding tests or for calling pharmacies for prescription refills. It is important that you learn the rules for the office you work in and follow them without exception. The general rule is that a medical assistant does not give out information or call in a prescription without the **expressed** direction of the physician.

Write messages requesting prescriptions or test results in legible handwriting. If a patient requests a prescription refill, you need to know the name and phone number of the pharmacy as well as the name of the medication, strength, and prescription number. You also should record a telephone number where the patient can be reached in case the physician needs to talk with the patient before prescribing the medication. The physician may need to examine the patient first and you would need to call and schedule an appointment.

Many physicians prefer to have prescriptions and refills faxed to the patient's pharmacy. This practice is very efficient because it usually requires only one phone call, the one initiated by the patient for the medication refill. The fax document provides a paper trail for the patient's chart and should be filed as soon as possible. The medical assistant needs to ask the patient a few questions to note on the fax form, such as birth date, social security number, medical insurance number, and current phone number. It is vital that all information be kept in strict confidence.

A brief entry should be entered on the progress notes of the chart regarding the date and the name of the medication that was faxed to the pharmacy (with: "See fax"). Add your initials to indicate that you completed the procedure.

Another expedient and efficient method of dealing with medications may be available in certain instances. Patient information and the prescription can be entered into the computer and sent directly to the pharmacist. The patients can then go to the pharmacy and pick up their medications.

Test Results

When a patient calls for test results, you should never give them without receiving the physician's instructions on what to report. You would never give information to other people about a patient without the written permission of the patient and the approval of the physician. Procedures 6–1 through 6–4 outline steps of answering the office phone.

Professional Calls

When a physician telephones to speak to your employer, politely ask the caller for his name and inform the physi-

cian. Professional **etiquette** dictates that a physician will not keep a **colleague** waiting unless the physician is involved with an emergency or a surgical procedure.

Any calls that come into your office for the purpose of giving x-ray or laboratory results need to be recorded accurately. Always record the name of the person making the report. It is best to read back everything you have written down to be sure it is correct and complete before allowing the caller to leave the line.

Business, Personal, and Legal Calls

Your employer should let you know how to handle calls from family members, business associates, and sales people. Calls from attorneys requesting information about a patient must be handled with great caution. Attorneys know the patient must give written permission to divulge information to anyone regarding their health, yet attorneys will call and ask for information. Pull the patient chart and look for authorization listing the name of the attorney and the signature of the patient. If you find it, you may answer questions about the patient. Some physicians may still want you to check with them before releasing information. If you do not find authorization listing the name of the attorney, you must tell the caller to send an authorization signed by the patient and then you will be able to release information. It is advisable to return a call from an attor-

---

PROCEDURE

6-1   Answer the Office Phone

PURPOSE: Answer the office telephone promptly and efficiently in a professional manner.

EQUIPMENT AND SUPPLIES: Telephone, paper, pen, computer—if available.

PERFORMANCE OBJECTIVE: In a simulated (or actual) situation, using proper grammar, answer the telephone by the third ring identifying the office and yourself.

1. Answer the phone promptly (by the third ring) in a polite and pleasant manner.

2. Identify the office and yourself by name.
   NOTE: Your voice must be clear, distinct. Speak at a moderate rate, expressing consideration for the needs of the caller.

3. Listen to and record the name and phone number of the caller, the reason for the call, and the date and time of the call.

NOTE: ■ Obtain the correct spelling and pronunciation of the name.
   ■ **Process emergency calls immediately.**
   ■ **Before placing a caller on hold, wait for a response.**
   ■ **If you must place the caller on hold, check each minute to let him know you remember he is waiting (a patient should never wait longer than three minutes).**
   ■ **Complete all calls that were interrupted and/or were placed on hold.**

4. Screen and complete as many calls as possible before adding names to the physician's call back list.

5. Respond to an untimely request to speak to the physician by taking a message for the physician to return the call or having advice relayed by you.

PROCEDURE

6-2 📋 Process Phone Message

PURPOSE: Process a phone message properly.

EQUIPMENT AND SUPPLIES: Telephone, pen, paper/phone message log or computer, calendar, timepiece.

PERFORMANCE OBJECTIVE: In a simulated situation (or actual situation) receive, evaluate, and document a phone message.

1. Answer the phone properly (refer to steps in Procedure 6–1).

2. Listen carefully to the caller and determine the caller's needs (refer to your medical office's triage manual).
   NOTE: Scheduling a routine appointment may be all that is necessary.

3. Document information regarding the message, including date and time of call, on a message pad or phone call log. You must remember to include:
   - whom the request is for
   - what it is concerning
   - when the information is needed
   - where to return the call

4. Repeat the message to the caller to **verify** the contents. **Rationale: This practice helps to avoid errors.**

5. End the conversation with the caller politely.
   NOTE: It is a good practice to allow the caller to hang up first.

6. Sign your initials after the message.

7. Pull the patient's chart and record/attach the message.

PROCEDURE

6-3 📋 Record Telephone Message on Recording Device

PURPOSE: To provide a clear and precise message with all necessary information to the caller in a pleasant tone of voice when you (and other staff members) are unavailable to answer the office phone.

EQUIPMENT AND SUPPLIES: Telephone message device, pen, paper/phone message log or computer, calendar, timepiece.

PERFORMANCE OBJECTIVE: In a simulated situation (or actual situation) produce, with all necessary information in a pleasant tone of voice, a clear, accurate, and precise phone message on the telephone message device.

1. Assemble all necessary items in an area away from noise and distractions.
   NOTE: Determine the amount of time allowed on the recording device for the message before you begin. Messages that are too lengthy and/or complicated are frustrating to callers. Try to keep only essential information in the message.

2. Write out the appropriate message, check for completeness and accuracy, and read and determine the length of the message.

3. Record the message according to the directions of the answering device.
   - Speak in a pleasant, clear, and articulate tone of voice.
   - Sit up straight and project your voice into the speaker.
   - Identify the office.
   - Avoid being too wordy and overly friendly.
   - Be complete and accurate with information (Figure 6–5).

4. Play the message back and evaluate the quality of the message. Listen and determine if the message is of good quality and is appropriate for all callers who are trying to contact your medical facility.

5. Set the device to play the recorded message when you are unavailable to answer the phone.

Thank you for calling the Central Park Medical Center. [(Optional) It is: day of the week, month and day, year, time of day.] I am sorry I cannot take your call at this time. I am either away from my desk or on another phone line. If this is an emergency, please call 555-0000 **immediately**, phone the emergency medical service in your area, or go directly to the nearest hospital emergency room. If this is a non-emergency and you wish to speak to a member of our staff, please call us between the hours of 8:00 AM and 4:30 PM, Monday through Friday. We will be glad to help you in any way we can. After the tone sounds, please leave your name, phone number, a brief message, and when you may be reached. Your call will be returned as soon as possible. Have a pleasant day.

FIGURE 6–5 Example of phone recorder or voice mail message

ney even if you have authorization so you can be sure to whom you are talking. Anyone can call and claim to be a patient's attorney. Unless you know the caller, you cannot be sure you are talking to the correct individual.

Only information that has been authorized by the patient in writing, with the patient's signature, may be given to another party. Otherwise, the patient record is considered confidential information, and you may be liable for your actions.

Difficult Calls

There are a few calls that will be very much of a challenge to you no matter when they are received. These can include a call from an angry patient, a prank call, an obscene call, and "**bogus**" business calls. These types of calls should be reported to the police department if they persist. As with any phone call you receive, you should be as tactful, professional, and courteous as possible.

When an angry patient phones you and begins to rant and rave about something that you know nothing about, you should first, as calmly as possible and in a soft tone, ask the person to please start from the beginning and tell you his concerns. In this way, you can either answer the patient's needs or direct him to the proper person or department so that the problem can be resolved. If the patient is speaking so loudly that you have to hold the receiver away from your ear, ask the person to please hold for a few

---

P R O C E D U R E

6-4 Obtain Telephone Message from Phone Recording Device

PURPOSE: To obtain accurate message(s) from the recording with all necessary information from the caller to correctly process requests.

EQUIPMENT AND SUPPLIES: Telephone message device, pen, paper/phone message log or computer, appropriate patients' charts.

PERFORMANCE OBJECTIVE: In a simulated situation (or actual situation), obtain all necessary and **pertinent** information from the phone message recording device.

1. Assemble all necessary items in an area away from noise and distractions.

2. Listen to the recordings and write out each message accurately.
   NOTE: You may have to listen to the recording more than one time in order to obtain complete information, as some voices may be difficult to understand. It is a good practice to ask another staff member to listen if you have difficulty.

3. Sign your initials after the message. The date and time of the message must also be written.

4. List all patients who leave messages so you can pull their charts.

5. Prioritize messages according to the nature of their seriousness and distribute to the appropriate staff member/ department to be processed.
   NOTE: If you are to obtain messages from an answering service, call the service and obtain the messages from a customer service representative. Obtain messages from various answering services offered by phone companies by following the instructions for specialized features. Then, follow the steps as outlined above. If the answering service sends you a fax or e-mails the phone messages, the hard copy is already available for you to process and file in the patient's chart. Make sure you can legibly read the information and verify with the sender if there is a question or if there is any discrepancy.

seconds while you pull his chart. This will allow for a little time for the patient to calm down. If the caller uses profanity, you should remind the caller that you will not continue the call unless you can be spoken to in a courteous manner. There are times that the only way to sensibly handle a situation like this is to ask the office manager, your supervisor, or the physician to speak to the patient. Another way that may be helpful is to take the complaint and phone number and ask if you may call the patient back after you determine the extent of the problem. Explain that you need to discuss the issue with the proper person and call back with an answer. Let the patient know when you can be expected to call so that the patient does not get even angrier waiting unnecessarily for an answer. Whatever the case may be, it should be noted on the patient's chart regarding the nature of the problem and the outcome.

Prank calls are not common, but if you need to deal with this, you should alert all office personnel so that no one will be caught off guard. Usually the prank is childish and not harmful. The best way to handle this type of call is to simply hang up. Being disconnected will discourage the prankster from repeating this call. Either blowing a whistle into the mouthpiece during the initial call or by simply hanging up may be sufficient to stop obscene calls. Alert all other office staff of the call. As stated earlier, if the calls persist, they should be reported to the police.

The phone company should be contacted to trace calls of this nature, and criminal charges may be brought against the offender. You should keep a record of the date and time of the calls until the phone company becomes involved. Most phone directories have a section that outlines the steps that should be taken in situations such as bothersome and harassing calls. Simply telling the caller that you have reported the problem may be enough to make them stop calling. Taking action as soon as the situation occurs is the most sensible course to take.

Another type of call that you should be aware of is the "bogus" business call. Occasionally you may receive a call from a fake business owner who claims to have a special deal on office or medical equipment or supplies. Beware of this type of practice because the party demands payment before goods are received, and the outcome is that no goods are ever delivered. Do not make any business deal with any new company without checking them out first. All business should be conducted with well-established, reputable companies with good references to ensure solid business practices.

Follow-up Calls

Often physicians advise patients to call the next day to report their progress. You should determine if you are to take the call, relay the message to the doctor (and record the patient's report on her chart), or if the physician wishes to speak directly to the patient when she calls. It is also a good practice to check with the physician to see if you should contact the patient if you do not receive the follow-up call from her by a predetermined time. Make sure that you have the current home, cell phone, pager, or work number(s) before the patient leaves your office so that you will be able to call her if necessary. It is also a good practice to make sure that the patient's chart has a current phone number of a relative or friend in the event that the patient cannot be contacted.

Physician Visits Outside the Office

When a patient calls and requests a house call, be sure you check with your physician employer before you schedule one. If your employer makes house calls, you should have a city map or county map to help locate any new patient scheduled.

Many physicians visit patients in hospitals and nursing homes on a regular basis. You need to establish a method of recording these visits and hospital calls. The physician should have a list of calls to be made each day along with a checklist of needed follow-up and charges for services.

Long Distance Calls

You may need to place long distance calls. If you are calling an area outside of your time zone, you should consult the telephone directory for the map of time zones (Figure 6–6) so you can establish the appropriate time to call. Take into consideration when it is lunch break in a different time zone so that you will not waste time trying to phone an office when the staff is not available to take your call. Be sure you know the code number needed to dial for your long distance service, in addition to the telephone numbers of the persons

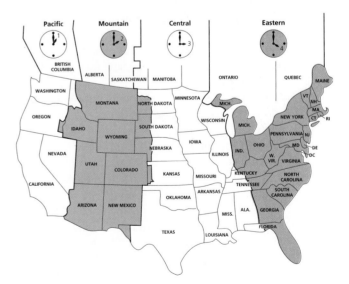

FIGURE 6–6 Make sure that you place long distance calls within regular business hours by referring to a time zone map such as this.

you need to call. A record book should be kept on all long distance calls made.

Call Monitoring

When your employer asks you to monitor a call either by an extension phone or speakerphone, listen quietly and take notes of the conversation. It is important to make certain the caller agrees to your listening and taking notes. It is illegal for you to do this without the consent of the caller. Another type of monitoring is to record the phone call so that it may be played back if necessary at a later time. This, also, is illegal to do without the party's written consent.

Refusal or Inability to Identify

Your office may have a specific method of handling individuals who call and refuse to identify themselves. A good general rule is to suggest that the individual write a letter to the physician and mark it *personal*, in which case the physician will receive it unopened. Most physicians do not wish to talk to unidentified callers during busy office hours.

The guidelines for handling the physician's telephone can be summarized as follows:

1. Answer the telephone as promptly as possible.
2. Keep a pad and pen next to the telephone at all times.
3. Verify the caller's name and correct spelling. If an adult calls about a child, make sure you have the correct last name. Do not assume the child's last name is the same as the caller's name.
4. Determine the reason for the call.
5. Handle as many telephone calls as you possibly can without disturbing the physician.
6. If the physician prefers to speak to a patient, call the physician to the telephone after asking who is calling. Pull the patient's chart and give it to the physician.
7. Whenever possible, if you cannot handle the call alone, take a message for the physician. The physician will tell you what to do or call the patient back as time allows (Figure 6–7).
8. Make a memorandum for the physician of every telephone call. Use printed telephone memorandum pads that show date of call, time of call, name of caller, telephone number, and message.
9. Always know where to reach the physician. If the message is urgent and the physician is not in the office, page or telephone at once and relay the message.
10. If the physician cannot be reached, have the message by your phone. When your employer checks in, you may relay the message.

11. Learn how much medical information the physician wishes you to give over the telephone. Patients frequently call the office because they have forgotten the physician's instructions about treatments or medications. If these instructions are clearly stated in the chart, or in a pre-approved triage manual, it may be possible for the assistant to repeat them to the patient.
12. When answering a second line, determine if it is an emergency or another physician before placing the caller on hold and returning to finish the first call.
13. End all telephone conversations on a friendly note. In general, let the caller be the first one to hang up or say "Goodbye."
14. Never promise a cure over the telephone or in person. Never say "I am sure the physician can help you."

If you have answered the phone and no one answers after you try twice to converse, simply hang up. Some phone systems may have caller ID, which may help in this type of situation. Immediately returning the call in this case may link you to a person in distress. **CAUTION:** Never tell anyone over the phone (or in person) that you are alone (even if you are) as this could possibly be an invitation for undesirable behaviors. For your safety, it is not wise to work alone when there is no one

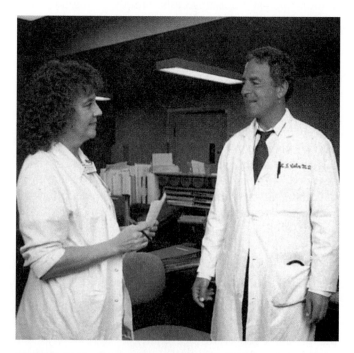

FIGURE 6–7 Phone messages that you cannot answer without the physician's advice should be completed as soon as possible between seeing patients.

near for assistance. If you must, and only if it is absolutely necessary for you to complete your responsibilities, a neighboring office staff or someone you trust should be informed of your being alone.

FINDING PHONE NUMBERS

You can save a great deal of time by keeping an up-to-date index of your most frequently called numbers by the telephone and by adding a list of e-mail addresses as you update phone numbers. In addition, when you need to use the telephone directory, it is helpful to know how it is organized.

The introductory section usually contains:

- Emergency numbers
- Community service numbers
- General telephone information
- Directory assistance information
- Rates for telephone calls
- Out-of-city area codes and time zones
- Money-saving tips on use of the telephone
- Directions for making international calls
- Rights and responsibilities
- Directory listings

You will find an alphabetic listing of individuals in the white pages. There may be separate listing of business and professional organizations in a second section of the white pages. An index of city, county, state, and United States government offices may be found in a separate section of pages. Local zip code numbers by street address are usually in the introduction or a separate section of the telephone book. This section can be taken out of the large phone book and kept on the top of the desk in a stand-up organizer for easy access. This makes your job less taxing and eliminates the need to lift a heavy book many times each day. There are also books of complete listings of all zip codes in the country available. This is a necessary reference to have in the office as it saves you from making frequent calls to the post office for information. Within the "rights and responsibilities" section of a telephone directory, you will find very helpful information regarding phone service and safety.

The contents section should be reviewed with each new updated directory as it will contain information which may have changed from the last edition. Another feature that most telephone companies now have are specialized services and equipment for the deaf. You may have an opportunity to pass this information on to patients who may need these services and not be aware of them. The yellow pages (or classified directory) list the name, address, and phone number of every business subscriber, grouped under product and service headings. The classified directory also contains an index that can help you determine the headings under which a specific type of product or service may be listed.

A CAAHEP CONNECTION

Communication skills are used continuously and are a vital part of the medical assistant's role. Instruction in telephone communications is extremely important and will be essential to your role as a member of the medical office staff. This is why it is included in the curriculum requirements for instruction.

ACHIEVE UNIT OBJECTIVES

Complete Chapter 6, Unit 1, in the workbook to help you obtain competency of this subject matter.

UNIT 2

Schedule Appointments

OBJECTIVES

Upon completion of the unit, meet the following terminal performance objectives by verifying knowledge of the facts and principles presented through oral and written communication at a level deemed competent, and demonstrate the specific behaviors as identified in the performance objectives of the procedures, observing safety precautions in accordance with health care standards.

1. Spell and define, using the glossary in the back of this text, all the **Words to Know** in this unit.
2. List and discuss ways that an office staff can establish the most desirable method of scheduling for their individual needs.
3. Explain what is meant by "establishing a matrix," and explain why it is important.
4. List and explain the various methods of scheduling.
5. Describe the advantages and disadvantages of each method of scheduling.
6. List and discuss the most important points to consider in determining appointment scheduling when someone calls the office.
7. Describe the importance of a triage manual for handling telephone calls.
8. Explain the most practical way to schedule a patient who is always late.
9. Explain and discuss the purpose of the rules for handling a canceled appointment.
10. List and discuss the goals of the physician, the medical assistant, and the patient regarding the appointment schedule.
11. List common abbreviations and their meanings used in making appointments.

12. Describe various ways of recording appointment schedules and give advantages and disadvantages of each.
13. State what information should be included in a procedure manual to help the medical assistant with making referral appointments.
14. Explain and demonstrate the procedures for making various appointments.

AREAS OF COMPETENCE (AAMA)

This unit addresses content within the specific competency areas of *Administrative procedures, Fundamental principles, Patient care, Professionalism, Communication skills, Legal concepts, Instruction,* and *Operational functions* that are identified in the Medical Assistant Role Delineation Study. Refer to Appendix A for a detailed listing of the areas.

■ WORDS TO KNOW

chemotherapy	matrix
commonality	obliterate
criterion	precertification
downtime	ramification
flex time	remote
gatekeeper	sequentially
geriatrics	unstructured
guarantor	utilization
increments	work-in

APPOINTMENT STRATEGIES

Ⓐ **Patient Reception Area:**
■ Scheduling

One of the most primary and vital functions in the course of managed care is the scheduling of appointments (Procedure 6–5). Managing time well for the physician and support staff will help keep patient flow at a satisfactory pace and promote a good professional working relationship. This may seem like an ideal situation that is unattainable. However, if there is genuine cooperation among all staff members, the schedule should flow well with some understandable exceptions due to emergencies and other unpredictable situations from time to time. Office hours may be scheduled with appointments made during specific times, or left as an open, **unstructured** block of time.

First, the entire staff must be made aware of the intended schedule of the physician(s) in the medical facility. An inservice or an orientation, whichever the case may be, is a practical way to inform employees about the schedule and enforce the established guidelines for "office hours." An organized routine helps the office staff as well as the patients with intended goals. In addition to providing the public with the routine hours when services are provided in printed form, the information should be posted at the entrance of the medical facility, on appointment cards, and on other printed materials. This information should also be placed in phone directories and wherever may be applicable. This way, everyone will know when the doctor is in and at what time business calls and

---

PROCEDURE

6-5 📋 Schedule Appointments

PURPOSE: Schedule appointments appropriately in a professional manner.

EQUIPMENT AND SUPPLIES: Appointment book and pen, computer and scheduling program, monitor, printer, and appointment cards.

PERFORMANCE OBJECTIVE: In a simulated situation, schedule an appointment for a patient according to accepted medical standards with consideration for the physician, staff, and needs of the patient.

1. Determine the means of scheduling: appointment book or computer entry.

2. Mark off the hours when the physician will be unable to see patients. Include daily hospital rounds, lunch hour, meetings, and vacation.

3. Attempt to give patients two choices of times for the appointment.
   NOTE: In black ink, record patients' names as well as phone number(s) so that you can easily and quickly get in touch with them if necessary.

4. Ask patients to schedule their next appointment before leaving the office.

5. Write patients' names in the schedule book, or enter the patient's name in appropriate space on appointment screen.

6. Complete an appointment card and give it to the patient. Be sure to record the appointment first in the appointment book and then on the appointment card.

7. Avoid over-scheduling and leave sufficient time for work-ins.

8. Allow time for the doctor to return phone calls. Patient charts should be pulled and given to the doctor for these calls.

appointments are taken. More discussion about an office policy manual is provided in Chapter 10.

After the office hours have been determined, the appointment schedule must be fashioned to meet the specific goals of the physician(s) and staff. Figure 6–8 outlines the goals that must continually be considered when scheduling.

The goals of the patient, the physician, and the medical assistant need to be considered. In general, the *goals of patients* are:

1. a minimum wait for an appointment
2. a minimum wait in the office
3. maximum time with the physician

The general *goals of physicians* are:

1. cost-effective use of time
2. to spend needed time with the patients
3. uninterrupted time
4. time for referrals, emergencies, and so on

The general *goals of the medical assistant* are:

1. a smooth-running office
2. to close the office on time
3. a lunch hour and breaks
4. patient and physician goals

FIGURE 6–8 Goals of the patient, the medical assistant, and the physician must be considered when preparing an appointment schedule.

Several styles of appointment books are available to schedule an entire year or more. A standard type of appointment book contains each day of the year printed with hours ranging from 8:00 AM to 5:00 PM, as shown in Figure 6–9. Individual medical facilities can have appointment books custom-made for their needs. Where several physicians' schedules are kept, the computer is the most desirable log of appointments as it eliminates the awkward use of several appointment books.

When you use computerized appointment scheduling, you totally replace the paper appointment book. You should certainly have an accounts receivable system well established before converting to appointment scheduling. This feature should not be added if you have a single terminal, but can be effective if you have several terminals. You also must consider how you would handle **downtime**, when, for whatever reason, the computer is not functional. This is a reality you need to plan for before it takes place so the office will run as smoothly as possible through the downtime. Downtime in this context refers to the time when the computer is basically not working and you are unable to enter or obtain information.

A computerized appointment system automatically locates the next available time, gives you a record of all appointments already made, allows you to locate a specific date and time, and prints copies of the daily schedule. These printed copies should be filed with the accounting records of the day as a legal document that you could be

FIGURE 6–9 Appointment scheduling styles

called on to produce in the event of an IRS audit of the office practice. Most computer systems can be used to print charge slips for the patients as they are seen. The patient's next scheduled appointment can be printed at the bottom of the charge slip, which is also a receipt of payment of the services of that day's office visit.

ESTABLISHING A MATRIX

The appointment book or computer program schedule must have a fixed **matrix**, which means that wherever there is a section of a page crossed out or a full page (or pages) crossed out with an "X," such as is shown in Figure 6–10, nothing should be scheduled. In a medical practice schedule, this usually means that in these spaces, services by the physician(s) will not be performed during this time. For instance, nothing should be scheduled between the hours of 8:00 AM and noon on Thursdays, and nothing scheduled before 9:00 AM and after 4:45 PM on Fridays because the physician(s) will not be in to see patients. It can also mean simply that no one should be scheduled in this time slot because it is reserved specifically for urgent conditions and **work-ins**. All staff members need to be aware of the exact meaning of this practice for consistency in scheduling, that is, an entire day with an X through it means that the doctor is out, an X through the afternoon time slots means that the doctor is out only in the afternoon, and an X from 11:00 AM to 11:45 AM or 2:45 PM to 3:15 PM usually means that this time is reserved for catch-up and for work-ins (whichever is needed). It may also be referred to as **flex time** and can also be useful for time to return phone calls to patients during the day as necessary. If there is an established "lunch" time each day from 12:00 PM to 1:00 PM, it should be crossed out also. Toward the end of the scheduled day, from 4:40 PM to 5:00 PM for instance, time is saved so that there will be room to take work-ins, if needed. Whether the physician will be away for a medical meeting, on vacation, performing surgery, involved in a community service, or whatever else, as soon as the doctor informs the staff, the entire time that is needed should be blocked out so that no one will be scheduled by mistake during this period. To be practical and efficient, time should be blocked out for the entire year ahead if it is regarding a routine day off, or at least as soon as possible as dates of activities are made known to you by the physi-

cian. When scheduling appointments using a computer program, you may easily block out days and specified hours during the daily schedule for those times when the physician(s) will be out of the office and appointments should not be made.

Whether you use an appointment book or a computer program for scheduling appointments, it is an efficient and practical habit to make a hard copy of each of the scheduled appointments for the day for pulling patient charts and for use in checking off the patients as they arrive for appointments. It also is a good practice to do this the day before to get ready for the arrival of patients the next morning. It is not good to pull medical records too far in advance as it makes files difficult to find when so many are out without guides. It is not practical to place a guide card in place of every record when pulling them for the daily schedule. As patients come in for appointments, the receptionist can cross through their names as they report in for their appointments and their records are pulled, or as they are taken in to be prepared to see the physician. An additional hard copy of the daily schedule can make it easier for all to work from so that the staff can keep track of patient flow and anticipate the needs of patients.

Another practice which may be helpful is to highlight in a color (or several) for specific types of appointments (i.e., yellow is urgent, green is recheck, blue is injection, and so on). A separate schedule, or section of the master schedule, for those professionals in your facility (physician assistant, medical assistant, insurance secretary, and so on) who take appointments for various services, apart from the physician's appointment schedule, should also be kept. Figure 6–10 gives an example of a multiple appointment schedule. Patients who only need to be given immunizations, have weight and blood pressure checked,

Tuesday, March 10, 20xx

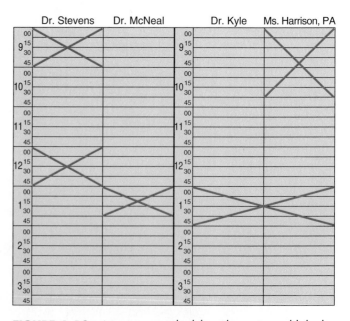

FIGURE 6–10 Appointment schedule with matrix established for three physicians and a physician assistant

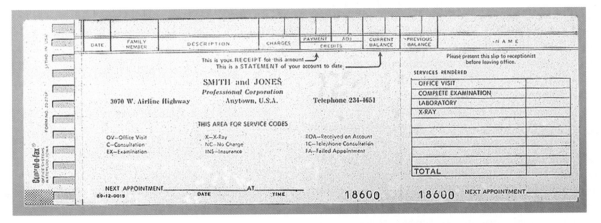

FIGURE 6–11(A) As shown on this pegboard system form, the receipt given to the patient has a space for recording the next scheduled appointment.

urinalysis rechecks, and so on, do not need to be seen by the doctor unless there is a problem. This should be done to avoid having all patients show up at the same time. In many cases the assistant, who reports the findings to the physician, is given instructions from the doctor and will then report back to the patient. This can save the physician valuable time that may be spent in providing managed care to others. This schedule should also have an established matrix. This is a sensible practice which helps to avoid possibly having to reschedule patients because of unplanned meetings, vacations, or lectures. Clear communication among the entire staff must be ongoing to prevent confusion, mistakes, and misunderstandings.

In cases where patients have a set, or standing, appointment, rescheduling should be done only when emergencies arise and it is absolutely necessary. The process of rescheduling involves calling each scheduled patient and offering an alternative appointment time as close to the original one as possible. This, of course, may crowd an already full schedule for a few days—or weeks—depending on the extent of the downtime created by the emergency. Downtime in this context refers to the time when the physician is called away from the routine schedule because of an emergency outside the office, usually with a hospital patient, or a personal emergency. The office staff may proceed with duties such as processing records, filing, inventory, and so on, that can be performed without the physician's presence.

Once the matrix has been established, the style of scheduling must be decided. There are several different ways to schedule. The preferred method of scheduling that is adopted for a particular medical practice is up to the physician and the staff. The choice should be determined only after creatively planning and carefully reviewing all of the options. In order for a schedule to run smoothly, many points must be taken into consideration. The medical assistant (receptionist or telephone secretary) must have excellent communication skills, a solid knowledge of the signs and symptoms of diseases and disorders, and an understanding of medical terminology and anatomy in order to proficiently perform telephone

---

Appointment for _Linda Parker_____

On _Thurs. 4/5_____ at ___9:30___ (AM/PM)

With Dr. Catherine Lang—Baldwin Family Practice Center
712 Central Parkway
Central City, XX Zip Code

Telephone 000/555-5000   Fax # 000/555-5001

If unable to keep this appointment please give 24 hour notice or a charge will be made for the reserved time.

FIGURE 6–11(B) An example of a typical appointment card to give the patient that has the date (and day) and time of the next scheduled appointment

triage and prepare an efficient schedule. Obtaining the most precise assessment of a patient's condition by speaking calmly and empathically to the patient over the phone and actively listening to what is being said is referred to as phone triage. Using this type of assessment technique should result in obtaining accurate information and yield in appropriate and complete care. When patients phone the medical facility with the request to see the doctor, the medical assistant must find out who the caller is (ask the correct spelling of the caller's name and address, and so on) and determine whether the person has previously seen the doctor. Refer to the procedures in this unit that will help you follow a pattern of order with this detailed task.

Patients who either stop at the desk after seeing the doctor or who stop in to make an appointment should be given the same courtesy that patients receive over the phone. Offer the person a choice between two dates and times, allow sufficient time for the person to decide, and then confirm it by repeating it to the person before writing (printing) it in the appointment book. Remember to write the phone number(s) of the patient in the schedule book next to the name (so that you can call the patient quickly, if necessary, without pulling the chart) and note briefly (using abbreviations) the nature of the office visit.

Write the time and date on an appointment card and politely hand it to the patient. If the pegboard system is used to record all patient transactions in the "write it once" fashion, you may record the next appointment in the space provided on the receipt section of the form. You should call attention to the space where the appointment is on the form when you hand the receipt to the patient. Figure 6–11A shows an example of the pegboard system form. Figure 6–11B shows an example of an appointment card that is given to the patient, which indicates the date, day, and time of the patient's next appointment. At this time you should also provide the patient with any appropriate printed instructions or educational materials regarding the patient's condition, further treatment, or scheduled studies. Keep in mind that all appointment cards or forms that are used for this purpose should have the full name of the physician, complete address, phone number, and type of practice printed clearly on them. If the practice is new or in a new location, it is a convenience to the patient to have a small map or instructions of how to get to the office. If there are other office locations, they should also be listed with complete information. Many appointment cards for professional services state that the patient must give the staff a 24-hour notice if a change in the scheduled appointment must be made. A verbal reminder to patients also helps to reinforce this policy. This can be very helpful in maintaining a smooth schedule.

A new patient must provide you with complete information not only so that you can prepare a chart for the initial appointment, but also in case it becomes necessary to reach the patient before the scheduled appointment. If data is on the computer, the needed information can also be called up immediately.

APPOINTMENT-MAKING SUGGESTIONS

As you gain experience in listening to patients' complaints over the phone, you will become more keen in assessing problems. Using a preapproved phone triage manual or a medical office handbook is a wise practice, as it reinforces continuity among staff members. All employees must be instructed to use the same format and ask the same questions every time of every patient who complains of similar symptoms. Following these pre-set guidelines that have been approved by the physician will help uncover serious conditions and lead to more efficient care of patients. Overlooking any of the questions or leaving out any part of a patient's symptoms is potentially a serious risk to both the patient and the medical practice. Also, you must be careful not to put words in the caller's mouth. Asking precise questions and waiting for a response from the patient is recommended. The medical assistant should not offer to speak for the patient, but tactfully encourage the patient to tell in her own words what the problem seems to be, and how long it has been going on. Next, the caller needs to let you know what has been done to relieve the problem, if anything. When writing

Medical Assistant: Good afternoon, Dr. Michael's office, this is Marla, how may I help you?

Caller: Hello, this is Mrs. Evans. I need to bring Kelvin in to see the doctor.

Medical Assistant: What seems to be the problem, Mrs. Evans?

Mrs. Evans: Well, I just got off work and I'm at the day care center to pick up the kids, and Kelvin feels feverish and has a runny nose.

Medical Assistant: Have you or anyone at the day care center taken his temperature?

Mrs. Evans: No, he just feels hot to me and he looks flushed.

Medical Assistant: Has he been sick or are there any other problems that you think seem to be bothering Kelvin?

Mrs. Evans: Kelvin gets an earache every time he gets a cold. He is telling me that his left ear hurts as we speak. I just wanted to see what you thought before we go home.

Medical Assistant: How long has Kelvin had a cold?

Mrs. Evans: For a few days I guess, but he hasn't had a fever until now.

Medical Assistant: Have you given Kelvin any medication for his cold?

Mrs. Evans: Just some decongestant cough formula twice a day.

Medical Assistant: Can you be here in a half hour, Mrs. Evans? We will work Kelvin in to see Dr. Michael as soon as possible.

Mrs. Evans: Oh, thank you, we will be right there!

Medical Assistant: You're welcome, Mrs. Evans, we'll see you soon.

FIGURE 6–12 A sample phone conversation between caller and medical assistant

down the information, be exact in how much and how often regarding medications, home remedies, and other treatments. Never leave out information that the patient tells you no matter how minor it may seem to you. The information disclosed to you by the patient should provide you with sufficient information necessary to determine how soon the appointment should be made. A sample phone call between the medical assistant and a patient is offered in Figure 6–12.

If the physician(s) in your medical facility cannot take new patients, as a courtesy, be prepared to suggest a physician in the area who may be able to take the caller. Ask the physician periodically which physicians may be taking new patients in the area so that you may send them referrals as necessary. This service is a professional courtesy also in cases where the physician cannot take any more patients because of a full capacity. Often a person's doctor is determined by the patient's insurance company

Methods of Scheduling

Clustering—This scheduling technique is frequently exercised in specialty practices as well as in the general and family practice office. A cluster, or group, of patients who have the same complaint, diagnosis, or other commonality are scheduled sequentially every 10 minutes throughout the morning or afternoon, or throughout a particular day of the week. Some specialists, such as pediatricians, prefer to use this method as a routine standard. Many patients can be provided with the necessary preparations, be examined by the physician, and have appointments completed quickly when clustering is used in scheduling.

Double-booking—Appointment times are given to two or more patients for the same time slot in this method of scheduling. Since most people have varying degrees of the concept of and the respect for time, the possibility of all patients entering the reception room at the same time for an appointment (for instance, at 2:00 PM) are remote. The usual course of events is that one of three will arrive between 1:40 PM and 1:45 PM, another at 2:00 PM, and the third, a little past 2:00 PM. This is precisely the reason that double-booking works out so well. For services that take a small amount of time, this is the ideal way to schedule. It is also a great help if there are patients who are "no shows" (those who do not come in for appointments with no courtesy call).

Open hours—For a very active practice, such as general and family practices, clinic settings, and student health centers, this method of scheduling is usually the most practical. Patients sign in, noting the time they arrive, and they are seen by the doctor in that order. Emergencies and urgent conditions must be given priority attention. However, as this occurs, there is usually a backup with patient flow. There may be procedures and treatments that are not anticipated when the patient first arrives. After the physician talks with the patient and performs the appropriate exam, further testing or treatment may be necessary. This process utilizes a considerable amount of time. There is no way to regulate the order of the seriousness of patients' problems. Whenever possible, the urgent medical problems are sent to the emergency room of the local hospital or an emergency medical service is called to provide immediate care.

Single-booking—This method is used when the appointment for the patient will take a considerable amount of time, as in consultations, counseling, patient education, or other types of therapy. The medical practices that would be more likely to use this method of scheduling are psychiatry, physical or occupational therapy, and other specialty services. Usually when there is only one patient or family scheduled each hour, the appointment is made for only 45 to 50 minutes of the hour. This allows for the

session to wind down comfortably as well as for the possibility of the session going overtime a few minutes. It also gives the professional conducting the services a short break in between patient care and to prepare for the next appointment.

Streaming—The focus of this method of scheduling is, as the word suggests, to keep a continuous flow of patients coming in through the facility and to avoid having alternating periods of idleness and crowding. Since most standard appointment books have a printed schedule of a 12-hour day in 15-minute increments, appointments are made to accommodate the specific needs of patients. New patients and those needing complete physical examinations, for example, require a long appointment in order to perform all the necessary preparations, examinations, and any diagnostic tests that may result. Specific medical problems, such as a child with an earache, a blood pressure recheck, or a dressing change, will routinely take no more than a maximum of 10 to 15 minutes. In some instances, some of the scheduled appointments that are allowed 15 minutes may in reality take only 5 minutes. This is the reason that scheduling by the streaming method seems to work out well most of the time.

Wave—This method of scheduling is used in many large medical clinics, family and general practice, and group practices because it runs most efficiently in a facility where there are several medical service departments and qualified personnel to provide managed care of patients. Appointments are made during the first 30 minutes of each hour. The number of patients that are scheduled depends on the type of practice and the amount of time needed for services. The remainder of the hour may be used for those patients who phone the same day and need to be checked by the physician. Since many patients are already scheduled in this type of scheduling, the times in the schedule are most likely filled. If there is a cancellation or a patient "forgets" to come in, the entire schedule is not ruined. Most often the staff is grateful for a little extra time to catch up on other duties.

Modified wave—The modified wave method of scheduling is the same as the wave method plus scheduling patients in the last half hour of each hour in 10- and 20-minute intervals according to the medical problems. For those patients that you know will need the most time with the doctor, the beginning of the hour is the logical choice of time. For patients who will most likely take only a few minutes, the last half hour seems to work best. Scheduling in this manner yields some flexibility so that patients who have urgent health problems or injuries can be worked in between already scheduled patients.

FIGURE 6-13 Methods of scheduling

or health maintenance organization (HMO) for full coverage of medical services. If the provider is not a member of a patient's medical insurance program, the patient must seek a physician who *is* in order for medical care expenses to be covered. All information must be determined before the appointment is made. This procedure is called **precertification**. This "pre-cert" must be done before certain procedures and treatments are performed to confirm that these services are, in fact, approved for guaranteed coverage and to determine what the percentage is. There are occasions when the patient must call the number printed on the back of their insurance card to precertify a service, such as an appointment for substance abuse or mental health counseling, so that the insurance company will cover the charges. If a person has no medical insurance and wants to see the physician, the patient must

understand that all expenses incurred must be paid for in cash at the time of service, or agree in writing as to the method of payment. Many medical facilities accept credit cards for the amount of service charges. Explain to the patient that this is not encouraged even though it affords the physician prompt payment of services. If a patient is receiving government assistance for medical treatment, this also must be docmented.

All staff members must be willing to work cooperatively and efficiently in order to provide quality care to patients. Included in the many choices for scheduling appointments are the following methods: clustering, double-booking, open hours, single-booking, streaming, wave, and modified wave. Figure 6–13 lists these methods of scheduling with a description of the purpose of each. Any one of these methods can be used exclusively or in combination with one or more to fit the specific individual needs of the practice. Even when appointment times have been assigned to patients, it is a good policy to have the patients sign in with their time of arrival. Some offices make it a practice of checking with all patients to determine if any of their personal information or insurance coverage has changed since they were last seen and to identify who they are scheduled to see (i.e., doctor, nurse, medical assistant, x-ray, or lab tech). This is a good way to identify new patients who need to complete initial forms for their chart. This way, current patient information is obtained as well as the order in which the patient should be taken in. It also is a more foolproof method of keeping track of patients so that no one is overlooked. A sign should be posted giving instructions for patients to "sign in" as they arrive. Periodic checking which patients are waiting will help in case a new patient has not signed in and registered with you. It must be stated that leaving the sign-in sheet out for all to read is a risk because it allows all patients to read everyone's name. You know that you would not leave the appointment book open for the general public to read because it would break the confidentiality of patients. The ideal way to keep this from being a potential problem is to write the information down yourself as patients arrive, or enter it into the computer, keeping the screen from the view of others. This should be discussed by the staff and an agreement made to determine how this is to be handled.

MAINTAINING THE SCHEDULE

After a period of time, through trial and error, each medical practice staff arrives at a schedule that works best for them. An assessment should be made of the efficiency of the schedule and appropriate changes should be made to better serve expedient patient flow. Management consultants suggest an evaluation of old appointment sheets for a 12- to 15-week period. The number of work-ins, cancellations, and no shows and the time spent with specific exams and complaints of patients will help determine the course of the revision of scheduling techniques. The time slots needed for various procedures, exams, and consultations can then be handled in short, medium, long, and extended appointment times. Often, a patient needs to have several procedures performed or must see one or more doctors in an office or a medical center. Coordinating all of these appointments for the patient on the same day is most thoughtful and will save the person from having to repeat unnecessary expense and travel which can be very tiring, especially to the elderly patient. The medical assistant may be expected to provide an explanation of different medical specialties, medical terms, instructions for procedures, exams, or treatments for patients who are unfamiliar with such matters. Sending the patient printed instructions regarding procedures and exams along with an appointment card prior to the scheduled appointment helps patients get prepared and reduces their anxiety. Further discussion and helpful information about diagnostic

examinations is provided in Chapters 15 and 16. Another thoughtful service to patients is to give simple but precise directions of how to get to your location. A map or printed instructions mailed to the patient before their appointment is appreciated by persons who are not familiar with your geographic area. An office brochure is a way to give new patients a brief explanation of your facility's policies and procedures regarding office hours, location and directions, when to call, whom to speak to for administrative business, the procedure for medication refills, and so on, and the philosophy of the practice. This way, all information is in one neat package. Educating the patients in these areas is most helpful in the elimination of repeat calls asking the same information.

Remember that patients who have to wait a long time before being seen by the physician become impatient and eventually angry, especially if the patient had a scheduled appointment. Understandably, this patient may wonder why an appointment was even made. Surveys have shown that patients usually do not mind as much as a half-hour wait, but tend to become angry if it is any longer. This could lead to medical-legal **ramifications** if it is not handled properly. Patients' time is as valuable to them as it is to you and the physician. Delays should be made known to patients tactfully as soon as they are realized. Patients need to be given the choice of waiting for as long as it may be, or rescheduling for another appointment time altogether. This is a considerate way to treat patients and prevents problems from starting. Announcing that there will be a delay as soon as you have been given the information (i.e., that the doctor is caring for a patient with an emergency at the hospital) is something that patients will understand and appreciate. It is far better to be honest with patients and let them know what the situation is from the start than to be silent. Patients appreciate your letting them know so that they can make a choice about waiting or returning at another time. A periodic announcement should be made to those patients who are waiting as to how much longer it may be before the doctor is able to see them.

Handling Patients Without Appointments

There may be a time when a patient who has an appointment brings along a family member or a friend to be seen. This complicates the schedule and presents a challenge in tact and diplomacy to the staff. When a patient arrives who has no appointment in a practice where it *is* necessary to have an appointment to see the physician, you need to explain this to the person as tactfully and as politely as possible. It is advisable to have a sign near the reception window that indicates the office hours and that patients are seen by appointment only. When the patient realizes that the doctor can spend a sufficient amount of time only with those patients who are scheduled, cooperation is usually attained. Patients who are persistent because of the nature of their problems should be referred to the office manager or physician. If a patient walks into your office with no appointment, the person should be referred to an appropriate medical facility according to the person's symptoms, if there is no way your schedule can accommodate him. The physician should be made aware of the situation before any definitive action is taken. The nature of the patient's problem will determine how quickly you should act. Often, the physician will make an exception and reinforce the policy for future appointment scheduling. If it is a serious emergency, you should automatically call for emergency medical service. In some cases, the physician may agree to take care of the emergency and then refer the patient to another physician for continuous managed care.

Canceled or Missed Appointments (No Shows)

If a patient cancels or does not show up for the scheduled appointment, it should be noted in the person's chart and the appointment time given to another patient as soon as possible. The physician should be notified about the patient's cancellation or "no show." The physician will advise you about further action as warranted by the patient's condition. For example, if a patient is being treated for a wound that requires follow-up care and a dressing change, the patient may cancel (or just not come) and the wound area could become infected. The patient might decide to sue the doctor for inadequate care. The record of the canceled appointment or no show is important in proving that the patient had an appointment but failed to follow the physician's instructions. The patient's name should be left in the appointment book with a single line drawn through it. It is also wise to phone the patient at home (and leave a message with someone or on the recorder if the patient cannot be reached) about the missed appointment. If patients cannot be reached by phone, mailing them a letter noting the missed appointment with a request that another appointment be arranged by calling the office. This procedure provides legal protection if a lawsuit is filed against the physician for failure to provide care for the patient. Having this process documented will show concern for the patient. It is difficult to prove negligence when such efforts to offer medical help have been made.

Appointment Book Maintenance

You should never erase a name or use liquid paper to **obliterate** a name in the book. Do not use pencil. There are those who, even though it not a suggested practice, use pencil in their appointment books. If this is the case, the entries should be written over at the end of the day in black ink. Having used pencil and possibly erasing from time to time during the course of the day may make the appointment book look messy, besides raising questions as to what names were erased and why it was done. Having a patient's name in the schedule book even though the appointment may not have been kept will help defend ef-

1.	NP	new patient
2.	CPE (CPX)	complete physical examination
3.	FU	follow-up examination
4.	NS	no show
5.	RS	reschedule
6.	C&C	called and canceled
	C	canceled
7.	Ref	referral
8.	Re✓	re-check
9.	PT	physical therapy
10.	Cons	consultation
11.	Inj	injection
12.	ECG	electrocardiogram
13.	Sig	sigmoidoscopy
14.	Surg	surgery
15.	Lab	laboratory studies
16.	BP✓	blood pressure check

FIGURE 6–14 The entire staff must know abbreviations (specific to the practice) and their meanings and use them consistently. Here is a sample list.

forts of providing the patient with the opportunity for medical care if ever the need arises. If there is no name on the appointment schedule because it has been erased, it is very difficult to prove that care was offered to the person. Management consultants advise that no altering of the schedule be done, as it may look as if one was trying to conceal information or fraudulently add it in at a later date. The appointment schedule is an official legal document and must be legible. For a cancellation, place a large letter "C" at the beginning of the person's name to indicate a cancellation, or "C&C" to indicate that the patient did call to tell you the reason the appointment had to be canceled. Some office personnel find it helpful to use a stamp to record in the chart the fact that the patient did not keep the appointment. The date, time, and reason (if known) for the missed appointment would be all that you would need to write, plus your initials. All staff members should be given a copy of the abbreviations common to your facility so that there is consistency with their use and the meanings are clear. A list of some common abbreviations that can be used in the appointment schedule is shown in Figure 6–14. A more extensive list of abbreviations is in the appendix of this text.

For legal concerns, all appointment schedule books must be kept for three years. It should be positioned out of the reach and eyesight of other patients and unauthorized persons.

MISCELLANEOUS APPOINTMENT SCHEDULING

In addition to routine scheduled appointments, emergency situations, and unexpected disruptions, there are other ancillary health professionals who may stop in to give the physician new information regarding medications, office equipment, medical supplies, and so on. A better way to deal with this before it becomes a routine disruption is to offer a regular appointment to the sales person or pharmaceutical representative (or detail person). Having a standing appointment (meaning at the same time and occurring regularly) for sales reps will give the physician the opportunity to acquire the most current information on products and have any questions answered immediately by the professional salesperson. Many reps bring in a variety of complimentary items on occasion, including lunch and other treats for the office staff. Leaving brochures and sample medications is another common practice of sales reps. You will have to organize and file or store all of the items which are left after the physician sees them. There is no need to schedule an extended amount of time for these individuals. Often the doctor chats briefly in the hallway and only a portion of the time blocked out for the appointment is actually used. Many physicians prefer not to see these sales people and ask that they talk to the office manager or medical assistant or just send information by mail only. If any new items are of particular use to the practice, information and samples may be left for the physician's perusal. If another doctor or a family member stops in to see the physician, you should politely interrupt and let the physician know so that the guest does not have to wait. A reminder to the physician-employer that the reception room has X number of patients waiting is a good idea before the meeting ensues. If the practice of surprise visits becomes a habit, it should be addressed in a staff meeting or in a private conference with the physician.

The medical assistant should note trouble spots in the schedule and report them to the physician or office manager periodically. This subject can be presented at staff meetings so that, with sharing ideas and suggestions, a better schedule may result. If the problem is that patients have had to wait far too long to see the doctor over a period of time (that is more often than not), then it is possible that there are more appointments made than the doctor can see in the set "office hours" and the simple remedy is that fewer appointments should be scheduled. It is vital to the success of a schedule that the medical assistant maintain open communication with the physician and staff regarding patient flow. The development of a team feeling should allow staff to be honest, consistent, loyal, and considerate and by all means to avoid gossip. A professional image is reflected through attitude, abilities, appearance, and ethics. When these characteristics are evident in a team spirit, cooperation and success will be obvious.

In certain situations where it seems that all efforts to improve scheduling have failed, it is smart to enlist an efficiency expert for an objective viewpoint. One who is not involved daily is better able to observe many points that could be changed for the better. The efficiency expert's expertise can make all staff members more aware

of how the schedule affects everyone throughout the office. The ideal schedule should provide a comfortable pace for the staff without making the patients feel rushed or slighted. *The importance of building good rapport with patients is invaluable; scheduling is where it begins.*

SETTING AND KEEPING REALISTIC SCHEDULES

Since the physician generally expects the medical assistant who schedules appointments to do so in time slots that are realistic for presenting complaints of the patients, a sample guideline for some typical office visits is presented in Figure 6–15. This is just a sample of the amount of time that may be spent with procedures and other services. The actual amount of time spent with patients will depend on the speed of the staff, the patient, and the physician, as well as how talkative all concerned are before, during, and after the service rendered. A good rapport is built with patients when the service is achieved, pleasantries are exchanged, and the time seems to pass quickly. Variations and rearranging of appointments may be necessary according to the way the course of events unfolds during any given day in the medical practice. Experience will be the best teacher in arriving at a successful schedule. Adding the patient's phone number next to his name on the appointment schedule makes it easy to contact the patient if it becomes necessary to alter the office schedule.

12	Lunch
12.15	
12.30	Carol Wang-Sig 555-0050
12.45	↓
1	Kenneth Franks BP✓ Lab
1.15	↓ 555-8846
1.30	Susan Steele-ECG
1.45	↓ 555-4495
2	Arnold Wing-CPE
2.15	
2.30	555-6483
2.45	↓
3	Work-ins
3.15	Peggy Watters Inj 555-9913
3.30	Walter Matthews PT
3.45	↓ 555-2237
4	Latasha Peters Cons
4.15	↓ 555-7702
4.30	Work-ins
4.45	Robert James BP✓ 555-4951

FIGURE 6–15 Sample time blocks for commonly scheduled appointments in a medical office

Helping to Maintain the Physician's Schedule

In addition to scheduling patients appropriately, the medical assistant has the responsibility to help the physician keep on time. If it looks as though the doctor is working faster than usual, calling in patients to be seen earlier to keep the patient flow moving at a steady pace is a sensible idea. On the other hand, sometimes there is an obvious slowing down on the part of the physician or other staff members, and the schedule is getting backed up. If the physician agrees that catching up is nearly impossible, the medical assistant should call patients and either delay their arrival time or reschedule them for another day. It is a necessary courtesy for you to explain tactfully to all patients who are waiting to see the physician when the schedule is getting behind because of an emergency. Remember that each patient has the right to feel that her time is just as important as anyone else's time, and therefore, you should offer to reschedule the appointment if the patient so chooses. A notation should be made in the patient's chart that because of an emergency the appointment was rescheduled and how long the patient had waited. Studies have shown that while a 10-hour day is 20% longer than an 8-hour day, the increase in productivity only rises 6% because of the increased likelihood of making errors. Therefore, overworking could prove hazardous to patients as well as to yourself and coworkers. The medical assistant may also want to work out a signal with the physician for those times when the patient gets too talkative and is taking more time than was allotted for the appointment. A suggestion is to interrupt by a signal over the speaker, such as "Excuse me doctor, you have a call on line five" (and there are only four phone lines). You may decide that a simple knock on the door or a particular signal on his or her pager can help the physician stay on task and help avoid getting further behind in schedule.

Handling Late Patients

There may be a few patients who seem to be late for every appointment. In this situation, you may schedule them just after you come back from lunch and work them in when they arrive, or you may decide to schedule them at the end of the day. If the person does not arrive for the appointment at the time it was scheduled, a reasonable time of waiting is documented, and attempts are made to reach the patient by phone to determine if she is still coming. Late arrivals can be told that they need to reschedule their appointment if it is impossible to work them in. Late and missed appointments should be documented in the chart. After the first offense, established office policy regarding late or missed appointments should be explained. If the appointment was at the end of the day, the patient should be advised regarding the length of waiting time established. With documentation in the chart, a pattern of late arrivals or missed appointments can be verified to discuss with the patient. If there are some extenuating circumstances such as transportation, child care, or work-associated problems, then a solution must be found to solve the problem. This type of problem may be alleviated if a printed sign posted in the reception area and a statement in the office information brochure state that patients who are late past a specific period of time must be rescheduled for the appointment. Providing printed information regarding office hours as well as posting them will help to avoid such situations from happening.

At certain times of the year there seems to be expected conditions that play havoc with a schedule, such as colds and flu in the winter months, injuries during winter and spring breaks from school, rashes and other ailments related to summer, and so on. These problems must be taken into account when preparing the daily schedule, especially the types of problems specific to the particular practice where you are employed. A pause of a few minutes between patient exams is acceptable. However, if there is too much slack time and more than a few minutes between patients happens too often, scheduling techniques need to be reviewed. Figure 6–16 offers a list of some helpful points to keep in mind when scheduling appointments. The saying "Time is money" is a good thought to consider. It should remind us to use time well and for the purpose intended. Efficient use of the physi-

---

The main points to remember in making appointments are:

1. Have the name exactly right.
2. Make the appointment for the next hour available.
3. Be sure the date and time are clearly understood.
4. Allow enough time for each appointment.
5. Check to see that no one else is scheduled at the same time for the same service.
6. Ask the time of day each patient prefers for an appointment: AM or PM?
7. When scheduling a series of appointments for the same patient, try to use the same day and time to make it easier for the patient to remember.
8. Offer a choice: "Would you like to come today at 3:00 or tomorrow at 9:00?"
9. If you have to refuse a request for an appointment at a certain time, explain why this is necessary and try to find another time that is convenient for the patient.
10. Enter the appointment in your appointment book or computer.
11. Complete an appointment card and hand it to the patient.
12. Try to allow extra time for emergencies each day.

FIGURE 6–16

cian's time and the entire staff's as well in treating patients is the main purpose of a schedule. Again, cooperation among the staff is required for a successful outcome.

APPOINTMENTS OUTSIDE THE MEDICAL OFFICE

When a patient develops a condition or requires an examination that your office cannot take care of, your employer will refer the patient to an appropriate colleague or facility. The office should have a page in the office procedures manual listing the names, addresses, and phone numbers of physicians your employer wishes to refer patients to in the different specialty areas. You should give at least two names. Keep handy for use the name, address, and phone number of facilities where you might refer patients (e.g., laboratories, x-ray facilities, and community clinics). Keep in mind that certain managed care plans require referrals (Procedure 6–6) to specialists within the plan with the approval of the primary care physician (**gatekeeper**). A list of these plans and participating physicians for handy referral is an excellent time saver.

When a patient is to be admitted to the hospital, it is important to know what admission information the hospital will require. Be prepared when you call to give the necessary information regarding the patient.

Hospitals have established guidelines for admitting patients. The purpose of these guidelines is to cut the cost of hospital care. If the care needed by the patient can be given in an outpatient facility, this must be the method used. Many insurance companies and government sponsored programs require a preadmission evaluation of the need for hospitalization of a patient. To determine the need for admission, a **criterion** statement would need to be composed by the admitting physician using specific terminology as to severity of the illness and an assessment of need. Definitions that may be given for these terms are:

acute onset—symptoms occurred within last six hours.
sudden onset—symptoms occurred within last twenty four hours.
recent onset—symptoms occurred within past week.
recently or newly discovered—symptoms not present on previous examination.

In some cases, in addition to terms describing the severity of the illness, the vital signs (temperature, pulse, respiration, and blood pressure), laboratory workup, any functional impairment, the physical findings, the need for monitoring, the medications needed, and the procedures, along with criteria for discharge, must be considered as part of the determination for need of admission.

PROCEDURE

6-6 Arrange Referral Appointment

PURPOSE: Schedule a referral appointment for a patient in a professional manner.

EQUIPMENT AND SUPPLIES: Patient's chart with referral request, phone directory, phone, pen, and paper.

PERFORMANCE OBJECTIVE: In a simulated situation, schedule a referral appointment for a patient by phoning the requested medical facility according to accepted medical standards with consideration for the physician, staff, and needs of the patient.

1. Obtain patient's chart with request for referral to other facility.

2. Use the phone directory to obtain phone number and address of the referral office.

3. Place the call to the referral office and provide the receptionist with:
   - your name and physician's name and address and phone
   - patient's name, address, and so on, and reason for the appointment

NOTE: It is a courtesy to also write the person's name down who schedules the referral appointment for the patient for any further questions the patient may have and for directions on how to get there.
   - indicate if you will send a confirmation letter of the referral request by mail or fax.
   - record appointment information on the patient's chart; also write the time, day and date, name, address, and so on, on paper for the patient to keep.

   NOTE: If the patient is standing before you while you make the referral appointment call, be sure to ask if the date is okay before you finalize the conversation. (If the patient is not present, you must phone the patient to confirm the appointment.)

4. Give the patient printed instructions regarding the appointment, as appropriate, and directions to the facility.

5. Initial the patient's chart, signifying the completion of the request.

In scheduling an admission, you may be asked to identify the attending physician for the admission, the service admitting under (i.e., whether medical, surgical, or obstetric), the admission date requested, and the type of reservation. The type of reservation might be: inpatient, admitting day surgery (ADS), ambulatory surgery (AS); patients who walk in, have surgery, and go home; or outpatient. Some hospitals furnish nearby hotel rooms for **chemotherapy** patients or other patients who need daily treatment for several hours but do not need to be admitted to a hospital room. Other information needed is listed here:

1. Full name of the patient (include birth name of married female patient if the woman has changed her name)
2. Age and date of birth
3. Sex of patient
4. Marital status
5. Social Security number
6. Address (including zip code)
7. Telephone numbers (home, pager or cell phone, and work) of patient and closest relative
8. Primary insurance **guarantor** and Social Security number of this individual
9. Employer of guarantor and work telephone number
10. Hospital insurance coverage along with verification if prior authorization granted
11. Name, address, and phone number of referring physician
12. The physician needs to furnish the diagnosis and plan of care for the **utilization** committee review.
13. If surgery is to be scheduled, you need to give the date of surgery, expected length of procedure in hours, name of procedure, type of anesthesia, units of blood needed, and whether x-rays will be taken.
14. When preadmission testing is to be carried out, you need to know the date, time, and names of tests, x-rays, ECG, and patient prep. If a generally required test is not ordered, you need to explain why it was not ordered.

The following conditions will generally justify inpatient hospital care for an otherwise outpatient procedure if the severity of the illness or intensity of service needed warrants it:

1. Severe myocardial insufficiency (with or without angina)
2. Chronic congestive heart failure
3. Chronic obstructive lung disease
4. Bronchial asthma
5. Diabetes
6. Thyroid disease
7. Hypertension

Guidelines are generally established with a detailed listing by current ICD–CM codes (International Classification of Diseases, Clinical Modification) for elective, outpatient procedures, for elective procedures that might require a preoperative length of stay, and for those procedures to be done on admission day.

FOLLOW-UP APPOINTMENTS

It is the medical assistant's responsibility to assist patients with their payments and any necessary follow-up or referral appointments after the physician has seen them.

The need for a follow-up appointment may be marked by the physician on the charge slip, or the patient may be told to inform you of this need. The patient should be given the choice of two appointment times, and only after the entry is made in the appointment book should an appointment card be prepared and given to the patient. This practice will prevent the possibility of forgetting to enter the patient's name in the book.

Physicians who treat patients who need regular follow-up but do not make appointments a year in advance may choose to send a recall notice. This notice could be a preprinted card sent to the patient as a reminder to call or write for an appointment. An example would be a reminder for an annual Pap test. Some offices find it helpful to send a reminder notice of appointments that were made far in advance. You might even ask the patient to address such a card at the time the appointment is made. The patient is handed an appointment card, which he may lose, and at the same time addresses a card with the appointment time marked on it. You place this in a file under the date when it should be mailed. This practice might be helpful for the forgetful **geriatric** patient or the busy executive who may forget to put the appointment on the calendar along with business appointments.

ACHIEVE UNIT OBJECTIVES

Complete Chapter 6, Unit 2, in the workbook to help you obtain competency of this subject matter.

UNIT 3

Written Communications

OBJECTIVES

Upon completion of the unit, meet the following performance objectives by verifying knowledge of the facts and principles presented through oral and written communication at a level deemed competent, and demonstrate the specific behaviors as identified in the performance objectives of the procedures, observing safety precautions in accordance with health care standards.

1. Spell and define, using the glossary at the back of the text, all the **Words to Know** in this unit.
2. List seven types of correspondence medical assistants may need to prepare.
3. Name instances when form letters may be indicated.
4. Produce a memo.

5. Demonstrate correct grammar, spelling, punctuation, and sentence structure to compose original letters.
6. Name six specific criteria for written communications.
7. Name and give examples of the eight parts of speech.
8. Identify the nine standards for producing a mailable business letter.
9. Explain the characteristics of business letter styles.
10. Use the formatting standards to prepare a business letter.
11. Use standard proofreading marks.
12. Describe 11 problem areas in written communications.

AREAS OF COMPETENCE (AAMA)

This unit addresses content within the areas of *Administrative procedures, Professionalism, Communication skills*, and *Legal concepts* as identified in the Medical Assistant Role Delineation Study. Refer to appendix A for a detailed listing of the areas.

A CAAHEP CONNECTION

Curriculum standards indicate the need to provide information regarding **Communication**, which includes *Fundamental writing skills, Application of electronic technology*, and *Responding to verbal communication*. The additional area of **Medical Terminology**, which includes *Application of terms, Structure of medical words*, and *Word building*, is also required. The content of this unit addresses these areas by discussing parts of speech, spelling rules, punctuation, and business letter composition. The Words to Know in this and other units address the areas of terminology and word building.

■ WORDS TO KNOW

adjective	interjection
adverb	mailable
apostrophe	misspelled
clause	modifies
communication	noun
compose	postscript
congratulations	preposition
conjunction	pronoun
context	proofread
contraction	punctuation
correspondence	signature
critique	stationery
denote	thesaurus
ellipses	verb
galley proofs	watermark
hyphen	

WRITTEN COMMUNICATION

A **Patient Reception Area:**
  ■ Correspondence—
    Letter

What is **communication**? One dictionary defines it as "the giving or receiving of information; a system for sending and receiving messages." You can communicate in many ways such as talking, gesturing, or writing. Written communication is often called **correspondence**. Again, the dictionary says correspondence is "communication by the exchange of letters." An individual who is hired by a newspaper or magazine to furnish news regularly from a certain place is called a correspondent. There are schools from which you can receive instruction in a particular sub-

ject by mail. They are known as correspondence schools. But in its broader sense, correspondence can be thought of as any exchange of information between persons. With this interpretation, correspondence or written communication could include the sending of notes, inneroffice communications (IOCs), form letters, information sheets, and business, professional and personal letters.

In a physician's office, written communication is often necessary:

■ to officially inform the staff of a policy or decision.
■ to contact professional colleagues.
■ to correspond with professional associations.
■ to request or respond to a medical consultation.
■ to engage in business communications with medical suppliers, financial consultants, attorneys, and insurance companies.
■ to send personal messages.

Inneroffice Communication (IOC)

This is an informal memo style communication that is usually specific to one concern. It is an effective way of being certain that everyone is aware of some event, policy, concern, and so on. If you want to ensure that everyone reads the memo, a copy must be given to each person, or a copy can be posted or circulated with an attached list of all people involved, who then must enter their initials next to their names to indicate they have read the IOC. An example might look something like Figure 6–17A and B.

Informal Notes

This type of correspondence is also informal in nature and would be indicated for times when "thank you's," **congratulations**, or similar expressions are desired. Usually, these are personal in nature. Often, these are written on a first-name basis.

SAMUEL E. MATTHEWS, MD
100 EAST MAIN STREET, SUITE 120
YOURTOWN, US 98765-4321

DATE: April 3, 20--
TO: Office staff
FROM: Doctor Sam
SUBJECT: New office computer system

Representatives from ABC Electronics will be at our office on April 10 and 11 to provide instruction on the use of our new equipment. Please see Joyce and schedule yourself into one of the four orientation sessions. After you have selected your time, enter your initials next to your name on the sheet at her desk to verify you have responded to this memo.

Thank you for your cooperation in this matter.

(A)

SAMUEL E. MATTHEWS, MD
100 EAST MAIN STREET, SUITE 120
YOURTOWN, US 98765-4321

After you have read the memo and selected a time for your orientation, please initial below on the line by your name. Your initials verify your response to the memo to attend one session presented by ABC Electronics on April 10 or 11.

_____	Amy Adornio	_____	Gerri Gore
_____	Betty Barry	_____	Harry Hecht
_____	Chuck Cukovich	_____	Inez Immel
_____	Diane Delong	_____	Jacki James
_____	Emily Everett	_____	Kelly Kendzierski
_____	Frank Flaherty	_____	Lisa Long

(B)

FIGURE 6–17 (A) Inneroffice communication (IOC); (B) IOC circulation sheet

Personal Letters

The physician may ask for assistance with personal correspondence. It is common for medical assistants to correspond with travel agencies, mail order catalogs, perhaps clothing suppliers, and specialty shops. A competent medical assistant should be able to **compose** (write) the necessary letter after receiving the specific information desired, so all the physician has to do is sign her **signature**.

Professional Letters

Physicians may need to write to their professional associations, licensing boards, and other physicians regarding some issue or concern affecting personal medical activities or their professional practice. Perhaps your employer holds an office in a medical society which requires communicating with the members or issuing the group's opinion on a particular subject to the community or media. Some physicians hold office on a hospital medical board which might necessitate issuing of written communication. Physicians who participate in research do a great deal of professional correspondence in regard to the experimental studies being conducted. Some physicians enjoy writing professional journal articles about a unique patient or explaining a procedure they have developed. Obviously, these specific writings require detailed dictating and perfect transcription.

Business Letters

The greatest amount of correspondence however, is of the business type required to manage the affairs of the practice. This would include the referrals, consulting, annual examination reminders, collection letters, school and work releases, suppliers of equipment and materials, and other correspondence necessary to the office operation. These types of letters can be individually composed or a form letter may be used. Prewritten form letters can be developed and stored electronically on disks of computers or word processors. When needed, the letter is pulled up, the appropriate date, name, address, amount due, and so on, is added, and it is sent without the need to prepare the total letter. Form letters are especially well suited for:

- return to work or school approvals (following surgery or illness).
- annual diagnostic examination reminders (eye examinations, Pap tests, mammogram, sigmoidoscopy).
- delinquent account reminders, usually in about three increasing levels of request intensity.
- office visit verifications (for work or school absence).
- athletic participation approvals.
- providing information to referred patients regarding appointment confirmation, office location, information needed, approximate time required for appointment, payment policy, and so on.

Several businesses offer prepared medical forms both in hard copy for completion or as software packages for computer use.

The *master* of each hard-copy form letter is stored in a file, and copies are made as needed. Specific information appropriate to the recipient is entered in the blank areas. This method requires a little practice to line up margins and lines so that it matches the rest of the letter.

Software form letters are very efficient and convenient. The appropriate form letter can be pulled up from the program, and the necessary specific information can be added and then printed out. When the same form letter will be sent to several people, specific information for each person can be added in a data format along with the name, address, and salutation and then merged to produce an individualized letter.

Information Sheets

Specific written instructions regarding the examinations and diagnostic tests performed in your office are very beneficial to patients. They help to reinforce what you have explained and serve as a reminder after they leave the office. They typically explain to patients how to prepare themselves for a particular test or what to expect when the test is performed. Usually there is a place on the form to enter the date and time the examination is scheduled. These information sheets can be prepared and stored in the files to be used as needed.

PREPARING WRITTEN COMMUNICATION

Almost every day, when the mail carrier arrives, there will be something received which requires a response. Your employer may want to review all the mail personally and request that you only open the envelopes and arrange everything neatly on the desk. Some physicians allow the mail to be opened and sorted, referring to only professional or personal material which requires their response; anything pertaining to the practice operation is handled by the office manager.

After a few days, the physician will need to devote some time to drafting responses to inquiries or responding to referrals. Some may use a dictating machine while others may prefer to dictate in person. Surgeons and other specialists who have a large number of referral patients will have the greatest amount of responses to compose. Usually a type of form letter is developed with the opening and closing paragraphs being a standard format and the middle of the letter specific to the patient. This format only requires minimal dictation, after the opening "Thank you for referring . . ." and the closing "If I can be of any additional assistance . . ." Of course, occasionally, written communication is required that is specific to a request or concern so the total correspondence is individualized.

Probably the most important criteria about any communication is that it be written using proper grammar and punctuation and have no **misspelled** words. It also must be spaced on the page properly and be neat and clean. Try not to use the same major word twice in the same or even consecutive sentence. The following information will assist you in producing attractive, error-free communications.

Spelling

Spelling is difficult for some people. If you are one of them you will have to try exceptionally hard until you master certain rules and habits. Here are some ideas that might help.

- If you have certain words that you cannot seem to spell correctly, try making a list of them to use as a quick reference.
- Make a mental picture of the word correctly spelled.
- Pronounce the word correctly several times.
- Write the word, dividing it into syllables and inserting accent marks.
- Write or type the word several times.
- Learn to use a general and medical dictionary when you are in doubt.
- If you use a word processor or computer software to compose correspondence, be sure to run your document on the spell checker. It will catch most errors. (Unfortunately you cannot rely on the checker completely because it is possible that the word is spelled correctly but you have entered the wrong word, a word "out of **context**." Examples of this are using "their" for "there," "cite" for "sight," "rite" for "right," "your" for "you're," and several others.)

There are 14 rules about spelling which are very helpful once you understand how to use them. Refer to Figure 6–18.

Parts of Speech

To compose effective, well-written communications, you need to be aware of the eight parts of speech and how they are used (Table 6–1).

Once you have the spelling and the parts of speech under control, it is time to put the words together in sentences. Written material should be composed of sentences of differing lengths and complexity to appropriately match the written matter being prepared. Patient referral or business letters require concise material while personal correspondence or medical articles can contain more variety. Be careful not to make run-on sentences containing too many clauses. The following information outlines sentence construction.

Sentence Structure

When writing letters, write in complete thoughts. A *simple sentence* consists of only one complete thought, that is, one independent clause with a subject and a verb.

Examples:

Physicians examine patients.
Physicians prescribe medication.
The receptionist scheduled appointments.

A *compound sentence* contains two or more independent clauses, separated by a comma.

Examples:

The physician dictates letters, and the medical assistant transcribes them.

Rule 1. Write *ie* when the sound is *ee*, as in:

achieve	piece
field	shield
grief	yield

EXCEPT after *c*, as in:

conceive	perceive
deceive	receive

OTHER EXCEPTIONS:

leisure	seize
neither	weird

Rule 2. Write *ei* when the sound is not long *e*, especially when the sound is long *a*, as in:

freight	veil
height	vein
sleigh	weigh

EXCEPTIONS:
friend
mischief

Rule 3. The prefixes *mis, il, in, im,* and *dis* do not change the spelling of the root word:

mis + spell = misspell
il + legal = illegal
il + literate = illiterate
in + audible = inaudible
im + mature = immature
dis + appear = disappear

Rule 4. Only one word in English ends in *sede: supersede.*
Only three words end in *ceed: exceed, proceed,* and *succeed.*
All other words of similar sound end in *cede,* as in:

concede
recede
precede

Rule 5. The suffixes *ly* and *ness* do not change the spelling of the root word:

sudden + ness = suddenness
final + ly = finally
truthful + ly = truthfully
lean + ness = leanness

EXCEPTIONS: Words ending in *y* preceded by a consonant change *y* to *i* before any suffix not beginning with *i*:
kindly + ness = kindliness
happy + ly = happily
happy + ness = happiness
Words ending in *y* preceded by a vowel also follow this rule.

Rule 6. Drop the *e* from the end of a word before adding the suffixes *al, ed, ing,* and *able*:

complete—completed—completing
care—caring
fine—final
love—lovable
observe—observable

EXCEPTIONS: Words ending in *ce* and *ge* usually keep the silent *e* when the suffix begins with *a* or *o* in order to preserve the soft sound of the final consonant:
notice + able = noticeable
change + able = changeable

Rule 7. Keep the final *e* before a suffix beginning with a consonant:

large + ly = largely
care + ful = careful
care + less = careless
state + ment = statement

EXCEPTIONS:
argue + ment = argument
true + ly = truly

Rule 8. With words of one syllable ending in a single consonant preceded by a single vowel, double the consonant before adding *ing, ed,* or *er*:

sit + ing = sitting
hop + ed = hopped
dip + er = dipper
run + ing = running
swim + ing = swimming

Rule 9. If a one-syllable word ends in a single consonant not preceded by a single vowel, do not double the consonant before adding *ing, ed,* or *er*:

reap + ed = reaped
heat + ing = heating

Rule 10. To make a word ending in *y* plural, check the letter before the *y*. If it is a vowel, just add *s*:

birthday—birthdays
day—days
ray—rays
toy—toys

If it is any other letter, change the *y* to *i* and add *es*:

city—cities
lady—ladies
study—studies
guppy—guppies
fly—flies

Rule 11. Most nouns (names of people, places, things, ideas) become plural by adding *s*:

boy—boys	desk—desks
dog—dogs	window—windows

Rule 12. The plural of nouns ending in *s, x, z, ch,* or *sh* is formed by adding *es*:

wax—waxes
dish—dishes
waltz—waltzes

Rule 13. The plural of most nouns ending in *f* is formed by adding *s*. The plural of some nouns ending in *fo* or *fe* is formed by changing the *f* to *v* and adding *s* or *es*:

gulf—gulfs	knifes—knives
belief—beliefs	life—lives

Rule 14. The plural of nouns ending in *o* preceded by a vowel is formed by adding *s*. The plural of nouns ending in *o* preceded by a consonant is formed by adding *es*:

patio—patios
ratio—ratios
tornado—tornadoes
hero—heroes

EXCEPTIONS:
eskimo—eskimos
silo—silos

FIGURE 6-18 Spelling reference rules

TABLE 6-1

THE EIGHT PARTS OF SPEECH

Speech Part	Description	Word Examples	Example of Use
Noun	The name of anything, such as: a person, a place, an object, an occurrence, or a state	assistant, office, attention, laboratory, Texas, computer	The *assistant* draws *blood* and takes it to the *laboratory*.
Pronoun	A substitute for a noun	she, her, he, him, his, which, some, everyone, it, their they, nobody	*He* called *her* to see if *she* knew if *anyone* else was going to the in-service program.
Verb	A word or word group that expresses action or a state of being	write, perform, cut, assist, attend, run, jump, enter am, is, are, will be, have been, feel, seem, appear	The assistant *measured* the patient's blood pressure and *entered* the findings on the chart.
Adjective	Describes, limits, or restricts a noun or pronoun	efficient, dedicated, tall, thin, dependable, irregular	Joyce is an *efficient* and *dependable* medical assistant.
Adverb	**Modifies** a verb, adjective, or another adverb. Adverbs commonly end in "-ly" and are used to answer questions.	How? What? When? Where? How often?	*Frequently* Jane arrives *early* for work and often stays *late*.
Preposition	Shows the relationship of an object to some other word in the sentence	of, with, without, for, above, below, on, from, between	*Between* you and me, Dr. Morrison's handwriting is, *without* a doubt, the most difficult *to* read.
Conjunction	Connects words, phrases, and clauses	and, but, or, for, because, if	We can work Jane in *if* she can be here by 1:00 *but* not at 3:00 as she requested.
Interjection	Used to express strong feeling or emotion. These words are usually followed by an exclamation point or a comma.	oh, hurray, ouch, wow	*Hurray!* We received the research grant.

Administrative medical assistants perform clerical duties, and clinical medical assistants perform clinical duties. Laboratory technicians analyze specimens, and medical assistants assist with physical examinations.

A *complex sentence* contains one independent clause and one or more dependent clauses. A dependent clause cannot stand alone as a sentence.

Examples:

The doctor, who is off on Thursdays, sees allergy patients in the morning. (An adjective clause)

Patients are sometimes quite apprehensive when they come to the office for diagnostic examination. (An adverb clause)

Physicians require that patients receive proper instructions for diagnostic procedures. (Noun clause)

A *compound–complex sentence* contains two or more independent clauses plus one or more dependent clauses.

Example:

Medical assistants should seek continuing education because medical technology is constantly changing, and the medical assistant must keep current with new procedures.

Punctuation Marks

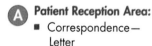 **Patient Reception Area:**
- Correspondence—Letter

To make sentences easier to read and to tell a reader when you come to the end of a thought, a variety of markings called **punctuation** are used. The most common are the comma, period, apostrophe, hyphen, and ellipsis. The following information describes the correct usage of these marks.

- A *period* is placed at the end of each sentence.
- A *comma* or period should appear before an ending quotation mark: "or."

There are four general rules for the use of a comma:

1. Use between main **clauses** connected by *and, but, so, for, or, nor,* and *yet.* If main clauses are short, no comma is needed.
2. Use following long introductory phrases or clauses that may begin with words such as *after, whenever, if, until, since,* and *once.*

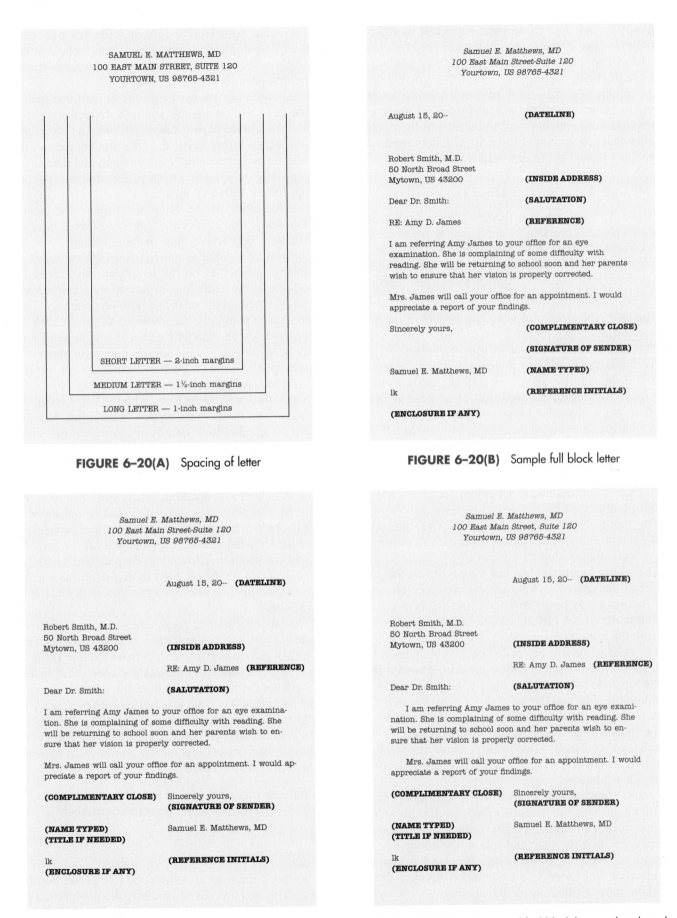

SAMUEL E. MATTHEWS, MD
100 EAST MAIN STREET, SUITE 120
YOURTOWN, US 98765-4321

SHORT LETTER — 2-inch margins

MEDIUM LETTER — 1½-inch margins

LONG LETTER — 1-inch margins

FIGURE 6–20(A) Spacing of letter

Samuel E. Matthews, MD
100 East Main Street-Suite 120
Yourtown, US 98765-4321

August 15, 20--   **(DATELINE)**

Robert Smith, M.D.
50 North Broad Street
Mytown, US 43200   **(INSIDE ADDRESS)**

Dear Dr. Smith: **(SALUTATION)**

RE: Amy D. James   **(REFERENCE)**

I am referring Amy James to your office for an eye
examination. She is complaining of some difficulty with
reading. She will be returning to school soon and her parents
wish to ensure that her vision is properly corrected.

Mrs. James will call your office for an appointment. I would
appreciate a report of your findings.

Sincerely yours,   **(COMPLIMENTARY CLOSE)**

          (SIGNATURE OF SENDER)

Samuel E. Matthews, MD   **(NAME TYPED)**

lk   **(REFERENCE INITIALS)**

(ENCLOSURE IF ANY)

FIGURE 6–20(B) Sample full block letter

Samuel E. Matthews, MD
100 East Main Street-Suite 120
Yourtown, US 98765-4321

                    August 15, 20-- **(DATELINE)**

Robert Smith, M.D.
50 North Broad Street
Mytown, US 43200   **(INSIDE ADDRESS)**

                    RE: Amy D. James **(REFERENCE)**

Dear Dr. Smith: **(SALUTATION)**

I am referring Amy James to your office for an eye examination. She is complaining of some difficulty with reading. She
will be returning to school soon and her parents wish to ensure that her vision is properly corrected.

Mrs. James will call your office for an appointment. I would appreciate a report of your findings.

(COMPLIMENTARY CLOSE) Sincerely yours,
                    (SIGNATURE OF SENDER)

(NAME TYPED)   Samuel E. Matthews, MD
(TITLE IF NEEDED)

lk
(ENCLOSURE IF ANY)   **(REFERENCE INITIALS)**

FIGURE 6–20(C) Sample modified block letter

Samuel E. Matthews, MD
100 East Main Street, Suite 120
Yourtown, US 98765-4321

                    August 15, 20-- **(DATELINE)**

Robert Smith, M.D.
50 North Broad Street
Mytown, US 43200   **(INSIDE ADDRESS)**

                    RE: Amy D. James **(REFERENCE)**

Dear Dr. Smith: **(SALUTATION)**

    I am referring Amy James to your office for an eye exami-
nation. She is complaining of some difficulty with reading. She
will be returning to school soon and her parents wish to ensure that her vision is properly corrected.

    Mrs. James will call your office for an appointment. I would
appreciate a report of your findings.

(COMPLIMENTARY CLOSE) Sincerely yours,
                    (SIGNATURE OF SENDER)

(NAME TYPED)   Samuel E. Matthews, MD
(TITLE IF NEEDED)

lk   **(REFERENCE INITIALS)**
(ENCLOSURE IF ANY)

FIGURE 6–20(D) Sample modified block letter with indented paragraphs

A **watermark** appears on bond paper and should read across the paper in the same direction as the typing. You can determine the correct watermark side by holding the paper to the light.

Be certain to make a copy of every business letter or report to be sent from the office. Copies of correspondence regarding patients need to be filed in their charts. Correspondence in answer to business letters need to be copied and placed in the appropriate file.

COMPOSE A BUSINESS LETTER

A letter can be prepared from dictated notes or from a dictation machine tape, or it may be composed by you at the keyboard. There are certain formatting standards which result in a mailable letter. The following are points to remember as you perform Procedure 6–7, "Compose a Business Letter."

Points to remember are:

- The date typed indicates when the content of the letter was dictated.
- The month is spelled out in full (traditional style is month/day/year; military style is day/month/year).
- The inside address should be copied exactly from the correspondence to be answered or as printed in the phone book or medical society directory.
- A courtesy title is used (Mr., Mrs., Miss, or Ms. If gender unknown, use Mr.).
- Do not use Dr. before the physician's name if MD follows.
- If a street address and box number are given, use the box number.
- The words North, South, East, and West preceding street names and Road, Street, Avenue, and Boulevard are NOT abbreviated.
- The words Apartment and Suite are typed on the same line as the address and are separated by a comma.
- Apartment may be abbreviated if the line is long.
- The name of the city is spelled out and is separated from the state by a comma.
- The state name can be spelled out or abbreviated (see Unit 4 for list of abbreviations) and is separated from the zip code by one space; there is no punctuation between the state and the zip code.
- A proper salutation is Dear followed by the title and the person's last name. If the correspondence is to a colleague or friend, a first name is appropriate (ask the physician). When writing to a business, use "Dear Sir" or "Dear Madam."
- To use a reference line, type "RE:," then the person's full name. This line goes two spaces *below* the salutation, flush with the left margin in block style. It may be lined up with the date and follow the address in the modified block style. It is a common error to type the reference line prior to the salutation because that is where most dictators name the person.
- Always double space between paragraphs, flush left with block style and indented five spaces with modified block.

- If a second page is necessary, stop the first page at the end of a paragraph, if possible. If not, include at least two lines from the broken paragraph on the bottom of the first page.
- The bottom margin must measure at least one inch.
- The last word on a page cannot be divided.
- When a second page is necessary, enter a second page heading in either vertical or horizontal format. The heading includes name, page number, and date.
- Capitalize only the first word of a complimentary closing; follow with a comma.
- The formality of the letter determines the closing: "Cordially" or "Sincerely" is considered informal, whereas "Very truly yours" is more formal.
- The sender's name is entered four spaces below the closing, exactly as on the letterhead; an official title follows on the same line, separated by a comma, or it can be typed on the next line with no comma.
- The typist's initials, in lower case, are placed two spaces below the sender's name. When the sender will not be signing the letter, both dictator's (in upper case) and typist's initials are used. Typists do not use their reference initials on letters they sign.
- When items will be enclosed with the letter, enter "Enclosure" or "Enc." one or two lines below reference initials; number and identify if more than one enclosure is included.
- If copies are sent to others, enter "cc" (for carbon copy) and the other receiver's name one or two spaces below the initials or last notation. When more than one individual is carbon copied, list their names alphabetically or by rank. When a copy is sent to another person without the knowledge of the recipient, it is known as a *blind copy*. No notation is placed on the recipient's letter, but *bcc* is placed on the file copy to **denote** it was sent.
- A **postscript** (PS) is entered two spaces below the last notation.
- When using a second page, a heading of the patient's name, page number and date, is entered either vertically or horizontally, one inch from the top. If the letter does not concern a patient, the receiver is listed.
- The letter continues on the third line after the heading; the page should contain at least two lines of a paragraph.
- Print a draft copy and proof it. Proofing on screen is difficult because you cannot view the total letter at one time. Make corrections on the stored copy, and print the letter on a letterhead.

Compose a business letter following the steps in Procedure 6–7, referring to the points to remember.

Proofreading

All written communication must be **proofread** before it is sent. This is a process of carefully reading printed material and marking errors for correction. The spell checker and immediate feedback of composition errors from word processing software will identify most of your common

PROCEDURE

6-7 Compose a Business Letter

PURPOSE: To prepare a mailable business letter.

EQUIPMENT AND SUPPLIES: Word processor or computer, paper, dictation machine or dictation tape, and transcriber.

PERFORMANCE OBJECTIVE: Given access to equipment and supplies, complete a mailable letter following the steps in the procedure within the number of attempts and time frame specified by the instructor. The final copy must meet mailable standards described in this text.

1. Move cursor down at least three lines below letterhead.

2. Enter the date. **NOTE: Be sure that the location is appropriate for the chosen style.**

3. Move to the fifth line below the date.

4. Enter the inside address.
   NOTE: Be sure the address is in the appropriate location for the style of letter. Use the appropriate courtesy title and enter the name exactly as printed on the received letterhead or as is in the phone or medical society directory.

5. Double space after the last line of the address.

6. Enter the appropriate salutation followed by a colon.

7. Double space.

8. Enter the reference line in the location appropriate for letter style. Type RE: Enter patient's name or person about whom the letter is written.

9. Double space.

10. Enter the body (content) of the letter.
    ■ Be sure the paragraph style is appropriate to the style of the letter.
    ■ Always double space between paragraphs.
    ■ If a second page is needed, end the first page at the end of a paragraph. If this is not possible, place at least two lines of the paragraph on the first page. Do not divide the last word on the first page.

11. When a second page is necessary, enter the second page heading in vertical or horizontal format.
    NOTE: Includes name, page number, and date.

12. Continue body of letter.

13. Enter a complimentary closing in letter style format.

14. Go down four spaces.

15. Enter the sender's name in letter style format exactly as printed on letterhead.
    NOTE: An official title follows the name on the same line separated by a comma, or it is placed directly below, with no comma required.

16. Double space.

17. Enter reference initials to indicate the typist.

18. Single or double space if enclosing materials.

19. Enter the preferred style enclosure.
    NOTE: Number and identify if there is more than one enclosure.

20. Single or double space if copies will be sent.

21. Enter cc and the recipient(s) name(s).
    NOTE: Enter bcc on file copy if sending a blind copy.

22. Double space.

23. Enter PS for postscript, if desired.

errors. However, it will still miss the correctly-spelled wrong word and out-of-context words. Watch for certain things that seem to be problems such as:

words ending in "s"	periods
combinations of punctuation	commas
capital letters	two-letter words
numbers	dashes
apostrophes	double letters in words
hyphens	

Proofreading requires concentration and attention to details in a step-by-step process. Career proofreaders use at least a three-read system. First they read through the material to make sure it makes sense and to check for errors in composition such as a misaligned margin, paragraph indents, spacing on the page, etc. Then they read for content, to make certain correct words, punctuation, and grammar are used. And last, they do a check of spelling. Because we can be fooled by what we think we see when we read normally, spelling is

⤳	Subscript	⌃	Insert comma
⤴	Superscript	⌄	Insert apostrophe
⌙	Paragraph indent	:⎮	Insert colon
no ⌙	No indent; run in	⊙	Insert period
⌐	Break; start new line	?⎮	Insert question mark
⌐	Move left	⤸ ⤸	Insert quotation marks
⌐	Move right	⌃	Insert semicolon
⌐	Move up	⹀	Insert hyphen
⌐	Move down	⌶	Insert em dash
⌐⌐	Center	⌶	Insert en dash
Sp	Spell out ((Wd) or (5))	∧	Insert
TR	Transpose letters (words) or	⨍	Delete
BF	Boldface type	#	Insert space
ROM	(Roman) type	⌒	Close up space
ITAL	Italic type	⨜	Delete and close up
CAP	Capital letter	#⃠	Close up, but leave normal space
LC	Lower case letter		
SC	Small caps	eq.#	Equal space between words
STET	Let it stand	‖	Align type vertically
WF	Wrong (font)	=	Align type horizontally

FIGURE 6–21 Proofreader's marks

checked by reading the content *backwards,* checking each word, one word at a time. Going through these steps should ensure an error-free communication. If possible, as a final precaution, have someone else **critique** the letter.

When you proofread a draft copy, you should use standard proofreader's marks to indicate changes that need to be made. Knowledge of these marks is very helpful if your employer writes for professional journals or other publications because materials that are submitted may be returned by the publisher with these markings and any other clarifications or changes the publisher may desire. The final draft, called **galley proofs**, will require very careful proofreading for any remaining errors before the material goes to print. The most common proofreading marks are shown in Figure 6–21.

Good transcription and composing skills and the ability to produce error-free communications are very desirable traits. It can make you an asset to the physician's practice. If you enjoy this type of work, it will probably be possible for you to specialize in communication preparation.

Medical assistants can be self-employed by establishing arrangements with physicians to pick up dictation tapes and return completed correspondence within a short time frame.

ACHIEVE UNIT OBJECTIVES

Complete Chapter 6, Unit 3, in the workbook to help you obtain competency of this subject matter.

UNIT 4
Receiving and Sending Office Communications

OBJECTIVES

Upon completion of the unit, meet the following performance objectives by verifying knowledge of the facts and principles presented through oral and written communication at a level deemed competent.

1. Spell and define, using the glossary at the back of the text, all the **Words to Know** in this unit.
2. Sort, open, and annotate incoming mail.
3. Describe how vacation mail might be handled.
4. Identify postal services that may be required by an office.
5. List points to remember in processing metered mail.
6. List six classifications of mail.
7. Describe two reasons to use a certificate of mailing.
8. Explain why you might use certified mail.
9. Describe purpose for use of registered mail.
10. Explain what restricted delivery means.
11. Explain the purpose of a return receipt.
12. Name six means of communication other than by mail.
13. Name six uses for a fax machine.
14. Describe the characteristics of an electronic address.
15. Define the term "computer virus."
16. List four guidelines to avoid acquiring a virus through e-mail.

AREAS OF COMPETENCE (AAMA)

This unit addresses content within the specific areas of *Administrative procedures, Professionalism, Communication skills, Legal concepts*, and *Operational functions* as identified in the Medical Assistant Role Delineation Study. Refer to Appendix A for a detailed listing of the areas.

WORDS TO KNOW

abbreviations	polling
annotating	postmark
cancellation	priority
certified	receipt
consecutively	recipient
domestic	registered
envelope	restricted
facsimile	standard
foreign	teleconference
guaranteed	thermally
judgment	transmitted
periodical	

INCOMING MAIL

The amount of mail coming into physicians' offices depends on the number of physicians. In smaller offices the task of handling the mail is manageable, but in large clinics it may be necessary to have a mail clerk who is responsible for sorting and delivering the mail within the clinic.

The office policy manual should give instructions regarding the handling of mail. If no manual is available, the office manager or the physician should be consulted. Following are some generally accepted practices.

SORTING MAIL

Incoming mail should first be sorted. Any mail marked *personal* should be placed on the physician's or office manager's desk unopened. Special delivery mail, Mailgrams, or special messenger mail should be opened immediately. (The Mailgram is a postal service offered jointly by the United States Postal Service (USPS) and Western Union.) Mailgrams are transmitted over Western Union's communication network to printers located in over 140 post offices, placed in special envelopes carrying the postal service emblem, and delivered the next day by regular carrier.

There are many different types of mail that come into a physician's office. Office policy will determine whether it is sorted and placed on the physician's desk or the office manager's desk or whether a combination of both occurs in relation to the type of mail received. The process will depend upon the number of physicians, the office management design, and the assignment of personnel. The actual processing of the mail may be done by the manager, the receptionist, or an administrative medical assistant. The following are some examples of mail that will be received:

Special delivery mail
Mailgrams
Special messenger mail
Correspondence from patients
Payments from patients
Payments from insurance companies
Insurance forms to be completed
Referral letters or reports from physicians
Laboratory reports
Hospital reports
Professional organization mail
Professional journals
Magazines
Newspapers
Advertisements
Promotional literature and samples from pharmaceutical companies

Mail may be sorted into categories, such as mail from patients, physicians, insurance companies, and miscellaneous sources. Other classes of mail, such as magazines, professional journals, and newspapers, should be separated from drug samples and advertisements.

OPENING MAIL

When opening mail, you will need a letter opener, paper clips, a stapler, and a date stamp. It is more efficient to stack all envelopes so that they are facing in the same direction. A quick tap on the desk will move contents away from the flap side of the **envelope**. Open each letter along the flap edge, being careful to remove all contents from each envelope. As the mail is removed be sure the contents contain the same name and return address shown on the envelope. Some offices want you to keep the envelope with the mail received, and certainly you should if it is needed to help identify the contents. Otherwise you may discard the envelopes.

Date-stamp the correspondence and attach any enclosures. If an enclosure is indicated on the letter but is missing, it is necessary to write "None" after the "Encl." notation and circle it to indicate need for follow-up.

A word of caution regarding mail: From time to time someone will use the mail to send material that is explosive, contaminated, or otherwise dangerous. It is possible that a disgruntled patient could seek to harm or at least frighten the physician or the office staff. Although this is probably highly unlikely, for your own safety and that of the office, you should be aware of what is considered to be a suspicious letter or package. The USPS has suggested that certain things would make a letter seem suspicious:

- It is unexpected or from someone you do not know.
- It is addressed to someone no longer at your address.
- It is handwritten and has no return address or bears one that you cannot confirm is legitimate.
- It is lopsided or lumpy in appearance.
- It is sealed with an excessive amount of tape.
- It is marked with restrictive endorsements such as *Personal* or *Confidential*.
- It has excessive postage.

Other suggestions regarding packaging that could make it seem suspicious are:

- A package wrapped with string (against postal regulations, could have been delivered by other means)
- Any sound coming from a package

If such a letter or package should arrive, what should you do?

- Don't handle a letter or package that you suspect is contaminated.
- Don't shake it, bump it, or sniff it.
- Wash your hands thoroughly with soap and water.
- Notify local law enforcement authorities.

PROCESSING INCOMING MAIL

Exercise your best **judgment** to determine which mail can be handled without the aid of the physician. This type of mail would include routine office expense bills, insurance forms, and checks for deposit. If cash is received in the mail, you should always seek a witness to verify the amount of money and have that person sign a receipt along with you to be sent to the patient. This helps avoid the possibility of the patient saying that more was sent than was actually found in the envelope. This can happen quite innocently with elderly patients who may have a poor memory.

If you are employed by a surgeon, the mail will contain copies of hospital summaries and operative notes. These can be filed directly in the patient chart. Often copies are sent to the referring physician. Other hospital, laboratory, or special examination reports received should be seen by the physician and initialed before they are filed. Requests regarding patients or other office matters should be placed in a designated area for the physician to see and respond to each day.

The medical assistant can perform a valuable, timesaving service for the physician by **annotating** the incoming mail, or identifying important points to be noticed. If any correspondence or a patient chart will be needed to answer mail, it should be pulled and placed with the mail to be answered.

Notifications of meetings, miscellaneous correspondence, and professional journals are placed under the stack of mail. Some physicians want to see all supply catalogs and pharmaceutical company descriptions of products. In other offices, many of these items are disposed of immediately, especially if they concern areas of practice the office does not provide. Items that may be needed for future reference should be placed in a designated file.

Drug samples that may be used should be placed in a designated area for future use. Samples that will not be used should never be placed in the trash because they could cause harm to individuals taking them without medical evaluation and advice. Often, community clinics and service organizations can make good, safe use of donated samples. The office should have a box to collect samples for this purpose.

VACATION MAIL

When the physician is away from the office for professional meetings or on vacation, the medical assistant may be asked to carefully read all mail and decide how each piece will be handled. You should discuss what to do with urgent mail before the physician leaves. The physician may want you to call to discuss, or in some cases, to copy and forward the mail. Never send the original. If the physician will be away for a long time, you may need to send urgent mail more than once. If so, be sure to number the envelopes **consecutively** and keep track of what you send so that you can be sure all the urgent mail is received. When responding to the person who sent urgent mail, you may also wish to send a brief note explaining the reason for the delay in answering. If the office will be closed temporarily or permanently, be sure to go to the post office and complete a form to have mail held or forwarded to another address. Never send this form by mail because it may be delayed. The USPS cannot take verbal orders for this purpose. Allowing mail to accumulate invites theft.

MAKE MAIL MACHINABLE

The United States Postal Service (USPS) uses optical character readers (OCRs) and bar code sorters (BCSs) to read the addresses on envelopes you mail. The BCS equipment is capable of sorting over 36,000 pieces of mail per hour, but only if envelopes are properly addressed.

Each piece of mail passes by the computer's scanner for a quick read of the delivery address. Then, it goes to the OCR's printer, which sprays on a bar code representing the zip code or ZIP + 4 code for the address. The bar code is a series of little lines you often see at the bottom of letters from utility companies, banks, retailers, and other businesses (Figure 6–22). Next, the mail piece goes to one of the OCR's sorting channels reserved for the proper delivery area. From there, the bar coded mail is fed to BCSs for the final separations. The BCS processes mail just as quickly and in much the same way as the OCR reads addresses, except its scanner recognizes only one thing—the bar code. As the bar code on your mail piece passes the BCS lens, it is quickly read and sent to the appropriate channel for delivery.

FIGURE 6–22 Example of a bar code (Courtesy of United States Postal Service.)

ADDRESSING ENVELOPES

A **Patient Reception Area:**
- Correspondence—
  No. 10 Envelope
  No. 6¾ Envelope

Addresses must be typed or machine printed in order to be processed by automatic equipment. A standard type font is also required. Script or executive type can not be used because the letters run together. The OCR must be able to see a clear space between each character and word, or it won't know where one word ends and the next begins. Capitalize everything, using plain block letters. Omit all punctuation, except the hyphen in the ZIP + 4 code. Use approved abbreviations whenever possible. Lines of the address should be formatted with a uniform left margin. Also, be sure your toner is producing good quality print so that there is adequate contrast to be scanned.

The letter mail must also be of a proper size. If smaller than 3½ × 6⅛ inches, it is not mailable. If the letter is over 6⅛ × 11½ inches, it is mailable but must be processed by hand.

ADDRESS BLOCK LOCATION

The shaded area in Figure 6–23 illustrates the area on the face of the mail piece where address information should be located to be read by the OCRs. The OCRs and BCSs register mail pieces on the bottom edge; therefore, all vertical measurements are relative to the bottom edge.

Where possible, the entire address (exclusive of the optional lines above the name of recipient line) should be contained in an imaginary rectangle which extends from ⅝ inch to 2¾ inches from the bottom of the mail piece, with 1-inch margins on each side. At a minimum, all characters of the last line of the address block—the post office (city), state and zip code or ZIP + 4—should be located within an imaginary rectangle which extends from ⅝ inch to 2¼ inches from the bottom of the mail piece with 1-inch margins on each side. Make sure the address is as complete as possible, including all apartment or suite numbers.

Care must be taken to make the lines straight, as slanted lines cannot be read by the OCR process. The only **abbreviations** permitted in the name of the city are those found in the "Abbreviations" section of the *National Zip Code Directory*. The OCR cannot read a nonstandard abbreviation.

No portion of the return address should appear in the OCR read area. Special notations for the recipient such as *PERSONAL* or *CONFIDENTIAL* should be typed in all capitals aligned with and two lines below the return address.

The zip code is critical to the rapid delivery of mail. The first number of the zip code refers to a region of the United States, from 0 for the East Coast to 9 for the West Coast and Hawaii. The next two numbers refer to the major post office in the region, and the final two identify the

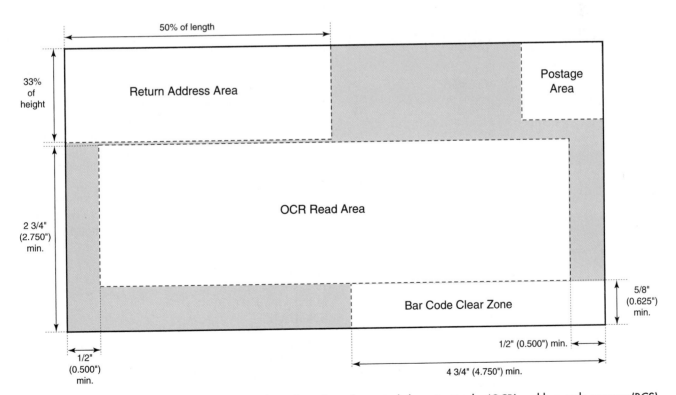

FIGURE 6–23 Designated zones for accurate reading of envelopes by optical character reader (OCR) and bar code scanner (BCS) (Courtesy of United States Postal Service.)

local delivery post offices. The ZIP + 4 coding allows even better use of automated processing in that the first two additional numbers denote a delivery sector, which may be several blocks, a group of streets, several office buildings, or other small geographic area. The last two numbers denote a delivery segment, which might be one floor of an office building, one side of a street, specific departments in a firm, or a group of post office boxes.

Annex	ANX	Park	PK
Apartment	APT	Parkway	PKY
Association	ASSN	Pike	PIKE
Attention	ATTN	Place	PL
Avenue	AVE	Plaza	PLZ
Boulevard	BLVD	Post Office	PO
Canyon	CYN	President	PRES
Causeway	CSWY	Ridge	RDG
Circle	CIR	River	RIV
Court	CT	Road	RD
Department	DEPT	Room	RM
East	E	Route	RT
Expressway	EXPY	Rural	R
Freeway	FWY	Rural Route	RR
Heights	HTS	Secretary	SECY
Highway	HWY	Shore	SHR
Hospital	HOSP	South	S
Institute	INST	Southeast	SE
Junction	JCT	Southwest	SW
Knolls	KNLS	Square	SQ
Lake	LK	Station	STA
Lakes	LKS	Street	ST
Lane	LN	Terrace	TER
Manager	MGR	Treasurer	TREAS
Meadows	MDWS	Turnpike	TPKE
North	N	Union	UN
Northeast	NE	Vice President	VP
Northwest	NW	View	VW
Palms	PLMS		

FIGURE 6–24 Examples of USPS-approved address abbreviations (Courtesy of United States Postal Service.)

Alabama	AL	Montana	MT
Alaska	AK	Nebraska	NE
Arizona	AZ	Nevada	NV
Arkansas	AR	New Hampshire	NH
California	CA	New Jersey	NJ
Canal Zone	CZ	New Mexico	NM
Colorado	CO	New York	NY
Connecticut	CT	North Carolina	NC
Delaware	DE	North Dakota	ND
District of Columbia	DC	Ohio	OH
Florida	FL	Oklahoma	OK
Georgia	GA	Oregon	OR
Guam	GU	Pennsylvania	PA
Hawaii	HI	Puerto Rico	PR
Idaho	ID	Rhode Island	RI
Illinois	IL	South Carolina	SC
Indiana	IN	South Dakota	SD
Iowa	IA	Tennessee	TN
Kansas	KS	Texas	TX
Kentucky	KY	Utah	UT
Louisiana	LA	Vermont	VT
Maine	ME	Virginia	VA
Maryland	MD	Virgin Islands	VI
Massachusetts	MA	Washington	WA
Michigan	MI	West Virginia	WV
Minnesota	MN	Wisconsin	WI
Mississippi	MS	Wyoming	WY
Missouri	MO		

FIGURE 6–25 Two-letter state abbreviations (Courtesy of United States Postal Service.)

The USPS will offer assistance in converting to ZIP + 4, but the confidential nature of medical office records means that patient interests would best be served by converting your own records. The customer service representative at the post office can answer your questions on the use of the *ZIP + 4 National State Directory.*

Now that you know how to address an envelope correctly, it is time to put it all together. The name of the intended **recipient** (business or individual) should appear on the first line. The line above the name of recipient line is an optional line for additional address information. When needed, it should be used to direct mail to the attention of a specific person when a business name has been placed on the name of the recipient line or to provide other information that will facilitate delivery (e.g., the name of a department within a company).

The line immediately below the recipient line is designated the *delivery address line.* The street address, post office box number, rural route number and box number, or highway contract number and box number should appear on this line. Mail addressed to multiunit buildings should include the apartment number, suite, room, or other unit designation immediately after the street address of the building, on the same line. When the length of the delivery address is such that it prevents the placement of the unit number or other designation on the same line, the number or designator should be placed on the line immediately above the delivery address line. When use of the building name in the address is necessary, it should also be placed on the line above the delivery address line (Figure 6–24).

For **domestic** mail, the post office (city), state, and zip code or ZIP + 4 should appear in that order on the bottom line of the address. However, if all three elements will not fit on that line, the zip code or ZIP + 4 may be placed on the line immediately below the post office and state, aligned with the left edge of the address block. The standard two-letter state abbreviations should also be used (Figure 6–25). The ZIP + 4 codes should always be printed as five digits, a hyphen, and four digits. The hyphen should be treated as any other character as far as spacing and stroke width are concerned.

Mail addressed to **foreign** countries should include the country name printed in capital letters (no abbreviations) as the only information on the bottom line. For example:

MR THOMAS CLARK
117 RUSSELL DRIVE
LONDON WIP6HQ
ENGLAND

Mail addressed to Canada may use either of the following formats when the postal delivery zone number is included in the address:

MRS HELEN SAUNDERS
1010 CLEAR STREET
OTTAWA ON K1AOB1
CANADA

MRS HELEN SAUNDERS
1010 CLEAR STREET
OTTAWA ON CANADA
K1AOB1

The post office will furnish additional information on mailing to foreign countries if assistance is needed.

COMPLETING MAILING

When you are satisfied that your letter and envelope are complete, place the flap of the envelope over the top of the letter and secure it with a paper clip. If enclosures are indicated, be sure these are included. It is a good idea to have a signature folder in which finished mail waiting to be signed is placed.

When the mail has been signed, fold it and place it in the envelope. A standard-size letter should be folded by bringing the lower third of the letter up and making a crease, then folding the top third of the letter down to about half an inch from the creased edge and making a second crease. The second crease goes into the envelope first. To fold a standard-size letter for a 6¾ envelope, bring the bottom edge to within half an inch of the top edge and crease. Fold from the right side about one third the width of the sheet and crease. Fold from the left edge to within half an inch of the second crease. Insert the left-edge crease into the envelope first.

If you have a large number of envelopes to seal you can speed up the process by placing eight or ten envelopes address side down with flaps open in a shingle fashion. Use a damp sponge to wet all the flaps at once and then starting with the one on top, turn down each flap and seal. Be sure that the sponge is not too wet as it will wet the envelopes and may spread the glue so that the letters stick together before you can seal them.

STAMP OR METER MAIL

The cost of sending mail is an expenditure that must be examined to be sure you obtain the most for your money. Your local post office can furnish you with current information. Postage rates, categories, and regulations are changeable, so you need to be current.

Mail may be either stamped or metered. Stamps may be purchased at a post office or obtained through the mail by using a specially printed envelope available through the post office. If you have a large volume of mail, it is preferable to use a postage meter. This machine can be leased from several authorized dealers, but the license to use it must be obtained from the USPS. A medical office can obtain a license by submitting an application to the post office where the metered mail will be deposited.

Postage meters contain a sealed unit that houses the printing die and two recording counters. One counter adds up all postage printed by the meter. The other counter subtracts and shows the balance of postage remaining in the meter. When you purchase an amount of postage, the post office will open the meter with a key, set the counter for the amount of postage purchased, and relock the meter. When the prepaid amount has been spent, the meter will lock automatically. The postage meter prints prepaid postage either directly on the mail or on adhesive strips

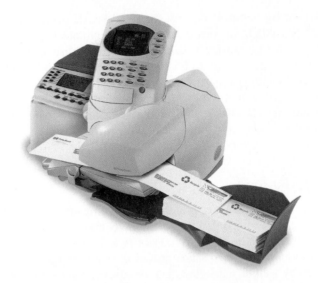

FIGURE 6–26 Postage scale and meter (Courtesy of Pitney Bowes, Inc.)

that are then affixed to the mail. The metered mail imprint, or metered stamp, serves as postage payment, **postmark**, and **cancellation** mark. All mail classes, amounts of postage, and quantity of mail may be metered. Metered mail, when bundled, can provide faster service than stamped mail because it is already postmarked and will bypass postal cancellation equipment.

To expedite the processing of metered mail, remember to: (1) change the date on the meter daily, (2) apply the correct amount of postage by weighing the mail before affixing postage, (3) check the imprint to be sure it is clear and readable, and (4) use fluorescent ink in the meter (Figure 6–26).

MAIL CLASSIFICATIONS

The USPS has many informative bulletins and booklets regarding the classifications, mailing standards, special mailing services, and other customer services that they offer. These are available at your local post office and through the USPS Internet site. Most mail from the physician's office will probably be first class, but a brief discussion of the classifications with their variations and additional methods of mailing is included for your information. If you have special mailing needs, it would be advisable to consult with your local post office for advice and up-to-date regulations because they tend to change periodically.

Express Mail

Express Mail is the fastest service and is guaranteed delivery 365 days a year. This is appropriate for important letters, documents, and merchandise. If mail for Express Mail Next Day Service is received at a designated Express Mail post office by 5:00 PM (usually), it will be delivered by noon or 3:00 PM the next day. If overnight is not possible to the destination, then a guaranteed second-day delivery service is available. Merchandise is automatically insured up to $500 and, for a fee, up to $5000. If you wish, you can waive the recipient's signature requirement so that the delivery can be left if the recipient is not there (unless it is insured above $500). Special envelopes, boxes, and tubes are provided free of charge. The rates vary by the amount of material mailed.

Priority Mail

Priority Mail provides preferential handling and expedited delivery of materials up to 70 pounds and 108 inches in combined length and width. Priority Mail stickers, labels, envelopes, and boxes are provided at no charge. Rates vary by weight. This classification of mail can be insured, *registered*, *certified*, or sent COD (collect on delivery).

First-Class Mail

First-Class mail is for sending letters, postcards, stamped cards, greeting cards, checks, and money orders. If the piece is heavier than 11 ounces, it is handled as Priority Mail. Additional services, such as certificates of mailing, certified, registered, COD, and *restricted* delivery, can be added to First-Class Mail. If the piece is NOT letter-size, it must be marked "First Class," or a large, green-diamond-bordered first-class mail envelope must be used. First-Class delivery is usually overnight in local cities and within two days to most states.

Periodicals

Periodicals classification applies only to printed materials from publishers and registered news agents approved for Periodical privileges. Magazines or newspapers mailed by others will use First-Class or Standard Mail (A) rates.

Standard Mail (A)

Standard Mail (A) is a classification used by retailers, catalogers, and other advertisers to promote products and services. Churches and other eligible nonprofit organizations can take advantage of the special rates of Standard Mail when mailing in excess of 200 pieces, each weighing less than 16 ounces, or for sending over 50 pounds per mailing. The mailing must be specially prepared for efficient handling. This classification will also permit anyone to mail a parcel weighing less than one pound.

Standard Mail (B)

Standard Mail (B) is for parcels weighing one pound or more. If a First-Class Mail piece is attached or enclosed,

you will pay for it in addition to the Standard Mail (B) parcel charge. Insurance to cover the value of articles mailed can be purchased. Parcels mailed under this classification can weigh up to 70 pounds. There are special rates for books or catalogs. The delivery time is slower, perhaps taking up to 9 days.

SPECIAL MAILING SERVICES

There are other special mailing services you may want to use when mailing personal or confidential patient information. These are in addition to the various classifications discussed.

Certificate of Mailing

A certificate of mailing is a receipt showing evidence that the piece was mailed. It is purchased at the time of mailing. This is helpful when you want to prove that something was mailed or a deadline was met. There is not proof of delivery, and no insurance against loss is provided with the certificate.

Certified Mail

Certified mail provides proof of mailing and delivery of the mail. The sender receives a mailing receipt when the item is mailed, and a receipt of delivery is kept at the recipient's post office. If the sender wishes, a proof-of-delivery return slip can be purchased. This service is available only for First-Class or Priority Mail. It does not carry insurance protection. This is appropriate to use if the physician is terminating services to a patient for some reason. A signed return receipt should be purchased to provide evidence to be placed in the discharged patient's chart.

Collect on Delivery (COD)

Collect on delivery (COD) is used when you wish to collect payment for merchandise and/or postage when the item is delivered. It can be used with First-Class, registered, Express, Priority, or Standard Mail. The receiver must have ordered the material. Fees include insurance coverage limited to $600.

Insurance

Insurance can be purchased for up to $5000 for regular Standard Mail and for mail sent at Priority or First-Class Mail rates. A *restricted* delivery, return *receipt*, or special handling service can be purchased for items insured over $50.

Registered Mail

Registered mail is the most secure option offered. It provides protection for valuables and important mail. Registered articles are placed under tight security from the point of mailing to the point of delivery. First-Class Mail or Priority Mail postage is required. Return receipt and restricted delivery is available. Insurance up to $25,000 can be purchased.

Restricted Delivery

Restricted delivery means that the mail is delivered only to a specific addressee or someone authorized to receive mail for the addressee. This can be used to be certain that only the patient receives specific communication, such as lab reports, a copy of a consultant examination, or any other personal material.

Return Receipt

Return receipt is the sender's proof of delivery. It can be purchased at the time of mailing for mail sent COD, Express Mail insured for more than $50, or registered, certified, or restricted mail. The receipt shows who signed for the item and the date it was delivered.

Other services are available should there be a need. Depending upon what you want to send, FedEx and UPS offer other alternatives.

If you have deposited mail and find you want it back, you will need to file a written application at the local post office, with an envelope addressed exactly as the one you wish returned. If the post office finds that the letter has left the local post office, the postmaster will telephone or telegraph the destination post office, at your expense, to have the letter returned to you.

If you have mail returned because the patient has moved and left no forwarding address, you can try contacting the patient's employer for a new address or talking with the individual who referred the patient. When a letter is returned after an attempt has been made to deliver it, you must prepare a new envelope and put on new postage before remailing it. The return of a letter sometimes happens if you have made an error, such as transposing numbers in an address.

ALTERNATIVE WAYS TO COMMUNICATE

There are many ways to receive and send information in today's technological society. Some common methods are fax, pager, cellular phone, voice mail, conference call, teleconferencing, e-mail, and the Internet.

Fax Machines

Facsimile (fax) machines (Figure 6–27) can be used by hospitals, physicians' offices, and clinics to send and receive information regarding patients over telephone lines. The machine makes it possible to send and receive letters, medical reports, laboratory reports, and insurance claims. Physicians may use the fax machine to send prescription

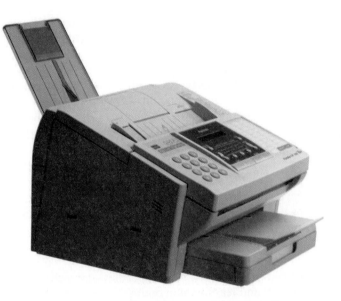

FIGURE 6–27 Fax machine (Courtesy of Panasonic Document Imaging Co.)

orders to pharmacies. The office may also use it for ordering office or medical supplies.

A fax machine is connected to a telephone line. The machine scans a document and converts the image to *electronic* impulses that are **transmitted** over the telephone lines. The receiving fax machine converts the impulse to make an identical copy of the original. Fax machines may print on **thermally**-treated or plain paper. The thermally-treated paper eventually fades when exposed to sunlight; therefore, you would usually photocopy an important document onto bond paper.

The fax machine is available with many special features. Certainly a concern in the medical office is the transmission of confidential material. It is possible to have a secret code that will lock out unauthorized **polling**. The fax machine may also be able to store multiple documents in memory and have automatic dialing with redialing when a busy signal is detected. The fax machine can be a *plain-paper* type using standard $8\frac{1}{2} \times 11$-inch copy paper or a type that uses a paper roll that is automatically cut to the length of each page of received message. If the recording paper runs out, the message is stored in memory and will be automatically printed out when new paper is loaded. A battery safeguards the document memory in case of power failure. The machine may be equipped with a white-line skip function that automatically skips over horizontal blank spaces on a document. This feature allows a standard document to be transmitted in as little as twelve seconds.

You will need to learn the specific procedure for operating the fax machine you will be using. However, there are general rules which are important to the use of any fax machine.

1. Always remove paper clips and staples from material to be scanned so you will not damage the fax machine.

2. Make a test copy if the document has color. Dark colors may block copy and can slow transmission.

3. Do not use correction tape or fluid on documents to be transmitted.

4. Do consider using typed words for numbers to avoid problems with interpretation.

5. If the material you are faxing is confidential, before sending it, call to alert the recipient to be watching for the material.

6. The first sheet of any transmission is called the fax page. It includes the date, name of recipient, recipient's address and fax number, and the number of pages being sent (including the fax page). The name and fax number of the sender will also be included. Any other special information required for routing instructions should be added.

7. Be familiar with error messages the fax machine may display and learn how to correct these problems. The machine may be equipped with built-in service diagnostic codes that can be automatically transmitted over telephone lines to a service provider. Most service calls can be resolved by telephone, therefore reducing costly equipment downtime and labor costs.

8. You may need to resend a message if noise or interference on the telephone line resulted in an unclear transmission.

9. Check to be sure the transmission is completed. It will indicate that the message was sent, identifying the date and time of transmission. Remove the original from the machine.

Pagers

Physicians commonly wear pagers so they can be contacted regardless of where they are or what they are involved in. A pager is a small electronic device that is activated by a telephone signal. When you wish to contact the physician, you simply dial the number. After it rings, a series of beeps will be heard and you then enter the phone number from which you are calling. Meanwhile, the pager being worn by the physician will be activated and will produce a beeping sound or, if the sound is turned off, will vibrate to alert the wearer of a call. The phone number of the caller will be displayed in the pager's small viewing area, and the physician can go to a phone and make the call. Some newer models have the ability to receive small messages which print out on the pager viewing area. An additional feature provided by some paging services allows voice messages to be left which can be retrieved by the receiver from any phone. Pagers are very beneficial and allow people to stay in contact even when they are not near a phone.

Voice Mail

Voice mail is another way to communicate. It is similar to a telephone answering machine, except voice mail can receive messages and place them in your "mailbox" even if

your phone is busy. Basically, if you call and the individual is either not there to answer or is talking on the line, a recording comes on. The message is usually spoken by the individual and typically changes daily. It may tell you the date and explain where the person may be. It may also give you the individual's schedule for the next couple of days. It will then typically request that you leave a message. When the individual checks the phone, an audible cue, such as an intermittent dial tone, alerts the individual to a message in the voice mailbox, or the phone may be equipped with a message light. Another advantage of voice mail is that the sender, with the proper software, can record a message and then direct it to several mailboxes. This is especially helpful within a company or association to notify several people of an event or a meeting. These messages can also be retrieved from any phone by accessing the voice mailbox using a personal identification number.

Cellular Phones

The ease and portability of cellular phones make them another option for communication. As phone technology makes them smaller and lighter, they are becoming a more easily-carried device. Slim, pocket-sized phones are now available, and some are slightly larger than a credit card. Of course their greatest advantage is the familiarity of use and the ability to give and receive information instantly. Perhaps their only disadvantage may be difficulty of reception within certain environments and within certain locations. The inconvenience of ringing at inappropriate times can be solved, for the most part, by adjustment of the ringer's volume.

Conference Calls

The telephone can be used to simultaneously conduct conversations with several people in various locations at the same time. This allows business to be conducted, meetings to occur, and professional or personal communication to be carried out. Conference calling saves time, travel, and money—all important in managing practice expenses. If your phone system is not equipped to allow multiple connections, conference calls may be arranged with the local phone service provider.

Teleconferencing

This means of exchanging information is like a conference call, but everyone can see and hear each other at the same time. They are linked together by way of telecommunications equipment. There are cameras, speaker phones, connection devices, and television monitors in each location. The phone company for the meeting originator will contact all other sites and network the phones together. With the aid of the phone, camera, and television, participants can see and talk to each other. A **teleconference** can involve several people in many different locations. Ideas can be presented, concerns expressed, and new techniques shown; teleconferencing is the next best thing to actually being together in a meeting, yet it conserves travel time and expense.

Telemedicine

In January 1997, *The Harvard Health Letter* reported on an exciting long-distance medical care that is happening and may become more routine. It enables physicians to "see" patients at other sites miles away from the physician's home base or office. It involves the use of electronic stethoscopes, digitized x-ray transmissions, and interactive video to examine, diagnose, and treat patients. In Kansas, nurses who make home visits to chronically ill patients began using interactive video to enable them to "see" more people. The home-care agency sets up a camera and a 13-inch TV in a participant's home. The nurse sends a "buzzer" sound to alert the patient that the call will occur in two minutes. The patient sits in front of the camera and talks with the nurse as together they perform a series of tasks by using digital equipment attached to the TV. The electronic stethoscope is placed on the chest to check the patient's heart; a blood pressure cuff gets a reading; a finger stick and the glucometer tests the blood sugar level; and the finger oximeter measures the amount of oxygen in the blood. Patients seem to like the approach and it has greatly boosted efficiency. When driving from patient to patient, only five people could be seen in a day; now the nurses are able to "see" three times as many patients.

Telemedicine enables primary care physicians to immediately consult with a faraway specialist while the patient is still in their office. For example, the cardiologist can listen to a patient's heart with the electronic stethoscope and assist the primary physician in diagnosing a murmur or irregularity. It has been adapted to permit "house calls" to people who find it physically difficult to visit care facilities or for those who live or are stranded by weather in remote areas. Health care reform may encourage this form of practice as a more efficient use of resources (e.g., skilled specialists). A California pilot program links physicians at Stanford University with patients at a nursing home, an urban clinic, and a multispecialty medical practice. This allows experts from the university to participate in the examination of high risk or problem cases. Through the use of high-resolution computerized images, it is possible for the specialist to view a skin rash, a fetal ultrasound, or the retina of the eye. The capabilities are endless. In 1996, doctors at the New England Medical Center in Boston conducted about 1,500 consultations with regional and overseas patients—one as far away as South America.

A new technology being used by cardiac surgeons at The Ohio State University Hospital sounds almost like science fiction. With the use of computers, an operative console, and a robot, a surgeon is able to perform surgery through very small incisions in the chest. The surgeon sits at the console in an adjoining room and manipulates the hand controls. The computer translates the motions into a language the robot can understand. The robot's thin *arms and hands* are fitted with very small instruments and actually perform the surgery. One procedure that can be done is a coronary bypass. The robot can harvest a vein from the inside of the chest wall and transplant it to the heart surface.

The most immediate advantage of this type of surgery is a great reduction in recovery time and patient discomfort because the opening is very small compared to when the hands of the surgeon must actually get inside the chest. Often, these patients are not good operative risks, and reducing the invasiveness of the procedure is very beneficial. It has been suggested that, with the proper technical equipment in place, it would be possible to perform procedures at great distances from the surgeon through the use of communication technology. Someday a surgical specialist in the United States could perform a procedure in the outback of Australia while sitting at a console dressed in jeans and a sweatshirt.

There are some issues to be settled regarding these forms of medical practice. Items such as costs to initiate and legal, ethical, and professional concerns need to be addressed. Some physicians see it as threatening since they would have to compete with many more physicians than just those in their local area. And, of course, there is the issue of malpractice liability. If the consult is out of state, whose state laws apply? Another factor is privacy when sending personal medical records through telecommunication systems. Congress recently passed legislation requiring federal health officials to develop specifications for a national computer network that will enable doctors, hospitals, insurers, and others to transfer patient records electronically. Now, a way to keep the records confidential must be found. Another big question is medical licensure since physicians are licensed only in the state they practice. Currently, 10 states are requiring that doctors who practice within their boundaries hold a state license, even if their presence is purely electronic. The AMA went on record recommending full licensure for each state except in emergencies and physician-to-physician consultation. Some states, however, feel a limited telemedicine credential would be sufficient. Some telemedicine physicians feel it is time for a national licensure to be established for physicians and solve the problem completely. This new form of medical practice will be interesting to watch develop.

E-Mail

This form of communication, "electronic mail," is carried out by a computer, appropriate software, and the Internet. Before you can send or receive messages you need to have an e-mail "address." E-mail can be exchanged within a company or clinic, or outside to anyone with a phone and an e-mail address. Electronic addresses have certain common characteristics. They begin with the person's name, some abbreviated form of it, or any other word the individual desires. Next may come the name or abbreviation of a business or company when it is a business address. Next comes the "@" symbol, which denotes the beginning of the individual's server's address. The name of the Internet service provider (ISP) follows, which is then followed with a "dot" and an abbreviation such as "com," "org," "gov," or "net" to designate commerce, organization, government, or the Internet.

It is desirable to pay for the registration of your e-mail address to ensure no one else can choose the same one. A registered name in known as a *domain name* and usually needs to be renewed every year. To communicate by e-mail, you will need some form of communication software on your computer and an electronic service provider for your computer to connect to the Internet. When you send a message, the software converts words into standard digital language and sends it via the phone line to your e-mail server's computers. There the server checks the "domain name" (that part that follows the "@" in the address) and forwards the message over the Internet to the recipient's e-mail server. The recipient's server files the message until the computer checks for e-mail messages and then delivers the message to the computer. Once again, the digital message is translated back into words that can be read. This all occurs in a matter of a few seconds.

E-mail allows for the almost instant exchange of information without the costs associated with long-distance phone calls. In addition, the advantage of transmitting written material makes it appropriate for transferring reports, documents, correspondence, and all forms of written communication. Not only can material from one computer be sent to another, but material can also be scanned from other sources and sent over the Internet. When you receive communication, you can "open" your e-mail and read the information. If you wish to save it, it can be printed or sent to your hard disk and stored.

The Internet/World Wide Web

This communication link allows you access to information from all over the world. It can be a great source of data from health organizations such as the American Cancer Society and the Centers for Disease Control and Prevention. Another capability through the Internet, which your physician may wish you to use, is the ability to schedule airline, hotel, and other services directly without going through various agents. Again, to access the "information super highway," as the Internet is called, you will need a computer, the appropriate software, and a modem. If you learn how to identify what you are looking for, you probably can find it. All you have to do is give the ISP computer your subject matter. You enter the appropriate key words into a "search engine" such as Yahoo or Alta Vista. In return, you receive a listing from which you can select a more specific entry. When this is viewed, it may be even further definable until you are able to pinpoint the topic you want. You can access a source's "home page" to obtain the source's general information. By identifying your topic more specifically, you can bring the appropri-

ate information to your screen to view. You can read it there, produce a hard copy with your printer, or store it on your disk.

The Internet contains a wealth of information, but there can be serious problems associated with some online sources. It is important for the health care worker to obtain accurate information and be able to direct patients to reliable sources. As an example, one of the most dangerous areas that patients may be tempted to take advantage of is the Internet site that conducts a minimal inquiry online and then prescribes and provides medications. This could cause serious consequences to the prescribed treatment and medications ordered by the physician.

You need to take certain precautions when reading and evaluating web sites. Remember, there is no official agency that reviews or evaluates the information. The controls over legitimate sites come from the sponsoring organizations or governmental agencies. You may want to follow some simple web site guidelines such as:

1. Check the source. Are there links to professional affiliations or are there professional credentials?
2. Be cautious about personal testimonies from "users"; they often are just receiving monetary compensation for making a statement.
3. Watch for dates of the information; the information may be very old and no longer valid.
4. Use your analytic skills to interpret *scientific* studies or reports. Who did the research? How many people were included in the study? Is the amount of time spent appropriate to arrive at the stated conclusions? Is there more than one study on the subject to give its results credibility?

As you become more familiar with technical reading and practice analyzing information, you will be able to make good decisions.

It is possible to enter, obtain, and exchange information, as well as conduct business transactions such as banking, all electronically. The amount of material available is mind boggling. It is possible to look at books, museums, association's publications, the world's encyclopedias, and on and on. However, there is some concern about the lack of security. With all the providers and information routing involved, interception of information is possible. Because of this and the nature of medical records and the need to provide for privacy of information, electronic communication may not be advisable in a medical office.

This new technology has made great changes in the way we access and exchange information. At present, the storehouse of historical data is unbelievable; the ability to have instant connection with virtually every person, business, university, organization, and even government is possible. It is important that you learn to use new technologies. When things change, you must change with it or be left behind and unable to compete in the new workplace.

According to information released by the Pew Internet & American Life Project, about 104 million Americans, or 56% of the adults in the United States, have Internet access. This form of communication is definitely becoming a preferred method of information exchange.

With the increased use and dependence on the Internet for communication and information gathering, you need to be aware of the very real threat that computer viruses pose. A virus is information that is sent electronically to interfere with or destroy your electronic files. There are standard methods of protection offered by employing firewalls and antivirus software (with the virus database kept up-to-date) to protect your computer while browsing and downloading files. You must be especially careful with respect to the use of e-mail. The following rules of thumb can help keep your computer virus-free:

1. Before opening an e-mail, look at the subject and who sent it. If you receive an e-mail from an unfamiliar source or with a suspicious subject (e.g., the subject is out of character with what you would expect to receive from the sender), do not open it! Delete and purge the suspicious e-mail immediately.
2. Never open an executable or script file (files with a "exe." or ".vbs" suffix) unless you are expecting to receive such a file from the sender. Opening these types of files is particularly dangerous because they can cause any number of actions, ranging from sending an e-mail to everyone in your address book to completely erasing the contents of your hard drive.
3. Use antivirus software to scan e-mails before opening them (either through your e-mail server on from you local mail application). Keep in mind that this is not entirely effective because new viruses are being created and deployed continuously and may not be detectable even if you have the most up-to-date virus database.
4. Last but not least, be aware that operating systems and the services and programs they run can be inherently open to attack. If you are computer-savvy, keep abreast of the latest patches and software upgrades that address security. Otherwise, consult with the administrator of your computer network to be sure you are protected.

ACHIEVE UNIT OBJECTIVES

Complete Chapter 6, Unit 4, in the workbook to help you obtain competency of this subject matter.

UNIT 5

Office Management Equipment

The medical assistant may be responsible for the operation of many pieces of business equipment while performing administrative duties. A variety of office machines contribute to the efficiency of an office. Some are rather simple, whereas others can be quite complicated, requiring specialized training and practice to master. This unit identifies a variety of equipment that could be found in a medical practice.

OBJECTIVES

Upon completion of the unit, meet the following performance objectives by verifying knowledge of the facts and principles presented through oral and written communication at a level deemed competent, and demonstrate the specific behaviors as identified in the performance objectives of the procedures, observing safety precautions in accordance with health care standards.

1. Spell and define, using the glossary at the back of the text, all the **Words to Know** in this unit.
2. Demonstrate the use of a calculator.
3. Explain why a check writer is used.
4. Demonstrate the use of a check writer.
5. List seven types of material that often is photocopied.
6. Demonstrate the use of a copy machine.
7. Give two reasons why records are microfilmed.
8. Explain when dictation on a tape should be saved.
9. Demonstrate the operation of a transcriber.
10. Define all the computer terms listed in the unit.
11. List four items known as computer hardware.
12. Explain why the backing up of computer data is necessary.
13. Demonstrate the basic operation of a computer.

> ### AREAS OF COMPETENCE (AAMA)
>
> This unit addresses content within the specific competency areas of *Administrative functions, Procedures, Practice finances, Communication skills, Legal concepts*, and *Operational functions* as identified in the Medical Assistant Role Delineation Study. Refer to Appendix A for a detailed listing of the areas.

WORDS TO KNOW

acronym	microfilming
calculator	payee
computer	processor
dictation	programmed
electronic	software
hardware	technology
maintenance contract	transcription
microfiche	

A variety of machines and equipment is required to manage the business operation of a medical office. Large multi-physician offices and clinics have more patients and employees and therefore require a greater number and larger capacity of equipment. Smaller offices and single-physician practices will likely have less-specialized equipment, and will concentrate on the essentials primarily because of costs and limited operating personnel. The following material discusses the types of common office management equipment found in a medical practice.

CALCULATOR OR ADDING MACHINE

There are many occasions when an accurate calculation of figures is necessary. Some examples are the totaling of charges when preparing a patient's statement, submitting an insurance claim for services rendered, preparation of banking deposits, and the reconciliation of a banking statement. The summation of the daily log of receipts and charges is easier and more accurate when calculating equipment is used. Of course, care must be taken to enter the figures accurately or the results will be incorrect. NOTE: when multiples of the same item are listed, it is often listed as a "single" cost, which must be mathematically converted to the total price. This is especially important when checking the accuracy of invoices for ordered items. If the **calculator** produces a hard copy, the entries can be easily reviewed. If it displays the amount digitally in the display window, each entry can be viewed for accurate keying when entered; but it would be wise to also repeat the calculation to see if you get the same answer twice. A simple 10-key calculator with a few additional function keys is adequate for general office management (Figure 6–28). Calculators are powered by various sized batteries, electricity, or even light from the sun or a lightbulb. Some models can use either electricity or battery. The term "adding machine" was used before the era of electronics and refers to equipment that performs many of the same functions as a calculator, but it is probably older and larger and may operate manually. Adding machines and printing calculators (Procedure 6–8) use a roll of narrow paper upon which the numbers are printed, similar to what you receive from the grocery store.

COPY MACHINE

The copy machine is extremely important to the efficiency of the office (Figure 6–29). A **photocopy** of correspondence, an insurance form, a patient's record, laboratory reports, or account information is often needed (Procedure 6–9). Most machines can be set to use either letter- or legal-sized paper. Frequently, prepared literature, information sheets, and initial information forms will require copying. Newer copy machine models can produce color copies, which greatly enhances informa-

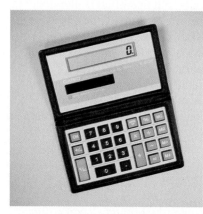

FIGURE 6–28 Ten-key calculator

PROCEDURE

6–8 Total Charges on Calculator

PURPOSE: To accurately total and record a list of numbers using a calculator.

EQUIPMENT: Calculator, a list of 20 charges to be calculated, an invoice or ledger card, pen or pencil.

PERFORMANCE OBJECTIVE: Provided with necessary equipment and materials, calculate a list of 20 charges, performing any necessary mathematical functions, and correctly determine the total amount. The same correct answer must be obtained twice within a maximum of three attempts.

1. Turn on calculator.
2. Clear machine.

Key Point: The digital display window or printed tape gives visual evidence that the machine is cleared.

3. Enter figures to be calculated and perform mathematical functions.
4. Total fees.
5. Double-check tape or refigure on digital display to be sure you get the same answer twice.
6. Record total.

tion materials. Some offices may use the copier for monthly billing. The accounting record is copied, folded, and inserted into an envelope and mailed, thereby eliminating preparation of a separate statement. Remember,

the copier is not for your personal use. Generally, if the equipment is owned, you will be permitted to make a few copies if necessary. Some machines are leased and have attached counters which record the number of times the camera flashes making copies. Offices are charged a rate reflective of their usage. With this arrangement, use of the copier is restricted. NOTE: Care should be taken to avoid copying material that carries a copyright protection, as this is considered illegal unless the permission to copy is obtained from the writer or publisher.

Routine maintenance will improve the quality of copies made. Offices should have service arrangements with suppliers of equipment and copy materials. Service representatives can demonstrate cleaning of the glass, feed rollers, and surfaces, and show you how to maintain the toner. Large copiers can be programmed to perform several functions such as enlarging or reducing copy size, stapling, sorting, off-set stacking, one- or two-sided copying, and insertion of cover sheets. A properly operating copier can produce a great variety of materials and is a valuable asset to the physician's office.

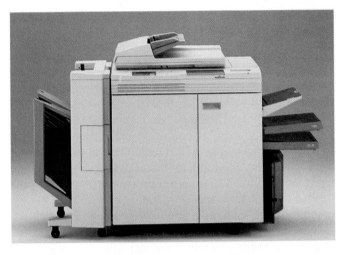

FIGURE 6–29 Copy machine

PROCEDURE

6–9 Operate Copy Machine

PURPOSE: To accurately prepare settings on a copy machine in order to produce a duplicate of the original in the size, number, and order desired.

EQUIPMENT: Copy machine, paper, and material to be copied.

PERFORMANCE OBJECTIVE: Given access to necessary equipment and supplies, demonstrate adjustment of settings to produce the specified copy or copies while operating the copy machine accurately following the steps in the procedure.

1. Assemble material to be copied.
2. Determine number of copies needed.
   Rationale:
   a. **You usually make one file copy of every letter you send. If copies are to be sent with the letter, you need additional copies.**
   b. **Two copies of the most medical legal reports are needed.**
   c. **If you are making copies of instruction sheets for patients, copy enough for a month's use at one time.**
3. Turn on copy machine.
   NOTE: Some offices leave the machine on all day because it requires a warm-up period before it can be used. If this is not your office policy, turn the machine off when finished.

4. Adjust settings for what you want to copy.
   Note:
   a. **Legal or letter size paper.**
   b. **Regular copy/lighter/darker may be adjusted on some machines.**
   c. **Regular, reduced, or enlarged copy.**
   d. **Number of copies.**
5. Check paper supply.
   Rationale: Assure adequate supply. Some machines will jam when supply becomes too low. Also, check paper type. The last person using the copier may have used colored paper, a different size, or letterhead paper.
6. Raise lid and place material to be copied, one sheet at a time, face down on glass.
   NOTE: On self-feeding models, place material on feeder tray. If more than one page, arrange in proper order.
7. Close lid.
8. Press button or key pad to activate copier.
9. Remove original(s) and copy/copies. Remove special paper, if used, from supply.
10. Return machine to "standard" settings if changed.
11. Turn off machine (if policy).

MICROFICHE OR MICROFILM

The medical assistant may need to be familiar with the microfilming process (Figure 6–30). Microfilming is a method of preserving material by reducing it to minute film images. **Microfilming** of office records can provide the necessary record security while using a minimum of storage space. The machine is easy to operate. Documents are placed on the scanner's feed tray. The machine automatically detects the size of the document and produces image data on the microfilm in the correct proportions. The film is contained on a reel that the machine automatically monitors to determine the amount of film remaining.

The digital microfilm scanner connected to the file printer (Figure 6-31), displays the image on the screen, and converts film images to letter- or ledger-sized laser quality printouts. With the appropriate interface board, the scanner can be connected to a computer that would allow the scanned images to be converted electronically over fax, e-mail, or the Internet, or stored on disks.

DICTATION-TRANSCRIPTION MACHINE

The most common units to be used in the physician's office are the desktop machines (Figure 6–32). Several kinds of units are available: a unit for **dictation** only, a unit for **transcription** only, or a combination unit that can be used for both purposes. Many physicians use a portable dictating machine that can be operated by battery or electricity. The physician may use this machine in the office, in the car, at home, or while attending meetings. Some physicians will dictate their notes following each patient's appointment rather than writing on the chart. When office hours are over, they will give you the tape so their observations, comments, and findings can be entered on the respective patient's chart.

The medical assistant can help the physician use the equipment more efficiently by tactfully discussing any problems encountered while transcribing. Tell the physician when the dictation is good. If you are experiencing difficulties due to dictation or mechanical reasons, explain precisely the problem and offer specific solutions. Sometimes a list of helpful hints to improve dictation and reduce the chance of error can be used to help both the physician and the transcriptionist. The list might include the following:

1. Check the machine to be sure it is recording.
2. Indicate date and what is being dictated (chart note, letter, research paper, report, and so on).
3. Recognize that you are talking to a person through the machine.

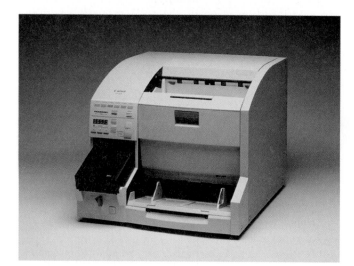

FIGURE 6–30 Microfilm machine (Photo courtesy of CanonUSA, Inc.)

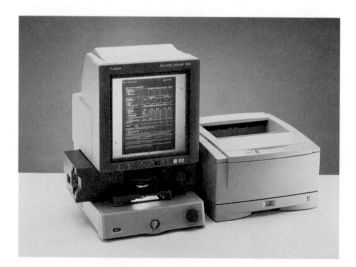

FIGURE 6–31 Microfilm reader-printer machine (Photo courtesy of CanonUSA, Inc.)

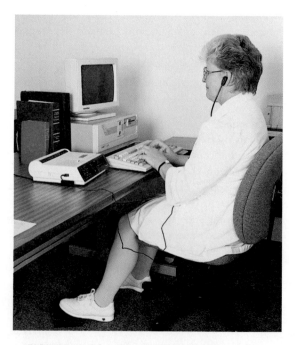

FIGURE 6–32 Dictation-transcription machine

PROCEDURE

6-10 Operate Transcriber

PURPOSE: To operate transcriber equipment in order to produce a printed copy from recorded material.

EQUIPMENT: Transcriber, dictation tape, headset, foot control, wordprocessor or computer, and paper.

PERFORMANCE OBJECTIVES: Given access to equipment and supplies, operate the transcriber correctly following all steps in the procedure. Complete an accurate transcription within a specified time period.

1. Turn on the transcriber.
2. Verify that headset with earphones and the foot control are attached to the unit.
3. Select dictation tape. **Rationale: Type rush reports or oldest dictation first.**
4. Adjust headset with earphones. **NOTE: Earphones should not be shared. Rationale: Prevents the spread of organisms.**
5. Insert tape. Press the play tab or the pedal to listen for the beginning of the dictation.
6. Listen for physician's instructions. **NOTE: The material to be typed will guide you in selecting the appropriate paper. It may be a chart note, a report, or a letter requiring letterhead paper.**

7. Adjust volume, tone, and speed controls for clearest communication reception.
8. Bring up word processing screen, set computer margins and tabulator stops as needed.
9. Enter the recorded information.
10. Alternately press and release foot pedal to listen and transcribe the recorded message. **NOTE: Consult a dictionary if a word is unfamiliar. If you are unable to understand a word or words, leave a blank, note the place on the tape and ask someone else to listen. If necessary, ask the dictating physician for assistance so you can complete the work.**
11. Turn off the machine and place accessory items in proper storage space.
12. Save the dictation on the tape. **Rationale: In case questions should arise before the physician will approve the report or sign the letter.**
13. Erase tape following the approval of the material or physician's signature on letter, so the tape can be used again.

---

4. Dictate the name of the patient and the name of the person or firm who will be the recipient of the message.
5. Dictate the street address, city, state, and zip code to which correspondence is to be sent and the number of copies needed.
6. Dictate punctuation such as "period," "comma," or "paragraph."
7. Encourage the physician to refrain from eating, drinking, or listening to loud music or television while the dictation is being done.
8. Speak in a normal, clear voice.
9. End with an appropriate message to indicate the dictation is completed.

The dictation machine that is carried out of the office must be kept in operating order at all times—you never know when the physician will put it to use. When it is in the office, check to be certain it is ready for use. Replace the batteries as needed and maintain a supply of erased tapes for reuse.

The transcription machine (Procedure 6–10) has a foot control that starts the machine. When the pedal is released the machine stops. It also has a backup pedal that allows you to relisten to the transcription if you need to hear it

again before you transcribe. You will learn how to press the pedal, listen, and then begin typing the sentences with a minimum of time. With practice and speed, you may be able to type and listen almost simultaneously. The machine has controls for automatic rewind and fast forward. The speed control can be adjusted to either slow down or speed up the voice message. The speed control should generally be adjusted for the normal voice quality for the physician making the dictation.

WORD PROCESSORS

The word **processor** may be an electronic typewriter with the added features of fast daisy-wheel printing, spelling checks, and spelling corrections similar to computer capabilities. These are equipped with insertable disk drive units for either line or add-on screen display. This allows you to store text on a microfloppy disk for later use. They may also allow an auto-cut sheet feeder and tractor feeder to be added.

Word processing software is available for all computers (Figure 6–33). These programs provide almost limitless composition of written and graphic materials. You have the ability to select from a number of print font

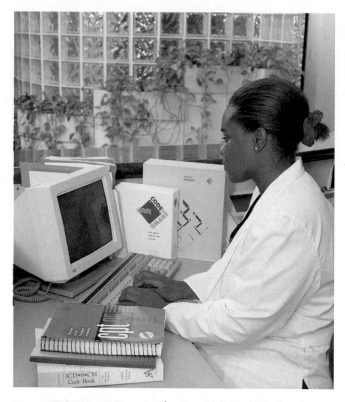

FIGURE 6–33   Word processing on a computer

styles and sizes, which can be bolded, italicized, underlined, superscripted or subscripted, printed with shadows, and more. You can vary line spacing and margins and set columns, borders, bullets, and tabs. You can rearrange content by highlighting, cutting, and then pasting it in the new location. It is possible to insert page breaks, use auto shapes that allow you to add text boxes, draw lines, input clip art or content from files, draw and insert tables, and much more. With practice you can not only create quality standard correspondence but also outstanding reports, articles, and presentations for your employer.

The ability to view the document while it's being developed is very helpful. By selecting the print preview screen, you can visualize the whole finished product for page placement and balance before actually printing it. This is especially important before printing a letter on letterhead paper.

THE COMPUTER

In a text titled *Computer Fundamentals for an Information Age,* authors Shelly and Cashman define a computer as follows:

A **computer** is an **electronic** device, operating under the control of instructions stored in its own memory unit, which can accept and store data, perform mathematical and logical operations on that data without human intervention, and produce output from the processing.

Computers come in a variety of makes, styles, sizes, capacities, and price ranges. However, they all perform about the same way. Some can be carried like a small notebook; others are large designated primary network machines. Many have the capacity to convey sound, and some are capable of responding to voice commands. The most recent development is a wireless mouse and keyboard known as "Blue Tooth Technology." It operates by radio frequencies. Clicking the mouse or input from the keyboard transmits signals to receivers in the computer ports, thereby eliminating the need for cumbersome cables. In reality, you could sit across the room in an easy chair with the keyboard in your lap and operate your computer, provided the screen was large enough to be seen.

Computer **technology** advances so rapidly that the last statement will seem outdated by the time this book is published. The computer has changed the way information is processed and stored. An individual with computer skills can be a valuable employee. With technology constantly changing, it is necessary to update and learn new applications almost continuously. It would be wise to take every opportunity possible to acquire additional skills.

Physicians are aware of the advantages of using computers in the office. Large clinics often have direct-line insurance reporting by computer: the necessary information is **programmed** into the clinic computer and travels directly to the insurance company computers. This eliminates paperwork, and the speed of processing claims is enhanced considerably.

Computer Terms

With the development of the computer came a whole new vocabulary of technical terms as well as new meanings for old words. In order to communicate with other users, it is important to understand and use computer language. The following are some of the most commonly used terms relating to the computer and its components. Become familiar with them quickly.

- **@**—The symbol that represents the word "at" that is used in e-mail addresses. It separates the user name from the name of the mail server.
- **attachment**—a file you send along with an e-mail message.
- **backup**—duplicate of data files made to protect information. Records should be backed up daily. Some experts recommend twice daily.
- **batch**—an accumulation of data to be processed.
- **boot**—to start up a computer.
- **bug**—an error in a program.
- **catalog**—a list of files on the storage media.
- **CD-ROM**—compact disk read-only memory. The term which indicates the computer is capable of playing compact disks.
- **characters per second**—term used to measure printer output.

- **CPU**—central processing unit, or the "brain" of the system. The memory is made up of **bits.** A bit is a single **BI**nary digi**T.** *Binary* refers to a situation in which there are only two choices: for example, yes/no, on/off, pass/fail. *Digit* refers to a single number. A bit is either 0 or 1. A **byte** is the fundamental group of bits that a computer will treat as a word. A byte consists of 8 bits. A 16-bit processor is twice as fast as an 8-bit processor. One **K** (Kilobyte) is equal to 1,024 bytes. A 64-K computer can handle 65,536 bytes. The greater the number of bytes, the greater the memory. Present day computers are at least 32-bit machines with 128 MB (one megabyte is one million bytes) of memory and a hard-drive storage capacity of 40 GB (one gigabyte is one billion bytes).
- **cursor**—a marker on the screen that shows where the next letter, number, or symbol will be placed (may be an underline dash or a blinking rectangle or square).
- **data**—information that can be processed or produced by a computer.
- **debugging**—finding errors and correcting them in computer programs.
- **disk**—a magnetic storage device made of rigid plastic material (floppy disk).
- **disk drive**—the device used to get information on and off a disk.
- **domain**—the naming convention used on the Internet. It is separated by periods in the name.
- **DOS**—(**D**isk **O**perating **S**ystem) a program that tells the computer how to use the disk drive.
- **dot matrix printer**—printer that uses dots to form letters and numbers.
- **download**—to retrieve information from a source, such as a computer, the Internet, or an e-mail, and transfer it to another computer
- **downtime**—a period of lost work time during which a computer is not operating or is malfunctioning because of machine failure.
- **electronic mail (e-mail)**—the transmission of letters, messages, or memos from one computer to another over telephone lines.
- **external memory**—recording on floppy disks.
- **file**—a single, stored unit of information that is given a file name from which it can be accessed.
- **floppy disk**—a flat, rigid, plastic square that looks like a coaster with a metal center. It stores content that has been entered into a computer. The disk permits taking information from one computer and transferring it to another. When the disk is inserted into the disk drive of another computer, the information can be transfered and used.
- **font**—a family or assortment of characters of a given size or style.
- **GB**—gigabyte; approximately one billion (1,000,000,000) bytes (1,073,741,824 bytes to be more exact).
- **hard copy**—the readable paper copy or printout of information.
- **hardware**—the electronic, magnetic, and electro-mechanical equipment of a computer system (keyboard, disk drive, monitor, and printer).
- **home page**—the first page of a document on the World Wide Web (www).
- **HTTP**—Hyper Text Transport Protocol; retrieves hypertext documents (web pages).
- **initialize**—to prepare a diskette to receive data. This is usually referred to as *formatting* the disk.
- **input**—data processed from peripheral equipment into the machine via the keyboard or the floppy disk for internal storage.
- **interface**—the hardware and software that enable individual computers and components to interact.
- **Internet**—network of computers that are all connected to each other.
- **ISP**—Internet Service Provider, a company that provides users with Internet access.
- **K**—computer-shorthand for 1,024 bytes; a term used to measure computer memory capacity.
- **KB (kilobyte)**—about one thousand (1,000) bytes.
- **keyboard**—an input device resembling a typewriter keyboard that converts keystrokes into electrical signals which are displayed on the screen as words or symbols.
- **main memory**—the internal memory of the computer.
- **MB (MegaByte)**—approximately one million (1,000,000) bytes (1,048,576 bytes to be more exact).
- **memory**—data held in storage.
- **menu**—a display of available machine functions for selection by the operator.
- **microcomputer**—a self-contained computer system that uses a microprocessor as the central processing unit. Often called a desktop or personal computer (also known as a PC). Has limited capacity for internal memory.
- **microprocessor**—a single chip where the computer computes.
- **minicomputer**—a computer significantly smaller in size, capacity, and software capability than its larger mainframe counterparts.
- **modem**—**MO**dulator/**DEM**odulator. A peripheral device that enables a computer to communicate with other computers or terminals over normal telephone lines.
- **monitor**—visual display unit with a screen called a cathode-ray tube (CRT).
- **mouse**—a handheld computer input device, separate from a keyboard, used to control cursor position on a VDT (video display terminal).
- **output**—what the computer produces after recorded information is processed, revised, and printed out.
- **peripheral**—anything you plug into a computer; for example, a printer, disk drive, CRT terminal, or printer.
- **printer**—a device that produces hard copy. It may be dot-matrix, letter-quality, or laser.
- **program**—a set of instructions written in computer language.

- **prompting**—messages issued to a user requesting information necessary to continue processing.
- **RAM**—**acronym** for **R**andom **A**ccess **M**emory. This is a temporary, or programmable memory. You can put new information into RAM. When you turn off the computer, this memory is gone.
- **ROM**—acronym for **R**ead **O**nly **M**emory. This is permanent memory. You cannot put new information into ROM. It has been determined by the computer manufacturer.
- **scanner**—a device for a computer that is similar to a mini copier. Items placed on the glass surface are *photographed* and show up on the computer screen.
- **scrolling**—moving cursor up, down, right, or left through information on a computer display to view information otherwise not visible.
- **search engine**—computer program that enables information to be retrieved from a database in response to a query.
- **security code**—a code the operator must enter in before procedure may be completed. Used to prevent unauthorized access to data in system.
- **server**—any computer that provides users with Internet services.
- **software**—computer programs necessary to direct the hardware of a computer system to perform specific tasks.
- **terminal**—a device used to communicate with a computer, usually a keyboard and monitor. Terminals depend on the main (host) computer for their operating abilities. An office may have several terminals and a main frame host computer, which is physically removed from any of them but connected by phone lines.
- **URL**—Uniform Resource Locator (URL) is the address or name of your web site's home page. URLs are all unique.
- **Web browser**—computer software that is used to navigate or move around the Web and connect you to an individual web site or Internet address.
- **write-protect**—process or code that prevents overwriting of data or programs on a disk.

Input into a computer is by means of a keyboard very much like that on a typewriter. There are added keys to give you expanded capability. You do not need to be an expert on computer technology or programming to make good use of a computer.

Any computer, like a typewriter, will occasionally require service. When this becomes necessary, contact is made with the supplier's service department and arrangements are made. Usually, a faulty system component must be taken in for service. Large business central systems will be serviced on site.

When discussing computers, reference is made to hardware and software. The **hardware** refers to the hard disk drive, the CPU, the monitor, and the keyboard. **Software** is the programs containing instructions to the computer that enable it to perform tasks. You interact with the soft-

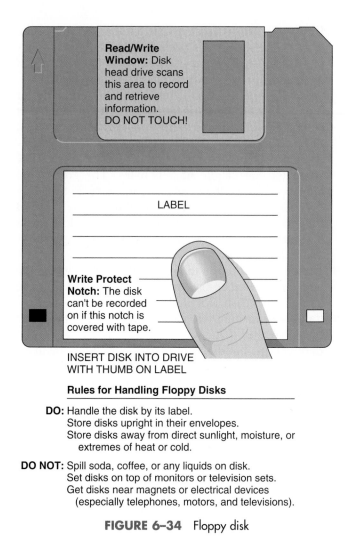

Read/Write Window: Disk head drive scans this area to record and retrieve information. DO NOT TOUCH!

LABEL

Write Protect Notch: The disk can't be recorded on if this notch is covered with tape.

INSERT DISK INTO DRIVE WITH THUMB ON LABEL

Rules for Handling Floppy Disks

DO: Handle the disk by its label.
Store disks upright in their envelopes.
Store disks away from direct sunlight, moisture, or extremes of heat or cold.

DO NOT: Spill soda, coffee, or any liquids on disk.
Set disks on top of monitors or television sets.
Get disks near magnets or electrical devices (especially telephones, motors, and televisions).

FIGURE 6–34 Floppy disk

ware to produce correspondence, maintain records, calculate financial statements, and many other tasks. Software is available on disks to be transferred to the computer's hard drive. A great deal of software is now available on CD-ROM. When you input data with a software program, you can enter it into the memory and store it on the hard drive or on a floppy disk inserted into the disk drive. Floppy disks are usually covered with hard plastic and are $3\frac{1}{2} \times 3\frac{1}{2}$ inches. Figure 6–34 provides guidelines for handling floppy disks. Disks come in different capacities and densities to match different hardware.

The information stored on a disk is called a *file*. It is necessary to assign a code to information to be saved on a file so that it may be *called up* from the storage disk by using the code. Computer manufacturers usually provide basic software programs that are compatible with the hardware. Many companies design special programs of software for use with specific computers. A computer is useless without the software instructions for accessing and inputting data.

The main storage component for a computer is its hard drive, an oxide-coated metal platter that is sealed inside a housing to ensure dust-free operation. The hard drive can store enormous amounts of information which can be retrieved almost immediately. PCs store their software programs as well as input data on their hard drive. In offices with several work stations, the individual computer or terminals can be networked with a service or mainframe computer. This central unit will contain the software programs and the data banks of information to be shared in the office. Each terminal can access information from the central computer, thereby freeing up hard-drive space at each work station. A properly networked system permits input and updating of records from all stations and allows the information to be accessed from all stations.

Electrical surges and power outages can destroy information currently being used by the computer if it has not yet been saved by the operator or automatically by the program. This is most likely to occur during a severe storm. Loss of data due to electrical surges and power outages can be prevented by the installation of a protective device known as an Uninterrupted Power Supply (UPS), which contains a battery backup system. An UPS is capable of sensing a surge or outage, and automatically switches to a backup battery to preserve the data. The size of the battery determines the length of time the equipment can be sustained. The primary purpose is to allow you time to save your document, exit the program, and shut down your system until the power is again stable.

It is very important to establish a "backup policy" to make copies of office programs and data. Often this is performed each night. Data on the hard drives of individual PCs can be copied onto floppy disks if the data is not too extensive. Computer hard drives can "crash," causing the loss of all programs and stored data. Programs and extensive data can be copied by a tape backup device which is a peripheral to the computer, thereby providing a durable copy of information. All central computer data should be backed up on tape daily. Some offices may even contract to have materials backed up in an off-site facility in order to protect against loss of files from fire or natural disaster.

COMPUTER PRINTERS

To produce hard copy, you must have a printer. Printers may be equipped with a single-sheet feeder or a tractor feeder that automatically advances the paper. Three types of printers are appropriate for a medical office: dot-matrix, ink-jet, or laser. The dot-matrix produces print made up of pin-head dots and can produce "near letter quality" printing. Depending on the type of printer you have, you may set "draft mode," and the printer will print more than twice as fast as it will on letter quality. Printer speed is expressed in terms of the number of pages printed per minute. An ink jet printer might print in three different modes. In draft, when less dots or less ink is used, the page can be printed faster. When printing in letter quality, when a professional looking finish is desired, all the dots or maximum ink coverage is used, and therefore the process is slowed. For example, the printer may print five pages a minute in draft, three pages a minute in "normal," and only print one page a minute in best or letter quality mode. The purpose of the draft setting is to

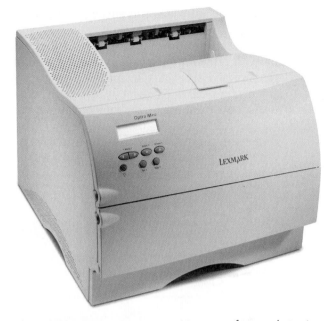

FIGURE 6–35 Laser printer (Courtesy of Lexmark, Inc.)

conserve printer toner or ink when printing a large number of pages of a document which is not in its final stages.

The print wheel in most cases will be bidirectional (prints from left to right and right to left) as this offers more speed. The letter-quality printers may have many print styles built in, and more can be loaded into the printer. Ink-jet printers produce letter quality copy by "spraying" letters onto the paper. A variety of type fonts allow great variation of print styles and many interesting features can be added to your office's print communications.

Laser printers are more expensive, but the print quality is comparable to typeset material. A toner cartridge inside the printer contains the printer's powered "ink" material that produces the type or graphic images. The cartridge will last for approximately 4000 pages of text. The laser printer can also have postscript capability, which allows infusion of many graphic applications to customize office correspondence, patient information sheets, reports, and professional papers (Figure 6–35).

COMPUTER SOFTWARE

Computer software capabilities are virtually limitless. Software companies are continually designing programs that make it possible to direct a computer to produce different prescribed outcomes. It takes anywhere from 12 to 24 months to research, write, and test a comprehensive software program. When the project is begun, the newest technology is used. By the time the project is completed and fully tested, the newest technology is now two years or more outdated. It is important to keep this in mind if you are in a position to recommend use of specific software.

Medical management software is available from many different companies. An example is the program available from MedWare. The software programs make it possible to keep patient information with no limit to the number of patients, except as limited by the capacity of the computer memory. It provides information needed for billing such as primary and secondary insurance. It is easy to look up patient treatment or payment history, print patient mailing labels, phone listings, or set up a recall/reminder system.

The number of procedure and diagnosis codes that may be entered is limitless (Figure 6–36). The codes may be searched by number or by description.

The computer program allows all posting charges and payments to be completed. The input screen is modeled from the standard insurance form (HCFA-1500) (Figure 6–37). The program allows the medical assistant to input the necessary information and then push one key to print a completed insurance form. The information in the computer may be retrieved at any time.

Reports can be prepared with a minimum of effort when data is regularly put into the computer. Accounts receivable may be printed by date or aging or alphabetically. Accounts receivable may be broken down between insur-

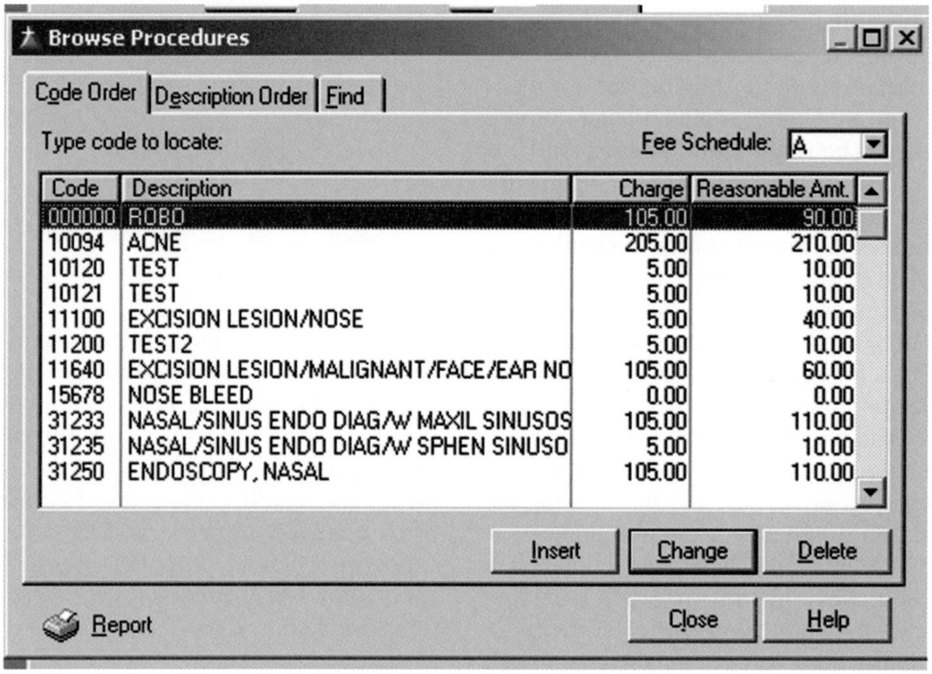

FIGURE 6–36   Diagnosis and procedure codes may be quickly called up alphabetically or numerically (Courtesy of MedWare.)

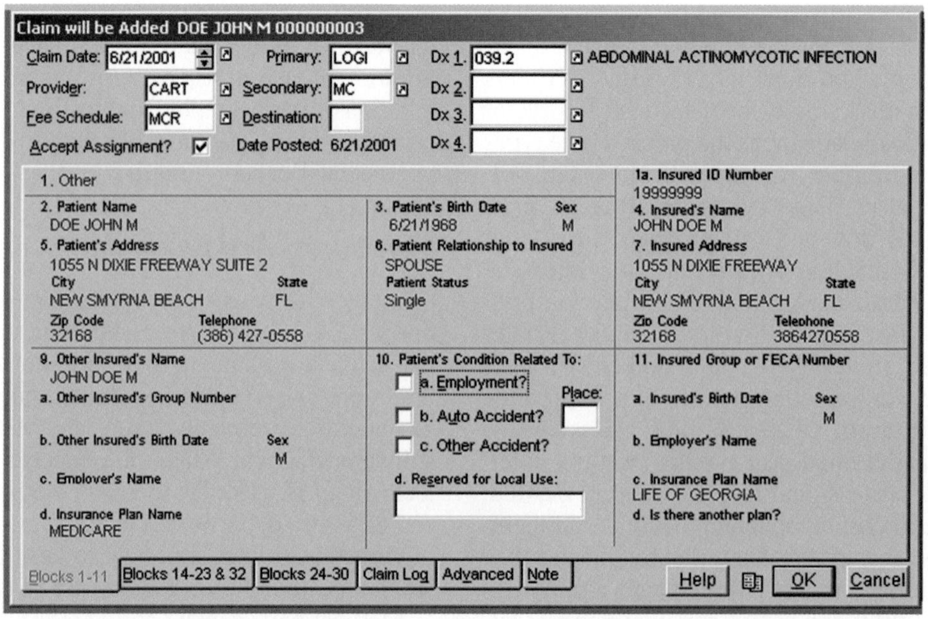

FIGURE 6–37   Screen modeled on the HCFA-1500 layout (Courtesy of MedWare.)

ance company and patient. A detailed summary of income between two given dates may be easily prepared. The report of charges between any two dates may be accessed in detail or summary. A day sheet can be easily prepared. Physicians may find a need for a statistical report of diagnosis and procedure code usage, which can be retrieved from the stored data. Reports can also be sorted and output by individual patient, physician or insurance company.

The patient entry screen provides for the entry of account information for each patient. All the data needed to properly bill the account is included.

The transactions entry screen is where all charge entries are done, including the entries for payments made at the time of service. During charge entry, a running total of the account is displayed at all times. When you have finished making entries for the patient, the account updates immediately. When you have finished your entries for each patient, you will be given the option of printing a patient statement. Prompt billing of patients means faster payment, and efficient, accurate submission of claims means a higher percentage of payment.

The medical office daily register report shows charges and receipts for daily records.

The utility menu screen gives you access to all the functions that let you set up and maintain the custom files to be used by the system, establish the format for your custom forms, and do the maintenance work to keep your system running efficiently. Once these files are established, the data in them is a keystroke away when the system is in use. For additional information on computer billing see Chapter 8, Unit 4.

These illustrations of computer screens are only a sampling of the many office procedures possible with computers. It is important to note that many of the software manufacturers make programs which are compatible with more than one brand of computer. Many of the software systems run on IBM® computers. MAI Systems Corporation has developed its own computer and software for medical offices. Healthcare Communications™ makes software exclusively for Macintosh™.

Some believe that in the future it will be common practice to use a hand-held scanner (like those used in department stores) to scan the bar code on the patient charge slip and thus automatically enter the code number of the procedure or illness and the charge for service. This would eliminate the possibility of error in typing the figures into the computer.

The computer should be useful for inventory control of office supplies, to personalize form-letter mailings for collections, to reschedule annual checkups, and to gather research data.

Some physicians find the computer essential if they are engaged in research and need to quickly identify all patients with a specific diagnosis. It is also valuable in the quick identification of patients taking a particular drug if the manufacturer should issue a warning about side effects.

You may be involved in the use of a computer for patient education. This is similar to the television programs used by some offices. The medical assistant may load the programs into the computer, discuss with patients what they will see, and ascertain whether patients have further concerns after they complete the viewing. Information programs have been developed for diabetes, cancer, pregnancy, health hazards of smoking, and many other subjects.

Most word processing software has a standard built-in dictionary that helps with spelling. Misspelled words are highlighted when the spell check is activated. You still must read carefully to be sure you typed the correct words for the message you wish to convey. You must be accurate in your proofreading. Medical dictionaries are also available as enhancements to the standard dictionary.

Continuous letterheads and new continuous envelopes make your work much faster. There is no need for a typewriter to address envelopes.

You have learned in this unit that using computers in medical offices can be extremely important in helping to complete your work. You should use any opportunity you have to practice with the computer. You should learn the vocabulary and how to read and understand an instruction manual. You need to practice on a typewriter if an extra computer is not available so that you will have accurate keyboarding skills.

All computer systems and word processors have instructions to help you utilize the equipment. Some instructions are in the form of books, known as documentation, which are helpful references for both beginners and experienced operators. With large programs requiring much information, it will probably be available online or on a CD, which can be easily accessed from your screen. Most computer dealers offer basic training with the purchase of new equipment and provide "pay for instruction" classes on the use of specific software applications for the general public. Many public schools and community colleges provide adult education classes which are very beneficial. Procedure 6–11 discusses basic operation of the office computer.

IMPORTANT STEPS IN SELECTING A COMPUTER SYSTEM

The medical assistant employed in an office that is planning to upgrade the computer system will be able to look forward to the experience if there is an opportunity to take part in the planning.

It is important to research the kinds of software available, the kinds of computers the software can be used with, the costs, how long the supplier has been in business, and the kinds of support offered after installation.

A good source for this information is *The Computer Talk Directory of Medical Computer Systems,* which is published semiannually by:

Computer Talk Associates, Inc.
482 Norristown Road, Suite 112
Blue Bell, PA 19422
610-825-7686

PROCEDURE

6-11 Operate Office Computer

PURPOSE: To operate a computer system to enter, revise, delete, save data, and print a hard copy of document.

EQUIPMENT: Computer, peripherals, printer paper, prepared material to be entered. (Suggest a list of 12 "patient" names to be scheduled from 1:00–3:00 PM on an electronic appointment sheet.)

PERFORMANCE OBJECTIVE: Given access to equipment and material to be entered, operate system following steps in the procedure to produce an accurate print copy of a schedule.
NOTE: This exercise is generic, loosley based on Word Perfect . . . Specific steps must be performed as required by available software and computer system.

1. Turn on power to computer.
2. Position cursor on appropriate program on main menu, key ENTER or click mouse.
3. Position cursor on scheduling software program, key EN-TER or click mouse.
4. Locate cursor or click on first cell to be completed.
5. Enter 1:00 PM appointment for first patient on list.
6. Enter remaining names at 15-minute intervals.

7. SAVE data.
   NOTE: If input is not saved, it will be lost when computer is turned off. Some programs save automatically at intervals. Others will save data as part of the EXIT process.
8. Exit scheduling program to main menu.
9. Exit from main menu.
10. Re-enter main menu.
11. Bring up scheduling software.
12. Locate cursor at 2:30 PM, enter patient as work-in who is currently scheduled for 1:30 PM.
13. Locate cursor at 1:30 PM, cancel appointment.
14. Scroll through schedule to view and proofread.
15. Turn on printer, allow time for test sheet, if appropriate.
16. Check paper supply.
17. Key or click on PRINT.
18. Select from available options.
19. PRINT document.
20. Exit program.
21. Exit main menu and system.
22. Turn off power to printer and computer according to office policy.

There are hidden costs to consider. A **maintenance contract** should be available. Investigate the costs and availability of insurance to cover theft, natural disasters (such as a tornado), and internal disasters (such as fire or flood damage). Determine the availability and cost of a consultant to supervise the training of the office staff.

It is always important to obtain cost estimates from at least three companies. The companies should also refer you to current users to help you determine the reliability of the software and hardware. Find out if the software company can furnish new formats when needed.

A CAAHEP CONNECTION

The standards specify the need for instruction in **Application of electronic technology** and **Basic medical office functions**. These skills, such as composing a letter or entering information into the computer, are very important to the operation of the physician's office. Possessing these and other current skills contribute to your employability, a curriculum area in the **Professional Components** standard called **Job readiness**.

RELATING TO ABHES

Chapter 6 discusses opportunities; the preparation, processing, and sending of various forms of office communications; mailing regulations; and the equipment involved in preparing office communications. This content is related to the ABHES accreditation requirements of **Manual and computerized records management** within the content area of **Medical Office Business Procedures/ Management**.

When the physicians decide what they want to accomplish with the system and the costs have been obtained, a decision must be made as to whether the return will justify the cost.

If the determination is made, the first task is to select software that will meet the needs of the office. It should meet the needs of the office in word processing, accounting and office management, and should permit a database for research. The software can then be matched with a compatible computer system.

ACHIEVE UNIT OBJECTIVES

Complete Chapter 6, Unit 5, in the workbook to help you obtain competency of this subject matter.

Medical-Legal-Ethical Scenario

On the advice of her family practice physician, Ruth had phoned a prominent neurologist's office. She had been experiencing severe headaches and pain radiating down her left shoulder and upper back. When the appointment was made, she was informed that a two-hour block of time would be required for the initial testing and consultation. She was also told that she must call at least 48 hours in advance if she could not keep her appointment, or she would be charged a missed appointment fee of $100. Three days before she was scheduled, she began to experience symptoms of the flu. Fearing she might not be able to make the appointment she phoned the office and spoke with a medical assistant named Mrs. Chan, and rescheduled her appointment for two weeks later.

When she went to her appointment, she was informed by Miss Sergio, the office manager, that she needed to pay her missed appointment fee herself since insurance would not cover the charges for a missed appointment. Ruth informed the manager that she had called in and talked with a Miss Chan and cancelled the appointment three days in advance. The assistant told her no such notation was made and the time went unused. She was also told Miss Chan was no longer there to verify her call, so they had no way to document her statement.

CRITICAL THINKING CHALLENGE

1. Refer to the Medical Assistant Role Delineation Study in Appendix A, and discuss the skills under Administrative Procedures, Legal Concepts, and Instruction that apply to this scenario.
2. Should Ruth be required to make the payment in order to continue her relationship with the doctor?
3. Do you think a patient might say they cancelled an appointment to avoid the charge?
4. Is a physician's time so valuable that a charge should be made for a missed appointment?
5. Why do you think Miss Chan is no longer there?

RESOURCES

Battenberg, E. (2001, February 26). Traffic control: Taking the mystery out of e-mail. Columbus, OH: The Columbus Dispatch Co.
United States Postal Service. (1995). Addressing for success. Washington, DC: Author.
United States Postal Service. (1998, March). Consumer's guide to postal services and products. Washington, DC: Author.
United States Postal Service. (2001, January). Quick service guide. Washington, DC: Author.

WEB LINKS   http://www.cc.nih.gov/ccc/ceg/info.html (Confidentiality Education Group [CEG])

This web site provides guidelines for faxing and e-mailing medical information.

http://www.usps.com (United States Postal Service)

This web site provides postal information.

Records Management

Medical records consist of a complete and detailed patient information form, health history, physical examination, diagnostic reports, and treatment notes that allow the physician to provide necessary care for patients. The records must be accurate, complete, and filed so that they may be quickly found when needed.

The confidentiality of the records must be maintained by careful management as they are used. Efficiency is essential to a well-run medical facility. Filing needs to be current at all times.

UNIT 1

The Patient's Medical Record

▇ OBJECTIVES

Upon completion of the unit, meet the following performance objectives by verifying knowledge of the facts and principles presented through oral and written communication at a level deemed competent, and demonstrate the specific behaviors as identified in the performance objectives of the procedures, observing safety precautions in accordance with health care standards.

1. Spell and define, using the glossary at the back of the text, all the Words to Know in this unit.
2. Describe the importance of the medical record as a legal document.
3. List examples of subjective information.
4. List examples of objective information.
5. Describe methods of recording progress notes.
6. Describe the correct procedure for making corrections of progress notes.
7. List the differences between a conventional record and the problem oriented medical record.
8. Explain the History Physical Impression Plan (HPIP) method of recording patients' medical information.
9. Describe the major sections of a medical record.
10. Explain the reason for a tickler file.
11. Explain the purpose of chart audits and their importance.

AREAS OF COMPETENCE (AAMA)

This unit addresses content within the specific competency areas of *Administrative procedures, Patient care, Professionalism, Communication skills, Legal concepts, Instruction*, and *Operational functions* as identified in the Medical Assistant Role Delineation Study. Refer to Appendix A for a detailed listing of the areas.

▇ WORDS TO KNOW

audit
charting
jeopardize
objective

procrastinator
progress notes
subjective

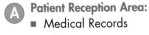

Ⓐ **Patient Reception Area:**
■ Medical Records

The patient history is the most important record kept in the medical office. The dates of any injuries, dates of treatment, and all notes regarding the condition of the patient must be accurate in every detail. In a lawsuit result-

ing from an injury, the patient chart information could win or lose the case.

Each office has its own method of charting patient information during visits. Some physicians ask the medical assistant to record the findings of a physical examination as it is being completed. Some physicians take the time to write all physical findings and progress notes for each visit. Many physicians prefer to dictate progress notes; then it becomes the duty of the medical assistant to type them, or process data using a word processor or computer. If dictating and transcribing the information is the preferred method, the printed document must be dated and placed in the patient's chart with a notation: e.g., *"As dictated by Dr. H.G. Brown."* Keep in mind that confidentiality is vitally important, especially where many staff members have access to patient files and when the patients and their families may have a clear view of the monitor screen at times. Safeguarding personal and private patient information is always necessary.

Computer generated patient records begin with entering the patient's general information for billing and scheduling. Computerized patient records also include the medical history appropriate for each particular type of medical practice. The extent of computer use in patient records is a decision made by the employer and the office manager. The issue of protection of patient confidentiality still remains a legitimate concern for both physician and patient. Extensive medical histories of patients who have conditions or diseases that may affect their insurance coverage, career, relationships, and so on are an important consideration. Some patients are reluctant to have their personal information accessible to so many people. Patients must be informed that there is a risk of a possible invasion of privacy of their medical information even though every effort is made to protect this confidence. A password should be made known only to a select few employees to access files. This helps to keep information confidential.

Software packages are available to fit the needs of the practice according to the types of functions desired. Computerized medical records and examination formats, as well as billing and insurance with Current Procedural Terminology (CPT) and International Classification of Diseases (ICD) codes and other helpful and time-saving programs, are designed to make processing and retrieving information easy and efficient in the daily practice of managed care of patients.

THE PURPOSE OF RECORDS

The complete medical record has several important purposes:

1. It serves as a basis for planning patient care and for continuity in evaluating the patient's condition and treatment. The combination of the personal and fam-

ily history with the findings of the physician must be combined with the results of laboratory studies, x-rays, and any indicated special tests. The review of all of these facts together help the physician determine the diagnosis and course of treatment. This would not be possible without a well-documented, accurate record. The patient history or family history may alert the physician to certain conditions such as a family history of diabetes or exposure to hazardous substances.

2. The medical record furnishes documentary evidence of the course of the patient's medical evaluation, treatment, and change in condition. The charting of progress notes is extremely important and should give an indication of the patient comments, physician's evaluation, prescribed treatment, and need for further follow-up.

3. The record furnishes evidence of communication between the physician and any other health professional contributing to the patient's care. The chart should include a record of reports from other physicians asked to evaluate the patient with special laboratory, x-ray, or diagnostic procedures.

4. It affords protection of the legal interests of the patient and the physician. The complete accurate record would be necessary if the patient wishes the physician to testify in an injury case. The complete accurate record is also necessary if the patient sues the physician for malpractice. The patient must always sign an authorization form before any information may be released. An authorization must indicate who is to be allowed to receive the information.

5. The medical record helps to establish a database for use in continuing education and research. The accurate record of patients is a useful resource for research concerning response to medications or procedures in every phase of medical treatment.

6. Insurance companies routinely send a representative to perform chart **audits** (inspections) of medical records of patients insured through their company. Medical offices receive an overall grade that reflects the thoroughness and quality of their record keeping. Offices that consistently score low **jeopardize** future contracts with those insurance companies.

The information in the medical record is classified as subjective or objective. The **subjective** information is supplied by the patient and includes routine information about the patient, past personal and medical history, family history, and chief complaint. The physician and various members of the health care team provide objective information (e.g., vital signs, exam findings, diagnostic tests, etc). The objective information includes examination, results of any laboratory studies, special procedures, x-rays, the diagnosis, treatment prescribed, and progress notes.

PARTS OF THE MEDICAL RECORD

The medical record is generally divided into the following sections:

- Administrative data
- Financial/insurance information
- Correspondence
- Referral
- Past medical records
- Clinical data
- Progress notes
- Diagnostic information
- Lab information
- Medications

Administrative Data and Financial/Insurance Information

Each patient should be asked to fill out demographic information on a patient data form during the first office visit. Ask the patient to complete the form by printing all blanks, such as full name, Social Security number (SS#), birth date, spouse's name, address, work and home phone numbers, insurance information, emergency contact information, etc. Demographic information should be updated at every visit. Make sure that the information is updated on the patient's chart and in the computer. Refer to Figure 7–1 for an example of a patient information sheet. Place an attractive sign in the reception area and at the checkout window that directs a simple question to patients such as, "Do we have your current address and phone number?" Another example of a sign to post is, "Please let us know if there are any changes we should make about your address, phone, workplace, etc." Some offices post a sign or notice on the back of the exam room door. This way a patient can read the reminder and let the medical assistant know of any changes. Another way to monitor patients' whereabouts is to make a copy of their driver's license during their initial office visit. This way you will be able to trace a patient if ever you have a return of the patient's mail. Even though this information should be obtained from patients at the reception window, it is not always possible. In a fast-paced medical practice there is sometimes no opportunity to do everything that should be done in perfect time. The medical assistant who realizes this will survive the hectic times that do happen in dealing with patients every day. Prioritizing matters of importance is the logical thing to do. Being prioritized and completing one task at a time will help reduce stress and help you be efficient.

Correspondence

This section of the medical record includes all correspondence received concerning the patient. Referral or follow-up letters from specialists, informational or request-of-information letters from insurance companies, and any

PATIENT INFORMATION SHEET
(PLEASE PRINT)

PATIENT INFORMATION

NAME: _____
      (LAST)   (FIRST)   (INITIAL)

ADDRESS: _____
      (STREET) (CITY) (STATE) (ZIP)

HOME PHONE: _____ RELIGION: _____

MARITAL STATUS: S M W SEP D

SS#: _____ BIRTHDATE:_____ OCCUPATION: _____

EMPLOYER: _____ WORK PHONE: _____

EMPLOYER'S ADDRESS: _____

YOUR INSURANCE COMPANY: _____
(If insurance is your HUSBAND'S or PARENT'S, please list below.)

INSURANCE CERTIFICATE OR I.D. #: _____ GROUP #: ____

HUSBAND and/or RESPONSIBLE PARTY INFORMATION:
(Give husband's information even if you are not covered under his insurance.)

NAME: _____
      (LAST)   (FIRST)   (INITIAL)

ADDRESS: _____
      (STREET) (CITY) (STATE) (ZIP)

HOME PHONE: _____ RELATIONSHIP TO YOU: _____

SS#: _____ BIRTHDATE:_____ OCCUPATION: _____

EMPLOYER: _____ WORK PHONE: _____

EMPLOYER'S ADDRESS: _____

INSURANCE COMPANY (Only if you are covered): _____

INSURANCE CERTIFICATE OR I.D. #: _____ GROUP #: ____

NEAREST RELATIVE (Not residing with you):

NAME: _____ RELATIONSHIP TO YOU: _____

ADDRESS: _____ PHONE #: _____

REFERRED BY: NAME: _____

ASSIGNMENT AND RELEASE WE DO NOT SUBMIT INSURANCE FOR ROUTINE OFFICE VISITS

I hereby authorize that my insurance benefits be paid directly to Katherine Lang, MD and I authorize the physician to release any information required. I acknowledge that I am financially responsible for any noncovered services. I further authorize release of these records for the purpose of medical care review by my insurance company. I permit a copy of this authorization to be used in place of the original.

SIGNATURE _____ DATE _____

FIGURE 7–1 Example of a new-patient information form. At each office visit this information should be verified and appropriate changes made in the patient's chart.

correspondence from the patient should be filed in the patient's chart as soon as possible from the date it is received.

Referral

Frequently, patients need to be sent to other facilities for specified diagnostic testing and to specialists for conditions beyond the expertise of the preferred provider. In or-

der for the insurance company to pay for these visits, the preferred provider generally will need to submit a referral to the hospital, specialist, etc., so that the patient's medical services are covered by their insurance. It is imperative that the referring physician sends the patient to a participating provider listed on the patient's insurance plan. Often explaining this to the patient is one of the most important duties of the medical assistant. Failure to comply with these conditions could make the referring physician responsible for the cost of the diagnostic tests, which could result in a costly mistake of thousands of dollars.

Past Medical Records

Physicians usually request medical records from prior physicians for reference purposes. Knowing the patient's medical history is quite helpful in providing quality health care.

Progress Notes

Progress notes are the chronologic listing of visits, prescription refills, all calls that pertain to the patient, and all calls that the patient has had with any member of the health care team. Any time a patient has an interaction with anyone in the medical office, it should be recorded in the patient's progress notes.

The progress notes should be arranged in chronologic order with the most recent date on top. If several notes are recorded on a page, the last on the page should be the most recent. The chart should be carefully dated for each visit. As discussed in the chapter on medical-legal considerations (see Chapter 3), each no-show, cancellation, telephone call, or prescription needs to be recorded as a progress note in the record of the patient, along with the date each took place, and signed by the individual making the entry.

The initial visit for any condition is usually written as a chief complaint on the progress note. It is a brief description of what is wrong with the patient. A history of the present illness, and any remedies taken by the patient are usually included. Home remedies should also be included. The patient's medication and drug allergies should be recorded and updated during each subsequent visit. Use standard abbreviations whenever possible when charting information. Using a + (plus) sign to indicate that the patient has the symptom and a − (minus) sign to indicate that the patient does not have that symptom provides valuable information for the physician (Figure 7–2). The level of pain that the patient experiences must also be recorded on the chart. Use the standard scale of 1 to 10, with 10 being the worst. The physician will complete the progress notes by listing all objective findings and assessment and plan for further treatment and by signing the chart once the patient's examination is completed.

Example 1:

Ms. Sabrina K. Lane, DOB 12/23/1977

01/15/XX Pt C/O urinary sx × 3 d +frequency, +burning, +pain/urination, +N/−E, +chills, −fever, −pus or blood in urine, −back or abdominal pain, −vag sx, LMP

01/05/XX − OTC meds, current prescribed meds: Ortho-Novum 7-7-7 and tetracycline. NKDA.

D. Brown, CMA

Example 2:

01/18/XX TC [telephone call]: pt called to tell Dr. Smith that the Macrobid makes her sick. Her sx are worse. Called in new Rx for Cipro 500 mg, BID to XYZ pharmacy per Dr. Smith.

D. Brown, CMA (KL)

Example 3:

01/20/XX TC: pt called and said that sx are better and that Cipro does not make her sick. Pt encouraged to continue Cipro and to follow up with an appointment in 1 wk per Dr. Smith.

D. Brown, CMA (KL)

Example 4:

01/27/XX Pt here for a F/U [follow-up] for UTI. Pt states that she took all of the Cipro and is presently asymptomatic.

D. Brown, CMA (KL)

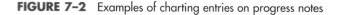

FIGURE 7–2 Examples of charting entries on progress notes

Diagnostic Information

All x-rays and non–lab-related testing should be placed in chronologic order in this section of the patient's chart.

Lab Information

All lab reports should be placed in chronologic order in this section of the chart. Notice in the charting examples that follow in this unit that the medical assistant signs her name and credentials after recording the procedure that she completed. In the parentheses are the physician's initials that signify that the physician has approved the orders that were completed.

Medications

Copies of prescriptions and documentation of any medications that are administered in the office are usually placed in this section of the chart. Administrative data is usually placed on one side of the chart and clinical data on the other side of the chart. This makes it easier and more expedient to locate each of the sections for information about a patient.

DATING, CORRECTING, AND MAINTAINING THE CHART

It is extremely important to record the date when documenting the patient's chief complaint or additional information on progress notes. In pertinent cases, such as car or industrial accidents, the time should also be recorded. You should make sure that you indicate AM or PM when noting the time. The date may be written in ink or stamped. Every time a patient is given a prescription over the phone or is given a report or advice should also be recorded with the date and time. Failure of a patient to keep an appointment should always be recorded by the date stamp on the chart. When it is necessary to start a new page, the patient's name and birth date should be written at the top of each new page. If office staff other than the physician are making notes on the chart, these should be signed by the person making the notation.

In making a correction on progress notes, a handwritten entry should have a single line drawn through it and the correction written above or following it. An indication of correction should be made in the margin and should bear the initials of the person making the correction. Using correction fluid or erasing the error is not recommended because it looks as if one were trying to cover up or completely eliminate what was written. This could raise suspicion if there is ever a legal question regarding a patient and treatment. Write or print in a neat and legible manner. Be careful to spell the patient's name correctly and learn how to pronounce them accurately. (If necessary, you should ask the person to give you a phonetic spelling with accent symbols to show how to pronounce the name correctly. Some examples of difficult names to pronounce, followed by their phonetic spelling, are: Gnomic, gno′-mic [no′-mic]; Coughlin, cog′-lin; Chappelle, cha-pell′; Skowronski, Sko′-ron-ski; Zielachowski, zi-la-chow′-ski.) Charting becomes a part of the permanent record and one should respect this fact. Using black ink will make much better photocopies of the record. When you finish with a patient's chart, always try to straighten up the forms and make the chart neat before filing it. Forms and other documents tend to shift with handling and they sometimes become folded or tattered, which eventually makes them difficult to read. After you have completed recording or filing additional information in a patient's chart, you should return it to the files as soon as possible. Having stacks of files pulled too far in advance of the patients' appointments is not necessary and is not practical. Patient charts should be filed when not in use for a specific purpose.

Typing should be corrected at the time of error by use of correcting ribbon or correction fluid. An error found at a later time is corrected in the same manner as in a handwritten record, but there should be no need to do this if typed material is carefully proofread.

In each medical specialty there are unique terms and phrases. You should make a correctly spelled list of these

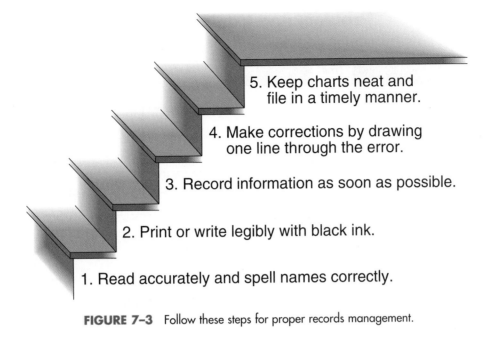

5. Keep charts neat and file in a timely manner.

4. Make corrections by drawing one line through the error.

3. Record information as soon as possible.

2. Print or write legibly with black ink.

1. Read accurately and spell names correctly.

FIGURE 7-3 Follow these steps for proper records management.

terms so you won't have to continually refer to a dictionary. These may be anatomical terms, surgical terms, appliances, medications, or simply English vocabulary the physician uses frequently. You will also find that the physician frequently uses abbreviations in handwritten notes or even in dictation, and knowledge of these is also useful. See Figure 7–3 for steps to follow.

TRACKING MEDICAL RECORDS

Every office or clinic has a system that works efficiently for them to track outstanding work that must be completed before releasing the chart to be filed. Many medical practice offices separate the charts at the physician's station or desk into specific stacks. Divisions may include:

- Charts to be filed
- Prescription refills
- Lab results
- Coding/financial corrections
- Charts awaiting dictation
- Referrals

The physician will work on these stacks throughout the day generally in the order of the most urgent to the least. It is the medical assistant's responsibility to track the stacks and complete any assigned work such as prescription call-ins, phoning patients with lab results, and sending completed charts to the central filing area. Time management is essential when working on these tasks. The assistant who works throughout the day to eliminate these stacks is the assistant who will get to leave at the usual closing time each day. Medical assistants who wait until all patients have been seen to file charts away will unfortunately end up staying overtime to complete their work.

Many fine physicians are **procrastinators** when it comes to completing paperwork in the office. It is the duty of the medical assistant to see that it gets done even if this requires daily reminders.

CALL-BACKS

As mentioned earlier in this unit, the medical assistant will make calls to patients, pharmacies, and labs. These are frequently referred to as *call-backs*. There will be some occasions where the medical assistant will be unable to complete all calls that need to be made. The following list categorizes calls that should take precedence.

1. All abnormal lab results, especially prothrombin time levels and other medication levels
2. Prescription refills
3. Patient concerns that were not handled at the time of the initial call

None of the above issues should ever be left until the following day without the direct approval of the physician. All phone calls should be documented, even if contact with the patient was not accomplished. Recording the time of the call is critical in these situations.

A helpful practice for keeping track of referral appointments, follow-ups, and re-checks is to use a small, recipe card–sized filing unit called a tickler file. A more in-depth discussion of tickler files will be presented at the end of the chapter.

THE PROBLEM ORIENTED MEDICAL RECORD

In the early 1970s Lawrence L. Weed, M.D., a professor of medicine at the University of Vermont's College of

Problem and Medication List

Patient Name: **DOB:**

Allergies: **Pharmacy #**

Date	Dx #	Chronic Problems	Dx #	Chronic Medications	Date		Refills					
					Start	Date						
					Stop	Initials						
					Start	Date						
					Stop	Initials						
					Start	Date						
					Stop	Initials						
					Start	Date						
					Stop	Initials						
					Start	Date						
					Stop	Initials						
					Start	Date						
					Stop	Initials						
					Start	Date						
					Stop	Initials						
					Start	Date						
					Stop	Initials						
					Start	Date						
					Stop	Initials						

Preventive	Date	Date	Date	Date	Date	Date
History Update Every 2 Years						
Breast Exam (plus Self Exam)						
Mammogram						
DEXA						
Diabetic Blood Sugar Monitoring						
Diabetic Foot Care						
Diabetic HbA1c						
Diabetic LDL						
Diabetic Retinal Exam						
Diabetic proteinuria						
Fasting Glucose						
Lipid Panel						
Pap/Pelvic						
Prostate Exam, PSA						
Rectal Exam						
Sigmoid/Colonos						
Stool for Occult Blood						
Testicular Exam (plus Self Exam)						

Immunizations						
Vaccination	Schedule	Date	Date	Date	Date
Hepatitis	As appropriate				
Influenza	At risk—q1y				
Pneumovax	At risk X 1				
Td Booster	PRN—q10y				

Education	Date	Date	Date	Date
Advanced Directives/ Power of Attorney				
Alcohol/Drug Use				
Birth Control/Menopause				
Diabetes				
Diet				
Exercise				
Smoking				
Stress				

FIGURE 7–4 A sample patient problem and medication list that also provides space for dates and details of preventive actions, patient education, and immunizations, as well as the patient's pharmacy phone number.

Medicine, originated a system of record keeping for patients that he named the problem oriented medical record (POMR). In the traditional medical record, the progress notes are recorded according to the source they come from—the physician, laboratory, or physician's assistant—with no special attempt to record a relationship between them. The POMR record begins with the standard database, which includes patient profile, chief complaint, review of systems, physical examination, and laboratory reports. The chart usually contains a page near the front cover that lists and dates chronic problems. The page may also contain such information as a medication list, a preventive care list, and an education section that dates when patient education was given to the patient (Figure 7–4). This allows the physician to review at a glance the patient's past history without having to read through each individual entry of the progress notes. Using this system, the physician can make an assessment of the patient's health status to date. It works especially well in group practice settings because it promotes the continuity of patient care among the group members. The physician will first record findings on the progress notes of the chart using the Subjective Objective Assessment Plan (SOAP) method that follows (Figure 7–5):

S —Subjective impressions
O—Objective clinical evidence
A—Assessment or diagnosis
P —Plans for further studies, treatment, or management

This process makes the chart easier to review and helps in follow-up of all problems the patient may have. Figures 7–6A and B are two methods of charting patients' medical information. Notice how similar they are. Following these formats in recording findings of patients yields better point-of-care service because there is a logical sequence to follow. There is less chance of overlooking a problem or a plan to treat patients.

Another similar system of recording medical information about patients is the History Physical Impression Plan (HPIP) method.

H—History (subjective findings)
P —Physical exam (objective findings)
I —Impression (assessment/diagnosis)
P —Plan (treatment)

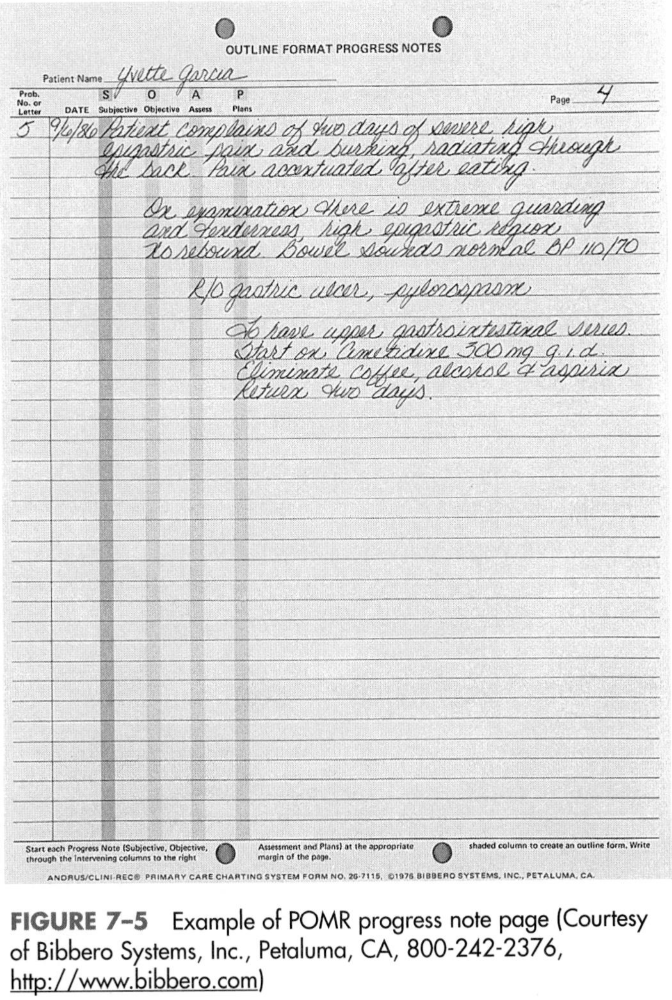
OUTLINE FORMAT PROGRESS NOTES

Patient Name *Yvette Garcia* Page *4*

Prob. No. or Letter | DATE | S Subjective | O Objective | A Assess | P Plans

5 9/6/86 Patient complains of two days of severe high epigastric pain and burning, radiating through the back. Pain accentuated after eating.

On examination there is extreme guarding and tenderness high epigastric region. No rebound. Bowel sounds normal. BP 110/70

R/O gastric ulcer, pylorospasm

To have upper gastrointestinal series. Start on Cimetidine 300 mg q.i.d. Eliminate coffee, alcohol & aspirin. Return two days.

Start each Progress Note (Subjective, Objective, Assessment and Plans) at the appropriate shaded column to create an outline form. Write through the intervening columns to the right margin of the page.

ANDRUS/CLINI-REC® PRIMARY CARE CHARTING SYSTEM FORM NO. 26-7115, ©1976 BIBBERO SYSTEMS, INC., PETALUMA, CA.

FIGURE 7–5 Example of POMR progress note page (Courtesy of Bibbero Systems, Inc., Petaluma, CA, 800-242-2376, http://www.bibbero.com)

Ms. Sabrina Katherine Lake DOB 12/23/1977
01/29/XX

Subjective	Pt states, "I've been feeling very tired and weak for the past month," LMP 01-15-XX very heavy flow. Exam: 6 # Wt loss since last visit 12/19/XX.
Objective	BP 112/70, Hb 10.4, Hct 31%. Decrease in muscle strength, pale.
Assessment	R/O anemia.
Plan	CBC with diff sent to lab, return in 1 week.

FIGURE 7–6(A) A labeled sample of the SOAP method of charting.

Mr. Dennis J. Roberts DOB 8/25/XX
3/4/XX

(H) Hx	C/O severe H/A Rt side of his head lasting several hours to up to 3 days; has had 4 in the past 6 wks, pain is increasing each time; takes ASA for pain.
(P) PX	Neurologic exam shows slight tremor in both hands.
(I) Impression	R/O encephaloma.
(P) Plan	CAT scan of cranium. Refer to Clearbrook Neurological Associates.

FIGURE 7–6(B) A sample of the HPIP method of charting as related to the SOAP.

Medical-Legal-Ethical Scenario

Mrs. Fields has an appointment for the doctor to check a severe burn on her right arm. When she came in, she asked the receptionist if the doctor could see her new neighbor who was with her. She explained that her neighbor was having some chest congestion and a productive cough. Darlene, the receptionist, politely told Mrs. Fields that she was sorry but the doctor was not taking any new patients. She told Mrs. Fields that there was a clinic or a hospital emergency room close where she could take her neighbor after the doctor sees her. As they were speaking at the receptionist window, the neighbor collapsed on the reception room floor. She was unconscious.

Critical Thinking Challenge

1. What should Darlene do?
2. What do you think Mrs. Fields should have done?
3. Who is responsible for the neighbor? And why?
4. Explain why Darlene should or should not make a chart for this woman.
5. Is it important that there is a record of this situation? Why or why not?
6. What would you have done first? Second? And so on.

CAAHEP CONNECTION

Relating to patient records, the medical assistant should have knowledge of *Medical Terminology, Medical law and ethics, Skills in communication*, and *Basic medical office functions*. The information in this chapter may impress upon you the importance of accuracy and efficiency in preparing, maintaining, and storing patient records.

ACHIEVE UNIT OBJECTIVES

Complete Chapter 7, Unit 1, in the workbook to help you obtain competency of this subject matter.

UNIT 2

Filing

OBJECTIVES

Upon completion of the unit, meet the following performance objectives by verifying knowledge of the facts and principles presented through oral and written communication at a level deemed competent, and demonstrate the specific behaviors as identified in the performance objectives of the procedures, observing safety precautions in accordance with health care standards.

1. Spell and define, using the glossary at the back of the text, all the Words to Know in this unit.
2. Explain basic filing methods.
3. List the steps used in filing.
4. Describe methods of removing and replacing patient files.
5. List the storage media used for "paperless" filing systems.
6. List and discuss the sections of a medical chart.
7. Describe purging files.
8. Explain ways to locate a missing chart.
9. Explain the pros and cons of alphabetical and numeric (digital) filing systems.

WORDS TO KNOW

accumulated	sequence
caption	subsequent
chronologic	supplemented
data	systematically
expedite	unproductive
illuminating	warranty
purge	

IMPORTANCE OF FILING

Assembling and filing the patient's medical record are necessary to good patient care. Records must be filed accurately and **systematically**. Accuracy in assembling and filing the patient's medical record is necessary in providing quality managed care. Carelessly filed records produce chaos in the office. Reports that are lost or filed in the wrong chart or hidden in stacks of unfiled material will result in many hours of **unproductive** time spent searching for them. An efficient office requires accurate filing daily. Not only does this maintain efficiency, it also reduces the chance of accidental loss of correspondence and reports.

FILING STEPS

Folders or cards are easily filed alphabetically or numerically, but the procedure for filing reports and letters requires several steps (Figure 7–7).

Step One: Inspect

Generally, the medical assistant is the first to *inspect* reports. The reports are divided into negative/normal and

Patient: Carol Sue Lamp ✓

City Hospital
Troy, Ohio

ROENTGEN FINDINGS

Examination of the pelvis. AP supine including the upper thirds of the femora bilaterally visualizes advanced degenerative arthritis of the right hip with narrowing almost to obliteration of the hip joint space and with degenerative changes and cystic formation affecting the articulating surfaces of the head of the femur as well as the acetabulum. The remaining pelvis and left hip appears essentially normal.

Impression: Advanced degenerative arthritis right hip, otherwise normal pelvis and left hip.

FIGURE 7–8 The check mark in the upper right-hand corner of this report shows that the physician has read this report and notified the patient, and it may now be filed in the patient's chart. Often a practice is for the physician to either sign or initial the report to signify that it has been read and can be filed.

positive/abnormal for the physician to read. It is the practice of some physicians to have the medical assistant send reports or phone patients about diagnostic reports if the reports are normal or negative. Many physicians prefer to review all reports regardless of the findings. After the physician reads a report, a check mark in the right upper corner of the document or a circle around the abnormal finding is made in red, and a notation is made about the follow-up (e.g., "Repeat mammography in 3 months," "Schedule an appointment for consultation," "Needs chest x-ray," etc.). A letter may be dictated or a referral may be necessary (Figure 7-8).

Step Two: Indexing

The second step is *indexing*. This requires that you make a decision as to the name, subject, or other **caption** under which you will file the material. Materials for patients should be filed under the patient name. Research papers can be filed under illness, procedure, treatment, medication, or author. A cross-reference may be helpful in finding things later (Figure 7–9). For example, a research paper might be filed under the title, *Diabetes,* and a cross-reference to the article placed under the author's name, *Allen, John.*

Step Three: Coding

Coding is the third step, and is done by marking the index caption on the papers to be filed. If the name, subject, or a number appears on the paper, you can underline or cir-

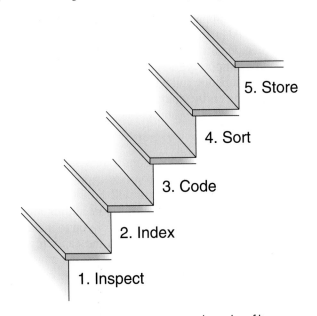

5. Store
4. Sort
3. Code
2. Index
1. Inspect

FIGURE 7–7 Steps to remember when filing

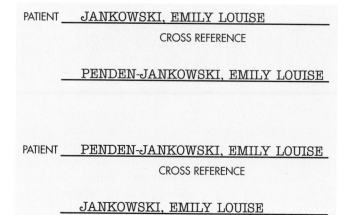

PATIENT ___JANKOWSKI, EMILY LOUISE___

CROSS REFERENCE

___PENDEN-JANKOWSKI, EMILY LOUISE___

PATIENT ___PENDEN-JANKOWSKI, EMILY LOUISE___

CROSS REFERENCE

___JANKOWSKI, EMILY LOUISE___

FIGURE 7–9 Example of a cross-reference card for efficient filing

Patient: <u>Marsha Leonard</u>

Tri-County Hospital
Miami, Ohio

ROENTGEN FINDINGS

Films of 8/31 _____. Review of the PA and lateral chest film of 8/31 _____ shows the traches to be shifted slightly to the left by a soft tissue mass in the right thoracic inlet in the superior mediastinal area. This probably represents tumor and is again seen on the lateral view lying in the anterior portion of the thoracic inlet on the right. Heart is otherwise normal. Lungs are otherwise clear.

FIGURE 7–10 Underlining the patient's name on a report is one way of signifying that the patient has been notified and that the report may be filed in the patient's chart.

cle it, preferably with a colored pencil or a color highlighter (Figure 7–10). (Your employer may have a preference as to the color to be used for the coding process.) If the name, subject, or other caption does not appear on the material to be filed, write the caption in the upper right-hand corner. The medical assistant (or whoever is reviewing the chart or report) should sign the chart (with first-name initial and full last name, e.g., J. Williams) or report signifying that the patient has been contacted. The physician should review all charts and place her initials in parentheses after the medical assistant's signature to signify that the physician is aware that orders were carried out. As soon as the recommendations have been completed and the patient has been informed, the chart is ready for sorting to be filed.

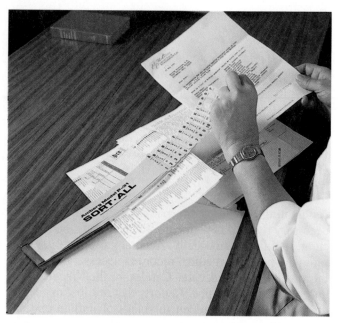

FIGURE 7–11 In this photo the medical assistant is using a desk sorter to alphabetize reports to make filing easier.

Step Four: Sort

The fourth step is to *sort* the material. A desk sorter may be used to put papers in alphabetic order after they have been coded. This speeds up the process of filing (Figure 7–11). Using this sorter or an expanding alphabetic file to sort reports, mail, and other items can provide a temporary file of these records until they can be placed in the patient's permanent chart. On days when it is especially hectic and all the filing has not yet been completed, this means of sorting can help you locate a particular report quickly. This can be a practical answer to more efficient filing because when all items are arranged alphabetically, it saves steps because each letter of the alphabet is in groups and filing goes much more quickly. Also, there are times when the patient's chart is in another department and mail, for example, can be placed in this temporary file for ease in obtaining information to answer a phone call without having to take time out to go and get the entire chart.

Step Five: Storing

The final step is *storing*. You must first locate the file drawer or shelf with the appropriate caption. Then find the folder in which the reports will be stored. Lift the folder and place it on a flat surface before adding any material. This procedure makes it easier for you to make sure the caption on the folder agrees with the caption on the paper to be filed. Place the papers with the heading to the left and the most recent material on top. Some offices attach laboratory reports to the folder in a "shingle" fashion (Figure 7–12). The first is attached at the bottom of the page and each **subsequent** report partially overlaps the previous ones.

LABORATORY REPORTS

PLACE TOP OF REPORT #13 HERE

PLACE TOP OF REPORT #12 HERE

PLACE TOP OF REPORT #11 HERE

PLACE TOP OF REPORT #10 HERE

PLACE TOP OF REPORT #9 HERE

PLACE TOP OF REPORT #8 HERE

PLACE TOP OF REPORT #7 HERE

PLACE TOP OF REPORT #6 HERE

PLACE TOP OF REPORT #5 HERE

PLACE TOP OF REPORT #4 HERE

PLACE TOP OF REPORT #3 HERE

PLACE TOP OF REPORT #2 HERE

PLACE TOP OF REPORT #1 HERE

INSTRUCTIONS: TO ATTACH REPORT, REMOVE PROTECTIVE TAPE BACKING, ALIGN REPORT AND PRESS DOWN FIRMLY. REPEAT PROCEDURE FOR SUBSEQUENT REPORTS.

INHEALTH
RECORD SYSTEMS

5076 Winters Chapel Road • Atlanta, Georgia 30360
1-800-477-7374 • 1-770-396-4994

FORM F260

LABORATORY REPORTS

FIGURE 7-12 This type of report is filed by shingle fashion with the most recent report on top. (Courtesy of INHEALTH Record Systems.)

FINDING A MISSING CHART

There are times when a chart seems nowhere to be found. There are a few steps to consider in locating the missing chart. First, go to the files where the chart you need should be, and look through several of the charts in front of and after this location. The chart may have been accidentally placed within one of the other charts near where it belongs. Second, check the name of the chart you need, and see if the chart was filed in the alphabetic section of the person's first name. Next, check the day's schedule, and see if the chart is out for the patient to be seen. If you know the person was seen earlier in the day or week and you cannot locate the chart, look on the day's schedule when the patient was last seen, and check in several of the charts of those seen before and after the patient. It could have been placed within one of those charts by mistake. If you still cannot find the chart, the other logical places to look are on the desk of the physician, in the insurance or billing department, with the lab technician or office manager, or on the cart of the charts being pulled for the day or charts to be filed.

FILING STORAGE

Every office that requires you to file paper records will have storage units for this purpose. Files come in many different styles, shapes, and sizes. There are vertical or lateral file cabinets, card index files, open shelf files, and tub files (Figures 7–13 and 7–14). To save space, many offices are using movable shelving systems (Figure 7–15). Automation has made its way to the medical office. Automated shelving units not only save space but also provide extra security for the medical records. The carriers rotate automatically, bringing requested files to your fingertips so that you avoid reaching, bending, or wasting steps. At any given time, the Lektriever 2000 (Figure 7–16) can give the operator access to 350 linear

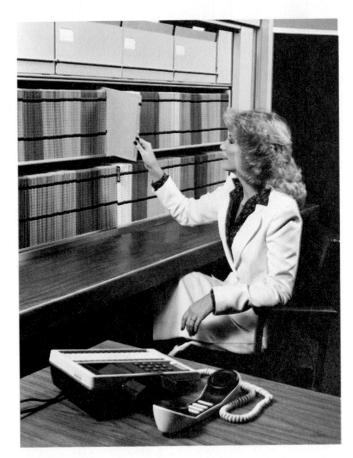

FIGURE 7-13 The medical assistant in this picture is retrieving a chart from lateral shelf files. (Courtesy of Kardex.)

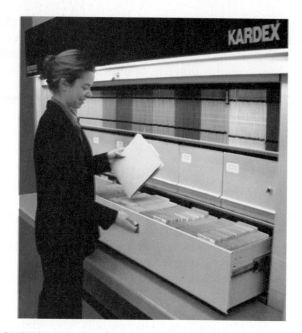

FIGURE 7–14 An administrative assistant is filing a patient's chart in pull-out drawer files. (Courtesy of Kardex.)

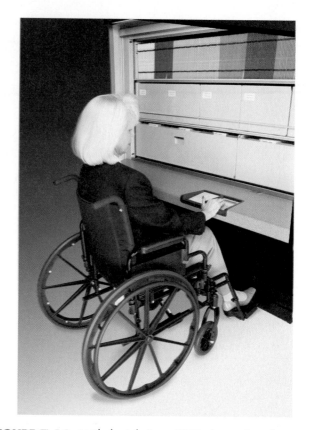

FIGURE 7–16 With the Lektriever 2000, the work surface is adjustable to standing or sitting position. It is ergonomically correct for all employees. (Courtesy of Kardex.)

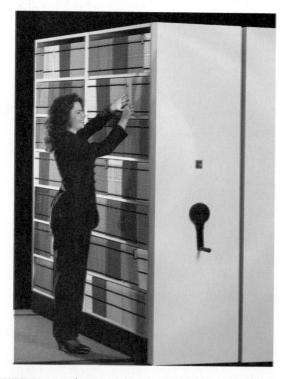

FIGURE 7–15 The Kompakt movable shelving provides maximum file space while taking up a minimum of floor space. (Courtesy of Kardex.)

up an accident scene. If you pull out more than one file drawer at a time in a vertical file cabinet, it can tip over and injure you. Be careful when pulling a file drawer out to reach material in the back because some drawers do not have a stop to prevent the entire drawer from falling out. **CAUTION:** There can also be the danger of a file cabinet tipping over and falling on you if you pull the entire top drawer out as far as it can open and do not have enough weight in the bottom drawer(s). This can be a problem especially with new file drawers as they are being filled with charts. It is best to start placing files in the bottom drawers first to avoid the possibility of injury as well as the avoidance of a potential mess of papers and forms if a drawer were to fall. You always should be mindful to keep all drawers, cabinet doors, step stools or any other source of a possible accident closed or out of the path of others.

FILING SUPPLIES

Filing supplies include guides, OUTguides or OUTfolders, folders, vertical pockets, index tabs, and various colored self-stick number and letter labels, as well as the standard office equipment such as stapler, staple remover, tape, etc. (Figures 7–17 and 7–18). A properly organized filing system will have many dividers or guides that identify sections within the file. The guides should be con-

inches of storage space. The work surface area is adjustable to a standing or sitting position, providing an ergonomically-correct work height for all workers.

Safety is an important consideration when you work with file cabinets. When you leave a file drawer open at floor level where someone can fall over it, you are setting

FIGURE 7-17   Example of OUTguide cards

FIGURE 7-18   Examples of top-cut and end-cut file folders

structed of heavy material to stand up under continual wear. They reduce the area to be searched and allow you to locate a folder more quickly. Some authorities recommend a guide for every 8 or 10 folders, but this would occupy a great deal of space. The number of guides used is a matter of personal preference and will be determined by each office.

An OUTguide or folder is used to temporarily replace a folder that has been removed. It is thick and may be of a distinctive size and color for easier detection. The use of OUTguides makes refiling much easier and also alerts the medical assistant to missing files. The OUTguide may also have lines for recording information, such as where the missing folder may be located, or it may have a plastic pocket for inserting an information card. In a large office with several physicians and employees, it is essential to know who has the folder when it is out of the file. Occasionally, a record may be sent to another physician or treatment facility and it is extremely important that this information be recorded. The OUTfolder is also useful in

providing a place to file material until the original folder is returned. Make sure you check with the physician before allowing a patient to take an entire chart. This is not an accepted practice and requires written permission and signatures with an expected date of return. It is only allowed in exceptional cases. A copy of, or a written summary of, a patient's health records is the usual procedure in sending information regarding a patient to another physician or health care facility.

A color coding system may be used to **expedite** both filing and finding of folders. Ordinary manila folders may be coded with colored strips or dots along the edge of the folder. The coding may be used to identify portions of the alphabet or patients of different physicians within an office. Color coding is also useful in identifying different types of insured patients. Everyone should have a key to the color coding through use of a procedure manual or posted chart.

A more sophisticated and efficient way of creating color-coded labels can be achieved by using your printer. Software programs are now available that can create color-coded indexing, text, bar codes, graphics, and full color images directly onto label paper or printable folders using your desktop color printer.

Offices that bar code their files can eliminate the need for OUTguides by scanning files prior to leaving the file area (Figure 7–19). The file clerk not only scans records when they leave the file area but also scans records in each department at least once or twice a day. This provides a great tracking system when the file leaves one

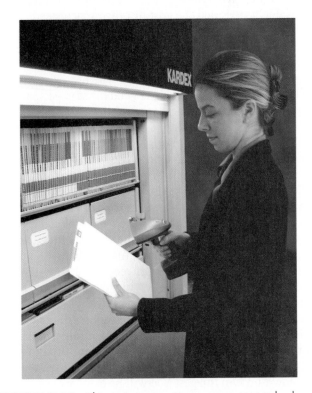

FIGURE 7-19   This assistant is using a scanner to track where charts are located in the office. (Courtesy of Kardex.)

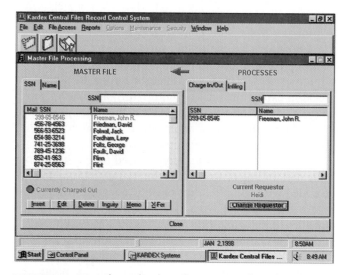

FIGURE 7–20 Charts that have been scanned can be viewed on the monitor to easily locate them. (Courtesy of Kardex.)

area and is moved to another area. When the clerk inserts the file name into the computer, the file name pops up and identifies in chronologic order each department that has had the file since its initial removal. A list of files is shown in Figure 7–20. This system not only reduces the search time but also greatly decreases the number of lost files.

PAPERLESS FILES

With computers outputting volumes of information at unbelievable speeds and the cost of office space steadily increasing, many offices have installed "paperless" filing systems. These systems record information for storage on such media as magnetic tape reels, cartridges, or cassettes; magnetic disks; and/or microforms. The use of such media has dramatically reduced the need for storage space. It is estimated that microforms (microfilm and microfiche) use less than 2% of the storage space required for traditional paper files. Microfiche is a rectangular sheet of clear film containing rows of tiny negatives. Each negative represents a separate page of a document or report.

Storage units used to house such paperless media are either card files, drawers, open shelves, or racks. Shelves or drawers are used to store boxed rolls of microfilm. Card files are used for microfiche and aperture cards. (Aperture cards are one tiny negative mounted on a data processing card.) These types of records require an **illuminating** and magnifying viewing device to read the stored information.

If you are hired to work with a paperless filing system, you will be taught how to use the special filing equipment on the job. You will learn about the camera used to produce reduced images on film and the viewers used to read the blown-up film images. You will be using word processors and duplicating equipment to handle **data** and print-

ers to produce hard copy from film images. There will be automatic storage and retrieval units to master. Paperless files have become common with the use of the computer. Storage of a vast array of information regarding patient records, employee information and payroll, scheduling, statistics regarding medical conditions, office management, taxes, inventory, and a host of other records can be filed and stored on a computer system with easy retrieval whenever necessary. This eliminates clutter and the need for filing space. Software companies provide advice for practical use to fit particular needs of the practice.

FILING SYSTEMS

Most filing systems are based directly or indirectly on an alphabetic arrangement. In alphabetic filing, the names of persons, firms, or organizations are arranged as in the telephone directory. This is the simplest and most commonly used method of filing. In numeric filing, the material is arranged in numeric order in the main file. The main file is **supplemented** by an alphabetically arranged card index. The number under which a given item is to be filed can be determined by referring to the alphabetic card index file.

A subject file is based on an outline or classification of the subject matter to which the material refers. In a physician's office, it is customary to maintain files of reference materials **accumulated** by subject matter.

In geographic filing, material is arranged alphabetically by political or geographic subdivisions such as country, state, city, and even street, and each subdivision is alphabetized.

Chronologic filing refers to filing according to date. Arranging documents with the most current date on top, is recommended.

When you are filing additional documents in a patient's chart, place them in order of dates with the most current date on top. Patient files are generally arranged in an orderly fashion in sections as follows (with the chart opened flat): progress notes are on the right with physical exam form under them; imaging reports and lab reports are shingled on the inside (right) back cover of the chart; and on the inside cover (left) are immunization records, medication list, and patient data. This is one way to organize a chart. Follow the office policy of your place of employment.

Files are also arranged by color-coding them in either alphabetic or numeric order or by category. Figure 7–21 shows movable file shelving that are color-coded. Each category (e.g., allergy patients, workers' compensation, charts of patients who are delinquent in payments, etc.) are assigned a different color. This is done to expedite patient care and processing of payment of services. This type of indexing also helps to reduce the time that it takes to file and retrieve patient charts. Misfiles are quickly spotted with this system. Also the colors of the charts are very bright and attractive. The office manager is generally the one who makes the decision about filing systems.

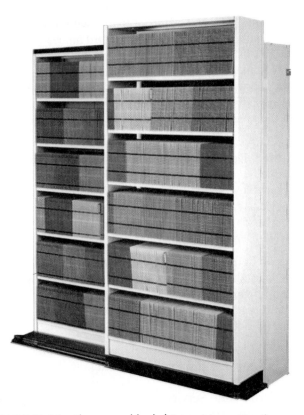

FIGURE 7–21 These movable shelving units are attractive space savers. (Courtesy of Kardex.)

HOW TO FILE ALPHABETICALLY

Ⓐ **Patient Reception Area:**
- Filing
- Subject Filing

The most common method of filing is alphabetic. Patient charts are filed in alphabetic order. They are also labeled with colorful numeric codes. In Procedure 7–1 are the steps necessary in filing alphabetically. The rules for filing material alphabetically must be learned. They are as follows.

RULE 1. In filing the names of persons, the surname or last name is considered first, the first name or initial second, and the middle name or initial third.

Example: John E. Brown is filed as Brown, John E.

RULE 2. Names are filed alphabetically in an A-to-Z sequence from the first to the last letter, considering each letter in the name separately and each unit separately. The following names are listed in correct filing order:

    Allard, Wm.
    Allen, E. S.
    Allen, Edna
    Allen, Wm. A.
    Allen, William C.
    Allens, M. R.

PROCEDURE

7-1   File Item(s) Alphabetically

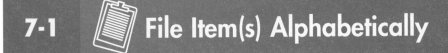

PURPOSE: To file and store patient file(s) or other items accurately in alphabetic order.

EQUIPMENT AND SUPPLIES: Items to be filed, cabinet for files.

PERFORMANCE OBJECTIVE: In a simulated situation, given the patient's file or other items, accurately file and store the file(s) and/or other items within an acceptable time limit according to accepted medical standards.

1. Use the rules for filing items alphabetically. **NOTE: Double check the spelling of the name for accuracy when using the cross-reference file. (Refer to Figure 7–22.)**

2. Determine the appropriate storage file.

3. If you are filing new material, scan the guides for the area nearest to the letters of the name(s) on the items that you have to file. **NOTE: When filing items such as lab reports or letters, be extremely careful to place them in the cor-** rect chart. Remove the chart, open it, and place the item in the chart with the top of the item toward the top of the inside of the chart on the appropriate left or right side. Be sure to place dated items in chronologic order with the most recent date on top.

4. Place the folder in the correct alphabetic order between two files. **NOTE: Be sure to insert the new file *between* two other folders and NOT within another folder where it could be lost.**

5. If you are filing material previously in the file, scan for the OUTguide. Remove the OUTguide after you have removed the file. **NOTE: Check to be sure it was marking the space for the file you just returned and not another.**

(Procedure 7–2 discusses pulling a file folder from alphabetic files.)

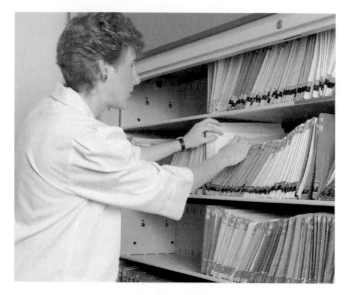

FIGURE 7–22 These charts are filed in alphabetical order and also have numerical codes.

- When the surnames of two persons are spelled differently, the first and middle names or initials need not be considered. See the first two names in the preceding list. The order of these two names is determined by the fourth letter in the surname.
- When a shorter surname is identical with the first part of a longer surname, the shorter name is listed first. The rule is sometimes stated as "nothing before something." See the fifth and sixth names in the preceding list.
- When the surnames are alike, the order in filing is determined by the first names or initials. When the surname and first names or initials are alike, the filing order is determined by the middle names or initials. See the fourth and fifth names in the preceding list.

- An initial is listed before a name beginning with the same letter. See the second and third names in the preceding list. This again is the example of "nothing before something."
- An abbreviated first or middle name is treated as if it were spelled out in full. See the fourth and fifth names in the preceding list.

RULE 3. A prefix (also called a surname particle), such as Mc, Mac, De, Le, and von, is considered as part of the surname.
  Examples:
    MacAdams, Bruce
    McAdams, Helen
    VonBergen, T. R.

RULE 4. In filing the name of a married woman, her legal name is used. The title Mrs. is disregarded in filing, but is placed in parentheses after the name.
  Example: Mrs. R. A. (Betty A.) Smith is filed as Smith, Betty A. (Mrs. R. A.).

RULE 5. Most firm names are filed as they are written. The apostrophe is disregarded in filing.
  Examples:
    Herb's Auto Service
    Walters Printing Company

RULE 6. Firm names that include the full name of an individual are filed with the name of the individual transposed.
  Example: Edward Wenger Company is filed as Wenger, Edward Company.

RULE 7. When the article *the* is part of a title, it is placed in parentheses and disregarded in filing.
  Examples: Sam the Barber is filed as Sam (the) Barber; The Family Steak House is filed as Family Steak House (The).

PROCEDURE

7-2 📋 Pull File Folder from Alphabetic Files

PURPOSE: To obtain the correct patient file(s) from the file cabinet.

EQUIPMENT AND SUPPLIES: Name of patient file to be pulled, OUTguide (card), pen, cabinet of patient files.

PERFORMANCE OBJECTIVE: In a simulated situation, given the patient's name, accurately prepare the OUTguide and pull the file, replacing the file with the OUTguide within an acceptable time limit according to accepted medical standards.

1. Find the name of the patient in the alphabetic file. Double check the spelling of the name for accuracy.

2. Complete the OUTguide with the date and your name. **NOTE: If you are pulling files for the day, OUTguides may not be necessary. When pulling files for another person, write that person's name and your initials.**

3. Pull the file(s) needed and replace with the OUTguide.

RULE 8. *And, for, of,* etc., are disregarded in filing but are not omitted.

Example: Adams & Smith Pharmacy is filed as Adams (&) Smith Pharmacy.

RULE 9. Abbreviations such as *Co., Inc.,* or *Ltd.,* in a firm name are indexed as though spelled out.

Example: Frank Smith Co. is filed as Smith, Frank Company.

RULE 10. Hyphenated surnames and hyphenated firm names are indexed as one unit.

Examples: Dunning-Lathrop & Assoc. Inc. is filed as Dunning-Lathrop (&) Associates, Incorporated; Lester Smith-Mayes is filed as Smith-Mayes, Lester.

RULE 11. Numbers are usually filed as though spelled out.

Example: 5th Avenue Store is filed as Fifth Avenue Store.

RULE 12. Professional or honorary titles are not considered in filing but should be written in parentheses at the end of the name for identification purposes.

Examples: Dr. Anne Lewis is filed as Lewis, Anne (Dr.); President John Kennedy is filed as Kennedy, John (President); Prof. William S. Smith is filed as Smith, William S. (Prof.).

■ Titles are filed as written when they are part of a firm name. Foreign or religious titles followed by one name are also filed as they are written.

Examples:
Dr. Scholl's Foot Powder
Prince Phillip

RULE 13. Terms of seniority, such as *Junior, Senior, Second,* or *Third,* are not considered in filing. If two names are otherwise identical, the address is used to make the filing decision in the order: state, city, street.

Examples:
Willard Keir, Sr.
Willard Keir, Jr.
Filed as:
Keir, Willard, Sr. (Cleveland, Ohio)
Keir, Willard, Jr. (Columbus, Ohio)

RULE 14. File the names of federal, state, or local government departments first by political division and then by name of department.

Example: Drug Enforcement Administration, Cincinnati, Ohio is filed as Cincinnati, City, Drug Enforcement Administration, Cincinnati, Ohio.

HOW TO FILE NUMERICALLY

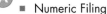 **Patient Reception Area:**
■ Numeric Filing

The second filing method used, especially in very large clinics, is the numerical system (Procedure 7–3). This system provides the most patient privacy, as all that is visible on the folder is the patient number. As mentioned before, a cross-index or cross-reference is required in the form of an alphabetic card file, and a number is assigned to each patient. You first locate the alphabetic card to determine the patient's number and then locate the numbered file.

Most offices use the same number of digits for each number assigned, and the numbers are always filed in or-

---

PROCEDURE

7-3 File Item(s) Numerically

PURPOSE: To file and store patient file(s) or other items accurately in numerical order.

EQUIPMENT AND SUPPLIES: Items to be filed, cabinet for files.

PERFORMANCE OBJECTIVE: In a simulated situation, given the patient's file or other items, accurately file and store the file(s) and/or other items within an acceptable time limit according to accepted medical standards.

1. Use the rules for numerical filing. **NOTE: Double check the spelling of the name for accuracy when using the cross-reference file.**

2. Determine the appropriate storage file.

3. Match the first two or three numbers with those already in the file. If using terminal digits, match the last two numbers.

4. Match the remaining numbers with those in the file. **NOTE: If you have assigned a number to a new patient, it should probably be at the very end of the file.**
(Procedure 7–4 discusses pulling a file folder from numerical files.)

PROCEDURE

7-4   Pull File Folder from Numeric Files

PURPOSE: To obtain the correct patient file(s) from the file cabinet.

EQUIPMENT AND SUPPLIES: Name of patient file to be pulled, OUTguide (card), pen, cabinet of patient files.

PERFORMANCE OBJECTIVE: In a simulated situation, given the patient's name or account number, accurately prepare the OUT-guide and pull the file, replacing the file with the OUTguide within an acceptable time limit according to accepted medical standards.

1. Find the name of the patient in the card file to obtain the account number. Double check the spelling of the name for accuracy.

2. Complete the OUTguide with the date and your name. **NOTE: If you are pulling files for the day, OUTguides may not be necessary. When pulling files for another person, write that person's name and your initials.**

3. Locate the corresponding section of the numeric file.

4. Scan the files for the number.

5. Pull the requested file and replace with the prepared OUTguide.

---

der from smallest to largest. If the zero (0) falls before another number, it is disregarded when filing. A system using six digits would begin 000001, 000002, 000003, and so on.

Some systems use the same terminal digit or digits to designate shelves or drawers. The patients are assigned numbers, which are separated into twos (2s) or threes (3s). The numbers are then read from the right hand group of numbers to the left hand group. After the last two or three digits are sorted together in numeric order, you next consider the middle digits and sort them in order. Finally, you consider the first group of digits and sort them in order.

For example, the numbers of charts in one series might end in 25 and another series might end in 35. Charts labeled 10-07-25 and 02-17-25 would then be filed separately from charts labeled 08-17-35 and 12-25-35. The order of the charts numbered above would be:

02-17-25
10-07-25
08-17-35
12-25-35

HOW TO FILE BY SUBJECT

In the medical office it is necessary to have files for business information. You must file financial records, copies of inventory, copies of orders, and records of supplies and equipment received. You should have a file for tax records, insurance policies, and canceled checks. The subject headings of the above would be relatively easy to

determine, but it is more difficult to determine where to file some general correspondence or reprints of medical research publications.

Very often reprints are filed with a cross-index, one file for the subject and one for the author with a listing of reprint subjects available. The miscellaneous folder is an important subject file. When you have one letter on a subject it should go into the miscellaneous file indexed by subject or names. The material in each subject file is filed in chronologic order with the most recent entry on top. When five papers are assembled in the miscellaneous file on one subject or person, a separate folder should be prepared and the material removed from the miscellaneous file.

HOW TO USE A CHRONOLOGIC (TICKLER) FILE

A **Patient Reception Area:**
■ Tickler Files

This file is commonly called a "tickler file" and is used as a follow-up method for a particular date (Figure 7–23). The file may be an expanding file, a card file, or even a portion of a file drawer. It consists of dividers with the names of all the months and dividers numbered from 1 to 31 for the days of the month. Some offices have patients fill out a card to be sent as a reminder to return for examination, testing, or injections. The patient addresses the card and the office retains it in the tickler file to be mailed by you at the appropriate time. You place the month card in the front of the file each month and check each day to see if anything needs to be done. Reminders for equip-

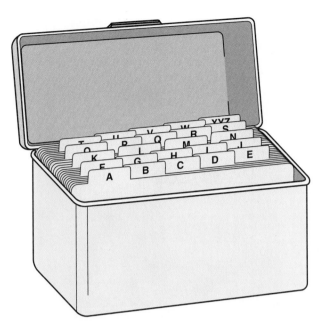

FIGURE 7–23 Using a tickler file (reminders) helps to plan and keep track of important dates, events, and duties.

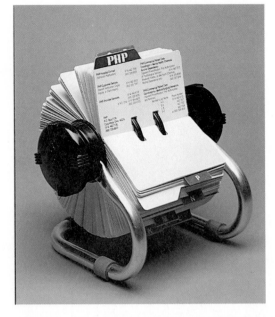

FIGURE 7–24 Shown here is a desktop rolodex file which takes up little space and provides fingertip access to important phone numbers.

ment servicing, carpet cleaning, completing monthly orders, making an appointment for a patient to have elective surgery, sending a reminder to a patient who needs to be seen for follow-up, and scheduling a speaker for an inservice are among the many types of reminders that can be included in this file. These 5 × 7-inch cards should have the party's name and phone number, the date and reason for the reminder, the referral facility phone number, etc. There should also be a line for the person who completes the task to sign and date that it was completed. The tickler file should be the responsibility of the administrative medical assistant who is generally the person who handles the reception of and check out duties for patients. This file should be checked every day at the same time. Once the reminder is sent, the card should be kept for a period of weeks, months, or however long your employer/office manager requires. This is a smart practice because it serves as a reference in case of a misunderstanding or a question about the way the patient or a referral was notified, when it was made, and who was responsible.

DESKTOP FILES

A convenient desktop file such as the one shown in Figure 7–24 makes it easy to flip to the phone number or address you need quickly. Other helpful materials that will fit neatly on the desktop are a list of frequently called referral facilities, pharmacies, labs, and hospitals. Using supplies that make your job easier is most practical. Being efficient in record keeping is a key factor in helping the workday go smoothly.

PURGING FILES

In all medical practices, at some point the shelves holding the *files* become full, and there is no room for any more charts. Periodically you must purge files of those patients who are no longer being seen by the physician(s). **Purge** means to clean out. You simply take out the inactive charts to make room on the file shelves or in drawers for new and active patients. Basically, you are moving files around to fit into other file cabinets or in storage boxes. Files are generally purged when the shelves become too full, at the end of each quarter, or biannually. Purging can also be done routinely with charts that have been inactive two years or more (depending on the office policy). When using the year tab stickers to make new charts, those files that are to be purged can be easily spotted. Purging can be time-consuming and should be accomplished over a given period of time. When you purge files, it must be accomplished in a systematic manner. There has to be a plan and a place to accommodate the inactive files. If inactive files are boxed, it is critical to label them accurately. Some practices have inactive patient charts on microfilm to be stored. Caution should be taken by those involved in moving volumes of files and charts to lift only a small amount at a time to prevent back strain and other injuries. Those who lift any heavy object should practice proper body mechanics, lift carefully, and lift only a reasonable number of charts at a time. Figures 7–25 and 7–26 show correct movement when lifting to prevent injury. A helpful means in moving great numbers of charts from one file-shelving unit to another is shown in Figure 7–27. This way you can easily transport a large number of files with

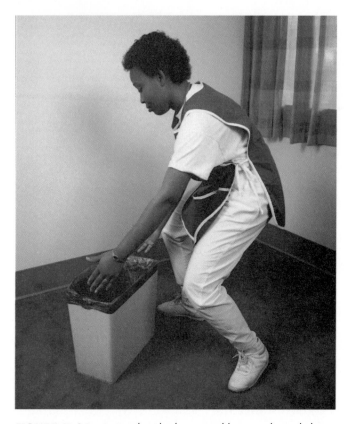

FIGURE 7–25 1. Bend at the knees and hips, and stand close to the object. Keep the back straight, and lift using the muscles in the arms and legs.

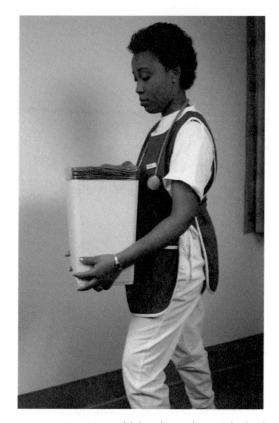

FIGURE 7–26 2. Hold the object close to the body.

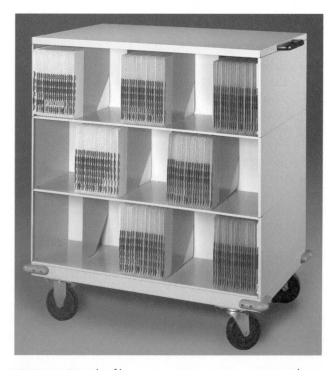

FIGURE 7–27 This filing cart is an easy way to transport large numbers of patient charts or to designate charts that need to be filed. (Courtesy of Colwell, a division of Patterson Dental Supply Inc., 800-637-1140.)

the wheeled cart and eliminate making so many trips to the inactive file cabinet or room.

Inactive files must be available because the patient may return. Transferring records of deceased patients should be delayed until all requests for forms have been completed. At that time, the files can be closed and may be placed in the deceased storage area. The transport file cart may also be used daily for charts that are ready to be filed, keeping them separated from those charts out for patient care and phone call-backs. The charts can be placed in alphabetic or numeric order for convenience for filing and if another team member needs one of the patient charts.

Security is necessary in keeping this stored information regarding patients confidential. The files should be locked when there is no one monitoring them. All records of patients are generally kept in medical practices no matter how far back the date goes. You can see that putting this information on disk or on microfilm to save space is often necessary to save the cost of additional storage space. You must check in your state for the regulations concerning files and the time you must keep them. Usually medical records are kept from three to seven years. In different states and countries this may vary. It is wise to ascertain the necessary time limit in keeping these documents in your state or country.

In addition to purging and storing files, all appointment books, laboratory logs, telephone message books, the facility's triage manual, and any other records pertaining to patient care should be kept and stored for future reference because patient information is valuable and could possibly be necessary in a medical-legal case.

All office records should be in closed files when not in use. Professional liability insurance policies, life insurance policies, canceled checks, wills, licenses, deeds, stocks, and bonds should be kept in a safe or in a fireproof box. Receipts for business and medical equipment and any warranties should also be kept in fireproof storage until you no longer have the equipment.

ACHIEVE UNIT OBJECTIVES

Complete Chapter 7, Unit 2, in the workbook to help you obtain competency of this subject matter.

Medical-Legal-Ethical Scenario

While Darius was on vacation last week, a temporary service provided a medical assistant, Judy, to assist in his place. Judy had a few years of experience and was a good medical assistant. However, in this fast-paced family practice, she was finding it difficult to keep ahead of things. In addition to Darius being on vacation, the receptionist called in sick. Francene, the clinical supervisor, asked Judy to bring in the next patient, named Geoffrey Stephens, while she answered the phone. Judy said she would but noticed that the patient's chart was not out. She quickly pulled Mr. Steven Jeffries' chart and recorded the patient's vital signs, weight, etc., on the progress note in the chart. Soon after, Dr. Lane came to the receptionist's window and said that she needed the chart for Mr. Geoffrey Stephens, not Steven Jeffries.

CRITICAL THINKING CHALLENGE

1. What did Judy's apparent haste cause to happen?
2. Do you think Judy had good intentions?
3. What do you think needs to be done to Mr. Jeffries' chart?
4. What do you think Francene said to Judy about this error?
5. Who should record the data on Mr. Stephens' chart?
6. What would you have done in this situation?
7. Would you call the temporary service to report Judy's error?
8. What do you think of the temporary service?
9. Would you call the temporary service again?

RESOURCES

Lindh, W.Q., et al. (2002). Comprehensive medical assisting (2nd ed.). Clifton Park, NY: Delmar Learning.

Kardex Systems, Inc., Marietta, OH 45750.

Mish, F.C. (Ed.). (1994). Merriam-Webster's collegiate dictionary (10th ed.). Springfield, MA: Merriam-Webster, Inc.

Smead Manufacturing Co., Hastings, MN 55033

WEB LINKS

http://www.kardex.com (Kardex® Information and Materials Management Systems)

Provides information on office products.

http://www.smeadsoftware.com (Smead Software Solutions)

Provides information on products that provide record management software.

Collecting Fees

The medical assistant must be concerned with the collection of fees from patients, as there are many expenses to be covered in the practice of medicine. The medical assistant needs to know the local clinics where limited-income, **indigent** patients can be referred for care at a reduced fee. The medical assistant can also help patients plan a payment schedule for a costly surgical procedure, therapy, or the birth of a baby. It is important to determine who is responsible for the payment of the physician's services. If it is not the patient, it may be the patient's employer, an insurance company, a school, or a government agency.

UNIT 1

Medical Care Expenses

◼ OBJECTIVES

Upon completion of the unit, meet the following performance objectives by verifying knowledge of the facts and principles presented through oral and written communication at a level deemed competent, and demonstrate the specific behaviors as identified in the performance objectives.

1. Spell and define, using the glossary at the back of the text, all the **Words to Know** in this unit.
2. Name the factors in determining fees for patient care.
3. List the types of patients who pay no fees or reduced fees.
4. Explain the pitfalls of reducing fees.
5. List the information that should be obtained for every new patient.

AREAS OF COMPETENCE (AAMA)

This unit addresses content within the specific competency areas of *Administrative procedures, Practice finances, Professionalism, Communication skills, Legal concepts,* and *Operational functions*, as identified in the Medical Assistant Role Delineation Study. Refer to Appendix A for a detailed listing of the areas.

◼ WORDS TO KNOW

complexity	pitfalls
indigent	subsequent
nominal	verify

Most physicians have traditionally been reluctant to discuss fees with patients. It is fairly common for the medical assistant to be the one who must answer these questions. When a patient is unhappy about medical costs, it is important to listen and try to explain why the charges are as stated. The physician should be told when a patient is unhappy with the cost of treatment, and it may be necessary for the physician to talk with the patient about the concern regarding cost of care.

Physicians must set their fees based on their professional financial profile and the fees appropriate for similar specialists in the community. In considering the fee for services to the patient, the physician considers the time spent with the patient, the **complexity** of the diagnosis, and the treatment. In addition, the cost of maintaining an office and staff is considered. The physician can also obtain usual and customary fee schedules from the local medical society or a medical practice management firm.

In some instances, you will find that insurance companies and government agencies establish a fee profile for the physician based on charges averaged over a period of time. This is one of the reasons it is so critical to learn to code patient visits accurately. When such a profile is established, it represents the highest payment the insurance company or government agency will make for the services listed in the profile.

PERSONAL DATA SHEET

The patient should complete a personal data sheet at the initial office visit (Figure 8–1). This information form can be custom-designed and purchased from a printing company, or you may design one specifically for your office practice by using the office computer.

At each subsequent office visit, it is important to verify and update the patient's current phone, address, employment, and insurance information. Often a patient may actually forget to inform you of a change because the nature of their visit is stressful. If you approach the patient in a polite and friendly manner to ask for the update,

PATIENT DATA SHEET

Patient's Name _____
Last   First   Middle

Address _____
City _____ State _____ Zip+4 _____
Date of Birth _____ Social Security Number _____
Home Phone _____ Pager/Cell Phone _____
Employer _____ Work Phone _____
Occupation _____
Address _____

INSURANCE INFORMATION

Subscriber's Name _____
Insurance Company _____
Policy Number _____ Group Number ____ Union/Local ____
If Group Insurance, Name of Policy Holder (e.g., employer, union)

_____

Insured's ID or Medicare Number (include any letters) _____
Effective Date of Insurance _____ Coverage _____
Exclusions or Exceptions _____

ADDITIONAL COVERAGE

Other Health Insurance? _____ Yes _____ No _____
Copy of Insurance Card(s)? _____ Yes _____ No _____
If Yes, Name of Policy Holder _____ Company _____
Plan Name and Address _____
Policy or Medical Assistance Number _____
Patient's Signature _____ Date _____
Subscriber's Signature _____ Date _____
(if patient is a minor)

FIGURE 8–1 Patient data sheet

the patient is generally cooperative. The following information should always be obtained:

- Patient's full name, correctly spelled.
- Date of birth. This is especially useful if your office treats two people with the same or similar names.
- Social Security number. This is used as the identification number with insurance carriers in many cases.
- Marital status.
- Current address and length of time at that address. (A person who moves frequently may lack stability in payment of bills.)
- Telephone numbers at home and at work or pager, cell phone, e-mail, and fax numbers.
- Name and relationship of person legally responsible for charges. Under normal circumstances parents are considered responsible for the charges of their children. However, if a third party is involved, an oral agreement is not binding and the individual who will pay the bill needs to sign a simple statement before care is given. This statement may be a form you have prepared or it may be a handwritten statement (Figure 8–2).
- Patient's occupation, with name, address, and phone number of employer. If a patient has a spouse, you should also obtain the spouse's occupation, name, and address, and phone number of employer.
- The name of the person who referred the patient to your clinic. This information can be valuable if the patient later moves without leaving a forwarding address.
- Health insurance information. Ask to see the patient's identification card (or cards, if they are covered by more than one plan). You need to make a copy of both sides of the card(s) on your copy machine to be sure you have all the information. Some states require a consent for release of information separate from the printed one on insurance forms. If this is the case in your state, be sure that this form also is completed at the time of the first visit (Figure 8–3). Be sure you have complete information regarding all insurance carried.

Jason E. Jackson, MD
8247 Central Avenue
Stockdale, NY 23456-7890
345-678-9100

Date: 6-17-XX Patient: Julia Renee Price

Party Responsible for Payment: Martina J. Burnette

I, *Martina J. Burnette*, agree to pay for all examinations and treatments for Julia Renee Price.

Margo Little 6-17-XX
Witness Date

FIGURE 8–2 Example of third-party liability statement

MEDICAL RECORDS RELEASE Date ________

I, Kendra Leigh Forest, 4406 Slate Run Drive, Bluestone MI, request that all of my medical records be released from:

Catherine R. Lang, MD
431 S. Water Street
Bluestone, MI 12345-6789
123/789-0123

To: Jason E. Jackson, MD
8247 Central Avenue
Stockdale NY 23456-7890
345/678-7890

Sonia D Philips 3-7-xx *Kendra Leigh Forest 3-7-xx*
Witness Date Patient Date

FIGURE 8–3 Records release form

- A copy of the patient's driver's license or the driver's license number. Patients who know that you have this information in their chart are more likely to take responsibility for their bills.

ACHIEVE UNIT OBJECTIVES

Complete Chapter 8, Unit 1, in the workbook to help you obtain competency of this subject matter.

A CAAHEP CONNECTION

Be sure to speak to patients about their financial status in private areas, away from earshot of others. If you are entering the data at the same time the patients are answering your questions taken from the patient information form, speak at a volume that can be heard, but which is not loud enough to carry into the reception area where others can hear. Often patients are asked to complete the form on their own, and then the information is entered into the computer by the medical assistant at a later time. (This practice is especially convenient if you are trying to care for several patients at once.) The patient data form can then be easily computer generated, and a copy is made quickly when needed. Have patients complete a new form annually to keep your records updated. This will also provide you with a current "signature on file" for processing insurance claims forms. Complete, current information makes your job easier. The insurance information section is completed for billing the physician's services to the insurance company.

UNIT 2

Credit Arrangements

OBJECTIVES

Upon completion of the unit, meet the following performance objectives by verifying knowledge of the facts and principles presented through oral and written communication at a level deemed competent.

1. Spell and define, using the glossary at the back of the text, all the **Words to Know** in this unit.
2. List some circumstances when you may need to discuss payment planning with a patient.
3. Describe credit arrangements that can be used to finance medical care.
4. Describe the reason for accepting credit cards as payment for services rendered.

AREAS OF COMPETENCE (AAMA)

This unit addresses content within the specific competency areas of *Administrative procedures, Practice finances, Professionalism, Communication skills, Legal concepts*, and *Operational functions* as identified in the Medical Assistant Role Delineation Study. Refer to Appendix A for a detailed listing of the areas.

WORDS TO KNOW

solicit   substantial

PAYMENT PLANNING

Ⓐ Billing and Collections:
  ■ Receipts
  Insurance:
  ■ Case Files

The medical assistant can assist patients who are going to have a baby, elective surgery, or extensive therapy by helping them develop a payment plan. When the patient knows in advance that there will be costly medical expenses, the medical assistant should review the patient's health insurance coverage. Some physicians use a cost estimate sheet to give the patient an idea of the cost for surgery or long-term treatment (Figure 8–4). The estimate may include the approximate cost of the anesthetist, any consultants, and hospital charges.

If it appears that the patient will need to pay a **substantial** sum out-of-pocket, the medical assistant should discuss with the patient the manner in which payments will be made. Even if the patient has medical insurance, there could be a substantial amount that their particular insurance company does not pay, or the co-pay is a sizable amount. Often

---

SURGERY COST ESTIMATE
Catherine R. Lang
123-789-0123

Patient _____ Date _____

Scheduled surgery time: _____

At _____ Hospital/Medical Center

On the day of your scheduled surgery you should arrive at _____ am/pm and go to the _____ floor.

Check with your insurance company for the cost that you are expected to pay (your co-pay) unless your insurance covers the total cost. Plan for budgeting payments for this service.

For your information, in addition to the hospital costs for your surgery without complications, you will be charged for the following:

• Operating Surgeon _____ $_____ to $_____
• Assisting Surgeon _____ $_____ to $_____
• Anesthetist _____ $_____ to $_____

The total cost of the surgery and related charges are based on the length of time for the procedure. Your costs will vary also with the length of time of your hospital stay. For the surgical procedure that you are having, the average length of stay in the hospital is ____ days. The hospital room charges depend on your preference of a semi-private or private room. Be sure to bring your insurance information with you the day of your surgery. You will be telephoned ahead of time by a hospital admissions clerk to discuss specific information and to give you a confirmed time for your surgery. This person may also ask you to come to the hospital a few days or a week before your surgery to do a series of blood tests and a preadmissions exam.

If you have any questions or concerns, please call us at the number at the top of this estimate.

FIGURE 8–4 Example of a surgery cost estimate and information sheet

---

the costs accumulate over a long period of time, as with physical therapy, and the amount the patient owes is quite significant. Assisting the patient in planning a reasonable payment schedule for these expenses will help the patient to be more at ease and have less worry about financial matters. The patient can concentrate on getting well. If the patient does not have current resources to pay the full amount in one payment, the medical assistant should offer the option of a fixed sum as a down payment and regular payments of a fixed amount on specified dates. The Truth in Lending Act, which is enforced by the Federal Trade Commission, specifies that when there is an agreement between the physician and a patient to accept payment in more than four installments, the physician is required to provide disclosure of finance charges. Most medical offices charge only a minimal amount for financing, but this makes no difference; the form still must be completed (Figure 8–5). The patient must sign this form in your presence and the disclosure statement must be kept on file for two years. If the physician makes no specific arrangement for more than four payments and bills each month for the full amount, rather than installment amounts, there is no need for the signed statement.

Catherine R. Lang, MD
431 S. Water Street
Bluestone, MI 12345-6789
123-789-0123

FEDERAL TRUTH IN LENDING STATEMENT
For Professional Services Provided

Patient _____ Date _____

Address _____

Parent/Guardian _____
1. Fee for Service $_____
2. Down Payment $_____
3. Unpaid Balance $_____
4. Amount Financed $_____
5. Finance Charge $_____
6. Annual Percentage Rate
   of Finance Charge $_____
7. Total Number of Payments (#s 4 + 5) $_____
8. Deferred Payment Price (#s 1 + 5) $_____

Total payment due (#7) is payable to Dr. Catherine R. Lang at the above address in monthly payments of $_____, the first of which is payable on _____, 20XX. Each subsequent payment is due on the 15th of each month until paid in full.

_____   _____
Date   Signature of Patient/Parent/Guardian

FIGURE 8–5 A federal truth in lending form

CAAHEP CONNECTION

Projecting professionalism and practicing good communication skills in conducting financial and other administrative procedures are critical components of the medical assistant curriculum. Good communication makes your job easier and helps you to establish a good rapport with coworkers and patients. It also is vital in dealing with financial matters because communicating with patients regarding their care and the cost of their treatment is a delicate matter. Your compassion and understanding will help patients to be more cooperative and receptive.

CREDIT CARD USAGE

Patients are currently using many methods of financing medical care. The AMA Code of Ethics includes several guidelines for physician participation in credit card programs. Physicians may not increase their charges for services to patients who wish to use credit cards; they may not encourage patients to use credit cards or use the credit card as a way to **solicit** patients; and physicians may only offer credit card payment as a convenience for patients.

The advantage of credit card use for paying for medical services is the monies are generally available to the physician within 24 hours of depositing. Also, it removes the responsibility from the physician for collection. This service does not come without cost to the physician, however. Generally, a fee of 1% to 3% is assessed to the physicians, based on the volume of credit cards used. Many physicians feel this is to their advantage because office time is not used for collection of any delinquent accounts.

Some banks have set up financing programs in which the bank sends the money directly to the physician after deducting a handling charge. It is important for the physician to be sure that any outside financing arranged for patients is managed in a professional manner and that no unreasonable pressure tactics are used. In larger cities the physician may want to check credit references before extending credit for a large surgical fee. Some large medical societies have Bureaus of Medical Economics that perform a collection service and also provide credit information.

If you should receive a request from a credit bureau, you can say when a patient's account was opened, the current balance, and the largest amount of the account at any time. **However, you will be in violation of the law if you make any statements regarding paying habits of the patient or the character of the patient.**

ACHIEVE UNIT OBJECTIVES

Complete Chapter 8, Unit 2, in the workbook to help you obtain competency of this subject matter.

UNIT 3
Bookkeeping Procedures

OBJECTIVES

Upon completion of the unit, meet the following performance objectives by verifying knowledge of the facts and principles presented through oral and written communication at a level deemed competent, and demonstrate the specific behaviors as identified in the performance objectives of the procedures.

1. Spell and define, using the glossary at the back of the text, all the **Words to Know** in this unit.
2. Transfer charges from charge slip to daily log.
3. Post charges from daily log to patient ledger card.
4. Type itemized statement.
5. Describe exceptions to usual billing procedures.
6. Describe the advantages of one-write bookkeeping system.

AREAS OF COMPETENCE (AAMA)

This unit addresses content within the specific competency areas of *Administrative procedures, Practice finances, Professionalism, Communication skills, Legal concepts,* and *Operational functions* as identified in the Medical Assistant Role Delineation Study. Refer to Appendix A for a detailed listing of the areas.

■ WORDS TO KNOW

assets	ledgers
bankruptcy	petition
bookkeeper	posted
chemotherapy	trial balance
journalizing	

BOOKKEEPING TERMS

Some of the basic terminology used in recording office business transactions includes:

- *Daily journal* or day sheet. All patient charges and receipts are recorded here each day.
- *Account.* A record for each patient, which will show charges, payments, and balance due.
- *Accounts receivable.* All of the outstanding accounts (amounts due).
- *Posting.* Transfer of information from one record to another.
- *Debit.* A charge, added to existing balance.
- *Credit.* A payment, subtracted from existing balance.
- *Balance.* Difference between debit and credit.
- *Adjustment.* Professional courtesy discounts, write-offs, or amounts not paid by insurance. If no adjustment column is included, discounts are listed in red in the debit column.
- *Debit balance.* Shows that the patient paid an amount less than the total due.
- *Credit balance.* Shows that the patient paid more than was due or is paying in advance. A credit balance is written in red ink, circled, or noted in parentheses.

A CAAHEP CONNECTION

In dealing with patients in the area of finances, you must be polite and understanding but firm in your request for payment of services. Working with patients to encourage their responsibility in payment is essential in the management of the practice.

Daily Log

Ⓐ **Billing and Collections:**
- Daily Log Sheet

The medical assistant should record the charges, or no-charge visits, for each patient on the daily log sheet (Figure 8–6). They should be itemized, and a total should be put in the charge column. Payments should be placed in the credit (paid) column. Payment types should be noted in the paid column for ease of balancing the daily log. Note the check or money order number, type of credit card used, or whether cash was paid. When a patient pays in any form a receipt should be given so the patient has a record of the payment. In particular, you should make sure that with a cash payment there must be a receipt given to the patient, and tell patients that it is not safe to pay accounts by mailing cash payments. The daily log sheet will reflect the names of all patients treated in the office each day and any payments received in the mail or from patients who come to the office just to pay the bill. Unassigned columns on the daily log may be used to distribute charges or receipts among partners or to distribute charges by departments, such as laboratory, x-ray, or physical therapy, or by medication type in cases such as **chemotherapy**.

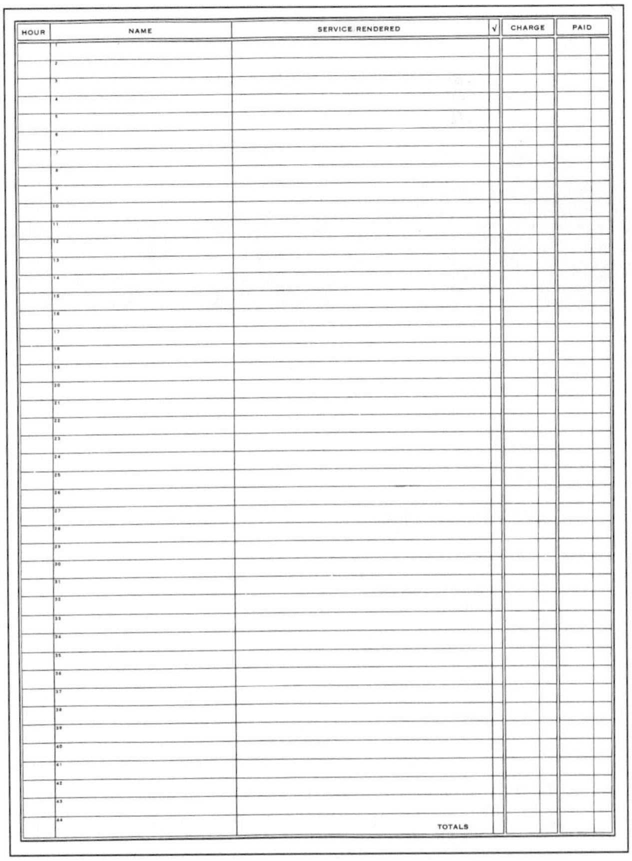

FIGURE 8–6 Daily log sheet

Patient Accounts

Many health care providers use computerized billing systems that allow for timely filing of encounters, and itemized statements, with immediate access to patient demographic information and account status. Often these systems can also generate reports that are used to improve the efficiency of the practice.

Some health care providers use ledger cards. The medical assistant who must transfer the charges from the day sheet to the patient account card should do this when there will be a minimum of interruptions (Procedures 8–1 and 8–2). The variety of ledger cards available makes it possible to increase efficiency by using the one which best suits your needs. It is a good policy to place a small check mark on the day sheet after each entry has been

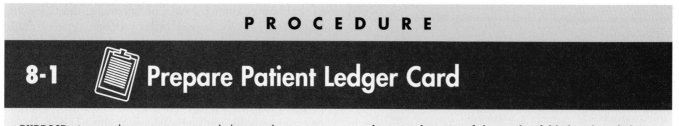

PROCEDURE

8-1 Prepare Patient Ledger Card

PURPOSE: Accurately prepare a patient ledger card.

EQUIPMENT: Blank ledger card(s), typewriter or pen with black ink, patient information sheet, or a computer.

PERFORMANCE OBJECTIVE: In a simulated medical office situation, prepare a patient ledger card following the steps in the procedure. The instructor will observe each step.

1. Type name of patient, last name first.
2. Type complete address with zip code. **Note: On a ledger card to be photocopied, the name and address are completed in the same manner as an address on an envelope**

because the copy of the card is folded and mailed in a window envelope.

3. Type name and address of person responsible for charges if different from patient.
4. Type telephone number of patient.
5. Type the name of the insurance company.
6. Type the name of the referring individual.
7. If this is a continuation of a previous card, carry forward any balance due.

PROCEDURE

8-2 Record Charges and Credits

PURPOSE: Accurately record charges and payments on patient ledger cards/computerized account.

EQUIPMENT: Ledger cards, typewriter or pen with black ink, daily log, or a computer.

PERFORMANCE OBJECTIVE: In a simulated medical office situation, record charges and credits following the steps of the procedure. The instructor will observe each step.

1. Pull ledger card for the patient.
   NOTE:
   ■ If you can record charges near your ledger file it will be efficient to do one at a time. Tilt up the card behind the one you are posting to use as a marker.
   ■ If you must post away from your ledger file pull all the cards you need at one time; then return all to the file when done.

2. Post all charges and credits for a patient and check them off on the day sheet before you go on to the next patient.
   NOTE:
   ■ Use small, neat figures.
   ■ Note the dividing line between dollars and cents. In some cases this is a darker line.
   ■ Never use dollar signs on account cards.

3. Charges are posted in the debit column.
   Key Point: If a balance is shown on the card add the new debit to get a new balance.

4. Payments are posted in the credit column and are subtracted from the balance due. **NOTE: If the credit is greater than the balance due, the difference is a credit balance and is shown in red.**

5. The balance column should always reflect the current status of the account.

posted to the account card. Then if you are interrupted you will know where to begin again in your posting job.

Statements

Statements (Procedure 8–3) must be accurate in every detail, from the name of the patient to the figures for charges and payments (Figure 8–7). If your office uses monthly billing, send out bills on the last day of the month. Your patients are more likely to pay if statements are received on a regular basis. If you have a large number of statements to send, cycle billing should be used. With this system, you divide your account cards into groups to correspond to the number of times you will be billing. You then maintain the same cycle each month so that patients learn when to expect your statement. You might send A through F on the tenth of each month, G through M on the twentieth, and N through Z at the end of the month.

Medical assistants are generally more involved with bookkeeping as entry level employees. A **bookkeeper** is one who records information. You may be required to keep a record of accounts receivable and payable. The office accountant will inform you of any records you need to provide to prepare summary reports of financial information, which are as important in the practice of medicine as in any well-run business. The accountant will analyze the figures and prepare reports that not only tell the present status of accounts receivable and payable, but compare current reports with other years or periods of time. A breakdown of the most cost-efficient procedures and least cost-efficient procedures may be revealed in such a summary. The accountant may be the person designated to prepare payroll checks and pay the quarterly amounts due to government agencies for taxes withheld.

The medical assistant who is going to do bookkeeping must be accurate in every detail. There is no "almost right" in bookkeeping. The work either is 100% correct, or it is incorrect and must be corrected. The bookkeeper must enjoy detail work and must make clear, legible figures using a fine-point, black ink pen. Care must be taken to record figures in correct columns as debit or credit and always in straight columns. Care must also be taken to place the decimal point correctly and always double-check figures on a calculator or adding machine. An adding machine tape is helpful in that you can double-check figures easily. Employees have been fired from their jobs because of carelessness with figures in simple math. You should practice adding and subtracting numbers without the use of paper or pen or computer. The bookkeeper who can independently compute answers

---

PROCEDURE

8-3 Generate Itemized Statement

PURPOSE: Accurately prepare an itemized statement.

EQUIPMENT: Ledger cards, typewriter (or computer and printer), appropriate stationery for statement.

PERFORMANCE OBJECTIVE: In a simulated medical office situation, generate itemized statements with 100% accuracy following the steps in the procedure. The instructor will observe each step.

1. Stack ledger cards beside the computer or typewriter.

2. Assemble statement forms and window envelopes.

3. Stamp the ledger card on the line below the last entry with a date stamp.

4. Type the name and complete address in an area that will show in window envelope.

5. If there is a balance from the previous month, list that first under services.

6. Type each service charge and payment for the current month.

7. The last line should show the current balance due.

   a. Generate itemized patient account statement from computerized billing system.

8. Fold and place the statement in envelope with the address showing through window in envelope.
   NOTE:
   ■ **You may want to stuff all the envelopes after you have typed all the statements.**
   ■ **Be careful to place only one statement in each envelope.**

9. Fan out several envelopes with flaps exposed.

10. Dampen a sponge and wipe over all flaps at once.
    NOTE: Be careful not to overwet.

11. Fold down flaps and seal.

Catherine R. Lang, MD
431 S. Water Street
Bluestone, MI 12345-6789
123-789-0123

Ms. Glenda Page
145 Central Avenue
Bluestone, MI 12349-6784
123-786-9876

| DATE | | DESCRIPTION | CHARGE | CREDITS | | CURRENT BALANCE |
				PAYMENTS	ADJ.	
		BALANCE FORWARD →				
4/12/XX	Sara	Allergy Injection	18.00			18.00
5/02/XX	Glenda	Exam	65.00	65.00		18.00
		UA	20.00			38.00
5/15/XX	Sara	Allergy Injection	18.00	20.00		36.00
5/18/XX	Sara	Exam	25.00			61.00
		Ace Wrap	10.00			71.00

276L   PLEASE PAY LAST AMOUNT IN THIS COLUMN ▲

THIS IS A COPY OF YOUR ACCOUNT AS IT APPEARS ON YOUR LEDGER CARD

FIGURE 8-7 An example of an itemized statement of a patient's account

quickly and accurately is considered an asset to any office. Chapter 18 of this text offers a basic math review.

BOOKKEEPING

As a bookkeeper, the medical assistant prepares the daily log or journal and posts charges and payments on the patient **ledger** card or enters the payment on the computer. The patient ledger card is a record of all charges or services rendered, any payments made by the patient or the insurance carrier, and any adjustments. If your office has a computer system that has software that includes a bookkeeping program, all charges and other information is entered into the computer. Make sure that you double check your entries to proofread for errors. Note that it is easy to transpose numbers as well as letters. The entries on the daily log are called **journalizing**. The entries should be kept in chronologic order. The total amount of cash and checks, including credit/debit card payments, should be recorded on a cash control sheet. This may be a daily record sheet or a monthly record showing an entire month with a line used each day to show income in cash and checks, any deposits made, and any amounts not deposited and therefore carried over to the next day.

When the balance is carried forward it is important to record it under "previous balance" for the next day, where it will be added to the total received to calculate "total on hand." This kind of record is also helpful in double checking your bank deposit slips. The cash and checks should equal the amount shown on the cash control sheet (Figure 8–8). This amount should also equal the amount of the bank deposit for the day.

An accounts receivable record should be kept daily. This record represents the total amount owed to the physician for services rendered. The total should be the same as the total of balances on all the active patient ledger records. The process of running such a total is called a **trial balance**. The accounts receivable balance is carried forward from month to month and added to the daily charges. The payments made by the patient and any adjustments are subtracted to determine the true account receivable each day.

This single-entry method of bookkeeping records all increases and decreases in the **assets** of the practice. Assets are anything that have value which are owned by a business. Examples of assets are office furniture, equipment, the building itself, and the land on which the building stands.

EXCEPTIONS TO USUAL PROCEDURES

There are a number of exceptions to the usual billing procedures. Many companies make arrangements for annual

CASH CONTROL SHEET

Date _____   Signature of Patient/Parent/Guardian _____

Day	Total Rec'd	Total Cash	Total Charges	Total Checks	Previous Balance	Total Available	Deposit	Balance Carried Forward
2	$2820.00	260.00	2820.00	2560.00	–0–	2820.00	2820.00	–0–
3	$ 600.00	–0–	600.00	600.00	–0–	600.00	–0–	500.00
4	$4750.00	650.00	4750.00	4100.00	500.00	6000.00	6000.00	–0–

FIGURE 8-8 Example of a cash control sheet

physical examinations to be completed by community physicians. In these cases, the statements are sent to the employer rather than the patient. Some physicians complete physical examinations for individuals applying for insurance coverage. In this case the bill is sent to the insurance company. Physicians who specialize in sports medicine and examine athletes may be paid by the school or team referring the patient.

When it is necessary to collect a bill owed by a deceased patient, the statement is sent to the estate of the deceased in care of any known next of kin at the patient's last known address. You do not address the statement to a relative unless you have a signed agreement that that person will be responsible for the bills. You may need to contact the probate court to obtain the name of the administrator of the estate if the patient died in a nursing home and had no known next of kin.

When your office receives an official notice that a patient has filed for **bankruptcy**, you send no more statements and can make no attempt to collect the account. The patient who has filed a wage earner's bankruptcy will pay a fixed amount to the court to be divided among the creditors. Your office may receive only a dollar at a time. Accept this and credit the account. You will be notified of a creditors' meeting in a straight **petition** for bankruptcy, but it is usually best just to be sure they have a copy of the statement and wait to see if you will receive any money. Sometimes the patient wishes to continue seeing the physician and will make payments on the account independently on a cash basis.

The physician may examine a patient in consultation in a legal claim, and in this case the person or agency requesting the consultation is responsible for the charges. The statement is sent with the consultation report. Other examples of third party billing are auto accidents, workers' compensation, and Medicaid.

Some offices send copies of charge slips to an outside billing service. In this case you need to be sure all charges and payments are sent so that the statements will be accurate and complete. The disadvantage of this system is that you do not have records in your office of current balances for your patients. In this case, if patients ask you a question about their account, give them reminders to refer to the outside billing service directly.

PEGBOARD SYSTEM

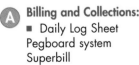

Billing and Collections:
- Daily Log Sheet
Pegboard system
Superbill

The pegboard system is referred to as the *write-it-once* system. Even though there are not as many pegboard systems in use today as in the past, it is a very efficient system. This system shows that you can make an entry on the ledger, the daysheet, and the charge slip simultaneously. For learning the basics of bookkeeping records, it is a vi-

sual tool that can help students comprehend the basics of how the financial side of a medical practice functions. The base or board has pegs, which you should place up and to the left. This log holds all of your daily entries; it becomes a listing of patients seen, as well as a complete financial record of charges made and payments received. You position a shingle of receipt/charge slips on top of the daily log, with the notches fitted over the pegs. Working downward from the top of the daily log, the shingle must be placed so that the charge/receipt slip nearest the top of the pegboard has its posting line directly over the first available line on the daily log. At the beginning of each day this will be at the top of the daily log. These forms are prenumbered in the lower right corner; be sure to use them in numeric sequence to preserve the strong audit trail designed into the system. The receipt/charge slip serves several functions. It is the charge slip for current fees; a receipt for any payment received either by check or cash; and a statement of account showing previous balance, today's charges, today's payments, and the new balance. It also shows the next appointment if there is one. After the pegboard system is completed you are ready for your first patient of the day (Figure 8–9).

When you check in a patient, pull the appropriate ledger card from your file tray. If the patient is new to your practice, prepare a ledger card. Post to the first available charge/receipt slip the existing balance (if zero, write —0—), and the patient's name. What you are writing on the charge/receipt slip is being written simultaneously on the daily log sheet. You then detach the charge slip portion at the perforation and forward it to the doctor with the patient's clinical record. The doctor will check the services received by the patient and give the slip to the patient to return to the receptionist. This gives the patient an opportunity to review the services and to ask any questions about the charge. The medical assistant will then position the ledger card so that the posting line of the receipt slip is directly over the first available line on the ledger card and post the receipt number, date, and professional services rendered, using the codes preprinted on the form. The total charges are figured from the charge slip and entered in the charge space on the receipt slip. This is the time to ask for payment. If there is no charge the entry is written *n/c*.

Post any payment received in the paid space on the receipt slip. If there is no payment, record as —0—. Post the new balance in the appropriate space and again, if zero, write —0—. In one writing you have created for the patient a combination receipt and statement. With the same one-write system, you have recorded the financial data you need on both the patient's ledger card and the daily log sheet. You are now ready to detach the receipt slip from the shingle at the perforation and remove it from the pegboard.

Arrange the patient's next appointment, if necessary, and record the date and time in the appropriate spot on the receipt slip. Also be sure to record the appointment in the

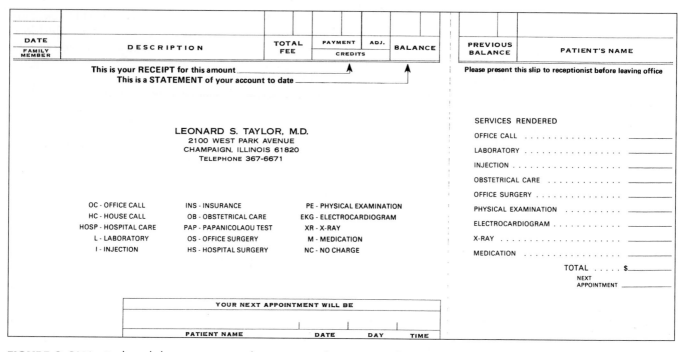

DATE FAMILY MEMBER	DESCRIPTION	TOTAL FEE	PAYMENT CREDITS	ADJ.	BALANCE	PREVIOUS BALANCE	PATIENT'S NAME

This is your RECEIPT for this amount _____
This is a STATEMENT of your account to date _____

Please present this slip to receptionist before leaving office

LEONARD S. TAYLOR, M.D.
2100 WEST PARK AVENUE
CHAMPAIGN, ILLINOIS 61820
TELEPHONE 367-6671

OC - OFFICE CALL
HC - HOUSE CALL
HOSP - HOSPITAL CARE
L - LABORATORY
I - INJECTION

INS - INSURANCE
OB - OBSTETRICAL CARE
PAP - PAPANICOLAOU TEST
OS - OFFICE SURGERY
HS - HOSPITAL SURGERY

PE - PHYSICAL EXAMINATION
EKG - ELECTROCARDIOGRAM
XR - X-RAY
M - MEDICATION
NC - NO CHARGE

SERVICES RENDERED
OFFICE CALL . . . . _____
LABORATORY . . . . _____
INJECTION . . . . _____
OBSTETRICAL CARE . . . . _____
OFFICE SURGERY . . . . _____
PHYSICAL EXAMINATION . . . . _____
ELECTROCARDIOGRAM . . . . _____
X-RAY . . . . _____
MEDICATION . . . . _____
TOTAL . . . . . $_____
NEXT
APPOINTMENT _____

YOUR NEXT APPOINTMENT WILL BE

PATIENT NAME	DATE	DAY	TIME

FIGURE 8–9(A) Pegboard charge, receipt, and appointment slip (Courtesy of Colwell, a division of Patterson Dental Supply Inc, 800-637-1140.)

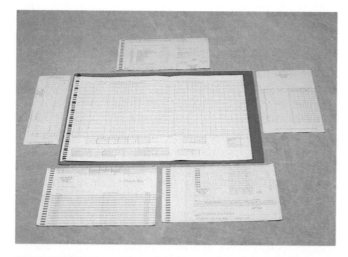

FIGURE 8–9(B) Pegboard, ledger card, and charge slip, ready to be assembled (Courtesy of Colwell, a division of Patterson Dental Supply Inc, 800-637-1140.)

appointment book before handing the receipt to the patient. Never write in the appointment space while the receipt is still attached to the shingle. The last step is to return the patient ledger card to its proper position in the file tray.

If payment is made other than when service is rendered, the receipt slip is used if the payment is made in person. If the payment is received in the mail, it is written directly on the ledger card and through it to the daily log sheet. The new balance is then posted on the ledger card after it is removed from the daily log sheet.

At the close of the day, remove remaining charge/receipt slips from the pegboard and verify that all receipt numbers are listed on the daily log. You will usually have several blank lines at the bottom of the sheet; on the last line write "End of (date)." Use a new log sheet each day. Add each column and post totals in spaces provided. Save your tapes and double-check the figures. It is a simple matter to have an up-to-date account of accounts receivable at all times with this system. The total owed to the physician by all patients is increased by the day's charges and reduced by the day's receipts. The total of the receipts should be the amount of the bank deposit each day. To protect the employees of the office against a possible bank error, the daily cash summary and the bank deposit slip should be initialed by at least two persons.

ACHIEVE UNIT OBJECTIVES

Complete Chapter 8, Unit 3, in the workbook to help you obtain competency of this subject matter.

UNIT 4

Computer Billing

OBJECTIVES

Upon completion of the unit, meet the following performance objectives by verifying knowledge of the facts and

principles presented through oral and written communication at a level deemed competent, and demonstrate the specific behaviors as identified in the performance objectives.

1. Spell and define all the Words to Know by using the glossary in the back of this text.
2. Describe the advantages of computerized billing.
3. Describe different ways to locate an account in a computer system.
4. Describe an account history.
5. List reasons why billing statements would/should be withheld.

AREAS OF COMPETENCE (AAMA)

This unit addresses content within the specific competency areas of *Administrative procedures, Practice finances, Professionalism, Communication skills, Legal concepts,* and *Operational functions* as identified in the Medical Assistant Role Delineation Study. Refer to Appendix A for a detailed listing of the areas.

■ WORDS TO KNOW

account history   alpha search

Billing is the most common use for a computer in the medical office. Many different computer systems and software packages are available. It is important to determine the needs of the office prior to purchasing. You may also:

■ visit medical offices in similar practice to discuss advantages and disadvantages of their system and software packages
■ ask personnel in other medical practices about their equipment, software and service
■ attend trade shows and demonstrations of medical practice software
■ have representatives from various companies present hands-on in-service presentations of their medical practice systems and software for all medical office personnel, including the physician(s)

Practice management software offers a variety of services, such as posting electronic claims, providing statistics on the number of patients seen per day (week, year), the diagnoses, and monthly and year-to-date billing information. Software should also provide Current Procedural Terminology (CPT) and International Classification of Diseases (ICD) codes for processing insurance claims efficiently. Although the system may provide CPT and ICD codes, care must be taken to ensure that the most current codes are used because these are updated annually. Careful and thoughtful consideration must be given before a new system is purchased. Cost is the primary concern. Often the existing hardware may need to be upgraded, thereby eliminating the additional expense of a complete new system. If the billing system software is self-contained for the practice, patients' questions may be answered by the administrative assistant who handles the billing. Making a back-up file disk of all transactions daily is necessary to keep billing records secure. Patients can have more personalized service if all transactions are done on site. If the billing is sent out to a billing service, patients must deal with yet another person for any billing questions or problems. With planning, each method can be equally efficient.

The computer terminology for a patient ledger is **account history**. This is simply a record of the information that should be obtained for every new patient. You need to know the name and address of the person responsible for payment of the account, all data regarding insurance, and all necessary information regarding family members under the same insurance. Generally, account histories follow the same organized plan you used for ledger records of patients. You may have a choice in determining how you will find an account entered in the computer system. When the system will accept a number only, you must maintain a cross-reference file of an alphabetical listing of patients along with their account numbers. The easiest and fastest method is called an **alpha search**. You type in the first few letters of the name and the screen will automatically list all names of patients starting with those letters. You select the name you wish to make an entry for and type in the appropriate entry. The account history automatically shows the balance of the account and the number of days the account has been due. The entire account activity is available to see on the screen or to make a printout for the patient.

Your system should allow you to remove inactive accounts from the computer just as you remove inactive ledger cards. When a physician's office converts to a computerized system, it is important to choose the CPT codes commonly used in the practice. They are then programmed into the computer along with the descriptions of the codes and the fees to be charged for each. The ICD diagnostic codes may be programmed into the computer for insurance claims use. The computer can be coded to indicate the source of the payment: insurance, cash, check, money order, or credit/debit cards. Adjustment codes can be used for returned checks, courtesy discounts, and any cancelled account balances.

Some computers can be programmed to create charge slips. When the patient hands a computer-generated or handwritten charge slip (also referred to as a "walk out" slip, or superbill) to the receptionist, the charge and payments may be entered on the patient account history. In some offices, the receptionist would check to be sure that the services rendered were indicated on the charge slips and then send them to the business office for processing in the computer. All charge slips must be accounted for each day. The computer can create a statement or receipt to be handed to the patient before leaving the office.

Computers can be programmed to lead you through the entry of every transaction by means of questions flashed on the screen or statements telling you what to do next. A medical assistant should be an accurate typist to operate a computer efficiently. If an error is posted on a transaction, there are ways to delete the transaction and start over again with a correct entry.

Computerized insurance claims can greatly improve cash flow. A claim can be completed in a matter of seconds for every patient visit. This is a great advantage for patients who pay cash and need to be reimbursed as soon as possible. When the physician accepts the insurance payment, the computer can be programmed to print "patient signature on file" in the signature portion of the claim, so that there is no need to have the patient sign the form. Where there is no such system, the form must be signed by the patient or sent to the patient for signature in the hope that it will be forwarded to the insurance company. A "patient signature on file" should be obtained annually and maintained in the patient's chart.

The computer can speed up monthly billing and can be programmed to withhold statements on accounts for which you do not need or wish to send statements. Some examples are government assisted patients, workers' compensation, or families of patients who have recently died. The computer statement is considered to be an efficient collection method for the office because it not only shows an itemized account of all transactions, but the age of the account can also be listed. The statement should show the portion of the amount due that is current, over 30 days, over 60 days, and over 90 days.

The computer can furnish you with a daily journal report. This report can be a record of cash control also, as a listing of checks and cash can be shown separately. All computer systems should be set up to record deleted transactions as a printed safeguard against anyone tempted to steal money by entering a transaction and then deleting it.

The computer can be used to print out monthly summaries of charges, payments, and accounts receivable. Year-to-date reports can be easily produced. You may print out a record of all outstanding accounts with an analysis of account age.

The computer can provide a detailed list of patients seen by each physician in a large clinic and the services rendered. It can be used to determine the number of patients seen with a specific diagnosis or for a particular procedure for research summaries.

The medical assistant can also program the computer to print a list of hospital and nursing home patients to be seen. Such a list improves the accuracy in recording all out-of-office patient charges.

When you have a computer system with many of the printout possibilities detailed here, you will find the business management of the office much more efficient. You will find you can complete all of these procedures in a fraction of the time required to do them by more conventional methods. For additional computer information and sample medical management computer screens, see the computer section in Chapter 5, Unit 3.

ACHIEVE UNIT OBJECTIVES

Complete Chapter 8, Unit 4, in the workbook to help you obtain competency of this subject matter.

UNIT 5
Collecting Overdue Payments

OBJECTIVES

Upon completion of the unit, meet the performance objectives by verifying knowledge of the facts presented through oral and written communication at a level deemed competent, and demonstrate the specific behaviors as identified in the performance objectives of the procedure.

1. Spell and define, using the glossary at the back of the text, all the **Words to Know** in this unit.
2. Define "aging of accounts."
3. Demonstrate use of the telephone for collection of accounts.
4. Compose collection letters suitable for a variety of situations.
5. Define the statute of limitations.

AREAS OF COMPETENCE (AAMA)

This unit addresses content within the specific competency areas of *Administrative procedures, Practice finances, Professionalism, Communication, Legal concepts,* and *Operational functions* as identified in the Medical Assistant Role Delineation Study. Refer to Appendix A for a detailed listing of the areas.

WORDS TO KNOW

aging of accounts	idle
antagonize	reputable
convey	skip
expended	specified
harassment	termination

Computers can help in analyzing accounts receivable for accounts past due. This process is known as **aging of**

M_____ Date _____

Address _____

Phone _____

Have you forgotten your payment you agreed to mail us last month? This is a gentle reminder that you owe a balance of $_____ that was due on _____.

We appreciate your cooperation in settling this account balance.

Catherine Lang, MD

FIGURE 8–10 A sample postcard collection payment reminder. Use of a bright, bold color attracts attention, so you can be relatively sure that the patient will read it.

accounts. It is basically a means of dividing accounts into categories according to the amount of time since the first billing date. Accounts are considered current if within 30 days of the billing date. Some medical assistants place a colored metal tag on accounts 60 days past due to indicate that a reminder was placed on the statement. At 90 days the tag color is changed and a letter is sent requesting prompt attention. Some offices use the numbers 1, 2, and 3 after the stamped date on the ledger card to indicate that past due notices were attached to the statement. The notices can be in the form of pressure-sensitive colored stickers that are progressively more severe in wording and in colors which are sure to attract attention (Figure 8–10). The first one might be a mild yellow, the second an orange, and the third and final one a red. No account should be referred to a collection agency unless the physician has given approval for this to be done. However, federal law requires that when you have stated you will turn the account over for collection you must follow through and do so if the bill is not paid. You cannot make **idle** threats.

A personal telephone call will often result in payment of overdue accounts. If you make collection calls, never do so without the consent of your employer, and confine your calling to your normal office hours. If you make calls early in the morning or late at night you can be held liable for **harassment.** Confine your calls to a place in the office where you will not be overheard by other patients. It is generally not a good policy to call a patient at work. If the patient has no home phone it may be necessary to call at work, but you should simply ask the patient to return your call at a time when he or she can discuss the problem with you. Remember that you will violate the confidentiality of patient-physician relationships if you talk to anyone other than the patient or the individual responsible for the charges. When the telephone is answered, use the full name of the patient in asking, "May

I speak to Jane Ann Jones, please?" Always ask if it is convenient to talk at this time; if it is not try to set a definite time when you may call, or ask the patient to call you at a **specified** time. If the phone is answered by someone other than the patient, identify yourself by name only. When the patient is on the phone, come directly to the point by saying that you are calling regarding the past due account. Approach the task with a positive attitude. Say that you are sure nonpayment of the bill is an oversight and, if not, that you want to help them make arrangements for payment. Make every attempt to establish a date when the bill will be paid, and make a notation on the ledger card indicating when that will be. Be sure you have a reminder file to help you follow up on promises to pay. If the patient indicates dissatisfaction with the results of medical care be sure that you **convey** this information to the physician.

Some physicians feel that collection cards or stickers are a sufficient reminder, but others prefer the use of collection letters (Procedure 8–4). Consult the office procedure manual or your employer regarding preferences for follow-up on the collection of accounts. You may want to compose a series of standardized letters that you can personalize as needed (Figure 8–11). When composing collection letters, avoid words that tend to **antagonize**, such as *neglected, ignored,* and *failure.* Words such as *missed, overlooked,* and *forgotten* are not quite so negative and seem more human. Decide whether you are going to use a series of three, four, or five letters. The last letter in the series will usually inform the patient that you must resort to a collection agency if you do not receive payment by a *specified* date. Use your knowledge of the patient to decide what type of letter to use. You would use a stronger-sounding first letter for someone with a poor payment record. For a patient who has an excellent payment record your first letter would be a gentle reminder. Every effort must be **expended** to collect as many accounts as possible without resorting to a collection agency, which charges a percentage of everything collected. Most offices avoid collection agencies if at all possible.

An example of a form letter that can be used to obtain an answer in writing of reasons for nonpayment of an account is shown in Figure 8–12. If you can get this kind of letter signed by the patients, you not only know the reasons for nonpayment, but you have a signed paper acknowledging the amounts they owe the physician. If you know the reason for nonpayment, it is easier to help work out a solution for payment. If the payment is not made within the prescribed period used by your office, the fact that you have a signed statement from the patient acknowledging the amount owed is helpful in a collection situation. The patient cannot deny the debt.

Each state has laws (called *statutes of limitations*) which establish the number of years during which legal collection procedures may be filed against a patient. If

PROCEDURE

8-4 Compose Collection Letter

PURPOSE: Compose collection letters appropriate for the aged accounts.

EQUIPMENT: Personal computer/typewriter, stationery, patient ledgers, envelopes.

PERFORMANCE OBJECTIVE: Using a typewriter or a personal computer, compose appropriate mailable collection letters for assigned accounts to be collected according to the procedure that follows.

1. Identify patients to whom an initial collection letter should be sent. **NOTE: If you categorize your collection accounts you will be more efficient. Complete all #1 letters before proceeding to all #2 letters, etc.**

2. Compose a rough draft with the first paragraph indicating *why* you are writing.

3. The second paragraph should indicate what response or reaction you expect.

4. Reread the rough draft to be sure you have written clearly, correctly spelled words (if using a spell check, be careful to proofread the letter to make sure you have not missed an error before you print from the computer or before you take the letter out of the typewriter), and correctly punctuated sentences.

5. Type the letter.
   NOTE:
   - **Follow standard letter form (block or modified block).**
   - **Proofread the letter.**
   - **Sign the letter with your name unless the physician wishes to sign. Remember to type your position below your name and your title (Mr., Mrs., Miss, or Ms.) before your name.**
   - **Do not use identification initials if you sign the letter.**

6. If using a computer software program that prints address labels, print those needed and affix to the envelopes.

7. Fold the letter, place in the envelope, seal, affix appropriate postage, and mail.

```
        Since your last office visit in May we haven't received any word
    of how you are feeling or any payments on your account.

        If arrangements can't be made to pay the full amount of $____ by
    June 12, please let us know so that the office can help you make arrangements
    for your payments.
    _____

        You have always paid promptly on your account in the past, so you
    must have accidentally overlooked the statements we've sent.  If that is
    the case, please accept this as a friendly note to remind you of your
    account due in the amount of  $_____.
    _____

        We can no longer carry your account on our books.  The balance of $_____
    must be paid within 10 days.

        Our collection agency receives all delinquent accounts on the 25th of
    each month.
```

FIGURE 8–11 Three different samples of possible wording for collection letters

Catherine R. Lang, MD
431 S. Water Street
Bluestone, MI 12345-6789
123-789-0123

May 23, 20XX

Ms Glenda Page
145 Central Avenue
Bluestone, MI 12349-6784
123-786-9876

Dear Ms. Page:

Our policy is giving our patients the best medical services possible. We also expect that payments for our services be made in a timely manner. Because your account is past due, and before it is turned over to a collection agency, we would like to hear from you about what can be done to settle your account. Please select your choice of how you would like to take care of your obligation by checking one of the following, sign and return to us within 3 days from its receipt. Your account balance is $_____.

☐ I would prefer to settle this account. Payment in full is enclosed.

☐ I would like to make regular payments of $_____/month until the account is paid in full. My first payment is enclosed.

☐ I would prefer that you assign this account to a collection agency. (Failure to return this letter will automatically result in this action.)

☐ I don't believe I owe this amount for the following reasons(s):

_____

Signature of patient   Date

Please indicate your preference above and sign and return this letter.

Thank you for your cooperation.

Sincerely,

Catherine R. Lang, MD

Catherine R. Lang, MD

FIGURE 8-12 Sample collection letter requesting statement from patient explaining how account will be settled

a patient is being treated for a chronic illness, there is no **termination** of the illness or treatment unless the patient dies or changes physicians. The last date of debit or credit on the patient account card is the starting date for that particular debt. If the last date was June 2002, a 2-year statute could be collected through June 2004. In written contracts the statute of limitations starts from the date due. Some states have a shorter time limit on the statute of limitations on single entry (single charge) accounts.

When statements you have mailed are returned marked *moved, no forwarding address,* you have to consider the possibility that the patient is a **skip** (collection agency slang), or has moved to avoid payment of bills. The first step is to check your records to make sure you mailed to the correct name, address, and zip code. If these are all correct, place a telephone call to see if perhaps the old phone number was transferred to a new address. You may call referring individuals to try to obtain a new address for the patient, although you must not indicate your reason for needing the new address other than that you need to verify it. You may call the patient's employer for information regarding address change, identifying yourself by name only and asking that the patient return your call.

Medical-Legal-Ethical Scenario

It was Clara's second day at the office. A coworker, Yvonne, was helping Clara get settled and showed her how to obtain a completed data sheet for each patient. After lunch Yvonne noticed that one of the charts of patients seen in the morning did not have a patient data form. When asked why, Clara said that the patient couldn't understand her, so Clara had let it go. Taking a closer look at the chart, they realized that the patient was new to the area and spoke very little English. Yvonne asked the physician about this, who said that the patient was only in for some medication for a rash on her hands and that a data sheet wasn't necessary. Looking up the charges and posting of accounts, Yvonne found that the patient had paid cash for the visit.

CRITICAL THINKING CHALLENGE

1. Does there seem to be a lack of continuity and communication among the office personnel?
2. What should have been done about this? Whose fault was it?
3. What should Clara have done when she realized the patient couldn't understand her?
4. Should the person who took care of the cash payment have alerted someone about having very little information about this lady?
5. What happens if the patient has a reaction to the medication?
6. Do you think this is a critical issue that should be discussed at a staff meeting?
7. What would you have done in this situation?

You may find the patient simply forgot to inform the post office of an address change. You may also find the patient has left his or her place of employment, in which case you should check with your employer about referring the account for collection. The longer you wait, the less chance you have to collect.

Your employer should have arrangements with a **reputable** collection agency. The office reputation can be severely damaged if the agency you work with uses unethical collection methods. When the decision to refer an account for collection has been made by your employer or the business/office manager, send the collection agency the full name of the patient, name of spouse or person responsible for the bill, last known address, full amount of debt, date of last entry on ledger card, occupation of debtor, and business address. Send no further statements, and refer any calls regarding the account to the collection agency. If you should receive any information regarding the account or any payments, you should forward it to the collection agency.

RELATING TO ABHES

Chapter 8 discusses medical expenses, bookkeeping, billing, and other content dealing with the collection of office fees. This content is related to the ABHES accreditation requirements of *Office machines, Transcriptions,* and *Computerized systems/medical data processing* within the content area of **Basic Keyboarding** and *Financial management* within the content area of **Medical Office Business Procedures/Management.**

ACHIEVE UNIT OBJECTIVES

Complete Chapter 8, Unit 5, to help you obtain competency in this subject matter.

RESOURCES

American Medical Association. (1979). The business side of medical practice. Chicago: Author.

Lindh, W. Q., Pooler, M. S., Tamparo, C. D., and Cerrato, J. U. (2002). Delmar's comprehensive medical assisting administrative and clinical competencies (2nd ed.). Clifton Park, NY: Delmar Learning.

Simmers, L. (2001). Diversified health occupations (5th ed.). Clifton Park, NY: Delmar Learning.

WEB LINKS

http://www.credit-to-cash.com **(ROK Associates Credit and Debt Management Limited)**

Provides general information on debt recovery.

Health Care Coverage

Insurance has long been the way for most people to have some semblance of security in the event of a personal or property loss of one type or another. The insurance industry is vast. It encompasses a wide variety of areas to cover all forms of anticipated losses such as life, health, home, and auto.

The high cost for health care has been, and still remains, a concern and the reason for all the attention throughout the nation. News of national health care insurance has been a primary issue for many years. Since the high cost of medical care is apparent to most everyone, health insurance has become a basic necessity. There have been efforts to research the insurance industry and determine if reasonable cuts and changes could bring about a plan for the citizens of this country that could provide quality health care at a more reasonable cost. This cost containment attempt was a good idea; however, in trying to cut costs, the physicians were penalized by having reimbursement fees reduced which, in turn, reduced the income of the physicians. This also affected the income of the practice. The rippling effects are reflected in employee benefits, as well as many other factors regarding the whole practice. The reality of where these changes in insurance coverage may take us is uncertain. Of real concern is the quality of health care. Cutting costs could mean that there may be a decrease in the number of diagnostic tests and procedures that a patient may have according to their health insurance plan. This could affect the health of the patient because it would deter the patient from having treatment simply because of the cost. The quality of patient care may also be affected by the realization that reimbursement is not likely for many medical services that may be considered unnecessary or experimental by the insurance company.

What is certain is that the traditional type of insurance that once covered the cost of our medical care is fast becoming extinct. Even though traditional private insurance is fading, there are still individuals who choose to pay high premiums so that they may have the flexibility to seek medical care from health care professionals of their choice. This is referred to as fee-for-service care. The different types of plans are mentioned in Unit 1 with their brief definitions, and will be explained further in Unit 2 of this chapter.

Health care reform has, in many cases, changed the way individuals select a physician. Often members of health insurance plans are required to select a physician from a published directory of participating physicians. The directory lists the physicians who have signed agreements with the insurance plan to provide care for their members. The physicians are listed by their area of practice and the county of location. Patients should call the office of their selected provider (physician) to determine if they are accepting new patients and to be certain the provider is currently participating with their health care plan. (The directory may not have the latest additions or deletions of providers.)

Both administrative and clinical medical assistants will find it necessary to keep abreast of changes in insurance billing and coding procedures and learn to **implement** them in a timely manner to guarantee the income of the practice. A discussion of the language of insurance, managed care, various medical care plans, and preparing claims for payment is offered in this chapter.

UNIT 1

Fundamentals of Managed Care

◼ OBJECTIVES

Upon completion of the unit, meet the following performance objectives by verifying knowledge of the facts and principles presented through oral and written communication at a level deemed competent.

1. Spell and define, using the glossary at the back of this text, all the **Words to Know** in this unit.
2. Describe the changes in health care coverage in the last two decades and the reasons for the change.
3. Explain the purpose of HMOs.
4. Explain the concept of managed care.
5. Distinguish the two major classes of health insurance.
6. Explain the reason for keeping patient insurance information confidential.
7. Define the terms listed in this unit.
8. List the different types of health insurance discussed in this unit.
9. Explain the **birthday rule**.

AREAS OF COMPETENCE (AAMA)

This unit addresses content within the specific competency areas of *Administrative procedures, Practice finances*, and *Legal concepts* as identified in the Medical Assistant Role Delineation Study. Refer to Appendix A for a detailed listing of the areas.

◼ WORDS TO KNOW

birthday rule
cessation
coordination of benefits
devastating
direct payment
encompass

implement
premium
primary
reimbursement
secondary

HEALTH MAINTENANCE ORGANIZATIONS

Managed care is a phrase regarding health insurance that became popular in the late 1980s in the United States. Initially, it was used in the early 1970s to convey the concept of promoting good health and preventive medicine. The contracts of these plans which were negotiated between the insurance company and the employer grew in popularity. This medical insurance coverage is a great employee benefit and has created much competition over the years. These insurance plans are referred to as health maintenance organizations (HMOs). The contracts offer people affordable health care plans because they are provided through their place of employment at a reasonable cost. The employer pays a large amount of the cost for the plan. The employee's cost is a reasonable group **premium** rate for health insurance coverage (a part of their employee benefits) that requires only a small co-payment at the time of the medical service. This is a good arrangement for individuals and families. These organizations employ physicians and other providers of medical care and patients visit them for their needs. Today, managed care is an organized system of medical team members and groups who provide quality and cost-effective care that **encompasses** both the delivery of health care and the payment of these services.

The initial purpose of HMOs is the containment of health care costs. Promoting wellness by offering members counseling about nutrition, exercise programs, stress management, weight control, low-fat diet, smoking **cessation**, drug rehabilitation, and the like, are efforts to keep people well and thereby cut the costs of medical care. Encouragement of annual physicals and PAP tests, breast self-exams, testicular self-exams, mammographys, prenatal programs, well-baby checkups and immunizations, and in general, requesting that people see their physician as soon as any problems are noticed, all help to reduce medical care costs.

The two major types of health insurance are individual and group. Any individual may buy individual health insurance by paying the required premium. Group health insurance generally costs less and is more comprehensive. The group may be employees, a union, or any other party. Complete coverage may or may not be paid by the employer. The employee may have to pay an additional premium to include other family members in the coverage. Most people have some form of health and accident insurance coverage because they realize that a serious illness or injury can be **devastating** to family or individual finances. Insurance seldom pays all medical costs.

There are many different types of medical care coverage plans, which are third-party payers. They will be discussed further in this chapter. A brief definition of each type can be found in the list of important words on the following pages that are used in working with patients and their various plans. Those you will be in contact with are Medicare, Medicaid, TRICARE (CHAMPUS) CHAMPVA, workers' compensation, HMOs, preferred provider organizations (PPOs), and private insurance companies.

One of the most helpful points that the medical assistant can stress to patients is to have them check their insurance policy regarding their coverage. Many times there is a misunderstanding or a lack of comprehension on the patient's part as to the type of coverage their insurance allows. If the patient seems to be confused, it is a good idea to suggest to them to phone the insurance company and speak to someone in customer service. This is helpful to the patient because he receives answers to questions. Even though it would be a kind gesture on the medical assistant's part to go over the policy with the patient, there is not sufficient time for this activity in a professional setting where other patients need attention. It is fair to let patients know that not all physicians are members of all plans. Each insurance company sends members a packet of information when the contract is issued. Periodic supplemental information should also be received by the patient in the mail. You can ask the patient to gather this together and look for a *provider of services* booklet. This will help the patient to find the names of the physicians who are participating members of the patient's HMO.

Primary and Secondary Insurance Coverage

When greeting the patient in the office upon arrival for an appointment, ask the patient for a current insurance

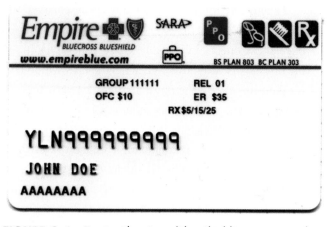

FIGURE 9–1 Empire Blue Cross/Blue Shield insurance card (Courtesy of Empire Blue Cross/Blue Shield.)

card(s). Make a copy of both sides of the card(s); it will be needed to complete forms or to request information regarding that patient and her coverage (Figure 9–1). Patients may have more than one insurance plan. Often families have coverage which is from each parent's place of work. Many insurance companies include a "nonduplication of benefits" or "**coordination of benefits**" clause in the policy. If both husband and wife have insurance, it will be necessary to determine who is considered the **primary** carrier (responsible for payment first) and who is the **secondary** carrier (responsible for payment after primary coverage). The charges are filed first with the primary carrier. After payment and an explanation of benefits is received, then the balance is submitted to the secondary carrier for payment. The charges are usually covered, or nearly so, with both plans. Responsibility for primary coverage will be based upon the language contained in the policies. For example, one spouse may have a good plan as a fringe benefit; then the other may decide to refuse the option to contribute to a plan and instead participate in a supplemental coverage that will become the secondary coverage. There can be many variables.

Covering dependent children is another variable. The primary coverage is usually responsible, but if both parents have equal coverage, another variable may be the determining factor. In this situation the **birthday rule** will apply. This rule states that:

- The parent whose birthday occurs first in the calendar year is primary, and the other parent's plan is secondary.
- If both parents have the same birthdate, the plan in effect the longest is primary.
- If the parents divorce and retain their plans, the parent with custody is primary.
- If a court order exists that dictates which parent is responsible for medical expenses, the court order supersedes the birthday rule.

More information regarding primary and secondary insurance coverage will follow later in this chapter.

Terms Used in Health Insurance

Accounts payable—The total amount owed by the practice to suppliers and other service providers.

Accounts receivable—The total amount of all charges for services rendered to patients which have not been paid to the physician.

Admitting physician—The physician who admits a patient to the hospital (not necessarily the patient's attending physician).

Advance directives—A printed and signed statement to direct those who will take care of medical decisions for a patient when the patient becomes unable to make decisions. (Also known as a living will.)

Assignment of benefits—The authorized signature of the patient for payment to be paid directly to the physician for services.

Attending physician—The physician who cares for a patient in the hospital (not necessarily the physician who admitted the patient).

Authorization to release medical information (release of medical information form)—A form that must be signed by the patient before any information may be given to an insurance company.

Balance billing—The amount of the charges to the patient for medical services that the insurance company did not pay.

Capitation—The health care provider is automatically paid a fixed amount per month regardless of provided services for each patient who is a member of a particular insurance organization.

Civilian Health and Medical Program of the Veterans' Administration (CHAMPVA)—Established in 1973 for the spouses and dependent children of veterans who have total, permanent, service-connected disabilities.

Claim—A request for payment under an insurance organization made by either the physician (medical assistant) or the patient.

Coding—Transference of words into numbers to facilitate the use of computers in claim processing.

Coordination of benefits (COB)—Procedures used by insurers to avoid duplication of payment on claims when the patient has more than one policy. One insurance becomes the primary payer and no more than 100% of the costs are covered.

Co-payment or Coinsurance—A specified amount which the insured must pay toward the charge for professional services rendered.

Current procedural terminology (Code CPT)—Coding system published by the American Medical Association.

Deductible—A predetermined amount that the insured must pay each year before the insurance company will pay for an accident or illness.

Diagnosis related group (DRG)—A system developed by Yale University to group together major diagnostic categories, organized by body systems, from which the 470 DRGs are drawn.

Effective date—The date when the insurance policy goes into effect.

Electronic claims—Also referred to as electronic media claims, electronic data interchange, and electronic claims processing.

Encounter form—See "Superbill."

Endorser—The one who writes his/her signature on the back of a check that is made out to another person.

Early and periodic screening, diagnosis, and treatment (EPSDT)—This program requires screening and diagnostic services to determine any diseases or disorders, as well as complete health care, in children from birth through 21 years. (Also called Healthchek.)

Explanation of benefits (EOB)—A printed description of the benefits provided by the insurer to the beneficiary.

Fee disclosure—The action of health care providers informing patients of charges before the services are performed.

Fee schedule—A list of approved professional services for which the insurance company will pay with the maximum fee paid for each service.

Fee slip—A printed (computer) form with the patient's information, listing the services and code numbers with the charges.

Gatekeeper—A term given to a primary care physician for coordinating the patient's care to specialists, hospital admissions, and so on.

Group insurance—Insurance offered to all employees by the employer.

Health Care Procedural Coding System (HCPCS Code)—An alphanumeric coding system devised by the federal Health Care Financing Administration (HCFA) as a supplement to the CPT code and distributed by the regional fiscal agents of Medicare, TRICARE (CHAMPUS) and Medicaid.

HCFA 1500—The standard claim form of the Health Care Finance Administration to submit physician services for third-party (insurance companies) payment.

Health maintenance organization (HMO)—A prepaid group practice serving a specific geographic area with a wide range of comprehensive health care at a fixed fee schedule; HMOs are interested in promoting wellness and good health, thus containing the cost of health care. These can be sponsored and operated by the government, medical schools, clinics, foundations, hospitals, employers, labor unions, hospital medical plans, or the Veterans' Administration.

Indemnity plan—a commercial plan in which the company (insurance) or group reimburses physician or beneficiaries for services.

Independent practice association (IPA)—A group of independent physicians who provide health care to a group of patients who pay an annual fee in advance.

Individual insurance—Insurance purchased by an individual for self and any eligible dependents.

International Classification of Diseases (current number), Revision, Clinical Modification (ICD-9-CM)—The coding system used to document diseases, injuries, illnesses, and mortalities.

Loss-of-income benefits—Payments made to an insured person to help replace income lost through inability to work because of an insured disability.

Managed care—A system of medical team members organized into groups to provide quality and cost-effective care that encompasses both the delivery of health care and payment of the services.

Medicaid—A joint funding program by federal and state governments (excluding Arizona) for low income patients on public assistance for their medical care.

Medicare fee schedule—A list of approved professional services that Medicare will pay for with the maximum fee that it pays for each service.

Medigap (Medifill)—Private insurance to supplement Medicare benefits for non-covered services.

Member physician—A physician who has contracted to participate with an insurance company to be reimbursed for services according to the company's plan.

National Committee for Quality Assurance (NCQA)—A nonprofit organization created to improve patient care quality and health plan performance in partnership with managed care plans, purchasers, consumers, and the public sector.

Out-of-area—HMO members are generally covered for emergency services out of their geographic area, but other coverages may not always be provided.

Patient status—Refers to patient's eligibility for benefits. Insurance companies frequently have stipulations that services be provided on an inpatient or outpatient basis; there are also requirements for prior authorization from the insurance company for certain services or procedures to be performed.

Point-of-service (POS) plan—An open-ended HMO, POS encourages their members to choose a primary care physician.

Preadmission testing (PAT)—Routine tests required for all patients before hospital admission to screen for abnormal findings that could interfere with the patients' hospital stay or scheduled procedure.

Pre-certification—Prior authorization must be obtained before the patient is admitted to the hospital or some specified outpatient or in-office procedures.

Preexisting condition—A condition that existed before the insured's policy was issued.

Preferred provider organization (PPO)—This plan offers different insurance coverage depending on whether the patient receives services from a contracting network or non-network physician. The benefits are higher if the physician provider is a member of the PPO (or is a network physician).

Premium—Monies paid for an insurance contract.

Release of medical information form (authorization to release medical information)—A form that must be signed by the patient before any information may be given to an insurance company.

Resource-based relative value scale (RBRVS)—Fee schedule based on relative value of resources that physicians spend to provide services for Medicare patients.

Service area—The geographic area served by an HMO.

Skilled nursing facility—A medical facility which is licensed (as defined by Medicare) to primarily provide skilled nursing care to patients.

Subscriber—The person who has been insured; an insurance policy holder.

Superbill—A printed form containing a list of the services with corresponding codes (encounter form).

Third-party check—A check from one person which is made out to a second person for payment of a third person.

Third-party payer—An insurance carrier, who is not the doctor or patient, who intervenes to pay the hospital or medical bills per contract with one of the first two parties.

TRICARE—Civilian Health and Medical Program of the Uniformed Services (CHAMPUS)—Established to aid dependents of active service personnel, retired service personnel and their dependents, and dependents of service personnel who died on active duty, with a supplement for medical care in military or Public Health Service facilities.

Usual and customary fee—The usual fee is the charge physicians make to their private patients; the customary fee is one within the range of usual fees charged by physicians in a given geographical and socioeconomic area who have similar training and experience.

Utilization management—A panel that tracks what their members receive and checks if their medical care meets the standards of the organization.

Utilization review—A review carried out by allied health professionals at predetermined times to assess the necessity of the particular patient to remain in an acute care facility.

Walkout statement—A printed form with the patient's charges and the amount paid for the services rendered which the patient takes with them.

Workers' compensation—Government program that provides insurance coverage for those who are injured on the job or who have developed work-related disorders, disabilities, or illnesses.

Please present your insurance card to the receptionist when you arrive for your appointment.
Thank you!

FIGURE 9–2 Sample of a sign that could be posted at the receptionist's window to help keep records current

Those who have Medicare may also have additional insurance coverage to supplement their insurance costs. Remember to ask for their current information and insurance card(s) because changes may occur from one visit to another. Posting a sign that says, "Please give your insurance card to the receptionist when you arrive—thank you," (Figure 9–2), will help with obtaining current information from all patients served. Current insurance information is imperative to correctly bill for services rendered.

The Insurance Paper Trail

An example of how the paper trail for services rendered to patients is initiated and progresses is provided in Unit 3. The importance of accuracy and completeness is made evident by this series of forms and billing statements generated by only one patient for a relatively minor procedure. The medical assistant must be careful in documenting all information. Legible writing or printing as well as exactness is critical in successful **reimbursement** for services. Another sign which will help in collecting fees for services is one that states clearly, "Payment for services is appreciated at the time of service" (Figure 9–3). Even if this payment is the co-pay amount, it can save time and work in ending the potential future paper trail. Submitting a claim form for the services to the patient's insurance provider will speed up the cash flow of the practice. Patients will comply with requests if they are made in a pleasant manner. It is the usual custom to have insurance payments and

We appreciate payment at the time of service.   Thank you!

FIGURE 9–3 Sample of a sign to inform patients that payment at time of service is expected

reimbursements sent directly (**direct payment**) to the physician. In those cases where the patient is reimbursed for medical services, the payment may be delayed because the patient may put off sending in the payment for one reason or another. This is referred to as indirect payment.

Included in this unit are many of the terms (with brief definitions) used in dealing with insurance claims. As medical terminology and anatomy are necessary for dealing with patients and procedures, so too is the terminology used in preparing insurance claims. You should familiarize yourself with these important words and their meanings to communicate needs and expectations of both patients and insurance companies. Your knowledge will help to expedite the processing of claims accurately and efficiently, thereby bringing payment for medical services to the practice in a timely manner. For those who prepare claims, it is necessary to keep current with any changes in policy, terminology, and procedures. There are newsletters, periodicals, and workshops offered to help in providing data to keep up with the latest information. It is to your advantage and that of the practice where you are employed to participate in these informative offerings. Knowledge in the important task of processing claims will lessen the frustration that is often associated with the complications of preparing and processing claims for patient services.

As with any patient information obtained concerning patients, the strictest confidence must be kept to safeguard their privacy. Under no circumstances should any information about a patient be given to anyone without specific instructions from the patient. This permission is granted only by patient authorization by the signature of the patient. The release of medical information form must be kept in the patient's chart for this purpose. Updating this periodically and as insurance carriers change is necessary for legal concerns. If information is given to a third party without the signed authorization of the patient, the one who gave the information may be charged with breach of confidentiality. A contract is legally binding. Those who enter into a contract have certain expectations. A contract is an agreement between two (or more) parties for certain services or obligations to be fulfilled. Where there is a concern as to the competence of the patient or if the patient is a minor, a guardian must sign for any information to be released as well as for any service to be completed. Refer to Chapter 3 regarding legal terms.

A CAAHEP CONNECTION

Standards for medical assistant instruction require knowledge of **Legal Guidelines** and **Medical Ethics** as well as the ability to prepare insurance forms. It is important at all times to practice risk management when dealing with confidential patient information.

ACHIEVE UNIT OBJECTIVES

Complete Chapter 9, Unit 1, in the workbook to help you obtain competency of this subject matter.

UNIT 2

Health Care Plans

OBJECTIVES

Upon completion of the unit, meet the following terminal performance objectives by verifying knowledge of the facts and principles presented through oral and written communication at a level deemed competent.

1. Spell and define, using the glossary at the back of the text, all the **Words to Know** in this unit.
2. Identify the original purpose of an indemnity type insurance plan.
3. Identify the health care philosophy of an HMO.
4. Name the types of HMOs and explain their differences.
5. Explain how a PPO differs from an HMO.
6. List five federal health care plans.
7. Name the three centers that were established by the changes in 2001.

AREAS OF COMPETENCE (AAMA)

This unit addresses content within the specific competency areas of *Administrative procedures, Practice finances*, and *Legal concepts* as identified in the Medical Assistant Role Delineation Study. Refer to Appendix A for a detailed listing of areas.

WORDS TO KNOW

accreditation	Medigap
annuity	periodic
capitation	preauthorization
comprehensive	premiums
connotations	quality assurance
deductible	restricted
indemnity	statutory
Medicaid	supplement
Medicare	utilization

COMMERCIAL HEALTH INSURANCE

A large segment of the population is covered by commercial insurance policies. These private, commercial insurance companies control the price of **premiums** paid and specify the benefits they will provide.

Blue Cross and Blue Shield health insurance plans are generally well known. Physicians helped originate them. Blue Cross was originally set up to pay for hospital expenses but now covers outpatient services as well. Blue Shield was originally used to pay for physicians' services. In the early years, Blue Cross and Blue Shield was an **indemnity** type plan with an annual **deductible** and co-payment. They have changed with today's health care demands and now also offer a variety of HMO, PPO, point of service (POS), and indemnity type plans.

Indemnity type insurance gives patients the option of the provider of their choice, and patients can see specialists without referrals. The patient assumes a greater financial responsibility for their health care. Indemnity plans require that the insured pay an annual deductible, usually between $100 to $250, before the carrier begins to pay any benefits, and then usually 80%. Physicians will often ask patients to pay at the time of service and provide them with a superbill or itemized statement to submit to their carrier for reimbursement.

The HMOs are plans set up to provide **comprehensive** health care with an emphasis on wellness and preventative medicine. The patient is encouraged to have annual physicals to identify health problems early. Some HMOs have the subscribers choose a primary care physician (PCP) to oversee their medical care. The PCP is responsible for referring the patient to a specialist if needed. Another cost containment measure with HMOs is preauthorization for all inpatient hospital stays, some outpatient surgeries, and referrals to physicians outside the panel of providers.

Determining Carrier Coverage

The terms *precertification, preauthorization,* and *predetermination* refer to a patient's eligibility for services. Many times these terms are used interchangeably, but there are technical differences, and they do not all mean the same thing.

- *Precertification* refers to the discovery as to whether a treatment (surgery, hospitalization, diagnostic test) is covered under the patient's insurance contract.
- *Preauthorization* relates not only if the services are covered, but also if the proposed treatment is medically necessary.
- *Predetermination* refers to the discovery of the maximum amount of money that the carrier will pay for primary surgery, consultation service, postoperative care, etc.

Even though these conditions are all similar because they affect the patient's ability to receive services, they are also specific and different in their application and effect on the patient's coverage.

Most HMOs require the patient to pay a co-payment at the time service is rendered, usually $5 to $20. The physician's office staff then files the claim with the insurance carrier for the balance due. Along with the physicians, the HMO also contracts with hospitals, laboratories, and other ancillary services, such as pharmacies. There are at least four different types of HMOs.

Types of HMOs

- **Staff model HMO** is where all services (physical therapy, radiology, and so on) are provided at the same location. The PCP is responsible for routine care and referrals. True emergency (life-threatening) care does not require preauthorization. If the patient is traveling outside the HMO geographic area, she must call and preauthorize any non-emergency care. Failure to do so will result in the HMO refusing payment of the services.
- **Group model HMOs** are multispecialty practices contracted to provide health care services to members. The physicians are reimbursed on a capitated basis. **Capitation** means that the physician is paid a set fee per patient on their patient listing each month, whether the patient is seen one or more times or not at all.
- **Open-ended HMOs** allow members greater freedom in their choice of care. They do not have a primary care physician and can self refer to specialists. If they choose to use a non-panel provider the benefit would be more like an indemnity plan with a deductible and coinsurance. If they choose a panel provider they would receive the HMO benefit.
- **Point-of-service (POS)** is another type of HMO and has gained in popularity in recent years. The organization consists of a network of physicians and hospitals that contract to provide an insurance company or an employer with services for their members or employees at a discount rate. This benefits the insurance company by reducing the cost of care, which in turn should reduce the cost of the insurance for the employer. The physicians benefit by gaining a group of patients from whom they can receive payments.

HMO Accredidation

To qualify as an HMO, an organization must present proof of its ability to provide comprehensive health care. To retain eligibility, the HMO must submit **periodic** performance reports to the Department of Human Services. The National Committee for Quality Assurance (NCQA) is responsible for assessing, measuring, and reporting outcomes of HMOs. They also provide the **accreditation** for HMOs after reviewing the HMOs' performance and procedures. It is important for the physician's office to keep complete and accurate records for their patients, maintenance records on all equipment, and records of medications dispensed from their offices; office safety procedures, office cleanliness/appearance, and accessibility are all components to the NCQA standards. There are four levels of accreditation.

1. Full accreditation is given for three years indicating excellent performance.
2. HMOs that are well equipped to make recommended improvements are given a one-year accreditation.
3. Provisional accreditation for one year is given if it appears that the potential for improving the HMO is there.
4. Accreditation is denied because the HMO does not meet the NCQA standards.

Independent Practice Associations

Independent practice associations (IPAs) are individual health care providers who join together to provide prepaid health care to groups and individuals who purchase coverage. This is a **restricted** health plan as only panel providers, hospitals, laboratories, and other ancillary services can be utilized for benefits to be paid. The IPA physicians can hire their own staff and maintain private offices. Primary care physicians are usually paid on a capitated basis while the specialists are paid on a fee-for-service basis.

Preferred Provider Organization

A preferred provider organization (PPO) is not an HMO. The PPO affords the patient the option of using network or non-network physicians and hospitals. Benefits are greater if a network physician/hospital is utilized. The patient assumes a greater financial responsibility if non-network physicians and/or hospitals are used. PPOs do not have a PCP, but do have more patient care management than an indemnity type plan because of the limitations of the provider panel. A PPO usually has deductibles and co-payment requirements, and the physician's office generally files the claim for services rendered.

Many physicians belong to multiple HMOs, PPOs, and IPAs, unless restricted by specific terms of an insurance carrier contract or because of certain regulations in their area.

MANAGED CARE DELIVERY SYSTEMS

With the advent of health care reform, managed care delivery systems are gaining prominence in the types of plans employers are offering employees. Managed care plans integrate the financing and appropriate delivery of services to covered persons by contracting with selected providers for comprehensive health care services, with specific standards for the specialty of the provider and programs for **quality assurance** and **utilization** review. The PCP or gatekeeper is responsible for coordinating all care for the patient. The patient must first consult with his PCP for a referral before seeking the services of a specialist. The PCP is encouraged to use the specialists listed with the HMO/IPA panel of physicians. There may be circumstances when a referral is necessary outside the panel as the specialty may not be part of the panel. Some managed care plans will allow a woman only one visit a year to her gynecologist for her annual well-woman exam and Pap smear. If there are any gynecologic problems prior to the next well-woman exam, she will need a referral from the PCP to see the gynecologist again. Managed care also encourages mammograms for the female patient based on the American Cancer Society guideline.

Well-child care is also promoted by the HMOs. This includes periodic visits for screenings of height, weight, vision, and hearing; neurologic exams; immunizations at appropriate intervals; and tuberculosis (TB) tine tests. Most managed care plans require that the patient pay a co-payment, usually between $5 to $20, at the time of service. The administrative medical assistant in the physician's office files the claim for reimbursement of charges for services rendered for the visit.

Managed care plans employ a large staff of provider/ professional relations representatives. These representatives periodically personally call on physicians' offices to provide new information, distribute new policy manuals, and answer questions that the staff or physicians may have regarding their particular company. Also, monthly newsletters are mailed to providers offices to keep them apprised of changes between representative's visits. Some managed care plans also offer periodic seminars on their policies and claim filing procedures.

GOVERNMENT HEALTH PLANS

Workers' Compensation

Employees in the United States have the benefit of being covered by workers' compensation laws. For many years the name of the coverage was known as workman's compensation but it was changed to avoid **connotations** of gender bias. Every state has these laws to cover employees who are injured while working or become ill as a result of their work. In addition to state statutes, there are federal statutes covering federal employees injured on the job—United States Longshoremen and Harbor Workers Compensation, Federal Coal Mine Health and Safety Compensation, and special benefits for workers in the District of Columbia. The state compensation laws cover those workers not protected by federal statutes. The employer pays the premium for workers' compensation insurance, with the premium based on the risk involved in performance of the job.

Physicians who treat patients under workers' compensation plans are usually required to register with the state Workers' Compensation Board on an annual basis. The code assigned to each physician will limit care to a particular medical specialty.

There are four principal types of state benefits: (1) the patient may have medical treatment in or out of a hospital; (2) if there is determined to be a temporary disability, the patient may receive weekly cash benefits in addition to medical care; (3) when a percentage of permanent disability is found, the patient is given weekly or monthly benefits, and in some cases a lump-sum settlement; or (4) payments are made to dependents of employees who are fatally injured. Benefits also include comprehensive vocational rehabilitation for severely disabled employees.

In most states the report of an industrial injury is initiated by the employer and sent to the physician who reports to the insurance company responsible for paying the claims (Figure 9–4). A few states have their own state fund for workers' compensation, and in these states the forms must be forwarded to the state office responsible. Time requirements for filing a claim vary. When the physician receives the form, it is considered authorization for treatment.

A patient who has an industrial injury should have a separate file set up for that injury and a separate account card. If the patient's record is required in a court case for settlement of the claim, there is no chance of violating the patient's confidentiality if other medical records are in a separate file. The patient is never billed in these cases unless treatment was given without authorization or was considered excessive by the Workers' Compensation Commission, in which case the patient may be billed for the portion denied by the commission. Patients who have a continuing partial or permanent disability are reevaluated at intervals and the physician must furnish a supplemental report.

The medical assistant must keep current files of procedures to be followed and forms to be used, as these are frequently changed. The public affairs section or office services section of your state workers' compensation carrier will furnish any needed information.

The complete and accurate preparation of forms will ensure prompt payment of services. The following details are necessary for reimbursement:

- An accurate claim number appears on all forms and bills.
- The patient's complete name, the date, and the nature of the treatments is included.
- The payee name, address, and number are listed on the form.
- Fees for laboratory or x-ray examinations with interpretations are attached.
- If a surgical billing, a copy of the operative report is attached.
- Fee totals are accurate.
- Forms and bills must be legible.
- The form is signed by the physician.

A bill may be disallowed if it is not filed within the **statutory** time limit. If the claim is rejected for late filing and your records prove your original billing was filed within the statutory time limit, that information should be submitted for reconsideration of the claim. Always retain a copy of your billing. A code number should identify each patient.

BWC
Better Workers' Compensation
Built with *you* in mind.

For faster service
Complete as much of all four sections of this form as possible. Type or print in black or blue ink.

First Report of an Injury, Occupational Disease or Death

Claim Number

WARNING:
Any person who obtains compensation from BWC or self-insuring employers by: knowingly misrepresenting or concealing facts, making false statements, or accepting compensation to which he/she is not entitled, is subject to felony criminal prosecution for fraud.

(R.C. 2913.48)

Injured Worker Info.

Last Name, First Name, Middle Initial			Social Security Number --	Marital Status ☐ Single	Date of Birth
Home Mailing Address			Sex ☐ Male ☐ Female	☐ Married ☐ Divorced	Number of Dependents
City	State	9-digit ZIP Code	Country if different than U.S.A.	☐ Separated ☐ Widowed	Department Name

Wage Rate $	☐ Hour Per: ☐ Year	☐ Month ☐ Week ☐ Other	What days of the week do you usually work? ☐ Sun ☐ Mon ☐ Tues ☐ Wed ☐ Thur ☐ Fri ☐ Sat	Regular Work Hours From :00 To :00

Have you been offered or do you expect to receive payment for this claim from anyone other than the Ohio Bureau of Workers' Compensation or the employer? ☐ YES ☐ NO	Occupation or Job Title

Benefit Application/Medical Release

I am applying for recognition of my claim under the Ohio Workers' Compensation Act for work-related injuries that I did not purposely inflict. I request payment for compensation and/or medical expenses as allowable. Direct payment(s) to the providers of any medical services are authorized. I understand that I am allowing any provider who attends to, treats or examines me	to release all medical, psychological, and/or psychiatric information that is related to my workers' compensation claim to the Ohio Bureau of Workers' Compensation, the Industrial Commission of Ohio, the employer listed in this claim, that employer's managed care organization, and any authorized representatives.	Telephone Number	Work Number
		Injured Worker Signature	Date

Injury/Disease/Death Info.

Date of Injury/Disease	Time of Injury 12:00 ☐ AM ☐ PM	If fatal, give date of death	Date Last Worked	Date Returned to Work
Accident Location (street address)		Date Hired	State Where Hired	Date Employer Notified
City		State	Was place of accident or exposure on employer's premises? ☐ YES ☐ NO	

Description of Accident (Describe the sequence of events that directly injured the employee, or caused the disease or death)	Type of Injury/Disease and Part(s) of Body Affected (For example: sprain of lower left back, etc.)

Treatment Info.

Physician/Health- Care Provider Name	Telephone Number	Fax Number	Initial Treatment Date
Street Address	City	State	9-digit ZIP Code

Diagnosis(es): Include ICD-9 Code(s)	Will this incident cause the injured worker to miss eight or more days of work? ☐ YES ☐ NO
	Is this injury causally related to the industrial incident? ☐ YES ☐ NO
Provider Signature	BWC Provider Number	Date

Employment Info.

Employer Name	Policy Number -0	CHECK IF ☑ Employer is Self-Insuring ☑ Injured Worker is Owner/Partner/Member of Firm
Mailing Address (Number and Street, City or Town, State, and ZIP Code)		County
Location, if different from mailing address		Manual Number
Telephone Number	Fax Number	Federal ID number

☐ **CERTIFICATION** - The employer **certifies** that the facts in this application are correct and valid.	☐ **REJECTION** - The employer **rejects** the validity of this claim for the following reason(s) below:	**FOR SELF-INSURING EMPLOYERS ONLY:** ☐ **CLARIFICATION** - The employer **clarifies and allows** the claim for the condition(s) below:

Employer Signature and Title	Date	**OSHA Case Number**

FROI-1 (Combines C-1, C-2, C-3, C-6, C-50, C-51, OD-1, OD-1-22)   BWC-1101 (Rev. April 3, 2000)   This form meets OSHA 101 requirements.

FIGURE 9–4 First report form for workers' compensation

Medicaid

Title 19 of the **Medicare** Act of 1965 provides for **Medicaid** agreements with states for low-income families, older persons, the blind, families with dependent children, and in some states, other specified individuals. The states establish eligibility requirements and these are constantly being reviewed. Eligible citizens are issued cards to identify their Medicaid status. As a general rule, prior authorization is needed to provide medical treatment except in an emergency. There are usually time limits for submission of claims. Again, the medical assistant must be aware of current rules for submitting claims. You should always check carefully to see if the card is current so that reimbursement for services can be obtained. Patients should receive the same standard of care as provided to privately insured patients.

Medicare

Medicare is a program of health insurance administered under the Social Security Administration for people over the age of 65 who meet the eligibility requirements and have filed for coverage. In addition, those who are disabled, receiving Social Security benefits, or in end-stage renal disease, are also eligible. Patients are issued a red-white-and-blue membership card to verify their coverage (Figure 9-5).

Part A Medicare is for hospital coverage, and any person who is receiving monthly Social Security benefits is automatically enrolled. The deductible amount has increased significantly. Many patients now feel it is necessary to carry a supplemental insurance plan to pay the deductible amount. One such plan by Blue Cross is called *MediFill*. The term **Medigap** is also used to describe this type of supplemental insurance program.

Part B of Medicare is for payment of other medical expenses, including office visits and the services of a physician in or out of the hospital. The premiums are automatically deducted for those who wish the coverage and are

on Social Security, railroad retirement, or civil service **annuity**. Other individuals who are eligible pay premiums directly to the Social Security Administration.

Remember that Medicare B is the coverage that will pay for visits to the physician's office. If you are to assume responsibility for completing the forms, be sure to enter the Medicare identification card number in your records for the patient. The number is the Social Security number followed by a letter. A husband and wife will have separate cards.

Medicare Administration and Claims Processing Physician providers and medical assistants need to keep current with the regulations governing health care and processing of claims. Professional organizations, inservice education providers, and insurance companies offer periodic training sessions and seminars to inform the medical community of changes. When Medicare and Medicaid were enacted originally in 1965 as part of the Social Security Act, they came under the Social Security Administration. In 1977, they were transferred to the Department of Health and Human Services and to the Health Care Financing Administration (HCFA). Changes occurred in attempts to improve the health care delivery system.

Beginning in September 1990, The Omnibus Budget Reconciliation Act (OBRA) of 1989 required that all physicians and suppliers submit Medicare claims for their patients. Physicians and suppliers are not responsible for filing the Medicare claim if the service is not covered by Medicare or for filing other health insurance claims. Claims must be filed within a year of the time the service is received by the patient. In some cases the Medicare insurance carrier will automatically send the amount not covered on to the private insurance carrier, which will pay the deductible and the 20% not covered, eliminating the need to fill out additional forms.

Physicians who sign a contract with Medicare to be a participating provider will receive payment directly from Medicare for services rendered. Physicians who choose not to be a participating provider can collect only the Medicare approved amount for the service rendered. They cannot balance bill the patient for the difference between what Medicare approves and what the physician charges. Non-participating providers are limited to 115% of the Medicare fee schedule for their services.

Patients who have Medicare Part B coverage are responsible for the first $100 of covered services annually; then, Medicare will reimburse the provider 80% of the approved charge. The patient or supplemental insurance would then be responsible for the remaining 20% of the approved charge.

Most Medicare patients will have some form of supplemental or Medigap insurance to cover the deductible and the 20% co-payment. Medigap is health insurance offered by private companies to persons eligible for Medicare benefits and is specifically designed to supplement Medicare benefits. Medicare generally forwards the

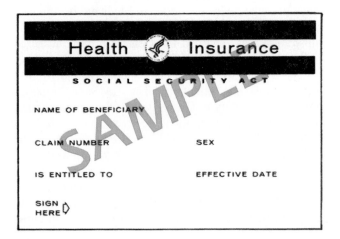

FIGURE 9–5 Medicare identification card (Courtesy of the Social Security Administration.)

claim information directly to the Medigap carrier, thus saving the office staff time. It is important to ask the patient about any supplemental insurance at the time of service. Make a copy of both sides of the Medicare and supplemental insurance cards for your records. (A copy of both sides of *all* insurance cards should be made at each visit.) If the patient does not have a commercial supplemental insurance and is unable to pay the co-payment, the patient may be eligible for Medicaid. In this case, Medicare would be the primary insurance and Medicaid would be secondary and balance billed for the co-payment.

Another variable with primary and secondary coverage occurs when a person qualifies for Medicare by virtue of age but remains employed. If the employee continues to work and is employed by a company with 20 or more employees, the group plan is billed primary and Medicare is billed as secondary. Health insurance coverage provided through employment group plans terminates when the employee retires and Medicare becomes the primary coverage. Supplemental coverage is often available through the company's retirement plan. However, if a Medicare beneficiary is retired but has a working spouse with health insurance, and the beneficiary is an eligible dependent on the spouse's policy, then the spouse's plan becomes primary and Medicare is secondary. Medicare is also secondary when patients are receiving Veterans Administration or workers' compensation benefits.

Physician payment reform (PPR) is another part of OBRA passed by Congress that made sweeping changes in the payment of physician services by Medicare Part B.

■ The PPR payment is based on a fee schedule, which is based on a resource-based relative value system referred to as the Medicare fee schedule (MFS).
■ Medicare volume performance standards (MVPS) have been established to track annual increases in Medicare Part B payments for physicians' services and levels for future years.
■ Various financial protections for the beneficiary have been developed.
■ Payment and medical policies used by Medicare carriers have been standardized.

Medicare is only permitted to pay for services or supplies that are considered medically reasonable and necessary for the diagnosis given. Medicare will not pay for routine physicals, cosmetic surgery, experimental, unproved, or investigational services. If the physician does provide a noncovered service, the patient must be informed in advance and an advanced notice statement must be signed by the patient. The notice must state the specific service, the date of service, and the specific reason the service is not covered. The following are some examples of advanced notice statements which can be used:

■ Medicare usually does not pay for this service.
■ Medicare usually does not pay for this injection.
■ Medicare does not pay for this service as it is considered experimental.

If the patient is not informed in advance of a noncovered service, the patient will not be responsible for payment and any money collected will need to be refunded.

Current Medicare requirements specify that nonparticipating surgeons must notify all patients in writing of their estimated charge, the estimated Medicare approved charge, and the difference between the two in advance of elective operations that involve charges over $500.

Another change occurred when HCFA designated a uniform health insurance claim form to standardize information requested and the method in which it was submitted. This form is known as the HCFA-1500 (Figure 9–6). Regulations were established requiring that all claims submitted by Medicare contractors after May 1, 1992, had to be on an original HCFA-1500 claim form. Photocopied forms would not be acceptable and would be returned regardless of whether the provider accepted assignment or not. Forms could be obtained by requesting the name of special printers from Medicare processing insurance companies.

The special bar code at the top of the HCFA-1500 form allows the claims processor to assign a unique identification number to the claim during microfilming. Effective March 1, 1996, Medicare adopted a national format for completion of claims. If claims are incomplete they are rejected and no payment is made. Additionally, after April 1, 1996, there are no appeal rights for rejected assigned claims. Medicare also encourages all providers to file claims electronically; this speeds up the claim turn-around time for the provider because data entry errors are eliminated when the information does not have to be transferred from a paper claim. Computer software companies provide regular updates as changes occur with Medicare.

In 1997 the State Children's Health Insurance Program (SCHIP) was included as part of the Balanced Budget Act. The program was an attempt to respond to the growing problem of families without health insurance coverage, which in reality means that many children do not receive even basic medical care.

The latest change in health care administration occurred in October 2001. A massive restructuring took place "to better serve the needs of Medicare/Medicaid beneficiaries and health care providers." The Health Care Financing Administration was renamed the Centers for Medicare and Medicaid Services (CMS). This change was part of a package of reforms to "change the agency and drive it to be responsive and effective." The CMS is "organized around three centers to clearly reflect the agency's major line of business: traditional fee-for-service Medicare, Medicare+Choice, and state-administered programs such as Medicaid and SCHIP." One center is known as the Center for Medicare Management and focuses on the traditional fee-for-service program. It is charged with responding to Medicare and Medicaid beneficiaries and health care providers to strengthen health care services and information availability.

The second center, The Center for Beneficiary Choices, focuses on providing beneficiaries with information on

PLEASE
DO NOT
STAPLE
IN THIS
AREA

CARRIER

HEALTH INSURANCE CLAIM FORM

| | PICA | | | | | | PICA | | |

| 1. MEDICARE | MEDICAID | CHAMPUS | CHAMPVA | GROUP HEALTH PLAN (SSN or ID) | FECA BLK LUNG (SSN) | OTHER | 1a. INSURED'S I.D. NUMBER | (FOR PROGRAM IN ITEM 1) |

X (Medicare #) | (Medicaid #) | (Sponsor's SSN) | (VA File #) | (SSN or ID) | (SSN) | (ID) | **090815621B**

2. PATIENT'S NAME (Last Name, First Name, Middle Initial)
JAMES   MICHAEL   J

3. PATIENT'S BIRTH DATE
MM | DD | YY   SEX
08 | 23 | 29   M **X**   F

4. INSURED'S NAME (Last Name, First Name, Middle Initial)
JAMES   MICHAEL   J

5. PATIENT'S ADDRESS (No., Street)
525 N SHORT ST

6. PATIENT RELATIONSHIP TO INSURED
Self **X**   Spouse   Child   Other

7. INSURED'S ADDRESS (No., Street)
525 N SHORT ST

CITY
YOURTOWN   STATE **US**

8. PATIENT STATUS
Single   Married **X**   Other

CITY
YOURTOWN   STATE **US**

ZIP CODE
12345-6790   TELEPHONE (Include Area Code)
(987) 654-0321

Employed   Full-Time Student   Part-Time Student

ZIP CODE
12345-6790   TELEPHONE (INCLUDE AREA CODE)
(987) 654-0321

9. OTHER INSURED'S NAME (Last Name, First Name, Middle Initial)

10. IS PATIENT'S CONDITION RELATED TO:

11. INSURED'S POLICY GROUP OR FECA NUMBER
NONE

a. OTHER INSURED'S POLICY OR GROUP NUMBER

a. EMPLOYMENT? (CURRENT OR PREVIOUS)
YES   **X** NO

a. INSURED'S DATE OF BIRTH
MM | DD | YY   M   SEX   F

b. OTHER INSURED'S DATE OF BIRTH
MM | DD | YY   M   SEX   F

b. AUTO ACCIDENT?   PLACE (State)
YES   **X** NO

b. EMPLOYER'S NAME OR SCHOOL NAME

c. EMPLOYER'S NAME OR SCHOOL NAME

c. OTHER ACCIDENT?
YES   **X** NO

c. INSURANCE PLAN NAME OR PROGRAM NAME

d. INSURANCE PLAN NAME OR PROGRAM NAME

10d. RESERVED FOR LOCAL USE

d. IS THERE ANOTHER HEALTH BENEFIT PLAN?
YES   **X** NO   If yes, return to and complete item 9 a-d.

READ BACK OF FORM BEFORE COMPLETING & SIGNING THIS FORM.
12. PATIENT'S OR AUTHORIZED PERSON'S SIGNATURE I authorize the release of any medical or other information necessary to process this claim. I also request payment of government benefits either to myself or to the party who accepts assignment below.

SIGNED **SIGNATURE ON FILE**   DATE

13. INSURED'S OR AUTHORIZED PERSON'S SIGNATURE I authorize payment of medical benefits to the undersigned physician or supplier for services described below.

SIGNED **SIGNATURE ON FILE**

PATIENT AND INSURED INFORMATION

14. DATE OF CURRENT: ILLNESS (First symptom) OR INJURY (Accident) OR PREGNANCY (LMP)
MM | DD | YY
06 | 16 | XX

15. IF PATIENT HAS HAD SAME OR SIMILAR ILLNESS. GIVE FIRST DATE MM | DD | YY

16. DATES PATIENT UNABLE TO WORK IN CURRENT OCCUPATION
MM | DD | YY   MM | DD | YY
FROM   TO

17. NAME OF REFERRING PHYSICIAN OR OTHER SOURCE

17a. I.D. NUMBER OF REFERRING PHYSICIAN

18. HOSPITALIZATION DATES RELATED TO CURRENT SERVICES
MM | DD | YY   MM | DD | YY
FROM   TO

19. RESERVED FOR LOCAL USE

20. OUTSIDE LAB? $ CHARGES
YES   NO

21. DIAGNOSIS OR NATURE OF ILLNESS OR INJURY. (RELATE ITEMS 1,2,3 OR 4 TO ITEM 24E BY LINE)
1. **401.1**   3. |____.___
2. |____.___   4. |____.___

22. MEDICAID RESUBMISSION CODE   ORIGINAL REF. NO.

23. PRIOR AUTHORIZATION NUMBER

| 24. A DATE(S) OF SERVICE | | B Place of Service | C Type of Service | D PROCEDURES, SERVICES, OR SUPPLIES (Explain Unusual Circumstances) CPT/HCPCS   MODIFIER | E DIAGNOSIS CODE | F $ CHARGES | G DAYS OR UNITS | H EPSDT Family Plan | I EMG | J COB | K RESERVED FOR LOCAL USE |
From MM DD YY	To MM DD YY										
06 18 XX	06 18 XX	11	1	99212	1	35 00	1				4567890123

25. FEDERAL TAX I.D. NUMBER   SSN   EIN
11-0000521   **X**

26. PATIENT'S ACCOUNT NO.
1234

27. ACCEPT ASSIGNMENT? (For govt. claims see back)
X YES   NO

28. TOTAL CHARGE
$ **35 00**

29. AMOUNT PAID
$ **00**

30. BALANCE DUE
$ **35 00**

31. SIGNATURE OF PHYSICIAN OR SUPPLIER INCLUDING DEGREES OR CREDENTIALS (I certify that the statements on the reverse apply to this bill and are made a part thereof.)

SAMUEL E MATTHEWS MD

SIGNED   DATE **06/20/XX**

32. NAME AND ADDRESS OF FACILITY WHERE SERVICES WERE RENDERED (If other than home or office)

33. PHYSICIAN'S, SUPPLIER'S BILLING NAME, ADDRESS, ZIP CODE & PHONE #
SAMUEL E MATTHEWS MD
100 E MAIN ST STE 120
YOURTOWN US   98765-4321
PIN# **4567890123**   GRP#

PHYSICIAN OR SUPPLIER INFORMATION

(APPROVED BY AMA COUNCIL ON MEDICAL SERVICE 8/88)   *PLEASE PRINT OR TYPE*

APPROVED OMB-0938-0008 FORM HCFA-1500 (12-90), FORM RRB-1500,
APPROVED OMB-1215-0055 FORM OWCP-1500,   APPROVED OMB-0720-0001 (CHAMPUS)

FIGURE 9–6   Completed and approved health insurance claim form

A CAAHEP CONNECTION

A medical assistant is expected to be knowledgeable of guidelines and requirements for health care and demonstrate the ability to properly code and complete insurance forms. This is a very important part of your employment in the office of a provider. In order for you to obtain this competency, the standards require that it be included in your program of study.

Medicare, Medicare Select, Medicare+Choice, and Medigap. It is also responsible for managing the Medicare+ Choice plan, consumer research and demonstration, and grievance and appeals functions.

The third center is The Center for Medicaid and State Operations, which focuses on programs administered by states which include Medicaid, SCHIP, insurance regulation functions, survey and certification, and the Clinical Laboratory Improvements Act (CLIA).

A 1999 survey of Medicare recipients determined that many beneficiaries and their caregivers did not understand Medicare costs, coverage, and the options available such as Medigap and Medicare+Choice. To help inform participants, several changes were implemented:

- Beginning October 2001, customer service representatives at the CMMS call center expanded their hours for providing information to a 24-hour, 7-days-a-week service. They can be reached at 800-Medicare (800-633-4227) to answer questions and to request written information through the mail.
- A web-based information site is available at http://www.medicare.gov.
- The center has budgeted $35 million for a Medicare Education Campaign, involving a national advertising effort in the Fall of 2002 to inform participants about expanded services.
- Information for physicians and their staff is accessible at http://www.hcfa.gov.

TRICARE (CHAMPUS)

As part of the United States Department of Defense, the Civilian Health and Medical Program of the Uniformed Services TRICARE (CHAMPUS) was established to aid dependents of active service personnel, retired service personnel and their dependents, and dependents of service personnel who died on active duty, with a **supplement** for medical care in military or Public Health Service facilities. The word *dependents* refers to spouses and dependent children only; this program does not cover active duty military personnel. All members of TRICARE (CHAMPUS) over the age of 10 are issued an identifica-

tion card. A patient who lives within 40 miles of a uniformed services hospital will need a *nonavailability statement* to be cared for in a civilian or physician's office. This simply means that the necessary services are not available at the service hospital or that for medical reasons it would be better to continue care under the civilian physician who has been treating the patient. Authorization is not necessary if the patient lives more than 40 miles from a military medical facility that could furnish the necessary care.

The Civilian Health and Medical Program of the Veterans' Administration (CHAMPVA) was established in 1973 for the spouses and dependent children of veterans who have total, permanent, service-connected disabilities. This service is also available for the surviving spouses and dependent children of veterans who have died as a result of service-connected disabilities. The local VA hospital determines eligibility and then issues identification cards. The insured members can then choose their own private physicians. There are deductibles and cost-sharing requirements your office needs to be aware of.

If your office needs additional information on military benefit programs, you can contact your local health benefits advisor (HBA) at the nearest military hospital or clinic or the office of TRICARE (CHAMPUS), in Aurora, CO 80045-6900. The TRICARE (CHAMPUS) phone number is 303-361-3907; the phone number for CHAMPVA is 303-782-3804.

Easter Seal/Crippled Children

All states operate Crippled Children's Services with federal support under Title V of the Social Security Act. The intent of this service is to locate disabled children under 21 or those who have potentially crippling conditions to see that appropriate health care is furnished. Part or all of this treatment may be paid for if the family's resources are not adequate. Some Crippled Children's Services are being changed to Easter Seal rehabilitation centers because of the stigma attached to the words *crippled children.* Some Easter Seal rehabilitation centers are now operated as private nonprofit organizations.

ACHIEVE UNIT OBJECTIVES

Complete Chapter 9, Unit 2, in the workbook to help you obtain competency of this subject matter.

UNIT 3
Preparing Claims

OBJECTIVES

Upon completion of the unit, meet the following performance objectives by verifying knowledge of the facts and

principles presented through oral and written communication at a level deemed competent, and demonstrate the specific behaviors as identified in the performance objectives of the procedures, observing safety precautions in accordance with health care standards.

1. Spell and define, using the glossary at the back of the text, all the **Words to Know** in this unit.
2. Explain why claim forms were developed.
3. Explain the meaning of primary and secondary coverage and how it affects coverage.
4. Name the two main classifications of codes and explain their basic difference.
5. Explain the meanings of both the "reason rule" and sequencing.
6. List four general coding rules.
7. Identify two things to be done <u>before</u> completing a patient's claim form.
8. Demonstrate completion of a claim form.
9. List six common errors made when filing claims.
10. Explain the purpose of an insurance log, listing six of the items to enter.
11. Name four pieces of information to have before calling to follow-up a delinquent insurance claim.
12. Explain the phrase "accept assignment."
13. Describe what action should be taken when a procedure is <u>not</u> covered by insurance.
14. Name five of the seven items necessary for adequate documentation on a patient's record.
15. Identify three ways to stay current with Medicare and other insurance company regulations.

AREAS OF COMPETENCE (AAMA)

This unit addresses content within the specific competency areas of *Administrative procedures, Practice finances, Professionalism,* and *Legal concepts* as identified in the Medical Assistant Role Delineation Study. Refer to Appendix A for a detailed listing of the areas.

WORDS TO KNOW

bundle	modifier
carrier	nomenclature
contributory	numeric
Current Procedural	preferred
Terminology	primary
encounter	reason rule
fee schedule	reimbursement
Health Care Financing	secondary
Administration	sequenced
International	specificity
Classification of	third-party
Diseases	reimbursement
Medicare	truncated

THE BEGINNING OF CLAIM FORMS

The preparation of claims for the purpose of receiving payment for medical services is a fairly recent development in the history of health care. For centuries, providers were paid directly with some form of money, bartered goods, or the exchange of services. With industrialization and the scientific advancement of medicine, this was no longer appropriate. At the same time people began receiving employment benefits such as vacations and pensions. Soon, other benefits such as health care were added and the new industry of health insurance exploded. The phrase "**third-party reimbursement**" was coined to indicate payment of services rendered by someone other than the patient. With this intermediate step came the need for some form of paperwork to serve as the means of reporting the health care provided to the source of payment: the claim form was developed. Today, the most common third-party reimbursers are federal and state agencies, insurance companies, and worker's compensation.

Originally, patients would provide the physician with forms obtained from their employer's benefits office for their insurance coverage. The patient completed their portion of the form and either signed or did not sign the section that authorized payment for services to be made directly to the physician. If it was not signed, the patient paid the charges and then the insurance company sent the payment to the patient. It was customary for physicians to charge a small fee to complete forms after the first one was done. Patients often had multiple coverage and could even "make money" with covered conditions. Medical findings, diagnoses, and treatments were described verbally in medical terminology and fees were paid as requested if they were reasonable. Third-party reimbursement was simple and fairly easy. The contract for services was primarily between the physician and the patient; controls were minimal. As time went by, medicine evolved into a very sophisticated science. Medical care became extremely complicated and technologic advances caused a rapid rise in medical costs. Premiums for insurance coverage skyrocketed. Unemployed and retired persons had to resort to community clinics in order to obtain health care.

THE HISTORY OF CODING

While medical care was evolving into a highly technical service, another need was surfacing. There needed to be some method of collecting health data so that physicians, scientists, and government agencies could assess the incidences and treatments of diseases. As early as the 1890s, a physician developed a classification of causes of death. From this beginning, the American Public Health Association recommended that this classification system be adopted by those responsible for recording deaths in Canada, Mexico, and the United States. It was decided that the classification should be revised every 10 years. In 1938, the fifth revision had evolved into the **Interna-**

tional **Classification of Diseases** (ICD). A few years later hospitals began trying to classify diseases and their medical records departments used a modified ICD version to code and index records.

The initial reason for classifying deaths was to provide a means of assessing statistically the prevalence of certain diseases or disorders or the incidences of fatal injuries. Later, codes were used in order to retrieve medical records by diagnosis or surgical procedure to be useful in medical research and education. As other applications became evident, the system provided a method of identifying the incidence of diseases and disorders being treated throughout the world. Reported prevalence provides statistics for assessing the status of people within and among various countries. As the need for greater **specificity** of medical conditions became desirable, the codes were revised, expended, and refined.

By 1978, the World Health Organization published the ninth version of the ICD (ICD-9) and in the United States the *International Classification of Diseases, 9th Revision, Clinical Modification (ICD-9-CM)* was issued and will remain in effect until the 10th revision is released. Currently, this is anticipated in October 2003. The 10th revision contains ICD changes made by the World Health Organization and the clinical modifications (CM) changes made by the National Center for Health Statistics in the United States. The new code book will serve every field of health care. Its full title will be *International Statistical Classification of Diseases and Related Health Problems*. The book will go beyond classification of disease and injuries to the coding of ambulatory care and risk factors encountered in primary care. It will also include additional clinical details about current diseases as well as those diseases discovered since the last revision. However, for the most part it will retain the same format. Some change will occur in the Injury and Poisoning chapter where injuries will be catalogued by the anatomic site instead of by type of injury. Another change involves the E codes that were used for external causes of disease. E codes will be used for endocrine system diseases while the external causes will be listed under V codes. The new code book will be published in three volumes and include the following:

Volume 1—The tabular listing of alpha-numeric codes as in ICD-9

Volume 2—An instructional manual that provides rules and guidelines of coding

Volume 3—An alphabetic index of the codes in the tabular list

The codes now allow for the expression of extensive verbal descriptions into a numeric system. Coding is, in reality, the transferal of verbal or written descriptions of disease or injury into numeric designations to achieve uniform data that can be easily entered into electronic processing and storage systems.

USE OF CURRENT ICD CODES

The ICD codes became useful for reporting all medical care on claim forms for Medicare, Medicaid, and other third-party payers of medical services. Later, the impact of The Catastrophic Coverage Act of 1988 on the physician's office changed the way physicians manage their practices. Since April 1, 1989, ICD coding is no longer an option; it is required on all Medicare and other government health care claims. The act mandates submission of an appropriate diagnostic code or codes for each service provided under Medicare B, or other coverage, for which payment is requested. Specific coding guidelines have been developed for physicians' offices. It is very important that coding be done properly. The physician's **reimbursement** is based upon the codes that are submitted.

The ICD codes are descriptive of the *disease* or *condition* presented by the patient. The ICD code selected by the physician must be as specific to the patient's diagnosed condition as possible. Another coding system based on the *procedures* and *services* the physician or the office staff provides for the patient are known as the Current Procedural Terminology (CPT) codes. These codes must be appropriate for the ICD code of the disease or payment will not be approved by the carrier. Accurate and precise coding not only helps to optimize reimbursement, it is essential for carrier acceptance. Mistakes not only cost the physician, but patients are also affected when services are not covered.

The coding systems established a way to communicate numerically with carriers and at the same time provided a means to collect numeric data for national and international purposes. It is a complex system, but with experience it becomes more manageable. One of the most important factors to remember is that the codes have to be sequenced in relation to the intensity and level of service provided. Basically this involves listing the primary reason for the office visit first and other reasons next in order of their importance. The staff person who processes claim forms needs to be a detail-oriented individual. This is a very important role in the medical practice and is not suitable for a beginning employee.

PERFORMING CODING FUNCTIONS

To become an accurate and efficient coder, three things are necessary: a working knowledge of medical terminology, an understanding of anatomy and physiology, and comprehension of ICD characteristics and terminology. Coding requires attention to detail. Work experience and a period of learning with the help of an experienced coder can be very beneficial. In this unit, only a brief introduction to the process is presented. This responsibility can best be learned by actual performance using the code materials provided by your employer. Because various companies produce manuals with the ICD codes, and different methods of organization of the information, specific directions are not practical. Some examples of manuals are *The Educational Annotation of ICD-9-CM, St. Anthony's ICD-9-CM Code Book for Physician Payment, ICD-9-CM Family Practice Easy Coder,* and *2001 Physician ICD-9-CM Volumes 1 and 2* by Medicode.

The standard codes were taken from the federal government's official **Health Care Financing Administration** (HCFA) material. Some coding books arrange diseases and injuries in two volumes.

Volume I—A tabular list, organized into 17 chapters, with conditions listed by body systems in one chapter and by conditions according to their causes in another chapter. Other information in Volume I is in supplementary classifications such as:

- V-codes—Factors influencing health status and contact with health service.
- E-codes—External causes of injury and poisoning.

Volume I also contains appendices of:

- M-codes—Morphology of Neoplasms.
- Glossary of Mental Disorders.
- Classification of Drugs by the American Hospital Formulary.
- Classification of Industrial Accidents According to Agency.
- List of Three-Digit Categories.

Volume II—An alphabetic index organized into three main sections:

- Section 1—Alphabetic Index to Diseases and Injuries.
- Section 2—Table of Drugs and Chemicals.
- Section 3—Index to External Causes of Injuries and Poisonings (for assigning E-codes).

Some references have a Section 4—Index to Procedures, while others have a Volume III, which is used by hospital coders to code procedures (physicians' offices use the CPT coding for their procedures so this section or volume is not used for coding in the medical office).

In addition, many code books have enhancement variations. Some are loose-leafed, and some have highlighting of codes to be avoided or ones that require additional information. Some carry additional explanations of diseases or disorders while others are color-coded to identify cautions, signs, symptoms, external causes, and so on.

ICD-9-CM 2001

One example of an ICD code book is published by Medicode. It contains both Volumes 1 and 2. The tabular section with disease classifications and increasing spe-

DISEASES OF MALE GENITAL ORGANS (600-608)

● **600 Hyperplasia of prostate**
Use additional code to identify urinary incontinence (788.30-788.39)

600.0 Hypertrophy (benign) of prostate ▼
Benign prostatic hypertrophy
Enlargement of prostate
Smooth enlarged prostate
Soft enlarged prostate

600.1 Nodular prostate
Hard, firm prostate
Multinodular prostate
EXCLUDES *malignant neoplasm of prostate (185)*

600.2 Benign localized hyperplasia of prostate
Adenofibromatous hypertrophy of prostate
Adenoma of prostate
Fibroadenoma of prostate
Fibroma of prostate
Myoma of prostate
Polyp of prostate
EXCLUDES *benign neoplasms of prostate (222.2)*
hypertrophy of prostate (600.0)
malignant neoplasm of prostate (185)

600.3 Cyst of prostate

◆ **600.9 Hyperplasia of prostate, unspecified**
Median bar
Prostatic obstruction NOS ▲

● **601 Inflammatory diseases of prostate**
Use additional code to identify organism, such as Staphylococcus (041.1), or Streptococcus (041.0)

601.0 Acute prostatitis
Sudden, severe inflammation of the prostate.

601.1 Chronic prostatitis
Persistent inflammation of the prostate.

601.2 Abscess of prostate
Pocket of pus within the prostate.

601.3 Prostatocystitis
Inflammation of the prostate and bladder.

▮ ***601.4 Prostatitis in diseases classified elsewhere***
Code first underlying disease, as:
actinomycosis (039.8)
blastomycosis (116.0)
syphilis (095.8)
tuberculosis (016.5)
EXCLUDES *prostatitis:*
gonococcal (098.12, 098.32)
monilial (112.2)
trichomonal (131.03)

◆ **601.8 Other specified inflammatory diseases of prostate**
Prostatitis: cavitary, diverticular
Prostatitis: granulomatous

FIGURE 9–7 Sample page of disease classification codes from ICD-9-CM 2001 code book (Courtesy Medicode Ingenix Company.)

cific codes is arranged numerically from 001, Infectious and Parasitic Diseases, to 999.9, Other and unspecified complications of medical care, not elsewhere classified. A partial page taken from *Diseases of the Genitourinary System,* specifically Diseases of Male Genital Organs (600–608) is shown in Figure 9–7. This book has some features that help ensure accurate coding:

- The red dot signifies additional digit(s) required for coding.
- The yellow diamond indicates this is a nonspecific code.
- The blue rectangle indicates this code is not a primary diagnosis.
- The black triangles indicate the start and end of a new section of codes.

The diagnosis with a proper code is easily recognized. Note the description of the conditions in 601.0 to 601.3. In addition to the codes, notice the blackboxed *EXCLUDES* feature that indicates other code numbers used for these conditions. New lines of information are identified with a solid black diamond, while a revised line is an outlined black diamond. This code book also includes anatomic illustrations of various body structures to aid in selecting codes.

Coding Rules

The general coding rules are:

1. Code correctly and completely any diagnosis or procedure that affects the care, influences the health status, or is a reason for treatment on that visit.
2. Code the minimum number of diagnoses that fully describe the patient's care received on that visit. The diagnosis must reflect the patient's need for treatment, x-rays, diagnostic procedures, or medications.
3. Code each problem to the highest level of specificity (3rd, 4th, or 5th digit) available in the classification (see Figure 9–7).
4. Sequence codes correctly so that it is possible to understand the chronology of events (e.g., the reason for the visit and care).

The <u>main rule</u> to remember is the "**reason rule**," which says that the reason for the patient visit (encounter) is coded <u>first</u>.

This is **primary**; other "side" issues are coded next, in order of importance. There is a situation when the main rule will not apply. Sometimes, after the patient has been examined, another condition is discovered that differs from the condition for which the patient had originally sought treatment. In this situation, the diagnosis that required the greatest amount of effort would be coded first. At first, coding is confusing and difficult, but with experience, it will become easier.

IDENTIFYING THE DIAGNOSIS

Identifying the diagnosis may be a difficult task for the beginning coder. Remember to follow the rules and suggestions above. Physicians usually help by marking indications on the patient's encounter form or superbill as well as recording diagnoses on the chart. However, it is necessary for the coder to read the chart, or if employed by a surgeon, the operative report, in order to determine any other codes that might apply or to carry those indicated to the next digit. Remember, this affects your rate of payment. Some code books provide cues in their listings. Forms with codes that should be carried to the 4th or 5th digit in order to make the diagnosis more specific, but are not, <u>will be rejected and returned</u>. To complicate matters further, the rules are always changing. In 1996, Medicare had made five "changes" by July 1 which affected how claims are filed. One referred to rebundling of codes when multiple procedures are performed and said that generally only reimbursement would be given for the <u>major</u> procedure. To

bundle refers to the process of considering several parts as a whole. At other times, Medicare will unbundle a multilevel procedure and allow billing on each portion. The **truncated** (cutoff) ICD coding ruling, which became effective July 1, 1996, stated that claims must be coded to the highest level of specificity or they will be rejected and the provider will be required to file a new claim.

The standardized <u>required</u> form will accept up to four diagnostic codes (see Figure 9–6, p. 223, line 21). Remember: you only receive reimbursement for procedures or services that relate to the identified diagnostic codes. Again, refer to Figure 9–6 line 21. The form asks you to relate the diagnosis code to the procedure and enter that in line 24 D and E. There must be a reason for the procedure to be done. For example, if a patient just wanted to know her blood type, but there was no <u>reason</u> (diagnosis) that the information was necessary, the procedure code would probably be rejected.

While the government was busy publishing the ICD code books, the American Medical Association developed and published *The Physicians' Current Procedural Terminology (CPT)* code book. This is a descriptive listing of codes for reporting medical services and procedures performed by physicians. NOTE: These two standard **nomenclature** code books (ICD, CPT) are published <u>annually</u> and are absolutely essential to the function of the medical office. Each year codes are added, deleted, changed or modified for the new editions. Books can be ordered in advance and are released in the Fall for use beginning on the following January 1. Claim forms <u>may</u> use the new codes after January 1 but <u>must</u> use them after April 1 or forms will be returned to the providers.

CURRENT PROCEDURAL TERMINOLOGY CODES

The Current Procedural Terminology (CPT) codebook has a systematic listing and coding of procedures and services performed by physicians. Each procedure or service is identified with a five-digit code which is used to report services. The main body of the material is listed in six sections:

1. Evaluation and Management (E/M)
2. Anesthesiology
3. Surgery
4. Radiology (including Nuclear Medicine and Diagnostic Ultrasound)
5. Pathology and Laboratory
6. Medicine (except Anesthesiology)

Within each section are subsections with anatomic, procedure, condition, or descriptor subheadings. The procedures and services with their identifying codes are presented in **numeric** order with one exception: the entire Evaluation and Management section is placed at the beginning of the listed procedures. These items are used by most physicians in reporting a significant portion of their services. At the end of the book are the appendix and the index. Following the index is a page listing instructions for the use of the CPT index. The index has four general categories. Each category has examples to assist the user in understanding the category.

Using the CPT Book

To determine a code, the name of the procedure or service that most accurately identifies the service performed is selected. This could be a diagnostic procedure, radiologic examination, or surgery. Other additional procedures performed or pertinent services may be listed including any modifying or extenuating circumstances. Any service or procedure which is coded <u>must be</u> adequately documented in the medical record. As with ICD codes, you can rely on the physician for assistance. Generally, services performed in the office are marked on the patient's encounter form. Care must be taken not to miss items like injections, urinalysis, or blood samples, or the need to use a **modifier** for prolonged E/M services. If you must code from operative reports, it will be necessary to review the description the surgeon dictated to be certain all pertinent codes have been identified.

The introduction in the CPT code book gives excellent instructions on the use of CPT terminology and coding. The book is divided into specialty sections, but codes from any section may be used to give an adequate description of a treatment or procedure rendered by a qualified physician. In reading the introduction, you will find guidelines are presented at the beginning of each section to define items that are necessary to interpret and report the procedure and services to be found in that section. In some instances a specific procedure or service may need to be slightly altered. Instructions and the appendix explain the use of modifiers. Some examples of when these would be used are if unusual events occurred, if a service was performed by more than one physician, or if a procedure had both professional and technical components. Other examples are listed.

If you cannot find a code listed for a procedure or service your employer has performed, a provision has been made for the use of specific code numbers for reporting unlisted procedures. In these instances a description of the service must also be provided.

It is important to use the current year's code book to check the codes you are using to be sure they have not been changed. A special appendix in the book provides a complete list of the codes deleted, revised, and added to the book. Another detail requiring attention is the superbill or encounter form. Usually they are preprinted with the most frequently used ICD and CPT codes listed to facilitate coding by the physician and insurance coder. When new books are issued, these frequently used codes especially need to be checked prior to the deadline. If changes have occurred, the slip may need reprinting.

Software companies have made it possible for a physicians' offices to design their own superbills in whatever format they choose. The software contains all the ICD and CPT codes, and the practice chooses the ones appropriate to their services. Once the superbill is designed, it can be printed out from a computer. Errors and fraudulent billing codes are reduced when completing a claim form. The software even warns the user that fourth and fifth digits are required. Updating the software when codes are revised will also allow the program to scan the designed superbill to identify code changes.

Features of the CPT Book

The CPT 2001 book uses symbols to indicate specific information about code numbers, much like those found in the ICD publications. Figure 9–8 is a sample of breast incision and excision codes that illustrate most of the symbols. In addition, notice the descriptive language and symbols that explain the specificity of the procedure:

* ∗   Service includes surgical procedure only
* +   Add-on code
* ▲   Revised code
* ●   New code
* ►◄   New or revised text

The AMA also makes available magnetic computer tapes and disk formats of the CPT manual. One tape presentation is the complete procedural text of the manual

Breast

Incision

19000∗	Puncture aspiration of cyst of breast;
+ 19001	each additional cyst (List separately in addition to code for primary procedure)
	(Use 19001 in conjunction with code 19000)
19020	Mastotomy with exploration or drainage of abscess, deep
19030	Injection procedure only for mammary ductogram or galactogram
	(For radiological supervision and interpretation, see 76086, 76088)

Excision

(All codes for bilateral procedures have been deleted. To report, add modifier '-50')

▲19100∗	Biopsy of breast; percutaneous, needle core, not using imaging guidance (separate procedure)
	(For fine needle aspiration, use 88170)
	(For ►image guided◄ breast biopsy, see ►19102, 19103,◄ 88170)
	(For radiologic guidance performed in conjunction with breast biopsy, see 76095, ►76360, 76393,◄ 76942)
▲19101	open, incisional
●19102	percutaneous, needle core, using imaging guidance
	►(For placement of percutaneous localization clip, use 19295)◄

FIGURE 9–8 Sample CPT-2001 codes showing procedures and symbols to denote new, revised, add-on, and surgical procedures only (CPT codes, descriptions, and numeric modifiers only are copyright 2000 of the American Medical Association.)

while the other is a CPT short description tape. The short description tape also contains the complete listing of procedural codes in the manual but each has an abbreviated narrative written in nontechnical terms. The disk version is identical in content to the short description tape.

Evaluation and Management Services Guidelines

The Evaluation and Management (E/M) section codes are divided into 17 categories of provider services beginning with *Office and Other Outpatient Services* and ending with *Other Procedures*. The E/M codes are related to medical services as opposed to surgical services. Figure 9–9 illustrates two of the five coding areas for a new patient office visit. The codes are important because they describe the nature of the physician's actions such as:

- Place of service
- Level of history and examination required
- Degree of decision making involved
- Extent of the patient's problem
- Amount of time the physician spent

Another classification which affects coding is whether the patient is new or established.

Within each category or subcategory of E/M services, three to five levels are available for reporting purposes.

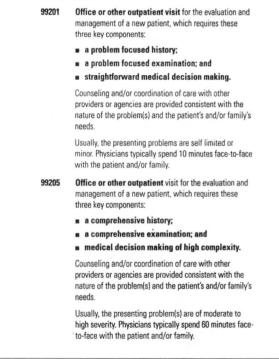

New Patient

99201   **Office or other outpatient visit** for the evaluation and management of a new patient, which requires these three key components:

- **a problem focused history;**
- **a problem focused examination; and**
- **straightforward medical decision making.**

Counseling and/or coordination of care with other providers or agencies are provided consistent with the nature of the problem(s) and the patient's and/or family's needs.

Usually, the presenting problems are self limited or minor. Physicians typically spend 10 minutes face-to-face with the patient and/or family.

99205   **Office or other outpatient** visit for the evaluation and management of a new patient, which requires these three key components:

- **a comprehensive history;**
- **a comprehensive examination; and**
- **medical decision making of high complexity.**

Counseling and/or coordination of care with other providers or agencies are provided consistent with the nature of the problem(s) and the patient's and/or family's needs.

Usually, the presenting problem(s) are of moderate to high severity. Physicians typically spend 60 minutes face-to-face with the patient and/or family.

FIGURE 9–9   Sample CPT-E/M codes for New Patient Office or Other Outpatient Services (CPT codes, descriptions, and numeric modifiers only are copyright 2000 of the American Medical Association.)

The levels include examinations, evaluations, treatments, conferences with or concerning patients, preventative pediatric and adult health supervision, and similar medical services. The levels encompass wide variations in skill, effort, time, responsibility, and medical knowledge required for the prevention or diagnosis and treatment of illness or injury.

In addition to the levels are descriptors which recognize seven components that are used in defining the levels of E/M services:

1. history
2. examination
3. medical decision making
4. counseling
5. coordination of care
6. nature of presenting problem
7. time

The first three are considered key components in selecting a level of E/M services. The next three and the nature of the presenting problem are considered **contributory** factors in the majority of **encounters** (contacts). It is <u>not</u> required that these services be provided at every patient encounter. The actual performance of any diagnostic test or study requires separate specific coding in <u>addition</u> to the appropriate E/M code. Several other items unique to the section are described in the E/M guidelines, which are fairly easy to read and understand. If you refer to the first page of the E/M section of the CPT code book, you will see codes for a new patient that show four levels of history and examination. Selecting the appropriate E/M and CPT codes is a complex clinical decision that is the responsibility of the physician.

COMPLETING THE CLAIM FORM

 Insurance:
- Case Files

Before claims are processed, be certain that you have a copy of the patient's insurance coverage card and have secured his or her signature on a form to permit release of information. This form will also have an "assignment of benefits" clause which authorizes benefits be paid directly to the provider.

Medical assistants who submit Medicare insurance claims with the stamped statement "Patient's signature on file" must be prepared to make these files available in the event they are audited by the insurance carrier. The only time a signature is not needed is when a patient has services performed without being physically present in the office. An example of this would be the laboratory where a specimen collected in the physician's office was analyzed. In this case, the insurance form should state "Patient not physically present for services." Signatures of welfare patients are not required if the state agency maintains records of the signatures. It was suggested by Nationwide Mutual Insurance Company in a *Medicare Newsletter* that an office have a form prepared for the signature of Medicare patients. This could be signed once and kept on file and it would not be necessary to obtain the signature of the patient on every form. The form should list the name and Medicare claim number of the patient along with the following statement:

> I request that payment of authorized Medicare benefits be made either to me or on my behalf to Dr. _____ for any service furnished to me by that physician. I authorize release of medical information about me needed to determine these benefits or benefits payable for related services.

The form should be signed by the patient and dated.

The HCFA has developed codes for Medicare that allow for uniformity throughout the country. The three levels of codes range as follows:

1. The CPT codes are established and updated by the American Medical Association. These are five digit numeric codes ranging from 00000 to 99999 for physicians' services, such as examinations, surgeries, radiology, and pathology. Most Medicare B coverage is covered by CPT codes.
2. The HCPCS codes are established and updated. These alpha-numeric codes range from A0000 to V9999 and are used for physician and nonphysician services not listed in the CPT.
3. Codes W0000 to Z9999 are reserved for local assignment. These codes are not present in CPT and are not common to all carriers.

Another important number necessary for completion of Medicare claims is the physician's National Provider Identification (NPI) number. In 1997, the NPI replaced the PIN, or physician's identifying number, and the UPIN, or unique physician's identifying number, previously used. The NPI is a ten-digit number; the first seven digits are unique to the physician, the eighth digit is a check digit, and the last two have to do with location. If your physician has more than one office, there will be a NPI for each practice location. The NPI will be used in blocks 24k and 33 of the approved form to identify who provided the service. When the physician refers a patient to another practice for services, the referring physician's NPI will appear in block 17a of the form. If this number is missing from the claim, the claim will be returned.

Medicare provides annual updated policy manuals and monthly newsletters to keep physicians and their staffs current on Medicare policy. Medicare also offers training session to new medical assistants and seminars to those who are already experienced with Medicare policy to keep up-to-date.

In processing Medicare insurance forms, you must use ICD codes for diagnosis, CPT codes for treatment, and HCPCS codes for any supplies or appliances used.

Today the patient has little or no responsibility for filing claims. The physician is <u>required</u> to file **Medicare** claims and it is normally an obligation when contracting as a provider with other carriers. Once the physician has billed the primary coverage and primary carrier has responded, either the carrier will automatically forward the claim to a secondary carrier, or the physician as a courtesy may choose to file for the secondary coverage. Often this is to the physicians' advantage as the supplemental amount is usually paid directly to them. After primary and secondary carriers have responded, the remaining approved balance can be billed to the patient for payment.

As stated previously, government sponsored health care claims must be filed on the approved insurance claim form (refer to Figure 9–6). Regulations also require that the form be an original; copies are not acceptable. Procedure 9–1 "Complete a Claim Form" will give you some practice in preparing a form. Physicians can obtain packages of 50 to as many as 1000 sheets through the AMA. Other suppliers, including the government, are available. The forms are designed for use with computer printers. In addition to government mandatory use, all other insurance companies will accept the form. This is helpful, especially with patients who have **secondary** coverage; it eliminates the need to complete two forms. Even if the secondary carrier has its own claim form, a copy of the approved form can be attached and will be acceptable.

It is very important to photocopy all completed forms before mailing in order to have a record. Some offices file claim forms in an insurance folder until payment is received; then, they are filed in the respective patient's chart.

MAINTAINING AN INSURANCE LOG

A method for monitoring the status and payment of insurance claims should be established. It is easy to forget about filed claims, and soon a sizeable amount of money is owed to the physician. Some practices use an insurance log (a book in which a list of insurance claims is kept). When a claim is filed, it is noted on a log. The log should have columns for recording pertinent information. The following would be helpful in monitoring claim status:

- the date the claim is filed
- the insurance company's name
- the patient's name
- the amount of the claim
- the amount paid
- the secondary company's name
- the date filed
- the amount billed
- the amount paid
- the date the patient was billed
- the follow-up date

Today, most offices use computer software designed for monitoring insurance claims. The information can be en-

P R O C E D U R E

9-1   Complete a Claim Form

PURPOSE: To accurately complete a claim form for processing.

EQUIPMENT: Appropriate form, patient record, account ledger/information, computer, and software.

PERFORMANCE OBJECTIVE: Given access to all necessary equipment and information, follow the procedure to complete an approved claim form without error within the instructor's prescribed time limit.

1. Check for a photocopy of the patient's insurance card.

2. Check the chart to see if the patient signature is on file for release of information and assignment of benefits.
   NOTE: If not on file, the patient must sign the form. It is best to have it signed before the form is completed. If the completed form is forwarded to the patient to be signed and sent to the insurance company, it is best to send a stamped and addressed envelope so there will not be a delay in forwarding the form to the insurance company.

3. Using Figure 9–6 as a guide, complete the following entries:
   A. Check appropriate box at top of form.
   B. Enter name of patient (be certain the name used on the form is the same as that on the identification card).
   C. Enter birthdate and check box for male or female.
   NOTE: Use six digits to write birthdate (e.g., 08/23/29).

4. Enter insured's name.

5. Enter patient's full address and telephone number.

6. Enter patient's relationship to insured.

7. Enter insured's full address and telephone number.

8. Enter patient's status.

9. Enter other insured's name and necessary information:
   - Other insured's policy or group number
   - Other insured's birthdate, and check box for male or female
   - Employer's name or school name
   - Insurance plan name or program name (Fill in "none" or N/A, for not applicable, so there is no doubt you have observed this section.)

10. Check the appropriate box regarding employment and accident. (Do not leave all these boxes blank.)

11. Enter insured's policy number and other necessary information:
    - Insured's birthdate, and check box for male or female
    - Employer or school name
    - Insurance plan name or program name
    - Is there another health benefit plan?

12. Obtain patient's or authorized person's signature.

13. Obtain insured signature or stamp "signature on file" if you have the record to prove it.

14. Record the date current illness began.

15. Record the date patient was first treated for same or similar illness.

16. Enter dates unable to work or state N/A.

17. Complete with name of referring physician or state N/A.

17a. Enter ID number of referring physician.

18. Complete with dates of hospitalization or state N/A.

19. Leave blank.

20. Mark appropriate box regarding lab.

21. Enter ICD codes on separate line for each diagnosis.

22. Complete if Medicaid.

23. Complete if applicable with medical authorization code.

24. Complete A through G with appropriate codes for services.
    NOTE: List each service separately with the most important listed first.

25. Add the physician's Social Security number or practice tax identification number and mark the appropriate box.

26. Add patient's account number if applicable.

27. Check one box regarding assignment.
    NOTE: Must be marked "yes" to accept assignment

28. Total charged.

29. Amount paid.

30. Any balance due.
    NOTE: Form will be rejected if not completed.

31. Obtain physician's signature and date.
    NOTE: Medicare will accept stamped signature.

32. Name and address of facility where services were rendered, if other than home or office.

33. Physician's name, address, and telephone number and specific identification numbers for Medicare or other group plan if applicable.

tered on the grid and brought up on the screen for review or printed out so it is possible to see the total file at once.

By looking at the log or the computer file, you can quickly see the status of each claim. If claims become delinquent, a carrier can be easily identified and contacted. As a general rule, claims are paid in a timely fashion after billing, usually within 30 to 60 days. At times, a carrier will deny ever receiving a claim. This is when a copy will be helpful because it will be necessary to refile. When claims are <u>not</u> approved or are rejected because of errors, you will be able to refile upon submitting additional information or documenting the charge. When a claim is returned after being denied, it may not be eligible for refiling.

DELINQUENT CLAIMS

If a claim has not been paid and you have not received a denial, it is time to follow up. Most carriers provide a toll-free telephone number on their claim form. Before you make the call, be sure you have the following information available: patient's name, identification number, group name or number, and if the patient <u>is not</u> the insured, the insured's (spouse's) name. Once the account is identified, they will request the date(s) of service and the total amount submitted. The carrier will then give you the status of the claim. If it is still in process, request an anticipated date of payment. If the claim is delayed pending additional information, be sure to follow up quickly and return the material requested. If the company has no record of receiving a claim, ask if you may submit a <u>copy</u> of the claim previously submitted and verify the mailing address. Also ask if you could direct the claim to a specific person to accelerate the process. It is helpful to have a specific contact person in case further discussion is necessary. If the carrier indicates that the claim has been paid, ask when the payment was made and to whom it was sent. If it was sent to the patient, you will need to send the patient a statement.

COMMON CLAIM ERRORS

In a recent survey of insurance companies, the following common errors were listed as causes of claim payment delays:

1. The patient's—not the policyholder's—Social Security number is used as the certificate number. The claim would be rejected for lack of membership.
2. The "Coordination of Benefits" section is not completed, thereby suspending the claim for additional information.
3. Use of incorrect ICD (International Classification of Diseases) codes.
4. Use of an incorrect or deleted CPT code could result in a decreased payment or a rejection.
5. Use of incorrect provider identification number could result in misdirection of payment.

6. Superbills attached to a claim form are sometimes illegible. Always attach additional information to the back of the claim, in the upper left-hand corner.
7. Member does not respond to the request for clarification of insurances covering injury or illness when another party might have responsibility.
8. Lack of operative report if procedure is unusual, complicated, or fee is unusual.
9. Incorrect spelling of patient's name.
10. Inconsistent use of patient's name; for example, middle name is used as first, nicknames are used instead of correct first name (i.e., Bill instead of William).
11. An incorrect patient birthdate is reported.
12. Use of an incorrect place of service code will suspend a claim.

ELECTRONIC CLAIM FILING

Many offices electronically process claim forms to the insurance carrier. The turn-around time is shortened, and there is a reduction in preparation time. The system does require that you purchase a software program that can be accessed by the carrier. A new service has evolved from this technology. Offices can now enter information and codes in a program and then submit it to an intermediary clearing house service. The service screens the forms for coding errors, returns those needing corrections, and forwards claims to the carrier via whichever program the carrier requires. The cost of the service is considered money well spent because the claims are "clean" when submitted and reimbursement is received within a couple of weeks. A hard copy of the claims is kept on file until electronic processing is completed.

ACCEPTING ASSIGNMENT

Medicare and other carriers enlist physicians to "sign up" as approved or **preferred** providers. Usually, the physician agrees to treat people enrolled in the program for an "agreed" rate for services. This rate is referred to as a **fee schedule**. In return for being willing to participate and accept a reduction in charges, the physician is assured a supply of patients enrolled in the health care program of the provider. Physicians often contract with many carriers in order to be able to provide services for a large group of current as well as future patients. (This concept was covered earlier in this chapter when carriers and managed care were discussed.)

Particularly with Medicare patients, the contracted provider agrees to accept the "approved amount" as their fee and the agreement is known as "accepting assignment." The difference between the amount charged and the fee received is "written off" by the physician as uncollectible. The physician or any other provider can charge the patient only for the part of the deductible that has not been met and the small leftover balance from the approved charge. The provider can also charge for any service <u>not</u> covered by Medicare. If your physician is making a charge for a noncovered service, be certain the patient understands that the charges will be his or her responsibility. It is a good idea to have a statement signed by the patient which states the fee is <u>not</u> covered so that the patient cannot later refuse to pay and claim noncoverage was unknown.

All physicians, whether they choose to participate or not, must abide by Medicare laws. When the doctor does <u>not</u> accept assignment, he must be paid directly by the patient who is responsible for the entire bill, even if it is higher than the Medicare-approved amount. However, even when a doctor does not accept assignment, the most that can be charged is 115% of what Medicare approves. Doctors and other providers who exceed limits can be fined.

MEDICARE AUDIT

The importance of complete records and documentation is never as critical as when the office is involved in a Medicare audit. Audits may be conducted if there is any question as to the amount of service rendered in exchange for the claims paid. Records are essential to provide evidence that diagnoses and treatments were appropriate and that the services paid for were actually provided. The level of service must also be documented. Failure to adequately document the level of service could cause a downcoding by Medicare and can result in the charge of "fraud" with a $2000 fine per infraction. Documentation is essential. Remember: when records are reviewed by third-party payers, "If it is not documented, it was never done." Office staffs should monitor physicians' records and inform them of what is needed if necessary. Not only does it ensure adequate documentation but it also ensures that the physician receives the maximum reimbursement due. Of the following seven items, at least five must be documented in the office medical records:

- Complaints and symptoms
- Duration and course of illness
- Details of illness
- Examination and findings
- Laboratory and x-ray values and findings
- Diagnosis or problem
- Treatment, injection, or advice

REIMBURSEMENT

Remember that Medicare reimburses the approved fee at the rate of 80% after the year's $100 deductible amount has been paid by the patient. Secondary payment is then sought to cover the 20% not covered. Many secondary carriers likewise will pay 80% of the 20% not covered of the approved amount, after the deductible is met. The remaining small percentage and the initial annual deductible is the responsibility of the patient. Figure 9–10 is a summary of the Medicare and secondary insurance "ex-

A CAAHEP CONNECTION

Medical assistants are an integral part of the physician's practice. Being able to communicate effectively with patients, insurance companies, employers, and other medical personnel is extremely important. Just as essential is the knowledge of legal and ethical guidelines to provide for patient's privacy. The accurate coding and filing of insurance forms is essential to prevent any question of improper billing. The necessity for documentation of services cannot be overstated. These factors are part of the risk management strategies involved in the operation of a medical practice and must be addressed in the curriculum of a CAAHEP-approved medical assistant program.

planation of benefits" reports, resulting from an actual minor medical situation, in the approximate order they were received. In this example, the patient is a 65-year-old female who had a suspicious mammogram which resulted in an incisional biopsy of two areas of microcalcification in the same breast. The procedure was performed in the same-day surgery department of a hospital.

The importance of detailed descriptions, procedure codes, and accurate records is very evident. With insurance payment of medical charges, there are several factors to be considered: annual deductibles, approved fee schedules, and percentages of approval rates which all influence the amount paid. Review the summary. Notice how much of the charges are approved and how much is the patient's responsibility. Follow the initial charges through deductibles, Medicare, secondary coverage, sometimes refiling, and finally, the patient's responsibility. This excessive amount of paperwork is a good example of why patients become so confused with insurance coverage and payment, and why medical assistants seem to never finish filing claims.

THE FUTURE OF INSURANCE CLAIMS

As long as there are third-party payers, the filing of some sort of claim will continue. Probably the greatest change will come in how the filing is done. Providers will take advantage of the electronic process. With the capability of computer programs, it is possible to use software that, given a diagnosis, automatically identifies coding, sequences it, and compares it to the treatment codes. An annual update for the software program is required to screen for any changed, added, or deleted codes. This eliminates much of the rejection and refiling problems. A built-in fee by the carriers for the physician's filing expenses would also be a helpful update.

DATE OF FORM	DATE OF SERVICE	SOURCE OF FORM	PROVIDER OF SERVICE	SERVICE PROVIDED—CODE	CHARGE	MEDICARE APPROVED	MEDICARE PAID	SECONDARY INSURANCE PAID	PATIENT RESPONSIBILITY	COMMENTS
1995 10/9	9/27	Medicare	Radiologist #1	Mammogram—7609L XA Both Breasts	$135.00	$65.91	-0-	-0-	$65.91	$65.91 applied to '95 deductible
11/2	10/3	Medicare	Surgeon	Office consult—99242	$105.00	$69.16	$28.06	-0-	$41.10	$34.09 applied to '95 deductible
11/10	10/11	Medicare	Primary physician	Office consult—99243 ECG—93000 Chest x-ray—71020-XA Blood draw—60001-	$130.00 54.00 69.00 7.00 $260.00	$85.85 26.49 32.84 3.00 $148.00	$119.14	-0-	$29.04	$3 chg paid at 100%—$145.00 applied to deductible and co-pay
11/30	10/17	Medicare	Radiologist #2	Place needlewire—19290 X-ray needlewire placement in breast—76096-26 X-ray specimen—76098-26	$175.00 133.50 20.50 $329.00	$69.93 29.21 8.08 $107.22	$85.77	-0-	$21.45	1995 deductible met
11/30	10/17	Medicare	Surgeon	Excision breast lesion—19125	$800.00	$348.16	$278.53	-0-	$69.63	—
11/20	10/17	Medicare	Anesthesia-#1	4.3 Anesthesia—00400—Chest skin surgery QKQS	$350.40	-0-	-0-	-0-	-0-	Requested information had not been received.
11/20	10/17	Medicare	Pathologist	1 Tissue exam—88305-26 1 Tissue exam—88307-26 1 Consult in surgery—88329	$165.00 230.00 70.00 $465.00	$50.35 86.47 38.52 $175.34	$140.28	-0-	$35.06	Deductible met Other insurance may pay
11/20	10/17	Medicare	Anesthesia-#2	4.3 Anesthesia—00400 QKQS Chest skin surgery	$111.25	-0-	-0-	-0-	$111.25	Charges denied, other insurance may pay
12/2	10/11	Insurance	Primary physician	Medical x-ray, testing	$260.00	$148.00	$119.14	$23.24	$5.80	Deductible met
12/14	10/3	Insurance	Surgeon	Medical	$105.00	$69.16	$28.06	$32.88	$8.22	—
12/15	10/17	Medicare	Hospital	Laboratory Radiology Pharmacy Surgical service	$155.00 399.00 182.88 2317.92 $3,054.80	$1,527.40	$916.44	-0-	$610.96	Deductible met
1996 1/5	10/3 and 10/17	Statement	Surgeon	Balance after insurance payments	$110.73	—	—	$32.88	$77.85	Remaining balance due
1/16	10/11	Statement	Primary physician	Balance after insurance payments	$260.00	$148.00	$119.14	$23.24	$5.80	Remaining balance due
1/27	10/17	Insurance	Hospital	Surgical services	$3,054.80	$1,527.40	$916.44	$610.96	-0-	Paid in full by insurance
2/12	10/17	Statement	Radiologist #2	X-ray services balance after insurance payments	$329.00	$107.22	$85.77	-0-	$21.45	Balance due
1/26	10/17	Insurance	Radiologist #2	X-ray services balance after insurance payments	$329.00	$107.22	$85.77	$17.16	$4.29	Remaining balance due

FIGURE 9–10 Summary of insurance explanation of benefits form and medical statements received in connection with one routine breast incisional biopsy procedure

MAINTAINING CURRENCY

Staying informed and up-to-date with Medicare is a never-ending process. Ideally, in each practice someone is designated the claims filer and is expected to maintain currency. This can be done in various ways. Medicare updates are discussed in bulletins sent monthly to the practice. Many practice specialty organizations will have newsletters, specific to their needs, to keep members informed. Other insurance carriers will send newsletters to their participating physicians describing any changes in their coverage or processing.

Seminars are conducted frequently. The annual major update seminar sponsored by your state medical association is practically a requirement in order for any practice to survive. Other seminars are conducted by private companies and can prove very informative. The content, of

Medical-Legal-Ethical Scenario

Maria was employed by Dr. Grey six months ago to process all insurance-related business. She had two years of experience with another physician and has attended updating seminars sponsored by her medical assistant association. Accepting the position with Dr. Grey seemed almost too good to be true. She is allowed to work a flexible, hourly schedule, which helps her manage her responsibilities as a single parent of two children. In addition, she was able to increase her salary and will be eligible to participate in the practice's profit-sharing plan after one year. She enjoys working with the three other office employees and often receives praise from them and the physician for her management of the insurance affairs.

About three months ago, Maria began to wonder about some charges listed on occasional encounter forms but dismissed the thought. Lately however, after more careful observation, she is almost certain the doctor is identifying charges that are not actually being done. For instance, he listed two hospital visits she is almost certain he did not make. She can also think of at least four instances last week when an office urinalysis was charged and not done. And 2 weeks ago, she knew an ECG was falsely charged. Subtler charge irregularities involved the listing of some office visits as comprehensive when in reality they were only focused. She was certain this occurred this week with Mrs. Lopez and Mr. Lee because neither one of them was in the office more than 10 minutes each. She likes her job very much and knows she is considered a valued employee, but she is concerned about this issue.

CRITICAL THINKING CHALLENGE

1. What should Maria do?
2. Is she liable for filing fraudulent insurance claims when in reality she just enters what the physician has indicated?
3. There is a phone number to report Medicare fraud (800-477-8477). Should she call and report her suspicion?
4. What do you think would be the ramifications if she approaches the physician with her observations?
5. Because this position is so perfect for her and she is paid well, should she just overlook the occasional irregularities? After all, physicians are only allowed to charge so much for services, and they need to add on a little to help make up the difference.
6. Do you think it is possible that the physician realizes her personal situation and might take advantage of her loyalty?
7. Look at the Medical Assistant Role Delineation Study under Administrative Procedures, Professionalism, and Legal Concepts to find related areas of practice dealing with this situation.

course, depends upon the amount of time and the expertise or focus of the presenting organization.

It is very important that you closely review any inservice advertisement. It should identify the content, perhaps include an outline, and if objectives are listed, give you a good idea of expected outcomes. Another assurance of its value is the approval for CEUs by the AAMA or the ARMA. If not preapproved, however, remember that you can submit information and request CEUs for educational seminars you attend, but approval is not ensured. Make certain you understand what is being offered and to what extent it will be presented so that your investment of time and money will be worthwhile.

ACHIEVE UNIT OBJECTIVES

Complete Chapter 9, Unit 3, in the workbook to help you obtain competency of this subject matter.

RESOURCES

American Medical Association. (2000). Current procedural terminology, CPT™ 2001 standard edition. Chicago, IL: Author.

Medicode (2001). Physician ICD-9-CM volumes 1 & 2. Los Angeles, CA: Practice Management Information Corp.

Mosio, M.A. (2001). A guide to health insurance billing. Clifton Park, NY: Delmar Learning.

Rowell, J., and Green, M.A. (2002) Understanding health insurance (6th ed.). Clifton Park, NY: Delmar Learning.

Thompson, T.G. (2001, June 22). Renaming and restructuring of Health Care Financing Administration (HCFA) to Centers for Medicare and Medicaid Services (CMMS) (Press Release). Washington, DC: U.S. Department of Health and Human Services.

WEB LINKS

http://www.ama-assn.org/cpt (American Medical Association)

Provides information on CPT coding.

http://www.cms.hhs.gov (Centers for Medicare and Medicaid Services— formerly the Health Care Financing Administration [HCFA])

Provides information on Medicare and Medicaid programs and services.

Medical Office Management

Many different methods are used to affect the overall management of the medical office. A one- or two-physician office that employs only a few people could assign someone to deal with all the office management duties. Most physicians find that a professional accounting firm or professional management company is best suited for the preparation of tax forms and financial statements and maintenance of salary records. Medical assistants with adequate office experience and management abilities are often selected to be the office manager. However, large group practices, clinics, and physician corporations with several physicians and many employees may choose an individual with a business background or degree in business to be the office manager or elect to use a professional management service, in addition to an accountant.

It would be impossible to include specific management instructions in this text to cover all variables because individual physician preference results in a wide array of possibilities. Therefore, this chapter discusses the general administrative duties and responsibilities of the medical assistant and also includes information regarding the role of an office manager. Regardless of who is serving as manager, you should be aware of the records the accountants will need. You will probably be responsible for maintaining certain financial and tax records.

The physician places great confidence in a manager to efficiently and accurately handle the business affairs of the office. The following units outline the skills and duties related to the fiscal and physical operation of a medical office and include such topics as:

- Processing received payments for banking
- Preparing checks for office expenses
- Maintaining office accounting records
- Maintaining employer records
- Maintaining office equipment
- Obtaining essential reference materials
- Attending office management update seminars

UNIT 1

The Language of Banking

OBJECTIVES

Upon completion of the unit, meet the following performance objectives by verifying knowledge of the facts and principles presented through oral and written communication at a level deemed competent.

1. Spell and define, using the glossary at the back of the text, all the **Words to Know** in this unit.
2. Differentiate between savings and checking accounts.
3. Explain the significance of the ABA and MICR codes.
4. Define the banking terms listed in this unit.
5. Differentiate among cashier's, certified, limited, postdated, stale, traveler's, and voucher checks.
6. Explain the difference between overdraft and overdrawn.
7. Explain the "stop payment" process.

AREAS OF COMPETENCE (AAMA)

This unit addresses content within the area of *Practice finances* as identified in the Medical Assistant Role Delineation Study. Refer to Appendix A for a detailed listing of the area.

WORDS TO KNOW

agent	negotiable
certified	overdraft
collateral	payee
currency	power of attorney
debit	promissory
deposit	transaction
endorsement	voucher
insufficient	warrant
limited check	withdrawal

This unit presents the most common banking terms and their definitions to help you understand financial transactions. The medical assistant must have a good working knowledge of banking and basic accounting procedures. These skills are not only important in the physician's office but also in the management of your own personal finances.

BANKING TERMS

(A) **Billing and Collections:**
  - Checkbook

- *American Bankers Association (ABA) number.* A code number found in the right upper corner of a printed check. It may be above the check number on a business check or below the check number on a personal check.

- *Agent.* An agent is a person authorized to act for another person. You are the agent for your employer in the office. Bank officials are agents for the bank.

- *ATM.* An automated teller machine (ATM) is a banking machine operated by inserting a credit or bank card and entering a personal identification number (PIN) code. Deposits, transfers, withdrawals, and other banking functions can be performed at the ATM location.

- *Bankbook.* In the case of a savings account it is called a savings passbook and contains a record of deposits, withdrawals, and interest earned, with the dates of all the transactions. This book must be presented with each deposit or withdrawal. At regular intervals, usually quarterly, interest earnings are credited to an account. These earnings should be entered in the passbook by the bank. Some banks indicate the passbook should be presented for interest entry at least once in a three-year period.

- *Bank statement.* A record of a checking account sent to the customer, usually on a monthly basis, showing the beginning balance, all deposits made, all checks drawn, all bank charges, and the closing balance. The customer's canceled checks are returned with the statement.

- *Cashier's check.* The purchaser pays the bank the full amount of the check. The bank then writes a check on its own account payable to the party specified. This type of check "guarantees" the recipient that the full amount of money indicated on the check will be paid on processing.

- *Certified check.* The bank stamps the customer's own check *certified* and then holds the certified amount in reserve in the customer's account until the check is cashed. This is a guaranteed check and so is always acceptable when a personal check is not.

- *Check register.* Also referred to as a check stub. It is a record showing the check number, person to whom check is paid, and amount of check, date, and balance. It is kept by the person writing the check as a record of the transaction.

- *Checking account.* A bank account against which checks may be written. The bank will issue the checks and deposit slips.

- *Currency.* Paper money issued by the government.

- *Debit.* An entry in an account of an amount owed that has been charged to the account.

- *Debit card.* A card similar to a credit card that withdraws money from the account to pay for the debit. Another type of debit card is used specifically to make purchases, in effect replacing a check. These are called check cards.

- *Deposit.* An amount of money (cash and/or checks) placed in a bank account.

- *Deposit record.* A record of a deposit that is given to the customer at the time of the deposit. It is important to keep the deposit record as proof of the deposit in case the bank fails to list the deposit on the bank statement.

- *Deposit slip.* An itemized list of cash and checks deposited in a checking account. It is important to keep a copy of all deposit slips.
- *Direct deposit.* When an amount is sent electronically by the payer directly into a savings or checking account of the payee.
- *Electronic fund transfer systems.* Methods of crediting or debiting accounts by computer without checks or deposit slips.
- *Endorsement.* The payee's signature on the back of a check. It is a transfer of title on the check to the bank in exchange for the amount of money on the face of the check.
- *Endorser.* The payee on a check. If the name is spelled incorrectly on the face of the check, it should be endorsed in the same way and then endorsed correctly.
- *Insufficient funds.* A bank term used to indicate that the writer of the check did not have enough money in the account to cover the check. An office usually has a policy regarding returned checks, which normally involves contacting the patient immediately and asking the person to pick up the check and bring a cash payment. These checks are sometimes described as *bounced,* and the account is called *overdrawn.*
- *Limited check.* A check that will be marked void if written over a certain amount. These checks are often used for payroll or for insurance payments. A check may also list a time limit during which it must be cashed. It must be cashed within the time limit or you will find it is not **negotiable**.
- *Maker.* The individual who signs a check or the corporation that pays it.
- *Magnetic ink character recognition (MICR).* This technique consists of characters and numbers printed in magnetic ink at the bottom left side of checks and deposit slips (Figures 10–1 and 10–2).
- *Money order.* Negotiable instrument often used by individuals who do not have checking accounts or to meet the requirement for purchasing an item or service. Money orders may be purchased for a fee from banks, credit unions, post offices, and many other money order service locations.
- *Negotiable.* Refers to the fact that something is able to be transferred or exchanged. On a check the words "Pay to the order of" are considered to make the check negotiable. In other words, the amount written can be transferred from the account of the payer to the payee.
- *Note.* Legal evidence of a debt. A **promissory** note is a written promise to pay. A **collateral** note is a written promise to pay with the additional requirement that the maker of the note must list marketable securities that may be sold by the creditor if the maker does not pay the note within the time limit promised.
- *One-write check writing.* System that makes it possible to make a record on a check register as you write a check. This is excellent for payroll because you can record deductions for the employee and office records in one writing.
- *Online banking.* Banking on the bank's Internet web site is called online banking. It is possible to check account information, transfer money, and pay bills over the Internet.
- *Overdraft checking accounts.* Accounts that allow checks to be written for a larger amount than is currently in the account. The **overdraft** is covered by the bank in the form of a loan for which interest is charged.

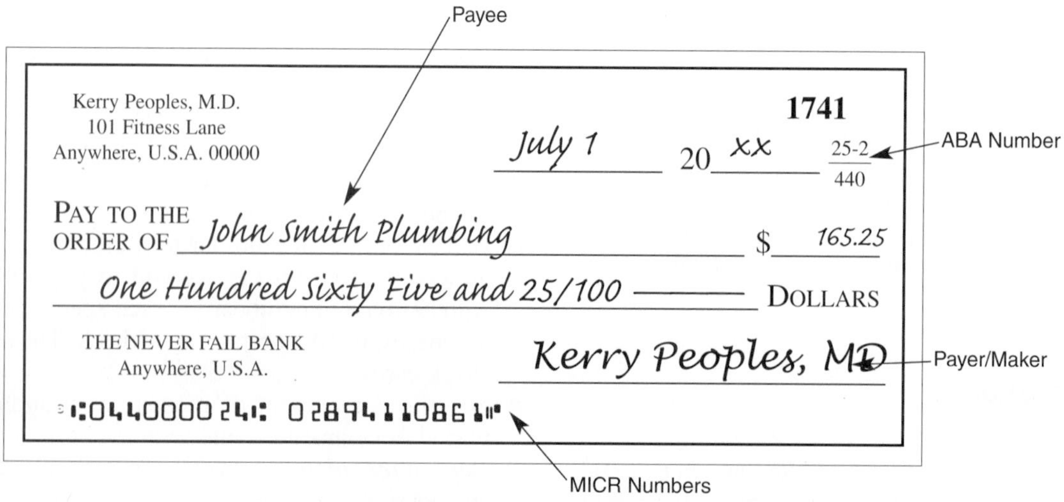

FIGURE 10-1 Check with MICR numbers

money while the patient watches to be certain it is correct. Enter the payment as cash on the ledger card, encounter form, walk-out statement, financial software, or other form of recording payment used. Prepare a written or computer-generated receipt as evidence of the cash payment.

The presence of cash in the office also presents another area of concern. Because currency and coin are instantly expendable, care must be taken to keep it secured. All cash money should be placed out of sight as soon as received, in a cash box, file drawer, or some other secure location. Care should be taken that your *place* is not in view of patients in the reception area. Usually, all daily proceeds are either locked in a safe or deposited at the close of the day.

FEATURES OF A CHECK

Checks have a long history. The first recorded use of a check was in 1374. They were rare before 1700 but became common after World War II. It is believed about 63 billion checks are processed in the United States every year, and that number is growing. With this great amount it is understandable why coding to make machine processing possible and electronic transfer of funds are increasingly necessary. With this increase in checks also comes the increase in the number of bad checks and fraud.

There are seven features you must examine to ensure a check is valid. You should question any missing or contradicting feature (Figure 10–3):

1. The date: Watch for a stale date (six months or older), a postdate (a future date), or a preprinted date requirement such as *void after 60 days*. A check with these features is not valid before or after a specific period of time.
2. Words of *negotiability*: A check must say "Pay to the order of" or "Pay to the bearer" to be negotiable.

3. The payee: The check must identify to whom the check is written. In the office, this will be the physician who receives checks as payment for care provided. A payee can also be a person or company that has rendered the practice a service for which a check is written.
4. The numeric amount: This is the amount in numbers that the check is written for.
5. The written amount: This is the amount written in words. It must agree with the numeric amount.
6. The drawee financial institition: This identifies where the check is payable. Checks issued by the government, traveler's checks, corporate checks, and money orders do *not* have a drawee institution printed on them because they are the drawee.
7. The signature: The signature is usually handwritten but can also be a reproduced facsimile.

There are five other features that banks have instituted to guard against fraud, but they are not necessary for validity. If they are missing, it is best to scrutinize the check very carefully.

1. The name and address of the maker: This is usually preprinted by the check printer.
2. A chronologic check number: This is printed at the right upper corner of the check.
3. The check routing symbol (ABA number): It is in fractional form and identifies the institution involved in the clearing process. This number was originated by the American Bankers Association. The purpose is to have a method of identifying the area where the bank on which the check is written is located, and to identify the bank within the area. It may be written as a fraction: $\frac{51-44}{119}$ on a business check, or 25-2/440 on a personal check.
4. Magnetic ink character recognition (MICR) numbers: These are numbers that aid in the clearing process.

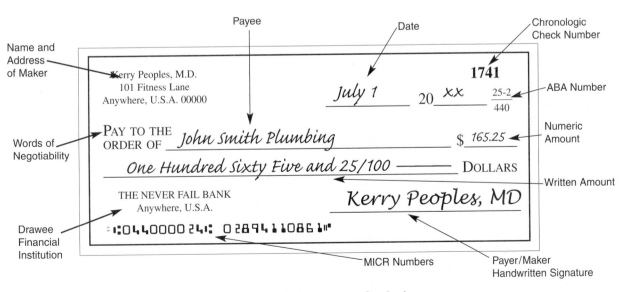

FIGURE 10-3 Features of a check

The numbers are printed with special magnetic ink and identify the Federal Reserve district and branch, the drawee financial institution, the maker's account number, and usually the check number. This information is specific to each checking account and is imprinted on each check and deposit slip by the company printing the checks. The first series of numbers is the routing information that identifies the bank and area. The second series identifies the account numbers. The last series corresponds to the check number. When the bank processes the check, additional magnetic ink numbers are printed across the bottom identifying the amount of the check. These characters and numbers can be read by high-speed machinery, which greatly enhances the bookkeeping procedures in the bank by simplifying the sorting of checks and the printing of individual monthly statements.

5. One rough or perforated edge: This is where the check is separated from a book or sheet of checks. This will not be found in government or traveler's checks.

1741 $ *165.25*

Date: *July* 20 *xx*

To: *John Smith Plumbing*

For: *Repair faucet leak*

Balance Forward	$ *8,645.89*
Deposits	—
Total	$ *8,645.89*
This Check	$ *165.25*
Balance Forward	$ *8,480.64*

FIGURE 10–4 Check stub

WRITING CHECKS

Billing and Collections:
- Checkbook

The medical assistant may often be required to write checks to pay for equipment, supplies, or wages. These are then given to the physician for signature before being mailed or otherwise distributed. Some physicians will give check-signature power to an office manager to eliminate the need for their personal signature. A signature **authorization** card obtained from the bank must be completed to allow someone other than the recorded owner of the account to execute checks. Some offices, as a means of monitoring expenditures and preventing employee embezzlement, require two signatures on a check or have a policy that the individual writing the check (e.g., bookkeeper) must have another authorized person (often the office manager) sign the check. This also provides an opportunity to question expenditures and maintain a sense of cash flow. Complete the check stub when the check is written in order to maintain a record of expenses and deposits as well as the current balance (Figure 10–4). Practice preparing checks by following Procedure 10–1, completing the exercises on the Administrative Skills CD in the back of the text, and using the workbook samples.

One area of expenditure that must be carefully monitored is payment of invoices for office equipment and supplies. When a statement is received from a supplier, it is essential to know that everything on the invoice and the amount or number of each item has in fact been received. The shipment must be compared to packing slips or invoices at the time it is received and notification of any discrepancy made to the supplier. Frequently, partial shipments are sent and some items are on back order. Payment of the total amount of the invoice would represent payment for goods not received. Some difficulty may also arise in trying to obtain materials not sent once you have paid in full for the shipment. The provider assumes everything was shipped as stated on the invoice because no questions were raised when the shipment was received.

If a mistake is made in writing a check, it is necessary to write "**VOID**" across the check and stub and write another check.

CHECKS RECEIVED FROM PATIENTS

The medical assistant should take certain precautions when accepting checks from patients:

- Be sure the check has the seven features that make a check valid and that no corrections have been made.
- Do not accept a **third-party** check unless the check is from an insurance company. A third-party check is generally one made out to the patient by someone unknown to you. Because you do not know how creditworthy the check writer is or have any personal information about the individual, it is unwise to accept a third-party check that person has written.
- You might have patients who want to write a check for more than the amount due so they can have some cash in hand. This is generally not a good policy, and it would be advisable to refuse such a check. When you accept the check as payment and give out an additional amount in office cash, you risk the check not being honored by the bank. Your office will lose not only the amount owed by the patient, but also will lose the cash given out.

P R O C E D U R E

10-1 Prepare a Check

PURPOSE: Accurately prepare a check and stub.

EQUIPMENT: Checkbook, pen with black or blue ink, computer and computer checks, or typewriter.

PERFORMANCE OBJECTIVE: In a simulated medical office situation, prepare a check and stub following the steps of the procedure. The check must be without error and contain the five essential factors, and the stub must be completed accurately within the time established by the instructor.

Note: The check must:
- Be dated
- Identify the payee
- Have the correct numeric amount
- Have the correct written amount
- Have appropriate signature

The stub must:
- Be completed before writing the check
- Be completed in black or blue ink or with computer
- Have check number entered if not preprinted
- Be dated
- Identify payee
- List amount of check
- Have balance from previous stub
- Have any deposit added to the balance
- Have new balance entered

1. Complete check stub
2. Enter the date on check.
3. Enter the name of the payee on check.
4. Enter numerically the amount of the check. **NOTE: Keep numbers close to the dollar sign so other numbers cannot be inserted to change the amount of the check.**
5. Write out the amount of the check in words beginning as far to the left as possible.
   NOTE:
   - **After writing the amount, fill in remaining space with a line to prevent insertion of words that would increase the amount.**
   - **All amounts are written in terms of dollars and fractions of dollars. A check for $10 is written "Ten and no hundredths (no/100)." A check for $12.65 is written "Twelve and sixty-five hundredths (65/100)."**
   - **When writing a check for less than a dollar, write the word "Only" and then the amount. ("Only ninety-five hundredths [95/100].")**
6. The check should be signed with the same signature(s) used on the authorization card when the checking account was opened.

- Do not accept a check marked "paid in full" or "payment in full" unless it does pay the account in full, including charges incurred on the day the check is written. If there is still a balance, you will be unable to collect if you accept and deposit such a check. People often write "paid in full" or "payment in full" on the memo line on the front of a check. Be sure to check this line because it is easy to overlook. When you receive a check, stamp it with the deposit endorsement (see below) to protect against theft.
- Do not accept a postal money order with more than one endorsement because two is the limit honored.

ENDORSEMENT

Ⓐ **Billing and Collections:**
- Checkbook

An endorsement is a signature or a signature plus other information on the back of a check. The endorsement of a check transfers all rights in the check to another party. Endorsements should always be made in ink and may be made with a pen or rubber stamp. The end of the check to be endorsed can be identified by holding the check on the right end as you look at it, turning it over, and endorsing the opposite or left end. All checks received in the office, whether in person or through the mail, should be protected by endorsement at the time received.

The two kinds of endorsement commonly used are blank endorsement and restrictive endorsement. A *blank endorsement* is a signature only. It should not be used until the check is to be cashed, because if the check is stolen with such an endorsement, someone else could endorse the check below your name and cash the check. A *restrictive endorsement* is used to endorse checks when they are received. It is a stamp or written information that states, "PAY TO THE ORDER OF (name of bank where check is to be deposited)" followed by the name of the physician. If such a check is stolen it could not be used in any way.

ENDORSE HERE:

X_____ *Your name* _____

_____

_____

DO NOT SIGN / WRITE / STAMP BELOW
THIS LINE, FOR FINANCIAL USE ONLY*

----

*FEDERAL RESERVE BANK REGULATION CC

FIGURE 10–5 Proper placement of signature endorsement

If the name of the payee is misspelled, it should be endorsed the same way followed by the correct signature directly below.

Effective September 1, 1988, federal regulations required all endorsements to be within 1½″ of the "trailing edge" of all checks. Checks on which the endorsement extends beyond the 1½″ area may be refused by the financial institutions for improper endorsement. To avoid processing delays, be sure to endorse all checks as described (Figure 10–5).

MAKING DEPOSITS

Ⓐ **Billing and Collections:**
  ▪ Checkbook

The medical assistant is also expected to deposit cash and checks received in the office. This may be a daily task or it may be as infrequent as once a week for a physician with a limited practice. Deposits should be prepared in a secure place out of people's view. Currency should be sorted with all bills of the same denomination placed together, facing the same directcion, with the portrait side up. Place in order from the highest to the lowest denomination (for example, 50s, 20s, 10s, 5s, and 1s). count the bills and enter the total amount on the currency line of the deposit slip (see Figure 10–2). Next, count the coins (if any) and enter the total on the coin line. If there is a large amount of coin, it should be placed in wrappers. Check to be sure all the checks have been endorsed. Arrange them facing up from the largest amount to the least. List checks by number, last name of maker, and amount on deposit slip or other form. Attach deposit slip to a computer-generated list or other listing of checks. Total the amount of the checks and enter on the slip. To avoid errors, total the actual checks and compare with the total listed amount. Total the deposits and enter amount on deposit slip. Make a copy of both sides of a deposit slip in case any question about the deposit should arise. When the deposit slip is finished, enter the amount in the checkbook and add it to the existing balance, enter it on the daily log sheet, or post it on the appropriate computer screen. Deposit slips (Procedure 10-2) are imprinted with the account number in MICR numbers that match those on the checks. These numbers make it possible for checks and deposit slips to be sorted and recorded by computer. Banks will accept a list of deposited items on something other than the bank-provided deposit slip as long as the bank deposit slip is attached (see Figure 10–2, p. 241).

Deposits are usually placed in a zippered bank bag to be taken to the bank. They can be taken inside and given to a teller or deposited in the night depository. Care should always be taken when transporting money. Be aware of your surroundings and do not put yourself in a questionable situation. If there is any chance you are being watched, do not leave your car. It probably is a good idea to vary the deposit day and time if possible so you do not become predictable.

DEPOSIT BY MAIL

Checks may be deposited by mail. You should avoid sending cash or currency by mail, but if you must, then send it registered. The deposit slip and money are prepared as for any deposit. The checks should be endorsed by restrictive endorsement only. If no stamp is available, the handwritten notation "for deposit only to the account of (name of your employer)" will suffice. You should request a receipt, as this record is necessary to prove a deposit was made. It is extremely important that you have an accurate record of all checks deposited with the check number, whom the check is from, and the amount of check so that you can follow up if necessary. It is a good idea to neatly arrange the checks on the photocopier glass and then photocopy them. If checks become lost in the mail, it will be necessary to notify all payees to stop payment and issue you new checks.

PROCEDURE

10-2 Prepare a Deposit Slip

PURPOSE: Accurately prepare a deposit slip.

EQUIPMENT: Deposit slip, pen with black or blue ink or typewriter, cash and/or checks to be deposited.

PERFORMANCE OBJECTIVE: Prepare a bank deposit slip, following the steps in the procedure. All cash, checks, and coin must be entered without error and the deposit accurately totaled within the time established by the instructor.

1. Separate money to be deposited by check, currency, and coin.
2. Total currency and record on deposit slip.
3. Record the total amount of coins on the slip.

4. List checks by number, name of maker, and amount. **NOTE: Money orders are listed as money order and name or MO and name.**
5. Total all checks listed on back and enter total.
6. Total currency, coin, and checks and enter on slip.
7. Make a copy of deposit slip for your office files.
8. Enter deposit total in checkbook.
9. Deposit at bank. **NOTE: Be sure you receive a record of deposit either personally or by mail if you make a mail or night deposit. This record is necessary to prove a deposit was made if the bank fails to give credit for it on the monthly statement.**

RECONCILING BANK STATEMENTS

An important part of banking is the reconciliation each month of the bank statement with the office records. You need to be sure that you and the bank agree as to the amount of money in the account. You will receive a statement that shows all banking transactions concerning the account along with the checks which the bank has received and processed. Most statements contain a section similar to Figure 10–6 that allows you to list outstanding checks and do other calculations to reconcile the amounts. Follow Procedure 10–3 and workbook exercises to practice reconciling a bank statement.

PETTY CASH AND OTHER ACCOUNTS

Since it is not reasonable to write checks for small office transactions, most physicians have a petty cash fund. The physician will determine the amount of the fund and for what it will be used. The fund is established by writing a check payable to "cash" or "petty cash." The check is then cashed and the money kept in a locked cash box. (All patient payments should be kept in a separate money box.) The money is often used for postage due letters, inexpensive office supplies, and small charitable donations.

A **voucher** form or expenditure list should be completed each time payment is made from this fund. When the amount in the fund is nearly **depleted**, another check is written for the difference between the original fund and the amount remaining. The expense records

RECONCILING THE BANK STATEMENT

Bank Statement Balance $_____

Less Outstanding Checks

#_____ $_____

#_____ $_____

#_____ $_____

#_____ $_____

#_____ $_____

#_____ $_____

#_____ $_____

Total _____ $_____

Plus deposits not shown $_____

CORRECTED BANK STATEMENT $_____

Checkbook balance $_____

Less bank charges $_____

CORRECTED CHECKBOOK BALANCE $_____

FIGURE 10–6 Reconciliation form

PROCEDURE

10-3 Reconcile a Bank Statement

PURPOSE: Accurately reconcile a bank statement.

EQUIPMENT: Bank statement and canceled checks, reconciliation worksheet, pen or pencil, calculator or adding machine.

PERFORMANCE OBJECTIVE: Given all necessary equipment, follow the procedure steps to reconcile a bank statement so that the checkbook balance equals the bank statement balance.

1. Compare the opening balance on the new statement with the closing balance on the previous statement. **NOTE: If they do not agree, contact the bank.**

2. List the bank balance in the appropriate space on the reconciliation worksheet.

3. Compare the check entries on the statement with the returned checks. **NOTE: The bank may have your checks in numeric order; if not, you should place them in order.**

4. Determine if you have any outstanding checks.
   NOTE:
   - An outstanding check is one you have written that does not appear on your bank statement and has not been returned by the bank.
   - Put a check mark on each check stub or register entry that matches an entry on your statement.

   - Any stub or entry not checked indicates an outstanding check, which you list on your worksheet in the column provided.
   - Total the outstanding checks.

5. Subtract from your checkbook balance items such as withdrawals, automatic payments, or service charges that appear on the statement but not in the checkbook. **NOTE: These items are indicated by a code such as *AP* for automatic payment or *SC* for service charge.**

6. Add to your checkbook balance any interest earned as indicated on your statement. **NOTE: Some banks pay interest if a specified minimum amount is maintained in the account.**

7. Add to the bank statement balance any deposits not shown on the bank statement (e.g., deposited since statement prepared).

8. The balance in your checkbook and the bank statement should agree. **NOTE: If they do not agree, subtract the lesser figure from the greater for a possible clue to the error and recheck all figures.**

DATE	DESCRIPTION	VOUCHER NUMBER	TOTAL AMOUNT	OFFICE EXPENSE	DONA- TIONS	MISC.	BALANCE
10/1	Fund established						25.00
10/5	Postage due	1	.40	.40			24.60
10/8	Parking fee	2	1.60			1.60	23.00
10/10	Coffee	3	2.98				20.02

FIGURE 10–7 Petty cash form

are kept in a file to verify the use of the petty cash fund. Figure 10–7 shows a petty cash fund ledger form to monitor expenditures.

ACHIEVE UNIT OBJECTIVES

Complete Chapter 10, Unit 2, in the workbook to help you obtain competency of this subject matter.

UNIT 3
Salary, Benefits, and Tax Records

OBJECTIVES

Upon completion of the unit, meet the following performance objectives by verifying knowledge of the facts and principles presented through oral and written communication at a level deemed competent.

1. Spell and define, using the glossary at the back of the text, all the **Words to Know** in this unit.
2. Explain the W-4, W-2, and I-9 forms.
3. Identify eight items that may be needed for payroll records and a personnel file.
4. Differentiate between hourly wage and a salary.
5. Identify the information required for payroll records.
6. List the four factors that affect the amount of federal tax withheld.
7. Differentiate between gross and net salary.
8. Describe salary benefits, identifying six examples.

▮ WORDS TO KNOW

accountant	gross
benefits	Internal Revenue Service
bereavement time	longevity
complimentary	net
deductions	productivity
disability	profit sharing
exemption	unemployment
fringe benefits	vested

EMPLOYEE REQUIREMENTS AND RECORDS

Ⓐ Finance:
- Payroll Forms

All employees in a physician's office must have a Social Security number. This is a nine-digit number which is obtained from the Social Security Administration. Forms to apply for a Social Security number can be obtained from local Social Security office, **Internal Revenue Service** office, and post offices. Each employee must also complete an Employee's Withholding Exemption Certificate (W-4 form) indicating the number of **exemptions** claimed (Figure 10–8). Any employee who fails to complete a W-4 form will have withholding figured on the basis of being single with no exemptions. A new W-4 form must be completed if there is a change in marital status or a change in the number of exemptions.

Recent federal legislation requires employees to complete an Employment Eligibility Verification Form I-9. The form is issued by the Department of Justice, Immigration and Naturalization Service. Its purpose is to ensure all persons employed are either United States citizens, lawfully admitted aliens, or aliens authorized to work in the United States. By law, this form must be completed before an individual can be officially hired. **Accountants** will not permit salary to be paid to individuals who do not have a form I-9 on file.

In addition to these federal requirements, forms must also be processed for state and local tax records. Local government tax is paid to the city where employment occurs regardless of where the employee lives.

All employees should have the following documents or information available when filling out initial payroll forms:

- Driver's license or other state picture identification
- Social Security card and a copy of Social Security numbers of all dependents

- If not a United States citizen, a green card or equivalent

Other documentation needed for your personnel file include:

- Immunization record
- Copies of any professional license, registration, or certification
- Evidence of pertinent diplomas degrees or certificates
- Evidence of professional liability insurance (if applicable)
- Verification of Occupational Safety and Health Administration/Clinical Laboratory Improvement Amendments (OSHA/CLIA) training

MEDICAL OFFICE REQUIREMENTS AND RECORDS

The physician's office must have a federal tax reporting number, which is obtained from the Internal Revenue Service. In states that require employer reports, a state employer number must also be obtained.

When payroll checks are prepared, a record must be kept showing Social Security, federal taxes, any state and city taxes, and insurance amounts deducted from earnings. Employees may be paid an hourly wage or a salary (a fixed amount paid on a regular basis for a prescribed period of time). The Federal Fair Labor Standards Act regulates the minimum wage and requires that overtime be paid to hourly wage earners at a minimum rate of one and one-half times the regular rate for hours over and above 40 hours per week. It is necessary to keep records of hours worked, total pay, and all **deductions** withheld for all employees.

All employees are expected to work the assigned number of hours per day, week and month. Any time off must be reconciled on the payroll records and the salary adjusted according to office policy.

Several office supply businesses furnish forms for payroll record keeping. There should be a page for each employee's payroll record. The heading should give the name, address, telephone, Social Security number, and date of employment. In columns there should be a record of date of check, hours worked (regular and overtime), **gross** salary, and individual deductions (including federal income tax, Social Security tax, and any state and local taxes). There might also be deductions for insurances or uniforms. The final column should show the amount of **net** pay; that is, the actual amount of the paycheck after deductions. When an accountant or management firm is employed to prepare payroll, office records must be given to them by a designated date(s) each month in order that payroll can be prepared and records maintained.

The amount of federal tax withheld is based on the amount earned, marital status, numbers of exemptions claimed, and length of the pay period. The Internal Revenue Service will provide the charts used to figure deductions for federal income tax and Society Security tax. State and local taxes are usually a percentage of gross

20XX Form W-4

**Department of the Treasury
Internal Revenue Service**

Purpose. Complete Form W-4 so that your employer can withhold the correct amount of Federal income tax from your pay.

Exemption From Withholding. Read line 7 of the certificate below to see if you can claim exempt status. *If exempt, complete line 7; but do not complete lines 5 and 6.* No Federal income tax will be withheld from your pay. Your exemption is good for one year only. It expires February 15, 1993.

Basic Instructions. Employees who are not exempt should complete the Personal Allowances Worksheet. Additional worksheets are provided on page 2 for employees to adjust their withholding allowances based on itemized deductions, adjustments to income, or two-earner/two-job situations. Complete all worksheets that apply to your situation. The worksheets will help you figure

the number of withholding allowances you are entitled to claim. However, you may claim fewer allowances than this.

Head of Household. Generally, you may claim head of household filing status on your tax return only if you are unmarried and pay more than 50% of the costs of keeping up a home for yourself and your dependent(s) or other qualifying individuals.

Nonwage Income. If you have a large amount of nonwage income, such as interest or dividends, you should consider making estimated tax payments using Form 1040-ES. Otherwise, you may find that you owe additional tax at the end of the year.

Two-Earner/Two-Jobs. If you have a working spouse or more than one job, figure the total number of allowances you are entitled to claim on all jobs using worksheets from only one Form

W-4. This total should be divided among all jobs. Your withholding will usually be most accurate when all allowances are claimed on the W-4 filed for the highest paying job and zero allowances are claimed for the others.

Advance Earned Income Credit. If you are eligible for this credit, you can receive it added to your paycheck throughout the year. For details, get Form W-5 from your employer.

Check Your Withholding. After your W-4 takes effect, you can use **Pub. 919,** Is My Withholding Correct for 1992?, to see how the dollar amount you are having withheld compares to your estimated total annual tax. Call 1-800-829-3676 to order this publication. Check your local telephone directory for the IRS assistance number if you need further help.

Personal Allowances Worksheet

For 20XX, the value of your personal exemption(s) is reduced if your income is over $105,250 ($157,900 if married filing jointly, $131,550 if head of household, or $78,950 if married filing separately). Get Pub. 919 for details.

A   Enter "1" for **yourself** if no one else can claim you as a dependent . . . .   **A** _____

B   Enter "1" if:
- You are single and have only one job; or
- You are married, have only one job, and your spouse does not work; or
- Your wages from a second job or your spouse's wages (or the total of both) are $1,000 or less.

. . **B** _____

C   Enter "1" for your **spouse.** But, you may choose to enter -0- if you are married and have either a working spouse or more than one job (this may help you avoid having too little tax withheld) . . . .   **C** _____

D   Enter number of **dependents** (other than your spouse or yourself) whom you will claim on your tax return . . . . .   **D** _____

E   Enter "1" if you will file as **head of household** on your tax return (see conditions under "Head of Household," above) .   **E** _____

F   Enter "1" if you have at least $1,500 of **child or dependent care expenses** for which you plan to claim a credit . .   **F** _____

G   Add lines A through F and enter total here. Note: *This amount may be different from the number of exemptions you claim on your return* ▶   **G** _____

For accuracy, do all worksheets that apply.
- If you plan to **itemize or claim adjustments to income** and want to reduce your withholding, see the Deductions and Adjustments Worksheet on page 2.
- If you are **single** and have **more than one job** and your combined earnings from all jobs exceed $29,000 OR if you are **married** and have a **working spouse or more than one job,** and the combined earnings from all jobs exceed $50,000, see the Two-Earner/Two-Job Worksheet on page 2 if you want to avoid having too little tax withheld.
- If **neither** of the above situations applies, **stop here** and enter the number from line G on line 5 of Form W-4 below.

- - - - - - - - - - - - - - - **Cut here and give the certificate to your employer. Keep the top portion for your records.** - - - - - - - - - - - - - - -

Form W-4

Department of the Treasury
Internal Revenue Service

Employee's Withholding Allowance Certificate

▶ **For Privacy Act and Paperwork Reduction Act Notice, see reverse.**

OMB No. 1545-0010

20XX

1 Type or print your first name and middle initial	Last name	2 Your social security number

Home address (number and street or rural route)	3 ☐ Single ☐ Married ☐ Married, but withhold at higher Single rate. **Note:** *If married, but legally separated, or spouse is a nonresident alien, check the Single box.*
City or town, state, and ZIP code	4 If your last name differs from that on your social security card, check here and call 1-800-772-1213 for more information . ▶ ☐

5	Total number of allowances you are claiming (from line G above or from the Worksheets on back if they apply)	**5**
6	Additional amount, if any, you want deducted from each paycheck	**6** $

7   I claim exemption from withholding and I certify that I meet **ALL** of the following conditions for exemption:
- Last year I had a right to a refund of **ALL** Federal income tax withheld because I had **NO** tax liability; **AND**
- This year I expect a refund of **ALL** Federal income tax withheld because I expect to have **NO** tax liability; **AND**
- This year if my income exceeds $600 and includes nonwage income, another person cannot claim me as a dependent.

If you meet all of the above conditions, enter the year effective and "EXEMPT" here . . . ▶ | **7** | 20

8   Are you a full-time student? (**Note:** *Full-time students are not automatically exempt.*) . . . .   **8** ☐ Yes ☐ No

Under penalties of perjury, I certify that I am entitled to the number of withholding allowances claimed on this certificate or entitled to claim exempt status.

Employee's signature ▶ _____   Date ▶ _____ , 20 ____

9 Employer's name and address (Employer: Complete 9 and 11 only if sending to the IRS)	10 Office code (optional)	11 Employer identification number

FIGURE 10–8 Form W-4, Employee's Withholding Allowance Certificate

earnings. The net pay (pay actually given to the employee) is the gross earnings minus taxes and other deductions. The physician must provide the employee with a statement of gross pay and deductions along with the check each pay period. The tax deductions withheld must be sent on a quarterly basis to the federal, state, and local government offices along with the reporting forms provided by the tax offices. The local, state, and federal governments supply the guidelines necessary to complete these reports.

A W-2 form, which is a summary of all earnings for the year and all deductions withheld for federal, state, and local taxes, must be provided to each employee by January 31st of each year. The Social Security Administration must receive a report of W-2 forms each year. The physician who has several employees may also need to submit reports to the state and federal government for **unemployment** taxes. This tax is not deducted from the employee's earnings for federal tax but may be deducted in some cases for state unemployment tax.

BENEFITS

Full-time employed medical assistants and other medical office employees can expect **benefits** in addition to their salary. These are sometimes known as **fringe benefits**. Benefits will vary according to the situation of the employee and the generosity of the physician(s). The following are examples of benefits that may be offered.

- Vacation. Usually a minimum of two weeks with pay after completing a year of full-time employment; increases with **longevity**.
- Holidays. A minimum of six paid holidays per year—New Year's, Memorial Day, Fourth of July, Labor Day, Thanksgiving, and Christmas.
- Sick time. Some companies will pay employees when they need to be out of the office because of illness. Most organizations pay for 3 to 5 sick days per year.
- Personal time. This is time that an employee can take off for physician or dental appointments and other personal matters without having to use vacation or sick time. Three days per year is the usual amount.

- **Bereavement time.** This is the time that an employee can take off when a family member or very close friend dies. The amount of time is usually based on the relationship of the employee with the deceased.
- Jury duty. Some organizations will pay employees when they are summoned to appear in court. The amount of time granted is based on the court order. It may be possible to get excused from duty if your position is considered critical to your employer.
- Paid time off (PTO). Some companies group holidays, personal days, and vacation time into one category called PTO benefits. Using a mathematical equation based upon the employee's date of hire, a percentage of PTO is accrued each pay period.
- Health insurance. Available; may require some co-payment and may not be provided if employee is covered by insurance with spouse's employment.
- **Disability** insurance. Will cover a percentage of the salary if the employee is unable to work because of a disabling condition.
- Life insurance. Usually for a set amount, for example, equal to a year's salary.
- **Profit sharing.** A form of pension plan to employees who meet certain requirements such as: at least 21 years old, work a minimum of 1000 hours in a year, and employed for at least a year to establish eligibility. Each plan will have its own requirements. For example an amount equal to a certain percentage of the employee's salary is deposited annually into the plan by the employer. This amount accumulates interest and grows tax free until it is withdrawn. The employee is normally responsible for the taxes due. There is usually a period of time, five years for example, before an employee becomes **vested** in the plan. This means the person must be employed at least five years before being eligible to receive the money in the account should employment be terminated. This type of benefit can add up to a nice sum. As an example, a person earns $10 per hour, $20,800 per year. If 10% of the salary ($2080) is placed into the plan for ten years, it would be valued at $20,800 plus the interest earned. Even if there were no increase in salary and therefore no increase in annual contributions, with an interest rate of only 5%, the amount would be approximately $23,000 at the end of 10 years—a very impressive fringe benefit.

Another benefit, which is often overlooked, is the medical care you may receive as an employee. Depending on the type of practice in which you work, you may realize a considerable amount of **complimentary** health care. It is also of benefit to be a physician's employee when you need referral to another physician or medical specialist.

Another nice benefit that some physicians may provide is complimentary lunches that are sponsored by drug companies to have an opportunity to present their products to the physician and staff.

Medical practices that offer a good benefit package in addition to a competitive salary usually have a much more stable staff. This, in turn, results in reduced expense and maintenance of a high level of **productivity** because training time for new employees is not needed.

ACHIEVE UNIT OBJECTIVES

Complete Chapter 10, Unit 3, in the workbook to help you obtain competency of this subject matter.

UNIT 4

General Management Duties

OBJECTIVES

Upon completion of the unit, meet the following performance objectives by verifying knowledge of the facts and principles presented through oral and written communication at a level deemed competent.

1. Spell and define, using the glossary at the back of the text, all the **Words to Know** in this unit.
2. Discuss refunds to patients.
3. Explain why no-shows are a concern.
4. Describe a method to ensure inventory supplies.
5. Identify office equipment requiring frequent attention.
6. Identify six organizations that might inspect a physician's office.
7. Describe a manager's responsibility to the employees.
8. Describe a manager's responsibility to the physicians.
9. List general facility responsibilities.

AREAS OF COMPETENCE (AAMA)

This unit addresses content within the specific competency areas *Administrative procedures, Practice finances, Professionalism, Legal concepts, Instruction,* and *Operational functions* as identified in the Medical Assistant Role Delineation Study. Refer to Appendix A for a detailed listing of the areas.

WORDS TO KNOW

calibration	inventory
delegation	maintenance
expenditure	management
extensive	negligent
fiscal	reimbursement

Many duties performed in a medical office can be categorized under the broad classification of general **management** duties. These are activities that coordinate and maintain the functions within an office. This unit identifies a wide range of miscellaneous duties to acquaint you with those "behind the scenes" activities needed to efficiently operate a successful medical practice.

DAILY AND MONTHLY ACCOUNT RECORDS

Medical offices use a variety of bookkeeping and accounting systems. Regardless of the system used, some method will be needed to maintain a sense for **fiscal** status. It is essential to identify expenditures and income totals to ensure the practice is earning sufficient income to meet office expenses, taxes, insurance premiums and benefits payments and to provide an income for the physician. In addition, it is necessary to build assets for equipment purchases, investments, and perhaps the hiring of additional employees when needed.

In a medical practice, a percentage of patients may be **negligent** in paying for services. This can represent a sizeable amount of lost income. If it is allowed to continue or increase in percentage, it can present a serious problem and must be dealt with by the manager. Because of this fact, many physicians now require payment when services are delivered. In long-term care situations, such as with obstetric patients, a standard fee to cover the anticipated form of delivery is established and the patient makes periodic payments prior to the delivery.

It is necessary to keep a record of accounts receivable. You can do this with a record page that allows you to begin the month with the amount carried over from the preceding month. Then each day you list charges and receipts and increase or decrease your total accounts receivable balance depending on whether your receipts or charges were greater. A trial balance, or total of all outstanding accounts, should be calculated each month. The total should agree with the accounts receivable balance.

The accounts payable records include all invoices for purchases, the checkbook, and the disbursement journal. All **expenditures** must be carefully entered in the disbursement journal. Office expenses must be separated from the physician's personal expenses. Office expenses are tax deductible but not all personal expenses are.

In an office where a computer is used for accounting transactions, you will receive instructions before being expected to perform the work. Every system has special features not found in other systems. The practice management software should allow calculations of daily, weekly, and year-to-date figures to provide reports for analyzing income sources. It should also provide lists of outstanding receivables and have the capability of generating a list of delinquent accounts.

Many offices send their billing and invoices to a computerized accounting service through a telephone-linked terminal. Still other offices prepare all accounting records in a batch and take them to an accounting service computer center to be processed.

When a personal accountant is employed, the records will be maintained and a report provided to the medical practice each month, which indicates the expenditures, balances, and accounts receivable.

In addition to those already mentioned, the 1099 forms issued by third-party payers, which indicate the total amount paid directly to the physician during the year, must be saved and given to the accountant for inclusion with the tax forms.

MISSED APPOINTMENTS

Another related area that a manager may need to address is missed appointments. A missed appointment policy should be distributed in new-patient packets either prior to or during the first office visit. If a patient does not show, no payment is received for that scheduled time of the day. In addition, another patient who needed to schedule an appointment was either scheduled at another time or referred if necessary. As an example, say there is one no-show for an average charge of $40. If this occurs three days in a week for 48 weeks during a year, $5760 income is lost. A policy of calling to remind patients of upcoming appointments can be established or a fee assessed for additional missed appointments after the patient has been notified in writing.

Any time a patient calls to cancel an appointment, it is critical that it is recorded in the patient's chart or entered into the computer system. This will document that the patient failed to keep an appointment and eliminate accidental billing.

OFFICE POLICY MANUAL

The office manager is responsible for developing and maintaining the policy and procedure manual for the office. An office manual may include policy on such topics as:

- Absenteeism
- Paid time off (PTO)
- Harassment
- Confidentiality
- Continuing education
- Chain of command
- Expected performance
- Employment evaluation

OFFICE PROCEDURE MANUAL

An office procedure manual will identify the common procedures performed in the office. The manual may include such procedures as:

- Opening and closing the office
- Laboratory tests
- Documentation requirements
- OSHA/CLIA requirements
- Basic clinical procedures
- Basic administrative procedures
- Emergency procedures

The office manager should address these manuals during the employee's orientation. Employees should always sign a statement that they have read and fully understand the information included in the manuals.

The office manager will usually be responsible for maintaining and updating the policy manual. When a new operational policy is adopted, it must be put into writing and added to the manual. As new procedures become necessary, the manager should also develop the written procedure guidelines and add them to the procedure manual.

STAFF MEETINGS

The office manager is also responsible for conducting staff meetings. The meetings should last from 30 minutes to one hour. Many times they are associated with lunch or a continental breakfast to use time more effectively. Employees should receive pay for staff meeting time.

To have a successful meeting, it is necessary to have an agenda or order of business so that you will be organized and know in advance what topics will be covered. If decisions are made that will affect office operation, be sure a written record in the form of minutes is kept so that you will have a reference for any necessary changes in the policy and procedure manual. The meetings should be informative and beneficial and should concern the operation of the office. The meeting should never be allowed to turn into a "gripe session." Discussing personal issues associated with individual employees should be avoided when the total staff is present. If an employee wants to discuss an issue that may be considered controversial, the manager will need to schedule a private meeting to determine the appropriateness of how the issue may affect the practice.

PATIENT INFORMATION BROCHURE

The office manager may be asked to compose a patient information brochure to be distributed to new and/or existing patients. This should be a brief explanation of office policies. A brief history of the physician(s) education and practice interests should be included as well as information on office hours, appointments, telephone calls, after-hours calls, accepted insurance plans, payment policies, and hospital affiliation(s).

This brochure should be printed on a good quality paper. If the practice has a logo, this could be placed on the cover of the brochure. The brochure can be as simple as a single sheet neatly folded or as complex as a booklet. An added touch would be a picture of the physician(s) and a map showing the office location. A brochure can be sent to a new patient as confirmation of an appointment or given to the patient at the initial appointment. The brochure will need to be updated as physicians or services are added or deleted from the practice.

Additional information that the patient should receive on the first office visit includes:

- Patient information form
- Patient medical history sheet
- Missed appointment policy

- Patient's Bill of Rights
- Office smoking policy
- After-hours policy
- Advance directive policy

These forms should be read and signed by the patient and then returned to the chart. Copies may be given to the patient for future reference.

PATIENT REFUNDS

Managers usually assume the responsibility of verifying overpayment to a patient's account before approving **reimbursement** to the patient. This situation occurs when both the patient and the insurance company pay the physician or an error in the amount due is made.

EQUIPMENT MAINTENANCE AND SUPPLY INVENTORY

A **Finance:**
- Purchase Orders

The manager or the medical assistant is expected to keep track of equipment **maintenance** and maintain an **inventory** of clinical and administrative supplies. An office that has been in operation for several years will have an established list of companies that supply its needs. You should not change to another company without consulting the physician. You should be alert to the best quality for the best price, however. You will be a valuable member of the health care team if you are able to control costs without sacrificing the quality of the products and supplies you use. New medical assistants will usually have to prove their capability to handle routine office affairs before being entrusted with maintaining an inventory.

The best method for organizing office supplies is to prepare a separate inventory record for each item used. These should be reviewed and updated in a systematic manner. Some high usage items may require a daily update, whereas a weekly update is sufficient for others. The inventory record should indicate the supplier's name, address, phone number, and the cost of the item. A file should be maintained of the maintenance contracts on equipment along with the names and phone numbers of service personnel to be called.

Good housekeeping rules must be followed in storage of supplies. The storage areas should be clean and dry. All medications should be stored in a cool, dark area to avoid deterioration. Narcotics should always be in a locked cabinet. Some laboratory supplies must be refrigerated. Supplies should be stored near the area where they will be used.

It is not possible to give quality care to patients with faulty office equipment. You must be aware of daily, weekly, or monthly maintenance that must be carried out to keep equipment in good working order. Always go through a troubleshooting checklist to see if you can correct a problem before requesting outside help. Maintenance personnel charge for plugging in a machine just as they do for repair service.

Autoclaves require regular cleaning to work effectively in sterilization procedures. The **calibration** of aneroid sphygmomanometers should be checked periodically. The mercury level of mercury manometers should be checked to ensure an accurate blood pressure reading (see Chapter 13, Unit 3). Electrocardiograph machines must be maintained. Light sources on sigmoidoscopy, otoscope, and ophthalmoscope equipment should be checked and replaced when necessary. There should always be a supply of batteries and light bulbs to be used in maintenance of equipment. Many insurance companies want to verify that maintenance on all equipment has been performed every one to two years. Logs should be maintained documenting calibration or equipment service when it is performed. A sample of a documentation schedule is shown in Figure 10–9. This listing combined with a means to date the performance would adequately satisfy the company.

A part of office maintenance that cannot be overlooked is linen supplies. Some offices use gowns, towels, pillow cases, and sheets, which must be sent to a laundry. If disposable items are used, there must be an adequate supply at all times.

RESPONSIBILITY FOR DECISION MAKING

In large practices, clinics, and corporations, it is advisable to divide the decision-making responsibilities among the physicians according to their area of interest or expertise. When decisions need to be made, the manager has to confer with only that physician or two instead of the total partnership. An example of division of responsibility is:

- Employment/personnel concerns
- Purchasing and office facility concerns
- Lab and radiology issues
- Fees, investments, and other financial matters

Decisions made by designated physicians are then usually discussed at a general meeting.

From time to time, the manager may also be involved in the review and the eventual negotiations required for agreement to a manage care contract. The manager can provide insight and make inquiries from a different viewpoint than the physicians. When the manager has been promoted from a medical assistant administrative or clinical position, she has a valuable understanding of the patient care requirements specified in the managed care contract.

The office manager may also be asked to contribute to the determination of fee schedules for patient care. The manager will have a continuing awareness of the costs involved for the physician to perform certain diagnostic studies or the cost of disposable products and supplies involved in certain procedures. When the costs of the products and supplies increase, the fees may have to be adjusted to accommodate the increased expense.

RESPONSIBILITIES TO EMPLOYEES

The manager in large practices often has the following responsibilities related to the support staff employees:

- Interview, hire, and terminate employees in concert with physicians if desired.
- Supervise or personally train employees. This applies to new personnel as well as updating current staff.
- Conduct staff meetings to inform, discuss, and exchange information.
- Make out work schedules.
- Arrange vacations and coverage if needed. Work in the position if necessary.
- Conduct performance evaluations, establishing probationary periods as deemed necessary.
- Consult physicians concerning salary increases and benefit changes.

RESPONSIBILITY FOR THE FACILITY

The physical structure of the office must be observed and maintained. The manager assumes responsibility for:

- Maintenance of office services such as cleaning and laundry
- Subscriptions to magazines and health-related literature
- Monitoring and paying utilities
- Suggesting improvements: repairs, decorating, and organization of rooms

A manager who has served successfully in the position may also be given the responsibility to handle renewals of business and profession insurance policies. This could also involve researching different providers and making comparisons of coverage and benefits to obtain the most coverage for the amount spent. Another area that is often the responsibility of the manager is the negotiation of leases and prices for equipment and supply contracts. Careful comparisons of equipment features, supply packaging amounts, and price will determine the best purchase option.

RESPONSIBILITIES TO PHYSICIANS

Physicians also need to be kept informed and aware of conditions affecting the practice. The manager has a great deal of obligation to the physicians. Some areas the manager must consider are:

- Assist in creating or updating business policies to increase efficiency
- Attend meetings pertaining to office management such as those sponsored by the medical association and other professional organizations

Type	Frequency
Housekeeping schedule	Daily
Refrigerator and freezer temperatures	Daily
Cold sterilization to check the efficacy of the solution	Daily
Autoclave controls such as Steri-Strips	Daily in most states
Calibration of equipment	Daily or each shift in applicable cases
Quality control for lab procedures	Daily
Inventory of controlled substances	Daily
Spore checks	Weekly or Monthly depending on the state
Checking for outdated sterilized instruments	Monthly
Checking for outdated samples in the drug sample closet, refrigerator, freezer, and drug cabinets	Monthly
Infectious waste logs	Monthly
Changing X-ray processing chemicals	According to manufacturer's instructions
Fire extinguisher gauge and pin inspections	Monthly
Eyewash station	Monthly
Emergency/crash kits	Monthly
Automated External Defibrillator (AED) or defibrillator units	Monthly
Lab proficiency testing	Quarterly
Evacuation drills	One or two times annually
Hazard communication training	Annually
Blood-borne pathogen training	Annually
Exposure control plan	Annually
Review of safety manual	Annually
OSHA form 200 posted (if more than 10 employees)	Annually
Laboratory policy and procedure manual updated/reviewed	Annually
Emergency preparedness drills	Annually
Radiology policy and procedure drills updated and reviewed	Annually or according to state guidelines
X-ray certificate current	Annually, depending on the state guidelines
Federal CLIA certificate updated	Every two years
CPR certification	Every two years
Equipment maintenance	Every one to three years

FIGURE 10–9 Documentation schedule

- Update physicians on Medicare, health plans, and insurance company policy changes, fee schedules, and reimbursement rates (for example, changes in Current Procedural Terminology (CPT) and International Classification of Diseases (ICD) codes or descriptors or the reduction in Medicare coverage affecting reimbursement when accepting consignment). Approximately 85% of a physician's income is from third-party payers, either directly or indirectly. It is critical that physicians learn to code their services correctly to obtain the full amount allowed for their care.
- Order CPT and ICD books annually. Review for deleted or added numbers.
- Hold physician meetings to discuss practice concerns.

RESPONSIBILITY FOR PREPARING FOR A SITE VISIT

Many different organizations inspect physicians' offices from time to time, including:

- Insurance companies
- CLIA
- Commission on Office Laboratory Accreditation (COLA)
- OSHA
- Local or state board of health
- Drug Enforcement Agency (DEA)

Many insurance companies will announce their visits in advance. Other organizations such as CLIA, OSHA, and boards of health do not always give advance notification. It is imperative that office managers familiarize themselves with the latest guidelines from each of these organizations.

PREPARING FOR AN INSURANCE SITE REVIEW

It is the responsibility of the office manager to prepare the office for the site visits. Responsibilities need to be delegated to the office staff. Good teamwork is essential when preparing for site visits. Many different areas are examined during the review. They can be divided into categories such as:

- Site guidelines
- Building/facility
- Service accessibility
- Pharmaceuticals
- Laboratory
- Equipment
- Medical records, general
- Medical records, content and structure
- Staffing issues
- Radiology
- Patients' rights
- Medical records, preventative medicine items

An accumulation of checklists used by reviewers from many of the large insurance carriers across the country have been compiled into tables and placed in Appendix E. These tables would be extremely useful to managers who are preparing for an insurance site visit.

MOVING THE OFFICE

Medical offices change locations for many different reasons. Some offices outgrow their space. Others find a facility that is more economical or in a better and more convenient location. The office manager is usually the one who coordinates the move. Prior to the change, communication with the practice owner is essential. Goals need to be clearly defined. The following content represents many of the responsibilities that arise as a result of an office move.

RESPONSIBILITIES AT EXISTING FACILITY

Responsibilities at the existing facility may include:

- Purging medical records
- Purging x-rays
- Arranging for storage of purged records
- Discarding or cleaning and storing items that are no longer relevant
- Obtaining a minimum of three written estimates from moving companies

Movers can have many hidden costs. Do not accept an estimate that reveals only one price. Have the company itemize each item for which you are being charged. At the time of the move, the moving representative might indicate that additional services can be provided. Determine what the additional services are and how much they will cost. If you decide to accept more services, get the new price in writing before allowing the movers to perform the services.

You will need to notify many businesses of your move. This is a good time to carefully evaluate which businesses you wish to continue to work with and which you want to replace. The following is a partial list of businesses you will need to notify several weeks prior to your move:

- Gas company
- Electric company
- Telephone company
- Waste management
- Vending machine company
- Carpet runners supplier
- Security company
- Landscaping/snow removal services
- Background music provider
- Equipment leasing companies
- Post office
- Directory assistance

- White business and yellow pages
- Biohazardous waste removal
- Medical bureau
- Cleaning company
- Periodicals companies

If there is more than one physician in the practice, each one will need to be listed with the post office, phone company, medical bureau, and so forth. If the practice has a name, information for that too will need to be changed. All companies that provide services will need to be notified and work together to make certain that the office has uninterrupted service throughout the entire move.

Other businesses that need to be notified of your move include the hospitals and insurance companies with which the practice has current contracts, state medical boards, laboratories, CLIA, COLA, x-ray board, and all physicians who send referrals or to whom the practice sends referrals.

The patients are the biggest group to be notified. This is most effectively done by sending a form letter to each one. The database in the computer should be able to produce names and addresses to merge with the form letter's text to make it seem more personal. Names and addresses can be printed directly on the envelope or onto mailing labels, which can be affixed to the envelope. The move should be announced to patients coming to the office as soon as it is known because of the need to make follow-up appointments. The move also can become part of the office's recorded phone message. An announcement in the local newspaper would also be beneficial.

Responsibilities at the New Facility

Many things will need to be taken care of at the new facility prior to the move. If the facility is new or requires some remodeling, it may be necessary to work with construction contractors. Interior designers can take care of the decorating. Furniture, window coverings, and other items for the new facility will need to be ordered. Equipment and supplies will need to be stocked, utilities turned on, and the phone system installed to operate properly. Moving an office is a very involved task that must be organized to be as efficient and smooth as possible. Moving also requires things to be up and running almost the same day.

The Day of the Move

The staff should be divided on the day of the move; part of the staff will remain at the old location, and part will go to the new location. Organization is imperative. Each team member will have specific responsibilities. Once everything has been moved from the old facility and all areas have been checked for any missed items and completely cleaned, they can join the other staff members at the new facility.

MANAGER'S REWARDS

The role of office manager can be as limited or **extensive** as the physician(s) feels comfortable in the **delegation** of authority. A trusted employee who performs well in the role of office manager becomes a tremendous asset to the practice. This role in large medical offices carries a great amount of authority and responsibility, but the rewards are worthwhile both financially and personally. It is a challenge you should look forward to accepting should the opportunity arise.

ACHIEVE UNIT OBJECTIVES

Complete Chapter 10, Unit 4, in the workbook to help you obtain competency of this subject matter.

A CAAHEP CONNECTION

Facility management is specified under **Administrative Procedures** in the standards. It is important for you to have an appreciation of the duties and responsibilites of an office manager and to understand their role in the operation of a practice. A competent manager can free up the physicians from the day-to-day office activities, permitting them to concentrate on providing patient care.

RELATING TO ABHES

Chapter 10 discusses the many responsibilities of managing the medical office, such as processing checks and currency, maintaining required financial and employee records, providing training and policy updates, and a great many routine and occasional managerial duties involved in the operation of an office. This content relates to the ABHES accreditation requirements of *Legal terminology pertaining to office practice* within the content area of **Medical Law and Ethics** and *Financial management* and *Equipment and supplies (including ordering/maintaining/storage/inventory)* within the content area of **Medical Office Business Procedures/Management.**

Medical-Legal-Ethical Scenario

Michelle has been the office manager for a three-physician practice for the past two years. Rosie, one of five medical assistants, has worked for the practice for five years. She is very professional, can be depended on to perform her responsibilities, and is well liked by the patients. Recently, a friend of hers who works in a surgeon's office has been trying to encourage her to come work with her. Michelle does not want to lose a good employee, yet she realizes Rosie's dilemma because she could earn another $100 a month if she were to leave. Michelle talked with the physicians about giving Rosie a raise, but they feel they do not want to set a precedent of counter-offering a salary. In addition, the pay scales are established in the policy manual, and increases are tied to longevity and performance, as well as figured on a percentage of the current salary. They were concerned that the other staff members might resent Rosie receiving "special" treatment. Still, Michelle wants to keep Rosie on the staff and realizes she must figure out another way to do so.

CRITICAL THINKING CHALLENGE

1. What are some options open to Michelle?
2. What do you think about establishing a different job description with perhaps a little more responsibility in order to justify a salary increase?
3. Could additional fringe benefits be established for employees such as Rosie, who have been employed for five years?
4. Is there any guarantee that Rosie would stay even if Michelle did manage to arrange a salary increase?
5. What really is important for job satisfaction?

6. How would being given more responsibility, a *title*, and a sense of control over some portion of the operation provide an incentive?

The CAAHEP standards identify Workplace Dynamics as an area of instruction. The Medical Assistant Role Delineation Study mentions work as a team member and serve as a liaison as necessary roles. Management of an office and its personnel requires many special skills.

RESOURCES   Simmers, L. (2001). *Diversified health occupations* (5th ed.). Clifton Park, NY: Delmar Learning.

WEB LINKS   http://www.btcc.com **(Bankers Training and Consulting Company)** Provides financial news and several links to other Web sites.

Structure and Function of the Body

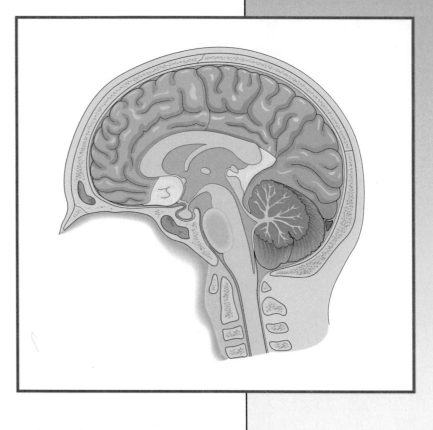

Anatomy and Physiology of the Human Body

The human body is a fantastic combination of parts that function in an organized manner, far more efficiently and effectively than any machine ever developed. This chapter describes the body's fundamental structure and the body systems and discusses how all the parts work together.

The diseases and disorders affecting the human body are a result of impairment, deterioration, or malfunction of one or more of its component parts. This chapter presents the anatomy of each body system and how that system physiologically functions within itself and with the other body systems. Following the presentation of each system will be a discussion of characteristic pathophysiological conditions and disorders, many of which result from the body's inability to adapt or defend itself. A basic discussion of the critical role of the immune system in maintaining a healthy state will help you to correlate your knowledge of the body's complex interrelationships. With this understanding, you will be able to see how the patient's concerns and complaints, the physician's examination, and the clinical findings fit together to indicate the diagnosis and the plan of treatment the physician prescribes.

The preparation of material relating to the structure and function of the human body is exciting yet at times quite technical. The inclusion of diagnostic examinations, diseases and disorders, and usual methods of treatment further complicates the content. In order to obtain the most recent information available, many medical newsletters and health-related association publications have been reviewed. Many professional colleagues revised the content and provided new information. Almost daily, the print and electronic media releases information on new research findings and results of studies that are rapidly changing the manner in which health care is provided. All this data is beyond the capability of any one individual to fully acquire or use. The speed at which scientific discovery occurs can be explosive once a specific "piece of the puzzle" is found. We realize that before this material is published, another discovery may cause the information to be inaccurate or obsolete. We encourage you to be alert to information about new findings. Evaluate it carefully. Look for *fact*, not "seems-to-be" results. Observe the persons studied in any research to see if it makes a reported finding seem valid for the total population. It is hardly significant when the findings are shown to be in a small group of people who are living in the same area or are all about the same age and sex. You live in a time when scientific capability is raising many ethical, moral, and legal questions. The possibility of altering our very cellular structure is at hand. Be inquisitive, be excited, be informed, and you will be knowledgeable.

UNIT 1

Anatomical Descriptors and Fundamental Body Structure

OBJECTIVES

Upon completion of the unit, meet the following performance objectives by verifying knowledge of the facts and principles presented through oral and written communication at a level deemed competent.

1. Spell and define, using the glossary at the back of the text, all the **Words to Know** in this unit.
2. Describe the anatomical position.
3. Apply the appropriate terminology to points of reference on the human body.
4. Locate the eight body cavities on an illustration.
5. Name the major organ(s) located within each body cavity.
6. Identify the regions of the abdomen.
7. Describe the basic characteristics of the cell.
8. Explain what happens when a mutation occurs.
9. Name the patterns of inheritance, and explain how they affect a trait.
10. Describe the six ways molecules pass through cell membranes.
11. Describe the identifying characteristics of the following genetic conditions: cleft lip, cleft palate, Down Syndrome, Spina Bifida, Klinefelter's Syndrome, Talipes, and Turner's Syndrome.
12. Explain DNA "fingerprinting."
13. Describe the four main types of body tissues.
14. Name the 10 systems of the body.

AREAS OF COMPETENCE (AAMA)

This unit addresses content within the specific competency areas of *Administrative procedures, Practice finances, Patient care, Communication skills,* and *Instruction,* as identified in the Medical Assistant Role Delineation Study. Refer to Appendix A for a detailed listing of the areas. (Note: Although *Anatomy and physiology* is not identified in the study, a basic knowledge of the body's structure and function is an essential foundation to the competent performance of many roles.)

WORDS TO KNOW

abdominal	hypertonic
abdominopelvic	hypochondriac
anatomic	hypogastric
anatomy	hypotonic
anterior	iliac
biochemistry	inferior
buccal	inguinal
cardiac	involuntary
carriers	isotonic
caudal	keloid
cavities	lateral
cell membrane	lumbar
centrioles	lysosomes
chromosomes	medial
congenital	membrane
connective	microscopic anatomy
coronal	midline
cranial	mitochondria
cytology	mitosis
cytoplasm	muscle
cytotechnologist	mutation
dehydration	myelin
diaphragm	nasal
diffusion	nerve
distal	neurilemma
DNA	neuron
dominant gene	normal saline
dorsal	nucleolus
edema	nucleus
elements	orbital
endocytosis	organ
endoplasmic reticulum	organelles
epigastric	osmosis
epithelial	osseous
etiology	pathophysiology
exocytosis	pelvic
extremities	peritoneum
filtration	phagocytosis
frontal	physiology
gene	pinocytosis
Golgi apparatus	posterior
gross anatomy	proximal
histology	pubic
histotechnologist	quadrant
homeostasis	recessive gene
horizontal	retroperitoneal

ribosome
sagittal
skeletal
smooth
spinal
striated
superior
syndrome
system

thoracic
tissue
trait
transverse
umbilical
ventral
voluntary
X-linked gene

ANATOMY AND PHYSIOLOGY DEFINED

 Library

Two terms are used in discussing the study of the human body: **anatomy**, which is the study of the physical structure of the body and its organs; and **physiology**, which is the science of the function of cells, tissues, and organs of the body. In other words, anatomy describes the framework and physical characteristics, whereas physiology explains how everything works together to support life.

Anatomy can be subdivided into various areas of study. For instance, the term **gross anatomy** refers to the study of those features that can be observed with the naked eye by inspection and dissection. As an example, the pathologist, when examining a tissue specimen, will describe its gross **anatomic** surface appearance and then proceed with the dissection and its description.

An area of study known as **microscopic anatomy** deals with features that can be observed only with the use of a microscope. Referring again to the pathologist, a fragment of a specimen can be properly prepared on a slide and observed with a microscope to complete the description of the specimen's characteristics and formulate an opinion as to its identity or state of condition.

There are two related areas of microscopic anatomy, **cytology**, the study of cell life and formation, and **histology**, the study of the microscopic structure of tissue. Pathologists are assisted by laboratory specialists known as **cytotechnologists** and **histotechnologists** who precisely prepare materials for microscopic examination and diagnosis.

Physiology is the study of the interrelationships of all the functioning structures of the body. When everything is in harmony and all biological indicators are within acceptable limits, the individual is referred to as being in a "steady state" or "normal." When the normal physiology is disrupted to the point of instability and begins to deteriorate, pathophysiological mechanisms are likely to occur and may result in the development of a disease condition. **Pathophysiology** is the study of mechanisms by which disease occurs, the responses of the body to the disease process, and the effects of both on normal function.

Pathophysiology attempts to bring together the clinical signs and symptoms present with the knowledge of the effects of the disease processes on the body, from the cellular level to the total human being. Often close observation of the clinical signs of a disease state has led to the discovery of physiological functions previously unknown. This is currently apparent in the great effort to understand the immune system to find a way to effectively control and eventually eliminate acquired immunodeficiency syndrome (AIDS) and cancer.

Fortunately, the healthy body has an enormous capacity to protect itself by compensating, defending, and adapting to the pathophysiological effects of disease. However, when this fails, appropriate medical intervention can often correct or at least control the disease process.

LANGUAGE OF MEDICINE

The members of the health care team must be able to accurately communicate information, findings, and instructions among themselves. Much of the language of medicine is precise and is specific to the field of health care. For instance, it is necessary to not only know about the human body but also to be able to physically and verbally locate body structures and be able to describe the site of a patient's complaint or injury. The following fundamental descriptive terminology will be essential to the understanding of body references.

ANATOMICAL DIRECTIONAL TERMS

Certain directional terms are universally used in describing anatomic structures. A body is said to be in anatomic position when standing erect, with arms down at the sides, and the palms of the hands facing forward (Figure 11–1). This means that when the person is facing you, his right side is on your left, as if you were looking in a mirror. When reference is made to a body structure or a specific area, it is in relationship to this anatomical position. The same is true when you are studying illustrations in this textbook or labeling a drawing in the workbook.

A CAAHEP CONNECTION

Anatomy and Physiology is recognized as a major component of a basic medical assistant program. The standards indicate that not only the study of the body's structure and function is essential but also content covering pathology, diseases, and diagnostic and treatment modalities. In addition, a similar emphasis is placed on the importance of medical terminology in the practice of medical assisting. This unit introduces and applies many medical and scientific terms and introduces the basic information necessary to understand the in-depth discussions of the systems of the body.

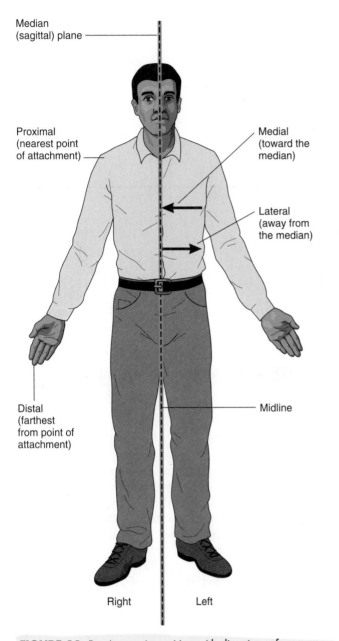

FIGURE 11-1 Anatomic position with direction references

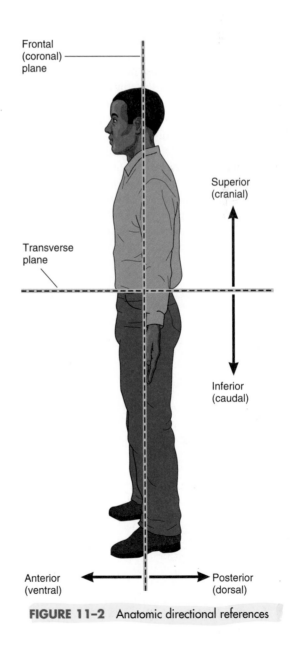

FIGURE 11-2 Anatomic directional references

other fingers and toes have proximal, middle, and distal sections.

If you draw a line vertically through the side of the body from the top of the head to the feet, you will make a front and back section (Figure 11–2). This line is known as the **frontal** or **coronal** plane. The front is known as the **anterior** or **ventral** section; the back is called the **posterior** or **dorsal** section.

Finally, drawing an imaginary line **horizontally** (across) the body creates a **transverse** plane. The portion of the body above the line is known as **superior** or **cranial**. The portion below the line is called **inferior** or **caudal**. It is not necessary that the body be divided into equal parts. The terms superior and inferior refer to any relationship of structures above or below a "line" and depend on where it is drawn. For example, with a transverse line at the waist, the chest is superior to the abdomen, but if at the neck, the chest is inferior to the head. All anatomic directional terms are ap-

Dividing the body vertically down the front will result in a right and left half. This imaginary line is known as the median or **sagittal** plane. The right and left designations always refer to right and left in anatomic position. Anything located toward the **midline** is said to be **medial**, whereas anything away from the midline is said to be **lateral**.

Two other terms are used to describe the relationship of the **extremities** or ends of the body, such as the arms and legs, to the trunk of the body. **Proximal** indicates nearness to the point of attachment, whereas **distal** indicates distance away from the point of attachment. These terms are also applicable when describing parts of the arms, legs, fingers, or toes. For example, the thumb and great toe have proximal and distal sections, whereas the

propriate only when describing the relationship of one structure to another.

These planes or sections can be applied to internal structures and to the body as a whole. *Incisions* (cuts) made on the body surface or into organs are often made along a plane. The surgeon's description of the operation will identify the location of the incisions made using referencing planes. A tissue specimen cut along the transverse plane is known as a *cross section*.

BODY CAVITIES AND ORGANS

The body is divided into two main **cavities**, an anterior or ventral cavity and a posterior or dorsal cavity (Figure 11–3). A dome-shaped **muscle** known as the **diaphragm** divides the anterior cavity into an upper **thoracic** cavity and a lower **abdominopelvic** cavity. The thoracic cavity (chest) has a wall of ribs that protects its vital organs—the heart, lungs, and the great blood vessels (Figure 11–4).

The diaphragm alternately contracts and relaxes to move the lungs, causing breathing to occur.

The abdominopelvic cavity has two parts, an upper **abdominal** portion and a lower **pelvic** portion. The abdominal portion extends from the diaphragm to the top edge of the pelvic girdle (bones). The organs found in the abdomen are the stomach, small intestines, most of the large intestine, the liver, spleen, pancreas, and gallbladder. The kidneys are located in the dorsal abdominal area but are behind the peritoneal **membrane** that lines the cavity and thus are technically outside the abdominal cavity. This space is referred to as **retroperitoneal**, behind the **peritoneum**. The pelvic cavity is surrounded by the pelvic girdle, which provides protection for the urinary bladder,

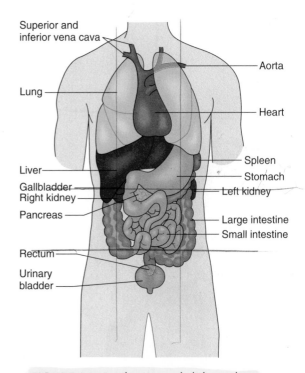

FIGURE 11–4 Thoracic and abdominal organs

the last portion of the large intestine, and the internal reproductive organs.

The cranial cavity is totally encased by the bones of the skull, which provides protection for the brain. The cranial cavity is joined at its base by the **spinal** cavity, which extends through the center of the column of vertebrae (bones). This bony structure contains the spinal cord and protects it from injury.

There are three other small cavities, the **orbital** for the eyes, the **nasal** for the structures of the nose, and the **buccal** or mouth.

Abdominal Regions

The abdomen is such a large area of the body that it is necessary to divide it into regions for purposes of identification or reference. There are two recognized methods of division. One creates **quadrants** known as the right and left upper quadrants (RUQ and LUQ) and the right and left lower quadrants (RLQ and LLQ) (Figure 11–5).

A more exacting division results in nine regions identifiable by location and an anatomical reference point. The three central areas are called **epigastric** (over the stomach), **umbilical** (around the umbilicus), and **hypogastric** (below the stomach; also called **pubic**). The six side areas are called the right and left **hypochondriac** (below the cartilage, referring to the ribs), the right and left **lumbar** (loin or side region; also called **lateral**); and the right and left **iliac** (referring to the ileum portion of the pelvic bone; also known as the **inguinal**, meaning groin, region) (Figure 11–6).

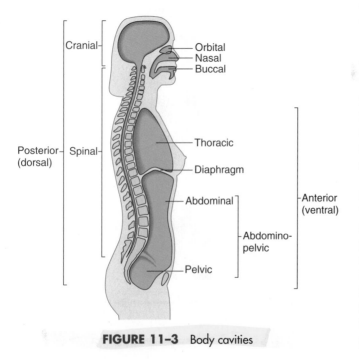

FIGURE 11–3 Body cavities

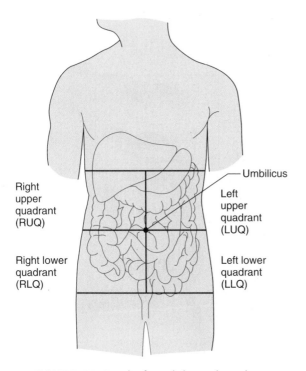

FIGURE 11–5 The four abdominal quadrants

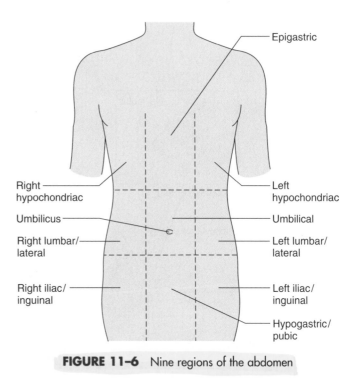

FIGURE 11–6 Nine regions of the abdomen

THE CELL

To understand the structure of the body, you must first learn about its basic building block, the cell. This fascinating wonder is a living, working, microscopic image of the body. It requires food and oxygen to survive, performs specific functions, produces heat and energy, and gives off waste products, and many can reproduce themselves to replace missing cells.

Cells vary greatly in size and shape as a result of their various activities. The body contains about 75 trillion cells. Some cells may be destroyed, but other cells, such as those of the skin or in the intestines, are lost as part of a natural process. These cells are replaced by new cells in line behind them within the tissue structure. Cells lost by injury may or may not be replaced, depending on the severity of the damage. If too many cells are lost and cannot be replaced, organ and eventually system dysfunction results. Cells come in different types to perform specific duties. Some secrete materials, some receive and transmit impulses, and some enable us to move. Still others carry nutrients and oxygen, clot blood, or destroy bacteria. Even though they are microscopic in size, their proper function is essential to life. No man-made apparatus can match the cell for structural architecture and the number of chemical reactions that occur in such a small space.

A conventional cell is composed of a fluid called **cytoplasm** and is surrounded by a cell membrane (Figure 11–7). The **cell membrane** separates the cell from the surrounding environment. It consists of protein and fat molecules. The membrane controls what enters and leaves the cell; therefore, it plays an important role in the health and welfare of the cell, which is discussed later. Enclosed within the membrane is the sticky semifluid material known as cytoplasm. It is a combination of protein, lipids (fat), carbohydrates, minerals, salts, and water (over 70%). Chemical reactions such as respiration and protein synthesis occur in the cytoplasm.

Within the cytoplasm of the cell are many minute bodies called **organelles** that perform amazing tasks. The organelles are the **nucleus**, **mitochondria**, **ribosomes**, **centriole**, **endoplasmic reticulum**, **Golgi apparatus**, and **lysosomes**. Scientists still do not understand how some functions are carried out but continue to investigate the processes. They do know some organelles physically separate the chemical reactions occurring in the cytoplasm because many reactions are not compatible. Organelles also control the time when reactions take place, such as producing or processing a molecule in one organelle and then later using the molecule in another reaction.

The *nucleus* is a dense mass within the cytoplasm. It is surrounded by its own nuclear membrane. Materials pass in and out of the nucleus from the cytoplasm through pores in the membrane. The membrane is continuous with the endoplasmic reticulum, which often has ribosomes attached. The nucleus is the control center of the cell. It regulates the chemical reactions and controls the process of **mitosis** (cell division) for reproduction.

Within the nucleus are the structures called **chromosomes**. Each member of a species has a specific number of chromosomes. Human beings have 46 individual or 23 pairs of chromosomes that store the hereditary material

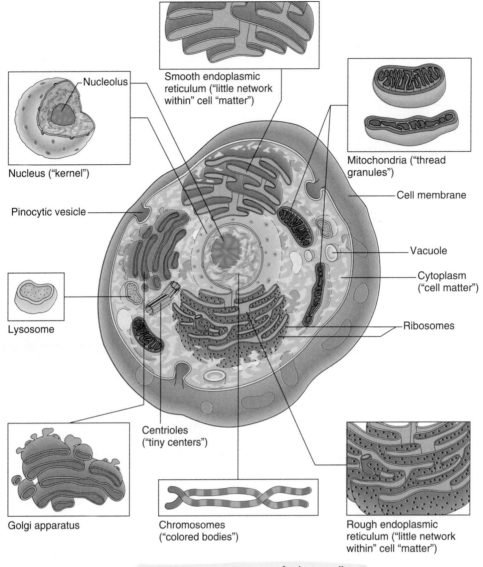

Nucleolus

Nucleus ("kernel")

Smooth endoplasmic reticulum ("little network within" cell "matter")

Mitochondria ("thread granules")

Cell membrane

Pinocytic vesicle

Vacuole

Cytoplasm ("cell matter")

Lysosome

Ribosomes

Golgi apparatus

Centrioles ("tiny centers")

Chromosomes ("colored bodies")

Rough endoplasmic reticulum ("little network within" cell "matter")

FIGURE 11-7 Structure of a basic cell

passed on from one generation to another. Twenty-two pairs of chromosomes are autosome (same in number and kind), and one pair are sex chromosomes, either both X if female or an X and a Y if male. One chromosome from each of the 23 pairs is contributed by the mother and one by the father. When the egg and sperm unite at fertilization, their chromosomes are united so that the new cell, a zygote, will also contain 23 pairs. The sex of the child is determined by whether it is combined with a father's cell carrying an X or a Y chromosome.

Chromosomes are rod-shaped structures composed of long strands of molecules known as deoxyribonucleic acid (**DNA**). DNA is the material within the chromosome that encodes the **genes** that are located at specific sites on the chromosome. The DNA carries all of the genetic information necessary for cellular functions. DNA is composed of sugar, phosphate, and four bases: adenine, cytosine, guanine, and thymine. The genetic coding makes it possible for the exact duplication of the cell.

Every individual has a different DNA code, but the code in all cells of the same individual are identical. It is the arrangement of the base pairs of the DNA code that makes for the differences. The genes are the units of instruction that produce or influence particular characteristics or traits and the capabilities of an organism. Genes are specific segments of DNA molecules that are located on the chromosomes in the cell nucleus. They act in pairs to dictate traits from eye color to the chemical reactions that determine not only cell structure but also function and, therefore, heredity. A gene consists of sequences of thousands of DNA base pairs. There appear to be 35,000 to 45,000 genes that compose the DNA of a cell. This great number of genes helps explain why there is so much variety in the human race, and yet each individual's structure is uniquely and identifiably their own. Consider that during meiosis, each parent's chromosomes are halved, "shuffled," and then combined at fertilization. The father and mother each contribute one half of the child's total number of genes to their offspring. The new being now has a unique combination of genes and, consequently, traits.

The nucleus itself will have at least one **nucleolus**. In a nucleolus, portions of ribonucleic acid (RNA) are assembled with proteins to make subunits of the ribosomes, which then pass through the nuclear pores of the nuclear membrane into the cytoplasm, to become a complete two-part ribosome to synthesize protein. Ribosomes are found circulating in the cytoplasm or attached to the endoplasmic reticulum.

Centrioles are the two cylinder-shaped organelles near the nucleus. During mitosis, the centrioles separate and form spindle fibers that attach to the chromosomes to ensure their equal distribution to the two new daughter cells.

Endoplasmic reticulum crisscrosses the cytoplasm in a network fashion. When attached to the nuclear membrane, it serves as a passageway for the transportation of materials in and out of the nucleus. If grouped together, they can store large amounts of protein. The difference between rough and smooth endoplasmic reticulum is the presence of *ribosomes* on the membrane. Ribosomes give the membrane a rough appearance.

Mitochondria are round or rod-shaped organelles that supply the cell's energy. There may be from one to over a thousand in each cell depending on how much energy that type of cell requires. Mitochondria have a double-membraned structure with the inner membrane folding into ridges. The cell is capable of respiration because the enzymes located in the ridges break down nutrient molecules and oxygen to provide carbon dioxide and water.

The *Golgi apparatus* is a stack of membrane layers that are believed to synthesize carbohydrates and combine them with molecules of proteins. The organelle appears to store and prepare secretions to excrete from the cell. Therefore, the cells of the gastric, salivary, and pancreatic glands have large numbers of Golgi apparatus.

Lysosomes are round or oval structures. They have a strong digestive enzyme that consumes protein molecules such as those found in old worn cells, bacteria, or foreign matter. This is a very important function of the body's natural immune system.

Pinocytic vesicles are pocket-like formations in the cell's membrane. These structures permit large molecules like protein and fat, which cannot pass through the pores of the cell membrane, to enter with the extracellular fluid into the vesicle. Then the "pocket" closes, forming a vacuole (bubble) in the cytoplasm. This process is called **endocytosis**. When liquid droplets, instead of protein or fat molecules, are enclosed, the process is known as **pinocytosis**, which means "cell drinking." A related term, **exocytosis**, refers to a similar process whereby substances are moved from the cell to the outside. On entering the cytoplasm, most vesicles fuse with lysosomes, and their contents are digested. Special white blood cells known as phagocytes rely on endocytosis to destroy harmful bacteria in the body. As you learn more about your body, you will begin to appreciate what a magnificent piece of "equipment" it is and how important it is that you care for it properly. You have the physical and mental power to have great impact on your health and your life.

Table 11–1 summarizes the organelles and their role in the function of the cell.

TABLE 11–1

SUMMARY TABLE OF CELL ORGANELLES

Organelle	Function
Cell membrane	Regulates transport of substances into and out of the cell.
Cytoplasm	Provides an organized watery environment in which life functions take place by the activities of the organelles contained in the cytoplasm.
Nucleus	Serves as the "brain" for the control of the cell's metabolic activities and cell division.
Nuclear membrane	Regulates transport of substances into and out of the nucleus.
Nucleoplasm	A clear, semifluid medium that fills the spaces around the chromatin and the nucleoli.
Nucleolus	Functions as a reservoir for RNA.
Ribosomes	Serve as sites for protein synthesis.
Endoplasmic reticulum	Provides passages through which transport of substances occurs in cytoplasm.
Mitochondria	Serve as sites of cellular respiration and energy production.
Golgi apparatus	Manufactures carbohydrates and packages secretions for discharge from the cell.
Lysosomes	Serve as centers of cellular digestion.
Pinocytic vesicles	Transport of large particles into a cell.
Centrosome and centrioles	Contains two centrioles that are functional during animal cell division.

PASSING MOLECULES THROUGH CELL MEMBRANES

As stated before, the cell membrane controls materials entering and leaving the cell. This is necessary for the cell to acquire substances from its environment to be processed for its use, for secretion, or for excretion of the waste materials. There are six processes by which materials pass through a cell membrane: **diffusion**, **osmosis**, **filtration**, active transport, **phagocytosis** and pinocytosis.

Diffusion is a process whereby gas, liquid, or solid molecules distribute themselves evenly through a medium. When the medium is a fluid and the molecules are solid, they are called solutes (Figure 11–8). When solutes and water pass across a membrane to distribute themselves, they will move from an area of higher concentration to an area of lesser concentration. Diffusion plays a vital role in the body. For example, higher concentrations of oxygen in the alveolus (air sac) of the lung cross the membrane into the lesser concentrated area of the red blood cell in the capillary (Figure 11–8). The blood cell, now with a high concentration of oxygen, circulates in the blood to a body cell with lower oxygen concentration and exchanges its oxygen for the cell's higher concentration of waste products. Hence, the body's cells "breathe" in a process called *internal respiration.*

Osmosis is a process of diffusion of water or another solvent through a selected permeable membrane, one through which some solutes can pass but others cannot (Figure 11–9). In the illustration, the membrane will only allow the salt and water to pass through; therefore, the salt leaves the greater concentrated area within the membrane to go to the lesser concentrated water. At the same time, the water leaves its higher concentrated area to enter the lesser concentrated area within the membrane. When the water molecules are equal on both sides, the

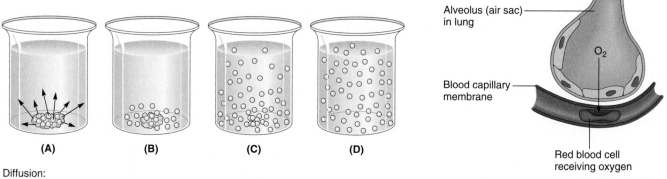

(A) **(B)** **(C)** **(D)**

Diffusion:

(A) A small lump of sugar is placed into a beaker of water, and its molecules dissolve and begin to diffuse outward. (B&C) The sugar molecules continue to diffuse through the water from an area of greater concentration to an area of lesser concentration.
(D) Over a long period, the sugar molecules are evenly distributed throughout the water, reaching a state of equilibrium.

Example of diffusion in the human body: Oxygen diffuses from an alveolus in a lung where it is in greater concentration, across the blood capillary membrane, and into a red blood cell where it is in lesser concentration.

FIGURE 11–8 The process of diffusion

Initial stage **10–12 hours later**

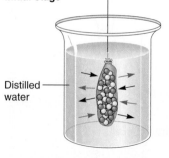

(A) Initially, the sausage casing contains a solution of gelatin, salt and sucrose. The casing is permeable to water and salt molecules only. Since the concentration of water molecules is greater outside the casing, water molecules will diffuse into the casing. The opposite situation exists for the salt.

Distilled water

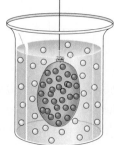

(B) The sausage casing swells because of the net movement of water molecules inward. However, the volume of distilled water in the beaker remains constant.

● Gelatin ○ Salt ● Sucrose

FIGURE 11–9 Osmosis is the diffusion of water through a selective permeable membrane. (A sausage casing is an example of a selective permeable membrane.)

Hypertonic solution

Hypotonic solution

Isotonic solution

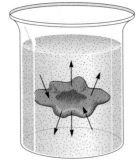

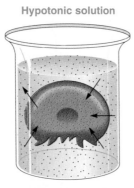

Water molecules

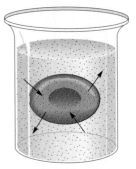

Hypertonic solution (seawater)
a red blood cell will shrink and
wrinkle up because water molecules
are moving out of the cell.

Hypotonic solution (freshwater)
a red blood cell will swell and burst
because water molecules are moving
into the cell.

Isotonic solution (human blood serum)
a red blood cell remains unchanged because
the movement of water molecules into and
out of the cell are the same.

FIGURE 11–10 Movement of water molecules in solution of different osmolalities

diffusion will stop. The pressure of the water molecules inside the membrane is then said to be at *equilibrium,* a state known as the *osmotic pressure.*

The osmotic characteristics of solutions are classified by their effect on red blood cells (Figure 11–10). If the solution is of the same osmotic pressure as blood serum, it is known as an **isotonic** solution. A 0.9% salt (NaCl) solution has the same salt concentration as that of the red blood cell and is called **normal saline**. If the osmolality is lower, the solution is **hypotonic**, and the blood cell will swell with water and burst. In a **hypertonic** solution, the cell will release its water and shrink.

Filtration is the movement of solutes and water across a semipermeable membrane as a result of a force such as gravity or blood pressure. The particles move from a higher to a lower area of pressure. The size of the pores of some membranes allow only small molecules to leave. This process occurs in the kidneys where small molecules of water and waste products are filtered from the blood in the capillaries, whereas the large protein molecules and red blood cells are retained (Figure 11–11).

Active transport refers to molecules moving across a membrane from an area of low concentration to an area of higher concentration. This is caused by the presence of adenosine triphosphate (ATP), a high-energy compound and a protein from the cell membrane. It appears as a "carrier" molecule, temporarily binding with another molecule on the outer edge of the membrane. The carrier crosses the membrane and releases its "passenger" into the cytoplasm. The carrier then receives more energy from the membrane and returns to the outer surface to transport another molecule. The carrier can also reverse the process and carry molecules from the inside to the outside.

Phagocytosis is known as "cell eating." White blood cells become phagocytes and engulf bacteria, cell fragments, or damaged cells (Figure 11–12). The white cell forms a vacuole by enfolding its membrane and enclosing

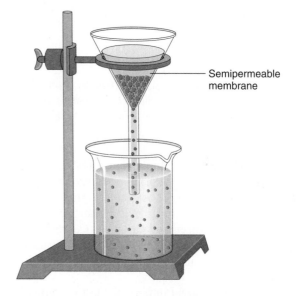

Semipermeable
membrane

Filtration: Small molecules are filtered through the semipermeable membrane, whereas the large molecules remain in the funnel.

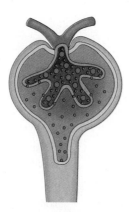

Example of filtration in the human body: Glomerulus of kidney, large particles like red blood cells and proteins remain in the blood, and small molecules like urea and water are excreted as a metabolic excretory product—urine.

FIGURE 11–11 Filtration is a passive transport process.

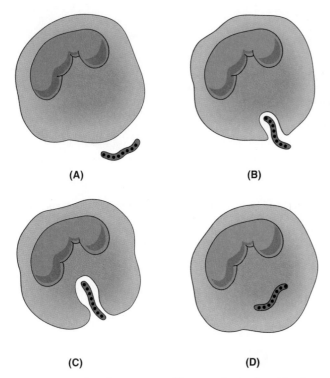

(A)

(B)

(C)

(D)

FIGURE 11–12 Phagocytosis of bacteria by a white blood cell. Phagocytosis can occur in the blood stream, or white cells may squeeze through capillary walls and destroy bacteria in the tissues.

the particle. When it is completely enclosed, digestive enzymes enter from the cytoplasm and destroy the trapped material. This process is extremely important to the body's ability to maintain a healthy state.

Pinocytosis, as discussed earlier, is called "cell drinking" and involves the engulfing of large molecules of liquid material. Once inside the cytoplasm, the fluid is digested by the cell.

Another area of great importance to the welfare of the human body is its chemistry. The study of chemical reactions within the body is called **biochemistry**. The basic building blocks of all matter are the **elements**, substances in their simplest form. There are 92 natural and at least 13 man-made elements. Of these, about 20 are in all living things. Four of these 20 elements make up 97% of all living matter. They are carbon, oxygen, hydrogen, and nitrogen. The remaining 16 elements are sodium, chlorine, magnesium, phosphorus, sulfur, calcium, potassium, iron, copper, manganese, zinc, boron, tin, vanadium, cobalt, and molybdenum. Because the last four elements occur in the body in such minute amounts, they are known as *trace elements.*

Many elements combine together in specific amounts to form new substances known as *compounds.* Some common compounds are water (hydrogen and oxygen), carbon dioxide (carbon and oxygen), salt (sodium and chloride), hydrochloric acid (hydrogen and chlorine), and sodium bicarbonate (sodium, hydrogen, carbon, and oxygen). Compounds can be classified in one of three groups: acids, bases, or salts. An acid compound will have positively charged ions of hydrogen and negatively charged ions of some other element. They have a sour taste such as found in some citrus fruits (limes and lemons). However, an unknown substance should not be tasted to determine its acidity; it should be tested by the special dyes contained in litmus paper. If acid is present, blue litmus paper will turn red.

A base compound is also called an alkali. A base substance will have negatively charged hydroxide ions and positively charged ions of a metal. Bases have a bitter taste and will turn red litmus paper blue. Table 11–2 lists some common acids and bases and identifies where they are found.

When an acid and a base are combined, they form a salt and water. A common example is sodium chloride (table salt), which is the result of combining hydrochloric acid with sodium hydroxide. When the water evaporates, the salt remains.

TABLE 11–2

NAMES, LOCATION, OR USE OF SOME COMMON ACIDS AND BASES

Name of Acid	Where Found or Used	Name of Base	Where Found or Used
Acetic acid	Vinegar	Ammonium hydroxide	Household liquid cleaners
Boric acid	Weak eyewash	Magnesium hydroxide	Milk of magnesia
Carbonic acid	Carbonated beverages	Potassium hydroxide	Caustic potash
Hydrochloric acid	Stomach	Sodium hydroxide	Lye
Nitric acid	Industrial oxidizing acid		
Sulfuric acid	Batteries and industrial mineral acid		

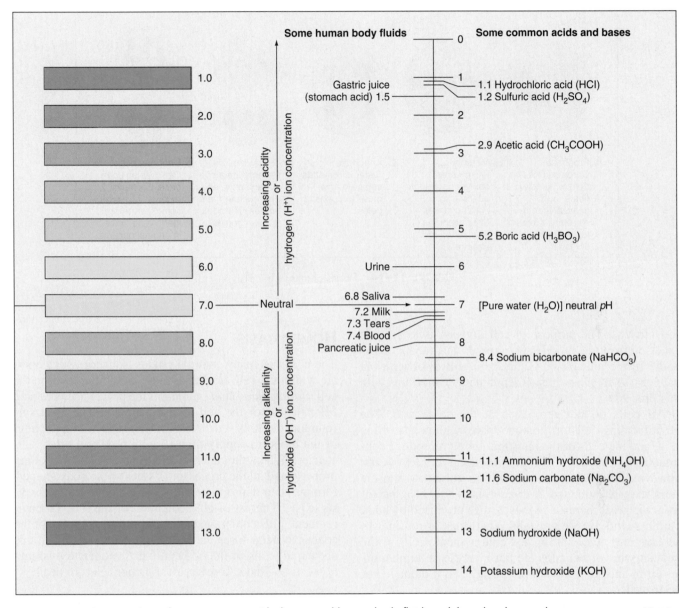

Some human body fluids

Some common acids and bases

Increasing acidity
or
hydrogen (H⁺) ion concentration

Increasing alkalinity
or
hydroxide (OH⁻) ion concentration

Neutral — 7.0

Gastric juice (stomach acid) 1.5
1.1 Hydrochloric acid (HCl)
1.2 Sulfuric acid (H_2SO_4)

2.9 Acetic acid (CH_3COOH)

5.2 Boric acid (H_3BO_3)

Urine

6.8 Saliva
7.2 Milk
7.3 Tears
7.4 Blood
Pancreatic juice

[Pure water (H_2O)] neutral pH

8.4 Sodium bicarbonate ($NaHCO_3$)

11.1 Ammonium hydroxide (NH_4OH)
11.6 Sodium carbonate (Na_2CO_3)

13 Sodium hydroxide (NaOH)

14 Potassium hydroxide (KOH)

FIGURE 11–13 *p*H values of some common acids, bases, and human body fluids and the color changes that can occur to a *p*H strip when tested

Frequently the determination of acidity or alkalinity of a body fluid or solution is desired. This measurement is referred to as the *p*H. A *p*H value of 7.0 on the *p*H scale indicates the solution has the same amount of hydrogen ions as hydroxide ions and therefore is neutral. An example of a neutral solution is water. A *p*H value between 0 and 6.9 indicates an acidic solution. The lower the number, the stronger the acid or hydrogen ion concentration. A *p*H value of 7.1 to 14.0 indicates the solution is basic or alkaline. The higher the number is above 7.0, the stronger the base or hydroxide ion concentration. The *p*H inside most cells is maintained between 7.2 and 7.4. The *p*H values of some common acids, bases, and human body fluids and their effect on a *p*H testing strip are shown in Figure 11–13.

CELLULAR DIVISION

The division of cells is known as mitosis and is controlled by the nucleus of the cell (Figure 11–14). When a cell is preparing to divide, the two pairs of centrioles, just outside the nucleus, move to opposite sides of the cell (A). Spindle fibers form and attach to the chromosomes, which "line up" in the center (B). The chromosomes divide and move toward the centrioles at different ends of the cell (C). The spindles then dissolve, and a nuclear membrane develops around each new set of chromosomes (D). For unknown reasons, the cell then pinches itself in two, thereby making two new cells (E) called daughter cells. Mitosis results in the formation of two daughter nuclei with the exact same genes as the mother

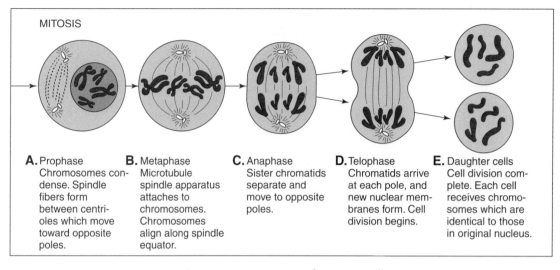

MITOSIS

A. Prophase
Chromosomes condense. Spindle fibers form between centrioles which move toward opposite poles.

B. Metaphase
Microtubule spindle apparatus attaches to chromosomes. Chromosomes align along spindle equator.

C. Anaphase
Sister chromatids separate and move to opposite poles.

D. Telophase
Chromatids arrive at each pole, and new nuclear membranes form. Cell division begins.

E. Daughter cells
Cell division complete. Each cell receives chromosomes which are identical to those in original nucleus.

FIGURE 11-14 *Stages of mitosis in cells*

cell nucleus. The purpose of cell division is to provide exact duplication of cells for growth and repair of the body. In the unit on immunity, you will discover what happens when an antigen (foreign matter) interferes with this process.

All cells do not reproduce at the same rate. The bloodforming cells of the bone marrow, the cells of the skin, and the cells of the intestinal lining reproduce continuously. Muscle cells only reproduce every few years; however, muscle tissue formed of voluntary muscle cells may be enlarged with exercise. This is apparent from the great increase in muscle size produced by body builders who use weights and repetitions of routines to achieve muscle definition and enlargement. Cells of the **nerve** tissue, or **neurons**, do not increase in number after birth, and some cannot be regenerated if damaged or destroyed.

There are many kinds of cells with different shapes and sizes. The characteristics shown previously in Figure 11–7 are common to most cells. However, cells like those in the blood (red, white, and platelets) and the nerve cells are very different and perform specialized functions. With this specialization, some of the other cell functions may be lost, such as the ability of some nerve cells to reproduce. Specialization also results in an interdependence among cells to enable them to carry out their activities. One type of cell that is very different is the sex cell (gamete), which is responsible for reproduction. During a process known as meiosis, the ovum from the female and the spermatozoon from the male each reduce their respective 46 chromosomes to 23, one half the normal amount. When fertilization occurs, the two cells combine to form a single cell called a zygote, which will then have the full set of 46 chromosomes, 23 from each parent. The zygote will subsequently, by mitosis, divide again and again until the new being is fully developed. This cellular activity will be more fully discussed in the unit on the reproductive system.

HOMEOSTASIS

The body has many control systems, some of which operate within the cell. It is important that the fluid within the cell *(intracellular fluid)* maintains the proper chemical and *p*H balance for the cell to maintain life. The fluid surrounding the cells *(extracellular fluid)* mixes with the fluid of the blood to supply the cell with food and other substances. When the internal environment is functioning properly and all the organs and tissues of the body are performing their appropriate tasks, a condition of **homeostasis** exists. This is a stable condition of the internal environment. This condition continues until one or more of the control systems loses the ability to maintain it. When this occurs, all cells of the body suffer. A moderate dysfunction causes illness; a severe dysfunction leads to death.

MUTATIONS AND TRAITS

Remember that the DNA is a code that provides information to the cell. It has been compared to the dots and dashes of the Morse code or the "0s" and "1s" of the computer binary code. When these symbols are arranged in different sequences, they form different words. The same is true of DNA. When DNA is being replicated, if some is lost, rearranged, or paired in error, the resulting change in instruction of the genetic code could lead to an improperly-functioning or missing protein when the DNA's code is translated. This is known as **mutation**. Genetic mutations can be caused by internal or external factors. Internal factors are those which occur during replication and abnormal metabolism. External causes include chemicals, x-rays, sunlight, and other radiations. A mutation is a change in a cell resulting from a chemical change in the structure of the gene. It is first reflected in the RNA copy, then in the enzyme or protein, and finally in the appearance of new **trait**. A trait is the recognizable result of the effect of a gene or group of genes.

Mutations may be either dominant or recessive. They may result in no change or can produce minimal or drastic alterations. They can be beneficial or lethal. Mutations provide an essential key for evolutionary change, even among humans.

Single genes may be involved in one of three patterns of inheritance as they produce recognizable traits. These are known as dominant, recessive, and X-linked. A **dominant gene** can produce a trait without regard to the nature of its pair member (Remember: There are two genes, one each from the mother and father). Dominant disorders are usually milder and result in structural defects rather than abnormalities in function. A **recessive gene** is one whose presence within the pair does not result in a recognizable trait *unless* both members of the gene pair are of a similar mutation; in this case, a recessive disorder would occur. Such people are known as **carriers**. The third pattern of inheritance is sex- or **X-linked** because the defective gene is carried on the X chromosome. In some instances, the pattern is dominant with direct inheritance, and in others it is recessive, depending primarily upon which parent has the defect and whether the child is male or female.

Another classification of traits deals with results caused by two mechanisms: multifactorial inheritance and chromosomal aberrations. Multifactorial inheritance refers to the fact that a trait appears as a result of the combined influence of a number of genes and environmental factors. The environment can be within the uterus before birth or in general following birth. The trait appears as a result of the accumulation of sufficient factors to raise the level of genes above a certain threshold, beyond which the trait develops. Examples of this are height and intelligence. Both are influenced prenatally by parental influence and postnatally by environment. Another example is pyloric stenosis, a narrowing of the opening from the stomach into the small intestines that interferes with the passage of food. It is linked to the possibility of a viral infection during pregnancy, and it is known that the child's sex is a factor. Development of the disorder is *influenced* by the fact that the threshold of the factor is lower in the male than in the female. Examples of environmental exposures that are classified as toxins include the use of alcohol (which results in small birth weights), liver dysfunction, and the condition known as fetal alcohol syndrome. Another toxin is the drug Diethylstilbesterol (DES), which can adversely affect sex organ development.

Chromosomal abnormalities are the result of either a group of genes occurring in excess or as a deficit of genetic materials. There is a difference in the general effects depending on whether the abnormality affects pairs numbered 1-22, called autosomes, or the X and Y chromosomes of the 23rd pair. Autosome genetic imbalance is invariably associated with mental retardation and exerts influence on the development of the physical structure of the early embryo and fetus. Incorrect numbers of X and Y chromosomes are among the most common chromosomal abnormalities. Chromosomal abnormality can occur as the result of abnormal cell division and from exposure to toxins.

GENETIC AND CONGENITAL DISORDERS

As we have learned, genetic and **congenital** disorders can result from improper sex cell division at the time of fertilization, from the inheritance of an altered gene or genes, from environmental factors, or from toxins. They cause structural defects, retardation, and physiological disorders. These are collectively called genetic or congenital disorders.

There is a difference between the two. The word congenital is defined as "occurring during fetal life; not hereditary." In other words, it is a "born with" condition. Genetic disorders result from initial cellular structure at conception. The more common disorders are discussed in the following content.

Cleft Lip

Description—The presence of a structural defect of the upper lip.

Signs and symptoms—It is characterized by a vertical split in the upper lip that often continues into the nostril. A cleft lip can be unilateral (one side) or bilateral (both sides) (Figure 11–15A).

Etiology—It is caused by the failure of the soft or bony tissues to unite during the eighth to twelfth week of gestation.

Treatment—Modern plastic surgery is very successful at closing the clefts and normalizing the infant's appearance.

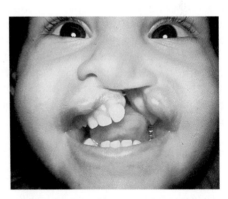

A

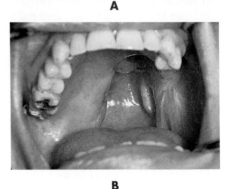

B

FIGURE 11–15 (A) Cleft lip, (B) cleft palate (Courtesy of Dr. Joseph Konzelman, School of Dentistry, Medical College of Georgia.)

Cleft Palate

Description—The presence of a structural defect in the roof of the mouth.

Signs and symptoms—It is characterized by an opening or hole to a total split of the palate. It is often associated with a cleft lip (Figure 11–15B).

Etiology—It is caused by the failure of the soft and bony tissues to unite during the eighth to twelfth week of gestation.

Treatment—Surgical intervention is necessary. The cleft can cause feeding problems for an infant because liquid is able to get into the nose and breathing passages. A temporary solution to the problem involves the use of various types of nipples or an inverted "spoon-like" feeder with a nursing nipple, which provides an artificial roof in the mouth. This allows the infant to suck milk until surgical repair can be done.

Color Vision Deficiency

Description—An inherited trait that makes perception of colors inaccurate. It is erroneously called "color blindness" because most people see some color; rarely do people see only black, white, and gray (Monochromatism).

Signs and symptoms—Most affected people see colors and do not realize they have a deficiency until they have a color vision test. The most common problem is distinguishing reds and greens, which can be a problem when driving an automobile. (See Ishihara color vision acuity color plates, Chapter 14, Unit 1.)

Etiology—The deficiency is caused by a defective gene carried on the X chromosome and occurs most frequently among men. Because men have only one X chromosome, it is more likely to be expressed. Women have two X chromosomes and are likely to have a normal gene that will dominate the defective one. Rarely the condition is caused by a severe lack of vitamin A or by retinal disease or cataracts.

Treatment—There is no treatment to correct the problem. Individuals with the deficiency must learn to compensate. It is estimated that seven million drivers in North America have the condition. The difficulty in recognizing traffic light colors and red taillights on cars accounts for some accidents. Studies have shown color defective drivers take much longer to respond to color signals. Traffic lights have been redesigned so red is at the top, amber in the middle, and green at the bottom. Experts suggest that adding a distinctive shape for each color would also be beneficial. White borders have been added to red stop signs to make them more visible. It has also been suggested that taillights be changed to green because it is the least sensitive color. Drivers must learn to compensate for their deficiency by allowing more distance from the car ahead and approaching intersections with extra caution.

Cystic Fibrosis (Sis'-tic fi-bro'-sis)

Description—A generalized dysfunction of the exocrine glands, affecting multiple organ systems. It is the most common fatal genetic disease of Caucasian children affecting 1 in every 2,000 live births. About 50% die by age 16, the rest survive up to age 30.

Signs and symptoms—May take years to develop. Includes sweat gland dysfunction resulting in salty tasting skin; wheezing; dry, non-productive cough; dyspnea; clubbed fingers; bulky, foul-smelling stools; and excessive appetite but poor weight gain.

Etiology—An autosomal recessive trait that probably causes an alteration in a protein or an enzyme.

Treatment—Treatment is aimed at helping the child lead as normal a life as possible. Salt is prescribed generously, and pancreatic enzymes and vitamins A, D, E, and K are added to food. Breathing exercises, aerosol therapy, postural drainage, and oxygen assist with breathing. Antibiotics are used aggressively when episodes of acute pulmonary infection occur. There is no cure.

A PEDIATRIC PERSPECTIVE

Recent research by Dr. Jeffrey Bartlett at Children's Hospital in Columbus, Ohio, may lead to a strategy to permit delivery of a normal copy of a gene to replace a defective one. He has been able to modify a non-pathogenic virus so that it will carry a "treated" gene to the epithelium of the airway cells. Patients with cystic fibrosis have defective fibrocystic genes that results in the development of the disease. This discovery will not only benefit these patients but effect many other gene therapy processes.

Down Syndrome (Sin'-drom)

Description—A well-known genetic **syndrome** (group of features) caused by improper cell division. Incidence in North America is about 1 in every 1,000 live births, depending on the mother's age.

Signs and symptoms—It is characterized by slanting eyes, a fold at the inner eye, a large tongue, pug nose, and microcephaly (small head). Other distinguishing features are a simian crease, (a single transverse palmer crease), slow dental development, small external ears, and a short neck. Mental retardation occurs in all cases, and there is some degree of growth restriction (Figure 11–16).

Etiology—Improper cell division results in the number 21 chromosome occurring in triplicate rather than as a pair, so the individual has 47 instead of 46 chromosomes per cell. Another form occurs when the long arm of chromosome number 21 breaks and attaches to another chromosome.

Treatment—There is no treatment to correct the disorder. Amniocentesis, a diagnostic test, is recommended

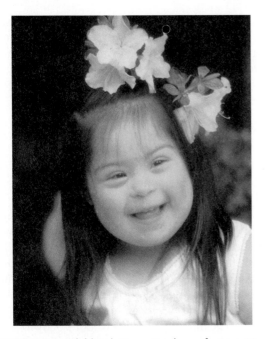

FIGURE 11–16 Child with Down Syndrome features (Copywright Marijane Scott, Marijane's Designer Portraits, Down Right Beautiful 1996 Calendar.)

when prenatal interviews indicate the possibility of a genetic problem. (See Unit 13.) It is also indicated in pregnancies of women past the age of 35. At twenty years of age, a woman has about 1 chance in 2,500 of having a child with Down syndrome, but by age 45, the risk rises to 1 in 40. Amniocentesis requires a small amount of amniotic fluid, which surrounds the fetus, to be withdrawn from the pregnant uterus. Skin cells from the fetus can be found floating in the amniotic fluid and can be grown in a culture for examination. The test can either relieve parental anxiety or can allow them time to prepare for managing a Down syndrome child. Early pregnancy termination can be achieved if findings are a cause of great concern for the parents.

Within a few years another option may be open to parents. In May of 2000, one of the scientific groups of the consortium working to decode the human genome completed the DNA sequence of the 21st chromosome. They learned it has only 225 genes and an approximate 33,827,477 decodable units of DNA. When scientists can identify the location and function of each gene on the chromosome, perhaps gene therapy could be devised to correct the abnormality. (See Discoveries in Human Genetics and New Genetic Techniques in this unit.) Other medical conditions have been traced to this chromosome, such as acute myeloid leukemia, Alzheimer's disease, epilepsy, Lou Gehrig's disease, and schizophrenia. This widely diverse group of seemingly unrelated diseases demonstrates the complexity of the human body.

Galactosemia (Ga-lakto-seem'-e-ah)

Description—An inherited metabolic disorder involving the digestion of milk and milk products. It occurs in about 1 in every 50,000 births.

Signs and symptoms—Usual signs are the failure to thrive, diarrhea, jaundice from liver damage, and severe vomiting. Other symptoms include enlargement of the spleen, cataracts, and a pseudo (false) brain tumor. Continued ingestion of galactose or lactose foods may cause mental retardation, progressive liver damage, and death.

Etiology—A recessive gene causes an inability to normally metabolize the sugar galactose, which is formed by the digestion of lactose in milk.

Treatment—Elimination of galactose and lactose from the diet will cause the side effects to subside. Infants must have breast or cow's milk replaced with a soybean-based formula. A galactose-free diet must be maintained throughout life. Screening of newborns is required in some states.

Hemochromatosis (Hem-o-kro-mat-o'-sis)

Description—A genetic condition of iron overload in the body. It is a common genetic disorder, affecting approximately 5 out of every 1,000 people. It is most prevalent in Caucasians of northern European descent. It has been overlooked in the past by physicians, but now more attention is being paid to its presence. Screening for the disorder is being recommended for all family members of diagnosed persons, but a team researching the disorder believes all young adult Caucasians should be screened at least once before age 40. The screening involves an inexpensive, simple blood test that detects the presence of a marker for iron status. Researchers found 70% to 80% of first-degree relatives (siblings, children, and parents) of diagnosed individuals were affected. Complications of cirrhosis of the liver, arthritis, diabetes, and congestive heart failure can be avoided by early intervention.

Signs and symptoms—Unfortunately, early signs are not observable. When complications arise, the signs and symptoms of those disorders are recognizable. Other signs may include increased skin pigmentation, usually bronze from increased melanin accumulation, but a metallic gray may also be visible from iron deposits in the skin. Other common abnormalities include depressed secretions from the pituitary gland, calcium deposits in cartilage, and iron deposits in the synovial fluid of the joints. Males may also have testicular atrophy and loss of libido.

Etiology—Complications arise because the body absorbs too much iron from foods as a result of a faulty metabolism. The absorbed iron is deposited in the tissues of the body. The slow accumulation of iron deposits in the cells causes tissue damage and the typical clinical features.

Treatment—The primary treatment is the removal of excess iron by withdrawing blood frequently until serum iron levels drop within normal range. It may take up to three years to obtain acceptable results. A drug, deferoxamine, mobilizes iron stores and promotes their excretion, but it is only about half as effective as blood withdrawal. Other systemic diseases that have developed must also be treated.

Hemophilia (He-mo-fil'-ee-ah)

Description—A sex-linked bleeding disorder carried by females but occurring only in males. Incidence is approximately 5 in every 40,000 live births.

Signs and symptoms—It is characterized by abnormal bleeding, which may be mild to severe, depending upon the degree of clotting deficiency. Typically there is easy bruising, hematomas, a tendency to nosebleeds, bleeding gums, and prolonged bleeding after injury or dental or surgical procedures. In severe cases, internal bleeding into joints, organs, and from major blood vessels is a cause for great concern. It is very dangerous when bleeding occurs within the brain, throat, or heart and can lead to shock and death.

Etiology—An inherited X-linked recessive trait with known transferral percentages. Female carriers have a 50% chance of transmitting the gene to each daughter, who then becomes a carrier, and a 50% chance of transmitting the gene to each son, who would develop hemophilia. The trait causes abnormal bleeding through the absence or deficiency of a clotting factor. A diagnosis is made following evidence from a clotting factor profile and a positive family history.

Treatment—The disorder is not curable but can be controlled to prevent anemia and severe deformities. Bleeding must be quickly stopped by administering the deficient clotting factors to raise the plasma levels so that the individual can form clots. Fresh, frozen plasma may be used if factors are not immediately available.

Klinefelter's Syndrome (Kline'-fel-ters)

Description—A sex-linked disorder which is caused by chromosome abnormality affecting, in varying degrees, approximately 1 in every 600 males.

Signs and symptoms—Mild cases probably go undetected. It usually becomes apparent at puberty when the penis and testicles fail to mature fully, often leading to sterility. Other symptoms are breast enlargement, mental retardation, sparse body hair, abnormal body build (long legs with a short, obese trunk), a tendency toward alcoholism, and often personality disorders.

Etiology—One or more extra X chromosomes resulting from abnormal meiosis. The severity depends on the number of extra X chromosomes—the more extra chromosomes, the more severe the disorder.

Treatment—If begun early, treatment with testosterone (the male hormone) may help reverse the feminine characteristics but will not reverse the sterility or mental retardation. Psychotherapy is indicated when sexual dysfunction causes emotional maladjustment.

Phenylketonuria (PKU) (Fee-nul-kee-toe-nur-ee-ah)

Description—A devastating, genetic metabolic disease, requiring early intervention to prevent its development and progress.

Signs and symptoms—The warning symptoms are not readily observable, so early detection and prevention are necessary. PKU disorders can be diagnosed from blood and urine tests. Newborn's blood is routinely checked at birth, but because enzyme levels may be normal at that time, a follow-up urine test is done at about the second week of life.

Etiology—The inability of the newborn's body to act upon an amino acid called phenylalanine. The newborn lacks the necessary liver enzyme, so the amino acid builds up in the blood and tissues causing brain damage, which results in profound retardation, seizures, and stunted growth.

Treatment—A restrictive diet is indicated to keep levels of phenylalanine low. This requires elimination of natural proteins from the diet and a milk substitute that does have a normal amount of other amino acids, carbohydrates, and fat until at least age five or six. The child must avoid breads, cheese, eggs, meat, poultry, fish, nuts, flour, and legumes. This must be carefully monitored to avoid brain damage.

Spina Bifida (Spi-na Bif'-i-da)

Description—A structural malformation of the spine in which the posterior portion of the spinal tissues fail to close during the first three months of pregnancy. These malformations occur in three forms: spinal bifida occulta, meningocele, and myelomeningocele. (See Spinal Cord Defects, Chapter 11, Unit 2, for more information. See also Figure 11–42.)

Talipes (Tal'-i-pez)

Description—A structural malformation of the feet, commonly called clubfoot (Figure 11–17).

Signs and symptoms—It is characterized by varying degrees of inward, outward, downward, or upward turning of one or both feet.

Etiology—The result of a deformed talus (foot bone) and a shortened Achilles tendon, apparently caused by a combination of genetic and in utero environmental factors. There is a strong heredity factor in some instances and an apparent arrestment of development during the ninth and tenth weeks of life when the feet are formed.

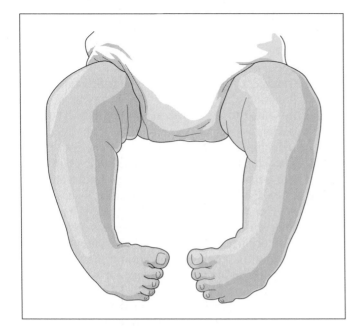

FIGURE 11–17 Talipes

Treatment—A distinction needs to be made between true and apparent clubfoot. X-ray reveals whether the talus and calcaneus bones of the foot are superimposed. Correction involves three stages: correcting the deformity, maintaining the correction, and long term observation. Surgical correction is done shortly after birth. Repositioning is maintained by a cast. After correction, proper alignment must be maintained through exercise, night splints, and special shoes. A deformity that resists manual correction or a neglected clubfoot will require surgical adjustment of the bone and tendons.

Turner's Syndrome (Turn-ers sin'-drom)

Description—A sex-linked disorder with a group of structural defects which affects about 1 in 10,000 newborn females.

Signs and symptoms—It is characterized by short stature, webbing of the neck, a low hairline, a wide chest with broadly spaced nipples, poor breast development, and underdevelopment of the genitalia. The ovaries fail to develop, making the female sterile. Often it is not recognizable until lack of menses and developing genitalia become apparent. The disorder also causes an abnormality of the aorta and edema of the legs and feet.

Etiology—The affected individual has only 45 chromosomes because the sex cells fail to divide correctly in meiosis, causing only one sex chromosome to be present in their cells.

Treatment—The use of estrogen (female hormone) after age 13, to prevent growth from stopping, will induce sexual maturation but doesn't reverse the sterility. Psychotherapy is indicated to deal with the emotional adjustment required to deal with the disorder.

DISCOVERIES IN HUMAN GENETICS

An article titled "Vital Data" appeared in the March 1996 publication of *Scientific American*. It reports that in 1990 a 15-year, $3 billion, federally-funded study called "The Human Genome Project" was formed to analyze human genetics at the molecular level. The project was launched because it seemed to promise the best hope for ultimately defeating not only diseases long known to be inherited but also those with more subtle links, like cancer. The planners estimated it would take several tens of thousands of technician years to find the sequence of all the DNA bases and the human genes and 390,000 pages to list them. The sequencing, it was believed, would reveal the possible functions and location of the estimated 100,000 human genes. But first it was necessary to devise "a genetic map," or diagram, which describes how thousands of known marker sequences in the chromosomes separate and recombine. They also needed physical maps to show the order along a chromosome of recognizable sequence sites. Using the maps, a researcher could compare a given condition's pattern of inheritance with that of the marker sequences. This makes it possible to determine where a gene that causes the condition might be located. Computers can then "match" the reams of data coming from sequencing machines onto the sites on a physical map. By comparing the two maps, it is possible to quickly find genes associated with an illness.

In February of 2001, two different scientific groups published the first drafts of the human genome in two leading scientific journals, *Science* and *Nature*. This accomplishment will likely revolutionize the understanding and treatment of disease. The studies indicate that humans have between 26,000 and 40,000 genes. The genome is the approximate 3 billion letter code of the human DNA that is the chemical sequence containing the basic information for building and running a human body. This chemical sequence determines every characteristic in the human body, from eye color to vulnerability to disease.

The number of genes discovered was surprisingly low, not much greater than the number found in other species, such as the fruit fly. The sequencing of the human genome was completed five years earlier than expected because of the significant development of new technologies. These same technologies are now being used to help diagnosis human diseases, design custom treatments, and even to identify criminals.

Although the newly discovered maps of the genome are considered to be just drafts, they are already providing breakthroughs in medicine. It is predicted that science will be able to zero in on the genetic factors involved in diabetes, heart disease, and other common disorders within the next 5 to 10 years. Cancer drugs are already being targeted at the molecular level of the disease. Companies have been formed that are taking blood samples from volunteers with known diseases to compare the codes and to identify the responsible genes.

In the course of this project, many other genetic technologies have been developed, such as gene therapy and gene transplantation. When genetic mutations are isolated, tests can be developed to identify their presence. Diagnostic technology has been developed that can simultaneously analyze DNA from patients for the presence of many different mutations on multiple genes. When the effects of mutations are known, test results can be a medical bonanza. It will be possible to indicate how likely a person is to develop a disease and, hopefully, determine a treatment or at least a method of control. In the course of the genome project, other genetic technologies like gene therapy and gene transplantation have been developed which will hopefully permit treatment of faulty genes. Although science is much closer to understanding defects in genes and the diseases that result, cures based upon changes in the genetic code may be years away while new drugs and ways to deliver corrected genes into defective cells are developed.

The exciting new technology is not without its critics. Abuses of the new science have already begun. Commercial value of certain DNA sequences are enormous. Efforts are being made by scientific companies to obtain "gene-based patents," which are certain to lead to vicious legal battles. Drug companies are spending hundreds of millions of dollars to identify genes connected to diseases because it will lead to molecules that are good targets for drugs and diagnostic reagents.

There is a potential problem with protecting against the misuse of individual genetic information. Discrimination in employment and life and health insurance has already surfaced. People with a genetic condition, or who are at risk for one, are often turned down for employment or insurance and some have lost their current jobs and coverage. They are declining the opportunity to have their children tested, even when it would be medically valuable, for fear of "labeling" them and therefore making their insurability or future employment questionable. There is concern that insurers might even classify the mutations as a pre-existing condition and refuse to cover any treatments related to that condition. Some testing is being done under false names, and researchers are being forced to obtain special legal documents called Certificates of Confidentiality that prevent courts from gaining access to data gathered in a study. Some adoption agencies are even requiring prospective parents to "pass" a genetic test before approving adoptions. Several states have enacted laws to limit descrimination based on genetic data. Congress is working on federal legislation to discourage or prevent insurance discrimination nationally.

On the positive side, mutated genes have now been identified for some diseases such as cystic fibrosis, polycystic kidney disease, some forms of Alzheimers and cardiovascular diseases, and hereditary forms of breast and colon cancers. Tests are becoming more commonplace. If someone is identified as having the mutated gene, the known percentages for its disease probability can be provided. With the near certainty for contracting specific inherited malignancies, some people have gone so far as to elect surgical removal of both breasts and entire colons in order to save their lives. Until unique new therapies can be developed, little else can be done.

Some researchers worry about uncontrolled testing and the interpretation of results. Many physicians are not well enough informed to be giving genetic advice. The psychological harm from DNA testing is also receiving growing attention. The fear of consequences and of discrimination overshadows the benefits. Genetic counselors believe that because of the potential for harm, children should not be tested for mutation-predicting diseases that will not develop until adulthood *unless* there is a possible medical intervention available. Yet the tests have gone on. One incident occurred reportedly because parents wished to avoid paying for a college education if their child was likely to develop an hereditary disease for which there is no cure. Truly, standards are needed. Leaders of the genome project acknowledged from the beginning that human genetics can be used to harm as well as to help. They have devoted millions of dollars to studying ethical, legal, and social questions. Yet, technical gains are outrunning the attempts of professional societies and government regulators to guide the use of the technology. Governments around the world are working on legislation to protect individual rights and confidentiality. Keep alert for reports. Watch for releases of information on this dramatic new medical field.

NEW GENETIC TECHNIQUES

Polymerase chain reaction is a technique being used in molecular biology to allow scientists to isolate, characterize, and produce large quantities of specific pieces of DNA from very small amounts of starting material that would otherwise be undetectable. Practical applications are applied to prenatal and postnatal diagnosis of genetic diseases, infectious disease (such as AIDS), and cancer. It assists in the matching of transplant recipients with donors, in the study of human genetic history and evolution, and in DNA fingerprinting by forensic scientists.

DNA fingerprinting is a detection and identification method that was first announced by a British geneticist in 1985. Except for identical twins, the DNA code for each individual is unique. Examination of blood, semen, and other body fluids at a crime scene can render positive identification when compared to the DNA molecules of the suspect. The evidence of a DNA match, in view of the great variance among the population, is considered to be a positive identification.

Genetic counseling provides information to a couple regarding their risks of having a child with a genetic disorder. Even "normal" couples face some risk with any pregnancy. About 3% of all live-born infants have a significant birth defect. Counseling is available to those couples who perceive their risk to be greater than the population in general. Information provided should include known risk statistics and offer available alternatives such as amniocentesis, pregnancy termination, adoption, artificial insemination (if the male has the risk factor), or information to permit understanding and acceptance of a pregnancy situation for which the parents agree no termination action will be taken.

Gene therapy is a new frontier in medicine. Persons who are born with a congenital disorder resulting from a defective gene could have a perfect gene inserted into their cells, preventing the development of or correcting the effects of the disease. This therapy began in 1990 when genetically engineered cells were infused into a four-year-old girl with a life-threatening immune deficiency. The infused cells were from her own blood into which researchers had inserted copies of a missing gene that produces the missing immune product. Again in 1991, gene therapy was used to treat cancer. Two patients who had advanced skin cancer were infused with their own white blood cells after they had been genetically altered to produce a tumor-killing protein. These early experimental attempts were the front-runners to the new exacting technology that will result from the genome project.

Genetic engineering is being used in the prenatal diagnosis of inherited diseases. The DNA pattern of cells from the parents, who may carry a gene for a congenital disorder, and the pattern of the fetus are compared. The disease status of the fetus can currently be determined in the following instances: thalassemia, Huntington's disease, cystic fibrosis, and Duchennes' muscular dystrophy.

Genetic engineering has allowed discoveries that could not otherwise have been made. An example is the discovery of oncogenes and tumor suppressor genes that play a role in causing some cancers. Scientists were able to cut the cancer-causing DNA into segments and identify the specific segments that were responsible for transforming normal cells into cancer cells. Much research remains to be done to achieve the promise of gene therapy and genetic engineering, but its value could be enormous.

There is always controversy when new techniques are introduced, but manipulating human cellular structure appears to have many ethical and moral issues to be resolved. On one hand is the opportunity to eliminate the devastating physical and mental conditions resulting from defective genes, and few people would deny the social and economic advantages of this capability. On the other hand, there are those who say man is playing "God," and that is not right. There is also the criticism that if you have enough money, you could "buy" perfect children of the sex, color, intelligence, and projected size you desired. When technology is known, regardless of ethical controls (which have yet to be developed), someone will always be operating outside the accepted practice for a price.

The reality of genetic identification discrimination hangs in the balance. Only the future will determine that outcome. As the director of the National Center for Human Genome Research said in *Scientific American,* "as the number of genetic tests grow, we are going to see it [genetic identification discrimination] happen on a larger scale, since we're all at risk for something."

TISSUES

As you are already aware, not all cells are alike. They may be transparent, as in the eye, or transmit electrical impulses or nutrients. Some have long thin fibers, and others produce secretions. When cells of the same type group together for a common purpose, they form a **tissue**. Tissues are from 60% to 99% water. The essential substances needed by the body are either dissolved or suspended in the tissue fluids. Therefore, water is indispensable to cell life, and lack of it causes death more rapidly than lack of any other substance, except oxygen.

Two common medical terms describe the opposites of tissue fluid balance. When there is too little fluid, the condition is known as **dehydration**. An abnormal accumulation of excess fluid, causing puffiness of the affected tissues, is known as **edema**.

Tissue Classifications

Tissues can be classified into four main types: **epithelial**, **connective**, nerve, and muscle.

Epithelial Epithelial tissues form the body's glands, cover the surface of the body, and line the cavities. Epithelium is the main tissue of the skin, which serves as a protective covering for the body. Epithelium also covers all the organs and lines the intestinal, respiratory, and urinary tract and uterus. Some epithelial tissues secrete fluids, such as mucus and digestive juices. Others selectively absorb nutrients, chemical elements, and water. The epithelium of the urinary bladder is uniquely arranged in folds to allow for expansion as the bladder fills.

Epithelial tissues in glands specialize to provide specific secretions for the body. Glands that secrete directly into the blood in the capillaries are known as *endocrine* or ductless glands.

Glands that produce secretions through ducts within the body are classified as *exocrine* (Figure 11–18). Two

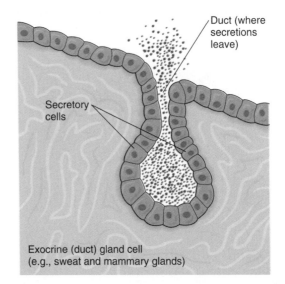

FIGURE 11–18 Epithelial cell tissue of an exocrine gland

glands, the liver and pancreas, produce both endocrine and exocrine secretions.

Connective Connective tissue forms the supporting structure of the body, connecting other tissues together to form the organs and body parts. There are several categories of connective tissue, but they can also be divided simply into soft or hard tissues. A soft type is adipose or fat tissue, which stores the body's reserve of food, fills the area between tissue fibers, insulates against heat and cold, and pads the body structures (Figure 11–19). Another form of soft connective tissue is stretchable and forms the subcutaneous layer of the skin. A soft but dense connective tissue in the form of tendons, ligaments, and organ capsules serves to support and protect organs and lend elasticity to the walls of arteries (Figure 11–20).

Blood and lymphatic vessels, lymph, the blood, and blood cells are forms of connective tissue. Cells in the blood carry nutrients and oxygen to the cells and pick up

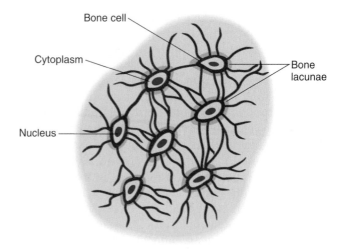

FIGURE 11–21   Hard connective tissue found in bone

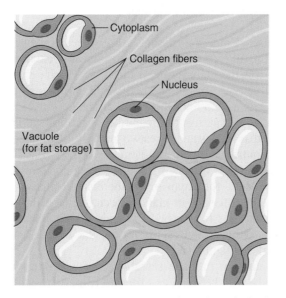

FIGURE 11–19   Adipose tissue throughout the body

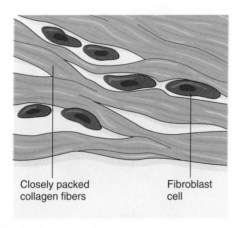

FIGURE 11–20   Dense fibrous connective tissue in ligaments and tendons

metabolic wastes for elimination. Lymph fluid consists of water, glucose, fats, and salt and is present in the spaces between the cells of the tissues and within the lymph vessels. Soft connective tissue plays a major role in the repair of damaged body tissue. The repair process involves new blood vessel formation and the growth of new connective tissue known as scar tissue. Excessive blood vessel development in the early stages results in a condition called "proud flesh." In instances of surgery or suturing (sewing) of a clean wound, the need for tissue regrowth and therefore the resulting scar are reduced because the cut edges are brought together closely by the surgical process. An excessive growth of scar tissue is called a **keloid**.

Hard connective tissue can be found in the cartilage and bones of the body. Cartilage is located between the bones of the spine (where it acts as a shock absorber and allows for flexibility) and in the ear, nose, and voice box (to provide shaping). Bone tissue is actually cartilage with the addition of calcium salts. This addition takes place gradually from birth until the tissue becomes hardened (Figure 11–21).

Bone tissue, which is also called **osseous** tissue, is not a lifeless material. Within most bone is a medullary cavity filled with yellow marrow, which is composed of fat, connective tissue, and blood vessels. Some long bones contain cavities filled with red marrow, which manufactures red blood cells. Because bone is a living tissue with a blood supply and nerves, it can easily repair itself when it is damaged.

Nerve Nerve tissue is found throughout the body. It serves as the body's communication network. The basic structural unit of the tissue is the neuron, which consists of a nerve cell body and fibers that resemble tree branches (Figure 11–22). The dendrites bring impulses to the cell body; the axon conducts impulses away. Neurons range from a fraction of an inch up to three feet in length.

There are three types of nerve cells or neurons. A *sensory neuron* in the skin or sense organs picks up a stimu-

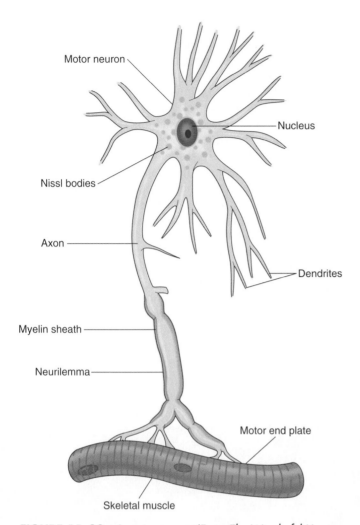

FIGURE 11–22 A motor neuron (From *The Wonderful Human Machine,* copyright 1979 by the American Medical Association.)

lus and sends it toward the spinal cord and brain. An *interneuron,* or *connecting neuron,* carries the impulse to another neuron. A *motor neuron* receives an impulse and sends a message, which causes a reaction.

Clusters of neurons form the nerve tissue. Nerves throughout the body join together to form the spinal cord, which in turn transmits electrical impulses to and from the brain. Nerves outside the brain and spinal cord are called *peripheral nerves.* The fibers of these nerves are covered with a fatty insulating material called a **myelin** sheath, which is then covered with a thin membrane called **neurilemma.** If a sheathed nerve fiber is damaged or cut, it can be surgically repaired, and a new fiber may form within the sheath, but nerve tissue recovers very slowly, if at all. Unfortunately, fibers of the brain, spinal cord, optic (eye), and auditory (ear) nerves lack sheaths and cannot be repaired by surgery when damaged or cut.

Muscle Muscle tissue is designed to contract on stimulation. Tissue that can be controlled at will with impulses from the brain is called **voluntary** muscle tissue. This type is found connected to the bones of the body and is called **skeletal** or **striated** muscle (Figure 11–23A). It gives us the ability to move our bodies.

Involuntary muscle action occurs without control or conscious awareness. There are two types of involuntary muscle tissue. One type, called **smooth** muscle tissue, is found within the walls of all the organs of the body except the heart. This type of tissue moves food and waste material through the digestive tract and changes the size of the iris of the eye and the diameter of arteries (Figure 11–23B). The other type of involuntary muscle tissue, called **cardiac** muscle tissue, is found only in the heart. Cardiac muscle fibers are joined in a continuous network and must contract together in a forceful, rhythmic action to pump blood throughout the body (Figure 11–23C).

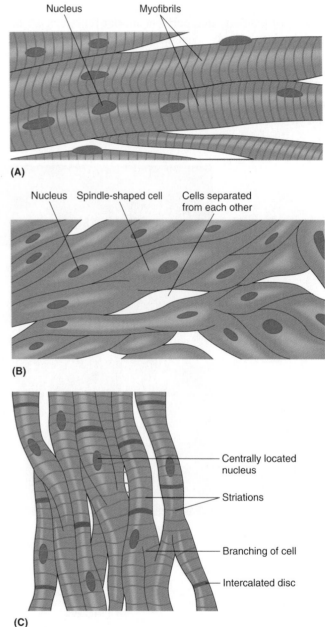

FIGURE 11–23 (A) Skeletal muscle tissue (striated voluntary) attached to bone, (B) smooth muscle tissue in walls of organs and blood vessels, (C) cardiac muscle tissue of the heart

ORGANS

The **organs** of the body are made of two or more types of tissue that work together to perform a specific body function. For example, the stomach is constructed with walls of smooth muscle tissue to "churn" the food; it is lined with one type of epithelial tissue, which secretes gastric juices, and covered with another type, which protects the organ; connective tissue fills the spaces between the other tissue fibers; nerve tissue controls the rate at which material is emptied from the stomach. (The roles of the organs will be discussed in more detail in the remaining units of this chapter.)

SYSTEMS

Organs of the body that perform similar functions are organized into a body **system**. Again as an example, the stomach joins with the mouth, throat, esophagus, and small and large intestines to make up the alimentary tract of the digestive system. The alimentary tract combines with the teeth, tongue, salivary glands, liver, pancreas, and gallbladder to form the total digestive system. The other systems of the body, which will be discussed individually, are the integumentary, skeletal, muscular, respiratory, circulatory, urinary, nervous, endocrine, and reproductive systems.

One additional "system" will also be discussed later in this chapter. The immune system is not normally considered, at least at the present time, a system. However, because the body's health and well-being directly depend on an intact and effective immune response, you should have a basic knowledge of its role in disease response. As scientists begin to better understand how it functions and what can be done to correct a malfunction, perhaps we can solve the mysteries of cancer, AIDS, and many other immunologically-based disorders. The basics of the complex subject of immunology are discussed in Unit 9.

Even a body system cannot function alone. All systems must combine their individual contributions for the health and well-being of the total human body. Figure 11–24 illustrates the body systems and briefly describes their functions.

Note: Figure 11–24 includes the lymphatic system. This system is usually considered to be part of the circulatory system. A summary of the fundamental construc-

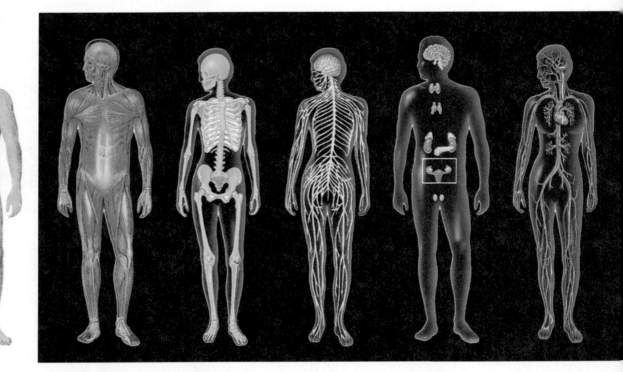

INTEGUMENTARY SYSTEM	MUSCULAR SYSTEM	SKELETAL SYSTEM	NERVOUS SYSTEM	ENDOCRINE SYSTEM	CIRCULATORY SYSTEM
Protection from injury and dehydration; body temperature control; excretion of some wastes; reception of external stimuli; defense against microbes.	Movement of internal body parts; movement of whole body; maintenance of posture; heat production.	Support, protection of body parts; sites for muscle attachment, blood cell production, and calcium and phosphate storage.	Detection of external and internal stimuli; control and coordination of responses to stimuli; integration of activities of all organ systems.	Hormonal control of body functioning; works with nervous system in integrative tasks.	Rapid internal transport of many materials to and from cells; helps stabilize internal temperature and pH.

FIGURE 11–24   The body systems (From Starr and Taggart, *Biology: The Unity and Diversity of Life*, 5th ed., copyright 1989 by Wadsworth Publishing Company.)

tion of the human body follows: it is composed of billions of cells, dividing individually, which are grouped together to form tissues that bind together to form organs to perform the functions of a system that cooperates with other systems to become the human body (Figure 11–25).

ACHIEVE UNIT OBJECTIVES

Complete Chapter 11, Unit 1, in the workbook to help you obtain competency of this subject matter.

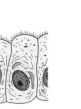 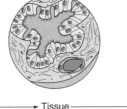 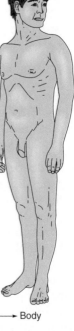

Cell ────────→ Tissue ────────→ Organ ────────→ System ────────→ Body

FIGURE 11–25 Fundamental cell to human body structures sequence

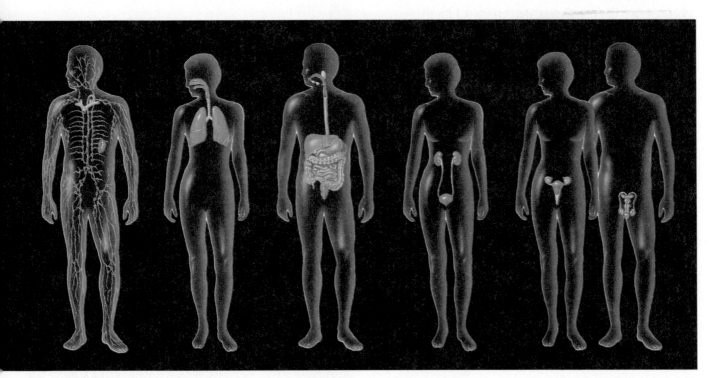

LYMPHATIC SYSTEM	RESPIRATORY SYSTEM	DIGESTIVE SYSTEM	URINARY SYSTEM	REPRODUCTIVE SYSTEM
Return of some tissue fluid to blood; roles in immunity (defense against specific invaders of the body).	Provisioning of cells with oxygen; removal of carbon dioxide wastes produced by cells; pH regulation.	Ingestion of food, water; preparation of food molecules for absorption; elimination of food residues from the body.	Maintenance of the volume and composition of extracellular fluid. Excretion of blood-borne wastes.	Male: production and transfer of sperm to the female. Female: production of eggs; provision of a protected, nutritive environment for developing embryo and fetus. Both systems have hormonal influences on other organ systems.

UNIT 2

The Nervous System

OBJECTIVES

Upon completion of the unit, meet the following performance objectives by verifying knowledge of the facts and principles presented through oral and written communication at a level deemed competent.

1. Spell and define, using the glossary at the back of the text, all the **Words to Know** in this unit.
2. Name the two main divisions of the nervous system.
3. Identify the two types of peripheral nerves and explain the function of the spinal nerves.
4. Describe simple and complex reflex actions.
5. Describe a synapse and the effects of various substances on its action.
6. Describe the purpose of the automatic nervous system, and explain the action of its two divisions.
7. Identify the main parts of the brain and their functions.
8. Name the coverings of the brain and spinal cord, and describe their purpose.
9. Describe the function of cerebrospinal fluid.
10. Name common diagnostic tests used to identify neurological disorders and possible reasons for their use.
11. List the functions of the hypothalamus.
12. Describe 25 diseases or disorders of the nervous system.

AREAS OF COMPETENCE (AAMA)

This unit addresses content within the specific competency areas of *Administrative procedures, Practice finances, Patient Care, Communication skills,* and *Instruction,* as identified in the Medical Assistant Role Delineation Study. Refer to Appendix A for a detailed listing of the areas. (Note: Although *Anatomy and physiology* is not identified in the study, a basic knowledge of the body's structure and function is an essential foundation to the competent performance of many roles.)

WORDS TO KNOW

action potential	cerebellum
angiography	cerebrospinal fluid
arachnoid	cerebrum
arteriography	coma scale
auditory	computerized axial
autonomic	tomography (CAT)
axon	cranium
central	dendrite

dura mater	parietal
electroencephalography	peripheral
(EEG)	pia mater
electromyography	plexuses
frontal	pneumoencephalograph
ganglion	pons
hypothalamus	positron emission
interneurons	tomography (PET
longitudinal fissure	scan)
lumbar puncture	sciatica
magnetic resonance	sensory
imaging (MRI)	skull x-ray
medulla oblongata	spina bifida occulta
meninges	subarachnoid
midbrain	subdural
migraine	sympathetic
motor	synapse
myelography	syndrome
occipital	temporal
olfactory	thalamus
optic	thorax
parasympathetic	ventricle

Ⓐ Library

The nervous system is the communication network that organizes and coordinates all the body's functions. It is a complex and somewhat difficult system to understand, and in most texts, it is not usually discussed early in the study of the body systems. However, in this text, it is being presented first. Hopefully, this will help you to better understand the involvement of the nervous system's regulatory action in the functioning of the other body systems as they are discussed.

You might think of the system as being something like your telephone system. You can make local, in-state, national, and international calls. You can easily call next door, but the further away you wish to call, the more number messages and the more "routing" of signals you need to complete your call. The phone picks up your voice (stimulus), converts it to impulses, and sends it along a charged line to a bundle of lines and on to phone company switching equipment. Every so often, the impulse is "boosted" to maintain your "voice." It may even be given special treatment and sent through space and bounced off a satellite, but the message is forwarded to its destination. Your nervous system operates in a similar but much more complicated manner. The system has two main divisions: the **central** nervous system (CNS), which consists of the brain and the spinal cord, and the **peripheral** nervous system, which includes all the nerves that connect the CNS to every organ and area of the body. The **autonomic** nervous system is a specialized part of the peripheral system and controls internal organs and other self-regulating body functions.

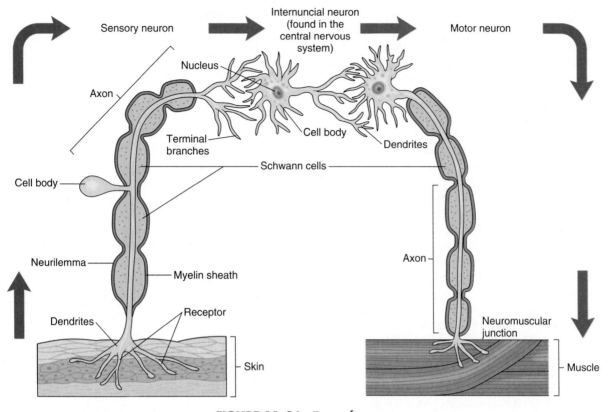

FIGURE 11-26 Types of neurons

Like in all systems, the basic functioning unit is the cell; in this system the unit is a nerve cell or neuron. As described in Unit 1, there are three types of neurons in nerve tissue: **sensory**, connecting, and **motor**. They receive stimuli or impulses, transmit impulses to other neurons, and deliver response actions to the muscles and glands. Connecting neurons are also called *associative* or *internuncial neurons*. Figure 11–26 illustrates the three types of neurons.

All nerve cells have a nucleus, cytoplasm, and a cell membrane. Scattered throughout the cytoplasm are little microscopic granular "dots" called Nissl bodies (see Figure 11–22). They may represent a store of nervous energy. The cell body has processes that are extensions of cytoplasm called **dendrites** and **axons**. A neuron may have many dendrites but only one axon. These extensions are also called *fibers*. Around the long thin axons of peripheral nerves are the Schwann cells. They form a tight protective covering called the myelin sheath and also play a part in the transmission of messages. The myelin is then surrounded by the neurilemma, an elastic sheath covering.

A nerve is composed of bundles of nerve fibers bound together by connective tissue. If a nerve is composed of fibers going from the sense organs to the spinal cord or brain, it is a *sensory* or *afferent nerve*. If it is carrying impulses from the brain or spinal cord to a muscle, organ, or gland, it is known as a *motor* or *efferent nerve*. Some

nerves have both kinds of fibers and are known as *mixed nerves*.

MEMBRANE EXCITABILITY

Nerves carry impulses by creating electric charges in a process known as membrane excitability. Neurons have a membrane that separates the cytoplasm inside from the extracellular fluids outside the cell, thereby creating two chemically different areas. Each area has differing amounts of potassium and sodium ions and some other charged substances, with the inside being the more negatively charged. When a neuron is stimulated, ions move across the membrane creating a current that, if large enough, will briefly change the inside of the neuron to be more positive than the outside area. This state is known as **action potential**. Neurons and other cells that produce action potentials are said to have membrane excitability.

To understand how impulses are carried along nerves or throughout a muscle when it contracts, we need to learn a little more about membrane excitability. Ions cross a membrane through channels, some of which are open and allow ions to "leak" (diffuse) continuously. Other channels are called "gated" and open only during action potential. Another membrane opening is called a sodium-potassium pump. By active transport, it maintains the flow of ions from higher to lower concentration levels across the membrane and restores the cytoplasm and extracellular fluid to their original value after an action potential occurs. This action is in response to an imbalance between the cytoplasm and the extracellular fluid. When diffusion takes place, particles move from an area of greater concentration to an area of lesser concentration.

The following simplified description explains how this whole process works.

1. A neuron membrane is "at rest." There are large amounts of potassium (K+) ions inside the cells but not very many sodium (NA+) ions. The reverse is true outside the cell in the extracellular fluid. Most of the open channels are for potassium to pass through, so it leaks out of the cell.

2. As the K+ ions leave, the inside becomes relatively more negative until some K+ ions are attracted back in, the electrical force balances the diffusion force, and movement stops. The inside is still more negative, and the amount of energy between the two differently charged areas is ready to work (carry an impulse). This state is called *resting membrane potential* (Figure 11–27A). The membrane is now polarized. The sodium ions are not able to move in because their channels are closed during the resting state; however, if a few leak in, the membrane pump sends an equal number out.

3. Now suppose a sensory neuron receptor is stimulated by something, such as a sound. This will cause a change in the membrane potential. The stimulus energy is converted to an electrical signal and if it is strong enough, it will depolarize a portion of the membrane and allow the gated sodium ion channels to open, initiating an action potential (Figure 11–27B).

4. The sodium ions move through the gated channels into the cytoplasm, and the inside becomes more positive until the membrane potential is reversed and the gates close to sodium ions.

5. Next, the potassium gates open, and large amounts of potassium leave the cytoplasm, resulting in the repolarization of the membrane (Figure 11–27C). After repolarization, the sodium-potassium pump restores the initial concentrations of sodium and potassium ions inside and outside the neuron.

   This whole process occurs in a few milliseconds. When this action occurs in one part of the cell membrane, it spreads to adjacent membrane regions, continuing away from the original site of stimulation, sending "messages" over the nerve. This cycle is completed millions of times a minute throughout the body, day after day, year after year.

But what happens when the impulse reaches the end of the neuron? You will recall that impulses travel across a neuron from the dendrites to the cell body and then to the axon. Here there is a minute space between the dendrites of the next neuron called a **synapse,** which the impulse must "jump" chemically. This space is technically called a

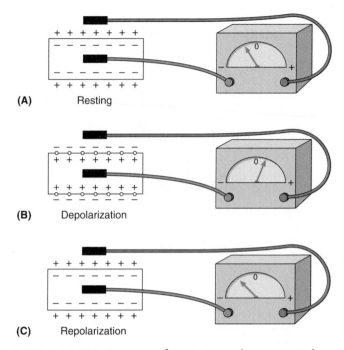

(A)　　　Resting

(B)　　　Depolarization

(C)　　　Repolarization

FIGURE 11–27 Sequence of events in membrane potential and relative positive and negative states:
(A) Normal resting potential—(negative inside/positive outside)
(B) Depolarization—(positive inside/negative outside)
(C) Repolarization—(negative inside/positive outside)

synaptic cleft. Impulses from the sending cell release chemical messengers called neurotransmitters into the cleft. These substances are signaling molecules that can cause a rapid change in the membrane potential of the receiving cell. These chemicals can either speed up or slow down the transmission. Normally nerve impulses travel about 200 miles per hour. The intake of alcohol, for instance, seems to aid the chemical that causes impulses to be blocked, and our reactions are therefore slowed down. Other chemicals, such as stimulant drugs and wartime nerve gases, cause the release of a chemical that allows the transmission of impulses to speed up, even to the point of causing a flood of impulses to the brain resulting in the possible breakdown of the body's ability to function.

Scientists have discovered that a number of mental disorders are the result of imbalances in brain chemistry. This has resulted in the design of new medications for treating specific mental disorders and behavior problems. The best known of the new drugs is probably Prozac. It inhibits the sending cell from reabsorbing the chemical serotonin. Research had indicated that depressed people had less serotonin than people who were not depressed, so by blocking its reuptake, the effect of a small amount of serotonin on the receiving cell is boosted (Figure 11–28).

A disease condition called tetanus results from the effects of the bacteria *Clostridium tetani* on the nervous and muscular systems. Bacteria invade the body through a puncture wound from a contaminated object or an animal

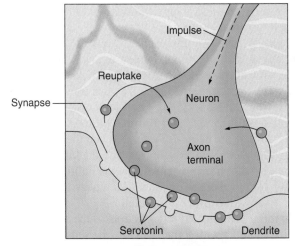

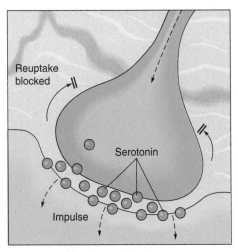

FIGURE 11–28 Transmission of a nerve impulse across a synapse is chemical. People who are depressed have less of the neurotransmitter serotonin. Note: The serotonin released from the axon before the medication is reabsorbed by the sending cell. With the presence of a serotonin uptake inhibitor, such as Prozac, the reabsorption is blocked or slowed to increase the effect of serotonin on the receiving cell.

bite. The tissues deep in the puncture do not receive oxygen, so they die off and the bacteria multiply. A substance is released by the bacteria, which is toxic to the motor neurons that innervate the muscles. A neuron normally stimulates muscle tissue through *balanced chemical messages,* which alternately contract and relax the muscle tissue. This balance is essential to our ability to maintain erect stature and movement. However, with the release of the neurotoxin from the bacteria, excitation is unbalanced, and the inhibitory synapses of the motor neurons of the brain and spinal cord are affected, thereby allowing excessive contraction of the muscles. (Without the control of the "inhibitor," the message goes on full permission to contract.) The muscles cannot relax, and there is a

prolonged, spastic paralysis of the muscles, which can result in death.

With these examples, it is apparent how the function of the nervous system affects the total welfare of the body. It is now important to learn how the nerves are organized in the communication network.

PERIPHERAL NERVOUS SYSTEM AND SPINAL CORD

The peripheral nervous system includes twelve pairs of cranial nerves that connect the brain directly to the sense organs (eye, ear, tongue, nose, and skin), the heart, the lungs, and other internal organs. Some cranial nerves, like the optic from the eye, have only sensory fibers, whereas others, like those to the heart and lungs, are mixed nerves containing both sensory and motor fibers. The peripheral system also includes 31 pairs of spinal nerves. The spinal nerves are both motor, to provide a function or movement, and sensory, to perceive stimuli; therefore, they are also mixed nerves (Figure 11–29).

All spinal nerves enter and leave the spinal cord, which is located within the canal created by an opening in each of the bones (vertebrae) of the spinal column. A cross-section of the cord would reveal a rounded white mass of myelinated nerve fibers with a notched area on the anterior surface (Figure 11–30). The white matter is mainly axons of **interneurons**. Some axons are grouped together into major sensory nerves going to a specific section of the brain. Others are grouped into major motor nerves going to their muscle or organ destination. Still others connect with each other up, down, and within the gray matter to provide control over activities that occur within the

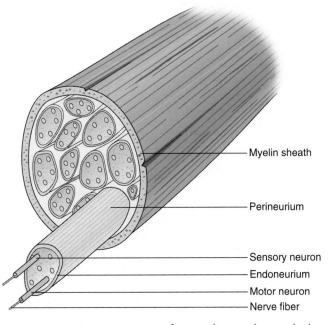

FIGURE 11–29 Cross-section of a spinal nerve showing both sensory and motor nerves (greatly enlarged)

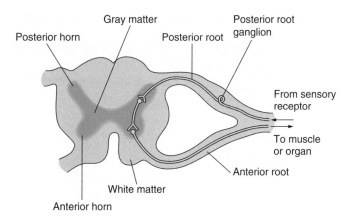

FIGURE 11–30   Cross-section of the spinal cord

cord itself. In the center of the white area is a gray area in the shape of an H, which is the nerve cell bodies and their fibers without the myelin covering. The gray matter is involved mainly with reflex connections in the spinal cord that deal with the reflexes involved in such things as walking or blinking.

A spinal nerve splits into two roots as it enters the cord. The rear root carrying sensory fibers to the cord enters at the rear horn of the H. The bulge on the rear root contains the sensory nerve cell bodies and is called a **ganglion**. The front root of the nerve leaves at the anterior horn of the H, carrying motor nerve fibers that have their cell bodies inside the gray matter of the cord. Neurons within the cord connect sensory to motor nerves.

Sensory neurons transmit messages from millions of special receptor cells to the spinal cord and on to the brain for interpretation and decisions. If a reaction is needed,

impulses from the CNS are transmitted to the appropriate muscle or organ over the motor neurons. Connecting interneurons route impulses throughout the body, permitting any nerve to communicate with any other nerve.

In very simple reflex actions where no interpretation or decision is required, the nerve impulse travels only to the spinal cord and back. The knee jerk test often used by physicians illustrates such a simple reflex and provides an evaluation of the nervous system. When the knee is hanging completely relaxed, the leg should kick up sharply when the tendon below the kneecap is lightly tapped (Figure 11–31). If there is no response, a nervous system disease or disorder can be suspected.

In more complicated reflex actions, such as a hand coming into contact with something hot, the sensory impulse is relayed through nerve cells to the spinal cord and up to the brain (Figure 11–32). There the impulse is interpreted, and the motor neurons carry the message back down the spinal cord and out the appropriate nerves. The eyes see the object, the hand will jerk away, and the voice may speak out.

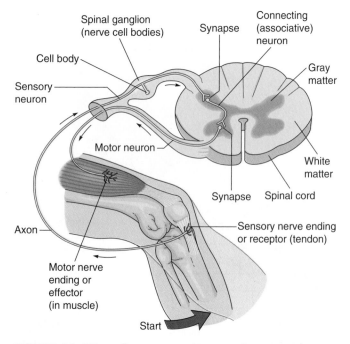

FIGURE 11–31   Reflex action. In this example, tapping the patellar tendon of the knee results in extension of the leg, producing the knee jerk reflex.

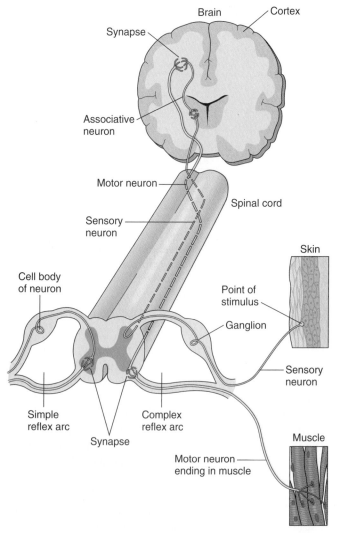

FIGURE 11–32   Complex reflex action (From *The Wonderful Human Machine*, copyright 1979 by the American Medical Association.)

Autonomic Nervous System

The autonomic nervous system is part of the peripheral nervous system. These nerves are involuntary and unconsciously regulate functions such as breathing, heartbeat, and digestion. The system consists of nerves, ganglia, and **plexuses** (networks of nerves). There are two divisions of the autonomic system. The **sympathetic** division accelerates activity in the smooth, involuntary muscles of the body's organs, and the **parasympathetic** division reverses the action and slows down activity. For example, the sympathetic nerves constrict blood vessels and speed up the heartbeat; the parasympathetic nerves dilate the blood vessels and slow down the heartbeat. These activities contin-

uously balance each other to maintain homeostasis in the body. However, this on or off mechanism does not apply to all organs because some do not have a dual nerve supply. Also, nerves in both divisions can have excitatory or inhibitory effects. At any given time, the actual effect depends on the net outcome of the two opposing signals.

The *sympathetic nervous system* begins at the base of the brain and runs down both sides of the spinal column in two tracts. These consist of nerve fibers and ganglia. The sympathetic nerves extend to all the vital internal organs, the blood vessels, the iris of the eye, and even to the sweat glands (Figure 11–33).

The *parasympathetic system* has two important nerves, the vagus and the pelvic nerve. The vagus extends from

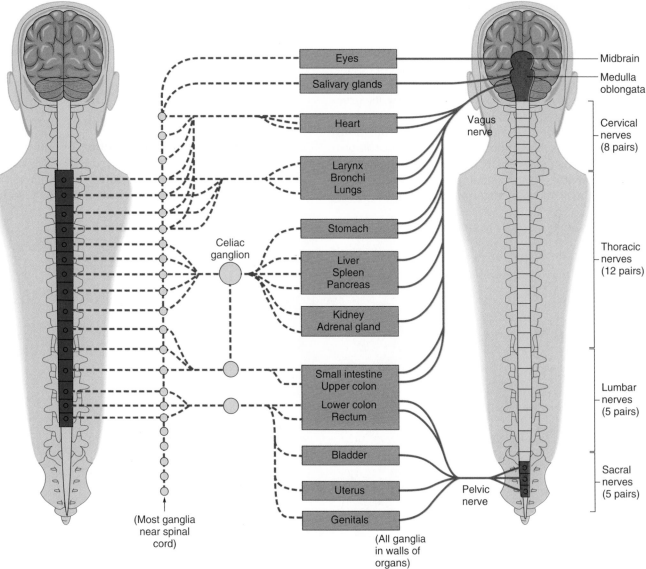

Sympathetic Outflow

Parasympathetic Outflow

FIGURE 11–33 Autonomic nervous system. Shown here are the main sympathetic and parasympathetic pathways leading out from the central nervous system to some major organs. As the lists of examples suggest, in some cases, the sympathetic and parasympathetic nerves operate antagonistically in their efforts on the organ. Keep in mind that both systems have paired nerves leading out from the brain and spinal cord. (From Starr & Taggart, *Biology: The Unity and Diversity of Life*, 5th ed., copyright 1989 by Wadsworth Publishing Company.)

the medulla oblongata of the brain and branches to the neck, chest, and upper abdominal organs. The pelvic nerve exits the spinal cord around the hip area and branches into the lower abdominal and pelvic organs. Both systems are strongly affected by emotions such as fear, anger, and stress.

The action of the autonomic system is extremely important to our ability to react in an emergency. It is frequently called our "flight-fright mechanism" because it accelerates our body functions to permit escaping or otherwise dealing with danger.

CENTRAL NERVOUS SYSTEM
The Brain

The brain is a large mass of nerve tissue with about 100 billion neurons. Scientists call it the most complex and challenging structure ever studied. This small organ, weighing only about three pounds, is a mass of interconnecting nerve cells that "talk" to each other continuously in both chemical and electrical language. The new discoveries in genetics and the ability to view its structure with new sophisticated equipment is allowing scientists to begin to understand how the brain functions. They are learning how groups of specialized cells produce memory, language, emotion, perception, and other complex activities. Understanding how a healthy brain operates allows them to determine what goes wrong

when disease strikes. The following discoveries are very exciting:

- Identifying disease-producing genetic mutations allows diagnosis of some inherited disorders and the ability to predict who will develop them. This knowledge will permit new therapies to alter the genes.
- Beginning to understand the programmed death of nerve cells that leads to degenerative diseases or expands the damage after a stroke may lead to new drugs to interfere with the process.
- Using the naturally-occurring chemicals that protect nerve cells from environmental destruction may prevent disease or reverse nerve injury.
- Understanding how brain chemistry affects mood and mental health is helping not only the patient with depression but hopefully others as well.

Scientists have found abnormal genes associated with Huntington's disease, Alzheimer's disease, amyotrophic lateral sclerosis, one form of epilepsy, Tay-Sachs disease (a disease affecting only the Jewish race), and two types of muscular dystrophy.

The Structure and Function of the Brain

The brain is protected and supported by surrounding membranes known as **meninges** (Figure 11–34). It is further protected by the **cranium** (skull). The brain surface has extensive deep furrows and folds and is divided into

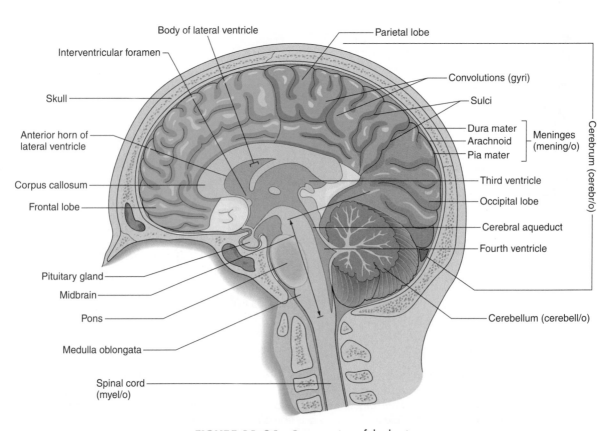

FIGURE 11–34 Cross-section of the brain

two hemispheres by a **longitudinal fissure**. The hemispheres are connected internally with nerve fibers and share information. The cerebral surface is covered with ridges and furrows known as *fissures* if they are deep or *sulci* if they are shallow. The elevated ridges between the sulci are called *convolutions*.

The brain is divided into five parts. The largest is the **cerebrum**, which controls sensory and motor activities. The cerebrum is further divided into lobes (Figure 11–35). The **frontal** lobe behind the forehead seems to be related to emotions, personality, moral traits, and intellectual functions. The frontal lobe is also the motor area for active voluntary muscle movements and two areas that control speech. The **occipital** lobe is the far back portion of the cerebrum. This area is associated with vision. The impulses of color and light received by the eyes are transmitted by the **optic** nerve fibers to the occipital lobe for interpretation. Between the frontal and occipital lobes is the **parietal** lobe; the motor area governing speech lies at its junction with the frontal lobe. It is the parietal lobe that receives impulses from receptors in the hands, feet, and tongue, among others, and sends impulses that cause movement in all these parts in response. This area also receives nerve impulses from sensory receptors for pain, touch, heat, and cold. A small **temporal** lobe lies on the side of the cerebrum. The **auditory** nerve association area is here, which provides us with the sense of hearing. The **olfactory** area, which provides our sense of smell, is within a small projection under the temporal lobe. It is connected by nerve fibers to receptors in the nasal cavity.

Beneath the cerebrum lies the part of the brain known as the **cerebellum**. This section is responsible for smooth muscle movement, muscle tone, and coordination of sensory impulses with muscular activity, particularly for equilibrium, walking, and dancing. If the cerebellum is

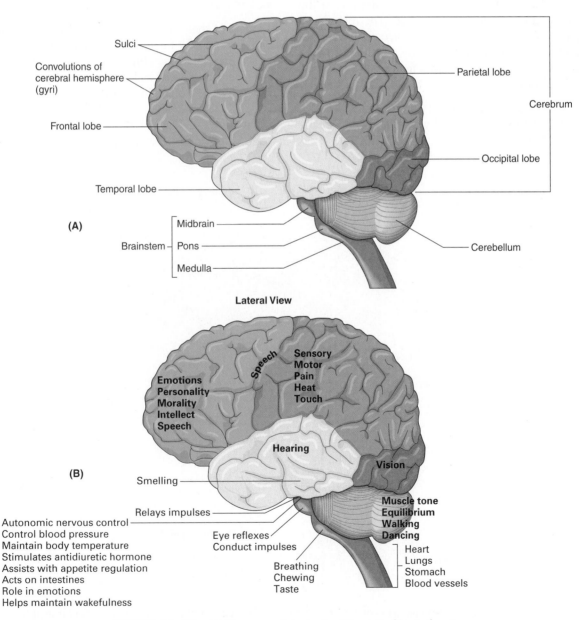

FIGURE 11–35 (A) The parts of the brain, (B) areas of brain function

damaged, many activities requiring coordination of muscles cannot be performed.

The **medulla oblongata** is the part of the brain that adjoins the spinal cord. The medulla influences, through the autonomic nervous system, the function of the heart and lungs, stomach secretions, and the size of the openings in blood vessels.

Just above the medulla is the **pons**. This part of the brain also helps to regulate breathing. It is the reflex center for chewing, tasting, and secreting saliva. A small part called the **midbrain** is superior to the pons. This area is the control center for some of the reflex movements of the eyes, such as blinking and changing the size of the pupil. It also conducts impulses between the brain parts above and below it.

In an area between the cerebrum and the midbrain are two major structures, the **thalamus** and the **hypothalamus**. The thalamus acts as a relay station for impulses going to and from the brain and those impulses from the cerebellum and other parts of the brain. The hypothalamus lies below the thalamus and is connected to the pituitary gland, midbrain, and thalamus by a bundle of nerve fibers. The hypothalamus performs many vital functions listed in the following:

1. Controlling the autonomic nervous system.
2. Controlling blood pressure by regulating the heartbeat and blood vessel constriction and dilation.

3. Maintaining body temperature.
4. Stimulating the production of an antidiuretic hormone to conserve water in the body and to cause thirst to maintain normal water balance.
5. Assisting in the regulation of appetite.
6. Increasing secretions and motility in the intestinal tract.
7. Playing a role in emotions such as fear and pleasure.
8. Helping maintain wakefulness when it is necessary.

The midbrain, the pons, and the medulla make up the brain stem. Doctors learned long ago that nerve fibers from the right side of the body cross over in the brainstem to the left side of the brain. The body's left side is likewise controlled by the right side of the brain. Therefore, when a person is paralyzed on the right side, there may be damage to the left side of the brain.

Meninges

Because of their common origin, the brain and the spinal cord are covered with the same meninges (membranes) (Figure 11–36). Three membrane layers make up the meninges. The innermost layer is called the **pia mater**, a delicate, tight-fitting covering containing blood vessels to nourish the nerve tissue. The middle layer, the **arachnoid**, is a delicate, lace-like membrane. The outer layer, called **dura mater**, is a tough, fibrous tissue which protects the CNS from being

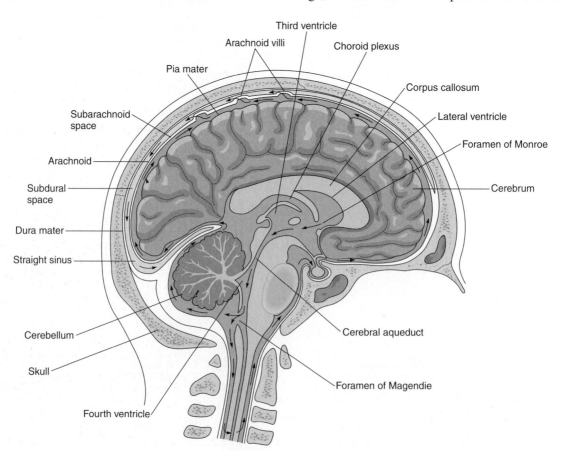

FIGURE 11–36 A diagrammatic representation of the meninges and the circulation of the cerebral spinal fluid from its formation in the choroid plexus until its return to the blood in the cranial sinus

damaged from contact with the bony surfaces of the skull and spine. The space between the dura mater and the arachnoid is called the **subdural** space. The **subarachnoid** space is between the arachnoid and the pia mater.

Cavities of the Brain and Spinal Cord

Within the brain are several hollow areas called **ventricles.** They extend into the lobes of the cerebrum and into contact with the other sections of the brain by means of small passageways. The central canal of the spinal cord is directly associated with the most inferior ventricle. There are also connections from the ventricles into the subarachnoid space of the meninges.

Cerebrospinal Fluid

The hollow cavities within the brain and spinal cord are filled with a liquid called **cerebrospinal fluid** (CSF). This fluid acts as a watery cushion or shock absorber to provide additional protection for the delicate tissues of the CNS. The fluid transports nutrients, primarily proteins, and carbohydrates to the brain and spinal cord. CSF is formed continuously within the ventricles of the brain at the rate of 450 mL (15 oz) per day. Only 150 mL are present at any one time in a normal adult. The fluid circulates within the cavities of the brain and spinal cord and the subarachnoid space, being reabsorbed into the blood vessels in special structures called *arachnoidal villi.*

DIAGNOSTIC TESTS

Diagnosis of neurological disorders and diseases may require the use of specific tests. Some of the more common tests and a few possible findings are as follows:

- **Arteriography**—(cerebral **angiography**)—A catheter (small tube) is inserted into an artery and threaded up to the carotid artery in the neck. A dye is injected through the catheter to show the cerebral blood vessels when x-rays are taken. This test can detect an aneurysm, hemorrhage, evidence of a cerebrovascular accident, and arteriosclerosis.

- **Coma Scale**—The Glasgow Coma Scale (GCS) is an assessment tool used to describe the level of consciousness (Figure 11–37). Terms often used to indicate this state are: semicomatose, stupor, lethargic, comatose, and others. The tool was developed in 1974 at the University of Glasgow to standardize what observers were reporting as evidence of the state of "coma" with head injury patients. The method is now acceptable in both European and American neurological centers as a quick, accurate, and simple tool for evaluating neurological status. The scale assesses three things: eye movement, verbal response, and motor response. The scale is based upon the need for more stimulation to induce a response in the patient. Paramedics may be trained to perform the grading at the accident scene or en route to alert the emergency room staff to the severity of the injury of the incoming patient. (This probably would not be encountered in the physician's office, but knowledge of the scale will be helpful in personal understanding and patient teaching.)

- **Computerized axial tomography (CAT or CT scan)**—A series of x-rays of layers of the brain to construct a three-dimensional picture. Useful for identifying tumors, bleeding, a blood clot, decrease in brain size, and brain edema. The machine is doughnut-shaped and was developed in the early 1970s. Today, CT scans can be equipped with spiral imaging to make images in seconds. The patient will have to remove earrings, any hair ornament, removable dental work, hearing aids, glasses, and any other item that might interfere with the test. After being positioned on the CT scan table, a special contrast material may be injected into the vein so that certain structures will appear on the CT scan images. The patient's head will then be positioned within the CT scan ring and immobilized with a band. The table moves slightly between each

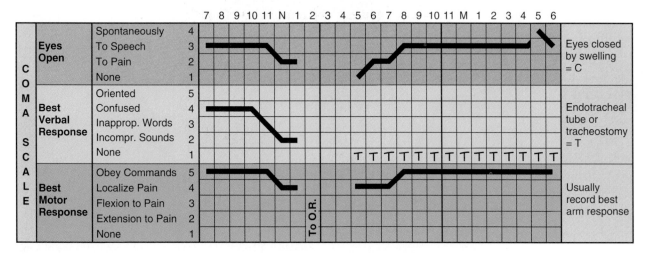

FIGURE 11–37 The Glasgow Coma Scale (GCS) includes three parts: assessment of eye opening, verbal response, and motor response. Each can be assessed hourly, given a numerical value, and plotted graphically.

scan. It takes about 15 minutes to complete a head CT scan. (See Chapter 16, Unit 4.)

■ **Electroencephalography (EEG)**—A brain wave test to detect abnormal electrical impulses that could be caused by a tumor, epilepsy, retardation, or psychological disorder. New technology has developed an ambulatory EEG monitor that helps diagnose neurological conditions, including fainting "spells" and seizures, by permitting continuous monitoring.

■ **Electromyography**—Needles are inserted into selected skeletal muscles. When the patient contracts the muscles, the nerve impulses are recorded, and the conduction time is measured to detect neuromuscular disorders or nerve damage. Electromyography is very useful to detect peripheral nerve problems such as with carpal tunnel syndrome (see Carpal Tunnel Syndrome, Unit 5).

■ **Lumbar puncture**—A spinal needle is inserted into the subarachnoid space between the vertebrae of the lower back, and CSF is removed for examination (Figure 11–38A & B). The procedure is indicated when infection is suspected, when there is hemorrhage from injury, or when the fluid pressure must be measured. When measurement is desired, a calibrated glass tube is attached to the needle, and the level of the fluid is observed and recorded.

■ **Magnetic resonance imaging (MRI)**—MRIs were pioneered in 1984. The machine resembles a large white tube and uses radio waves and powerful magnets to make pictures. When images of the brain and spine are needed, they are the machine of choice, usually as a follow-up of a CT scan finding. Their main advantage is that they can image from numerous angles. (See Chapter 16, Unit 4.)

■ **Myelography**—A lumbar puncture is performed, removing CSF and instilling a dye to outline the structures on the x-ray. This will show irregularities or compression of the spinal cord. If air is instilled following removal of CSF to visualize cerebral cavities, the procedure is called a **pneumoencephalograph**. It is used less frequently because of new technology.

■ **Positron emission tomography (PET scan)**—A newer form of imaging, which allows visualizing the physiological performance of the body. An "agent" is labeled or "mixed with" a radioactive substance. Agents can be many things, such as glucose or any number of hormones. After the material is injected into the blood, images are recorded to measure where the material ends up in the body. The images are further enhanced by the use of color, which can be selected by the operator. The brighter the shade of the color, the greater the amount of uptake. The PET scan has been useful with conditions such as epilepsy and Alzheimer's Disease.

■ **Skull x-ray**—To identify fractures and dense areas that indicate a tumor or increased pressure within the skull.

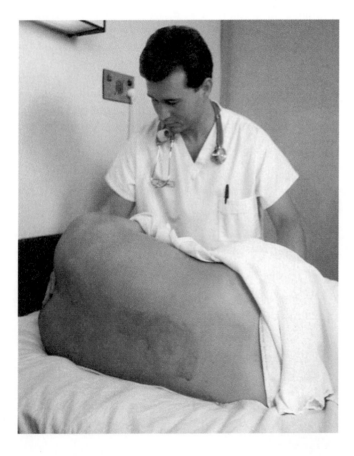

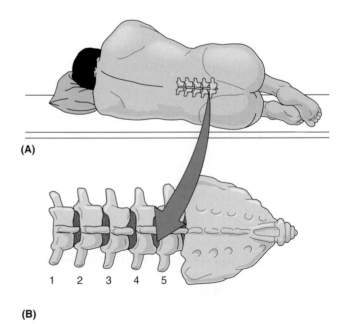

FIGURE 11–38 (A) Positioning of patient, (B) site of lumbar puncture

DISEASES AND DISORDERS
Alzheimer's Disease (Alz'-hi-merz)

Description—This is a progressive, degenerative disease that attacks the brain and results in impaired memory, thinking, and behavior. It affects an estimated four million American adults. It is the most common form of dementia (loss of mental function). More than 100,000 die annually, which makes it the fourth leading cause of death in adults, after heart disease, cancer, and stroke.

Signs and symptoms—Evidence of the disease includes a gradual memory loss, a decline in ability to perform routine tasks, impairment of judgment, disorientation, personality change, difficulty in learning, and loss of language skills. The individuals eventually become totally incapable of caring for themselves. Unfortunately, these are the same symptoms of other neurological disorders.

Etiology—The exact cause is unknown. Suspected causes include a genetic predisposition, a slow virus or other infectious agent, environmental toxins, and immunologic changes. The underlying cause of Alzheimer's Disease is the gradual extinction of certain brain cells. Brains from people who have died from Alzheimer's have been studied and show abnormalities called amyloid plaques and neurofibrillary tangles. About 20% of all cases are inherited, and these people tend to develop symptoms earlier in life than others. Scientists have also recently discovered several mutated genes that can cause the inherited form.

Treatment—There is no cure for Alzheimer's Disease. Scientists are working on preventing the death of nerve cells. Unlike other types of cells, nerve cells cannot reproduce themselves—they were meant to last a lifetime. It is normal for some brain cells to be gradually lost, but when a large population of a certain type die over time, it causes problems. Researchers are looking at neuroprotectors to keep cells alive even when there is a stroke or spinal cord injury. Cells manufacture several neuroprotectors on their own. It is their hope to develop neuroprotective drugs that could guard brain cells against damage and death or perhaps even help them regenerate. In the meantime, appropriate medication continues to be used to lessen agitation, anxiety, and unpredictable behavior; improve sleeping; and treat depression. Physical exercise, social activity, good nutrition, and health maintenance are important. A calm and well-structured environment may help maintain the patient's sense of well-being. It is especially important to support and assist the family in dealing with this devastating disease. The course usually runs from 2 to 10 years, but it can take as long as 20 years. The toll on the caretakers is unbelievable.

Currently, positive diagnosis of Alzheimer's is not possible until following death when the brain can be examined for the telltale signs of amyloid plaque; therefore, there is no way to rule out other degenerative diseases. Recently, a cell abnormality in Alzheimer's patients has been found and may lead to early diagnosis and treatment. The cells were grown and tested in the laboratory and showed collapsed potassium channels in their membranes, a finding which occurred only in the Alzheimer patients. Preliminary results are fairly reliable, and if after extensive clinical tests it appears to be diagnostic, it could save millions of dollars annually in diagnostic evaluations. Within the next 20 years, as the population ages, the incidence of the disease is expected to rise from the current level of about 4 million to approximately 12 million.

Although there's not yet a proven way to reverse or stop the disease, some promising treatments are being tested. A vaccine (AN-1792) is undergoing clinical tests in humans. The drug donepezil (Aricept), the herb ginkgo, and vitamin E have shown a slight slowing in the progress of the disease. In view of this, a recent panel's findings seem very important. After reviewing the current research on Alzheimer's, they came up with three "keys to cognitive vitality": (1) build reserve brain capacity, (2) acquire more knowledge, and (3) protect your brain from various forms of damage. It is possible to reduce the risk of Alzheimer's by following the eight steps to keep the brain function sharp:

1. Establish a brain reserve; think of it as a brain bank.
2. Exercise the body, it improves blood supply to the brain.
3. Eat well; it will protect against four potential causes: inflammation, oxidative stress, elevated homocysteine levels, and small strokes.
4. Consider a daily aspirin; some studies have identified it as a link to reduced risk.
5. Get enough folic acid through fortified foods or supplements because it keeps down serum levels of homocysteine. Alzheimer's patients have a higher than normal level.
6. Maintain a positive attitude because it may help hold off cognitive decline.
7. Avoid tobacco and excess alcohol. Smokers are more than twice as likely to develop Alzheimer's. Alcohol appears to be protective if only consuming one to two drinks per day.
8. Treat chronic conditions that can affect cognitive function such as hypertension, heart disease, high cholesterol, diabetes or depression.

The Alzheimer's Association publishes a list of 10 warning signs of the disease of which you should be aware. They are as follows:

1. Recent memory loss that affects job skills.
2. Difficulty performing familiar tasks.
3. Problems with language.
4. Disorientation of time and place.
5. Poor or decreased judgement.
6. Problems with abstract thinking.

7. Misplacing things (putting things in an inappropriate place, such as iron in the refrigerator).
8. Changes in mood or behavior.
9. Changes in personality.
10. Loss of initiative.

With the identification of genes that are believed to be involved with Alzheimer's, gene engineering and manipulation may effectively correct or replace the defective gene to stop the progression and restore former function.

Amyotrophic Lateral Sclerosis (ALS) (Am-e-o-tro'-fick) (Skleh-roh'-sis) (Lou Gehrig's Disease)

Description—ALS is a common motor neuron disease causing degeneration of the upper motor nerves in the medulla oblongata and the lower nerves in the spinal cord. It results in atrophy (wasting away) of the muscles. The onset occurs between the ages of 40 and 70 and is usually fatal within 3 to 10 years resulting from aspiration pneumonia or respiratory failure. The rate of incidence is two to seven people for every 100,000. It affects men four times as frequently as women.

Signs and symptoms—The symptoms are muscular atrophy and weakness, especially of the hands and forearms, plus problems with speech, chewing, and swallowing. If the brainstem is involved, respirations will be affected, and occasional choking and excessive drooling will result. Mental deterioration does not usually occur; therefore, the patient is acutely aware of the progressive physical deterioration, so depression caused by the consequences of the disease may happen.

Etiology—About 10% of the cases are from an inherited autosomal trait. Other causes are from vitamin E deficiency (which damages cell membranes), metabolic interference in the production of nucleic acid by the nerves, an autoimmune disorder, and the effects of a nutritional deficiency of the motor neurons.

Treatment—No effective treatment is available, only methods to control symptoms and provide emotional and physical support. Recent findings have uncovered a defective gene that produces excessive copper-containing enzymes that appear to lead to the death of nerve cells in the brain and spinal cord that control muscle movement. Experimental drugs appear capable of stopping the degenerative process by binding the copper in the enzyme, therefore prolonging the life of nerve cells containing the mutant enzyme.

Bell's Palsy (Pawl'-ze)

Description—This disease affects the seventh cranial nerve of the face. It occurs suddenly and will usually spontaneously subside within one to nine weeks.

Signs and symptoms—The affected nerve causes weakness or paralysis on one side of the face which causes the mouth to droop, on the affected side, resulting in the drooling of saliva. There is a distorted sense of taste and an inability to close the affected eye. Occasionally, pain in the area of the jaw's angle may be present.

Etiology—The cause is unknown for certain, but most scientists believe it results from a viral infection that inflames the facial nerve.

Treatment—Early treatment with steroids and an antiviral medication, such as valacyclovir (Valtrex), may shorten the course. Prednisone is usually prescribed in a high dose and then quickly reduced over 7 to 10 days. Moist heat applied to the face and jaw helps relieve any pain, but care must be taken to avoid burning the skin. It may be advisable to protect the eye with an eye patch while outdoors or if exposed to dust or pollutants.

Cerebral Palsy (Se-r-e'-bral)

Description—This disorder is associated with birth and involves both nerves and muscles. It is the most common crippler of children. Cerebral palsy appears in about 15,000 live births per year, 25% of which are either small or premature, weighing less than 5½ pounds. There are three forms of cerebral palsy: spastic, athetoid, and ataxic. About 70% of those affected have the spastic type.

Signs and symptoms—Characteristics of the spastic form are hyperactive tendon reflexes, rapid alteration between muscular contraction and relaxation, contracture tendency (permanent muscle shortening), and underdevelopment of the affected extremities. Approximately 40% of the children affected are also mentally retarded, 25% have seizures, and 80% have speech impairment.

Etiology—Cerebral palsy is probably caused by conditions that resulted in a lack of oxygen to the brain, hemorrhage, or brain damage. Prenatal conditions that may be associated with cerebral palsy include rubella (German measles), toxemia, maternal diabetes, and malnutrition. At the time of birth, such difficulties as forceps delivery, breech presentation, premature placental separation, premature birth, and either a too rapid or too prolonged labor are considered possible factors.

Treatment—There is no cure for cerebral palsy, only supportive treatment including physical, occupational, and speech therapy; psychological assistance; braces or splints; perhaps orthopedic surgery for severe contractures; muscle relaxors; and, when indicated, barbiturates and anticonvulsants to control seizures.

Encephalitis (En-sef-ah-ligh'-tis)

Description—This is a severe brain inflammation resulting from the lymphatic system infiltrating the brain tissue and causing edema and nerve cell destruction. The onset is sudden and acute.

Signs and symptoms—Symptoms include fever, headache, and vomiting with progression to stiff neck and back, drowsiness, and eventually restlessness, convulsions, and coma.

Etiology—It is usually caused by a virus-bearing mosquito or tick. It can also be contracted from viruses that cause polio, herpes, or mumps or following measles, rubella, or a vaccination.

Treatment—The disease is treatable with supportive drug therapy to control restlessness and convulsions, reduce edema, and relieve headache. Antiviral agents are ineffective except against herpes virus encephalitis.

Epilepsy (Ep'-i-lep-si)

Description—This seizure disorder affects 1% to 2% of the population. It is associated with abnormal electrical impulses from the neurons of the brain.

Signs and symptoms—The disorder is characterized by either petit or grand mal seizures. Petit mal seizures are of short duration and mild. Grand mal seizures may last up to five minutes with convulsions, loss of control of bodily functions, and unconsciousness.

Diagnosis is made based on evidence of seizure characteristics, a positive EEG (electroencephalogram), and various x-ray procedures.

Etiology—It is believed to be caused by either abnormal brain chemistry or several other possibilities, including birth trauma, anoxia (lack of oxygen), meningitis, encephalitis, ingestion of toxins (mercury, lead, carbon monoxide), brain tumor, PKU, and head injury.

Treatment—Treatment consists of drug therapy to control the seizures and psychological support.

Essential Tremor

Description—The involuntary shaking of the hands and head, which is made worse by action or movement. It effects between three and four million people in the U.S., usually beginning in the 30s or 40s with mild symptoms and becoming troublesome by the 50s. This common and benign condition is often confused with Parkinson's disease even though symptoms differ.

Signs and symptoms—Initially, mild shaking is noticed when trying to hold silverware to eat, thread a needle, drink from a glass, or perform writing tasks. The hands shake when trying to make movements, and the head may move in a yes-yes or no-no motion. The voice may also become shaky. Symptoms may worsen, but fortunately they can be controlled with medication. With Parkinson's, the hands shake at rest, and head motions are very infrequent. Also, writing with essential tremor results in large and scrawled letters, whereas Parkinson's causes progressively smaller and shakier handwriting within a piece of correspondence.

Etiology—The cause is unknown, but it is generally accepted to be a disorder of the nervous system. It is usually inherited, and each child of a person with essential tremor has a 50% chance of developing the disorder.

Treatment—The disorder can be treated with the beta-blocker propanolol (Inderal) or an antiseizure medication such as primidone (Mysoline). These can be taken daily, or some choose to use only on accessions such as dining out. The severity of tremors is reduced about 60% by the drugs. Without relief, other antiseizure drugs and tranquilizers can be tried. If the tremors become severe, a device can be implanted in the brain that delivers a mild electrical stimulation to block the signals causing the tremor. An unusual treatment may be the therapeutic use of alcoholic beverages. Essential tremor is usually relieved by alcohol and in fact can be used as a low-tech way to rule out other causes of tremor. Some doctors hesitate to recommend alcohol as a treatment because of the potential for abuse, but with no history of alcoholism, liver, or kidney disease, one to two drinks a day can relieve the tremor.

Headache

Headaches are commonly classified as vascular, muscle contraction (tension), or traction–inflammatory. Both muscle contraction and traction–inflammatory types cause dull, persistent aching and a feeling of a tight band around the head, with tender spots on the head or neck. Most chronic headaches result from tension that may be caused by emotional stress, fatigue, or environmental conditions. Other causes include inflammation of the sinuses, diseased teeth, and muscle spasms of the neck and shoulder.

Vasodilators, such as nitrates, alcohol, and histamine, expand arteries, causing pressure against the brain's nerve endings, and are often the causative factors. Many people are affected by anything aged or fermented, such as cured or processed meats and wine, especially red wine. Other foods or additives cause headaches by the vasoconstricting action of amines in such things as MSG, chocolate, and aspartame. A condition known as hypoglycemia (low blood sugar) can result in vasodilation and headaches but can be easily avoided by eating three meals a day, preferably five smaller ones.

Headache—Migraine (My'-grain)

Description—This is a severe throbbing pain which occurs more frequently in people with compulsive personalities and within families. About 16 to 18 million Americans suffer from **migraines**; approximately 75% are women.

A PEDIATRIC PERSPECTIVE

Children as young as two years old can have migraines.

Signs and symptoms—It is frequently characterized by prodromal (beginning) symptoms which may include fatigue, visual disturbances (such as zig-zag lines and bright lights), sensory symptoms (such as tingling of the face and lips), and sometimes motor symptoms like staggering. Usually the extreme pain is accompanied by sensitivity to light, nausea, and vomiting. It is usually on one side of the head, can occur suddenly, and will last from a few hours to a few days. They usually happen on weekends and holidays.

Etiology—The headache is caused by the initial constriction and then dilation of the blood vessels in the brain. There are "triggers" that seem to initiate migraines, which must be avoided if possible. They are chocolate, red wine, bright light, sleeping late, and the most common, fluctuating hormone levels (which explains why women are so disproportionately affected).

Treatment—It cannot be prevented, but medication can reduce frequency and intensity. Ergotomine, especially with caffeine, seems to be fairly effective if taken early; it is available in suppository form if vomiting prevents oral administration. There is no cure for migraine headaches, only control. Drugs known as beta blockers and tricyclic antidepressants appear to be very effective in prevention.

The drug Sumatriptan (brand name of Imitrex) is considered to be nearly "diagnostic" in that if the headache is a migraine, the medication is effective. It is non-narcotic and will stop a full-blown migraine. Previously, the drug required injecting, but now it is available in an oral and nasal spray form. The Sumatriptan in pill form will stop the migraine within two hours for 50% to 70% of the sufferers and by injection within one hour with effectiveness rate up to 80%. A second dose, by either means, is usually necessary within 24 hours to keep the migraine from returning. Another drug called dihydroergotamine mesylate (DHE), usually given only in emergency rooms, is now available in a nasal spray form. The spray DHE is effective in 60% to 70% of the people within three hours. People usually repeat the spray every 20 to 60 minutes, up to six or eight times, in order to get full relief. There are specific limitations and significant side effects that must be considered.

It seems to be best to lie quietly in bed in a darkened room until the symptoms subside. Limited relief may be obtained from regular analgesics, and some people feel an ice bag to the head and a wet cloth over the eyes and forehead are beneficial. Usually, it is just a matter of waiting out the episode.

When headaches are frequent, unusual (such as causing awakening in the middle of the night), persistent, or become increasingly more intense, medical attention should be sought. It may be important to rule out the presence of pathology such as an aneurysm, abscess, intercranial bleeding, or tumor.

Herpes Zoster (Her'-pees Zos'-ter) (shingles)

Description—This is an acute unilateral inflammation of the dorsal root ganglion (see Unit 4).

Signs and symptoms—It is characterized by fluid-filled vesicle lesions on the skin and severe pain from the affected nerves. The onset is characterized by fever and discomfort followed by severe deep pain, itching, and abnormal skin sensations. The vesicles erupt in about two weeks, spreading around the **thorax** or vertically on the extremities. The episode may last from one to four weeks.

Etiology—Shingles is caused by the same herpes virus that causes chickenpox. The virus has reactivated after lying dormant in the ganglion since a previous episode of chickenpox. Why this occurs is not clear; however, it may follow trauma, malignancy, and local radiation. Occasionally, there is no known factor.

Treatment—Treatment consists of medication, sometimes even narcotics, to relieve the pain and itching, plus an antiviral to reduce length of viral shedding.

Hydrocephalus (High-droh-sef'-ah-lus)

Description—This excessive accumulation of CSF within the ventricles of the brain occurs most frequently in newborns. The increased fluid compresses the brain tissue against the skull, resulting in brain damage.

Signs and symptoms—Hydrocephalus is characterized by an abnormally enlarged head, distended scalp veins, fragile, shiny scalp skin, a high-pitched, shrill cry, irritability, and vomiting.

Etiology—Hydrocephalus results from either the overproduction of cerebral spinal fluid or the lack of its absorption. Either results in excessive fluid and the enlargement of the brain. Because the newborn skull is not completely hardened, it expands to accommodate the extra fluid, resulting in the characteristic appearance.

Treatment—Surgery is the only treatment for hydrocephalus. A shunt (passageway) is inserted into a ventricle in the brain to drain off excess fluid into either the peritoneal cavity of the abdomen or the atrium (upper chamber) of the heart for absorption by the body (Figure 11–39A). The ventriculoperitoneal (VP) shunt is the most common (Figure 11–39B).

Meningitis (Men-in-ji'-tis)

Description—This is an inflammation of the meninges of the brain and spinal cord. Mortality is 70% to 100% if bacterial meningitis is left untreated.

Signs and symptoms—Meningitis is characterized by a high fever, chills, headache, vomiting, and specifically by positive Brudzinski's and Kernig's signs (Figure 11–40). Brudzinski's sign is demonstrated by the flexing of the hips and knees when the head and neck of a dorsal recumbent person are raised and pulled forward. Kernig's sign is demonstrated by pain and resistance when the knee is straightened after flexing at the thigh and knee.

Diagnosis of meningitis is confirmed by a lumbar puncture that shows elevated pressure, cloudiness from

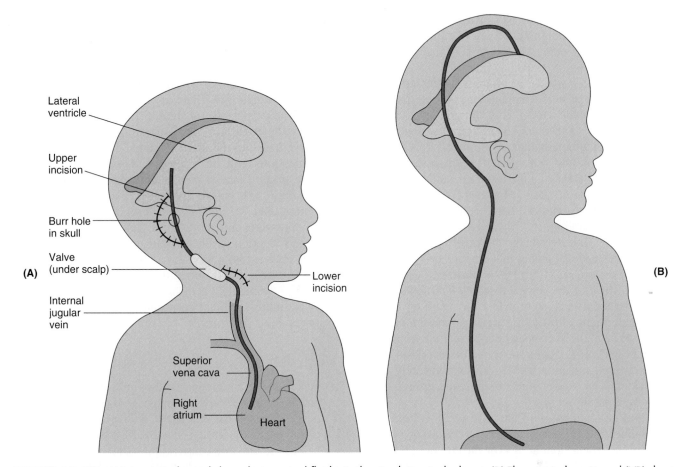

FIGURE 11-39 (A) A ventriculoartial shunt drains spinal fluid into the circulation in the heart. (B) The ventriculoperitoneal (VP) shunt drains spinal fluid into the peritoneum.

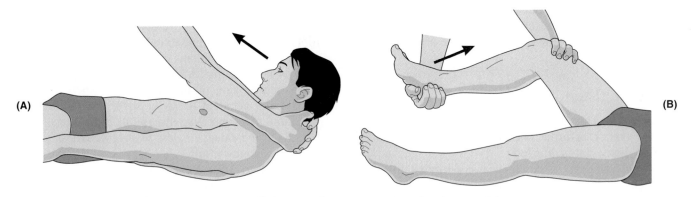

FIGURE 11-40 Two telltale signs of meningitis: (A) Brudzinski's sign, (B) Kernig's sign

the excess white cells, and identification of the causative organism after culturing.

Etiology—Meningitis is usually caused by a bacterial infection from the ears, sinuses, or lungs (pneumonia) or an abscess of the brain. Aseptic meningitis may result from a virus or other microorganism. At times, the cause is unknown.

Treatment—Treatment consists of antibiotics, medication to reduce cerebral edema, pain relievers for headache, and an anticonvulsant. Isolation may be indicated in certain instances.

Multiple Sclerosis (MS) (Skleh-roh'-sis)

Description—This is a tragic disease that attacks young men and women in the prime of life. It affects the central nervous system and is usually first diagnosed between the ages of 20 and 40. It is estimated that

500,000 Americans have MS or a related disorder. It causes a heavy economic burden of affected families because a great many people with MS are unable to work.

Signs and symptoms—The symptoms expressed depend upon the site of nerve damage but include paralysis, numbness, double vision, foot dragging, loss of balance, extreme weakness, hand tremors, speech and hearing difficulties, bladder and bowel problems, and "pins and needles" sensations. The disease is further characterized by spontaneous remission which may last for months or years. However, it is usually progressive, with a series of unpredictable attacks, and increasingly disabling.

Etiology—The disease attacks the myelin sheaths of the nerves, destroying patches that are replaced by scar tissue that distorts or interrupts the passage of nerve impulses. Much of the current research is based upon the idea that the disease is probably the result of a reactivated, dormant, slow-acting virus; an autoimmune response; or both. There is evidence that environmental factors play a role, but genetic factors may also determine a predisposition to MS. Viruses currently being considered are those from measles, mumps, chickenpox, and parainfluenza.

Treatment—Treatment consists of adrenocorticotropic hormone (ACTH) and steroids to relieve symptoms and hasten remission. Drugs for the emotional swings, urinary problems, and muscular spasticity are used as required. Bed rest to prevent fatigue is important during acute phases. The new drug Avonex, an interferon, is being used to treat relapsing forms of the disease.

The use of physical therapy is helpful. It does not restore lost strength, but it does help relieve some of the stiffness in the muscles and helps slow the deterioration. It also appears to have a positive psychological effect.

Neuralgia (Nu-ral'-je-ah)

Description—This is a term used to describe general nerve pain. It is further classified in relation to the area of the body that is affected.

Signs and symptoms—Neuralgia causes severe pain along the course of the involved nerve or nerves.

Etiology—This results from pressure on nerve trunks, faulty nerve nutrition, toxins, inflammation of the nerve, or changes in the root ganglia.

Treatment—Medications, the use of heat, physical therapy, rest, or stretching, depending upon the nerve involved, help relieve the pain.

Paralysis

Paralysis is a term used to describe the temporary or permanent loss of function in a portion of the body, especially the loss of sensation or voluntary motion. Any voluntary movement depends on the integrity of the motor neurons—the upper neurons in the brain, the lower neurons in the spinal cord, and those passing to the muscle. Paralyses are divided into two general groups: spastic, if caused by upper motor neurons, and flaccid, if caused by lower motor neurons. There are many forms of paralysis, but for the purpose of this unit, the term is being used to identify the condition following an injury or destruction of nerve tissue in the brain or spinal cord. Three general classifications will be discussed. **CAUTION:** It is extremely important to prevent damage to the brain and spinal cord. The possibility of a stroke, which damages the brain, can be reduced with proper exercise, healthy blood pressure and cholesterol, refrain from smoking, and the reduction in stress. Injury can be prevented with proper instruction, applying safety principles, the use of protective gear, not driving after drinking, and using seat belts. Unfortunately, once damage has occurred, it is usually irreversible. Spinal cord damage is devastating and changes one's life *forever.*

Hemiplegia (Heh-mih-plee-jee-ah)

Description—Hemiplegia is the unilateral (one-sided) paralysis that follows damage to the brain. Because nerves cross in the brainstem, damage to the right side of the brain causes left-sided paralysis, whereas damage to the left side causes right-sided paralysis.

Signs and symptoms—Hemiplegia produces unilateral weakness or paralysis of the arm, leg, face, and tongue. It may be sudden, if caused by a stroke or injury, or gradual, if caused by a tumor or disease. The paralysis begins as flaccid but often progresses to spastic. Hemiplegics often have difficulty understanding oral or written language, may develop muscle shortening and foot drop, have a decreased level of consciousness, and may experience problems eating.

Etiology—Hemiplegia is caused by any injury to the brain or one side of the spinal cord such as: cerebrovascular accident (CVA or stroke), a tumor, CNS infection, a degenerative disease, or trauma (see CVA, Unit 8). If the damage is less severe, weakness instead of paralysis may result.

Treatment—Early treatment involves preventing further involvement and lessening the effects of the damage, which varies with the cause. Later treatment focuses on prevention of complications such as muscle contractions, foot drop, and spastic muscular movements. The use of physical and speech therapy, orthopedic devices, and modifications in the surroundings are important to rehabilitation and promoting independence (Figure 11–41).

Paraplegia (Par-a-ple'-jee-ah)

Description—This is the loss of motor or sensory function in the lower extremities, usually from trauma,

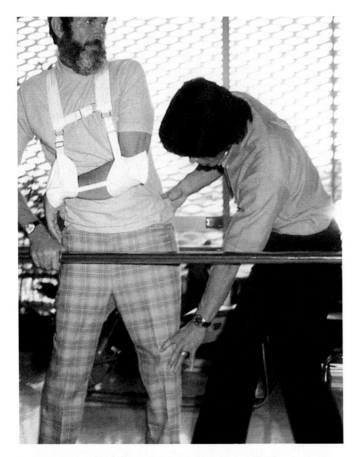

FIGURE 11–41 Physical therapy can be helpful for the hemiplegic patient following a stroke on the right side of his brain that affected the left side of his body.

with or without involvement of the abdominal and back muscles. The paralysis may be permanent or temporary, spastic or flaccid. Almost half of the 10,000 to 12,000 spinal cord injuries each year result in paraplegia. It occurs twice as often in males as in females with the highest incidence between the ages of 16 and 35.

Signs and symptoms—The onset of total or partial paralysis is immediate in most patients, with the loss of motion, sensation, and reflexes below the level of damage. With complete spinal cord injury, there is lack of sensation or voluntary muscle control that persists for 24 hours; any return of functional muscle activity below the injury is unlikely. There is usually loss of bladder, bowel, and sexual function. With incomplete damage, the patient can still sense the perianal area, flex the toes, and control the bladder and bowels.

Etiology—Paraplegia usually results from trauma that occurs with automobile, motorcycle, and sporting accidents; gunshot wounds; and falls. Conditions such as spina bifida and scoliosis may also cause paralysis.

Treatment—It is important that treatment starts at the time of the accident. The patient must be strapped on a board before any movement occurs to prevent additional spinal cord injury. The spine must be realigned

and any fractures reduced. Compression of the cord and nerves must be relieved. Surgery may be required to repair fracture dislocations and remove bone fragments. A urinary catheter is installed to drain urine. Extensive care to maintain the skin, monitor fluids, and promote good nutrition and medications to prevent infection and control muscle spasms are required. Rehabilitation to promote as much activity as is possible begins early. Psychological support is very important. The final extent of paralysis cannot be accurately evaluated until one year following the injury.

Quadriplegia (Quah-drih-plee′-jee-ah)

Description—The devastating permanent paralysis affecting all body systems, the arms, the legs, and all of the body below the level of the injury to the spinal cord. The injury is usually the result of a trauma. It affects about 150,000 Americans, most being men between the ages of 20 and 40.

Signs and symptoms—Quadriplegia is evidenced by the flaccid appearance of the arms and legs and the loss of sensation and movement below the level of the injury. If the cord is damaged above the fifth cervical vertebrae of the neck, body systems also will be dramatically affected. This type of injury would produce symptoms such as:

- Low blood pressure from the blocking of the sympathetic nervous system
- Low body temperature caused by dilated surface blood vessels, which allows heat to escape
- Slow heart rate caused by absence of sympathetic system inhibiting action
- Respiratory system involvement, which may require mechanical support

Etiology—Paralysis results from spinal cord injury in the cervical vertebrae. It is usually the result of automobile, motorcycle, or sporting activities accidents; gunshot wounds; or falls. Diving and gymnastics are common causes. The dangers of horseback riding became apparent in 1995 with the extensive injury to actor Christopher Reeve, which in a few seconds changed his life forever.

Treatment—Again, treatment begins at the scene of the accident with immobilization of the neck and spine. Following hospitalization, tongs or a halo traction are attached to the skull to pull the neck into alignment and stabilize the spine. Treatment is aimed at reducing the edema (swelling) of the spinal cord, thereby relieving pressure on the spinal nerves. An artificial airway will be required if injury is above the fifth vertebra, and ventilation assistance will be necessary. After about 10 days, surgery is done to fuse vertebrae and remove any fragments. Unfortunately, many functional problems will occur. Some of the more common are:

- Maintaining open airway and adequate respiration
- Providing adequate fluids and nutrition

- Excessively slow heart rate and resulting low blood pressure
- Low body temperature, perhaps to less than 90° F, which will require warming with blankets
- Extremely high blood pressure, which may lead to heart failure and intracranial bleeding when injury is above the fourth vertebra

The greatest challenge comes from the enormous change in the individual's life. If there is an airway, the patient may not be able to even speak. Paralysis requires extensive emotional, physical, and social support, not only for the affected individual but also for their entire family and circle of friends.

Extensive research continues to find ways of restoring function to damaged nerves. A great deal of discussion regarding the possibilities of stem cell applications is giving these individuals some glimmer of hope.

Parkinson's Disease

Description—This is a common progressive crippling disease affecting about one in every 100 people over age 60, which translates to about 60,000 new cases annually in the United States. It affects men more often than women. It progresses for about 10 years until pneumonia or another infection results in death.

Signs and symptoms—The main symptoms are the muscle rigidity and unilateral tremor of the hand, described as "pill-rolling." The disease produces a high-pitched, monotone voice and a masklike expression. As it progresses, the condition is characterized by severe muscle rigidity, a peculiar gait, drooling, and a progressive tremor. The body becomes bent forward, with head bowed. The steps become faster and faster with increasing forward body inclination, which often results in falling.

Etiology—The cause of Parkinson's disease is unknown; however, it has been established that a deficiency in dopamine prevents affected brain cells from functioning properly. Some researchers have noted some forms may be caused by a viral infection experienced many years earlier.

Treatment—There is no known cure for the disease, although a drug called Levodopa relieves most of the symptoms until the necessarily increased dosage begins to cause serious side effects. In selected patients, surgical procedures can either freeze, electrically coagulate, or radioactively destroy a small area of the brain to prevent the involuntary motions.

Surgical options are appropriate only for those in good health, who are relatively young (under age 70), no longer able to tolerate medication, and have specific symptoms. A thalamotomy, which destroys a specific group of cells in the thalamus, is appropriate for 5% to 10% of patients with severe tremor of the hand and arm. It results in immediate improvement in 80% to 90% of the patients. A pallidotomy destroys a specific group of cells within the globus pallidus (movement center of the brain). It is used for patients with slow movement, tremor, imbalance, and drug side effects. The results are about the same as with thalamotomy. Note: The surgery will not cure the disease; it only relieves the symptoms and decreases need for medication. The disease will progress.

Again a well-known person is giving urgency to research into treatment and a cure for this debilitating disease. Popular actor Michael J. Fox was diagnosed with Parkinson's disease in 1991, many years before he reached the "average age" of incidence. The involvement of well-known people like Christopher Reeve and Michael J. Fox in forming foundations for research and education into these tragic conditions is having a very positive impact on the urgency for answers and treatments.

Reye's Syndrome

Description—This acute childhood illness is characterized by fatty infiltration of the liver and increased intracranial pressure (ICP). Further damage from fat infiltration occurs in the kidneys and possibly the muscle of the heart. The **syndrome** (group of symptoms) affects children from infancy to adolescence, occurring equally in males and females, but affects whites more than blacks.

The syndrome prognosis depends on the degree of CNS depression from ICP. At one time, mortality was 90%; now with early treatment and ICP monitoring, the rate has been reduced to 20%. Death usually results from cerebral swelling, respiratory arrest, or coma.

Signs and symptoms—The symptoms occur in stages of severity, beginning with vomiting, lethargy, and liver dysfunction and then progressing to hyperventilation, delirium, hyperactive reflexes, and coma. The condition worsens as symptoms of rigidity; deepening coma; large, fixed pupils; seizures; and eventual respiratory arrest occur.

Etiology—Reye's syndrome almost always follows within one to three days of an acute viral infection, such as upper respiratory infection, type B influenza, or chickenpox. A correlation exists between the use of aspirin with children and the incidence of influenza and chickenpox. Even though it may not be causative, aspirin is not recommended for any pediatric patient.

Treatment—Proper treatment is essential. With increased ICP, the prime concern is to reduce the pressure and brain edema to prevent damage. Aggressive action involves medications to reduce body fluid, prevent seizures, and maintain appropriate levels of vitamin K, ammonia, and glucose. If the condition worsens, the ICP is monitored, and mechanical ventilation may be necessary. As a final effort, coma may be induced with barbiturates, dialysis may be used to extract fluids and built-up elements, and a section of skull may be removed to relieve brain compression.

Sciatica (Sigh-a'-ti-kah)

Description—**Sciatica** is the inflammation of the sciatic nerve of the leg. It is usually unilateral and is more common in males and in mid-age.

Signs and symptoms—A sharp, shooting pain that may begin gradually or abruptly and runs down the back of the thigh. It may seem to originate deep within the buttocks. It is often intensified with movement. The pain may become worse at night or when the atmosphere changes with the approach of a storm. It may be difficult to achieve comfort while sitting or standing.

Etiology—Primary causes may be exposure to wet and cold. The nerve may have been injured or irritated by impingement by the spinous processes of the spine. Gradually occurring pain can result from unequal leg length, causing improper vertebral alignment. The nerve may become damaged by strain or accidental stretching during strenuous activities.

Treatment—Activities causing discomfort will need to be curtailed temporarily. Treatment consists of bed rest, heat, medication for pain, and sometimes the use of traction. Some people find that the application of cold instead of heat is beneficial. An adjustment to a shoe may be helpful in leveling the legs. Often, the use of specific stretching exercises, begun gently, will gradually solve the problem. The discomfort may persist for an extended period of time. It may become chronic and cause atrophy (wasting away) of the affected muscles. Surgery may be indicated in severe cases that do not respond to conservative measures.

Spinal Cord Defects

Description—Spinal cord defects result from failure of tissues to properly close during the first three months of pregnancy. They occur most frequently in the lumbosacral area.

The incidence is approximately 5% of live births or about 100,000 infants per year and is highest among persons of Welsh or Irish descent.

Signs and symptoms—**Spina bifida occulta** (Spi'-na bif'-i-da oc-cult'-ah) is the most common type of the defects. It is characterized by the incomplete closure of one or more vertebra but without protrusion of the spinal cord or meninges (Figure 11–42). There is usually a depression, a tuft of hair, a port wine nevi, or a combination of these signs over the defect. In spina bifida with meningocele (men-in'-jo-ceel), a protruding sac contains meninges and CFS. With myelomeningocele (mie-lo-men-in'-jo-ceel), the meninges, CFS, and a portion of the spinal cord or distal nerve roots are within the sac. The defects usually occur in the lumbosacral area but are occasionally found in the thoracic and cervical areas. Neurological symptoms range from minimal weakness of the feet and some bladder and bowel problems to permanent neurological dysfunction, such as paralysis, inability to control the bladder and bowels, hydrocephalus, clubfoot, and sometimes mental retardation.

Etiology—A congenital defect caused by the failure of the neural tube of the embryo, which becomes the brain and spinal cord, to close properly. Normally, by about the twenty-third day, it is completely closed, except for the openings at each end. A recent finding revealed that lack of folic acid is a contributing factor. All pregnant women

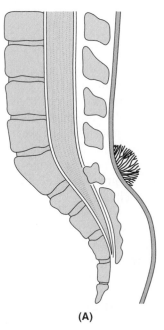
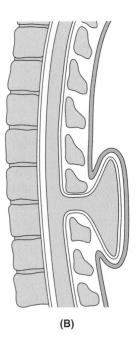
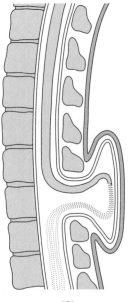

(A) (B) (C)

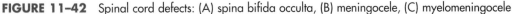

FIGURE 11–42   Spinal cord defects: (A) spina bifida occulta, (B) meningocele, (C) myelomeningocele

should take a supplement containing the element as soon as pregnancy is known. Ideally, it should be started prior to conception. Viruses, radiation, the environment, and genetic factors may also be responsible.

Treatment—Treatment and prognosis depend on the extent of the defect. Spina bifida occulta usually requires no treatment. If CSF and meninges are involved, surgical closure is required to prevent further injury. Unfortunately, the neurological conditions cannot be reversed. With hydrocephalus present, a shunt will be implanted to relieve the fluid pressure. Supportive measures to promote independence may involve leg braces, crutches, walkers, and wheelchairs. Note: With paralysis and spinal cord defects, there are bladder and bowel concerns.

Subarachnoid Hemorrhage (Sub-a-rak'-noid)

Description—This is a collection of blood in the subarachnoid space, usually caused by the spontaneous rupture of a weakened blood vessel.

Signs and symptoms—The patient may complain of a sudden, severe headache and experience nausea and projectile vomiting. This may be accompanied by motor disturbances, seizures, and deviations in sensory perception, particularly in vision.

Etiology—Precipitating factors include hypertension, oral contraceptives, malformations of cranial blood vessels, and family history.

Treatment—Treatment varies with the causative factor. With hypertension, efforts would be made to lower the blood pressure. If contraceptives are suspected, they would be discontinued.

Subdural Hematoma (Sub-dur'-al He-ma-to'-ma)

Description—This is a collection of blood within the subdural space. It is usually a slow process in which the gradually accumulating blood causes progressive symptoms.

Signs and symptoms—There are disturbances in motor activities and a progressive facial weakness on the side opposite the hematoma. With progression, there may be seizures and a decreased level of consciousness. Because the blood accumulates slowly, symptoms may not occur until days after the injury.

Etiology—Hematoma results from blood leaking into the subdural space as the consequence of a head injury.

Treatment—Surgical intervention is indicated to remove the pressure on the brain tissues caused by the hematoma when symptoms and intracranial pressure reach a significant level.

Tourette Syndrome (Tur'-et)

Description—Tourette syndrome (TS) is a neurological disorder characterized by "tics"—the involuntary, rapid, sudden movements that occur repeatedly in the

same way. The onset is before the age of 21. The incidence in the United States has not been determined, however, the National Institutes of Health estimate there are 100,000 people with the affliction, and may be as high as one in every 200 if chronic and transient childhood tics were included.

Signs and symptoms—The most common first symptom is a facial tic, such as rapidly blinking eyes or twitches of the mouth. Another tic involves the voice, which may result in barking noises and tongue clicking. Some people vocalize socially unacceptable words and echo things just heard. People with TS do have some control, repressing the symptoms until a more socially accepted time; however, this causes a more severe outburst when expressed. Tics of the limbs may also be an initial sign. Motor tics may cause jumping, touching other people or things, twirling about, and self-injurious actions such as hitting or biting oneself. There is no diagnostic test to confirm TS; only history and observation can be used to diagnose.

Etiology—The cause of TS has not been definitely identified. There is evidence that it is caused by the abnormal metabolism of at least one brain chemical called dopamine. Others are suspected. Genetic studies show that TS is from an inherited dominant gene that can produce different symptoms in different family members.

Treatment—Most persons are not significantly affected to require treatment. There are medications to control the outburst when necessary. The dosage must be determined individually. Psychotherapy can assist a person and her families to cope with the strange condition. Relaxation techniques and biofeedback help reduce stress that causes tics to increase. Affected people may be ridiculed and rejected. Children can be excluded from school activities and experience difficulty in interpersonal relationships.

Transient Ischemic Attack (Trans'-e-ent Is-kem'-ick)

Description—A transient ischemic attack (TIA) is a recurring stroke-like event that lasts from a few seconds to hours, then disappears after 12 to 24 hours. It is considered to be a warning sign of impending stroke. The age of onset varies but rises dramatically after age 50. It is highest among blacks and men. TIAs have occurred in 50% to 80% of patients who experience a stroke from a blood vessel blockage.

Signs and symptoms—It is characterized by symptoms such as double vision, slurred speech, dizziness, staggering gait, and falling. TIA is a warning sign of impending thrombotic CVA (stroke from a blood clot).

Etiology—A microemboli (tiny circulating mass) is released from a thrombus (blood clot) and probably interrupts blood flow in the tiny arteries of the brain. This causes symptoms similar to those of a stroke to develop; however, they are transient (passing quickly) in nature.

Treatment—Treatment includes the use of aspirin and anticoagulant to reduce blood clot formation and to minimize the risk of thrombosis and the resulting CVA.

Trigeminal Neuralgia (tic douloureux) (Tri-gem'-in-al Nu-ral'-je-ah)

Description—This is a disorder of the fifth cranial nerve, on one side of the face.

Signs and symptoms—It produces episodes of excruciating facial pain on stimulation of a trigger zone. It frequently follows exposure to heat or cold, a draft from air, smiling, or drinking hot or cold liquids. The episodes may last from one to 15 minutes, recurring from several times daily to a few times a year. Persons with the disorder live in fear of the next attack. It occurs mostly in people over the age of 40, in women more than men, and more frequently on the right side of the face.

Etiology—The exact cause is still under investigation. However, such things as compression on nerves by tumors, an aneurysm, and an afferent reflex condition can cause it. Occasionally it is associated with multiple sclerosis or herpes zoster. The pain is probably the result of an interaction or short-circuiting of touch and pain fibers.

Treatment—Treatment consists of oral medication and/or the injection of alcohol or phenol into the nerve branch. With frequent, severe attacks, a surgical procedure is indicated that severs the nerve, thereby relieving the pain but also resulting in loss of sensation to the innervated area. Care must be taken afterward to protect the affected eye, avoid burns from hot food, guard against dental decay, and avoid biting the inner cheek and lip.

Tumor

Description—Tumors can occur anywhere in the body. However, those in the brain that are malignant are especially difficult to treat. There are several types with differing age and sex preferences, but almost all limit life from six months to six years following diagnosis. They are slightly more common in men than women, with an incidence of 4.5 per 100,000 people. They are most prevalent between the ages of 40 and 60 in adults and between 2 and 12 in children. They are one of the most common causes of death from cancer in children.

Signs and symptoms—Tumors cause changes in the CNS because of the destruction of tissue; the compression of the brain, cranial nerves, and blood vessels; cerebral swelling; and increased intracranial pressure. Specific symptoms vary with the type of tumor, its location, and the extent of involvement. Common symptoms are nausea, vomiting, headache, seizures, facial nerve palsies, dizziness, visual and hearing changes, weakness, and many others. The symptoms are usually insidious (slow) and often misdiagnosed.

Etiology—The cause of brain tumors is unknown.

Treatment—A resectable tumor is removed, a non-resectable tumor is reduced if possible. The type of therapy depends upon the cellular structure, its sensitivity to radiation, and its location. Surgery, radiation, chemotherapy, and releasing of ICP by diuretics or shunting are the usual treatments.

ACHIEVE UNIT OBJECTIVES

Complete Chapter 11, Unit 2, in the workbook to help you obtain competency of this subject matter.

UNIT 3
The Senses

OBJECTIVES

Upon completion of the unit, meet the following performance objectives by verifying knowledge of the facts and principles presented through oral and written communication at a level deemed competent.

1. Spell and define, using the glossary at the back of the text, all the **Words to Know** in this unit.
2. Name the senses of the human body, identifying the corresponding organ(s) responsible for perception.
3. Identify on an anatomical illustration the structures of the eye, ear, nose, tongue, and skin.
4. Trace the path of a visual image from the cornea to the visual center of the brain.
5. Explain the effects of the lens and cornea upon the focusing of images.
6. Trace the path of sound from the entrance of the ear to the auditory center of the brain.
7. Explain the balance function of the inner ear.
8. Describe the anatomy of the olfactory organ, and explain how an odor is perceived.
9. Name the taste sensations, and identify the corresponding areas on the surface of the tongue.
10. Name the types of contact receptors found in the skin.
11. Describe seventeen diseases or disorders of the eye, eight of the ear, three of the nose, and three of the mouth and tongue.

AREAS OF COMPETENCE (AAMA)

This unit addresses content within the specific competency areas of *Administrative procedures, Practice finances, Patient care, Communication skills,* and *Instruction,* as identified in the Medical Assistant Role Delineation Study. Refer to Appendix A for a detailed listing of the areas. (Note: Although *Anatomy and physiology* is not specifically identified in the study, a basic knowledge of the body's structures and function is an essential foundation to the competent performance of many roles.)

■ WORDS TO KNOW

accommodation	Ménière's disease
amblyopia	myopia
aqueous humor	optic disc
astigmatism	organ of Corti
auditory	otitis
cataract	otosclerosis
cerumen	papillae
choroid	polyps
cochlea	presbycusis
conjunctiva	presbyopia
cornea	pupil
enucleation	receptor
epistaxis	retina
eustachian tube	retinopathy
fovea centralis	sclera
glaucoma	semicircular canals
hyperopia	sensorineural
incus	stapes
insidious	strabismus
iris	tinnitus
lacrimal	tympanic membrane
lens	vitreous humor
malleus	

The human being is able to communicate with the surrounding environment because of a miraculous network of nerves coordinated with the organs of the five special senses, which allow us to see, hear, taste, smell, and touch. Knowledge of the environment requires the cooperation of three factors: the sense organs to perceive, intact cranial nerves to transmit, and a functioning area of the brain to interpret the received stimuli.

A stimulus is anything the body is able to detect by means of its **receptors**. Receptors are the peripheral nerve endings of sensory nerves that respond to stimuli. They are not all alike and do not respond to the same kinds of stimuli. Some respond to environmental chemical energy from ions or molecules that are dissolved in body fluids. These are chemoreceptors and are associated with the sense of taste and smell. Changes in position or pressure or the effects of acceleration create mechanical energy, which is detected by mechanoreceptors. These are associated with touch, hearing, and equilibrium. The detection of energy from light is possible as a result of the photoreceptors in the eyes. Thermoreceptors detect radiant energy from heat and are in the skin or connective tissue.

The stimulus, regardless of its form, is converted into energy. If the stimulus is sufficient enough to cause an action potential in the neuron, the message will travel along the sensory nerve to the brain. The reason messages are interpreted differently (such as being hot, a color, or an odor) is that certain nerves always end up in the same specific part of the brain. In other words, the sensation of heat or pain and the "seeing" of a color actually occurs in

the brain, not at the point of stimulus. The ability to distinguish between hot, cold, red, or blue, for example, is the outcome of messages being received in an appropriate section of the brain, undergoing routing, being compared with stored past experiences and producing the interpretation of the stimulus.

The primary organs of the senses are familiar: the eye and the sense of sight; the ear and the sense of hearing; the tongue and the sense of taste; the nose and the sense of smell; and the skin and the sense of touch. However, these organs cannot perform their functions without the cooperation of the corresponding nerves and the section of the brain.

Ⓐ Library

THE EYE AND THE SENSE OF SIGHT

The structure of the eyeball is frequently compared to that of a camera. The outside of the camera is made of a strong plastic or metal to protect its interior structures. Well-protected, the eye is located within the bony orbital cavity of the skull. For additional protection, the outside of the eye is covered with tough, white fibrous tissue called the **sclera** (Figure 11–43). The sclera helps maintain the shape of the eyeball. Six extraocular or intrinsic (outside) muscles are attached to the sclera and anchored in the skull; these contract or relax as pairs to move the eyeball within its cavity. This permits the eyes to roll up/down, in/out, and in combinations of these directions, thereby permitting a large field of vision without moving the head (Figure 11–44). Under the sclera is another covering called the **choroid**, which contains the blood vessels that serve the tissues of the eye. This layer has a nonreflective pigment that makes it dark and opaque and prevents light from reflecting within the eye.

Focusing the Image

Both the eye and the camera have a lens to focus an image onto a surface for "recording." In the camera this surface is the film. In the eye it is the **retina**. In the camera, the distance between the film and the camera lens is adjusted to bring the picture into focus before it is recorded on the film. In the eye, the shape of the elastic **lens** is automatically altered by ciliary muscles of the ciliary body to focus objects onto the retina. When the ciliary body contracts, the lens becomes rounder in a process known as **accommodation** for permitting near vision. With relaxation, the lens thins out to accommodate focusing on distant objects. The shape of the lens is convex on both the anterior and posterior surfaces. The shape is quite rounded in childhood but becomes more convex with age until it is nearly flat in the elderly, causing difficulty accommodating for near vision.

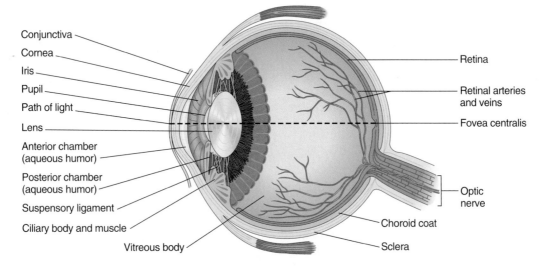

Conjunctiva
Cornea
Iris
Pupil
Path of light
Lens
Anterior chamber (aqueous humor)
Posterior chamber (aqueous humor)
Suspensory ligament
Ciliary body and muscle
Vitreous body

Retina
Retinal arteries and veins
Fovea centralis
Optic nerve
Choroid coat
Sclera

FIGURE 11–43   Cross-section of the eye

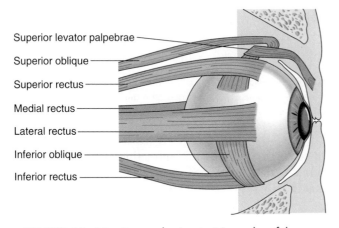
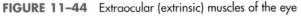

Superior levator palpebrae
Superior oblique
Superior rectus
Medial rectus
Lateral rectus
Inferior oblique
Inferior rectus

FIGURE 11–44   Extraocular (extrinsic) muscles of the eye

Controlling Light

The aperture of the camera is similar to the **iris** of the eye; the size of their openings is adjusted to allow varying amounts of light to enter. The iris is the colored circular muscle that surrounds the central opening called the **pupil**. The amount of melanin (color) and its location in the iris determines the color of the eye. When melanin is present only in the posterior area, the iris appears blue; if melanin is scattered throughout, eye color ranges from green to brown to black, depending on the amount of pigment. In the eye, the two intrinsic (inside) muscle structures of the iris regulate the amount of light that enters the eye. When the light is bright, the circular muscle fibers of the iris contract, reducing the size of the pupil, thereby permitting less light to enter. If it is dark or dimly lit, the pupil will dilate (enlarge) as the radial muscle fibers of the iris contract to pull it outward, permitting more light to enter.

The Cornea

The **cornea** is a transparent extension of the sclera that lies in front of the pupil. This covering has no blood vessels to interfere with vision, so the tissue is nourished by lymph fluid circulating through the cellular spaces. It has both pain and touch receptors, which cause it to be extremely sensitive to any foreign body that touches its surface. If an injury to the cornea results in scarring, vision will be impaired.

The curvature of the cornea "corrects" some of the unclear image that the edge of the lens projects. If the cornea develops an abnormal shape, vision becomes blurred, and the result may be a disorder known as **astigmatism**.

Surface Membranes

A mucous membrane called the **conjunctiva** lines the inner surfaces of the eyelids and covers the anterior sclera surface of the eye. At the margin of the cornea, the conjunctiva merges with the transparent epithelium covering that protects the cornea. The conjunctiva and cornea are lubricated by tiny glands that secrete an oily substance. Further protection for the eye is provided by **lacrimal** glands, which secrete tears to moisten and cleanse the surface of the membrane.

Cavities and Humors

The eyeball is divided into two main areas separated by the lens and its supporting ciliary body structures. The more anterior area is subdivided into the anterior chamber, which is between the cornea and the iris, and the posterior chamber, which lies between the iris and the lens. A salty, clear fluid known as the **aqueous humor** fills and circulates between the chambers. It maintains the curvature of the cornea and assists in the refraction process.

The eyeball behind the lens, sometimes called a vitreous chamber or vitreous body, is filled with a thick, jellylike substance called the **vitreous humor**. This material not only aids in refraction but also maintains the shape of the eyeball. Injury with the loss of an appreciable amount of the humor may cause damage to the eyeball, which could necessitate surgical removal of the eye by a procedure called **enucleation**.

The Retina

The inside layer of the eyeball is the retina, a multilayered nervous tissue. Specialized nerve cells called rods and cones transmit the stimuli focused on the retinal surface through the optic nerve to the visual center in the brain where the image is "seen." The cones, about seven million in number, are sensitive to colors and function only in well-lighted environments. Most of them are located in a depression on the posterior surface of the retina called the **fovea centralis**, the area of sharpest vision. There are about 100 million rods in the more peripheral areas of the retina. The rods are very sensitive to light and permit us to see, without color, in dimly-lit or nearly-dark surroundings.

Optic Disc   Two other types of nerve cells in the retina relay impulses from the rods and cones. The axons of one type form the fibers of the optic nerve. Where the optic nerves exit the retina, there are neither rods nor cones, so this area is referred to as the **optic disc** or blind spot.

The Path of Light

The process of sight begins with the passage of light rays through the cornea; on through the aqueous humor, the pupil, and the lens into the vitreous humor; and finally focusing at the back of the eyeball on the retina. Here the image is picked up by the rods and cones, transformed into nerve impulses, and transmitted over the optic nerve to the thalamus. Here some of the fibers cross over to the nerve tract of the other eye. From the thalamus, other neurons relay the impulses to the visual center in the occipital lobe of the cerebrum, where the impulses are "developed" into pictures and "seen."

Refraction Error

Each part of the eyeball refracts (deflects) the light to cause the image to focus on the retina (Figure 11–45A). However, this does not always occur correctly. When the image is improperly refracted and focuses in front of the retina (B), the person is said to be nearsighted, or to have **myopia**. When the image focuses behind the retina (C), the person is said to be farsighted, or to have **hyperopia**. These conditions may result from abnormal curvature of the lens or cornea, or from an abnormally-shaped eyeball. Note that images are inverted when they pass through the lens because of the curvature deflecting the image. Eye-

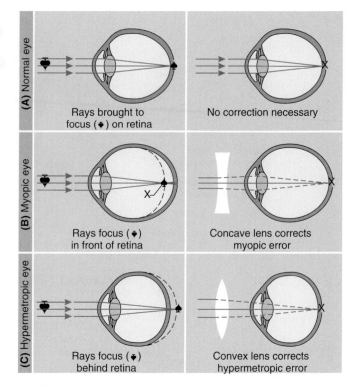

FIGURE 11–45   The refraction of an image: (A) normal vision, (B) nearsightedness, (C) farsightedness and the type of lens required to correct the vision

glasses provide a means of refracting light to correct abnormal deflection of the image. They perform artificially what the eyes' structures fail to do.

DISEASES AND DISORDERS OF THE EYE

Age-related Macular Degeneration (Mack'-u-lur De-jen-er-a'-shun)

Description—A disease that affects the macula, the most sensitive part of the retina, and alters the center of the visual field. Ten million Americans have some loss of vision from age-related macular degeneration (AMD). It is the leading cause of blindness in the United States.

Signs and symptoms—This is a gradual loss of central vision; however, side or surrounding vision is often maintained. There is a blurred, distorted, dark, or empty area in the center of things viewed. If both eyes are involved, it makes things like threading a needle and reading virtually impossible. The condition can be easily diagnosed by having the patient look at a square grid that resembles graph paper but has a small dot in the center. The appearance of crooked lines or other visual symptoms around the dot is diagnostic.

Etiology—It is caused by damage to the blood vessels supplying the retina. A recent study of the diets of 2,000 people from 45 to 84 years old showed a relationship between dietary fat and AMD. Signs of the disease were 80% more common with those people who had consumed the most saturated fat within the past 10 years. Researchers believe that the saturated fat clogs the arteries and reduces the amount of blood that reaches the retina. This form of degeneration is also known as "dry," "atropic," or "involuntional" macular degeneration and represents about 90% of the macular-related disease. Another form known as "wet" degeneration accounts for about 10% of cases and results from abnormal blood vessels forming at the back of the eye. This type of vision loss is usually rapid and severe. The vessels leak blood and fluid that can result in dense scar tissue.

Treatment—There is no cure for the dry form of degeneration; however, assistance with ways to cope with the visual impairment is available. There are various optical devices including magnifying, closed circuit TV, large-print reading materials, and special lighting to assist with vision. The wet form can also be helped with low-vision optical devices, but if it is caught early, it can be treated with laser surgery. The laser beam is focused to seal the leaking blood vessels. The surgery does make a permanent dark "spot" at the laser area, but it will retard damage and preserve more sight overall.

Scientists are perfecting an artificial retina that will permit limited vision of light and large objects. The technology involves the use of a bionic silicon chip and is being used with retinal pigmentosa, a genetically-induced form of blindness. It is anticipated that it may be applicable to macular degeneration as well. Researchers also believe that a dietary regime that protects against heart disease may preserve vision in later life.

Amblyopia (lazy eye) (Am-ble-o'-pe-a)

Description—**Amblyopia** is a condition known as lazy eye because it causes the turning eye to become "lazy." It is most prevalent in children under the age of five.

Signs and symptoms—Observation reveals one eye turns inward, causing blurred vision. The brain suppresses the visual impulses from the inward-turning eye.

Etiology—Amblyopia is caused by any condition that affects normal use of the eyes and their development. The three major causes are strabismus because of misaligned eyes, unequal focus caused by refractive errors, and cloudiness in the normally clear eye tissues. Strabismus is the most common cause because the crossed eye "turns off" to avoid double vision and becomes amblyopic. (See strabismus on page 312 in this unit.)

Treatment—The condition is treated by covering the "good eye," thereby stimulating the development of the "lazy eye." For a good prognosis, therapy should begin before the age of eight; otherwise, eventual blindness of the affected eye may result. Sometimes surgery is required to correct the eye.

Arcus Senilis (Are'-cuss Se-nill'-us)

Description—The condition accompanies normal aging and is included in this discussion because it is so prevalent. It results in a thin grayish-white arc or circle not quite at the edge of the cornea. If it is present in young people, it may suggest hypercholesterolemia (high level of cholesterol in the blood).

Blepharitis (Blef-ar-i'-tis)

Description—This is an inflammation of the edges of the eyelids involving the hair follicles and glands. The condition is usually associated with seborrhea of the scalp (dandruff).

Signs and symptoms—The person experiences itching and burning sensations, which cause her to blink continuously and rub the eyes, resulting in red-rimmed eyelid margins. The person afflicted develops greasy scales and sticky, crusted eyelids. Ulcerated lid margins, loss of lashes, and the presence of nits (with pediculosis) are possible.

Etiology—There are excess secretions from the hair follicles of the eyelids. It may also develop from pediculosis of the brows and lashes.

Treatment—Treatment depends on the cause. It consists of frequent shampoos of the hair and daily cleansing of the eyelids with a mild shampoo to remove the scales. Steroid creams can also be used. If pediculosis is present, the parasite must be removed.

Cataract (Cat'-a-rack)

Description—This gradually developing opacity (cloudiness) of the lens occurs most frequently in persons over 70 years of age as part of the aging process.

Signs and symptoms—The condition causes a painless, gradual blurring and loss of vision. The pupil turns from black to a milky white as the lens becomes visible. People with cataracts frequently complain of seeing halos around lights or being blinded at night by oncoming automobile headlights (Figure 11–46).

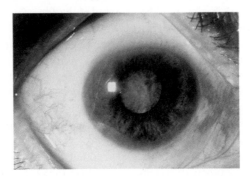

FIGURE 11–46 Cataract (Courtesy of National Eye Institute, NIH.)

Etiology—The probable cause of **cataracts** is a change in the composition of the proteins of the lens.

Treatment—Cataracts are treated by surgical removal of the lens and postoperative substitution of cataract eyeglasses. Other options are possible for some patients. Contact lenses can be fitted and provide much better correction than glasses. Frequently an intraocular lens (IOL) is implanted directly behind the cornea when the cataract surgery is performed. A new "taco" style lens is inserted in a folded-over state through a very tiny incision popping open after it is implanted. Cataract surgery is now being done on an outpatient basis, with the patient detained only an hour or two.

Sometime after surgery, the capsule that held the lens in place, which is now behind and supporting the IOL, may become clouded, once again obstructing the path of light into the eye. This problem can be easily solved without invasive surgery, using a laser beam to make a tiny opening in the capsule, which lets in light and restores vision.

Conjunctivitis (Pinkeye) (Con-junk-tiv-i'-tis)

Description—This condition is caused by inflammation of the conjunctiva. It usually begins in one eye, spreading rapidly to the other from contamination by a wash cloth or by the hands. Because it is highly contagious, other family members should not share towels, wash cloths, or pillows with the infected person.

Signs and symptoms—Conjunctivitis causes redness and a "blood shot" appearance. Pain, swelling, and occasionally a discharge from the eyes may be present.

Etiology—It is usually caused by an infectious organism, such as bacteria (streptococcus or staphylococcus) or a virus (herpes simplex). Allergic reactions and environmental irritants can also cause the condition.

Treatment—Bacterial conjunctivitis responds to antibiotics and sulfa drug therapy; the herpes viral type does not.

Corneal Abrasion (Core-ne'-al A-bray'-zun)

Description—A scratch or trauma to the cornea, usually from a foreign body in the eye. Even if the eye waters profusely to cleanse the surface, the scratch (abrasion) remains. Vision may be affected if the location and extent of injury are significant.

Signs and symptoms—The presence of redness, tearing, and irritation that cause excessive blinking.

Etiology—It is most often caused by dirt or small pieces of wood, metal, or paper that become embedded under the eyelid or an injury from a fingernail. Abrasions may also occur from falling asleep while wearing hard contact lenses.

Treatment—Foreign bodies embedded in the cornea require removal following application of a topical anesthetic. Treatment consists of antibiotic eyedrops or ointment and application of a pressure eye patch to prevent blinking. Corneal epithelium heals rapidly within 24 to 48 hours.

Corneal Ulcers (Core-ne'-al All'-sirs)

Description—An acute disease involving the cornea of the eye.

Signs and symptoms—The first signs are pain, aggravated by blinking, and excessive tearing. Blurred vision results from the ulcerations, the corneal surface appears irregular, and exudate (pus) may be present. Instillation of an ophthalmic dye will permit confirmation of the diagnosis.

Etiology—Corneal ulcers result from bacterial, viral, or fungal infections.

Treatment—A culture of the drainage to determine the causative organism will indicate appropriate medication. Broad-spectrum antibiotics are used initially to prevent corneal scarring and the resulting impairment of vision. Certain bacterially-caused ulcers progress so rapidly that, without proper treatment, the cornea will perforate (be pierced with holes), and vision in the eye will be lost within 48 hours.

Diabetic Retinopathy (Die-a-bet'-ick Reh-tin-op'-athe)

Description—This form of vascular **retinopathy** results from juvenile or adult diabetes. Approximately 75% of patients with juvenile diabetes develop diabetic retinopathy within 20 years after the onset of diabetes. Incidence in adults with diabetes increases with the length of time a person is diabetic. About 80% of patients with diabetes of 20 to 30 years' duration develop retinopathy. It is the leading cause of acquired blindness in adults.

Signs and symptoms—Symptoms result from an edematous retina, which causes light to scatter. Tiny capillary walls thicken and show evidence of dilation, twisting, and hemorrhage. This causes glare, blurred vision, and reduced visual acuity. If diagnosed and treated early, prognosis is good for simple forms; in extensive forms, prognosis is poor, with 50% becoming blind within five years.

Etiology—The condition is a result of an interference with the blood supply to the eyes.

Treatment—Treatment consists of sealing holes that have developed in the retina and coagulating the leaking vessels with a laser beam. If new abnormal vessels have grown onto the retina and into the vitreous body, it is possible for the retina to detach from the choroid layer, resulting in vitreous hemorrhage and blindness. With this advanced condition, open surgery will be required.

Glaucoma (Glaw-co'-ma)

Description—This condition of excessive intraocular pressure results in atrophy (wasting away) of the optic nerve.

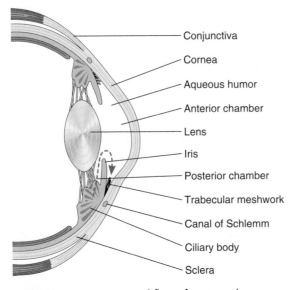

- Conjunctiva
- Cornea
- Aqueous humor
- Anterior chamber
- Lens
- Iris
- Posterior chamber
- Trabecular meshwork
- Canal of Schlemm
- Ciliary body
- Sclera

FIGURE 11–47 Normal flow of aqueous humor

Glaucoma causes severe visual impairment and eventually blindness. It occurs in 2% of adults over age 40 and accounts for 15% of all blindness in the United States. It is the most easily prevented cause of blindness.

There are several forms of glaucoma, such as chronic open-angle (most common) and acute or chronic closed-angle. Each form has its own parameters. All types of glaucoma may cause severe visual defects because the increased intraocular pressure within the eyeball causes pressure against the blood vessels of the retina, reducing the blood supply and destroying retinal nerve cells. Glaucoma is diagnosed with evidence of increased intraocular pressure as measured by a tonometer and confirmed by viewing, through an ophthalmoscope, characteristic changes in the optic disk.

The condition results from either an overproduction of the aqueous humor produced by the epithelium of the ciliary body or the obstruction of its outflow circulating mechanisms to the canal of Schlemm for absorption into venous circulation (Figure 11–47).

Glaucoma—Chronic Open-angle

Etiology—With this type of glaucoma, the circulating aqueous humor cannot drain because of a blockage of the trabecular meshwork, the canal of Schlemm, or the aqueous veins.

Signs and symptoms—The symptoms are **insidious** (gradual), bilateral, and often not recognized until late in the disease. They include mild aching, a loss of peripheral (side) vision, seeing halos around lights, and difficulty seeing at night or in darkened places.

Treatment—Treatment is aimed at reducing the production of aqueous humor by the use of medications and eyedrops to encourage the circulation. With inadequate response, a surgical procedure to create an opening for the aqueous outflow is indicated.

Glaucoma—Acute Close-angle

Etiology—This type results from obstruction resulting from anatomically narrow angles, shallow chambers, and a thickened iris that closes the passages. There is a rapid onset of symptoms and it is considered an emergency.

Signs and symptoms—There is pain and redness of the affected eye with a feeling of pressure. The pupil is moderately dilated and nonreactive to light. There is blurred and decreased visual acuity and sensitivity to light. Unless the pressure is relieved quickly, blindness will occur within three to five days.

Treatment—Usual treatment consists of aggressive drug therapy and a peripheral iridectomy (removal of a piece of the iris) to permit outflow of the aqueous humor.

Laser surgery is a quick, less expensive, and relatively painless solution to both open- and closed-angle glaucoma. In open-angle, if medication is ineffective, a laser beam is directed to open the trabecular meshwork. In closed-angle, the laser makes a tiny opening in the iris to allow the fluid to drain. A second treatment may be necessary in closed-angle glaucoma. Laser eye surgery is more effective in the early stages of the disease.

Hordeolum (Stye) (Hor-de′-o-lum)

Description—This localized infection of a gland of the eyelid produces an abscess around an eyelash.
Signs and symptoms—The eye is red, painful, and swollen.
Etiology—The causative organism is staphylococcus.
Treatment—Treatment consists of applying warm, wet compresses to relieve pain and promote drainage and the use of eye drops or ointment to treat the infection.

Iritis (I-righ′-tis)

Description—An inflammation of the iris.
Signs and symptoms—Iritis produces moderate to severe eye pain, photophobia, and a small nonreactive pupil caused by the spasm of the iris.
Etiology—It is often caused by an improperly-healed corneal abrasion, especially if damage is from a sharp object.
Treatment—Prompt treatment is required to prevent complications. The pupil is dilated with mydriatics to allow the eye to rest to prevent the formation of posterior synechiae (adhesions of the iris to the lens). Corticosteroid drops are used to reduce the inflammation.

Myopia (My-op′-eah)

Description—This condition is a defect in vision that is also known as nearsightedness. Objects can be seen distinctly only when close to the eyes. The rate of incidence is believed to be around 11 million Americans.
Signs and symptoms—There is a blurring of vision when looking at objects beyond immediate surroundings.

Etiology—The primary cause is a misshapen eyeball. When the cornea is too convex, objects are refracted in front of the retina.

Treatment—Myopia is normally treated with the application of glasses or contact lenses to alter the refraction of images and to bring them to focus on the retina. A procedure called radial keratotomy (RK) provides an alternative method of correction. It is a surgical procedure that requires extreme precision. Small cuts are made in the cornea to flatten it so that the focal point is corrected. It can be done only after the individual has passed young adulthood because myopia may worsen into the early 20s. The newest form of RK is a computerized procedure using an excimer (or cold laser).

This variation of keratotomy procedure is called photorefractive keratectomy (PRK). It removes a thin layer of tissue from the surface of the cornea to flatten and reshape it to the desired correction. The actual laser treatment takes only 15 to 40 seconds. One eye at a time is usually done in order to evaluate the results before treating the second eye. PRK is appropriate for people who have stable vision with low to moderate myopia and no other eye problems.

The newest method, which provides an alternative to surgery, reshapes the corneas with cornea-flattening *reverse-geometry* contact lenses. The lenses are worn at night for about 60 days and reportedly produce dramatic improvement with results equal to radial keratotomy.

Presbyopia (Pres-be-op'-e-ah)

Description—This condition is characterized by inability of the lens to accommodate for near vision. **Presbyopia** occurs as part of the normal aging process.

Signs and symptoms—The first symptom is usually the inability to read smaller print without straining and the use of a bright light. With advancement, all normal size print is out of focus at the normal reading distance.

Etiology—Presbyopia is caused by the loss of elasticity of the lens. It is no longer able to adjust to focus images on the retina properly.

Treatment—The condition can be corrected by the fitting of contact lenses or eyeglasses.

Ptosis (Toe'-sis)

Description—Ptosis is the drooping of the upper eyelid.

Signs and symptoms—This condition is evident upon observation. Eyes appear to be only partially open. The individual has a "sleepy" appearance.

Etiology—Ptosis may be a congenital condition or the result of aging, the presence of an excess fatty fold, or a neurological factor.

Treatment—Treatment may be required if vision is restricted or the appearance is cosmetically undesirable. A surgical procedure on the eyelid muscles will correct the disorder, or a device can be attached to the eyeglass frame to elevate the eyelid.

Retinal Detachment (Ret'-ih-nal)

Description—This disorder is characterized by the separation of the retina from the choroid layer of the eyeball.

Signs and symptoms—Diagnosis can be made from the patient's complaints of seeing floating spots, flashes of light, and a gradual vision loss. Confirmation is possible after pupil dilation and ophthalmoscopy reveal a gray and opaque retina with indefinite margins in the affected areas. Folds, tears, and a ballooning inward of the retina may be seen.

Etiology—The separation may occur with aging, which causes the normal vitreous support to shrink away. This results in a small hole or tear that permits the humor to seep between the layers and cause separation. Other causative factors include severe high blood pressure, diabetes, trauma, and other systemic diseases.

Treatment—Treatment consists of limiting eye movements with a patch, bed rest, sedation, and appropriate positioning of the head. Spontaneous reattachment is rare. A coagulation laser beam can repair simple tears in the retina by "spot welding" the area with several rows of "welds," but once separation has occurred, other treatment will be necessary. Both heat and cold therapies are used to create a sterile inflammatory reaction that causes the retina to readhere. A tight band is placed around the eyeball, inside the sclera layer, which makes the choroid "indent" against the retina to maintain its closeness. Various surgical procedures to reattach the retina to the choroid can be performed.

Strabismus (Stra-biz'-mus)

Description—This is a condition in which one eye deviates with the gaze being abnormally inward or outward, higher or lower than the other eye (Figure 11–48). An abnormally-inward gaze (convergent or "crosseye") is

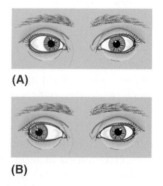

(A)

(B)

FIGURE 11–48 Strabismus: (A) convergent or esotropia, (B) divergent or exotropia

DISORDERS OF THE EYE

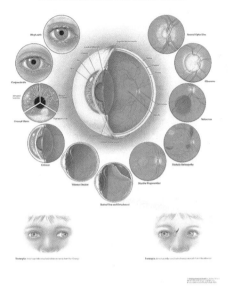

FIGURE 11–49 Disorders of the eye (Courtesy of Colwell, a division of Patterson Dental Supply Inc., 800-637-1140.)

also called esotropia, and an abnormally-outward gaze (divergent or "walleye") is also known as exotropia.

Signs and symptoms—This condition is obvious upon examination. The deviation and absence of coordinated eye movement cause complaints of double vision and the inability to see objects clearly. **Strabismus** is frequently associated with Down syndrome, cerebral palsy, and mental retardation.

Etiology—The disorder results from eye muscle imbalance or attempts to compensate for farsightedness.

Treatment—Conservative initial treatment consists of a patch on the normal eye, corrective glasses, and specific eye exercises. Surgery to adjust the muscles that control eye placement and movement may be indicated. If strabismus develops before age five, the deviated eye may be suppressed, resulting in amblyopia that could cause loss of vision if not treated.

Figure 11–49 illustrates many disorders of the eye.

Eye Protection

The National Society for the Prevention of Blindness, Inc., promotes many programs stressing the importance of protecting eyes from injury. Many occupations require the use of goggles or safety glasses. The society recommends the use of impact-resistant glass or plastic in all eyeglasses and sunglasses. A 1972 federal ruling requires that the lens be able to withstand the impact from a $\frac{5}{8}$-inch-diameter steel ball dropped from a height of 50 inches. Individuals with sight in only one eye should use industrial-quality safety lenses and frames. When engaging in do-it-yourself work, sports, or hobbies that involve

visual hazards, protective eye wear should be worn. It should be noted that contact lenses do not provide protection for the eyes, and the use of protective eye wear is necessary.

If injury should occur, initial treatment is important in order to prevent further damage. If something is splashed or blown into the eye, it should be rinsed thoroughly, for several minutes if caustic, with the eye held open. If caustic, rinse for several minutes. A physician should examine the eye as soon as possible. Foreign bodies which are not embedded may be removed with a wet fold of a tissue or a moistened cotton swab. Objects that are embedded into the surface require medical attention. See Foreign Bodies, Chapter 19.

THE EAR AND THE SENSE OF HEARING

The ear is capable of receiving vibrations in the air and translating them into the sounds we recognize: the more vibrations per second, the higher the frequency, or pitch, of the sound, the stronger the vibration, the louder the sound.

The Outer Ear

Vibrations are picked up by the pinna (auricle) of the outer ear and directed down the external **auditory** canal to the **tympanic membrane** (eardrum) (Figure 11–50).

The Middle Ear

The sound waves vibrate the membrane and the **malleus** (hammer) attached to its inner surface. The malleus in turn "strikes" the **incus** (anvil), which moves the **stapes** (stirrup). These three small bones and the space around them are called the middle ear. The middle ear communicates the vibrations to the inner ear by the stapes pushing against the fluid in the vestibule of the inner ear through the oval window.

The middle ear is connected by means of the **eustachian tube** to the throat. The tube is responsible for equalizing air pressure in the middle ear with the outside atmospheric pressure. Unfortunately, infections from the throat often pass through the tube into the middle ear. Rapid changes in altitude, harsh blowing of the nose, or a forceful sneeze may cause temporary air pressure inequities.

The Inner Ear

The vibrations from the middle ear continue through the coiled **cochlea**, which contains the **organ of Corti**, a collection of specialized nerve cells (Figure 11–51). These cells transmit the impulses to the auditory nerve, which passes them on to the auditory center of the temporal lobe of the cerebrum for interpretation.

The inner ear also contains three **semicircular canals**. These structures are responsible for maintaining equilib-

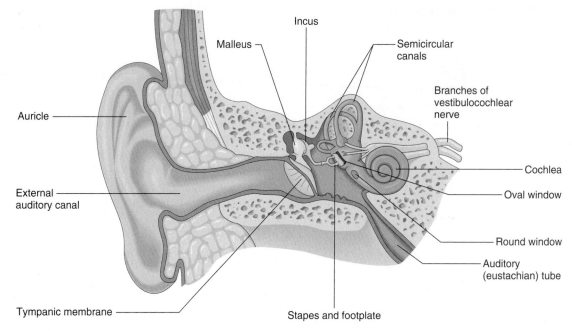

FIGURE 11-50   The ear

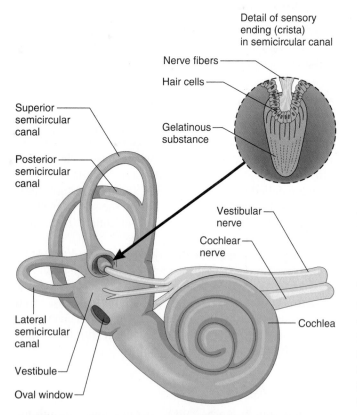

FIGURE 11-51   The inner ear (From *The Wonderful Human Machine*, copyright 1979 by the American Medical Association.)

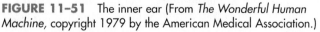

rium (balance). Inside the canals, hairlike nerve cell receptors are embedded in a gelatin-like material. When the head moves, the material pushes against the receptors, which transmit to the brain the change in position.

Another nerve receptor network in the semicircular canals is similarly constructed inside two small sacs. The gelatin surface here is covered with a layer of tiny limestone grains. When the head moves, the grains shift, causing the hair cells to send out impulses.

The inner ear, therefore, carries out two important functions for the body: It transmits vibrations to the auditory nerve so that we can hear, and its semicircular canals allow us to maintain our balance.

DIAGNOSTIC TESTS

Routine diagnostic examinations for the ear, such as audiometry, Weber, and Rinne, are discussed in Chapter 14.

Electronystafmograph

The electronystafmograph (ENG) is a special examination that evaluates balance function. Because eyes and ears work together through the nervous system, measurement of eye movements are used to evaluate the balance system. The test is performed in a darkened room with electrodes placed near the eyes. Wires from the electrodes attach to a recording machine. Warm and cool water or air are gently introduced into each ear canal. Patients are asked to identify locations of visible objects when shown. Coordination is evidence of balance function and will be affected by the involved ear.

CT Scan

A CT scan of the brain with special emphasis on the inner ear can be used to identify pathology.

DISEASES AND DISORDERS OF THE EAR

Auditory Canal Obstruction

Description—This refers to anything in the ear canal that in some manner occludes the opening.

Signs and symptoms—Symptoms vary with the obstruction. Insects may produce sounds or movement, or objects can cause discomfort, a degree of hearing loss, or annoyance.

Etiology—The auditory canal can be obstructed by impacted **cerumen** (ear wax) or a foreign body such as a bean, pea, pebble, bead, or insect. Children often put objects into their ears.

Treatment—Treatment consists of a removal technique appropriate to the obstruction. Cerumen can be removed by gentle scraping with a cerumen spoon and/or irrigation by syringe or an aerated water jet (see Chapter 14). Irrigation should be stopped immediately if it causes pain. Removal of insects can be accomplished easily after killing with an instillation of 70% alcohol. Similar objects can also be removed after irrigation with alcohol if they cannot be reached with forceps. Water must be avoided if it may cause swelling of the object, such as a bean or pea.

Hearing Loss

Description—This is a condition of reduced ability to perceive sound at normal levels.

Signs and symptoms—The loss can be gradual or sudden. The person has difficulty perceiving sounds in their environment. Hearing loss is classified as conductive if it is caused by the inability to carry sound waves through the ear structures. It is known as **sensorineural** if it is the result of nerve transmission failure within the inner ear or the auditory nerve. Some hearing loss can be caused by a combination of factors. The gradual loss of hearing that occurs normally as part of the aging process is known as **presbycusis**.

Etiology—Conductive loss may be caused by an obstruction from a buildup of cerumen (wax), a foreign body, swelling within the auditory canal, middle ear infection, or otosclerosis.

Sudden loss of hearing without prior impairment is considered a medical emergency because prompt treatment may restore hearing. Common causes are acute infection, head trauma, brain tumor, toxic drugs, or metabolic and vascular disorders.

Hearing loss can also be noise-induced and can be temporary or, over time, permanent. It follows prolonged exposure to noise in excess of 85 to 90 db (see Chapter 14). It is common among people who work in constant industrial noise, military personnel, and rock musicians. This loss is preventable with the enforcement of the use of protective devices, such as ear plugs, as mandated by law in occupational exposure.

Bone and air conduction hearing loss is assessed by the Rinne and Weber tests. An audiometer can be used to give a pure tone audiometry examination to measure the threshold and degree of loudness at which sound can be perceived (see Chapter 14).

Treatment—The form of treatment depends upon the causative factor. Removal of obstructions will correct that associated loss. With sudden loss, treatment may involve medication, surgery, or antidotes to toxins. Loss caused by aging can usually be improved with the use of modern hearing aids; providing sound amplification is all that is required. A new cochlear implant can improve severe hearing loss that is not benefitted by a hearing aid. The implant involves a mini-microphone behind the ear, a calculator-sized processor that can be worn on a belt, a receiver surgically implanted in the ear, and electrical contacts that run through the cochlea. To be approved for the implant, patients must have an intact auditory nerve and a hearing loss where less than 30% of speech is understood, even with a hearing aid. Most will gain at least modest communication ability; some are even able to use a phone. Implant failure rate is about 2% and unfortunately causes patients to lose any natural hearing they may have had prior to the surgery.

Ménière's Disease (Ma-nears')

Description—This disease is a disorder of the inner ear, usually affecting only one ear; however, 15% of patients may have both ears affected. It typically begins between the ages of 20 and 50, affecting men and women equally.

Signs and symptoms—The condition known as **Ménière's disease** is characterized by severe vertigo (dizziness) and **tinnitus** (ringing in the ears). Violent attacks may last from 10 minutes to hours and cause severe nausea, vomiting, and perspiration. Often the vertigo causes loss of balance and results in the person falling. The off-balance sensation may last for days. There is intermittent hearing loss early in the disease, but over time a fixed loss commonly develops, probably as a result of the degeneration of hair cells in the cochlea and vestibule.

Etiology—The cause is unknown, but it probably results from an abnormality in the fluids of the inner ear.

Treatment—Treatment consists of drugs to reduce fluid, antihistamines, and mild sedation. Anti-vertigo and anti-nausea medications may be used. Patients are advised to avoid caffeine, smoking, and alcohol. Excessive fatigue and stress may aggravate the disease. Patients who experience vertigo without warning are advised not to drive or engage in any type of potentially-hazardous activity because of the possibility of an accident. If attacks are not controlled conservatively and become disabling, a surgical procedure may be indicated. Options range from a shunt to remove excess fluid to the cutting of the balance nerve (which will usually control the vertigo while still maintaining hearing) to a labyrinthectomy and eighth nerve resection (which destroys both the balance mechanism and hearing on the affected side, but will control the attacks). There is only a cure for vertigo, not for Ménière's disease.

Motion Sickness

Description—A condition that occurs when engaging in activities involving movement, such as riding in automobiles, boats, planes, or amusement rides.

Signs and symptoms—This is characterized by loss of equilibrium, perspiration, headache, nausea, and vomiting brought on by irregular motion.

Etiology—The disorder probably results from excessive stimulation of the inner ear receptors or confusion in the brain between the visual stimulus and movement perception.

Treatment—Treatment consists of avoiding the causative motions, lying down, and closing the eyes. When avoidance is not possible, the head should be kept still and vision focused on distant and stationary objects. Medications to prevent nausea and vomiting, such as valium, scopolamine, and antihistamines, are usually beneficial if taken prior to the trip. Symptoms can also be controlled by applying medication in a patch form to the skin behind the ear.

Otitis: Externa (O-ti'-tis)

Description—An infection of the external auditory canal.

Signs and symptoms—**Otitis** causes pain and hearing loss.

Etiology—Otitis externa can result from contaminated swimming water (swimmer's ears); cleaning the canal with bobby pins or introducing an organism on a cotton swab; regular use of earphones or plugs which can trap moisture, creating optimal growing conditions; and scratching the ear canal with a fingernail.

Treatment—It is best treated with pain medication and antibiotic ear drops, following thorough cleaning.

Otitis: Media

Description—An infection of the middle ear often associated with respiratory infections.

Signs and symptoms—Otitis media is characterized by a severe, deep, and throbbing pain; fever; hearing loss; nausea and vomiting; and dizziness. The tympanic membrane may be reddened and bulge into the external canal. Excessive pressure may cause it to rupture, resulting in drainage into the canal. Recurring episodes may scar and thicken the membrane, causing a conduction hearing loss. Holes and tears from a rupture will also cause a loss of hearing.

Etiology—Otitis media usually occurs from an organism that has caused a sore throat or cold. However, it can also be caused by obstruction of the eustachian tube that results in a negative pressure within the ear that "pulls" serous fluid from the blood vessels into the middle ear.

Treatment requires antibiotics, such as penicillin or erythromycin (with a sulfa drug if allergic to penicillin), in addition to pain medication. A myringotomy (incision of the tympanic membrane) is indicated if bulging and severe pain are present.

Note: Young children and infants are prone to ear infections. Anatomically, their eustachian tubes slant horizontally, which allows fluid to collect more easily and become a medium for bacterial growth. Infants who are allowed to take a bottle while lying down may get fluid and bacteria into their eustachian tubes from reflux or from obstruction causing negative pressure to extract fluid.

Treatment—With chronic fluid collection caused by obstruction, it may be necessary to insert a tiny polyethylene tube through the tympanic membrane to temporarily equalize the pressure. This procedure is known as a tympanoplasty. Tubes usually fall out after about six months. **CAUTION:** Untreated middle ear infection can lead to severe complications, such as mastoiditis, brain abscesses, or meningitis. With today's antibiotics, these complications are rare. Sudden hearing loss, headache, dizziness, chills, and fever are possible warning signs. The physician should be consulted immediately if the child has had a recent cold or sore throat.

Otosclerosis (O-toe-sklur-o'-sis)

Description—The most common cause of conductive deafness is **otosclerosis**. It is characterized by the formation of spongy bone that immobilizes the stapes in the oval window of the vestibule, disrupting the conduction of vibrations from the tympanic membrane to the cochlea.

Signs and symptoms—Otosclerosis is a condition characterized by the slow and progressive loss of hearing and may be accompanied by tinnitus.

Etiology—It appears to result from a genetic factor and often occurs among family members. Incidence in Caucasians is at least 10%, affecting twice as many females as males, usually between 15 and 30 years of age.

Treatment—Treatment for otosclerosis consists of surgically removing the stapes (stapedectomy) and inserting an artificial substitute, which results in partial to complete return of hearing. An appropriate type of hearing aid may be of some assistance if a stapedectomy is not possible.

Presbycusis (Senile Deafness) (Prez-bi-ku'-sis)

Description—This hearing loss is an effect of aging. It is sensorineural in nature.

Signs and symptoms—The deafness normally manifests itself through the loss of high-frequency sounds. It is usually accompanied by an annoying tinnitus. The patient has difficulty understanding the spoken word and may become depressed because of inability to communicate.

Etiology—The loss is caused by the deterioration of the auditory system and a loss of the hair cells in the organ of Corti.

Treatment—Presbycusis is irreversible but can be somewhat overcome with an effective and properly-fitting hearing aid.

THE NOSE AND THE SENSE OF SMELL

The sense of smell is caused by the olfactory organ in the top of the nasal cavity (Figure 11–52). The nerve fibers in the organ are chemoreceptors that respond to stimuli from ions or molecules dissolved in the moisture from the mucous membranes. The organ is connected by nerve fibers, which run through tiny holes in the skull bone above the nasal cavity, to the olfactory center in the brain. The nerve fibers connect with hair cells in the mucous membrane of the nose. These odor detectors can "smell" something only after it is dissolved in the mucus secretions.

DISEASES AND DISORDERS OF THE NOSE
Epistaxis (Epi-stack'-sis) (Nosebleed)

Description—Bleeding from the nose.

Signs and symptoms—The presence of blood coming from the nose is evidence of epistaxis. However, blood originating from the nose may be expectorated from the mouth or swallowed into the throat. Symptoms other than visible blood may be lightheadedness, a drop in blood pressure, rapid pulse, dyspnea, pallor, and other indications of shock.

Etiology—This usually occurs after injury, either external or internal, such as a blow to the nose, nosepicking, or foreign body insertion. Less frequent causes of **epistaxis** are chronic conditions, such as nasal or sinus infection that results in capillary congestion and bleeding, or the inhalation of irritating substances. Predisposing systemic factors include high blood pressure, anticoagulation drugs, chronic aspirin use, and blood diseases, such as anemia, hemophilia, and leukemia.

Treatment—Treatment varies depending on the cause, location, and severity. Even moderate bleeding is considered severe if it persists longer than 10 minutes after pressure is applied. Initial first aid treatment may consist of: elevating the head; compression of nostrils against the septum continuously for 5 to 10 minutes; application of ice or cold compresses to nose and back of neck; preventing the swallowing of blood (to determine the amount lost); avoiding talking or blowing the nose; and observing for amount of blood loss and signs of shock.

Advanced treatment includes: For anterior bleeding, apply epinephrine-saturated cotton ball or gauze to the bleeding site and use external pressure, followed by cauterization by electric cautery or silver nitrate; for posterior bleeding, the insertion of a nasal pack for 48 to 72 hours may be required. Small catheters are passed through each side of the nose into the mouth. Rolled gauze packs are attached to the catheters and drawn back through the mouth and up into the posterior nasal cavity where they become lodged, creating pressure against the leaking blood vessels. If necessary, anterior bleeding can be treated by packing for 24 to 48 hours. Other treatment may include supplemental vitamin K, blood transfusions, and surgical ligation (tying) of the bleeding artery.

Nasal Polyps (Pol'-lips)

Description—These benign growths, usually multiple and in both sides of the nose, often occur in large enough numbers and size to distend the nose and obstruct the airway.

Signs and symptoms—A patient usually complains of obstruction and "something" in the nose. They experience difficulty breathing. Diagnosis is made by visual observation through a nasal speculum or by x-rays of posterior nasal passages and the sinuses.

Etiology—They are caused by prolonged mucous membrane edema associated with allergies, chronic sinusitis, rhinitis, and recurrent nasal infections.

Treatment—If infected, treatment with antihistamines, cortisone, and antibiotics will temporarily reduce the size of the **polyps**. However, surgical removal is the treatment of choice and is usually necessary.

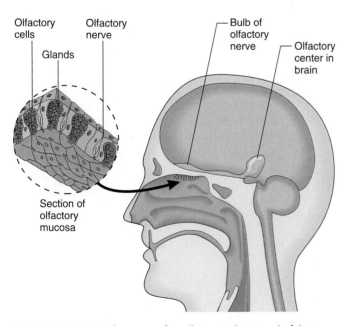

FIGURE 11–52 The sense of smell (From *The Wonderful Human Machine*, copyright 1979 by the American Medical Association.)

Rhinitis (Allergic) (Rye-in-i'-tis)

Description—Rhinitis is a reaction to airborne allergens.

Signs and symptoms—It causes sneezing, profuse watery discharge, itching of the eyes and nose, conjunctivitis, and tearing. Many symptoms are the result of the body's attempt to dilute or remove irritants coming into contact with its mucous membranes.

Etiology—Any antigen occurring in the environment can be an irritant and cause allergic rhinitis. Some of the most common are dust, ragweed, perfumes, and cat dander.

Treatment—Treatment consists of eliminating environmental antigens when possible, the use of antihistamines and systemic corticosteroids. Long-term management includes injections of the offending allergens to cause desensitization, the use of air conditioning, and, if severe and persistent, relocation to a safe environment.

THE TONGUE AND THE SENSE OF TASTE

The ability to taste flavors is located in the receptors of the taste buds on the tongue. They are located at the tip, sides, and back, grouped by the taste that can be perceived (Figure 11–53). The sweet area is at the tip, the salty areas are next along the sides, followed by the sour areas and another area of salty perception. The large **papillae** (raised areas) at the back transmit the bitter sensations. Like the sense of smell, taste is possible because of the chemoreceptors that receive stimuli from ions or molecules and initiate the impulses. As with smell, taste is not possible unless the substance is moistened. This moisture is supplied by the salivary glands in sufficient quantities to affect taste.

DISEASES AND DISORDERS OF THE MOUTH AND TONGUE

Candidiasis (Thrush) (Can-di-de-a'-sis)

Description—This disease is a fungal infection of the mucous membranes of the mouth and throat. The organism can cause infection in other locations, such as nails, skin (diaper rash), vagina, and the gastrointestinal tract.

Signs and symptoms—Evidence of the disease is cream-colored or bluish-white patches of exudate on the tongue, mouth, or throat that cannot be scraped off (Figure 11–54). The infected areas may swell, causing respiratory distress in infants. Occasionally they are painful, but they usually cause a burning sensation in the throat and mouth of adults.

Etiology—It is caused by a fungal organism of the Candida species. These organisms are normally present in the body but cause infection when their sudden growth is permitted by some change, such as an illness, a suppressed immune system, drug abuse, or from the use of broad spectrum antibiotics that alters the body's normal flora, which permits Candida to increase. Infants may acquire thrush during birth or from unclean bottle nipples.

Treatment—Initial treatment is aimed at improving the underlying cause, then swabbing the mouth with an oral mystatin suspension or oral antifungal medication.

A PEDIATRIC PERSPECTIVE

If the mother is breast-feeding, she must also treat her nipples with an antifungal medication.

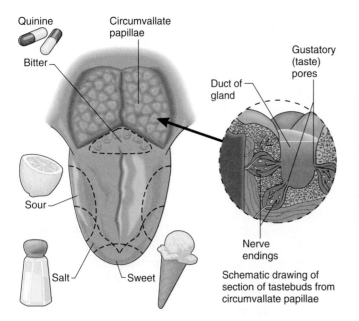

Quinine

Bitter

Circumvallate papillae

Duct of gland

Gustatory (taste) pores

Sour

Nerve endings

Salt

Sweet

Schematic drawing of section of tastebuds from circumvallate papillae

FIGURE 11–53 The sense of taste (From *The Wonderful Human Machine,* copyright 1979 by the American Medical Association.)

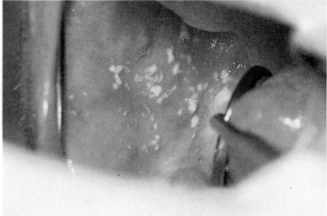

FIGURE 11–54 Candidiasis (Thrush) (Courtesy of Dr. Joseph Konzelman, School of Dentistry, Medical College of Georgia.)

Glossitis (Gloss-i'-tis)

Description—Inflammation of the tongue.

Signs and symptoms—The condition results in a red, swollen tongue, pain on chewing, difficult speech, and occasionally an obstructed airway.

Etiology—It is caused by an organism, irritation, injury, or nutritional deficiencies. Agents such as tobacco, alcohol, spicy foods, and jagged teeth may cause glossitis.

Treatment—Treatment includes topical anesthetic mouthwash, systemic pain medication, good oral hygiene, and the avoidance of alcohol and hot, cold, or spicy foods.

Oral Cancer

Description—In recent years, a significant increase in the incidence of oral cancer has been noted. There seems to be evidence that some people have switched from cigarettes to smokeless forms of tobacco in an effort to alleviate the development of lung cancer.

Signs and symptoms—Any lesion or growth within the mouth is not normal and should be examined by a physician or dentist. They can be of varying shapes and types and may present no evidence of pain or discomfort.

Etiology—No one knows for certain the exact cause for cancer, but there are strong correlations between substances and the development of malignant lesions. Normal cells are affected by something in their environment that causes their normal growth-limiting control to fail and excessive cell production to begin. The use of products such as chewing tobacco and snuff causes extensive disease of the gums, tongue, and other oral structures and often results in the development of cancer within the oral cavity.

Treatment—The use of surgical excision as a treatment depends upon the form of cancer developed with or without surgical excision. Quite disfiguring results arise from removal of part of the mouth, and often speech is affected when the tongue is involved. Chemotherapy and radiation are appropriate.

THE SKIN AND THE SENSE OF TOUCH

The sense of touch requires direct contact with the body through contact receptors (Figure 11–55). The sense of touch involves mechanical energy, such as pressure or traction, which activates mechanoreceptors. Radiant energy, such as heat or cold, activates thermoreceptors. The design of the receptor varies with its location on the body. Touch receptors are most concentrated in the fingertips. Pain receptors are simply bare nerve endings in the skin and other organs. Separate skin receptors perceive heat and cold. Each of the contact receptors in the skin has its own perceptive function enabling us to feel the many different sensations of pain, touch, pressure, heat, cold, trac-

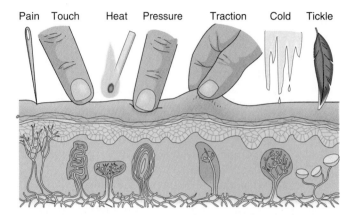

Pain   Touch   Heat   Pressure   Traction   Cold   Tickle

FIGURE 11–55 The sense of touch (From *The Wonderful Human Machine,* copyright 1979 by the American Medical Association.)

A CAAHEP CONNECTION

The standards specifically identify **Anatomy and physiology; Diseases, disorders, and treatments;** and **Medical terminology** as essential components of a medical assistant program. This unit contains content in all of these areas and provides the knowledge necessary to understanding that portion of the human body related to the senses. The addition of A Pediatric Perspective allows you to consider the implications of treatments for this stage of growth and development.

tion, and tickle. This sense aids us in protecting ourselves, identifying injury, feeling pleasure, and maintaining contact with our environment. The skin is the subject of the next unit.

ACHIEVE UNIT OBJECTIVES

Complete Chapter 11, Unit 3, in the workbook to help you obtain competence of this subject matter.

UNIT 4

Integumentary System

OBJECTIVES

Upon completion of the unit, meet the following performance objectives by verifying knowledge of the facts and

principles presented through oral and written communication at a level deemed competent.

1. Spell and define, using the glossary at the back of the text, all the **Words to Know** in this unit.
2. List the five functions of the skin.
3. Explain how the skin regulates body temperature.
4. Describe how the body cools its surface.
5. Name the three layers of skin tissue and the characteristic structures of each layer.
6. Describe the process that causes wrinkles.
7. Explain what causes a suntan to develop.
8. Describe the distinguishing features of basal cell and squamous cell carcinoma lesions.
9. Identify the ABCD rules and other warning signs of melanoma and the factors that contribute to its development.
10. Explain what causes blushing, birthmarks, moles, and albinism.
11. Identify 20 diseases or disorders of the skin.

AREAS OF COMPETENCE (AAMA)

This unit addresses content within the areas of *Administrative procedures, Practice finances, Patient care, Communication skills,* and *Instruction* as identified in the Medical Assistant Role Delineation Study. Refer to Appendix A for a detailed listing of the areas. (Note: Although *Anatomy and physiology* is not identified in the study, a basic knowledge of the body's structure and function is an essential foundation to the competent performance of many roles.)

WORDS TO KNOW

acne	melanin
albino	melanocytes
alopecia	papule
carbuncle	pediculosis
constrict	perception
dermatitis	pigment
dermis	psoriasis
dilate	pustule
eczema	receptors
epidermis	sebaceous
erythema	sebum
follicle	slough
folliculitis	subcutaneous
furuncle	transdermal
herpes simplex	urticaria
herpes zoster	verrucae
integumentary	viral shedding
keloid	vesicle
lesion	wheals
Lyme disease	whorl
macule	

A CAAHEEP CONNECTION

The standards specify the importance of **Anatomy and physiology** and the need for a strong foundation in medical terminology. A fundamental knowledge of the integumentary system is essential to understanding clinical procedures, diagnostic testing, examinations, and the proper medical terminology involved to accurately code insurance forms and coordinate patient care information to other health care professionals.

Ⓐ **Library**

The word **integumentary** refers to an external covering or skin. You may never have thought of the skin as a "body system," but according to the definition of a system in Unit 1, the skin with all its structures qualifies: it is many tissues (nerve, connective, muscle, epithelial), forming organs (sweat and oil glands), to perform a function. The skin is not usually listed as one of the body's systems, however. Most anatomists classify the skin as an organ. When listed in this category, it becomes the largest organ of the body. An average adult has about 3000 square inches of skin surface. The skin makes up about 15% of the total body weight, which would be approximately 20 pounds of a 145-pound person. The skin varies in thickness from very thin on the eyelids to quite thick on the soles of the feet.

The skin is so important to survival that the loss of even a small percentage of its vital function is a cause for concern. If about one-third of the skin of a healthy young adult is lost, death may result. Skin covers all the body's surface, preventing the tissue fluids from escaping and foreign materials in the environment from entering. At the openings to the body, such as the nose, mouth, or anus, it joins with the mucous membranes that line the openings into the respiratory and digestive systems to make a continuous internal and external covering.

FUNCTIONS

The skin performs five important functions for the body: protection, perception, temperature control, absorption, and excretion. The skin protects against the invasion of bacteria by serving as a barrier. It is effective, however, only as long as it remains intact. A cut or scrape of the surface allows bacteria to enter. It also protects the delicate underlying tissues from injury by the damaging rays of the sun. Equally important, it protects the body's tissues from loss of fluid. This is of great concern when large areas of skin are lost as a result of burns, for example, which allows fluids to escape and bacteria to enter.

The skin serves as an organ of **perception** in cooperation with the nervous system and the sense of touch. A square inch of skin contains about 72 feet of nerves and hundreds of **receptors** registering pain, heat, cold, and pressure.

In that same square inch are about 15 feet of blood vessels, which provide nutrients and oxygen and also regulate the body's temperature. This function is of such importance to the body that the skin receives approximately one-third of the blood circulating throughout the body. When the body's temperature control center in the brain senses the body is becoming too warm, the nervous system sends messages to the surface vessels to **dilate**, which allows heat from the blood to escape through the skin's surface and therefore cool the body. If heat must be retained, the vessels are ordered to **constrict** to reduce the loss of heat so that body temperature can be maintained at an adequate level. This important function is discussed in greater detail in Chapter 13, Unit 3, Vital Signs.

The skin also contains sweat glands, which are likewise controlled by the heat regulator in the brain. When the air temperature rises, the body produces sweat, which evaporates from its surface to provide a cooling effect and thereby reduce the amount of heat within the underlying blood vessels.

The skin is capable of absorbing some materials from its surface through the hair **follicles** and the glands. This function can be of use to the physician in treating certain conditions. Perhaps the two most common applications are antimotion sickness medication in a patch form, which is placed on the skin's surface behind the ear, and in a medicated paste form, which is placed on the chest to treat certain heart conditions. A trend seems to be developing toward a greater amount of medications being administered through the skin. Primarily the advantages are "timed release," which spreads medication evenly over a long period, thereby eliminating repeated dosage and the digestive system side effects from certain oral drugs. This form of drug administration is called **transdermal**.

Several substances known as lipid-soluble (e.g., vitamins A, D, E, and K and the sex hormones) and almost all gases (e.g., oxygen, hydrogen, and nitrogen) can pass through the skin. It is interesting to note that carbon monoxide cannot pass.

The skin's function of excretion consists primarily of eliminating water and salt plus a minute amount of other waste products. Excessive fluid loss as a result of strenuous activity or a highly-elevated temperature can be a matter of concern. Fluid must be replaced to maintain a proper fluid balance. The skin also combines the ultraviolet rays from sunlight with compounds normally present in the skin to produce vitamin D.

A great number of microscopic skin structures are located within an area of only one square centimeter. This is illustrated in Figure 11–56 as a small circle on the back of the hand. It seems inconceivable that this large group of anatomical structures could be located in such a small

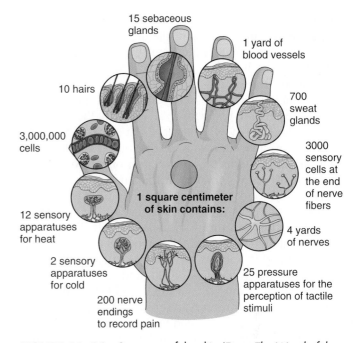

FIGURE 11-56 *Structures of the skin (From The Wonderful Human Machine, copyright 1979 by the American Medical Association.)*

area. These microscopic wonders perform an invaluable service for the body.

STRUCTURE OF THE SKIN

The skin is composed of three layers: the **epidermis** on the top, the **dermis** in the middle, and the **subcutaneous** layer on the bottom (Figure 11–57). The subcutaneous layer is filled with fat globules, blood vessels, and nerves. The dermis contains blood vessels, nerves, hair follicles,

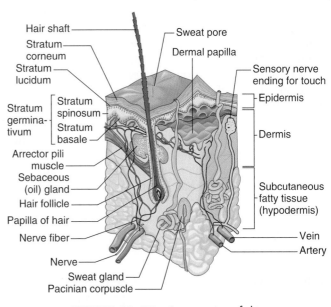

FIGURE 11-57 Cross-section of skin

and sweat and oil glands. This layer is usually referred to as the "true skin." The top of the dermis is covered with cone-shaped papillae, which create an uneven surface. The epidermis is full of ridges that fit snugly over the papillae on top of the dermis. These ridges form the **whorls** and patterns on the fingertips that we call fingerprints. Because no two people have exactly the same pattern of ridges, they will not have the same fingerprints, making this characteristic a suitable means of identification. Similar patterns of ridges appear on the soles of the feet and are used for identification of newborns. New cells are formed deep in the epidermis. Here rapid cell division pushes cells toward the surface of the skin to replace those that wear away, die, and flake off. The process from division to flaking off takes about 28 to 60 days. Because of the skin's ability to reproduce cells rapidly, it can repair itself quickly following cuts and abrasions.

The skin is strong, soft, flexible, and elastic in young people because of the presence of keratin in the epidermis and collagen fibers in the dermis. With age, elastic fibers in the dermis increase in size, and collagen in the dermis degenerates. The support for the epidermis is decreased, and as a result, wrinkles occur. This is especially noticeable in areas where there is more facial movement, such as around the eyes and mouth.

The skin has four appendages. These are the sweat glands, oil glands, hair and nails. The dermis contains the sweat and **sebaceous** (oil) glands. Sweat glands are tiny coiled tubes deep in the dermis and corkscrew tubules leading to the surface. Oil glands are located in or near hair follicles over the entire skin surface, except for the palms of the hands and the soles of the feet.

A sebaceous gland produces an oily substance that helps prevent the hair and skin from becoming dry and brittle. Unfortunately, oil glands often become plugged by cell overgrowth. The gland continues to produce oil, which fills the duct and results in development of a blackhead or pimple. This results in a condition known as **acne**.

Every hair has a root, which is inside a follicle (shaft) that extends deep into the dermal layer. With long hair, the root extends into the subcutaneous layer. Attached to each follicle is a small involuntary muscle. With certain emotions or sensations of coldness, the muscle contracts, causing the hair to stand erect and producing what we call "goose flesh." An inner layer of cells in the shaft of hair contains a **pigment** that gives the hair its color. Hair that is white has cells that contain little pigment.

The hair and nails are composed of hard keratin (soft keratin is found in the epidermis). The keratins are similar but the hard keratin is more permanent and does not **slough** (drop) off, which means they must be cut occasionally.

Skin Color

A brown-black pigment called **melanin** is produced by cells called *melanocytes,* which are present in the epidermis. They protect the underlying tissues from damage by the sun. The amount of melanin affects the color of the skin as does another pigment, carotene, which is yellow. In light-skinned people, melanin is found at the bottom of the epidermis. In people with darker skin, it is found throughout the epidermis. The presence of blood vessels in the dermis also contributes to the coloration of the skin. When the skin is exposed to the sun, it may become reddened because of dilation of the superficial blood vessels. The condition is known medically as **erythema**, but it is commonly known as sunburn. If it is not severe, the skin will acquire a brown coloration or suntan, which is produced by the melanin pigment increasing and moving to the surface to protect the underlying tissues. New melanin will replace the old in the lower cell layer. Freckles are actually small areas of melanin pigment.

Skin coloration is affected by many factors. When we blush, the rich supply of blood vessels causes reddening of the skin caused by dilation. Birthmarks may be caused by coloration from a concentration of blood vessels or from patches of skin pigment. Moles are also pigmented patches. A person whose skin has little or no pigment to give it color is said to be an **albino**. An albino's hair also lacks pigment and will be pale yellow or white. Because pigment is also lacking in the coloration of the eyes, the sun and artificial light cannot be filtered out. Therefore, the eyes of a person with albinism are a red color as the result of translucent irises and are very sensitive to light. People with this disorder must wear sunglasses or tinted lenses for comfort and to prevent eye damage.

THE SKIN AS A DIAGNOSTIC TESTING SITE

The skin is often used to test and diagnose disorders and diseases of the body, specifically in the area of allergies. Because of its natural capacity to defend the body from foreign substances, it makes an excellent medium for testing the reaction to minute amounts of allergens. Following injection of common substances, usually on the back or inner surface of the forearm, the skin will form varioussized areas around the injection sites, reacting to those materials that initiate an allergic response. Physicians can then identify causative substances and recommend measures to reduce the problems associated with the allergic disorder. (See Chapter 16, Diagnostic Procedures.)

Skin Appearance

Conditions of the skin cause changes in its appearance. These changes are known as **lesions** and manifest themselves as specific eruptions. Table 11–3 identifies the most common types of lesions.

DISEASES AND DISORDERS
Acne Vulgaris (Ack'-knee Vul-gar'-is)

Description—This inflammatory disease of the follicles of the sebaceous glands mainly affects adolescents.

TABLE 11-3

DIFFERENT TYPES OF SKIN LESIONS, THEIR CHARACTERISTICS, SIZE, AND EXAMPLES

Type of Skin Lesion	Characteristics	Size	Example(s)
Bulla (blister)	Fluid-filled area.	Greater than 5 mm across	• A large blister
Crust	A collection of dried serum and debris.	Varies in size	• Impetigo or eczema
Excoriation	Area missing the epidermal layer.	Varies in size	• Scrape or burn
Fissure	Linear crack from epidermis to dermis.	Varies in size	• Athlete's feet
Macule	A round, flat area usually distinguished from its surrounding skin by its change in color.	Smaller than 1 cm	• Freckle • Petechia (small hemorrhage spot)
Nodule	Elevated solid area, deeper and firmer than a papule.	Greater than 5 mm across	• Wart
Papule	Elevated solid area.	5 mm or less across	• Elevated nevus (mole)
Pustule	Discrete, pus-filled raised area.	Varying size	• Acne
Ulcer	A deep loss of skin surface that may extend into the dermis that can bleed periodically and scar.	Varies in sizes	• Venous stasis ulcer
Tumor	Solid abnormal mass of cells that may extend deep through cutaneous tissue.	Larger than 1-2 cm	• Benign (harmless) epidermal tumor • Basal cell carcinoma (rarely metastasizing)
Vesicle	Fluid-filled raised area.	5 mm or less across	• Chickenpox • Herpes simplex
Wheal	Itchy, temporarily elevated area with an irregular shape formed as a result of localized skin edema.	Varies in size	• Hives • Insect bites

Signs and symptoms—The acne may appear as a closed comedo or whitehead if it does not protrude from the follicle and is covered by the epidermis. If it protrudes and has black coloration caused by the melanin or pigment from the follicle, it is known as a blackhead or open comedo. Eventually, the enlarged plug leaks or ruptures, spreading into the dermis and resulting in inflammation and the development of pustules and **papules**.

Etiology—The cause if multifactorial (many factors). Research has determined that dietary habits appear to be less of a factor than originally thought. Present findings seem to suggest that hormonal dysfunction and an oversupply of **sebum**, oil from the sebaceous glands, are the probable underlying causes. It collects at the openings to the glands, hardens, and closes off the natural flow of oily secretion, causing blackheads or cysts to develop. Sometimes the area will become filled with leukocytes that cause pus to accumulate and pimples develop. Trapped bacteria within the follicle are also a contributing factor.

Treatment—Usual treatment for severe acne includes a topical antibacterial product either alone or in combination with a topical retinoid product. Antibiotics applied to the skin are helpful. Systemic antibiotics decrease bacterial growth within follicles. Accutane is reserved for use in those patients with severe scarring acne. Oral contraceptives are used in women.

Alopecia (Al-o-pech'-ea)

Description—This is loss of hair, usually occurring on the scalp. There are two types of **alopecia**: a scarring type, which causes irreversible hair loss, and a nonscarring type, which usually is reversible.

Scarring Alopecia

Signs and symptoms—The main symptom is the continual loss of hair, resulting in gradual thinning and the eventual absence of hair.

Etiology—This is usually an irreversible loss of hair resulting from the destruction of the hair follicles. It is caused by physical or chemical trauma or the chronic tension on the hair shaft from brading or tight rolling of the hair. Certain diseases like lupus erythematosus, bacterial or viral infections, and skin tumors may also cause this type.

Treatment—This depends upon the cause. A change in the way the hair is cared for and the control of infection could prevent further loss but may not restore lost follicles.

Nonscarring Alopecia (several forms)
Male-pattern baldness

Signs and symptoms—The most common form of non-scarring alopecia is the evidence of hair loss with male-pattern baldness. It often begins around age 30 with a receding front hairline and loss of hair on the top and back. In some men, the areas eventually meet leaving hair only on the sides (Figure 11–58A and B).

Etiology—It seems to be primarily caused by aging and the level of androgen (male hormone). There is a tendency for genetic influence, and it will often be dis-

played among male family members. Women may also exhibit the male pattern but at a lesser degree.

Treatment—There is no known "cure"; however, the use of Rhogain seems to prevent further loss and encourage regrowth in some men. Surgical grafting of hair follicles from other parts of the scalp have proved successful.

Physiologic

Signs and symptoms—A normal temporary hair loss which may occur immediately following or up to four months after giving birth.

Etiology—Prolongation of the growing phase.

Treatment—None required.

Areata (idiopathic)

Signs and symptoms—This type is self-limiting and reversible, occurring among both sexes from young to middle age adults. It usually affects small patches but can involve the entire scalp and body.

Etiology—Unknown, but some feel it may be linked to stress.

Treatment—None. Regrowth is normally spontaneous. Topical steroid creams may also be used.

Trichotillomania

Signs and symptoms—This hair loss is characterized by patchy, incomplete areas of hair loss with many broken hairs, primarily on the scalp, but can also involve other areas, such as the eyebrows. It is more common in children.

Etiology—This loss is the result of it being pulled out because of compulsive behavior.

Treatment—Some form of psychotherapy may be necessary. Dressings over the areas aid in behavior change to encourage normal growth.

Chemotherapy related

Signs and symptoms—There is a sudden loss of most of the hair.

Etiology—Certain chemical agents destroy the cells of the hair, which result in the massive loss of hair over a two- or three-day period soon after the initiation of the drug. Normally, some fine hair will remain but is very sparse.

Treatment—Fortunately, about three months after treatments end, hair will begin regrowth, sometimes a different color or texture.

Cancer

Description—The skin may be the site of different forms of cancerous lesions, such as basal cell carcinomas, squamous cell carcinomas, and malignant melanomas. Nevi (moles) are considered to be potentially malignant and require careful observation.

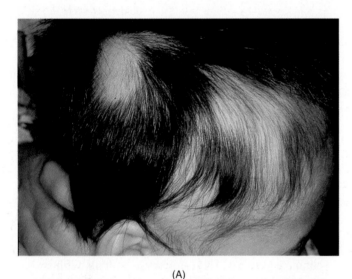

(A)

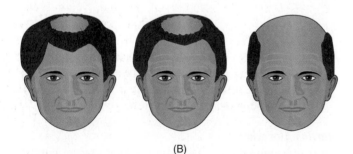

(B)

FIGURE 11–58 (A) Alopecia, (B) male-pattern baldness (**A,** Courtesy of Robert A. Silverman, MD, Clinical Associate Professor, Department of Pediatrics, Georgetown University.)

Signs and symptoms—Bleeding, itching, or a change in color, size, shape, or texture of a mole suggests a possible conversion to a malignant state. A new non-healing lesion that bleeds easily should also raise suspicion.

Basal Cell Carcinoma

This is a slow-growing, locally-destructive skin tumor. They occur where there are abundant sebaceous follicles, especially on the face. It is more prevalent in persons over the age of 40, especially those who are blond and fair skinned (Figure 11-59). It is the most common malignant tumor affecting Caucasians. There are basically three types of basal cell carcinoma lesions, each with its own distinctive characteristics and usual location. They are diagnosed by appearance and surgical biopsy.

1. *Nodulo-ulcerative* lesions occur most often on the face and are small, smooth, pinkish, and translucent papules. As they enlarge, the centers become depressed and the borders elevated and firm.
2. *Superficial* basal cell carcinoma are often multiple and commonly occur on the chest and back. They are oval or irregularly-shaped with sharply-defined, threadlike borders that are slightly elevated.
3. *Sclerosing* basal cell lesions occur on the head and neck. They appear yellow to white, are waxy, and do not have distinct borders.

Etiology—Basal cell carcinoma is caused primarily by prolonged exposure to the sun.

Treatment—Treatment depends upon the extent of the lesion. It can include surgical excision, irradiation, chemosurgery, or curretage and electrodesiccation.

Squamous Cell Carcinoma (Skwa-mus)

Description—This is an invasive tumor with metastatic potential. Its incidence is highest in fair-skinned Caucasian males over the age of 60. Living in sunny climates, working in outdoor employment, and smoking greatly increase the risk of development.

Signs and symptoms—This form of carcinoma is commonly found on the face, the ears, the back of the

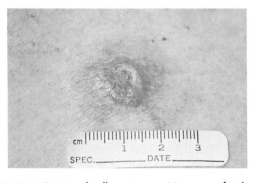

FIGURE 11–59 Basal cell carcinoma (Courtesy of Robert A. Silverman, MD, Clinical Associate Professor, Department of Pediatrics, Georgetown University.)

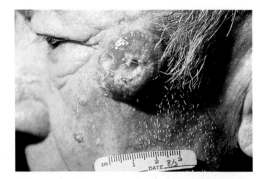

FIGURE 11–60 Squamous cell carcinoma (Courtesy of Robert A. Silverman, MD, Clinical Associate Professor, Department of Pediatrics, Georgetown University.)

hands, and other sundamaged areas. The lesions have a tendency to metastasize, with those located on unexposed skin having the greater incidence. Lesions of the lower lip and ears are exceptionally metastatic (Figure 11–60).

Etiology—This type is predisposed by sunlight, the presence of premalignant lesions, x-ray therapy, environmental carcinogens, and chronic skin irritation.

Treatment—The treatment varies with the size, location, and invasiveness of the lesion. Options include wide surgical excision, scraping and electrodesiccation, radiation, and chemosurgery.

Malignant Melanoma (Mah-lig'-nant Mel-an-o'-ma)

Description—A neoplasm that develops from the pigment-producing **melanocytes**. The peak of incidence occurs between 50 and 70 years of age. The incidence is more common in women. There are four clinical types: superficial spreading melanoma, nodular melanoma, lentigo maligna melanoma, and acral lentiginous melanoma. Superficial lesions may be curable with wide local excision. Deeper lesions may metastasize through the lymphatic and circulatory systems. Prognosis depends on the depth of the lesion, as measured in millimeters by the pathologist.

The American Cancer Society releases facts about the incidence of malignant melanoma. In 1993, 32,000 people were diagnosed; about 6,500 died. This incidence translated into 1 in every 105 United States residents (compared to only 1 in every 1,500 in 1935). According to a Harvard Medical College article in September 2001, the incidence of melanoma is now 1 in every 74 people. The American Academy of Dermatology views this prevalence as an undeclared epidemic.

Signs and symptoms—The information and photos in Figure 11–61 show the ABCD rules and appearance signs of melanoma.

Etiology—The major cause of malignant melanoma is exposure to the sun. The sun produces ultraviolet rays,

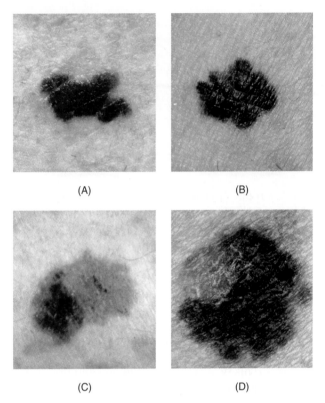

(A)   (B)

(C)   (D)

FIGURE 11–61 The signs of melanoma: (A) asymmetry, (B) border irregularity, (C) color, (D) diameter (Courtesy of the American Academy of Dermatology.)

mainly UVA and UVB. UVBs cause sunburn, premature aging of the skin, and skin cancers. Most sunscreens provide a degree of protection against this ray. However, recent evidence suggests that the UVA rays may also be damaging the skin, perhaps aiding the cancer-forming ability of UVB.

The Cancer Society cited the primary reasons for the melanoma increase to be weekend-packed leisure time, which results in intense bursts of exposure to UVB, the loss of the ozone layer protection, UVA rays not being blocked by sunscreens, and the tendency of people to purposely lie flat in the sun for hours at a time, which allows deeper penetration of the rays. People most at risk are those who have had severe blistering sunburns prior to age 20.

Other contributing factors are blond or red hair, fair skin, blue eyes, and a tendency to sunburn. Persons who work or spend many hours outdoors or who live in places with intense year-round sunshine are also at risk. Arizona has the highest incidence reported in the United States.

Treatment—Surgical resection is always required with a melanoma. If it is deep, the resection is at least two inches beyond the primary lesion's borders and into the deep tissues. Closure often requires a skin graft. Large lesions may also require chemotherapy. If there is metastasis, radiation may be used to relieve pain, but it will not prolong survival.

WHAT IS THE DIFFERENCE BETWEEN A MELANOMA AND AN ORDINARY MOLE?

A normal mole is an evenly-colored brown, tan, or black spot in the skin. It is either flat or raised. Its shape is round or oval, and it has sharply-defined borders. Moles are generally less than 6 mm in diameter (about the size of a pencil eraser). A mole may be present at birth, or it may appear spontaneously, usually in the first few decades of life. Sometimes several moles appear at the same time, especially on sun-exposed areas of the skin. Once a mole has fully developed, it normally remains the same size, shape, and color for many years. Most moles eventually fade away in older persons.

Almost everyone has moles, on the average of about 25. The vast majority of moles are perfectly harmless. A sudden or continuous *change* in a mole's appearance is a sign that you should see your physician. However, a melanoma is more complicated than a mole.

Here's the simple **ABCD** rule to help you remember the important signs of melanoma:

A. Asymmetry. One half does not match the other half (Figure 11–61A).

B. Border irregularity. The edges are ragged, notched, or blurred (Figure 11–61B).

C. Color. The pigmentation is not uniform. Shades of tan, brown, and black are present. Red, white, and blue may add to the mottled appearance (Figure 11–61C).

D. Diameter greater than 6 mm. Any sudden or continuing increase in size should be of special concern (Figure 11–61D).

Other Warning Signs of Melanoma

Change in the surface of a mole—scaliness, oozing, bleeding or the appearance of a bump or nodule; spread of pigment from the border into surrounding skin; redness or a new swelling beyond the border; change in sensation—itchiness, tenderness, or pain.

(The above information reprinted, with permission, from a brochure titled *Why You Should Know About Melanoma*, distributed by the American Cancer Society and developed in cooperation with the American Academy of Dermatology.)

The best treatment for melanoma is prevention. Skin cancer is preventable. Sun avoidance is the best defense.

Dermatologists recommend avoiding sun altogether from 10:00 AM to 3:00 PM (perhaps from 8:00 AM to 6:00 PM if the ozone condition worsens), and using a sunscreen of at least 15 SPF that will block both UVA and UVB during exposure. Sunlamps, tanning pills, and tanning salons should be avoided.

The practice of monthly self-examination should be established to observe for any developing lesion so that it can be caught in the early stages. While standing in a brightly-lit room in front of a full-length mirror and using a hand mirror, completely examine the body. Check under arms, on backs of legs, on feet, and between toes. Examine the back of the neck, and part the hair to check the scalp. If any growth, mole, sore, or discoloration appears suddenly or begins to change, it needs to be seen by a physician.

Cellulitis (Sel-u-li′-tis)

Description—The acute diffuse or spreading inflammation of the skin and subcutaneous tissue.

Signs and symptoms—It is characterized by localized swelling, pain, heat, and redness (Figure 11-62).

Etiology—The cause of cellulitis is usually the streptococcus or staphylococcus aureus bacteria. It is potentially dangerous.

Treatment—It is usually treated successfully with oral and topical antibiotics.

Dermatitis (Der-ma-ti′-tis)

Description—The term means inflammation of the skin and can refer to any form of skin condition such as: seborrhea, eczema, contact **dermatitis** (from irritants),

exfoliative dermatitis (large pieces of peeling skin), or stasis (from lack of blood supply).

Signs and symptoms—Common symptoms are dry skin, redness, itching, edema, formation of lesions, and scaling.

Etiology—Dermatitis is often caused by allergens, such as wool, detergent, cosmetics, pollen, or foods, such as eggs, milk, seafood, or wheat products. Irritants to the skin, lack of moisture in the environment, harsh soaps, and long, hot showers also contribute to dermatitis.

Treatment—It is treated by avoiding known allergens and irritants; using emollients, hydrocortisone creams and ointments, systemic steroids, and antihistamines; and taking other dermatitis-specific measures.

Eczema (Ek′-ze-ma)

Description—This noncontagious skin disease can be acute or chronic.

Signs and symptoms—This condition is characterized by dry, red, itchy and scaly skin. There may be the presence of a watery discharge if it becomes chronic (Figure 11-63).

Etiology—Several things may initiate **eczema**, such as diet, cosmetics, clothing, medications, soaps, occupational or environmental substances, and emotional stress.

Treatment—Treatment consists primarily of removal of the causative agent where possible and the local application of ointments to alleviate the symptoms. Topical steroids are indicated to reduce inflammation, and antibiotics are used if secondary infection is present. The

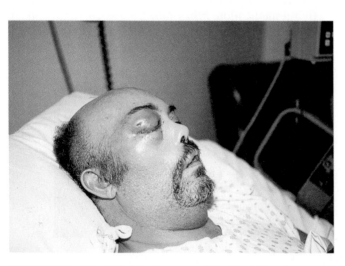

FIGURE 11-62 Cellulitis (Courtesy of Dr. Mark Dougherty, Lexington, KY.)

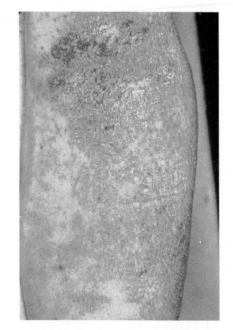

FIGURE 11-63 Eczema (Courtesy of The Centers for Disease Control and Prevention [CDC].)

noncortisone cream *tacrolimus* (Protopic) is the most effective remedy yet developed, usually providing results within several weeks. This and other eczema medications are available by prescription only.

Folliculitis (Fol-ick-u-li'-tis)

Description—This is an infection of the hair follicle with the formation of a pustule. It is known as **folliculitis**. It can be of a superficial form, involving only the surface area around a single follicle, or deep, involving the total hair follicle.

Signs and symptoms—The presence of redness and pustules around a single follicle on the scalp, arms and legs, and on the face of bearded men (Figure 11–64).

Etiology—The most common cause is *Staphylococcus aureus*.

Treatment—Treatment consists of thorough cleansing of the area, the application of moist heat to promote drainage from the lesion, and the use of topical antibiotics. Systemic antibiotics are usually indicated.

Furuncles (Fur'-uncles)

Description—Folliculitis may lead to the development of **furuncles** (boils).

Signs and symptoms—They are hard painful nodules that enlarge over several days' time until they rupture, releasing pus and dead cells through one draining point. The area remains red and swollen for a short time, but the pain lessens.

Etiology—Furuncles may be caused by irritation, pressure, friction, or infection with *Staphylococcus aureus*.

Treatment—Treatment consists of the measures used for folliculitis with moist heat to relieve pain and encourage "ripening" of the lesion. Often, incision and drainage are required to allow complete expulsion of the material.

Patients must be cautioned not to squeeze a boil because it may rupture into the surrounding tissues. Systemic antibiotics are necessary if there is surrounding erythema or a fever. A patient with recurring furuncles should see a physician to rule out any underlying cause, such as diabetes.

Carbuncles (Kar'-bunk-le)

Description—A **carbuncle** begins as a nodule, then enlarges to involve several adjacent hair follicles.

Signs and symptoms—It is characterized by deep follicular abscesses of several follicles with multiple draining points. It is extremely painful and usually associated with fever and general malaise.

Etiology—Usually caused by a persistent staphylococcal infection and often follows a furuncle.

Treatment—Carbuncles require treatment with systemic antibiotics in addition to the localized heat applications and drainage. Wash cloths, towels, bed sheets, and clothing used by the infected person must not be shared with other family members to prevent spreading the bacteria.

Herpes Simplex (Her'-pez)

Description—This viral infection is equally prevalent among males and females and occurs throughout the world. **Herpes simplex** I is most often associated with lesions in the oral and nasal area. Herpes simplex II is associated with genital lesions. Incubation period following exposure is from 4 to 10 days. A prodrome (symptom of approaching disease) of pain, tingling, and itching signals the oncoming **vesicle**.

Signs and symptoms—The presence of small, grouped, painful, clear vesicles on an erythematous base (Figure 11–65).

Etiology—It is caused by the herpes virus.

Treatment—The most effective treatment is an oral antiviral medication. It has shown some decrease in pain, new lesion formation, and a shortened period of viral shedding and healing time. Some relief from minor

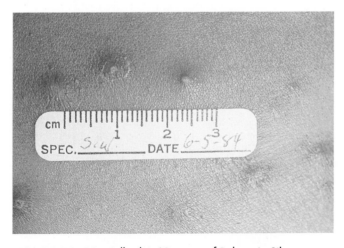

FIGURE 11–64   Folliculitis (Courtesy of Robert A. Silverman, MD, Clinical Associate Professor, Department of Pediatrics, Georgetown University.)

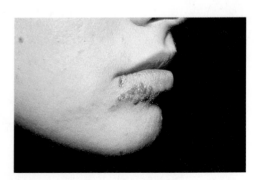

FIGURE 11–65   Herpes simplex virus I (Courtesy of Robert A. Silverman, MD, Clinical Associate Professor, Department of Pediatrics, Georgetown University.)

outbreaks may occur with the application of various over-the-counter topical preparations.

(Note: The term **viral shedding** refers to that period of time when a virus is the most active and most contagious.)

Herpes Zoster (Her'-pez Zos'-tur)

Description—**Herpes zoster** is an acute infectious process also known as shingles (Figure 11–66).

Signs and symptoms—It causes severe neuralgic pain along the area of the involved nerves. It is characterized by fever, malaise, and the eruption of vesicles in the painful area, which spread unilaterally around the back, chest, or back of neck or vertically on the extremities. (See Unit 2.)

Etiology—It is caused by the varicella zoster virus, which also causes chickenpox.

Treatment—Usually the patient requires an analgesic and antipyretic to reduce fever and relieve pain. Antiviral drugs decrease acute pain, new lesions formation, viral shedding, healing time, and rates of dissemination (spreading).

Hirsutism (Hur'-su-tis-m)

Description—This disorder usually appears in women and children. Excessive body hair develops in an adult male pattern of growth.

Signs and symptoms—The most common symptom is growth of facial hair, but other masculinization signs,

such as deepening voice, increased muscle mass, menstrual irregularity, and breast size reduction, may be exhibited.

Etiology—There may be a family history of the disorder, or it could be related to an endocrine problem resulting from either pituitary dysfunction, ovarian lesions, or adrenal gland enlargement.

Treatment—Treatment consists of hair removal by shaving, depilatory creams, or waxing as well as bleaching to minimize the appearance of hair. Electrolysis will permanently destroy the hair follicles but is slow and expensive. Laser hair removal may be effective. A new topical cream is available to treat increased hair growth on the face. If hormonal causes are evident, treatment may involve counteracting or controlling endocrine secretions in specific situations.

A PEDIATRIC PERSPECTIVE

Referral to an endocrinologist is necessary to reduce or prevent masculinization and encourage appropriate sexual development.

Impetigo (Im-pe-tag'-o)

Description—This is a contagious, superficial skin infection that is usually seen in young children.

Signs and symptoms—If the cause is streptococcal, the small red **macule** (flat area with definite edges) turns into a vesicle (raised lesion containing serous fluid) and then to a **pustule** (lesion with purulent material) within a relatively short time. (The terms macule, vesicle, and pustule refer to any skin lesion that demonstrates these descriptive characteristics, not to impetigo alone.) When the lesions break, a characteristic yellow crust develops from the exudate (drainage) (Figure 11–67).

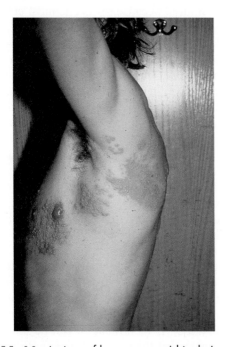

FIGURE 11–66 Lesions of herpes zoster (shingles); note how vesicles follow a nerve pathway. (Courtesy of Robert A. Silverman, MD, Clinical Associate Professor, Department of Pediatrics, Georgetown University.)

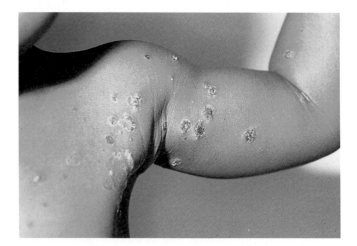

FIGURE 11–67 Impetigo (Courtesy of Robert A. Silverman, MD, Clinical Associate Professor, Department of Pediatrics, Georgetown University.)

Other sites develop from contact with the lesions or the drainage. The staph lesion is characterized by a thin-walled vesicle that forms a thin, clear crust from the exudate. Both forms characteristically have a clear central area and definite outer rims. The lesions appear primarily on the face, neck, and other exposed areas of the body. Contamination of others is prevented by avoiding contact through wash cloths, towels, and bed linens. Scratching of the lesions must be prohibited.

Etiology—It is caused by streptococcus or *Staphylococcus aureus* bacteria.

Treatment—Good hygiene is essential. The exudate can be removed by washing with soap and water two to three times a day. An oral systemic plus a topical antibiotic is indicated.

Keloid

A scar that developed excess dense tissue as it progressed through the healing process is known as **keloid**. (See Chapter 11, Unit 1.)

Lyme Disease (Lime)

Description—A tick-borne disease named after Old Lyme, Connecticut, where it was first reported in 1975. It has since been reported in 45 states, but over 90% of the cases occur within distinct areas: the East Coast from Massachusetts to Maryland, the upper midwest, the South and Southeast, and northern California and Oregon. Incidence is increasing dramatically. In 1986, only 700 cases were reported. In 1988, there were 5,000 reported. In 1994, New York alone reported 3,098 new cases. The disease is spreading primarily because people are moving into suburban and rural areas, and the explosive deer population is moving into habitated areas. Both humans and pets can become infected. Note: If you live or work in one of the high incidence areas, find out more about Lyme disease.

Signs and symptoms—The early stage of **Lyme disease** is usually marked by flu-like symptoms: fatigue, chills, fever, headache, muscle and joint pain, and swollen lymph nodes. In 60% of the cases, there is a characteristic circular, red skin lesion caused by the spirochete (corkscrew-shaped bacterium) migrating through the skin in all directions. This can appear from three days to one month after a bite. It enlarges to as much as several inches across and develops a clear center giving it the appearance of a bull's eye; hence the name, "bull's eye rash." Diagnosis is difficult in the remaining 40% who do not develop the rash and therefore may not get diagnosed and treated early. Their first symptoms are usually arthritis, fatigue, and memory loss. Later, nervous system symptoms develop. These may include numbness and pain, Bell's Palsy, poor motor coordina-

tion, insomnia, irritability, heart arrythmia, headaches, and depression.

Etiology—Lyme disease is caused primarily by the bite of a spirochete-infested deer tick. It is an unusual three-host tick with a two-year life cycle. It begins when adult ticks feed and mate on deer and then drop off to lay eggs. The eggs hatch and the young ticks, called nymphs, attach and feed on small rodents that carry the spirochete and infect the tick. The mice carry the nymphs through the woods and fields and into human habitats: the grass, shrubs, wood piles, garages, and homes. From contact they attach and feed on dogs, squirrels, and humans. Bites seem to occur most often between May and September. The tick, in its unfed state, is about the size of a pinhead. It looks like a pear-shaped crab and has eight legs. Ticks insert their barbed mouth parts into the skin, deposit spirochetes, suck blood until satisfied (usually two to four days), and then drop off. The longer a tick feeds, the larger it becomes and the greater the chance for infection. If the tick is removed before the first 24 hours, you probably will not become infected. (Not all ticks carry the spirochete; approximately 30% to 60% of northeastern ticks test positive.)

Treatment—The best treatment is prevention. Avoid tick-infected areas especially from May through September. Dress in light-colored clothing to make ticks more visible—they are not easily seen. Long sleeves and long pants tucked into light-colored socks or boots are highly recommended. Spray clothing with a tick repellent, and allow to dry before wearing. Applying a repellent containing up to 30% DEET directly to the skin (according to directions) is advisable for adults but unsafe for children because of its chemical composition. Check your entire body at the end of the day, paying particular attention to ankles, knees (especially backs), groin, armpits, under breasts, scalp, ears, and the back. Check all pets *before* bringing them into the house. *Do not* let pets sleep in or on the bed. Before washing, put outdoor clothing in the clothes dryer on the highest temperature for 30 minutes to kill hiding ticks. They can survive laundering.

If a deer tick is found, remove it and show it to a doctor, or send it to health authorities for positive identification. (See "How to Remove a Tick.") Its size is important because it is evidence of the length of time attached. Ticks that are to be tested should be put in a clean glass container and placed in the refrigerator until they are sent to health authorities. Results take about two weeks. Ticks, dead or alive, can be tested using a polymerase chain reaction test that detects the DNA of the spirochete, which will identify the type of tick, confirm the spirochete's presence, and therefore determine treatment. If identification can be made without testing, dispose of the tick by dropping it in 70% alcohol or diluted bleach. Do not "treat" ticks that are going to be tested.

If symptoms or a positive test result indicate Lyme disease, a course of antibiotics are prescribed for three weeks with one week off and then another three-week course of antibiotics, which effectively treats the infection. If diagnosis is not made until later-stage disease, then other systemic conditions require treatment in addition to antibiotics. Recent discovery of a specific antibody in patients with the disease may lead to immediate diagnosis and earlier treatment. Current blood tests are not conclusive. Dogs, cats, cattle, and horses can also become infected and treated with antibiotics if detected early. Prevention in dogs is possible with a good tick collar and a vaccine. Two human vaccines have been tested that may provide protection for uninfected people when available.

HOW TO REMOVE A TICK

Removal is done with forceps or tweezers at the mouth parts. Pull gently until it releases its hold. The entire head should be removed. If tweezers are not available, cover with a tissue. Never use bare fingers. A ruptured tick can release infectious material onto a cut in the skin and transfer its disease. If a part remains, see a physician immediately. After removal, wash the area and your hands thoroughly and treat the area with 70% alcohol. If a test is desired, mail a container with the tick and a check for $45 to Imugen, 220 Norwood Park South, Norwood, MA 02062. Call ahead to verify price: 800-246-8436. Results take about two weeks.

Pediculosis (Pe-dik-u-lo'-sis)

Description—There are three types of **pediculosis** resulting from three varieties of parasitic lice: capitis from head lice, corporis from body lice, and pubis from pubic lice. The lice feed on human blood and lay eggs known as nits on body hairs or fibers of clothing. The nits hatch and will die in 24 hours unless they feed on a host. Nits mature in two to three weeks.

Pediculosis Capitis

Description—It is the most common form and is found primarily among children, especially girls. It spreads through shared combs, brushes, clothing, and hats.
Signs and symptoms—It is identifiable as an oval, grayish, dandruff-like fleck that cannot be shaken off. Its symptoms are itching and scalp abrasions with matted, foul-smelling hair in severe cases.
Etiology—Pediculosis is caused by parasitic forms of lice that are found in overcrowded conditions and with poor personal hygiene.
Treatment—Treatment consists of gamma benzene hexachloride (GBH) cream rubbed into the scalp at night, then rinsed out with GBH shampoo the next morning.

Treatment is repeated the second night. A fine-toothed comb dipped in vinegar helps remove nits from the hair.

A PEDIATRIC PERSPECTIVE

Parents have the option of purchasing over-the-counter medication if they choose, it is similar to prescription medication and provides effective treatment.

Pediculosis Corporis

Description—Pediculosis corporis lives in clothing seams except when feeding on the host.
Signs and symptoms—Initially, small red papules appear, which itch. The resulting scratching causes rashes and wheals to develop.
Etiology—Prolonged wearing of the same clothes, overcrowding, and poor hygiene. It is spread through shared clothing and linens.
Treatment—Pediculosis corporis can be removed by bathing unless infestation is severe. Clothing and bed sheets must be washed, ironed or dry cleaned. A prescription medication may be ordered if necessary.

Pediculosis Pubis

Description—Pediculosis pubis, commonly called crabs, is found attached primarily to pubic hair.
Signs and symptoms—The lice cause itching, which results in skin irritation from scratching.
Etiology—It is transmitted through sexual intercourse or contact with infected clothes, bedding, or towels.
Treatment—Pediculosis pubis is treated with a prescription medication and left on for 24 hours or with shampooing the affected area. Treatment must be repeated in one week. The sexual partner must also be treated or reinfection will occur. This type of infestation is also treated with a prescription drug.

Poison Ivy

Description—This is a dermatitis caused by contact with the poison ivy plant.
Signs and symptoms—Initially, poison ivy causes moderate itching and burning that is soon followed by small blisters. As blisters increase, some break and skin is covered with a coating of serum. Marked discomfort and intense itching may be present (Figure 11–68).
Etiology—It is caused by the sap of the three-leafed poison ivy plant, fresh or dry.
Treatment—The best treatment is prevention. Learn to recognize and avoid contact with the plant. Specially susceptible people can be given injections to prevent its development. Different preparations are available to control the itching and to "dry up" the lesions. Treat-

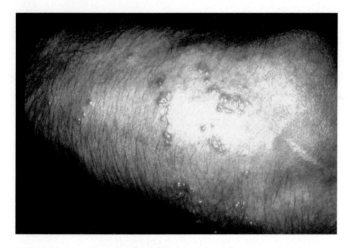

FIGURE 11–68 The fluid-filled vesicles of poison ivy (Courtesy of Centers for Disease Control, Atlanta, GA.)

ment depends upon the extent of involvement. Oral steroids or topical steroid cream is usually sufficient.

Psoriasis (So-ri'-ah-sis)

Description—This is a chronic inflammatory condition which is recurrent, with alternating periods of remission or increased severity. The episodes are affected by the environment (cold weather causes flare-ups), endocrine changes, pregnancy, and emotional stress.

Signs and symptoms—**Psoriasis** is a chronic disease characterized by red papules which are covered with silvery scales (Figure 11–69). The lesions are dry,

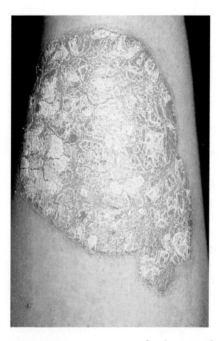

FIGURE 11–69 Psoriasis (Courtesy of Robert A. Silverman, MD, Clinical Associate Professor, Department of Pediatrics, Georgetown University.)

cracked, and encrusted, sometimes covering large areas of the body. The scales either flake off or build up, covering the lesion.

Etiology—The appearance is caused by the overgrowth of skin cells. Normally, a cell takes 14 days to move from the basal layer to the surface, where after another 14 days of wear it is sloughed off. The life cycle of a psoriatic skin cell is only four days during which it produces a surface of immature cells causing a thick and flaky appearance.

Treatment—Psoriasis cannot be cured, but it may be controlled. Initial therapy is with topical hydrocortisone preparations. Then, topical retinoids, vitamin A or D creams, topical tar, and salicylic acid preparations are also used. Ultraviolet light in a controlled, prescribed setting slows the cell turnover. Oral medications in the form of anti-metabolites, retinoids, and immunosuppressives are used in extensive severe cases.

Rosacea (Ro-za'-se-a)

Description—It is a chronic skin eruption that makes the face, especially the nose and cheeks, look flushed. It occurs most often in Caucasian women between 30 and 50 years old. It also occurs in men but is usually more severe and associated with rhinophyma (dilated follicles with an enlarged red nose).

Signs and symptoms—There is the characteristic coloration of the face that may also exhibit papules and pustules like acne but without the comedones.

Eitology—The condition results from the dilation of small blood vessels that causes the flushed, red appearance. The exact cause is unknown. Stress, infection, vitamin deficiency, and endocrine problems do aggravate the condition. Certain foods, such as spicy things and hot beverages, also cause problems. It is also affected by alcohol, physical activity, sunlight, and extreme temperatures.

Treatment—Topical use of cortisone ointment to reduce erythema may be helpful. Oral doses of tetracycline given in decreasing amounts as symptoms subside, and electrolysis may destroy the large or dilated blood vessels.

Ringworm

Description—This fungus may affect the scalp (tinea capitis), the body (tinea corporis), or other areas, such as the groin, beard, or feet (tinea pedia, or athlete's foot).

Signs and symptoms—On the body, it is characterized by flat lesions, which are dry and scaly or moist and crusty. When they enlarge, clear central areas develop, leaving an outer ring from which it gets its name. On the scalp, small papules occur causing scaly patches of baldness (Figure 11–70).

Etiology—Fungi dermatophytes.

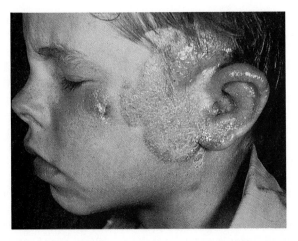

FIGURE 11–70 Ringworm (tinea corporis) of the face and scalp (Courtesy of Robert A. Silverman, MD, Clinical Associate Professor, Department of Pediatrics, Georgetown University.)

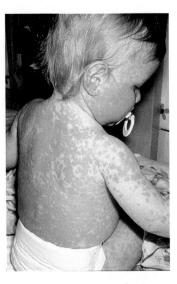

FIGURE 11–71 Urticaria (Courtesy of Robert A. Silverman, MD, Clinical Associate Professor, Department of Pediatrics, Georgetown University.)

Treatment—Treatment consists of systemic medication and/or the topical applications of antifungals. Because the disease is contagious, care must be taken to prevent its spread by refraining from sharing bed linens, combs, and towels.

Scabies (Ska'-bees)

Description—This skin infection is caused by the itch mite.

Signs and symptoms—The condition causes an itching that becomes intense at night. The lesions are characteristically threadlike red nodules, approximately ⅜ inch long. They occur between fingers, at the inner wrist area, on the elbows, in axillary folds (armpit), about the waist, on genitalia (external sex organs) of males, and on the nipples of females. The infection is spread by skin contact or sexual activity.

Etiology—It is caused by the itch mite, which has burrowed into the skin to lay eggs. The larvae emerge to mate and then reburrow under the skin. It can be associated with overcrowding and poor personal hygiene.

Treatment—Treatment consists of an application of pediculicide such as the prescription drug Elimite, which must remain on the skin from 6-8 hours or overnight. The treatment is then followed with a bath. An antipruritic (against itching) or steroid may be applied topically to help reduce the itching.

Urticaria (Hives) (Ur-ti-care'-re-ah)

Description—This is a self-limiting reaction to allergens. **Urticaria** often occurs during especially stressful or emotional times or during a viral infection.

Signs and symptoms—The reaction produces distinct, raised **wheals** surrounded by a reddened area. They may be few in number or cover the entire body. They may or may not cause itching, burning, and tingling (Figure 11–71).

Etiology—Urticaria are caused by allergy to drugs, food, insect stings, and occasionally inhaled allergens from animal hair, cosmetics, and flour. Non-allergic urticaria can be caused by the body's release of histamine for unknown reasons.

Treatment—Urticaria is treated by eliminating or limiting the causative allergen or, when that is not possible, by gradual desensitization through interdermal injection of the allergen. An antihistamine is used to reduce itching and swelling. A tranquilizer may be required when the causative factor is emotional stress.

Verrucae (Warts) (Ver-ru'-ki)

Description—This is a benign (noncancerous) viral infection of the skin.

Signs and symptoms—Common **verrucae** are characterized by a rough, elevated, rounded surface, usually on the extremities, especially the hands and fingers. They can also occur on the elbows, knees, and face and scalp.

Etiology—Warts are caused by a family of viruses known as human papillomavirus, which is spread by direct contact. It invades skin cells where the surface is broken and "encourages" the creation of more infected cells. In most cases, the body's immune system eventually eliminates the wart. It is estimated that a wart will die off within about five years. Plantar warts occur primarily at pressure points on the soles of the feet. Condyloma accuminatum (venereal warts) are moist, soft, pink to red warts occurring singly or most often in large clusters on the penis, vulva, or anus. They grow rapidly in groups, often accumulating into large clusters. Genital warts spread by sexual contact and are highly contagious. They may be associated with an increased risk of cervical cancer in women.

Treatment—Treatment of warts varies with the type, size, and location. Common types often disappear spontaneously. When removal is necessary, they can be destroyed by methods using electricity, acid, liquid nitrogen, or solid carbon dioxide. Genital warts must be treated promptly. Partners must also be evaluated by a physician for evidence of the virus and treated if present or the infection will be reacquired upon renewed contact.

Wrinkles

As people age, the skin begins to develop wrinkles, particularly on the face and back of the hands. This is primarily caused by years of exposure to the environment and the diminishing layer of collagen beneath the skin. Many forms of treatment can be performed to remove or reduce their presence and at least temporarily improve the patient's appearance. Because there is such an interest in the procedures, a brief discussion of the most common forms of correction follows.

Dermabrasion This is the controlled scraping of the top layers of the skin to remove scars from acne or accidents and to smooth out fine facial wrinkles, such as those around the mouth. Local anesthesia and a sedative are used during the procedure. It involves the use of a high-speed, hand-held rotary instrument with a rough wire brush or diamond impregnated burr. Afterwards, the skin is treated with ointment, a wet dressing, a dry treatment, or some combination. There is redness, swelling, and some pain, tingling, burning, or itching, which is controlled by medication. The side effects subside within a few days.

Microdermabrasion This is a non-invasive, non-surgical procedure. A controlled spray of fine aluminum oxide crystals is applied to remove the outer layer of the skin. This gives the skin a fresher appearance. There are varying depths of treatment available. It may improve the appearance of fine wrinkles, superficial age spots, and sun-damaged skin.

Chemical Peel This is known as chemosurgery and can be done at three levels: light, medium, and deep. Medium and deep peels require the use of medication during the treatment to relieve tension and discomfort. They involve the application of varying concentrations of an acid that strips away old, damaged skin cells, causing the body to replace them with healthy new ones. With deeper peels, collagen is stimulated which "pumps-up" the new skin.

A light peel affects only the top layer and can be done in about an hour. It produces only mild redness and will make the skin appear softer, reduce the size of pores, pro-

duce a more even coloring, and may reduce some fine lines. It may need repeating to achieve desired results.

A medium peel affects surface and some underlying cells. It also stimulates collagen and elastin, the fibers that act as the skin's support structure. This results in much smoother skin and the reduction of wrinkles. Some precancerous lesions may be removed. It takes from 7 to 10 days for the swelling, redness, and peeling to subside after the application.

A deep peel requires a strong acid and destroys all the top layers of skin and sometimes a part of the dermal layer. This results in removing all the signs of skin aging except deep forehead furrows and the nose-to-mouth grooves from sagging. Pigmentation problems and precancerous lesions can be removed. The procedure requires expert application and produces considerable pain for 12 hours, which requires medication, followed by discomfort for a few days. There is considerable swelling, redness, and peeling for a few weeks. It also results in the loss of pigment which causes a waxy, lighter face that may not match the body.

Laser Resurfacing This is the newest form of repair and involves the use of a controlled, pulsed laser beam to vaporize the skin's surface. The depth of the beam can be set to go light on the thin skin around the eyes and deeper into thicker skin around the mouth. Surface blemishes, sun-damaged skin, and the wrinkled surface is removed. It also stimulates the development of new cells and collagen for new, smoother, younger-looking skin and produces a tightening effect on the skin as it removes or reduces the wrinkles. Small areas to be treated can be injected with local anesthetic; full face treatment may require general anesthesia. Immediate visual change can be observed as the beam penetrates the skin, leaving behind a puff of mist and a fine ash which is "vacuumed" away as the skin tightens and the wrinkle disappears. The odor of burnt flesh is apparent. The procedure's immediate results are like a bad sunburn with some swelling of the area. The burned skin is tender, very red, and oozes fluid initially. Crusts form which can be gently removed. The area is covered with antibiotic ointment to relieve any surface drying and to prevent infection. Medication is prescribed for pain relief. The swelling and excessive redness subsides within a few days. It may take a few weeks for all the coloration to fade. The results are usually considered well worth the discomfort and temporary inconvenience.

Plastic Surgery This term is derived from a Greek word meaning to mold or give form. Plastic surgery is also known as cosmetic surgery and involves the reshaping of the facial features to improve appearance. The procedure demands a skillful surgeon to achieve the desired results. The procedures can remove "bags" under the eyes, lift drooping upper lids, and tighten up skin around the eyes. The repair of both upper and lower lids is known as quadrilateral blepharoplasty. The procedures to raise sagging jaws and forehead and pull back the sides of the face is commonly referred to as "a face lift." These procedures can be performed under general or local anesthesia in connection with sedation. Pain, marked swelling, and bruising will require medication for a few days. The recovery time varies but most swelling and significant bruising are sufficiently gone after two to three weeks to allow the patient to go out in public.

ACHIEVE UNIT OBJECTIVES

Complete Chapter 11, Unit 4, in the workbook to help you obtain competency of this subject matter.

UNIT 5

The Skeletal System

OBJECTIVES

Upon completion of the unit, meet the following performance objectives by verifying knowledge of the facts and principles presented through oral and written communication at a level deemed competent.

1. Spell and define, using the glossary at the back of the text, all the **Words to Know** in this unit.
2. Name the two divisions of the skeletal system and the bone groups in each division.
3. Describe the structure of the long bones.
4. Explain how long bones grow.
5. Identify the elements which make up bone tissue.
6. Identify the major bones of the body.
7. List the six functions of the skeletal system.
8. Name the divisions of the spinal column and the number of vertebrae in each division.
9. Describe fontanels and explain why they are essential.
10. Describe the structure of the rib cage and its primary function.
11. Identify three kinds of synovial joints, and give examples of each.
12. List the parts of a synovial joint, and identify the purpose of each part.
13. Name the seven types of fractures and the characteristics of each.
14. Outline the treatment of a fracture.
15. Describe the healing process of a fracture.
16. Define the term *fatty embolus,* explaining its origin and what might occur.
17. List situations predisposing to amputation.
18. Define the phantom limb sensation.
19. Describe four diagnostic examinations.
20. Explain why the symptoms of carpal tunnel syndrome occur.
21. Name the three types of spinal curvatures, describing their physical characteristics.
22. Identify 20 diseases and disorders of the skeletal system.

WORDS TO KNOW

alignment	laminectomy
amputate	ligament
appendicular	lordosis
arthritis	marrow
articulation	metacarpal
axial	metatarsal
bunion	osteoporosis
bursa	patella
callus	periosteum
cancellous	phalanges
carpal	phalanx
cartilage	phantom limb
cervical	prosthesis
clavicle	radius
coccyx	reduce
comminuted	sacrum
compound	scapula
cranium	scoliosis
depressed	simple
diarthrosis	skeletal
dislocation	spinal fusion
embolus	spiral
epiphysis	sprain
femur	sternum
fibula	symphysis pubis
fracture	synovial
greenstick	tarsal
humerus	tibia
ilium	traction
impacted	ulna
intervertebral	vertebrae
ischium	xiphoid
kyphosis	

 Library

The **skeletal** system consists of organs called bones. It may be difficult to think of bones as living, functioning organs, but they use food and oxygen and perform functions just as other organs do.

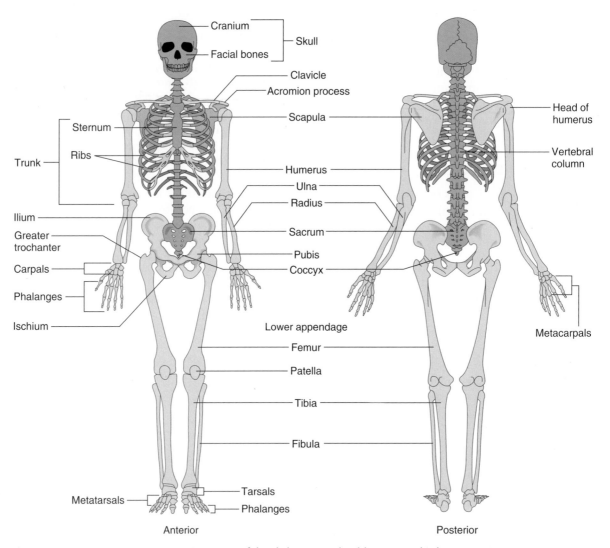

FIGURE 11–72 Bones of the skeleton (axial in blue, appendicular in gray)

The skeleton is divided into two sections. The spinal column, skull, and rib cage make up the **axial** skeleton. The bones of the arms, hands, legs, feet, shoulders, and pelvis make up the **appendicular** skeleton (Figure 11–72).

The primary purpose of the skeletal system is to support the body. This support must be strong yet not heavy. Bone is said to be as strong as cast iron, yet it is much lighter and more flexible. The skeleton must be flexible enough to endure pressure, stress, and shock without shattering.

BONE STRUCTURE

Over 20% of the weight of bone is water. Two thirds of the remainder are minerals and one third, organic matter. The main minerals are calcium, phosphorus, and magnesium. The organic matter is primarily collagen, a type of protein fiber that forms the matrix (intercellular substance) of the bone.

The ends of long bones have articulating (connecting) surfaces that fit together with other bones to form joints

(Figure 11–73). These ends are separated by cartilage to facilitate movement. The ends and parts of the shaft are filled with a meshlike network of spongy **cancellous** bone. The openings in the spongy bone are filled with red **marrow**. The inside of the shaft of the bone is filled with a fat or yellow marrow. Dense bone makes up the outside of long bones.

A tough membrane called **periosteum** covers the surface of the bone. Blood vessels and nerves pass through the periosteum and into the bone through a network of openings called Haversian canals. Some larger vessels pass directly into both the yellow and red marrow.

NUMBER OF BONES

At birth, a baby has 270 bones. As the child grows, some of the bones fuse together so that in adulthood there are only 206. For example, at the lower end of the spinal column, five **vertebrae** have fused to form the **sacrum**, whereas the last four have fused into the **coccyx** (tailbone) (Figure 11–74). The smallest bones in

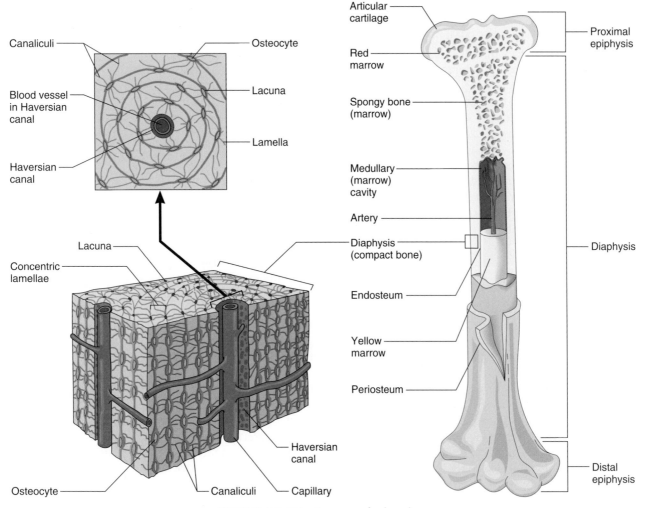

FIGURE 11–73 Structure of a long bone

the body are the malleus, incus, and stapes of the middle ear.

FUNCTIONS OF THE SKELETON

The skeleton serves at least six functions for the body. One, as previously indicated, is to support the body. The bones provide a framework for the distribution of the body's fat, muscles, and skin.

Two, the bones also serve to protect the body's vital organs. The brain and spinal cord are both located within bony cavities. The cranium also provides protection for the inner ear and parts of the eye. The heart and lungs are positioned within the rib cage. The internal reproductive organs and the urinary bladder lie within the bony pelvis.

Third, the bones are the points of attachment for skeletal muscles. When the muscles contract, they allow the joints of the skeleton to rotate, bend, or straighten, thereby providing for movement and flexibility. Fourth, the bones, along with the muscles, give shape to the body.

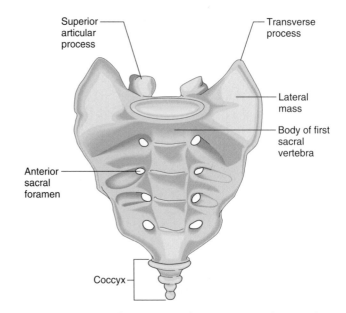

FIGURE 11–74 The sacrum and coccyx (From *The Wonderful Human Machine,* copyright 1979 by the American Medical Association.)

A fifth and vital function of bone is the formation of the red and white blood cells and the platelets. The red marrow in the spongy areas of the long bones, the ribs, and the vertebrae produces millions of red blood cells a minute. This rate is necessary to replace the cells, which live only a few weeks. When the body needs more red cells than the red marrow can produce, some of the yellow marrow is converted to red.

Finally, bones store most of the body's supply of calcium. Calcium is needed by the heart to beat, by the muscles to contract, and by the blood to clot. When the calcium in the body is inadequate for all its needs, the blood takes calcium from its storage in the bone. The bone minerals are constantly being borrowed and replaced through the blood flow within the body.

SPINAL COLUMN

The spinal column is a stack of vertebrae that supports the head and keeps the trunk erect. As noted earlier, it provides protection for the spinal cord, which descends from the brain through its canal. The bones of the column are separated by **intervertebral** cartilage disks between their rounded front portions, the vertebral bodies (Figure 11–75). The disks permit the column to bend or twist and also absorb much of the shock received from walking, running, or jumping. The vertebrae in the column are named for the area of the body in which they are located: **cervical** (neck), thoracic (chest), lumbar (back), sacral (posterior pelvic girdle), and coccygeal (tailbone) (Figure 11–76).

The spinal nerves enter and leave the spinal cord through foraminae (openings) between the vertebrae. The disks maintain adequate spacing between vertebrae to prevent damage to the spinal nerves from bone-to-bone contact.

Typical vertebrae, as shown in Figure 11–75, have descriptive parts, mainly the large solid part called the *body,* the winglike side projections called the *transverse processes,* a posterior projection called a *spinous process* (the part you can feel if you arch your back), and the *foramen* through which the spinal cord passes. Other processes called *articular* are where parts of two vertebrae touch.

THE SKULL

The skull is the bony structure of the head. It consists of a cranial and a facial portion. The **cranium** is actually a fusion of eight cranial bones, with the vital function of protecting the brain from injury (Figure 11–77). The main bones of the cranium are: the frontal (the forehead and upper eye sockets), two parietal, two temporal, and the occipital (back of the skull). The facial bones are: the mandible (lower jaw), the maxillae (upper jaw), the zygomatic (cheek bones), and the several small bones about the eyes, nose, and palate.

The cranium is not solid bone at birth. Spaces between the bones are soft incomplete bone to allow for the molding of the skull during the birth process and for enlargement of the skull as growth occurs. A large diamond-shaped anterior area where the frontal and parietal bones meet and a triangular space posteriorly where the occipital bone meets the parietals are known as *fontanels,* or "soft spots," and can easily be felt. Other smaller fontanels are located along the sides of the skull. Without these areas for growth, the brain could not increase in size during

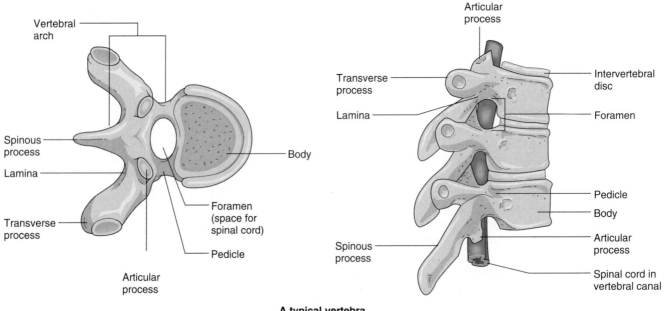

A typical vertebra

FIGURE 11–75 Vertebrae structure

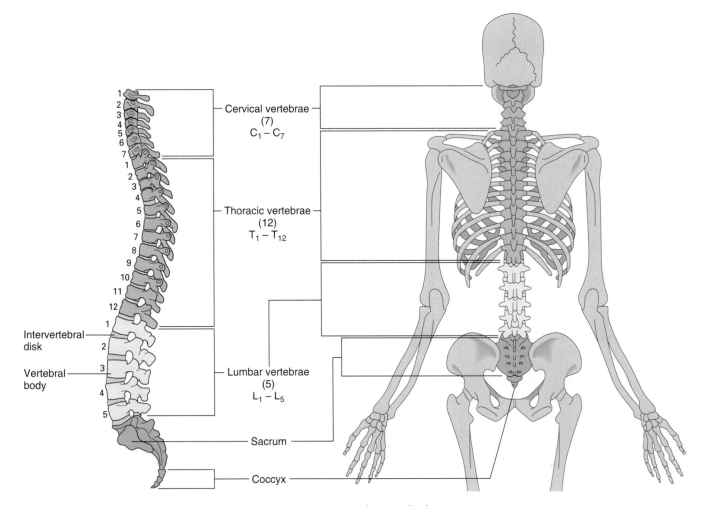

FIGURE 11-76   The spinal column

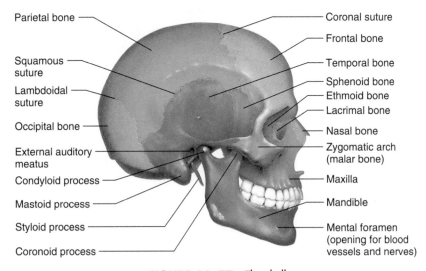

FIGURE 11-77   The skull

late pregnancy and early infancy. The fontanels gradually close, turning the membrane and cartilage into solid bone after about two years. The irregular lines marking the former growth areas are called *sutures*.

The skull does not grow remarkably when compared to the rest of the body. It makes up about one fourth of the total length of the infant's body but only one eighth of the adult's total length.

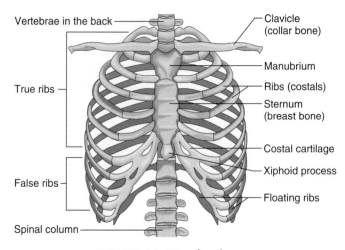

FIGURE 11–78 The rib cage

THE RIB CAGE

Thoracic vertebrae serve as the posterior attachment points for 12 pairs of ribs (Figure 11–78). The top 10 pairs are also attached by cartilage strips to the **sternum** (breast bone) anteriorly. The flexibility of the cartilage attachment allows the rib cage to move when the lungs are inflated to breathe. The bottom two pairs of ribs are called floating ribs because they are attached only to the spinal column and not the sternum.

The rib cage is sometimes described in terms of true and false ribs. When this division is made, the first seven pairs of ribs are considered "true" ribs because of their posterior and direct anterior attachment. The last five pairs are "false" ribs because they attach anteriorly to the cartilage of the rib above or have no anterior attachment.

Three other bony features of the thoracic area should be mentioned. They are the **clavicle** (collar bone), located anteriorly, and the **scapula** (shoulder blade), located pos-

teriorly. The inferior portion of the sternum is a small bony process called the **xiphoid** process.

LONG BONES

The long bones of the body are found in the extremities. To a great extent, the long bones of the lower extremities determine our height. Long bones are generally shaped like hollow cylinders to be strong with the least amount of weight. A typical long bone has three distinct regions: diaphysis, epiphysis, and metaphysis. The mid shaft (diaphysis) is connected to the ends (**epiphysis**) by a transitional segment (metaphysis). Early in life the epiphysis is mainly **cartilage**. Later the cartilage becomes a strip or "growth plate" which permits new tissue growth and bone length. At maturity, growth stops and the cartilage is replaced by bone.

The **femur** (thigh bone) is the longest bone in any species, extending from the hip joint to the knee. (Refer to Figure 11–72.) The thickness of the femur wall depends on the size and needs of the species. For example, large animals, such as the bear, have a thick, heavy femur to support their weight and accommodate slow movements, whereas the deer has a very thin and light femur to permit speed. The **tibia** (shin bone) and **fibula** complete the long bones of the leg. The small bone at the knee is known as the **patella**.

The long bones of the upper extremities are the **humerus** of the arm and the **radius** and **ulna** of the forearm. The radius extends from the thumb side of the wrist to the elbow, whereas the ulna extends from the little finger side to the elbow joint.

BONES OF THE HANDS AND FEET

The bones of the hands and feet are similar in structure (Figure 11–79). The wrist has eight bones, known as

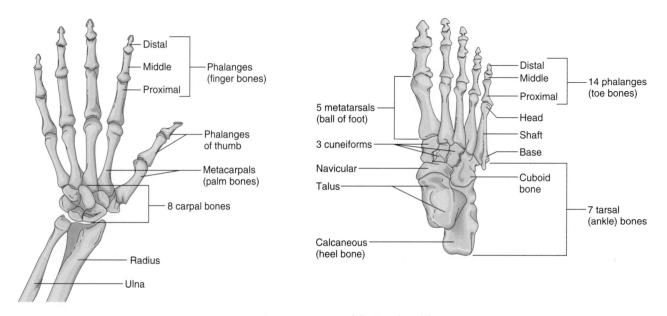

FIGURE 11–79 Bones of the hand and foot

carpals, whereas the ankle has seven, called **tarsals**. In the palm area of the hand, there are five **metacarpals** that correspond to the five **metatarsals** of the instep of the foot. The **phalanges** (fingers and toes) are further subdivided into individual sections called a **phalanx**. There are three phalanx sections in each finger and toe, except in the thumb and great toe, which have only two. The section of a phalanx is identified as distal, middle, or proximal by its relationship to the metacarpals or metatarsals.

THE PELVIC GIRDLE

The pelvic girdle provides the structure for the hip area. Two large bones called *os coxae* (hip bones) are joined posteriorly with the sacrum. The top blade-shaped portion is called the **ilium** (Figure 11–80). The anterior lower portion is called the pubis, and the point of attachment (right and left pubis) is called the **symphysis pubis**. The posterior lower portion of the bone is called the **ischium**. The hip bone provides the recessed area where the head of the femur fits. The anatomical name for the socket is *acetabulum*.

JOINTS

The place where two or more bony parts join together is known as an **articulation** or joint. Strong, flexible bands of connective tissue called **ligaments** hold long bones together at joints. Ligaments can stretch and often become torn as a result of injury.

There are three main types of joints, classified primarily by their degree of movement. A movable joint, such as the knee or elbow, is called **diarthrosis** or **synovial** joint. A partially-movable joint, like where ribs attach to the spine or between the vertebrae, is known as *amphiarthrosis* or *cartilaginous*. An immovable joint, such as a cranial suture, is called *synarthrosis* or *fibrous*.

Most of the body's joints are diarthrotic. They may have three distinct parts, articular cartilage, a **bursa** (saclike capsule), and a synovial cavity. The articulating joint surfaces of bones are covered with the articular cartilage, which provides a slippery, smooth surface and enables the joint to absorb shock. An articular capsule of tough, fibrous tissue encloses the articulating surfaces and is lined with a synovial membrane, which secretes synovial fluid into the cavity, lubricating the joint and reducing friction.

The joint is surrounded with ligaments, tendons, and muscles that hold the joint together but still allow for movement. Some synovial joints have cushionlike sacs called bursa, which form from the synovial membrane and are filled with synovial fluid. These are generally located between tendons and bones. In addition, synovial membranes may also form sheaths that wrap around the tendons. Bursae and tendon sheaths cushion and lubricate

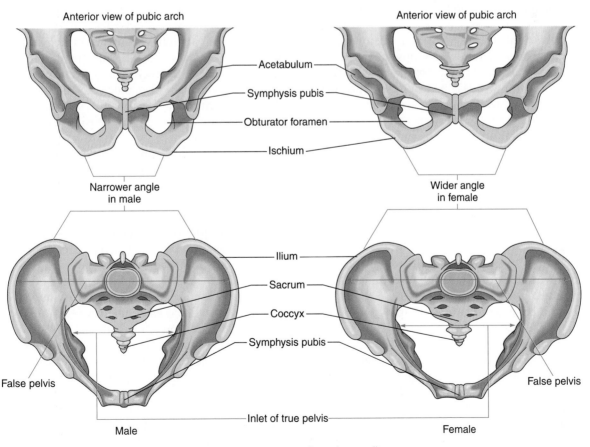

Anterior view of pubic arch

Anterior view of pubic arch

Acetabulum

Symphysis pubis

Obturator foramen

Ischium

Narrower angle
in male

Wider angle
in female

Ilium

Sacrum

Coccyx

Symphysis pubis

False pelvis

False pelvis

Inlet of true pelvis

Male

Female

FIGURE 11–80 The pelvic girdle

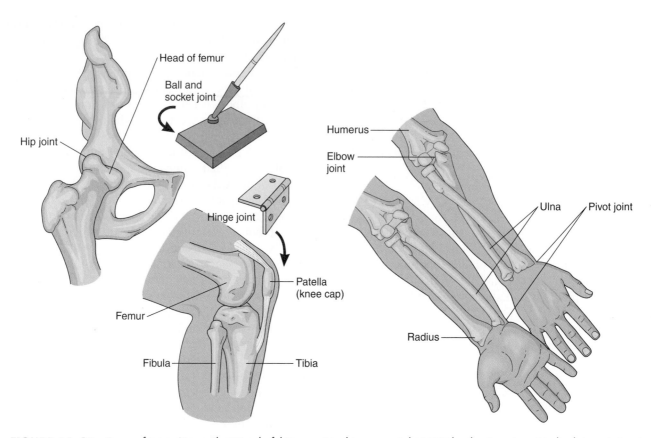

FIGURE 11–81 Types of joints (From *The Wonderful Human Machine,* copyright 1979 by the American Medical Association.)

tendons and help reduce friction between the tendons and the bone.

The synovial joints of the body have been copied by man to develop many useful devices (Figure 11–81). The ball and socket joint found in the hip or shoulder can be seen in the movement of a desk pen set. The action of the fingers, knees, and elbows is like that of a hinge. An unusual pivot joint appears at the wrists and elbows. When the palm of the hand is up, the radius and ulna are side by side. As the palm is turned down, the radius crosses over the ulna in a pivoting action. This type of motion is independent of the elbow's hinge action. Joints found in the wrists and ankle are formed by bones with curved surfaces, which allow for various angular movements.

FRACTURES

The bones of children contain a high percentage of cartilage and are much more flexible than those of an adult. Frequently, the bone will crack under pressure but will not break all the way through. This type of break is known as a **greenstick fracture**.

A complete bone break in which there is no involvement with the skin surface is known as a **simple** or "closed" fracture (Figure 11–82). When broken bone protrudes through the skin's surface, it is known as an open fracture, formerly called a **compound** fracture. This causes additional concerns because of the possibility of

infection to the area. A more involved type of fracture is called **impacted**, which indicates that the broken ends are jammed into each other. A **comminuted** fracture is one with more than one fracture line and several bone fragments. A **depressed** fracture may occur with severe head injuries in which a broken piece of skull is driven inward. A **spiral** fracture may occur with a severe twisting action, such as in a skiing accident, causing the break to wind around the bone.

A common injury among children is the Colles fracture. This involves the breaking and dislocating of the distal end of the radius, causing a characteristic bulge at the wrist. Often, the ulna is also fractured, resulting in a greater wrist deformity and a limply-hanging hand. It is a common fracture of children from injuries while skating, riding bikes, and climbing. It is generally the result of falling on an outstretched hand.

In treating fractures, immobilization of the affected part and prevention of shock are the main concerns. The extremity is splinted extending above and below the area of fracture. Elevation of the part and application of a cold pack or ice help prevent swelling. When there is also extensive damage to the surrounding tissues, especially to the exterior, control of bleeding may be indicated. This may require direct pressure over the wound.

When long bones are broken, they are usually pulled by the muscles attached to their surfaces into abnormal positions, often causing overlapping of their broken parts.

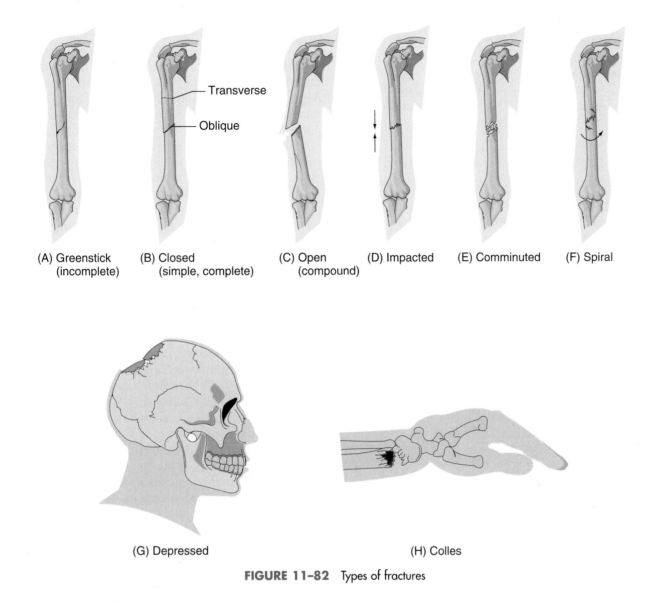

(A) Greenstick (incomplete)   (B) Closed (simple, complete)   (C) Open (compound)   (D) Impacted   (E) Comminuted   (F) Spiral

Transverse

Oblique

(G) Depressed   (H) Colles

FIGURE 11–82   Types of fractures

Before the bone can be set, **traction** (pulling)—either manually or by a system of ropes and pulleys—must be used to stretch the muscles and pull the bone pieces back into **alignment**. This procedure is known as **reducing** the fracture. Once the ends fit together properly, a splint or cast can be used to maintain the position until the bone has healed. Occasionally, an external fixator is used to maintain alignment of the fracture. An external fixator is a device that includes a frame through which pins or wires are attached to the bones.

With involved fractures, such as compound or comminuted, an additional surgical procedure is often necessary either to repair the skin and surrounding tissues or to place all the small bone fragments in position. This procedure is called an *open reduction* because it involves an opening into the fractured bone through the skin and overlying tissues to achieve alignment of the bone. Typically, open reduction includes the placement of pins, wires, plates and/or screws to hold the fracture in the proper position. When the hardware is used internally, it

is covered by the normal soft tissues of the body and is known as an internal fixation.

Bone Healing Process

When a fracture occurs, a collection of blood (hematoma) forms around the fracture site. The hematoma begins an inflammatory reaction that initiates the healing process. A fibrous bridge is formed between the fracture fragments. Some of the cells in this fibrous mesh differentiate into cartilage cells and begin to accumulate calcium, forming a **callus** (Figure 11–83). As time passes, the callus turns first to cartilage and then to bone. Certain bone cells build the new bone tissue, whereas others remove the cartilage and then slowly smooth the repaired section back to its approximate original size.

A complication that may occur after a fracture of long bones is a fat **embolus**. An embolus is a mass of foreign material circulating within the blood vessels. This potentially-fatal complication may follow the release of fat droplets

Normal bone repair

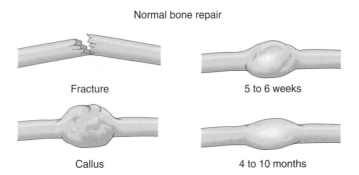

Fracture

5 to 6 weeks

Callus

4 to 10 months

FIGURE 11–83 Normal bone repair (From *The Wonderful Human Machine,* copyright 1979 by the American Medical Association.)

from the marrow of the long bones. The trauma of the event can also cause the body to release catecholamines, which in turn activate fatty acids. The fatty acids can develop into a fatty embolus and circulate in the blood, interfering with circulation in the lungs or even the brain. This interference may cause hypoxia (lack of oxygen), a change in the mental status, and even death.

Usual symptoms and signs include apprehension, sweating, fever, rapid heart rate, pallor, difficulty breathing, bluish discoloration of the skin, convulsions, and coma. If the complication occurs, it is usually within 24 to 48 hours but may occur as late as three days after the fracture.

AMPUTATION

Severe trauma, a malignant tumor, lack of circulation, or complications of other conditions, such as diabetes, may result in the need to **amputate** an extremity. The change in the patient's body image and function causes emo-

tional and physical difficulties in coping with daily activities. Following amputation, a condition often occurs known as **phantom limb**, the sensation that the missing extremity is still present. It is often described as an itching or tingling sensation. This may last for quite some time but will usually subside eventually. It is considered normal to experience the sensation.

When the amputated stump has healed sufficiently, a **prosthesis** (artificial part) may be fitted. Lower limbs are either attached directly to the remaining extremity, fastened by means of straps or belt to the waist, or hung from the shoulder. The method depends to a great extent on the amount of the remaining extremity. Upper limbs may be replaced by a "hook" device that can be opened and closed to grasp objects. A prosthesis that closely resembles a real arm and hand is often desired, even though it lacks the flexibility of the "hook."

DIAGNOSTIC EXAMINATIONS

■ Arthroscopy—This endoscopic procedure permits direct visual inspection of a joint, most often the knee (Figure 11–84). In an arthroscopic examination, a surgeon makes a small incision in the patient's skin and then inserts pencil-sized instruments that contain a small lens and lighting systems to magnify and illuminate the structures inside the joint. Light is transmitted through fiber optics to the end of the arthroscope that is inserted into the joint. By attaching the arthroscope to a miniature television camera, the surgeon is able to see the inside of the joint through this very small incision. It is frequently used to evaluate injuries suffered by athletes. Arthroscopy is useful in detecting **arthritis**, torn meniscus, cysts, or loose pieces of tissue. The television camera attached to the arthroscope displays

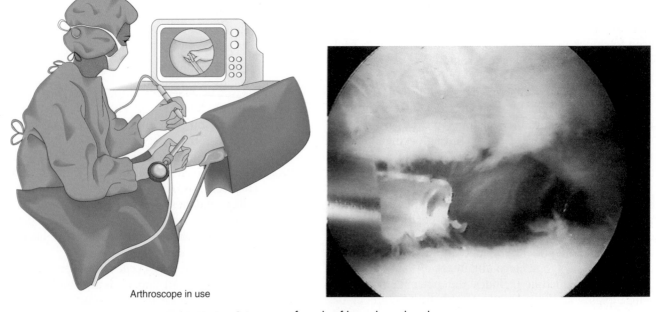

Arthroscope in use

FIGURE 11–84 View of inside of knee through arthroscope

the image on a television screen, allowing the surgeon to look throughout the knee to determine the amount or type of injury. Many surgical procedures can be performed through the scope, thereby eliminating open surgery.

- Bone Scan—This is a precise nuclear medicine procedure using small amounts of a radioactive substance that are injected into a vein to help diagnose the presence of disease based on structural appearance. A scintillation or gamma camera positioned over the area obtains images by detecting the substance in the bones and recording it on a computer or film. Usually the procedures is done in two parts. The injection is given first, and the medium is carried in the blood to the skeleton and distributed throughout the bones. After the injection, the patient may leave the area for about two hours while the bones thoroughly absorb the medium. After the time has passed, the patient returns and is placed on the imaging table, and the camera is positioned over the patient. It slowly moves up or down a framework over the body, taking the images for at least 30 minutes. It is important that the patient remains still throughout the scanning process.
- Computed Tomography (CT) Scan—A special x-ray in which the x-ray tube moves around the patient. A computer takes the information and reconstructs a cross-sectional (axial) "slice" of the patient. Multiple slices are taken that allow the physician to determine the anatomy in three dimensions.
- Magnetic Resonance Imaging (MRI)—The process uses strong magnets which cause all of the protons in the field to "line up." Radio waves are then passed through the patient, causing the protons to resonate. A computer takes this information and constructs images in any plane. This technology has three advantages over CT scans: (1) There is no ionizing radiation (x-ray) used, (2) soft tissues are seen in more detail, and (3) images can be constructed in any plane (not just axial). The major disadvantage is that the technique is expensive. There are also some factors that prevent many patients from being candidates for the procedure, such as obesity or claustrophobia.
- X-ray—A frequently used test that evaluates the condition of bones in cases such as dislocations, sprains, and fractures. X-ray can also be used to determine bone structure changes like those occurring in some metabolic conditions such as acromegaly (gigantism), **osteoporosis**, or with Paget's disease.

DISEASES AND DISORDERS
Arthritis (Arth-rite'-is)

Introduction—The word arthritis means joint inflammation. There are more than 100 different forms of arthritis. Currently it infects about 40 million Americans, the larger percentage being women. The most common forms are osteoarthritis, rheumatoid arthritis, gout, fibromyalgia, and lupus. It is important to identify the type a patient has because different types require different approaches to treatment.

Osteoarthritis (Os-te-o-arth-rite'-is)

Description—This common form of arthritis results in progressive deterioration of joint cartilage, most often at the hips and knees. It affects many people as they grow older. Symptoms result from the breakdown of cartilage between bones and the bones themselves. It is also known as degenerative joint disease. There is no cure.

Signs and symptoms—It is accompanied by joint pain, stiffness, aching (particularly with weather changes), "grating" during joint motion, and fluid around the joint.

Etiology—Osteoarthritis was believed to be caused by joint wear-and-tear from years of use. However, recent research suggests that a mild, slow-moving inflammation or a metabolic disorder is the root of the problem.

Treatment—Osteoarthritis is best treated with aspirin and other non-steroidal anti-inflammatory drugs (NSAIDS), intraarticular joint injections of steroids, and reducing pressure on joints through the use of a cane, crutches, or a cervical collar. Two very popular drugs being used to treat arthritis are Vioxx and Celebrex. They are from a class of drugs called COX-2 inhibitors, which means they block an enzyme that causes inflammation but not the enzyme that controls production of a prostaglandin that protects the lining of the stomach. They are effective in relieving discomfort without the significant risks of the gastric side effects of Tylenol or the NSAIDS (e.g., ibuprofen, naproxen, and Feldene).

If the COX-2 drugs do not work, new injectable drugs containing hyaluronic acid can be used. The acid is a gooey fluid found in joint cavities that normally lubricates and absorbs shock. A series of several injections is necessary but can provide relief for up to a year. Initially, the injections were approved for the knee joint only. Other promising therapies involve transplanting cartilage cells harvested from the patient's own healthy knee cartilage. They are grown in a culture and then injected into the injured area to make new tissue. A third therapy uses stem cells harvested from the patient and grown and implanted in defects where cartilage is worn. A fourth removes a cylindrical plug of cartilage and bone from a healthy area within the knee and fits it into a drilled hole in the damaged cartilage. All these rely on the body's ability to repair itself if given the necessary materials. Occasionally, disability and uncontrollable pain will require surgical intervention. This can range from scraping deteriorated bone fragments from the joint to replacing joint bone parts with prosthetic appliances (artificial joints).

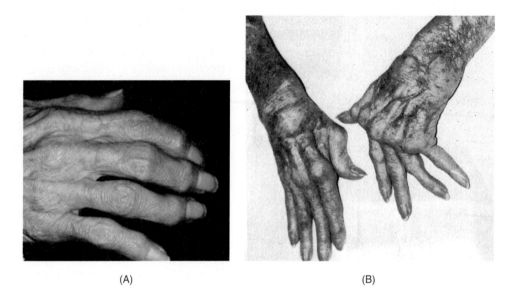

(A)   (B)

FIGURE 11–85   Comparison of (A) osteoarthritis and (B) rheumatoid arthritis of the hands and joints

Rheumatoid Arthritis (Room'-a-toid)

Description—A chronic systemic inflammatory disease attacking joints and surrounding tissues, this is an intermittent disease with periods of remission. It is three times more common in females than males, most often striking between the ages of 35 and 45.

Signs and symptoms—The disease attacks the joint synovial membrane, causing edema and congestion. Tissue layers become granulated and thicken, eventually involving the cartilage and destroying the joint capsule and bone. Scar tissue formation, bone atrophy, and malalignment cause visible deformities, pain, and often immobility (Figure 11–85).

Etiology—Rheumatoid arthritis is caused by a fault in the immune system that causes it to attack the joint membranes. The attack not only triggers inflammation but also stimulates the abnormal growth of cartilage and bone. It can affect persons of all ages.

Treatment—Treatments include anti-inflammatory and disease-modifying drugs, exercise, heat or cold, saving energy, joint protection, and sometimes surgery. Injections of cortisone directly into the joint may help to relieve pain and swelling; however, repeated frequent injections into the same joint can produce undesirable side effects. Researchers using genetic engineering techniques developed a drug called cA2 that blocks the immune system action. Maintaining a normal weight lessens stress on joints. Range of motion and low-impact aerobic exercise is beneficial and helps maintains flexibility. Warm water exercise is especially easy on joints. Figure 11-86 illustrates arthritis inflammation at various sites throughout the body.

A PEDIATRIC PERSPECTIVE

Juvenile Rheumatoid Arthritis (JRA) is characterized by fevers, joint pain, and redness over the joint areas. Laboratory testing to confirm diagnosis and referral to a specialist provides the best outcomes for the child with this disease.

ARTHRITIS-JOINT INFLAMMATION

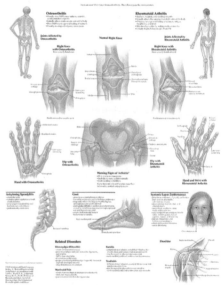

FIGURE 11–86   Sites of arthritis joint inflammation (Courtesy of Colwell, a Division of Patterson Dental Supply, Inc., 800-637-1140.)

Bursitis (Burr-sigh'-tis)

Description—This is a painful inflammation of the bursa. A bursa is a sac located around a joint and containing lubricating fluids that allow muscles and tendons to move freely over bony surfaces. Bursitis occurs most frequently at the hip, shoulder, or knee. It is usually associated with middle age.

Signs and symptoms—The most common sign is pain upon movement and limited motion of the affected joint. The pain can be gradual or sudden. Symptoms vary according to the joint involved.

Etiology—It usually occurs in middle age and is the result of recurring trauma that stresses or pressures a joint. It can also be the result of an inflammatory joint disease. A chronic form develops from repeated attacks of acute bursitis or repeated trauma and infection.

Treatment—Treatment consists of joint rest, often immobilization, a pain medication, and joint injection with a steroid combined with an anesthetic. It may be necessary to remove joint fluid by aspiration (withdrawal through a needle) and institute a program of physical therapy to preserve joint motion.

Carpal Tunnel Syndrome

Description—This condition results from the compression of the median nerve at the wrist. The carpal tunnel is a passageway for nerves, blood vessels, and flexor tendons to the fingers and thumb. It is formed by the carpal bones and the transverse ligament. The tendon sheaths become inflamed, causing swelling, which presses the median nerve against the transverse ligament.

Signs and symptoms—There is pain, tingling, numbness, and weakness of the hand. It involves only the thumb and index and middle finger. The patient will be unable to make a fist.

Etiology—Persons most likely to develop the syndrome are those who use their hands strenuously in grasping, twisting, or turning actions, such as assembly line workers and packers. Other systemic conditions that cause the carpal tunnel to swell are diabetes mellitus, pregnancy, menopause, hypothyroidism, and benign tumors.

Diagnosis can be made based on an examination that reveals decreased sensitivity of the first two fingers and the thumb on pricking with a pin and an electromyogram showing delayed motor nerve conduction. Patients may also have an *atrophy* (shrinking) of the muscle on the palm side of the thumb because of decreased innervation.

Treatment—If the syndrome is of short duration, treatment will consist of immobilizing the hand and forearm in a splint, local injections of corticosteroids, and systemic anti-inflammatory medication. It may be necessary to seek new employment if a work-related connection is determined. If conservative treatment does not correct the problem, a surgical procedure may be indicated to section the transverse ligament and "free-up" the nerve.

Congenital Hip Dysplasia (Con-jen'-i-tal Dis-play'-zhe-a)

Description—This abnormality of the hip joint is present at birth. It is the most common hip disorder of children, affecting one or both joints. It is present in three forms: unstable, with the hip in place but easily dislocated by manipulation; incomplete dislocation, with the head of the femur on the edge of the acetabulum; and complete dislocation, with the head totally outside the hip socket.

Signs and symptoms—Signs of hip dysplasia include the appearance of one leg being shorter than the other or one hip being more prominent. If both hips are involved, the child has a characteristic "duck waddle" or, if one hip only, a limp.

Etiology—The exact cause of dysplasia has not been proven. It is believed that hormones that relax maternal ligaments at the time of labor may also cause the infant ligaments to relax around the hip joint capsule. There is also an association of dislocation and a breech delivery.

Treatment—Early treatment is essential to normal development. In infants, a splint device is used for three to four months to maintain proper positioning. Older babies may be placed in traction, or the hips may be reduced and a cast applied for a period of four to six months.

Dislocation

Description—Displacement of bones at a joint so that the regularly meeting surfaces are no longer in contact is a **dislocation**. This occurs most frequently at joints of the finger, shoulder, knee, and hip.

Signs and symptoms—It is extremely painful and is often accompanied with joint surface fractures. Dislocation produces deformity around the joint, changes the length of the involved extremity, interferes with motion, and causes joint tenderness.

Etiology—Dislocation can be congenital, or it may follow trauma or disease of the surrounding joint.

Treatment—Prompt reduction (relocation) is essential to limit damage to surrounding tissues. Following reduction, a splint, cast, or traction (depending on the joint involved) to immobilize the area is indicated. Two to eight weeks will be needed to allow surrounding ligaments to heal completely.

Epicondylitis (Tennis Elbow) (Ep-i-kon-dil-i'-tis)

Description—This is an inflammation of the forearm extensor tendon at its attachment to the humerus.

Signs and symptoms—Pain occurs at the elbow and becomes intense. There is tenderness over the area where the radius articulates with the humerus.

Etiology—The condition probably begins as a tear and is common among people who grasp things forcefully or twist the forearm. Untreated epicondylitis can become disabling.

Treatment—The condition is best treated with an injection of a steroid and a local anesthetic, aspirin, an immobilizing splint, heat, and physical therapy. If the disorder is not treated, it may result in a disability.

Gout (Gouty Arthritis)

Description—This metabolic disease results in severe joint pain, especially at night. It most often affects the great toe but can involve other joints. The pain results from deposits of urates (uric acid salts), which are overproduced and/or retained by the body. Often gout is associated with another disease, such as leukemia, because of cell destruction by chemotherapy. Gout may also follow drug therapy that interferes with urate excretion.

Signs and symptoms—Gout can be a progressive disease, initially causing severe pain and a hot, tender, inflamed joint. This attack will be followed by a symptom-free period of approximately six months to two years, when a second episode will occur. Additional attacks usually involve other joints of the feet and legs. Eventually the condition becomes chronic (ongoing), involving many joints that are persistently painful and become degenerated, deformed, and disabling.

Etiology—The exact cause of gout is unknown, but it seems linked to a genetic defect in purine metabolism that causes overproduction of uric acid, retention of uric acid, or both. This interferes with urate excretion, leading to urate deposits that cause local tissue destruction.

Treatment—Gout is best treated with medication to suppress uric acid formation and promote excretion of the urates. Dietary restrictions must be followed, such as avoiding alcohol, primarily beer and wine, and purine-rich foods, such as liver, sardines, kidneys, and lentils.

Hallux Valgus (Hal'-lux Val'-gus)

Description—Common in women, this is a lateral deviation of the great toe with enlargement of the first metatarsal head and a **bunion** formation. A bunion is a bursa with a callus formation.

Signs and symptoms—The bursa becomes inflamed, filled with fluid, and tender. The overlying skin will be red.

Etiology—It may be congenital but is usually acquired from degenerative arthritis or the prolonged pressure on the foot from narrow, high-heeled shoes. Hallux valgus will cause bone deformity, and the change will alter the person's weight-bearing pattern.

Treatment—Early treatment with proper shoes, the use of padding and straightening devices, and exercises may correct the situation. A severe deformity and disabling pain will require surgical removal of the bunion.

Herniated Disk (Ruptured Disk) (Hern'-e-a-ted)

Description—In this situation, the soft gel-like material within an intervertebral disk has been forced through its outer surface. The extruded material may cause pressure on a spinal nerve exiting the spinal cord or may impinge on the spinal cord itself.

Signs and symptoms—The classic symptom is severe lower back pain, frequently radiating deep into the buttocks and down the back of the leg. It is usually unilateral (one sided). Sensory loss results from nerve compression, and the patient experiences numbness, muscle spasm, motor difficulty, and eventually weakness and atrophy of the leg muscles.

Etiology—A herniated disk may result from severe trauma or strain, but it is frequently related to degeneration of the intervertebral joints. It occurs most often in the lumbar or lumbosacral regions. Herniated disk usually occurs in adults, mainly men, under age 45. In elderly people with disk degeneration, herniation can occur from a minor trauma.

Treatment—Conservative treatment consists of prolonged bed rest, often with pelvic traction, heat applications, and specific exercises. A **laminectomy** is indicated if there is neurological involvement that does not improve with conservative therapy. This procedure involves removing a portion of the lamina (flattened portion of the vertebral arch) to remove the protruding disk material.

If pain still persists, a surgical procedure, **spinal fusion**, is performed to stabilize the adjoining vertebrae. A spinal fusion is typically accomplished by placing a screw/rod assembly into the spine to achieve a stable internal fixation. A piece of bone for a graft can be harvested from the pelvis or obtained from the bone bank. It is placed within a prepared space in the vertebra in conjunction with the hardware to achieve a solid fusion. When the bone heals, the joined vertebrae can no longer move independently to impinge on the nerve or spinal cord.

Kyphosis (Roundback, Humpback) (Ki-fo'-sis)

Description—This is a bowing of the back, usually at the thoracic level, resulting from improper vertebral alignment (Figure 11–87A). There are two types of **kyphosis**: adolescent and adult.

Signs and symptoms—With adolescent kyphosis, the condition is essentially without symptoms except for the visible curving of the back. Some adolescents may have mild pain, fatigue, localized tenderness, stiffness

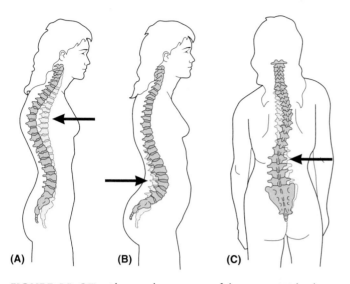

FIGURE 11–87 Abnormal curvatures of the spine: (A) kyphosis, (B) lordosis, (C) scoliosis

in the involved area, and tightening of the hamstring muscles of the posterior thighs because of compensating posture. In adult kyphosis, there is the characteristic rounded back, possible pain, weakness of the back, and fatigue.

Etiology—In children and adolescents, kyphosis may be caused by growth retardation or the result of rapid growth periods with improper epiphysis development. Poor posture and excessive sports activity can also result in curvature. In the adult form, it is caused by aging and the degeneration of intervertebral disks or the actual collapse of vertebrae resulting from osteoporosis.

Treatment—Kyphosis as a result of poor posture during childhood can be treated by therapeutic exercise, a firm mattress, and a Milwaukee brace to straighten the spine until spinal growth is complete. If neurological damage or disabling pain occurs in adolescents and adults (which happens rarely) a surgical procedure may be indicated, which involves posterior spinal fusion, bone grafting, and casting to straighten the severe curvature. With full skeletal maturity and debilitating curvature, a posterior spinal fusion can be accomplished with the use of a stainless steel Harrington rod mechanism to align the vertebrae.

Lordosis (Lor-doe'-sis)

Description—This abnormal anterior convex curvature of the lumbar spine is commonly referred to as swayback (Figure 11–87B). The body's spine normally curves in at this point; however, if it is exaggerated, it is considered to be **lordosis**.

Signs and symptoms—The obvious visual symptom is the excessive inward curvature of the lumbar portion of the back.

Etiology—It is usually the cause of poor posture. The wearing of high heels causes the inward positioning of the lower back to counteract the position of the feet to maintain balance.

Treatment—This condition can be improved, or at least prevented from progressing by appropriate exercises, improving posture, and having proper footwear.

Lumbar Myositis (Lum-bar My-o-sigh'-tis)

Description—An inflammation of the lumbar region muscles of the back.

Signs and symptoms—Low back pain.

Etiology—It is common and is primarily caused by a straining of the back muscles.

Treatment—The condition is best treated with rest, mild analgesics, and muscle relaxers. When improved, a program of stretching exercises is prescribed to condition and strengthen the muscles.

Osteoporosis (Os-te-o-pore-o'-sis)

Description—A metabolic bone disorder, characterized by acceleration of the rate of bone resorption while the rate of bone formation slows down, which results in a loss of bone mass. The loss of calcium and phosphate from the bone allows it to become porous, brittle, and prone to fracture. There are two forms of **osteoporosis**: primary and secondary. Primary is also known as senile or postmenopausal osteoporosis because it affects primarily elderly, postmenopausal women. Of the 25 million older Americans with osteoporosis, only five million are men. Secondary osteoporosis can occur following prolonged steroid therapy, bone immobilization or lack of use (with paralysis), malnutrition, excessive alcohol intake, scurvy, and hyperthyroidism. It is usually discovered following injury from bending to lift something.

Signs and symptoms—The individual hears a snapping sound and then feels instant pain in the lower back. The sound and pain are from the collapse of a vertebra. Other common signs of osteoporosis are slowly developing kyphosis with loss of height, fractures of the forearm or hip from minor falls, and additional spontaneous vertebral fractures. Figure 11-88 illustrates the progression of spinal curvature caused by osteoporosis and the resulting loss of height.

Etiology—The cause of primary osteoporosis may be the combination of aging, prolonged inadequate dietary intake of calcium, faulty metabolism because of estrogen deficiency, and/or a sedentary lifestyle. Females with small, thin frames are more likely to develop it. Males with low levels of testosterone are also more prone. The use of tobacco and a family history of osteoporosis also increases the risk.

Treatment—The condition is treatable to prevent additional fracturing by increasing exercise, giving an estrogen

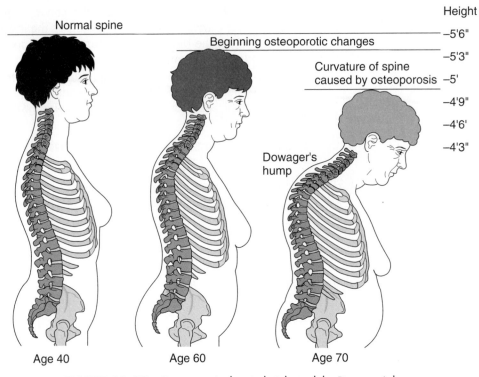

FIGURE 11–88 Osteoporosis: loss in height and the Dowager's hump

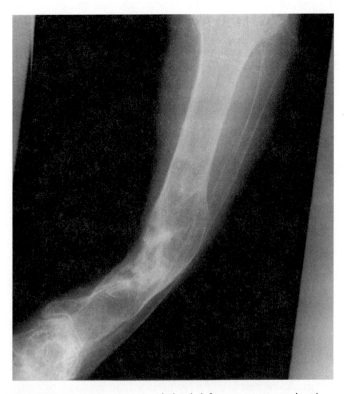

FIGURE 11–89 A severe skeletal deformity associated with osteoporosis

supplement, and taking calcium and vitamin D to support normal bone metabolism.

Today there are four new approved treatments. A drug called Miacalcin, which decreases bone loss, has been in use in injectable form but is now available as a nasal spray. Fosamax, Slow Sodium, and Citracel are also able to increase bone mass.

The most significant development is the ability to determine the disease before fractures occur. There are seven different techniques for measuring bone density in various body locations. The most used form of densitometry is called dual energy x-ray absorptiometry (DEXA). It can measure bone density and also estimate fracture risk. The procedure is relatively fast, uses a low level of radiation, and is fairly inexpensive. Another even simpler method screens for the rate of bone loss with a urine test called Osteomark, or the NTX test. The purpose of all procedures is early detection so that preventive therapies can be prescribed. Figure 11–89 shows the severe skeletal condition associated with osteoporosis.

Recently, scientists in Philadelphia, using new biotechnology equipment, believe they have discovered the cause of postmenopausal osteoporosis. They have linked the condition to a defect on chromosome 7, leading them to think that it may be possible to develop a test that will predict who will develop osteoporosis so that preventive measures may be taken long before the symptoms would become evident.

The National Osteoporosis Foundation is trying to educate people about the condition because osteoporosis is a "silent" disease, meaning there are no warning symptoms. Often, by the time it is diagnosed, there has been significant loss of bone strength leading to irreversible damage and probable disability. A risk analysis assessment provides a means of determining the probability of developing osteoporosis.

RISK ANALYSIS

Yes (4)_____	No (0)	I smoke cigarettes.
Yes (4)_____	No (0)	I drink alcoholic beverages [3 oz. or more a day].
Yes (2)_____	No (0)	I drink alcoholic beverages [1 to 2 oz. a day].
Yes (0)_____	No (3)	I often drink/eat dairy foods.
Yes (0)_____	No (3)	I exercise regularly.
Yes (4)_____	No (0)	I have an eating disorder.
Yes (2)_____	No (0)	My diet is high in red meat.
Yes (2)_____	No (0)	I often drink three or more cups of coffee or two or more cola beverages a day.
Yes (4)_____	No (0)	There's a history of osteoporosis in my family.
Yes (4)_____	No (0)	I have a small-boned frame.
Yes (2)_____	No (0)	I am older than 40.
Yes (4)_____	No (0)	I am older than 70.
Yes (3)_____	No (0)	I am a post-menopausal woman who began menopause before age 45.
Yes (4)_____	No (0)	I have taken steroid (cortisone) medications.
Yes (4)_____	No (0)	I have had or have an overactive thyroid gland.
Yes (3)_____	No (0)	I have chronic kidney disease.
_____	**Total Risk Points**	

0 to 8 points You have a very low risk of osteoporosis. As you grow older, be sure to consume adequate amounts of calcium and exercise regularly.

9 to 16 points Your risk is moderate. To reduce it, consume more calcium, exercise regularly, and ask your doctor if you should take other steps.

17 or more points Your risk is high. Ask your doctor to help you develop a bone-protection plan.

Scoliosis (Sko-le-o'-sis)

Description—A lateral curvature of the spine, usually in the thoracic region, associated with rotation of the spinal column. It may also be lumbar or involve both (see Figure 11–87C). The thorax usually curves to the right while the lumbar curves left. Because the body has to maintain balance, the cervical spine will also curve left, which gives the spine an "S" curve appearance.

There are different types of **scoliosis**. An infantile type of transmitted scoliosis occurs primarily in boys from birth to age three and causes left thorax and right lumbar curves. Another type, known as juvenile scoliosis, affects both sexes between the ages of four and ten. The third type, called adolescent, primarily affects

girls between 10 and maturity of the skeleton and results in varying types of curvatures.

Signs and symptoms—Adolescent scoliosis can be easily diagnosed. Classic symptoms are uneven hemlines or unequal pants legs, one hip appearing to be higher than the other, and one shoulder appearing higher and perhaps the scapula more pronounced.

Etiology—Different types have different causes. Some are from congenital defects of the vertebra, muscular dystrophy, paralysis, or a transmitted trait that develops during the growth process. Others are the result of poor posture or uneven leg lengths. Most scoliosis is of idiopathic (without apparent cause) origin.

Treatment—Treatment includes observation, exercises, and a brace. With curvature beyond 60 degrees, an immobilizing cast or preoperative traction system is followed by surgical correction using posterior spinal fusion and insertion of a Harrington rod for stabilization. Note the parent teaching aid box titled "How to Detect Scoliosis."

HOW TO DETECT SCOLIOSIS

Parents:

To check your child for scoliosis (abnormal curvature of the spine) perform this simple test. First, have your child remove his or her shirt and stand up straight. As you look at the child's back, answer these questions:

- Is one shoulder higher than the other, or is one shoulder blade more prominent?
- When the child's arms hang loosely at his or her sides, does one arm swing away from the body more than the other?
- Is one hip higher or more prominent than the other?
- Does the child seem to tilt to one side?

Ask your child to bend forward, with arms hanging down and palms together at knee level. Can you see a hump on the back at the ribs or near the waist?

If your answer to any of these questions is "yes," your child needs careful evaluation for scoliosis. Notify your doctor.

Sprain

Description—The complete or incomplete tear in the supporting ligaments of a joint.

Signs and symptoms—**Sprains** are characterized by pain, swelling, and a black-and-blue discoloration. The ankle is the most common site.

Etiology—Sprains follow a severe twisting action of a joint.

Treatment—Care of sprains should follow the easy to remember R.I.C.E. method—Rest, Ice, Compression, and Elevation. Treatment consists of (1) controlling pain and swelling by elevating the joint and applying ice intermittently for the first 12 to 24 hours, (2) immobilization using an elastic wrap or, if very severe, a soft cast, and (3) the use of crutches to eliminate stress on the joint. If healing does not occur normally in three to four weeks, the torn ligaments may require surgical repair, especially if sprains recur.

Subluxation (Sub-luks-a'-shun)

Description—The partial or incomplete dislocation of the articulating surfaces of joint bones.

Signs and symptoms—There is joint deformity, impaired motion, pain, and change in length if an extremity is involved. Common sites are shoulders, elbows, wrists, knees, fingers and toes, hips, and ankles. Diagnostic x-ray is usually indicated to rule out or confirm accompanying joint fracture.

Etiology—Subluxation is caused by an injury or a disease process of a joint. Often with an injury there is also involvement of the surrounding nerves, blood vessels, ligaments, and soft tissues that results in pain, swelling, and joint deformity.

Treatment—Treatment consists of reduction as soon as possible to minimize swelling and muscle spasms, which make reduction difficult. The use of medication to control muscle spasm and pain and possibly a splint or cast to provide joint immobilization and support while ligaments heal depend on the joint involved.

Temporomandibular Disorders (TMD) (Tem-poro-man-dib'-u-lar)

Description—This is a condition of the jaw that is described as a feeling that the jaw has come unhinged. For unknown reasons, 90% of sufferers are women.

Signs and symptoms—The symptoms include a grinding or clicking sound and pain and discomfort when opening the mouth. Jaw muscles become sore, chewing is difficult, and pain spreads to the facial and neck muscles. Symptoms persist continuously. Headaches, toothaches, and earaches may also be part of the disorder.

Etiology—The cause is not certain. Some feel it is emotional stress, others that the joint is very complicated and is a manner of many factors adversely affecting the joint. Teeth grinding and clenching cause muscle spasm and can be caused by it. A malocclusion of the teeth can throw the jaw out of line. Bad posture that thrusts the chin forward can strain the neck and jaw muscles. Certain orthopedic problems, such as arthritis and bone degeneration, can contribute. Other causes may be excessive chewing of gum or chewy foods or a blow to the jaw. A common cause is prolonged gripping of a phone between the shoulder and cheek or carrying a heavy shoulder bag that strains neck and shoulder muscles.

Treatment—First is self treatment, such as a soft diet and an analgesic for the pain, and eliminating activities known as causes. Hot or cold compresses, gentle exer-

---

A CAAHEP CONNECTION

Curriculum standards for preparing medical assistants specifically identify the knowledge of **Anatomy and Physiology, Diagnostic and Treatment Modalities,** and **Diseases and Disorders** as being essential components. It also requires content in the structure, application, and definitions of medical terminology. This chapter addresses these standards, and this unit particularly identifies content regarding the skeletal system.

---

cises, controlling yawns (with the hands), and resting of the jaw may help. If malocclusion is present, a simple grinding of teeth surfaces by a dentist may correct the problem. Bite splints or plates fitted over the teeth can also stabilize the bite and eliminate night grinding. Taking muscle relaxers and eliminating the source of stress may be necessary.

REPLACING BONE

When bone is destroyed by injury, cancer, or some other infectious process, doctors may use bone taken from other places in the body. However, there is a limit to the amount that can be "borrowed." When desperate, bone can be salvaged from cadavers, but the problems of inflammation and infection are a concern. Surgeons have discovered that coral from the ocean is uniquely compatible with bone and makes an excellent framework upon which bone cells can construct new bone. Certain species of coral have an almost identical physical makeup as bone. It unites, almost without seams, with the human skeleton. In addition, it does not activate the body's inflammation or immune responses. Once the surgery has healed, the strength of the resulting bone composite is excellent. The coral is available in blocks of different sizes, which doctors carve into the shapes they need for surgery.

ACHIEVE UNIT OBJECTIVES

Complete Chapter 11, Unit 5, in the workbook to help you obtain competency of this subject matter.

UNIT 6
The Muscular System

OBJECTIVES

Upon completion of the unit, meet the following performance objectives by verifying knowledge of the facts and

principles presented through oral and written communication at a level deemed competent.

1. Spell and define, using the glossary at the back of the text, all the **Words to Know** in this unit.
2. Explain how muscular activity increases body heat.
3. List six functions of skeletal muscles.
4. Name and describe the three types of muscular tissue and the purpose of each.
5. Describe the purpose of a muscle team, and give an example.
6. Explain what muscle tone means.
7. Describe the structure and function of a tendon, and identify the body's strongest tendon.
8. Explain the terms *origin* and *insertion.*
9. Describe a muscle sheath and a bursa and the purpose of each.
10. Identify the muscles of respiration, and describe how their function results in breathing.
11. Name the major skeletal muscles of the body.
12. Describe the smooth muscle action of peristalsis.
13. Explain the structure and function of a sphincter.
14. Describe four disorders or diseases of the muscular system.

AREAS OF COMPETENCE (AAMA)

This unit addresses content with in the areas of *Administrative procedures, Practice finances, Patient care, Communication skills,* and *Instruction,* as identified in the Medical Assistant Role Delineation Study. Refer to Appendix A for a detailed listing of the areas. (Note: Although *Anatomy and physiology* is not specifically identified in the study, a basic knowledge of the body's structure and function is an essential foundation to the competent performance of many roles.)

■ WORDS TO KNOW

abduction	hiccough
Achilles tendon	insertion
adduction	intercostal
anchor	latissimus dorsi
aponeurosis	muscle team
atrophy	muscle tone
biceps	musculoskeletal
contracture	origin
cramp	pectoralis major
deltoid	peristalsis
dystrophy	quadriceps femoris
extensor	sartorius
fascia	sheath
flexor	spasm
gastrocnemius	sphincter
gluteus maximus	sternocleidomastoid
hamstring	strain

tendon	torticollis
tendonitis	trapezius
tibialis anterior	triceps

Ⓐ Library

There are approximately 600 muscle organs in the human body. Muscles are composed of muscular tissue, which is constructed of bundles of muscle fibers about the size of a human hair. The larger the muscle, the greater the number of fibers. Muscles perform their duties by alternately contracting and relaxing. All muscle activity is influenced by the nervous system. Motor neuron axons innervate several muscle cells within a muscle. Signals from the brain go through the axons and cause all the cells under their control to contract at the same time. That group of cells and its motor neuron are called a *motor unit.* When only one stimulus acts on the unit causing a contraction, it is called a *twitch.* This quick, simple contraction naturally occurs occasionally as a spontaneous event in a muscle. Scientists can study these units by using an electrical stimulus, which will also activate the motor unit. A muscle contraction is a quick progression of events following a stimulus—a very brief interval before the contraction begins, then it intensifies to a peak, and decreases to relaxation. If a second stimulus is received before the first is completed, the contraction will strengthen. When repeated stimulation occurs without a relaxation time, the muscle is maintained in a state of contraction called *tetanus* (not to be confused with the disease of the same name). This occurs when we experience muscle **cramps** and **spasms**.

At all times, motor units are alternately either contracted or relaxed; there is no other state in which they exist. The units that make up the muscles are contracted in sufficient number to meet whatever need is necessary. During sleep, for instance, only a few would be contracted at a given time, yet during strenuous activity, a great number would be called on to contract, a process known as *muscle recruitment.*

Some muscles work in partnership with the bones and can be controlled voluntarily by the motor nerves of the peripheral nervous system. Other muscles function continuously without the slightest conscious concern. The autonomic nervous system directs their activities to provide the body with essential services. It is the action of these muscles that causes us to breathe and our blood to circulate.

MUSCLE FUEL

All body tissues must have food and oxygen to survive. The muscles receive an ample supply of both because of their importance to the body's safety and well-being. The body stores carbohydrates in its muscles in the form of a starch called *glycogen.* When muscles function, they use the stored glycogen, changing it to glucose, as their source of energy. Heat is released as this fuel is used, thereby warming the body. Strenuous exercise burns a great deal of stored glycogen and therefore often results in overheating the body.

FUNCTIONS OF MUSCLE

In addition to providing heat and the ability to move, muscles support the structures of the body and hold the body upright. The muscles along the back, shoulders, and neck hold the trunk and head erect while permitting great flexibility in movement.

The structure of the skeletal muscles protects the blood vessels and nerves that lie throughout the body. The contraction of lower leg muscles aids in the return flow of blood to the heart by squeezing the veins of the legs. Muscles also provide protective padding to shield delicate internal organs and structures from injury.

Visually, the muscles add greatly to our appearance by giving shape to the body. Body-building enthusiasts spend years developing the degree of muscle enlargement and definition they feel is desirable. Muscle fiber, and therefore the muscle, hypertrophies (grows larger) with exercise; the number of fibers does not increase, however.

MUSCLE GROWTH

Muscle tissue changes slightly with age. During infancy, muscles have little connective tissue, often being attached to the bone directly. With maturity, the connective tissue increases as do the elastic fibers. Muscles grow in relation

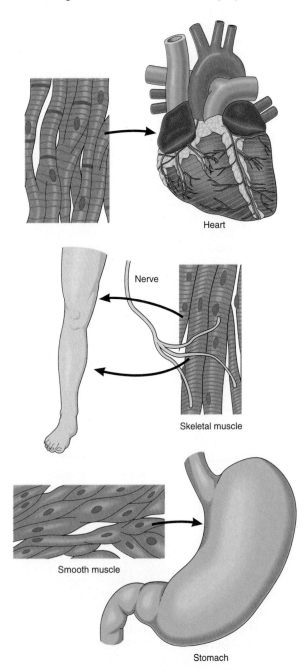

Heart

Nerve

Skeletal muscle

Smooth muscle

Stomach

FIGURE 11–90 Types of muscle tissue (From *The Wonderful Human Machine*, copyright 1979 by the American Medical Association.)

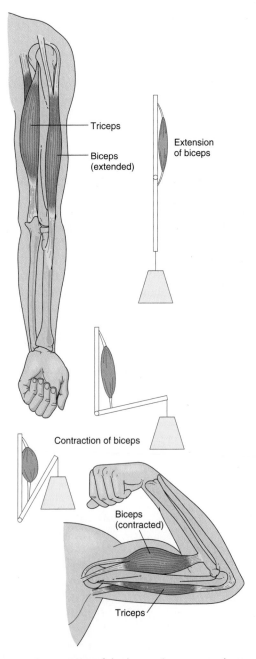

Triceps

Biceps (extended)

Extension of biceps

Contraction of biceps

Biceps (contracted)

Triceps

FIGURE 11–91 Action of the biceps/triceps muscle team (From *The Wonderful Human Machine*, copyright 1979 by the American Medical Association.)

to the structures to which they are attached. Muscles of the eye, for example, grow very little, whereas the large muscles of the lower extremities grow considerably.

TYPES OF MUSCLE TISSUE

There are three types of muscle tissue (Figure 11–90). First, there is the *skeletal* type. Skeletal muscles are attached to bones and therefore permit movement. Because we have some control over movements, this type of muscle tissue is also called voluntary. Skeletal muscle cells are long and strong, some reaching lengths up to 12 inches. These cells are held together by connective tissue to form a muscle bundle. The bundles in turn are enclosed in a tougher connective tissue **sheath** to form the muscle organs such as the **biceps** of the arm. The larger the muscle organ, the greater the number of fibers.

The second type of muscle tissue is *smooth.* Smooth muscle tissue is made of small, delicate muscle cells and is found throughout the internal organs of the body, except for the heart. Smooth muscle activity occurs continuously in such actions as breathing, moving food through the intestinal tract, changing the size of the pupil of the eye, and dilating or constricting blood vessels. These muscles function without conscious direct control, so they are also called involuntary.

The third type is *cardiac* muscle tissue. As the name implies, this type is found in the heart. These cells are joined in a continuous network without sheath separation. The membranes of adjacent cells are fused at places called *intercalated disks.* A communication system at the fused areas will not permit independent cell contraction. When one cell receives a signal to contract, all neighboring cells are stimulated and they contract together to produce the action of a heartbeat. This type of muscle tissue is also involuntary, which is fortunate. It would be a full-time job to consciously contract the heart muscle 70 times a minute, 100,800 times a day.

SKELETAL MUSCLE ACTION

When muscles contract, they become shorter and thicker. A good example is the skeletal muscle of the upper arm, the biceps. When the biceps contract to bend the elbow, the shorter and thicker muscle causes a bulge in the upper arm (Figure 11–91).

The skeletal muscle that bends a joint is called a **flexor**, whereas the action of straightening the joint is done by the **extensor** muscle. The extensor muscle that straightens the elbow is the **triceps**. The flexor and its partner, the extensor muscle, form what is known as a **muscle team** to bend and straighten joints (Figure 11–92). Muscles also contract to move extremities away from the body's center line, which is known as **abduction**, or toward the center line, which is known as **adduction** (Figure 11–93).

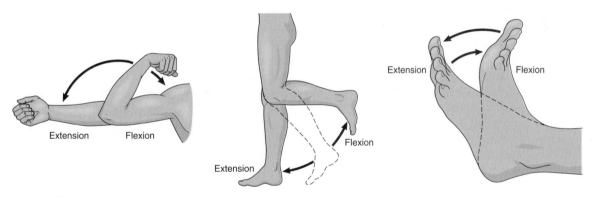

FIGURE 11–92   Flexor/extensor muscle team action

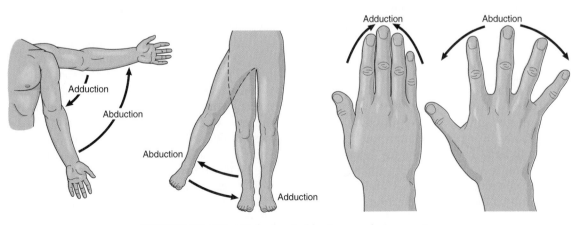

FIGURE 11–93   Abduction/adduction muscle team action

MUSCLE TONE

Most skeletal muscles are partially contracted at all times to maintain the body's erect position. It is believed that some fibers contract while others rest and that they then exchange places. This constant state of contraction is known as **muscle tone**. Physicians frequently refer to muscle tone when examining patients. Evaluation of muscle tone aids in determining the status of the CNS and the motor function of the peripheral nerves.

Loss of muscle tone can occur when muscles are not used, as with severe illness, elderly people, paralysis, or temporarily when an extremity has been immobilized in a cast. With prolonged lack of use, muscles will **atrophy**, which is a progressive wasting away of the muscle tissue. Another muscular condition that develops from lack of use is called **contracture**. Here flexor muscles become shorter and permanently bend the joints. This is a common condition with paralyzed or unconscious patients. The most common sites are the fingers, elbows, knees, and hip joints.

MUSCLE ATTACHMENT

Skeletal muscles are attached to bone in various ways. In some instances the connective tissue within the muscle is attached directly to the bone periosteum. Some muscular connective tissue sheaths extend to form a strong fibrous structure known as a **tendon**, which is attached to rough surfaces on a bone. Tendons are extremely strong and do not stretch. A one-inch thick tendon reportedly will support nine tons of weight. Because of this characteristic, a bone will sometimes fracture before the tendon attached to it will separate. The thickest and strongest tendon in the human body is the **Achilles tendon**, which attaches the **gastrocnemius** muscle in the calf of the leg to the heel bone.

A similar type of connective tissue is called a ligament, but it does not perform the same function. A ligament is a flexible, fibrous tissue that supports organs and connects bone to bone at joints. Ligaments, unlike tendons, do stretch.

Another form of muscular attachment is by **fascia**, a sheetlike, tough membrane that forms sheaths to cover and protect the muscle tissue. The term **aponeurosis** designates either a fascia or a flat tendon type of muscle attachment.

Origin or Insertion

When skeletal muscles join bones that meet at joints, one of the bones becomes the **anchor** on which the muscle has its **origin**. The bone to be moved becomes the **insertion** end for the muscle. For example, the biceps has its origin at the shoulder and its insertion on the radius. When the biceps contracts, being firmly anchored at the shoulder, it pulls upon the insertion location on the forearm, and the arm flexes (bends).

The terms origin and insertion can also apply to muscle attachments other than at joints. Essentially, the end nearest the center of the body is described as the origin, whereas the distal end is referred to as the insertion. Usually the origin is relatively immobile, whereas the insertion is into a movable structure.

SHEATHS AND BURSAE

To protect the moving parts of the muscles, muscle groups are separated from each other by membranes called *sheaths* to reduce the friction from movement. Within muscle groups, individual muscles are also separated by membranes. The tendons that extend from the muscle group are also enclosed in lubricated sheaths to protect them from damage by rubbing against other tendons, bone, or cartilage.

A sheath that is shaped like a sac and has a slippery fluid lining is known as a bursa. A bursa functions as a water cushion to minimize pressure and friction over bony prominences and under tendons. The most common bursae are located at the elbow, knee, and shoulder.

MAJOR SKELETAL MUSCLES

The muscle most important in breathing divides the chest cavity from the abdominal cavity. This muscle is called the *diaphragm* (Figure 11–94). It is a dome-shaped muscle with tendons that attach it in the back to the spinal column, in the front to the tip of the sternum, and along the sides to the cartilage edge of the ribs. When the muscle contracts, it becomes shorter and therefore flatter, creating a vacuum that causes the lungs to draw in air. When the muscle relaxes, it returns to its dome shape and forces air out of the lungs. The diaphragm also plays a role in coughing, sneezing, or laughing. Spasmodic contractions of the diaphragm, followed by spasmodic closure of the space between the vocal cords, cause the common **hiccough**.

The orbicularis oculi and orbicularis oris are circular muscles around the eye and mouth (Figure 11–95). Their contraction enables us to squint or wink and to whistle or pucker the mouth. The **sternocleidomastoid** and the **trapezius** are the major muscles of the neck and upper back that hold the head erect and assist with its movement (Figure 11–96). The trapezius not only supports the head but extends down the back and shoulders, giving us the ability to raise and throw back the shoulders.

The **pectoralis major** is the main upper chest muscle. It extends from the sternum to the head of the humerus, enabling us to flex the arm across the chest. The **intercostal** muscles lie beneath the pectoralis major, between the ribs. These serve as accessory muscles to the diaphragm by enlarging the thoracic cavity during inspiration.

The abdomen is covered by three main muscle layers that run in different directions to make a strong wall to protect the abdominal organs. The external oblique is

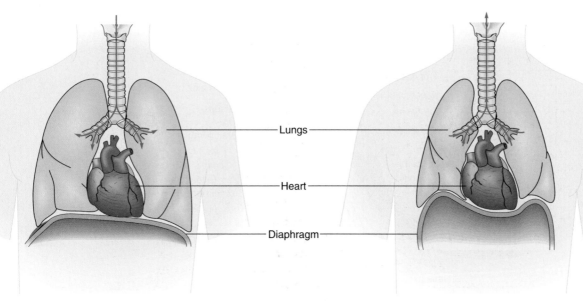

Diaphragm contracted

Diaphragm relaxed

FIGURE 11–94   The action of the diaphragm muscle

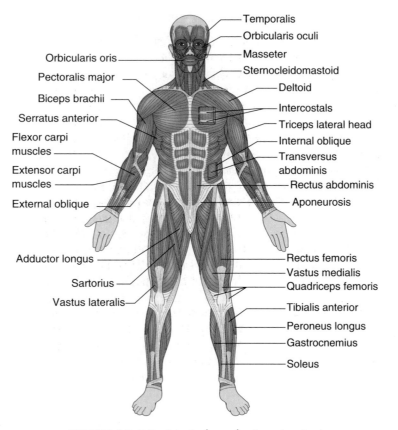

FIGURE 11–95   Principal muscles (anterior view)

first, the internal oblique is beneath, and the transversus abdominis is the innermost layer. A long, narrow muscle, the rectus abdominis, extends from the pubis to the bottom of the rib cage in the center of the abdomen. It overlies and is surrounded by connective tissue layers from the other three muscles.

The back is covered by a large muscle called the **latissimus dorsi**. Its main function is to extend and adduct the arm, as when swimming. Thick vertical groups of four different muscles overlap and extend from the sacrum and lower vertebrae to the occipital bone and upper cervical vertebrae to support and move the spinal column.

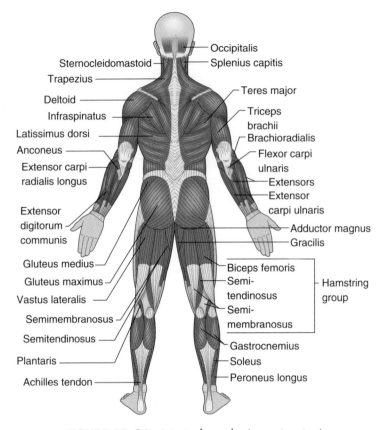

Occipitalis
Splenius capitis
Sternocleidomastoid
Trapezius
Teres major
Deltoid
Triceps brachii
Infraspinatus
Brachioradialis
Latissimus dorsi
Flexor carpi ulnaris
Anconeus
Extensors
Extensor carpi radialis longus
Extensor carpi ulnaris
Extensor digitorum communis
Adductor magnus
Gracilis
Gluteus medius
Biceps femoris
Semitendinosus
Gluteus maximus
Semimembranosus
Hamstring group
Vastus lateralis
Semimembranosus
Gastrocnemius
Semitendinosus
Plantaris
Soleus
Peroneus longus
Achilles tendon

FIGURE 11–96 Principal muscles (posterior view)

The shoulders are protected by a triangle of muscle called the **deltoid**, which abducts the arm. The deltoid, if of adequate size, may be used for small injections of medication that must be given intramuscularly.

Lower Extremity Muscles

The muscles of the lower extremities involve about one half of the body's total muscle mass. The buttocks are formed by the large **gluteus maximus** muscles, which support much of the body's weight and enable us to stand erect. The upper outer quadrant of the buttocks is the site of choice for intramuscular injections, especially for large amounts of a slowly absorbing material.

The front of the thigh has the longest muscle of the body, the **sartorius**. It anchors on the iliac spine and crosses diagonally down the front of the thigh to insert on the medial surface of the tibia. The sartorius flexes the hip and knee joints to turn the thigh outward, making it possible to sit cross-legged on the floor. The **quadriceps femoris**, with four separate parts (rectus femoris, vastus lateralis, vastus medialis, and vastus intermedius), makes up the bulk of the anterior thigh musculature. It is a powerful extensor of the knee and is used when we rise from a sitting position, kick a ball, or swim.

The **tibialis anterior** is in the front of the leg. When it is flexed, it is possible to walk on your heels with the rest of the foot off the ground. It also serves to invert the foot, turning it toward the other foot.

The posterior thigh is the site of the **hamstring** group, which includes the biceps femoris, semitendinosus, semimembranosus, and a portion of the adductor magnus. Their primary function is to flex the knee by pulling on the insertion at the fibula and tibia. The tendons are easily identified by palpation behind the knee. The gastrocnemius is the main muscle in the calf of the leg. Its tendon, the Achilles, has been mentioned. Contraction of the gastrocnemius permits you to stand to tiptoe because it acts as the flexor of the plantar surface (sole) of the foot.

Muscles of Expression

A number of muscles in the face enable us to show our feelings. The frontalis (forehead) can be raised to express surprise or lowered to show a stern glance. Raising one side of the obicularis oris about the upper lip will result in a sneer. The obicularis oris also allows us to whistle, kiss, smile, grin, grimace with pain, or pout.

The obicularis oculi around the eyes help complete the frown and enable us to squint or wink. The large muscle of the lower jaw, the masseter, in cooperation with other smaller muscles, opens and closes the mouth to express emotions of surprise and disbelief but also is powerful and is responsible for our ability to chew and grind the food we eat.

MUSCLE STRAIN AND CRAMPS

Occasionally, too much stress is applied to skeletal muscles while exercising or participating in athletic activities. This may result in a **strain**, but the muscles will recover with a period of rest. Athletes frequently "pull" their hamstring group during strenuous competition. Another frequent occurrence is a muscle cramp or spasm, caused by a muscle that has contracted but cannot relax. It can usually be relieved by stretching the muscle or causing it to bear weight.

Muscle Fatigue

Prolonged strenuous exercise can result in muscle fatigue. Muscles require large amounts of oxygen to sustain the conversion of glycogen stored in the muscle into energy (adenosine triphosphate or ATP), a function of the many mitochondria within muscle cells. Vigorous exercise is believed to cause an oxygen deficit within the muscle because the body cannot take in and circulate oxygen fast enough to keep up with the demand. When this occurs, lactic acid begins to accumulate, the glycogen is depleted, and the muscle's supply of ATP runs low. The muscle loses its ability to contract effectively and finally becomes incapable of reacting at all to the stimulus to contract. This occurs primarily in marathon runners who sometimes even collapse from muscle fatigue. Most of us simply stop our activities long before this happens.

Oxygen debt is "paid back" by the rapid and deep breathing that follows exercise. When the accumulated lactic acid is removed and the amount of oxygen is restored to once again produce ATP, the muscle can again respond to a stimulus and contract.

SMOOTH MUSCLE ACTION

Smooth, involuntary muscles can be found throughout the internal organs and structures of the body. They are controlled automatically by signals from the autonomic nervous system.

In the esophagus (the structure that connects the mouth with the stomach), the muscle tissue changes from voluntary muscles at the top that assist in swallowing, to smooth, involuntary muscles that move the food to the stomach. A two-layer muscle structure in the lower esophagus continues into the stomach and intestines. One layer of smooth muscle is circular and contracts to narrow the tube. Another layer is longitudinal and contracts to shorten the tube. The alternating action of both layers, contracting and relaxing, works the food through the body in a wavelike action called **peristalsis** (Figure 11–97). The stomach has a third layer in the muscle wall because of its need to break up and churn the food that is swallowed, which must be in a near-liquid state before it can be passed on to the small intestine.

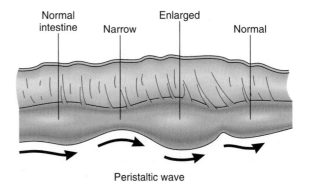

FIGURE 11–97 Peristaltic action (From *The Wonderful Human Machine*, copyright 1979 by the American Medical Association.)

Sphincters

Throughout the digestive system and inside the blood vessels of the body are smooth, donut-shaped muscle structures called **sphincters**. These pinch shut intermittently to control the flow of food, liquid, or blood. Sphincters in the digestive system are capable of remaining contracted for hours if necessary. Both ends of the stomach have sphincter muscles to hold the contents securely inside while muscular action and chemical processes digest food. When the food is in the proper state, the lower sphincter opens slightly to allow small amounts of the liquid to escape into the small intestine.

An example of smooth muscle sphincter action that can be easily observed is the pupil of the eye. When available light is decreased, the radial muscles of the iris contract to enlarge the pupil, permitting more light to enter, thereby increasing the ability to see. When light is focused on the eye, the circular sphincter muscles of the iris that surround the pupil contract, making the pupil smaller, thereby limiting the amount of light striking the retina. The physician will usually check light reflex action of the eyes in assessing the condition of the brain and autonomic nervous system.

DISORDERS AND DISEASES

Bursitis/Tendonitis (See Unit 5) (Bur-sigh'-tis/Ten-done-i'-tis)

Description—**Tendonitis** is a painful inflammation of the tendon and tendon–muscle attachments to bone, usually at the shoulder, hip, heel, or hamstrings. Bursitis is an inflammation of the bursa that covers and lubricates the muscles and tendons, and occurs most often at the shoulder, elbow, or knee.

Signs and symptoms—Pain at joints or at the muscle attachment that results in limited motion.

Etiology—Tendonitis normally follows a sports-related activity that damages the muscle–tendon structure. It can also result from misaligned posture and other **musculoskeletal** disorders.

Treatment—With injury, apply ice initially for the first 12 to 24 hours. Later, applications of heat will usually aid in relief of the joint pain. If calcium deposits have formed within the tendon, it becomes weak, and the condition will be aggravated by heat. The calcium deposits are visible on x-ray to confirm the diagnosis. Application of ice packs will help relieve discomfort from calcified tendonitis.

Both conditions may be treated by resting the joint, oral doses of pain medication, and intraarticular injections of a mixture of corticosteroid and a local anesthetic. If fluid has accumulated within the area, it may require aspiration prior to the injection treatment. When pain has subsided, a physical therapy regime may be indicated to maintain joint function and prevent muscular atrophy.

Epicondylitis (Tennis Elbow) (See Unit 5) (Ep-e-con-dill-i'-tis)

Description—This is inflammation of a forearm tendon at the attachment on the humerus at the elbow.

Signs and symptoms—The initial elbow pain gradually worsens and often involves the forearm and the back of the hand when an object is grasped or the elbow is twisted. There is tenderness over the head of the radius and the projection of the humerus at the elbow joint.

Etiology—Epicondylitis probably begins as a partial tear of the tendon from its attachment.

Treatment—Injection of the area, as with tendonitis, is effective. Immobilization, heat therapy, and manipulation of the tendon attachment are used before resorting to surgical excision of the tendon for recurring and continual inflammation.

Fibromyalgia Syndrome (Fi-bro-my-al'-ja)

Description—Fibromyalgia is a chronic musculoskeletal condition characterized by widespread pain. It was once called fibrositis. It affects people of all ages. It is estimated that at least 3.7 million people have the syndrome. Fibromyalgia occurs frequently in people with autoimmune and arthritis disorders.

Signs and symptoms—The prime symptom is widespread pain and the presence of tender points or trigger points at specific sites on the body (Figure 11–98). Diagnosis is considered positive when 11 of the 18 points are painful. Besides pain and muscle stiffness, patients may experience fatigue, an inability to concentrate, sleep disturbances, dry eyes and mouth, frequent urination, irritable bowel syndrome, headaches, numbness or tingling in the arms or legs, bursitis, tendonitis, and depression. All are symptoms of an alteration in the body's sympathetic nervous system.

Etiology—The cause is unknown. There seems to be some familial tendency, but a genetic connection has not been proven. It appears to be affected by many

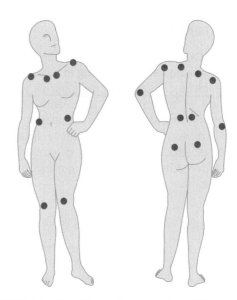

FIGURE 11–98 The tender point sites of fibromyalgia

things, such as the weather, stress, and a poor state of physical fitness. Symptoms come and go, but the syndrome persists.

Treatment—There is no cure, only methods to make it possible to cope with the symptoms. The use of biofeedback, massage, warm showers or baths, gentle aerobic exercise, and adjustments to reduce stress are helpful. Other treatments include injection of the tender points, spraying the skin with ethyl chloride and then stretching the muscles, physical therapy, ultrasound, heat and cold applications, a jacuzzi, and medication to relax muscles and relieve pain. Currently used drugs include low doses of tricyclic medications, such as Elavil and Flexeril. Other similar drugs are used that increase the level of serotonin, a neurotransmitter. When the serotonin level is low, there is an increase in depression, sensitivity to pain, and difficulty with sleeping. The best course of treatment is becoming physically fit, achieving a good body weight, and acquiring restful sleep.

Muscular Dystrophy

Description—This group of congenital disorders results in progressive wasting away of skeletal muscles. There are several types of muscular **dystrophy**.

Duchenne's Dystrophy represents about 50% of all the cases. The onset is in early childhood with death occurring after 10 to 15 years. It is usually first recognized when the child is about one year of age.

Signs and symptoms—Initially, the leg and pelvic muscles are affected, making all activities involving the lower extremities difficult. Children are usually confined to a wheelchair by ages 9 to 12. The disease progresses from skeletal to smooth muscles, affecting the heart and diaphragm and eventually resulting in cardiac or respiratory failure.

Etiology—Duchenne's is an X-linked chromosome disorder affecting only males.

Treatment—None available. However, orthopedic appliances, exercise, physical therapy, and surgery to correct muscle contractures can help preserve mobility.

Erb's or Juvenile Muscular Dystrophy progresses slowly and occurs later in childhood or adolescence. It affects both sexes. It does not reduce life expectancy.

Signs and symptoms—Erb's main symptoms are weakness of the upper arm and pelvic muscles. Other symptoms include winging of the scapulae, lordosis with protruding abdomen, waddling gait, poor balance, and the inability to raise the arms.

Etiology and Treatment—Same as Duchenne.

Mixed Dystrophy does not appear to be inherited and affects both sexes. It generally begins between ages 30 and 50. Progressive deterioration is rapid and is usually fatal within five years after onset.

Signs and symptoms—This type affects all voluntary muscles.

A positive diagnosis can be made from a typical medical history and evaluation of voluntary muscle movements. Confirmation is possible by a biopsy of the muscle tissue, which shows characteristic deposits of fat and connective tissue.

Torticollis (Wryneck) (Tor-ti-col'-lis)

Description—The neck deformity that bends the head to the affected side and rotates the chin toward the opposite side. It can be congenital or acquired.

Signs and symptoms—The obvious positioning of the head.

Etiology—Torticollis is caused by shortening or spasm of the sternocleidomastoid neck muscle. The congenital form usually follows a difficult (breech) birth and occurs mostly in firstborn females. It is thought to develop from malposition before birth, prenatal injury, or the rupture of muscle fibers with resulting scar tissue development. Acquired **torticollis** results from muscle damage by disease, a cervical spine injury, or muscle spasms.

A PEDIATRIC PERSPECTIVE

Infants less than six months of age with poor neck control can rupture the sternocleidomastoid muscle. The muscle heals over time and pain relievers, such as Tylenol, can be used.

Treatment—Treatment of the congenital type consists of stretching the shortened muscle through passive exer-

---

A CAAHEP CONNECTION

This unit stresses the **Anatomy and physiology** and **Medical terminology** as it relates to the muscular system. This area of content is identified in the standards as essential to the curriculum for medical assisting. The ability to understand the structure and function of the body is essential to the performance of many skills and to the communication of instructions to patients.

---

cises and positional arrangement of the head during sleeping. Surgical correction of the muscle can be accomplished if conservative methods are not effective. Acquired torticollis is treated by correcting the underlying cause whenever possible. Application of heat, cervical traction, a neck brace, exercise, psychotherapy, and massage are indicated.

ACHIEVE UNIT OBJECTIVES

Complete Chapter 11, Unit 6, in the workbook to help you obtain competency of this subject matter.

UNIT 7

The Respiratory System

OBJECTIVES

Upon completion of the unit, meet the following performance objectives by verifying knowledge of the facts and principles presented through oral and written communication at a level deemed competent.

1. Spell and define, using the glossary at the back of the text, all the **Words to Know** in this unit.
2. Describe the source and importance of oxygen.
3. Trace the path of oxygen to the internal cell.
4. Describe the structure and function of the nose, pharynx, epiglottis, larynx, trachea, bronchus, bronchiole, and alveolus. *[handwritten: → read only]*
5. Explain how voice sounds are produced.
6. Differentiate between external and internal respiration.
7. Describe the structure and function of the pleural coverings of the lungs and chest cavity.
8. Describe the relationship of the diaphragm and brain to breathing.
9. Describe five normal occurrences that alter breathing patterns and explain why they occur.

10. Identify diagnostic examinations for respiratory assessment.
11. Explain the role of surfactant in the lungs.
12. Differentiate between perfusion and ventilation scans.
13. Describe the diseases or disorders of the respiratory tract.

AREAS OF COMPETENCE (AAMA)

This unit addresses content within the areas of *Administrative procedures, Practice finances, Patient care, Communication skills,* and *Instruction,* as identified in the Medical Assistant Role Delineation Study. Refer to Appendix A for a detailed listing of the areas. (Note: Although *Anatomy and physiology* are not specifically identified within the study, a basic knowledge of the body's structure and function is an essential foundation to the competent performance of many roles.)

■ WORDS TO KNOW

allergic rhinitis	laryngitis
alveoli	larynx
angiography	Legionnaires' disease
apnea	liter
arteriography	lung
asthma	orthopnea
atelectasis	oxygen
bleb	perfusion
bronchi	pharynx
bronchiole	pleura
bronchitis	pleurisy
carbon dioxide	pneumonoconiosis
chronic obstructive	pneumonia
pulmonary disease	pneumothorax
cilia	pulmonary
cyanosis	pulmonary edema
diaphoresis	pulmonary emboli
dyspnea	respiratory
emphysema	rhinitis
empyema	septum
epiglottis	sinusitis
epistaxis	spirometer
expectorated	spontaneous
expiration	sputum
fibrosis	sudden infant death
hemothorax	syndrome
hiccoughs	surfactant
hiccup	trachea
histoplasmosis	tracheotomy
hypoxia	tuberculosis
influenza	upper respiratory
inspiration	infection
intubation	ventilation
laryngectomy	vital capacity

Ⓐ Library

Oxygen (O_2) is provided continuously by plants on land and in the sea. Plants use sun, water, and **carbon dioxide** (CO_2) to make oxygen, which they release into the air. Humans breathe O_2 and exhale CO_2 and water. This cycle provides the means for supporting life.

Oxygen in the air is essential to the survival of living cells. An adult human being carries two quarts of O_2 in the blood, lungs, and tissues. This supply is adequate for about four minutes. The respiratory system is responsible for taking in air, removing the oxygen, and sending it through the blood to the cells of the body. The oxygen concentration of inhaled air is about 21%.

The respiratory system must also take from the blood the waste product CO_2 and exhaust it from the lungs. Exhaled air still contains about 16% oxygen. When the level of CO_2 in the blood rises to a certain point, the respiratory center in the brain is triggered and a breath is taken. This function is so vital to life that its interruption for just a few minutes will result in death.

THE PATHWAY OF OXYGEN

The Nose

Air enters the body through the nose (Figure 11–99). Here the air is filtered, warmed, and moistened by the structures within the nasal cavity. The nose is divided by a wall of cartilage called the **septum**. Near the middle of the nasal cavity, on each side, are a series of three scroll-like bones called conchae or turbinates. The conchae are covered with mucus-producing epithelium, which adds moisture to the air, and are supplied with abundant blood vessels, which warm the air. Just inside the nostrils are hairs called **cilia**, which trap particles in the air so that they do not enter the lungs.

The mucus from the lining also helps trap dust and bacteria. When irritating substances come in contact with the lining, extra mucus is produced to dilute the irritant. This is why sneezing occurs and the nose "runs." Both actions are methods of removing irritants.

Ciliated mucosa in the posterior portion of the nose and in the pharynx (throat) help propel inhaled particles into the back of the pharynx to be swallowed. Particles in the trachea and bronchi must first be propelled upward past the epiglottis, in an action called *mucus streaming*. The particles can then be directed toward the esophagus and swallowed. The constant beating action of the cilia and the flow of the mucus secretions cleanse the air passages. This beneficial function is temporarily halted by the effect of smoking, which paralyzes the cilia and mucus streaming action, thereby allowing foreign particles to enter the lungs. The paralysis lasts for several minutes.

The sinuses of the head are lined with the continuation of the nasal membranes (Figure 11–100). This explains why **sinusitis** occurs frequently with nasal infections.

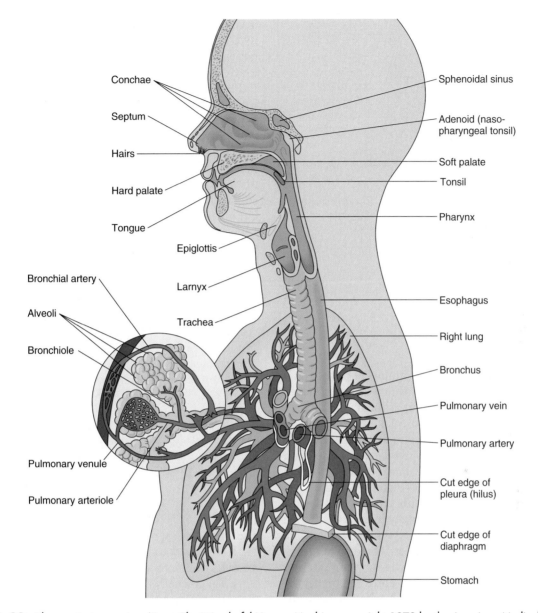

FIGURE 11-99 The respiratory system (From *The Wonderful Human Machine,* copyright 1979 by the American Medical Association.)

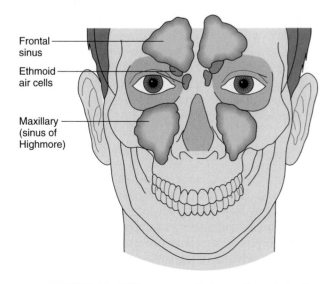

FIGURE 11-100 Paranasal sinuses (frontal view)

The Pharynx, Larynx, and Epiglottis

After the air is filtered, warmed, and moistened in the nose, it enters the **pharynx**. The pharynx serves as a passageway for both air and food. Except for an occasional mistake, it is not possible to swallow food and breathe at the same time. When this does occur, the result is choking, which can be very serious.

Normally, when food is swallowed, a cartilage "lid" called the **epiglottis** is pushed by the base of the tongue to cover the opening into the **larynx**. At the same time, the larynx moves up to help close the opening. With the opening to the larynx covered by the epiglottis, food is directed down the esophagus into the stomach.

When air passes under the open epiglottis, it enters the larynx, commonly called the voice box. The larynx is a tube with a series of nine separate cartilages to maintain its opening (Figure 11–101). The thyroid cartilage is the

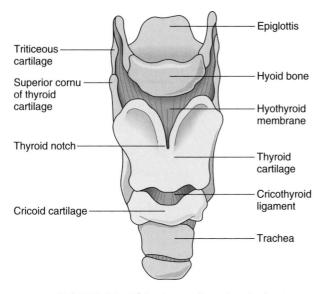

Triticeous cartilage

Superior cornu of thyroid cartilage

Thyroid notch

Cricoid cartilage

Epiglottis

Hyoid bone

Hyothyroid membrane

Thyroid cartilage

Cricothyroid ligament

Trachea

FIGURE 11–101 Larynx (anterior view)

largest and is located anteriorly. Its prominent projection is known as the Adam's apple, and its action can be observed when a person swallows. The larynx is lined with mucous membrane, which also forms two folds called the vocal cords. The cords are attached to the front of the larynx wall by cartilage. Muscles attach to the cartilage, and when they contract or relax, the vocal cords move either toward or away from the center of the larynx (Figure 11–102).

During breathing, the vocal cords are near to the wall of the larynx so that air can pass freely in and out. During speaking, the vocal cords move across the larynx and are held tense by the contracting muscles. The degree of tension and the length of the cords determine the pitch of the voice. The tighter and longer the cords the higher the pitch. The pressure on the air being expelled from the lungs determines the volume or loudness of the voice as

it vibrates the vocal cords. Note that speech is most easily accomplished during the exhaling of air. Inhaling does not create sufficient air pressure, nor can it be sustained long enough to produce speech.

Part of the mucous membrane lining of the larynx is loosely attached and of a different type of epithelium. With a severe infection, it may become swollen, actually preventing respirations. In this emergency situation, an airway may be achieved by **intubation** (passing a tube through the mouth, larynx, and into the trachae) or by making an external opening into the **trachea**, called a **tracheotomy**, and inserting a tube to permit air to enter.

A PEDIATRIC PERSPECTIVE

The respiratory structures of infants or small children, when compared to that of an adult, is relatively smaller in proportion to their relatively larger tongue and epiglottis. This difference results in a much easier obstruction of their airway. It takes a much smaller object or amount of material to completely occlude the opening. For this reason, parents must be taught to never let infants or small children have access to any object, food, toy, or piece of toy that measures smaller than the width of the infant's or child's little finger. This is a relative size in relation to the airway opening and provides a progressive measurement as the infant grows.

The Trachea, Bronchi, and Bronchioles

The next passageway for air is the trachea (Figure 11–103). It is commonly called the windpipe and extends from the neck into the chest, directly in front of the esophagus. The trachea is held open by a series of C-shaped cartilage rings. The wall between the rings is elastic, enabling the trachea to adjust to different body positions.

About the middle of the sternum, the trachea divides into two sections called the right and left **bronchi**. The structure of the two main bronchi is similar to that of the trachea, with incomplete cartilage rings to maintain the air passageway. Each bronchus divides and subdivides into many increasingly smaller bronchi, each with the cartilage-ringed structure, until they are barely visible without a microscope. These tiny air passageways have walls of muscle cells and are called **bronchioles**.

The Alveoli

Each bronchiole ends in a grapelike cluster of microscopic air sacs called **alveoli**. It is estimated that the body contains about 500 million alveoli, approximately three times the amount necessary to sustain life. The membrane walls of the alveoli are only one cell thick and are surrounded by a network of microscopic blood vessels called capillaries (Figure 11–104).

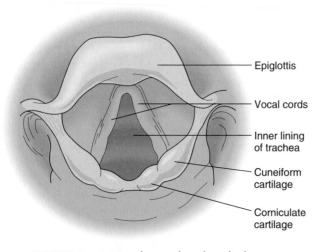

Epiglottis

Vocal cords

Inner lining of trachea

Cuneiform cartilage

Corniculate cartilage

FIGURE 11–102 The vocal cords in the larynx

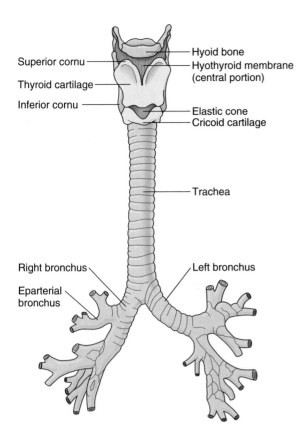

FIGURE 11-103 The larynx, trachea, and bronchi

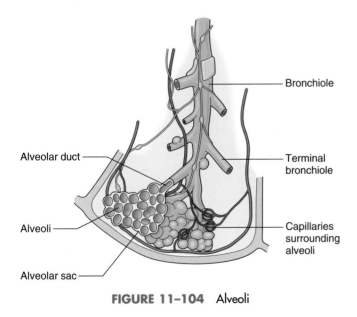

FIGURE 11-104 Alveoli

RESPIRATION

The structure of the **respiratory** apparatus has been compared to an upside down tree, with the trunk, branches, twigs, and leaves corresponding to the trachea, bronchi, bronchioles, and alveoli.

On **inspiration**, air enters the body, eventually arriving in an alveolus. Here O_2 passes through the wall of the

alveolus into the surrounding capillary as CO_2 leaves the capillary and enters the alveolus. When **expiration** occurs, CO_2 exits from the bronchial tree and is exhaled from the body. The process of getting O_2 from the nose to the alveolus and into the capillary and the return of CO_2 to the nose is known as *external* or *pulmonary respiration* (Figure 11–105A).

At the same time, oxygen from the alveolus is circulating through the body to every cell. First, the oxygen enters the capillary surrounding the alveolus, then it circulates through a venule, a vein, back to the heart, out an artery, to an arteriole, and into a capillary next to a tissue cell. Here the O_2 in the blood is given to the cell while CO_2 from the cell is picked up by the capillary. The exchange of O_2 and CO_2 at the cell is known as *internal* or *cellular respiration* (Figure 11–105B).

Oxygen and carbon dioxide in the alveolus and the cell exchange by the process of *diffusion*. Remember that materials move across a membrane from an area of higher concentration to an area of lower concentration. In the alveoli of the lung, O_2 concentration is greater than in the

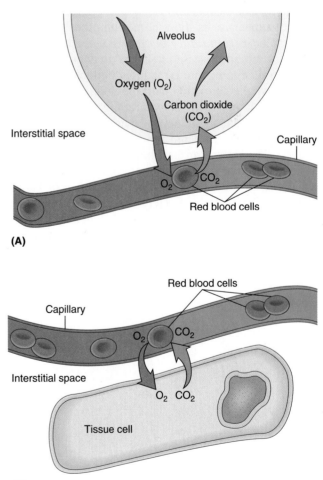

FIGURE 11-105 Simplified external (pulmonary) and internal (cellular) respiration: (A) external respiration in the lungs and (B) internal respiration at the cell

surrounding capillary, so it diffuses into the blood. At the same time, CO_2 is in higher concentration in the blood than in the alveolus, so it leaves the blood, enters the alveolus, and is exhaled during the next respiration. At the tissue cell, the O_2 content in the capillary is greater than that within the cell, so the O_2 leaves the blood and enters the cell. On the other hand, the CO_2 level within the cell is greater than in the capillary, so CO_2 diffuses out of the cell into the blood. This process of external and internal respiration is continuous throughout the life span of a person.

THE LUNG AND THE PLEURA

The structures of the bronchial tree are contained in an organ known as the **lung**. The tissue of the lung is so filled with the alveoli that it is spongy and extremely light. It will float if placed in water. Prior to birth and breathing, the lung is solid and will sink in water. At birth, the lungs begin to fill with air, inflating the alveoli. The degree of inflation depends on the presence of **surfactant**, a fatty molecule on the respiratory membrane. The surfactant maintains the inflated alveolus so that it does not collapse between breaths. Surfactant is not present in sufficient amounts to cause adequate inflation in premature infants and sometimes also in those born with other conditions. This results in *respiratory distress syndrome* (RDS) or hyaline membrane disease (described in detail later). The lungs continue to mature throughout childhood, with additional alveolar formation until the young years. Smoking at an early age retards the maturing of the lungs, and the additional alveoli are never developed.

The lung is divided into a right and left lung (Figure 11–106). The right lung has three lobes: upper, middle, and lower. The left lung has two: upper and lower. The heart lies on the medial surface of the left lung in a space called the *cardiac notch.* Each lung with its blood vessels and nerves is enclosed in a membrane called the visceral **pleura**. A membrane also lines the thoracic cavity and is called the parietal pleura. The airtight space between the

pleural membranes is known as the pleural space or cavity. It contains a lubricating fluid to prevent friction as the membranes rub together during respiration. The "space" is virtually nonexistent in healthy lungs because the lungs fill the thoracic cavity within the rib cage, pressing the visceral against the parietal pleura. However, as will be discussed later, certain conditions and diseases cause an abnormal presence or fluid or air within the pleural space.

THE MUSCLES OF BREATHING

The action of the diaphragm and the muscles of the rib cage were discussed in Unit 6. The diaphragm is the principal breathing muscle, and when it contracts, it produces a vacuum within the thoracic cavity, causing air to be drawn in. When this begins, there is a negative pressure within the lungs; the pressure inside is less than the atmospheric pressure outside. When the inside pressure exceeds outside atmospheric pressure, it becomes positive and causes expiration to again equalize inside/outside pressure. When the diaphragm returns to its relaxed state, air is forced out of the lungs (Figure 11–107).

Breathing action is controlled by the respiratory center in the brain. An increase of CO_2 or a lack of O_2 in the blood will trigger the center. Because we can somewhat voluntarily control breathing, it is possible to force rapid respirations and deplete the CO_2 in the blood, temporarily interrupting breathing and possibly losing consciousness. Children will occasionally hold their breath to frighten their parents and receive concessions. Usually, there is no need to be overly concerned because sooner or later a breath has to be taken. If consciousness is lost, the

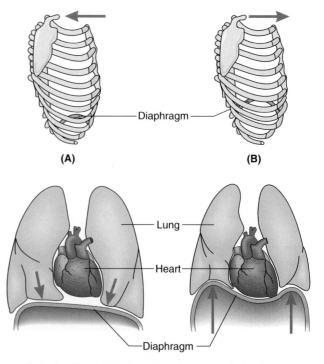

FIGURE 11-107 Position of diaphragm and ribs during (A) inspiration and (B) expiration

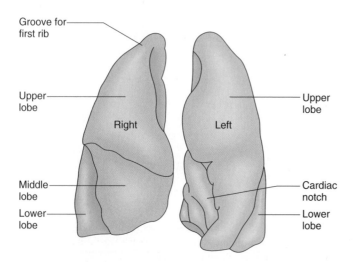

FIGURE 11-106 Anterior lung surface

automatic system resumes control, and breathing returns to normal.

Other situations can alter a breathing pattern for perfectly normal reasons, such as:

- Coughing—When a deep breath is taken followed by a forceful exhalation from the mouth to clear something from the lower respiratory structures.
- **Hiccoughs** (also spelled **hiccups**)—Caused by a spasm of the diaphragm and a spasmodic closure of the glottis (space between the vocal cords). It is believed to be the result of an irritation to the diaphragm or the phrenic nerve, which innervates the diaphragm.
- Sneezing—Occurs like a cough except air is forced through the nose to clear the upper respiratory structures. Usually results from mucous membrane contact with an irritant.
- Yawning—A deep prolonged breath that fills the lungs.
- Crying (or laughing)—Alters the breathing pattern in response to emotions.

DIAGNOSTIC EXAMINATIONS

- Arterial blood gases—Blood taken directly from an artery to evaluate the exchange of O_2 and CO_2 in the lungs. The test measures the partial pressures of both gases and determines the *p*H of the blood. The PaO_2 (partial pressure of oxygen) indicates how much oxygen the lungs are delivering to the blood. The $PaCO_2$ (partial pressure of carbon dioxide) indicates how efficiently the lungs eliminate carbon dioxide. The *p*H determines the acid–base level, which indicates the hydrogen (H^+) ion content. If acid, there is excess hydrogen ion; alkalinity indicates a deficit. Results aid in the medical management of many disorders and conditions, such as CNS depression from drugs or injury, pneumonia, **chronic obstructive pulmonary disease** (COPD), respiratory distress, certain kidney diseases, and many others.
- Bronchoscopy—The insertion of an instrument called the bronchoscope into the trachea and bronchial tree to view the airways, obtain a secretion or tissue sample, or remove a foreign body.
- Chest CT scan—A very sensitive computer-generated image that gives much more detail of the lungs and other structures in the chest than a chest x-ray.
- Chest x-ray—A radiological examination to determine the general health of lung and surrounding tissues or to identify a disease process, such as pneumonia.
- Lung **perfusion** scan—An examination of the lung following intravenous (IV) injection of a radioactive contrast medium to provide a visual image of pulmonary blood flow. It is useful in diagnosing blood vessel obstruction, such as **pulmonary emboli** (blood clot in an artery).
- Lung scan—A diagnostic x-ray known as a high-speed CT scan. The scan is done with an electron beam tomography scanner (Figure 11–108A). The examina-

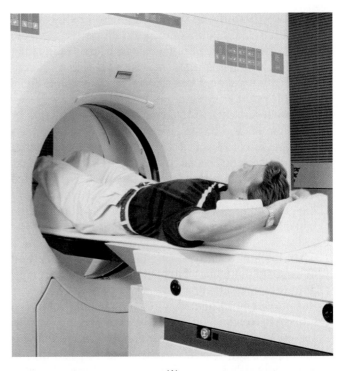

(A)

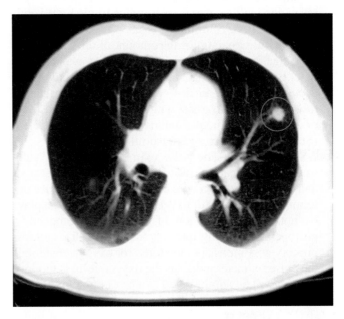

(B)

FIGURE 11-108 (A) High-speed CT scanner, (B) lung scan showing a nodule in the left upper lobe (Courtesy of CAT SCAN 2000.)

tion is four times more sensitive in detecting lung cancer than conventional x-rays. It can be used as a screening examination to identify disease long before symptoms occur. Unfortunately, about 85% of lung cancer is discovered after it has begun to spread. The high-speed scan takes only a few seconds and does not require removal of clothing. Figure 11-108B is a photo of a lung scan showing a nodule in the left upper lobe.

- Lung **ventilation** scan—An examination following the inhalation of a mixture of air and radioactive gas from a mask and bag. The test indicates the areas of the lung that are ventilated during respiration. It is used in conjunction with a lung perfusion scan to evaluate for a possible pulmonary embolus.

- Pulmonary **angiography/arteriography**—A radiological examination of the pulmonary circulation following the injection of a radiopaque iodine material through a catheter that is placed in the pulmonary artery or one of its branches. The catheter is inserted into a vein at the inner surface of the elbow or in the groin and passed through the veins and through the first half of the heart into the pulmonary artery. The test aids in diagnosing pulmonary emboli, especially when the lung scan was not conclusive. It is also used to evaluate pulmonary circulation in certain heart conditions before surgery.

- **Pulmonary** function tests—To measure lung volume in a normal breath, lung capacity when forcing air into and out of the lungs, and other variables during a specified time. Many non-invasive tests can be performed in a specialized hospital pulmonary laboratory; however, the most common test and one that is appropriate to the physician's office uses a **spirometer** to measure ventilation function. Spirometry is used to evaluate a patient's **vital capacity**, or the amount of air available in the lungs for respiration. It is also used to evaluate how quickly a patient can get air out of the chest and thus is useful to test for air-flow obstruction. Spirometry is most often used to assist with the diagnosis of asthma or chronic obstructive pulmonary disease (COPD). (See Chapter 14 for additional information.)

- Pulse oximeter—The pulse oximeter is a small electronic device that fits over the end of the index finger and is connected by a wire to a machine. The device determines the amount of oxygen in the blood and displays it digitally in the window of the machine. Frequently, postoperative patients and patients with cardiac and respiratory conditions are monitored for oxygen content. If the pulse oximeter indicates the oxygen level is too low, oxygen will be administered at a proper amount to supplement that being circulated by the body.

- **Sputum** analysis—A laboratory examination of material coughed up from the bronchial tree and/or trachea. If properly prepared, it can aid in the diagnosis of infectious organisms or cancer cells.

- Thoracentesis—Withdrawing of fluid from the pleural space by needle aspiration following local anesthetic (Figure 11–109). Fluid may be present as a result of excessive production or inadequate reabsorption of the pleural fluid that may be associated with cancer, tuberculosis, or a blood or lymphatic disorder. A specimen is often withdrawn for analysis to determine the presence of organisms, malignant cells, blood, or lymph fluid properties.

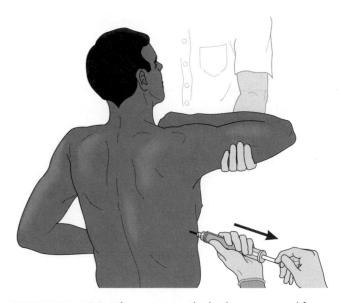

FIGURE 11-109 Thoracentesis. Fluid is being removed from the pleural cavity.

DISORDERS AND DISEASES

Allergic Rhinitis (Rye-ni'-tis)

Description—A reaction of the eyes, nose, and sinuses to airborne allergens.

Signs and symptoms—Sneezing, profuse watery nasal discharge, itching of the eyes and nose, red and swollen eyelids, and nasal congestion.

Etiology—**Allergic rhinitis** may be seasonal, as with hay fever, or perennial, caused by dust, mold, cigarette smoke, and animal mites.

Treatment—Treatment consists primarily of administering antihistamines and decongestants and avoiding the allergens. The use of air conditioning filters allergens, keeps down dust, and removes excess moisture from the air. The use of steroid nasal sprays to reduce inflammation may also be helpful. Desensitizing injections of the allergens before or during the season may be indicated for long-term management. In severe or persistent cases, it may be necessary to relocate to a relatively pollen-free environment.

Asthma (Az'-ma)

Description—**Asthma** is a chronic disorder characterized by swelling, inflammation, and constriction of the bronchi and bronchioles.

Signs and symptoms—Wheezing, coughing, and shortness of breath are the most common symptoms. With a severe attack, there can be significant bronchospasm (narrowing of the bronchioles), and mucous production, markedly limiting air-flow. This can result in respiratory distress, causing anxiety and a feeling of suffocation. Following an acute episode, accumulated mucous is coughed up and **expectorated**.

Etiology—Asthma is commonly caused by an allergic reaction to allergens, such as pollen, dust, animal hair, certain foods, and a number of other substances. However, it can also result from non-specific irritants to the airway, such as cigarette smoke and other unknown causes.

Treatment—Determination of the offending allergens can sometimes be accomplished with a series of skin tests. Minute amounts of the most common causative agents are introduced just below the skin by a needle prick or applied as patches to the skin surface. The presence of a reddened area about a site after a specified time is evidence of sensitivity. (See Chapter 16, Unit 1.)

The treatment of choice for asthma is prevention by eliminating allergens. When this is not possible, drugs to prevent or control attacks, such as inhaled steroids, long-acting bronchiodilators, and a "substance" blocker, are used. This "substance" is a byproduct of the liver that is known to precipitate asthma attacks. These drugs may be taken orally or administered with an inhaler. Other drugs are used to provide quick relief of an episode. The bronchodilating drugs Albuterol and Ipratropium open airways almost instantly and are considered rescue medications. The goals of asthma treatment are to prevent or reduce symptoms, maintain normal activity levels, and prevent flare-ups of asthma. During severe attacks, O_2 may be administered at approximately two **liters** per minute to ease breathing and increase O_2 within the arteries.

Atelectasis (A-te-leck'-ta-sis)

Description—This is the lack of air in the lungs caused by the collapse of the microscopic structures of the lung; **atelectasis** may occur following abdominal or thoracic surgery or with pressure from pleural effusion (fluid, air, pus, blood, or lymph) in the pleural cavity.

Signs and symptoms—Symptoms vary with the cause of collapse and the degree of hypoxia. There is generally some **dyspnea**. With extensive collapse there is severe dyspnea, anxiety, **cyanosis, diaphoresis** (profuse perspiration), tachycardia (rapid pulse), and retraction of intercostal muscles.

Etiology—It can be chronic, caused by mucous plugs in the bronchial tree in patients with cystic **fibrosis** and in heavy smokers with obstructive pulmonary disease. Bronchial occlusion can also result from cancer or inflamed tissues. Acute (sudden) atelectasis may occur with any condition that causes pain on deep breathing, such as rib fractures, traumatic injury, surgical procedures, or pleurisy.

Treatment—Treatment includes chest percussion, postural drainage, frequent coughing, and deep breathing exercises or intermittent positive pressure breathing (IPPB).

Bronchitis (Braun-ki'-tis)

Description—**Bronchitis** can be an acute or chronic disease with inflammation of the bronchial walls with distortion and narrowing of the airways. Chronic bronchitis is a condition in which excessive mucous is secreted in the bronchi during several months a year for several years in a row. The typical patient is middle-aged or older, often with a long history of cigarette smoking. Acute bronchitis is associated with an infection. It occurs abruptly and lasts several days or weeks.

Signs and symptoms—The presence of mucous and a productive cough with dyspnea upon exertion. Chronic bronchitis sufferers also produce thick mucous with a constant "smoker's cough," have recurring respiratory infections, and may have weakness and weight loss. Wheezing and prolonged expiration time may be observed.

Etiology—Acute bronchitis is caused by a viral or bacterial respiratory infection. Chronic bronchitis is caused by damaged cilia, enlarged mucous glands, and chronic inflammation. The severity of chronic bronchitis is related to the amount and duration of smoking.

Treatment—Acute bronchitis is managed with expectorants to help remove excessive mucous and by avoiding smoking. Antibiotics are sometimes needed. Chronic bronchitis requires bronchodilators, respiratory therapy to loosen mucous secretions, smoking cessation, and corticosteroids in some cases. Adequate fluid intake is important.

Chronic Obstructive Pulmonary Disease (COPD)

Description—This is a condition characterized by chronic obstruction of the airways, usually by a combination of respiratory disorders. It is a progressive disease. Symptoms occur gradually and become worse with age. COPD is the most common chronic lung disease affecting an estimated seventeen million Americans. It affects males more often than females, probably because until recently men were more likely to smoke heavily.

Signs and symptoms—The first signs are a decline in the ability to exercise or do strenuous work. A productive cough will begin to develop. These symptoms worsen with time, and eventually the patient develops dyspnea on minimal exertion and has frequent respiratory infections, hypoxemia (lack of oxygen in the blood), and grossly abnormal pulmonary function studies. Thoracic deformities develop (usually a barrel chest from muscular changes caused by struggling to breathe). Eventually there is overwhelming disability, severe respiratory failure, and death.

Etiology—The primary cause of COPD is long-term cigarette smoking, which impairs the ciliary action, causes inflammation in airways, destroys alveolar walls, and results in the formation of scar tissue around the bronchioles. COPD is the result of emphysema, chronic bronchitis, asthma, or any combination of these disorders. It can also develop from chronic respiratory infections and allergies.

Treatment—Treatment consists of methods to halt the progression of the disease and control its present state. Prime emphasis is placed on stopping smoking and avoiding other respiratory irritants. The main focus of treatment involves the use of bronchodilators, prompt treatment of respiratory infections, effective breathing and coughing instructions, proper diet, the use of O$_2$ as indicated, and exercise rehabilitation programs.

Emphysema (Em-fa-see'-ma)

Description—This is the irreversible enlargement of the air spaces in the lungs caused by the destruction of the alveolar walls. **Emphysema** results in the inability to exchange O$_2$ and CO$_2$ in the affected areas and to exhale stale air from the lungs. The lungs may actually be enlarged, but at the same time they are not efficient because of the decreased surface area for exchanging oxygen and carbon dioxide. Figure 11–110 is a photo of a CT scan showing the **blebs** (bubbles) of destroyed alveoli around the outer lung areas of a patient with emphysema. These are visible as large white-edged black areas.

Signs and symptoms—Emphysema is characterized by a chronic cough, weight loss, barrel chest, the use of accessory muscles to breathe, pursed lips, cyanosis, and eventually respiratory failure, heart enlargement and failure, and death.

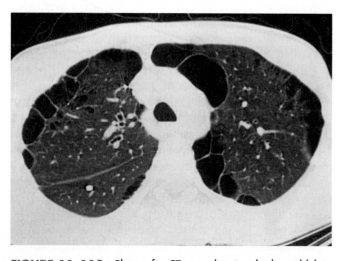

FIGURE 11–110 Photo of a CT scan showing the large blebs (bubbles) of emphysema. They are identifiable as the large dark areas with white borders on the outer edges of the lungs. (Courtesy of Philip T. Diaz, MD.)

Etiology—The prime cause is cigarette smoking. Emphysema can also develop from chronic infection or irritation from environmental factors.

Treatment—The treatment is the same as for COPD: smoking cessation, the use of bronchodilators, prompt treatment of respiratory infections, effective breathing and coughing instructions, proper diet, and the use of O$_2$ as indicated.

Epistaxis (Nosebleed) (Ep-i-stack'-sis)

Description—(See Unit 3.) Epistaxis is the loss of blood through the nose.

Signs and symptoms—The visible presence of blood coming from the nose or the patient experiencing bleeding posteriorly into the throat.

Etiology—Nosebleeds usually follow injury, either external or internal, such as a blow to the nose, nosepicking, or foreign body insertion. Less frequent causes of **epistaxis** are chronic conditions, such as nasal or sinus infection that results in capillary congestion and bleeding, or the inhalation of irritating substances. Predisposing systemic factors include high blood pressure, anticoagulation drugs, chronic aspirin use, and blood diseases, such as anemia, hemophilia, and leukemia.

Treatment—Treatment varies depending on the cause, location, and severity. Even moderate bleeding is of concern if it persists longer than 20 minutes after pressure is applied. Symptoms of severe blood loss may include lightheadedness, a drop in blood pressure, rapid pulse, dyspnea, pallor, and other indications of shock. Initial first aid treatment may consist of: elevating the head; compressing nostrils against the septum continuously for 5 to 10 minutes; applying ice or cold compresses to nose; preventing the swallowing of blood (to determine the amount lost); avoiding talking or blowing the nose; and observing for the amount of blood loss and signs of shock.

Advanced treatment includes: for anterior bleeding, applying epinephrine-saturated cotton ball or gauze to the bleeding site and the use of external pressure, followed by cauterization by electric cautery or silver nitrate; for posterior bleeding, the insertion of a nasal pack for 48 to 72 hours may be required. If necessary, anterior bleeding can be treated by packing for 24 to 48 hours. Other treatment may include supplemental vitamin K to aid in blood clotting, blood transfusions, and surgical ligation (tying) of the bleeding artery.

Histoplasmosis (His-toe-plaz-mo'-sis)

Description—This is a fungal infection, occurring worldwide. In the United States, histoplasmosis occurs in three forms: primary acute, progressive disseminated, and chronic pulmonary.

Signs and symptoms—Symptoms vary with the form contracted. The primary acute form resembles a severe cold. The progressive involves the liver, spleen, and lymph glands, and it may cause inflammation of the heart muscle, the pericardium (covering membrane), and the meninges of the brain and spinal cord. The chronic form resembles tuberculosis, causing a productive cough, dyspnea, weakness, and cyanosis.

Etiology—**Histoplasmosis** is caused by an organism found in droppings from birds or bats, or in soil near their roosts, as in barns, caves, chicken coops, around buildings, and under bridges. It may also come from cat feces because of ingested birds.

Treatment—The acute form generally does not require treatment. With the progressive disseminated or chronic pulmonary forms, a high dose or long-term treatment with an antifungal such as amphotericin B or itroconozole is indicated. Surgery to remove pulmonary nodules and a shunt to relieve intracranial pressure may be necessary. Oxygen can be given to reduce respiratory distress. Additional treatments are indicated if other severe conditions develop.

Hyaline Membrane Disease (HMD) (Hi'-a-lin)

(See Respiratory Distress Syndrome.)

Influenza (flu) (In-flu-n'-za)

Description—This acute, highly contagious respiratory infection usually occurs in colder months and in infrequent epidemics (widespread incidence, not of local origin). It is more prevalent in school children aged 6 to 14 and adults over age 40. **Influenza** can be fatal to the elderly or people with chronic heart, lung, or kidney disease. Influenza viruses have the ability to alter their influence on the population. As people develop immunity to a virus after coming into contact with it, the virus alters its composition and a new strain results to which people have little or no resistance. Hence an epidemic or pandemic (present in many areas of the world at the same time) can develop.

Influenza viruses are classified into three types:

- Type A—The most lethal, occurring every two to three years with a major new strain developing every 10 to 15 years
- Type B—Occurring every four to six years, resulting in epidemics
- Type C—Endemic (of local origin) and causing infrequent cases

Signs and symptoms—Symptoms of flu are the sudden onset of chills and a fever of 101° to 104°F (38° to 40°C), headaches, muscle aches, a nonproductive cough, and **rhinitis**. Pneumonia is the most common complication, developing three to five days after infection begins.

Etiology—The disease is directly transmitted by droplets inhaled from an infected person's sneezing or coughing or by indirect contact with contaminated objects, such as a drinking glass.

Treatment—Treatment consists of bed rest, adequate fluid intake, and aspirin or similar medication to relieve the pain and fever. Antibiotics have no effect on the virus and should not be used unless there is secondary bacterial infection. Flu immunizations, which provide protection for three to six months, are recommended for the high-risk population. However, the vaccine is only 75% effective.

Laryngectomy (Lar-in-jeck'-tom-e)

This is not a disease or disorder but a surgical solution to a life-threatening situation. It is the surgical removal of the larynx and is usually performed to treat throat cancer caused by smoking. The earliest symptom of internal disease of the larynx is persistent hoarseness. With involvement externally, it is a lump in the throat or pain, or burning when drinking hot liquids or citrus juices.

Diagnosis can often be made by viewing the larynx with a laryngoscope. This examination is often followed with radiological studies to confirm the diagnosis. With positive diagnosis, the larynx may be partially or totally removed. With total removal, a permanent opening called a stoma is made in the neck through which air can be taken in and exhaled (Figure 11–111). Coughing results in material being expelled through the stoma.

A great deal of patient support is necessary to assist in developing alternative methods of communication prior to surgery. The patient may need psychiatric assistance to cope with the loss of speech, sense of smell, ability to blow the nose, and related problems. Much support can be obtained from organizations established to aid in rehabilitation of **laryngectomy** patients. Local chapters of the "Lost Chord Club," made up of persons who have lost their larynx, volunteer their services to speak with new patients and help them learn techniques of producing speech. The American Cancer Society and the International Association of Laryngectomies also provide assistance with speech methods that use esophageal air that is swallowed and released slowly, the artificial larynx, and other mechanical devices.

The individual in Figure 11–111 has a Blum Finger voice prosthesis inserted into the stoma. By placing his finger over the opening in the prosthesis, he is able to produce a good quality of speech. A "patch" of thin foam is worn over the opening to prevent inhaling foreign materials. The foam is porous and permits easy exchange of air.

Laryngitis (Lar-in-ji'-tis)

Description—This inflammation of the vocal cords occurs in both acute and chronic forms.

Signs and symptoms—Acute **laryngitis** usually begins as hoarseness, with either minimal or complete loss of voice. There may be some pain when talking or swallowing, a

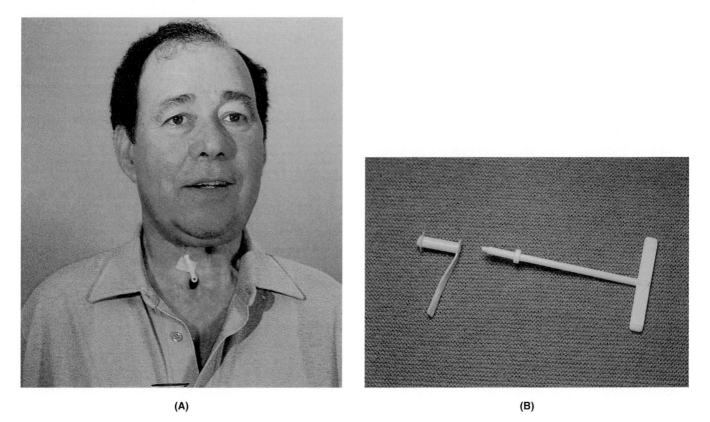

(A)   (B)

FIGURE 11-111 Laryngeal stoma following laryngectomy with (A) an inserted Blum Finger prosthesis and (B) an inserter

dry cough, fever, and malaise. With chronic laryngitis, the only symptom is persistent hoarseness.

Etiology—Acute laryngitis usually results from an infectious process, excessive use of the voice, inhalation of smoke or fumes, or accidental aspiration of chemicals. Chronic laryngitis develops from other preexistent chronic conditions (such as sinusitis, bronchitis, and allergies) or from smoking, abuse of alcohol, and continual exposure to irritants.

Treatment—Laryngitis is treated by resting the voice, using medication for underlying infection, if present, and eliminating coexistent causes (in the case of chronic laryngitis).

Legionnaires' Disease (Le'-jun-airs)

Description—This is an acute bronchopneumonia that derived its name from a highly-publicized incident in which 182 people developed the disease at an American Legion Convention in Philadelphia in 1976. **Legionnaires' disease** usually occurs in late summer or early fall.

Signs and symptoms—Symptoms are nonspecific and include diarrhea, lack of appetite, headache, chills, weakness, and an unremitting fever that develops within 12 to 48 hours. Temperature may reach 105°F (40.5°C). A cough then develops, which becomes productive, with grayish sputum. Other symptoms are nausea, vomiting, confusion, dyspnea, and chest pain. Severe symp-

toms are evidence of complications and include low blood pressure, irregular heartbeat, respiratory failure, kidney failure, and shock (which is usually fatal). Smokers are three to four times more likely to develop Legionnaires' disease than nonsmokers.

Etiology—It is caused by the bacteria Legionnaire Bacilli and is transmitted through water that is contaminated with the bacteria. In past epidemics, it was spread through air conditioning systems and cooling towers. It does not spread person to person.

Treatment—Treatment consists of antibiotics, medication to reduce the fever, maintaining fluid balance, and measures to support adequate respiration, such as oxygen and mechanical ventilation.

Lung Cancer

Description—This is the leading cause of cancer deaths among men and women, despite the fact that it is largely preventable. It is the progressive cellular degeneration of lung tissue. It usually develops within the wall or lining of the bronchial tree. There are different types of lung cancer: squamous cell, small-cell, adenocarcinoma, and large-cell. Approximately 169,500 new cases of lung cancer were estimated in 2001.

Signs and symptoms—There are often minimal symptoms that are usually not associated with cancer, such as cough, fatigue, and shortness of breath. This frequently results in diagnosis at the late stages when the disease is far advanced, offering little hope for survival. The symptoms of squamous and small-cell carcinomas are smoker's cough, sneezing, dyspnea, hemoptysis, and chest pain. Symptoms of adenocarcinoma and large-cell types include fever, weakness, weight loss, and anorexia.

Etiology—It is attributed to inhalation of carcinogens in tobacco and the environment. The inhalation of carcinogens causes damage to the cells of the lungs, which then causes uncontrolled abnormal growth when these cells become cancerous. There is a correlation between the risk of cancer and the number of cigarettes smoked daily, the depth of inhalation, the age at which smoking began, and the nicotine content of the tobacco. An individual over 40 who began smoking as a teenager and has averaged a pack a day for at least 20 years is most susceptible. Lung cancer can take 20 to 30 years to develop. Less than 10% of lung cancers occur among nonsmokers.

Other inhalants that increase *susceptibility* to cancer are industrial air pollutants, such as asbestos, arsenic, iron oxides, chromium, radioactive dust, vinyl chloride, and coal dust. There also is an indication that there is a familial tendency link to lung cancer. The combination of industrial pollutants and cigarettes is very risky. For example, asbestos workers who also smoke increase their risk of developing lung cancer by 60 times.

Involuntary smoking, which the nonsmoker receives "second hand" from a spouse or others, is less concentrated but still contains the same harmful substances. For example, wives exposed to husbands who smoke 20 or more cigarettes a day at home have double the risk of lung cancer when compared to wives of nonsmokers. Children of smoking parents are also affected. They are more prone to respiratory and middle ear infections.

The prognosis for lung cancer patients is very poor because by the time a diagnosis is made, two thirds of the patients have passed the stage where it might be curable. Only 13% of all lung cancer patients (all races and all stages) live five or more years after diagnosis. This is primarily the result of delayed diagnosis because of lack of symptoms. The disease metastasizes to many other sites within the thoracic cavity and throughout the entire body.

Treatment—Treatment consists primarily of surgical excision when appropriate, radiation, and chemotherapy. Often the disease is advanced before treatment begins, and little more than alleviation of symptoms is possible. The best treatment is obviously prevention. Quitting smoking or never starting is the best defense against lung cancer.

Figure 11–112 is a reprint of a brochure distributed by the American Cancer Society that illustrates the effects of emphysema and cancer on the tissues of the lung.

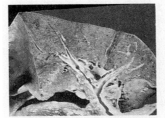

NORMAL LUNG

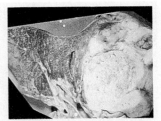

CANCER

The lung is our breathing machine. It draws in air, filters it, separates out life-giving oxygen for the body's use and expels what is left over—mostly carbon dioxide. The normal adult lung is about the size of a football.

When we inhale, air enters the lung through tubes, or passageways, called bronchi. These bronchi are lined with vibrating hairlike structures called cilia, which whip back and forth some 900 times a miunute, to help keep solid pollutants in the air from entering the lung. The air is carried down through smaller and smaller bronchi into tiny air sacs which are uniform in size. This is where the oxygen/carbon dioxide exchange takes place.

Unfortunately, damage to the lung often takes place before there are any symptoms.

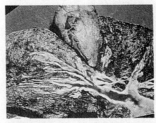

EMPHYSEMA

Emphysema is a disease which destroys the lung's elasticity, and therefore its ability to inhale and exhale properly.

Tissue affected by emphysema can never be repaired or replaced and the disease, progressing slowly but steadily, turns its victims into respiratory cripples. Patients spend years gasping for breath, and when death comes, it frequently is due to an overworked heart.

Emphysema changes the lung's normal appearance. Some of the air sacs burst and collapse, creating tiny craters in the lung, while others balloon in the body's desperate struggle to obtain oxygen and expel carbon dioxide.

Emphysema used to be a relatively rare disease, but today it is becoming increasingly common. It has been strongly associated with the cigarette habit because of the intense air pollution caused by cigarette smoke in the lungs.

Cancer ravages the lungs with an army of wildly multiplying cells. It begins most often with the constant irritation of the lining of the bronchi by cigarette smoke.

Under the onslaught of this irritation, the hairlike cilia which filter the air we breathe disappear from the lining of the bronchi. Although extra mucus is secreted to substitute for the cilia and trap pollutants, this mucus itself becomes a problem. It remains trapped until finally forced out of the lung by a "smoker's cough."

If a smoker quits before cancerous lesions are present, the bronchial lining will return to normal. If not, the abnormal cell growth spreads, blocking the bronchi and then invading the lung tissue itself.

In the latter stages of lung cancer, abnormal cells break away from the lung and are carried by the lymphatic system to other vital organs, where new cancers begin.

Because lung cancer is difficult to detect early, it is very difficult to treat successfully. It is often fatal. Yet if no one smoked cigarettes, 83% of lung cancers would eventually disappear.

Research now shows that even involuntary smoking exposures result in enough inhaling of smoke to increase the risk of developing lung cancer as well as other respiratory illnesses and risk to the fetus during pregnancy. A new study found that women exposed to husbands who smoked 20 or more cigarettes a day at home had double the risk of lung cancer compared to women married to nonsmokers.

It has been said that if the effects of cigarette smoking appeared on our skin instead of in our lungs—where it can't be seen—no one would smoke. Now you have seen the ugly inside story.

Call your local Unit of the American Cancer Society for information on how to quit smoking.

AMERICAN CANCER SOCIETY®

FIGURE 11–112 Normal and diseased lung tissue (Reprinted by the permission of the American Cancer Society, Inc.)

Pleurisy (Plu'-ri-see)

Description—This is an inflammation of the visceral and parietal pleura in the thoracic cavity. **Pleurisy** develops as a complication of viral infections, pneumonia, tuberculosis, chest injury, and other factors.

Signs and symptoms—Sharp, stabbing pain is experienced on respiration because of irritation of the pleural nerve endings as the lungs move, rubbing against the inner chest wall. As a result, lung movement on the affected side may be limited, and dyspnea occurs.

Etiology—Pleurisy pain is caused by the inflammation or irritation of sensory nerve endings in the parietal pleura. It begins suddenly as a complication of pneumonia, a viral infection, or other causes.

Treatment—In the case of a viral infection, treatment is generally symptomatic, with bed rest and medications to reduce the inflammation and relieve the pain. If fluid collects within the pleural space (see pleural effusion below) a thoracentesis is indicated to prohibit lung compression by the fluid or to determine, by laboratory examination, a causative agent (see Figure 11–109).

Paroxysmal Nocturnal Dyspnea (PND) (Pear-ox-siz'-mal Knock-turn'-al Disp-ne'-a)

Description—This is a symptom associated with chronic lung disease or left ventricular failure (heart disease).

Signs and symptoms—It occurs at night. Individuals awaken from sleep with a feeling of suffocation. They often run to open a window and gasp for air. Just sitting upright will help some people because of the effect of gravity on fluid in the lungs.

Etiology—This is associated with chronic lung disease and left ventricular heart failure probably caused by the accumulation of fluid in the lungs.

Treatment—The episode will often resolve within a few minutes; however, the symptom of PND indicates a serious underlying condition that requires treatment.

Pleural Effusion (Plur'-al E-fu'-zun)

Description—This is the presence of excess fluid in the pleural space.

Signs and symptoms—When the effusion becomes symptomatic, it compresses lung tissue and reduces the lungs' ability to exchange O_2 for CO_2, and **hypoxia** (lack of O_2) results. If the fluid is a result of an infectious process, exudate (pus) and dead tissue may be present, and the effusion is known as **empyema**.

Etiology—Pleural effusion results from the overproduction or the inadequate reabsorption of the pleural fluid. Some effusions result from chronic diseases, such as congestive heart failure, liver disease, tuberculosis, malignancy, lupus, and rheumatoid arthritis.

Treatment—Oxygen is administered to increase concentration to the remainder of the lung. Drainage of the material by thoracentesis and insertion of chest tubes may be necessary. Antibiotics may be required if the effusion is infectious in origin. Effusion that contains blood is called a **hemothorax** and will require drainage to prevent fibrothorax (scar tissue) formation.

Pneumonoconiosis (New-mo-no-cone-e-o'-sis)

Description—These are lung diseases developed after years of contact with environmental or occupational causative agents. Basically, there are three types of **pneumonoconiosis**: silicosis, asbestosis, and black lung disease.

Signs and symptoms—Some symptoms, common to all forms of pneumonoconioses, are rapid respirations, dry cough, dyspnea upon exertion which increases, pulmonary hypertension, right ventricular involvement, and recurrent respiratory infections.

Silicosis occurs from exposure to silica sand dust in occupations such as sand blaster and foundry worker, in manufacturing of ceramic and sandstone products and construction materials, and in mining of gold, lead, zinc, and iron. Nodules develop where specific disease-fighting cells have ingested the silica particles but then are unable to dispose of the ingested material. The cells die, causing the release of an enzyme that attracts more cells to assist in destroying the invading material. A fibrous (scar) tissue results, and the process continues until large areas of the lung tissue are destroyed.

Asbestosis can develop 15 to 20 years after regular exposure to asbestos has ended. Asbestosis is most prevalent in the construction, fireproofing, and textile industries and in brake and automotive occupations dealing with clutch linings. The general public may also develop the condition from exposure to fibrous dust or the waste piles of asbestos factories. Asbestosis is the result of inhaling minute asbestos fibers, which enter the bronchioles and penetrate the alveolar walls. The fibers become encased, and fibrosis of the lung tissue develops, obliterating the air passages. Fibers also cause fibrotic changes in the parietal pleura.

Coal Worker's or Black Lung Disease is a progressive nodular type found in two forms: simple, which produces small lung lesions, or complicated, which produces masses of fibrous tissue. The development usually occurs after 15 years or more of exposure and depends to some extent on the amount of dust, the type of coal mined, the silica content, and the location of the mine.

Initially, the body's fighting cells ingest the dust and become filled, forming macules in the terminal bronchioles, which are surrounded by dilated alveoli. The supporting tissue atrophies (wastes away), resulting in permanent dilation of the small airways. When the disease changes from a simple to a complicated form, one or both lungs can become involved. The fibrous tissue masses enlarge, causing destruction of the alveoli and airways.

Treatment—Treatment of all types is essentially the same: avoid respiratory infections, use bronchodilators to aid in respiration, supplement oxygen when indicated, and other use respiratory therapy to improve removal of bronchial secretions.

Pneumonia (New-moan'-e-ah)

Description—This is an acute infection of the principal tissues of the lungs, which may impair the exchange of O_2 and CO_2. Chances for recovery from **pneumonia** are good for persons with normal lungs, but pneumonia is a very common cause of death in debilitated (weakened) patients.

Pneumonia is classified in several ways: by microbiological origin (bacterial, viral, or fungal), by location (bronchial or lobar), or by type (primary or secondary).

Signs and symptoms—Symptoms include coughing, sputum production, pleural chest pain, chills, and fever.

Etiology—Pneumonia can be caused by inhaled pathogens, an inhaled chemical, or an infection spread from another area of the body. It often occurs with a chronic weakening illness (such as cancer or AIDS) or following surgery. It is also associated with malnutrition, smoking, COPD, advanced age, and with a decreased level of consciousness.

Treatment—Treatment consists of bed rest, antibiotics for bacterial pneumonia, adequate fluid intake, respiratory support measures (such as oxygen or mechanical breathing therapy), and medication for pain.

Pneumothorax (New-mo-thor'-ax)

Description—In this condition, air or gas has accumulated between the parietal and visceral pleurae, causing some degree of collapse of the lung tissue. Figure 11–113 shows an accumulation of air at the bottom of the right chest which has collapsed a portion of the lower lobe.

Signs and symptoms—The primary symptoms of pneumothorax are sudden, sharp pain made worse by breathing or coughing, and shortness of breath. As the degree of collapse increases, respirations become more stressful, the pulse becomes rapid and weak, and the patient becomes pale or cyanotic. Death may result without prompt treatment.

Etiology—If it is **spontaneous**, air has leaked from the lung tissue as the result of a disease process or a ruptured blisterlike lesion. A traumatic **pneumothorax** results from a penetrating chest wound (as by a knife or gunshot), from thoracic surgery, or as a complication from the insertion of tubing into the blood vessels of the chest. Fractured ribs can penetrate the thorax, causing collapse of the lung. Because the atmospheric pressure outside is greater than that within the pleural cavity, the air compresses the lung tissue as it enters. Frequently, blood is also present with an injury, and if it is located between the pleura, it is referred to as a hemothorax.

In tension pneumothorax, air enters the pleural space but is unable to leave by the same route. Each inspiration results in additional trapped air being sucked in. Eventually, pressure is exerted against the large chest veins, interfering with blood flow returning to the heart. If severe, the great vessels of the chest and the heart may be pushed toward the uninjured side of the chest. This is a medical emergency.

Treatment—Treatment varies with the degree of collapse. If the pneumothorax is spontaneous, small in size, and not association with dyspnea, or if there are apparent signs of increasing difficulty, it may be treated with bed rest and careful monitoring of vital signs. With greater than 30% collapse, the lung is slowly reexpanded by low suction through a tube inserted into the chest. If there is evidence of trauma, the tissue must be repaired, the chest closed, and the wound drained by means of chest tubes.

Pulmonary Fibrosis

Description—Scaring of the lung tissue, making the lungs stiff and small. This condition is often progressive and usually fatal.

Signs and symptoms—The most common symptom is shortness of breath on exertion. As the disease progresses, even minimal exertion such as talking causes dyspnea. A dry cough is also common. Signs include tachypnea, cyanosis, and a crackling sound when auscultating the lungs.

Etiology—Chronic exposure to dust (see pneumoconiosis) and chronic inhalation of certain allergens can cause fibrosis. It also results from some medications, especially chemotherapeutic agents. Radiation therapy to treat cancer in the chest may also cause fibrosis. Often no cause can be found, and the etiology is called "idiopathic."

Treatment—Steroids and immunosuppressive agents are used to decrease lung inflammation. Oxygen is often needed. Lung transplant offers hope for a cure, but the condition is often fatal.

Pulmonary Edema (Pull'-mon-airy E-deem'-ah)

Description—This is the accumulation, within the tissues of the lungs, of fluid that has escaped from the blood vessels caused by increased pressure in these vessels. **Pulmonary edema** is common in these vessels with heart disorders causing left ventricular failure.

Signs and symptoms—Symptoms include dyspnea on exertion, coughing, **orthopnea** (ability to breathe only in an upright position), and rapid pulse and respiration.

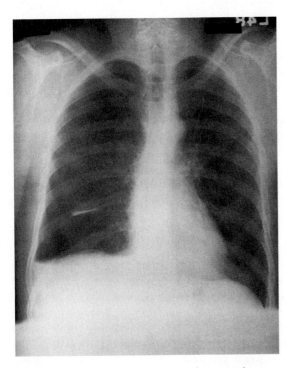

FIGURE 11–113   An example of pneumothorax

With progression, respirations become more labored, noisy, and rapid. A cough that produces frothy, bloody sputum may develop. As the condition worsens, the patient becomes cold, clammy, and cyanotic. Confusion and a depressed level of consciousness occur in cases of severe heart failure.

Etiology—Pulmonary edema usually results from left ventricular heart failure resulting from arteriosclerosis, hypertension, or a faulty valve that causes increased pressure within the left atrium and blood vessels of the lungs. The pressure causes fluid to "squeeze" out of the blood and into the lung tissue.

Treatment—Treatment consists of procedures to decrease the accumulated fluids and improve the exchange of O_2 and CO_2. Diuretics (water pills), nitroglycerin, and high concentrations of oxygen may be indicated.

Pulmonary Embolism (Pull'-mon-airy Em'-bow-lism)

Description—Obstruction of a pulmonary artery or arteriole by a circulating thrombus (blood clot) is called a pulmonary embolism.

Signs and symptoms—The obstruction causes dyspnea, chest pain, rapid heart rate, a cough, and a low-grade fever. The symptoms vary with the extent of obstruction. In massive embolism, with over 50% obstruction of arterial circulation, death can occur rapidly.

Etiology—Predisposing factors include long-term immobility, which permits slow-moving blood to clot within the vessels, varicose veins, surgery, pregnancy, vascular injury, obesity, fractures, and many chronic pulmonary and circulatory diseases.

Treatment—Treatment consists of measures to maintain adequate heart and lung function while the obstruction is being resolved, usually within 10 to 14 days. Medication is given to inhibit the blood from forming additional clots and to break up the present occlusion. Supportive oxygen therapy is used as needed. If the embolus is caused by purulent material from an infectious process, then aggressive antibiotic therapy is indicated.

Respiratory Distress Syndrome (RDS) (Formerly known as Hyaline Membrane Disease)

Description—This is a mysterious condition that kills apparently healthy infants. Those between birth and 8 months of age are at highest risk. The death is unexplainable even after autopsy. RDS attributes to approximately 40,000 newborn deaths annually in the United States. The condition occurs more frequently in infants born to smoking or diabetic mothers. Other maternal conditions, such as hemorrhage and infection, may also precipitate RDS.

Signs and symptoms—RDS most commonly presents symptoms within the first three to five minutes of breathing. Normal breaths become rapid and shallow. The nostrils flare, and the intercostal and substernal muscles are used to help with respirations, as evidenced by the retraction of the sternum. A "grunting" type of noise generated by the infant's attempt to breathe signals respiratory failure.

Etiology—RDS is caused by the lack of a lipoprotein called surfactant in the lungs. This substance maintains the openness of the alveoli at the end of expiration. Without adequate surfactant, many of the alveoli collapse, resulting in poor oxygenation of the infant.

Treatment—Urgent aggressive treatment is needed, preferably in a large hospital's neonatal intensive care unit to improve the outcome. Oxygen therapy, insertion of an endotracheal (breathing) tube, a ventilator, and the use of artificial surfactant are treatment priorities. Infants who have had RDS are more likely to have an increased incidence of respiratory infections after discharge from the hospital.

Sinusitis (Sign-u-si'-tis)

Description—Sinusitis is the inflammation of the paranasal sinus cavities.

Signs and symptoms—Symptoms include nasal congestion, low-grade fever, headache, pain over cheeks and upper teeth, pain over eyes or eyebrows, and a nonproductive cough.

Etiology—It usually results from the common cold organism or chronically from persistent bacterial infection.

Treatment—Treatment consists of analgesics for pain, medication to decrease secretions, steam inhalations to encourage drainage, and application of heat to relieve pain and congestion. Antibiotics are sometimes required in severe or chronic cases. Surgical drainage of the affected sinus cavity may be necessary in persistent, severe conditions.

Snoring

Description—Is the presence of noisy breathing while asleep. About 45% of normal adults snore at least occasionally, and 25% are habitual snorers. It is more prevalent among males and people who are overweight. It tends to grow worse with age.

Signs and symptoms—The snorer breaths loudly during sleep, particularly when lying on the back. It disturbs not only the sleep of the snorer but also disrupts family life. An exaggerated form is known as obstructive sleep apnea, when loud snoring is interrupted by frequent episodes of totally obstructed breathing. If this lasts over 10 seconds and occurs more than seven times an hour, it is considered a serious problem. Some patients have 30 to 300 obstructed events a night, resulting in a low blood oxygen level that causes more forceful heartbeats to "catch up" circulation. This can lead to irregular heart rhythm, elevated blood pressure, and heart enlargement.

Etiology—The noisy sounds of snoring occur when there is an obstruction to the flow of air through the back of the mouth and nose. This is the collapsible portion of the airway where the tongue and upper throat meet the uvula and soft palate. These structures strike against each other and vibrate during breathing. People who snore have at least one of the following:

- Poor muscle tone in the tongue and throat muscles, which allows the tongue to fall backwards into the airway. Often this occurs after the use of alcohol or sleep medication.
- Excessive bulkiness of throat tissues, such as tonsils and adenoids. Rarely, cysts or tumors can be the cause. Overweight persons also have bulky neck tissues.
- Excessive length of the soft palate and uvula may narrow the opening into the throat. A long uvula makes matters worse.
- Obstructed nasal airways, as when the nose is stuffy or blocked, cause the person to pull in air harder, creating an exaggerated throat vacuum that pulls the floppy throat tissues together and makes noise. Allergy season causes many to snore because of blocked nasal passages. The deformity of a deviated septum may also be the contributing factor.

Treatment—The majority of snorers can be helped by trying the following:

1. Lose weight and exercise daily to develop good muscle tone.
2. Avoid tranquilizers, sleeping pills, and antihistamines before bedtime.
3. Avoid alcohol within four hours of retiring.
4. Avoid heavy meals within three hours of retiring.
5. Avoid getting overtired.
6. Establish regular sleeping patterns.
7. Tilt the entire head of the bed up four inches on blocks.
8. Allow the nonsnorer to get to sleep first.

The very heavy snorer who interrupts family life needs a thorough physical examination. Sleep lab studies help determine how serious the snoring is and how much the person's health is being affected. Treatment may be only the management of an allergy or infection. Corrective surgery can alter contributing nasal and throat structures. Using a nasal mask overnight to deliver air pressure into the throat is helpful if other measures are not possible.

Sudden Infant Death Syndrome (SIDS)

Description—This is a mysterious condition that kills apparently-healthy infants. It is unexplainable even after autopsy. **Sudden infant death syndrome** kills about 8,000 infants annually in the United States. It occurs more frequently in winter, in poorer families, to mothers under 20, and among underweight babies. There is a slight increased risk to twins or triplets, those who received no prenatal care, and with mothers who smoked or took drugs during pregnancy. Death occurs rapidly, silently, and unexpectedly, usually during sleep.

Etiology—Study of the syndrome suggests that the infant may have had undetected respiratory dysfunctions that

caused prolonged periods of **apnea** (absence of breathing), resulting in extreme hypoxemia (lack of oxygen in the blood) and serious irregular heartbeat. Although the true cause is unknown, there is an increased risk of SIDS occurring with infants who sleep on their stomachs. In 1992, the American Academy of Pediatrics advocated a program called "Back to Sleep" that simply referred to placing babies on their backs to sleep. Since the acceptance of the sleeping position, the incidence of SIDS has declined by almost 50%. Several characteristics of the syndrome are diagnostic of SIDS, but an autopsy must be performed to rule out other causes of death. Child abuse must always be ruled out.

Treatment—The use of the proper sleep positioning and ongoing research to find other causes is the only thing that will save lives. Parents need a great deal of support to deal with the death because they often feel they were somehow to blame. There is a National Sudden Infant Death Foundation with local chapters of parents whose babies have died of the syndrome. Many local health organizations provide counseling and information services. These resources can be of great assistance.

Tuberculosis (TB) (Too-berk-u-low'-sis)

Description—An acute or chronic, highly contagious infection causing nodular lesions and patchy infiltration of the lung tissue is known as **tuberculosis** (TB). The body reacts to the invading causative organism by converting the destroyed tissue into a cheeselike material. This material may localize and become fibrotic, or it may develop into cavities within the lung tissue. The cavities are filled with the multiplying bacilli, and the infected debris spreads throughout the tracheobronchial tree.

On initial contact with the tubercular bacillus, most people's immune defense system kills the organism or walls it off in a nodule. These dormant organisms may become active later, causing an acute phase.

Signs and symptoms—Symptoms of primary infection include fatigue, weakness, lack of appetite, weight loss, night sweats, and low-grade fever. On reactivation, symptoms may also include a productive cough characterized by purulent mucus, which is occasionally mixed with blood, and chest pains.

Etiology—Tuberculosis is caused by the bacillus organism mycobacterium tuberculosis. Currently there is an increase in incidence of TB primarily because of the relationship of AIDS, the use of drugs, and the influx of third world immigrants. Certain conditions tend to increase the incidence of TB, such as low income, homelessness, alcoholism, being a prisoner, being HIV positive, and being a resident in a long-term care facility.

Treatment—Treatment consists of isolation until the contagious phase has passed. Care must be taken in handling the nasal and expectorated discharges. Bed rest and an adequate diet are very important. Medication specifically for TB must often be continued for six months or more to effect a cure. After two to four weeks, the disease is no longer infectious, and the person can resume a normal lifestyle.

Upper Respiratory Infection (URI)

Description—This term is used to refer to symptoms associated with the common cold.

Signs and symptoms—The disease is usually self-limiting after a one- to four-day incubation period. It is characterized by sore throat, nasal congestion, headache, burning and watery eyes, fever, and general lethargy. A cough may be present, which is nonproductive and hacking, often at night. Symptoms usually persist for a week before subsiding. Secondary bacterial infections affecting the lower respiratory tract are uncommon.

Etiology—An **upper respiratory infection** (URI) may be caused by several different viruses and be transmitted by respiratory droplets, contaminated objects, or hands. Children are the main transmitters of the organism.

Treatment—There is no cure for the common cold. Symptomatic treatment includes aspirin, fluids, and rest. Decongestants can relieve congestion, and throat lozenges can relieve soreness. Antibiotics are not indicated unless there is a chronic illness or complications.

Is It a Cold, Allergy, or the Flu? It is sometimes difficult yet always important to determine whether symptoms suggest a common cold, an allergy, or the flu because

A CAAHEP CONNECTION

A medical assistant curriculum must include content on **Communication** by using **Electronic technology** and community resources. Search the internet for local health organizations providing counseling and support for parents and other family members affected by SIDS. In the curriculum area of **Psychology**, it states you should learn about **Developmental stages of the life cycle**. In this unit and others, there is content that is applicable to infants, children, youth, and the elderly.

treatment and the course of the disease vary according to the diagnosis. Look at Table 11–4. It summarizes the differences between a common cold, the flu, and an allergy. The main symptoms to compare are fever, cough, muscle aches, nasal discharge, and fatigue.

ACHIEVE UNIT OBJECTIVES

Complete Chapter 11, Unit 7, in the workbook to achieve competency of this subject matter.

TABLE 11–4

HOW TO TELL A COLD FROM THE FLU OR AN ALLERGY

While the common cold, influenza, and allergies share some traits, they differ in several others. This table will help you spot the distinguishing features.

Symptoms	Common Cold	Influenza (Flu)	Allergy
Fever	Uncommon; slight	Prominent; high (typically 102°–104°F); sudden onset; lasts 3–4 days	None
Headache	Rare	Prominent	Common
Muscle aches	Slight	Prominent, often severe	None
Fatigue, weakness	Mild	Extreme; sudden onset; may last several weeks	None
Runny, stuffy nose	Common	Occasional	Common
Sneezing	Common	Occasional	Common
Sore throat	Common	Occasional	Occasional
Cough	Sometimes; mild to moderate	Common; often severe	Occasional
Red, itchy eyes	Rare	Uncommon	Common
Itchy nose	No	No	Common
Nasal discharge	Thick and clear to yellowish green	Uncommon	Watery and clear
Response to antihistamines	Poor	Poor	Good to excellent

UNIT 8

The Circulatory System

OBJECTIVES

Upon completion of the unit, meet the following performance objectives by verifying knowledge of the facts and principles presented through oral and written communication at a level deemed competent.

1. Spell and define, using the glossary at the back of the text, all the **Words to Know** in this unit.
2. Name the four main parts of the circulatory system.
3. Describe the anatomy of the heart, identifying the internal and external structures.
4. Differentiate between pulmonary, systemic, and portal circulation.
5. Describe the heart sounds, including the actions producing the sounds and where they can be auscultated.
6. Locate the pacemaker, explain its action, and tell how the heart rate is influenced by the body.
7. Explain how the cardiac conditions of heart block and fibrillation relate to the pacemaker.
8. Explain the purpose of an artificial pacemaker and how it functions.
9. Name the five types of blood vessels and their purpose and structure.
10. Describe the function of a capillary bed.
11. Trace the pathway of blood through the pulmonary and systemic circulation.
12. Explain the function and structure of the lymphatic system.
13. Name the components of whole blood and the role of each.
14. Describe the clotting process.
15. Name the blood types, and explain their importance to recipients of transfusions.
16. Explain the importance of the Rh factor in pregnancy and transfusions.
17. Identify nine cardiovascular tests and the reasons for giving them.
18. Describe 26 diseases or disorders of the circulatory system.

AREAS OF COMPETENCE (AAMA)

This unit addresses content within the specific competency areas of *Administrative procedures, Practice finances, Patient care, Communication skills,* and *Instruction*, as identified in the Medical Assistant Role Delineation Study. Refer to Appendix A for a detailed listing of the areas. (Note: Although *Anatomy and physiology* are not specifically identified within the study, a basic knowledge of the body's structure is an essential foundation to the competent performance of many roles.)

WORDS TO KNOW

accelerator	ischemia
acute phase	leukemia
adenitis	leukocyte
ambulatory	lubb dupp
anemia	lymph
aneurysm	lymphatic system
angina	lymphocyte
angioplasty	metastasize
anticoagulant	mitral
aorta	MUGA scan
arrhythmias	murmur
arterioles	myocardial infarction
arteriosclerosis	(MI)
artery	myocardium
atherosclerosis	nodes
atrium	pacemaker
AV node	papillary muscles
bicuspid	pericardium
bradycardia	phlebitis
capillary	plasma
cardiac	platelet
cardiovascular	portal
cerebrovascular accident	Rh factor
chronic leukemia	SA node
compatible	semilunar
congestive heart failure	septum
coronary	sickle cell anemia
cross-match	spleen
diastole	stasis ulcer
electrocardiograph	systole
(ECG)	tachycardia
embolism	thrombophlebitis
endocardium	thrombosis
erythrocyte	transfusion
exudate	transient ischemic attack
fibrillation	tricuspid
heart block	vagus
hemoglobin	valve
hemorrhage	varicose
Holter monitor	vein
hypertension	vena cava
hypotension	ventricle
infarction	venule

 Library

The circulatory system transports oxygen and nutrients to the body's cells, and it transports carbon dioxide and other waste products from the cells to be eliminated from the body. The blood, which flows through a closed circuit of vessels, is the transportation vehicle. A very efficient muscle, the heart, is the force behind the system. A few minutes' interruption of the circulatory system can result in death.

The circulatory system is composed of four main parts: (1) a pump, the heart; (2) the plumbing, the blood vessels; (3) the circulating fluid, the blood; and (4) an auxiliary fluid system, the **lymphatic system**. Each day the heart pumps the equivalent of 4,000 gallons of blood, at 40 miles per hour, through an estimated 70,000 miles of blood vessels. To achieve this, the heart must forcefully contract, squeezing out blood, at an average rate of 72 times per minute or about 100,000 times each day. In a year's time, the heart will contract 40 million times, resting only a fraction of a second between beats. To appreciate this phenomenal organ, alternately open and close your fist a little more often than once a second for just one minute by the clock. You will notice that not only your hand but also your forearm muscles begin to tire. Scientists have estimated that the work of the heart is about equal to the energy needed to lift a 10-pound weight three feet off the floor twice a minute for a lifetime. The condition of the blood vessels and the composition of the blood are major factors in the amount of force the heart must exert to circulate the blood.

THE HEART

The heart is about the size of a clenched fist and is located behind the sternum, between the lungs, with two thirds of it on the left side of the chest. It is constructed of several layers of muscles arranged in both circular and spiral fashion. When the muscles contract, blood is squeezed out of the heart chambers. During the relaxation phase, the heart fills with blood entering from the great **veins**. There is a considerable difference in the size of the heart during the phases, as shown in Figure 11–114.

The contraction phase is known as **systole**, and the relaxation phase is called **diastole**. Systole is the period when the heart exerts the greatest pressure on the blood. This corresponds to the beat phase of the heart and can be heard over the heart with a stethoscope or felt as the pulse in an **artery**. The systolic pressure can be determined by measurement with blood pressure equipment and is represented by the larger or top number of the blood pressure reading. Diastole is the period of least pressure and is the time when the heart rests. This phase cannot be felt as a beat, but the diastolic pressure can be heard and determined by measurement. It is represented by the smaller or bottom number of the blood pressure reading.

External Heart Structures

The outer wall of the heart is surrounded by a sac called the **pericardium**. Like the pleura of the lungs, the pericardium has one layer called the parietal, which lines the sac, and another layer called the visceral, which covers the heart itself. The pericardial fluid between the layers prevents friction when the heart beats. The heart structure does not receive its blood supply from the blood pumped through its interior but from a number of small blood vessels that cover the surface of the heart (Figure 11–115). These blood vessels, called the **coronary** arteries and veins, carry oxygen, nutrients, and waste products to and from the heart muscle. The right and left coronary arteries enter the top of the heart from the **aorta**. Blood from the coronary veins returns to the right atrium by a small opening called the coronary sinus.

The muscle wall of the heart is called the **myocardium**. The wall of the left lower chamber is thicker because it must pump blood through the entire general or systemic circulation, as discussed later.

Internal Heart Structures

A tissue known as **endocardium** lines the interior surface of the heart (Figure 11–116). The lining also covers the heart valves and the interior surface of the blood vessels to allow for the smooth flow of blood. Internally, the heart is a double pump, divided into a right and left side by a muscular wall called a **septum**. The septum prevents the blood on the right side from mixing with that on the left. The sides are further divided into upper and lower chambers. The right upper chamber is called the right **atrium**, and the lower is the right **ventricle**. The left side is similarly divided into a left atrium and left ventricle.

The chambers are separated by one-way **valves** that keep the blood flowing in the right direction. The **tricuspid** valve is between the right atrium and ventricle, and the **bicuspid** or **mitral** valve is between the left atrium and ventricle. **Papillary muscles** are attached by cords to the undersurfaces of the valve cusps or leaflets. When the atria contract, the papillary muscles also contract to pull open the valves, allowing the blood from the atria to enter the empty ventricles. Then the muscles relax, which allows the valves to close as the atria refill. The closed valves prevent the blood from reentering the atria when the ventricles contract.

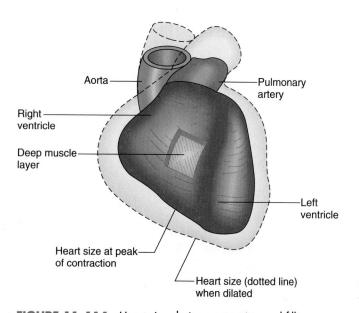

Aorta

Pulmonary artery

Right ventricle

Deep muscle layer

Left ventricle

Heart size at peak of contraction

Heart size (dotted line) when dilated

FIGURE 11–114 Heart size during contraction and filling actions (From *The Wonderful Human Machine*, copyright 1979 by the American Medical Association.)

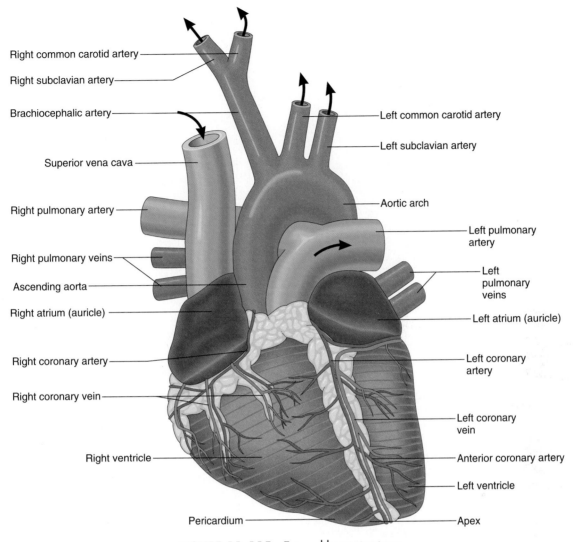

FIGURE 11-115 External heart structures

When the ventricles contract, blood is forced out to the great arteries of the body. The right ventricle sends the blood through a **semilunar** valve into the pulmonary artery on its way through the pulmonary circulation in the lungs for a supply of oxygen. The left ventricle forces the blood past a semilunar valve into the aorta to be distributed throughout the general or systemic circulation of the body.

A specific sequence of events occurs within the body as the blood is circulated. Blood flow occurs in two distinct patterns: *pulmonary circulation* between the heart and the lungs and *systemic circulation* between the heart and the rest of the body. Figure 11–117 and the following material describe the flow of blood through the pulmonary system.

Pulmonary Circulation

1. Deoxygenated (without O_2) blood carried in the superior vena cava from the arms, neck, and head and carried in the inferior vena cava from the lower ex-

tremities and internal organs (except the heart itself) enters the right atrium. Circulation from the heart also empties into the atrium by way of the coronary sinus.
2. The right atrium contracts, squeezing blood through the tricuspid valve, which is opened by the papillary muscles, into the right ventricle. Then the valve closes.
3. The right ventricle contracts, sending blood out through the semilunar valve into the pulmonary artery. (Remember, this artery carries deoxygenated blood but is still an artery because it is leaving the heart.)
4. The pulmonary artery divides into a right and left branch, one going to each lung. The division continues into smaller arteries, arterioles, and then to the capillaries in the alveolar sacs. Here the deoxygenated blood gives up its CO_2 and picks up O_2.
5. With a fresh supply of O_2, the capillaries join the venules, then become veins and reenter the heart as four pulmonary veins, two from each lung, emptying

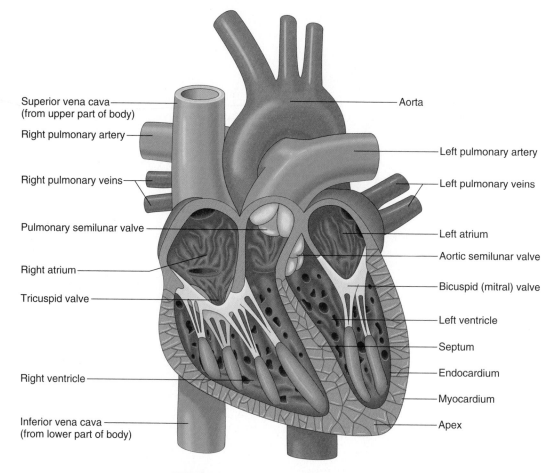

Superior vena cava
(from upper part of body)

Right pulmonary artery

Right pulmonary veins

Pulmonary semilunar valve

Right atrium

Tricuspid valve

Right ventricle

Inferior vena cava
(from lower part of body)

Aorta

Left pulmonary artery

Left pulmonary veins

Left atrium

Aortic semilunar valve

Bicuspid (mitral) valve

Left ventricle

Septum

Endocardium

Myocardium

Apex

FIGURE 11–116 Internal heart structures

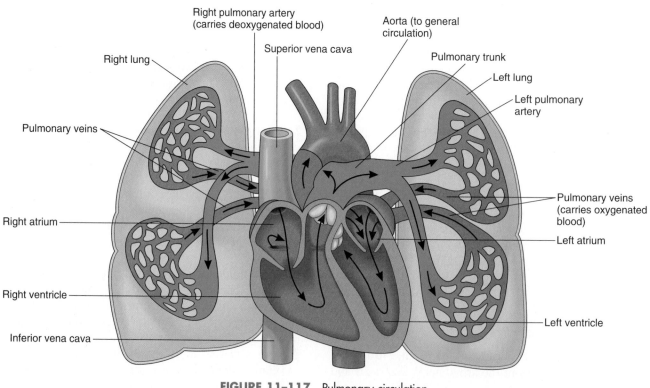

Right pulmonary artery
(carries deoxygenated blood)

Superior vena cava

Aorta (to general
circulation)

Pulmonary trunk

Right lung

Left lung

Left pulmonary
artery

Pulmonary veins

Right atrium

Right ventricle

Inferior vena cava

Pulmonary veins
(carries oxygenated
blood)

Left atrium

Left ventricle

FIGURE 11–117 Pulmonary circulation

into the left atrium. (This is the only time veins carry oxygenated blood, but they are still veins because they are returning to the heart.)

6. The left atrium contracts, forcing blood through the mitral or bicuspid valve into the left ventricle, and the valve immediately closes.

7. The left ventricle contracts forcefully, sending blood racing out of the heart past the semilunar valve into the aorta.

The action of the chambers of the heart just described occurs simultaneously in both sides of the heart. In other words, both atria contract at the same time, as do the ventricles. The chambers must work in unison, or blood being pushed forward would have no place to go (this situation does occur in certain cardiovascular disorders and will be discussed later). The total action just described occurs each time the heart beats.

Heart Sounds

The physician listens at specific locations on the chest wall to hear specific functions of the heart. Figure 11–118 illustrates the anatomical location of the valves and the corresponding auscultatory areas. When a stethoscope is used to listen to the heartbeat, two distinct sounds can be heard. They are referred to as the **lubb dupp** sounds. The lubb sound, which is heard first, is caused by the valves slamming shut between the atria and the ventricles. The physician refers to this sound as the S_1. It is heard loudest at the apex of the heart.

The dupp, heard second, is shorter and higher pitched. It is caused by the semilunar valves closing in the aorta and the pulmonary arteries. This sound is known as the

S_2. It is loudest at the second intercostal space on each side of the sternum. With a little practice, the valves' condition and level of function can be evaluated from their sounds.

Certain conditions cause changes in the action of the heart valves. Normally, the right heart valves close a fraction of a second before the left because of the lower pressure in the right side of the heart. When the ventricles are distended, an audible vibration may occur, which is referred to as an S_3 or a ventricular gallop. Occasionally, just before S_1 at the end of diastole, the atria may contract, forcing blood into an already filled ventricle. This causes a rise in the ventricular pressure and vibrations known as atrial gallop or S_4.

The Pacemaker

The normal heart beats rhythmically as long as the cells receive the correct balance of sodium, calcium, and potassium and an adequate supply of oxygen and nutrients. Another essential element is the "spark" from the group of nerve cells in the right atrium called the sinoatrial or **SA node**, also called the **pacemaker** (Figure 11–119). The node generates the electrical impulse that starts each wave of muscle contraction in the heart. The impulse in the right atrium spreads over the muscles of both atria, causing them to contract simultaneously,

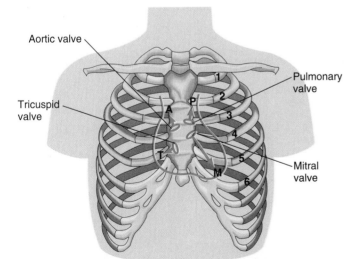

FIGURE 11–118 Anatomical location of the heart valves and the accompanying auscultatory location. Valves are shown as oval structures and the auscultatory location by the letters A, T, M, and P. The rib levels are numbered.

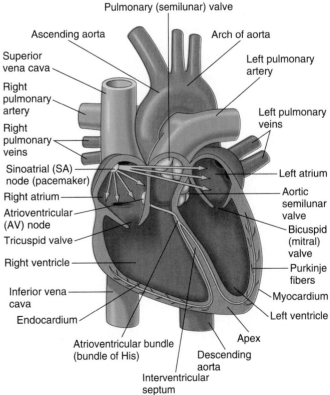

FIGURE 11–119 SA and AV nodes and the conduction pathway of the heart's electrical impulse

sending blood into the ventricles. The impulse apparently triggers the atrioventricular or **AV node**, located between the atria and the ventricles, even though there is no direct connection between the nodes. The AV node has nerve fibers which extend through the septum and are called the *bundle of His.* The bundle divides into a right and left branch, infiltrating the muscles of each ventricle with a system of Purkinje fibers. The AV node causes the contraction of the ventricles.

Rhythm Disorders

The self-generating impulse of the heart is one of the body's miracles. Even if the heart were removed from the body, it would continue to beat as long as it was supplied with the necessary nutrients. In a **cardiac** condition known as **heart block,** there is an interruption in the message from the SA node to the AV node. The interruption can occur in varying degrees. The abnormal rhythm patterns can be viewed on an **electrocardiograph** (heart action recording or **ECG**). *First degree block* is characterized by a momentary delay at the AV node before the impulse is transmitted to the ventricles. *Second degree block* can be of two forms. One occurs in cycles of delayed impulses until the SA node fails to conduct to the AV node, then returns to near normal. A second form is characterized by a pattern of only every second, third, or fourth impulse being conducted to the ventricles. This causes a marked decrease in heart output and usually progresses to the third degree. *Third degree heart block* is known as "complete heart block." There is no impulse carried over from the pacemaker. Because the heart is essential to life, there is a built-in safety factor. The atria continue to beat at 72 times per minute while the ventricles contract independently at about half the atrial rate; this is adequate to sustain life but results in a severe decrease in cardiac output.

Other rhythm disorders are known as **arrhythmias** (any deviation from the normal electrical rhythm of the heart). Premature contractions cause arrhythmia and occur when an area of the heart (not the SA node) "sparks" and stimulates a contraction of the rest of the myocardium. This area is known as an ectopic (abnormal place) pacemaker. There are three types of premature contractions, each identified by the area of its location: atrial, ventricular, or AV junctional.

Atrial are known as *premature atrial contractions* (PACs) and cause the atria to contract ahead of the anticipated time. *Premature junctional contractions* (PJCs) have the ectopic pacemaker focused at the junction of the AV node and the bundle of His. Usually PACs and PJCs are of no clinical significance and are caused by nicotine, caffeine, fatigue, or tension.

Premature ventricular contractions (PVCs) are a different matter. They originate in the ventricle and cause contraction ahead of the next anticipated beat. They can be benign or deadly. If frequent (5 to 6 per minute) or in

pairs, they may require immediate intervention to decrease the irritability of the cardiac muscle to maintain cardiac output. If the PVCs occur every other beat, it is a *bigeminal rhythm;* if they occur every third beat, it is a *trigeminal rhythm.* PVCs can be caused by electrolyte and acid–base imbalance, drug therapy, myocardial infarction (see diseases), or oxygen deficit.

Artificial Pacemaker

When the natural pacemaker of the heart fails to maintain a normal heart rate and cardiac drug therapy designed to cause effective, regular beats fails to correct the situation, an artificial pacemaker may be indicated. The device consists of a small battery-powered pulse generator with electrode catheters (Figure 11–120). The electrodes are inserted into a vein and threaded through the vena cava, one to the right atrium, the other into the right ventricle at the apex. The procedure is accomplished while observing the path of the electrodes by fluoroscopy. The action of the heart throughout the procedure, and for at least the first 24 hours following, is monitored carefully by frequent electrocardiograph (ECG) tracings. The stimulation threshold of the pacemaker to maintain myocardial contractions is determined by noting the number of milliamperes (MA) that produce the desired QRS complex (ECG tracing of contraction). This MA and the desired rate can be set in the pacemaker with a handheld radio transmitter.

It should be noted that when the heart is totally dependent on artificial pacing, the heart rate may always be that which is artificially set. Newer artificial pacemakers can increase the rate to meet the needs of increased activity by sensing body motion.

A pacemaker can be attached temporarily to the chest wall, upper arm, or waist. It can also be "permanently" inserted surgically into a muscular pocket on the chest wall.

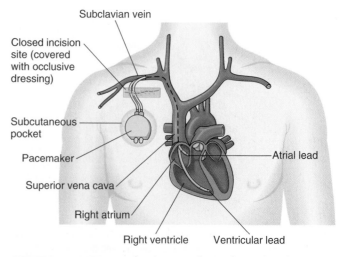

FIGURE 11-120 Artificial pacemaker with atrial and ventricular leads

Permanent units are self-contained and will operate for about 3 to 12 years. Pacemakers can also be of either the fixed or the demand type. Fixed units fire continuously at a predetermined rate. Demand types sense the person's own rate and fire only when required. An external unit can be programmed to change the mode of firing of some implanted types. Battery failure requires replacement of the entire generating unit.

Pacemakers are of benefit to patients with a slow, irregular heart rhythm, complete heart block, or a slow ventricular rate resulting from congenital or disease conditions.

In another malfunction of the impulse mechanism known as ventricular **fibrillation**, the rhythm breaks down and the muscle fibers contract at random without coordination. This results in very ineffective heart action and is a life-threatening condition. An electrical device called a *defibrillator* is used to discharge a strong electrical current into the patient's heart through electrode paddles held against the bare chest wall. The shock should interfere with the uncoordinated action and allow the SA node to resume its control.

A type of artificial pacemaker, known as an implantable cardioverter defibrillator, can also affect the rhythm of the heart. The defibrillator is used to reestablish effective heart action with patients who have episodes of potentially-fatal fibrillation. This device consists of a small power pack about the size of a pager. It is implanted in the chest wall near the clavicle and attaches to electrode tubes that are threaded through veins to permanent positions in the heart, much like an artificial pacemaker. It includes a microcomputer that monitors the heart's rhythm and responds with a low-energy "shock" for a minor problem or gives a high energy jolt, similar to one given with external defibrillator paddles, to automatically correct fibrillation. Use of the implanted defibrillator is becoming more common, especially with patients who have an increased risk of heart rhythm problems following a heart attack. In 2001, over 60,000 Americans were implanted with the sophisticated electronic device.

Controlling the Rate

Two nerves, the **vagus** and the **accelerator**, have fibers in the muscle of the heart and have some control over the natural rate of the heartbeat (Figure 11–121). The vagus nerve, also called the decelerator, slows down the heart rate, whereas the accelerator nerve increases the rate. The nerves, however, are stimulated by many things. Heart rate can increase as the result of fear, anger, or excitement and can decrease with severe depression. The amount of oxygen, carbon dioxide, and electrolytes (sodium, potassium, magnesium, phosphates, and chlorides) present in the blood affect the rate of the heart. A heart rate which is consistently rapid (over 100 beats per minute) is known as **tachycardia**. When the rate is consistently slow (less than 60 beats per minute) it is referred to as **bradycardia**.

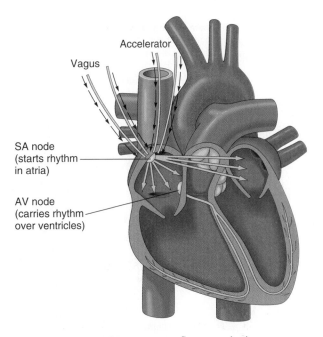

FIGURE 11–121 Nerves influencing the heart rate

THE BLOOD VESSELS

Blood vessels are divided into three main types: arteries, veins, and **capillaries** (Figure 11–122).

Arteries

An artery always carries blood *away* from the heart and usually carries fresh, oxygenated blood. The one exception is the pulmonary artery, which leaves the right ventricle of the heart on its way *to* the lungs to pick up oxygen. Arteries are constructed with layers of elastic fibers that allow the walls to expand and recoil in response to the injection of blood when the ventricles contract. In the systemic circulation, this action causes a wavelike effect within the arteries, which can be felt as the pulse at the pulse points of the body. Figure 11–123 shows the main arteries of the human body. In areas where arteries lie over firm or bony structure, such as at the wrist, the side of the neck, or the inner elbow surface, the pulse can be felt if the artery is pressed against the underlying structure.

The major arteries of the body are:

Aorta—the large artery exiting the left ventricle of the heart and extending down the center of the body. All other arteries branch off the aorta.

Carotid—extends up the side of the neck into the head.

Pulmonary—extends from the right atrium to the lungs.

Brachial—extends down the arm.

Radial—extends on the thumb side of the forearm.

Ulnar—extends on the little finger side of the forearm.

Common iliac—branches off the abdominal aorta and extends down through the pelvis.

Femoral—extends through the thigh.

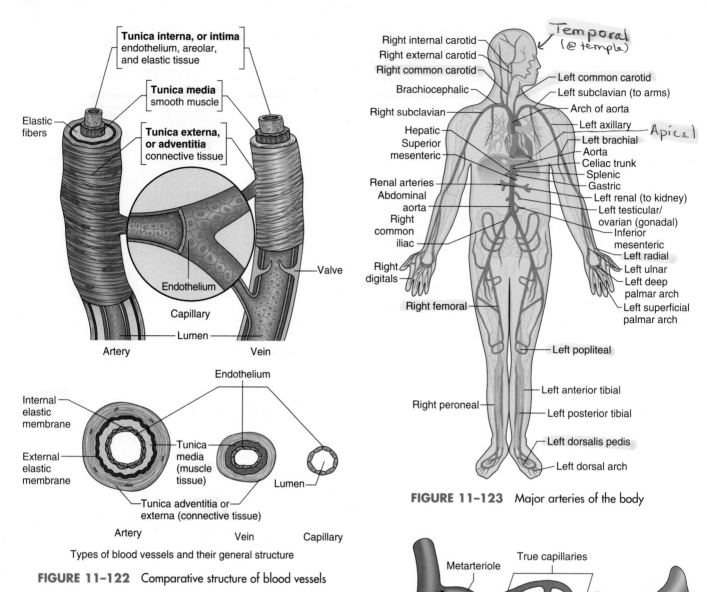

FIGURE 11-122 Comparative structure of blood vessels

FIGURE 11-123 Major arteries of the body

Tibial—extends from the femoral through the lower leg. Dorsalis pedis—extends along the top of the foot.

As the arteries divide and branch off into smaller and smaller vessels, they become known as **arterioles**. Eventually, the arterioles join the microscopic blood vessels known as capillaries. When the blood enters the vast network of capillaries, called a capillary bed, it is so dispersed that the rate of flow is reduced to a slow trickle, permitting time for O_2 and nutrients to enter the tissue cells in exchange for CO_2 and waste products (Figure 11–124).

Capillary walls are thin, one-cell structures that allow the passage of molecules into the fluid-filled tissue spaces surrounding the cells. The molecules pass through the fluid to enter either the cell or the capillary. Tiny openings in the capillary walls permit white blood cells to leave the blood and enter the fluid of the tissue spaces to destroy bacteria. **Plasma** also seeps through the capillary walls, adding to the amount of tissue fluid. Excess fluid, certain waste products, and other substances are removed by an

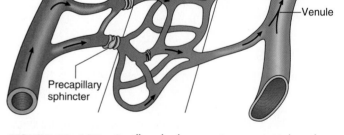

FIGURE 11-124 Capillary bed connecting an arteriole with a venule

adjoining capillary of the lymphatic system, an action that will be discussed later in this unit.

The vast number of capillaries within the body would be more than capable of holding all the body's supply of blood. Therefore, an automatic system is in effect that permits a group of cells being served by one section of a capillary bed to receive blood for only a short period of time. Then another section is served, and the first section must wait for another turn. This control is maintained by a series of capillary sphincters that open and close the entrances to the capillary beds.

Body cells, in order of importance, have a predetermined priority for receiving the available blood supply. At any given time, only two of the three major body functions can be served. The brain and other central nervous system structures always have first priority. Next come the skeletal muscles that enable us to move and therefore provide a degree of protection to the body with the flight/fight options. Last is the supply to the internal organs of the digestive system. This means that if you have eaten recently and you decide to run, swim, or exercise strenuously, your stomach may complain with cramps because the muscles are not getting enough blood supply to digest its contents.

When the blood leaves the capillary bed, it is carrying CO_2 and waste products from the cells to be circulated to the proper organ for disposal. Capillaries join with **venules**, which are tiny branches of the veins. As they return blood toward the heart, venules join together forming veins that eventually enter the heart from the lower body by the inferior **vena cava** and from the upper body by the superior vena cava.

Veins

Veins are similar to arteries in construction, except the walls are thinner and they lack the elastic fiber lining that lets arteries alter the size of their openings. The pressure that is present in arteries is absent in veins, and therefore they can collapse when they are not filled. The major veins of the body are shown in Figure 11–125.

The major veins of the body are:

Tibial—from the feet to the thigh.
Saphenous—in the thigh from the knee into the pelvis.
Femoral—in the thigh from the knee into the pelvis.
Common iliac—from the saphenous and femoral to the inferior vena cava.
Inferior vena cava—all lower body veins to the right atrium of the heart.
Jugular—from the head and neck.
Brachial—from the arm to the brachiocephalic.
Cephalic—from the arm to the brachiocephalic.
Superior vena cava—all upper body veins to the right atrium of the heart.
Pulmonary veins—from the lungs to the left atrium.

Veins carry deoxygenated blood back to the heart to be sent to the lungs for exhaling of CO_2 and to pick up a new supply of O_2. Every time the heart beats, blood is forced through the arteries and arterioles to the capillaries, where the pressure from the heart is dissipated in the vast capillary network. With each successive beat, additional blood is forced through the capillaries into the venules

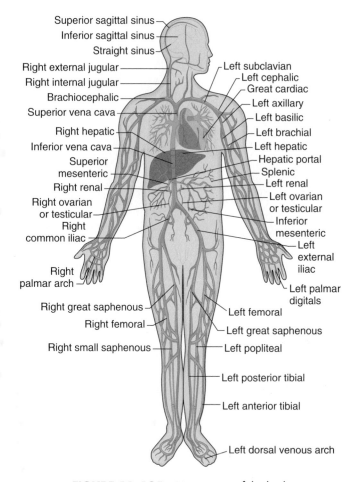

FIGURE 11-125 Major veins of the body

and veins, which move it back toward the heart. Special valve structures are located throughout the veins to maintain the flow of blood in the proper direction (Figure 11–126). Veins in the lower extremities especially contain many valves because they are returning blood "uphill" so to speak. During the relaxation phase of the heartbeat, the venous blood could flow back toward the capillaries, but

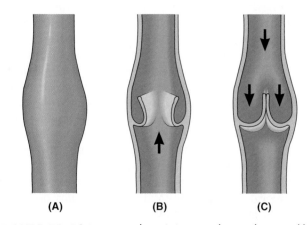

FIGURE 11-126 Vein valves: (A) external view showing dilation at site of valve, (B) vein opened and valves opened, and (C) valves closed to prevent backflow of blood

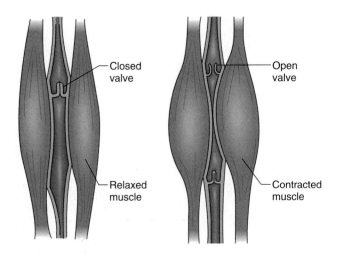

FIGURE 11-127 How muscles help move blood through internal veins

the valves close as relaxation begins, and the blood is trapped in the veins until the following beat forces it to move forward.

Another factor helps move blood in veins back to the heart. The veins of the extremities are located in and around the large skeletal muscles. When the muscles contract, they squeeze the veins, thereby aiding in the movement of the blood (Figure 11–127).

Blood flows to every cell in the body through the systemic circulation. Refer to Figures 11–123 and 11–125 as you read the following description of the flow through the major arteries and veins.

Systemic Circulation

1. As the blood leaves the left ventricle, it enters the huge aorta. Immediately, the right and left coronary arteries to the heart exit from the aorta at its arch. Other great arteries, the common carotid, the subclavian, and the innominate (which becomes the brachial and radial arteries of the arm), also exit from the arch, divide into right and left branches, and supply blood to the head, neck, and upper extremities.
2. As the aorta descends through the body, the thoracic and abdominal portions give origin to the large arteries supplying the organs of the thorax and abdomen.
3. When the aorta reaches the level of the fourth lumbar vertebra, it divides into two large common iliac arteries with the external branch descending down the legs and the internal branch leading to the pelvic organs and genitalia (external sex organs).
4. The external branch of the iliac artery becomes the femoral artery in the thigh and continues down the leg as the tibial branch.
5. Eventually all systemic arteries throughout the body subdivide until they become arterioles and then join the capillaries. In this circuit, the capillaries deliver

the O$_2$, water, and nutrients to the body's cells and pick up the cells' CO$_2$ and wastes.
6. Upon leaving the capillaries, the blood is considered deoxygenated. The capillaries join venules, which eventually become veins.
7. The major lower extremity veins are the anterior and posterior tibial, the small and great saphenous, the popliteal, and the femoral. These join with pelvic veins and enter the inferior vena cava.
8. The major veins of the upper extremities are the basilic, median, and cephalic. These join with the subclavian, internal and external jugular, the innominate, and the sinuses from the head to enter the superior vena cava.
9. The superior vena cava and inferior vena cava empty into the right atrium of the heart and systemic circulation is completed.

Portal Circulation

The preceding was a simplified description of the body's general circulation. However, there is another "circuit" that leaves and reenters the system just described. It is called the **portal** circulation (Figure 11–128). The details of its function are beyond the scope of this text, but it can be described in general terms.

As the aorta descends through the abdomen, arteries branch off to the internal organs: the stomach, liver, spleen, pancreas, kidneys, etc. Each organ receives substances on which it reacts. These substances may be sugar, salt, hormones, a toxic chemical, nutrients, or waste products from the cells of other organs. Everything you eat, drink, inhale, or inject into your body eventually enters the circulatory system.

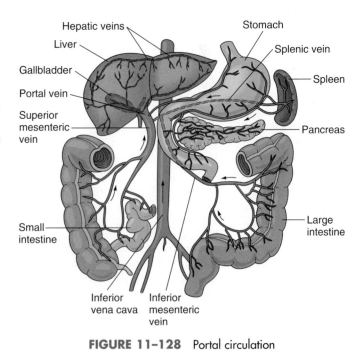

FIGURE 11-128 Portal circulation

The blood leaving certain organs (ones without a pair) empties into the special portal circulation and eventually becomes the portal vein. This vein goes to the liver to permit the blood from the large and small intestines, stomach, pancreas, and spleen to come into contact with the liver's specialized cells. Many life-preserving functions are performed by these liver cells. For example, here nutrients that enter the blood from the digestive system are altered, stored, or released into the main circulatory system as needed. After passing through the liver, the blood is carried by the venous system to the inferior vena cava and is recirculated.

THE LYMPHATIC SYSTEM

The lymphatic system consists of **lymph** (a straw-colored fluid similar to blood plasma), lymph **nodes**, lymph vessels, and the **spleen**. In addition, the lymphatic tissue, which produces **lymphocytes** (a type of blood cell), is often considered to be part of the system. This includes the tonsils, the thymus gland, and the intestinal lymphoid tissue.

Lymph

Lymph is composed of blood plasma that filters out of the capillaries, lymphocytes, hormones, and many other substances that are the products of cellular activity, such as water, digested nutrients, salts, oxygen, carbon dioxide, and urea (Figure 11–129). It is a continuous-forming process. Lymph fills the spaces between the cells and is also referred to as intercellular or *interstitial fluid.* Lymph acts as the "bridge" between cells and capillaries. Lymph is moved through the lymph vessels primarily by contraction of the skeletal muscles. There is no pump like the heart to move lymph. Lymph vessels are constructed like veins, however, with valves to prevent the backflow of fluid.

Lymph Vessels

Vessels carrying lymph are located throughout the body, somewhat like veins. Lymphatic capillaries absorb fluid and other substances from the tissues and return it to the circulatory system (Figure 11–130). However, it is a one-way system only, from the cells toward the heart. There are no separate vessels bringing lymph to the cells.

The vast network of lymph capillaries joins to form small lymph vessels that in turn form larger vessels called *lymphatics.* Lymphatics eventually form two main ducts. The right lymphatic duct receives lymph from the right side of the head, the right arm, and the upper right trunk. The thoracic duct receives lymph from the rest of the body (Figure 11–131).

Lymph Nodes

Lymph nodes are small, round or oval structures located usually in clusters along the lymph vessels at various places in the body. Lymph enters the nodes from four afferent lymph vessels, filters through a mesh of sinuses, and leaves by way of a single efferent vessel. Lymphocytes, a type of white blood cell, are derived from stem cells in the bone marrow. They enter the blood stream and go to the lymph tissue to "live." Their action is essential to the immune system of the body. When needed, they divide by mitosis, greatly increasing in number. Phagocytes, another type of white blood cell, can also be found in lymph nodes. The structure of the nodes and the cell's

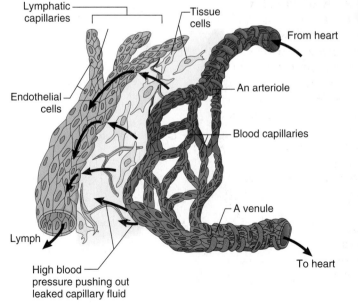

FIGURE 11–129 Leaked blood capillary fluid enters the lymphatic capillaries and becomes lymph.

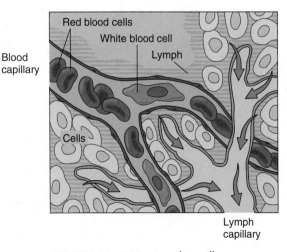
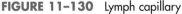

FIGURE 11–130 Lymph capillary

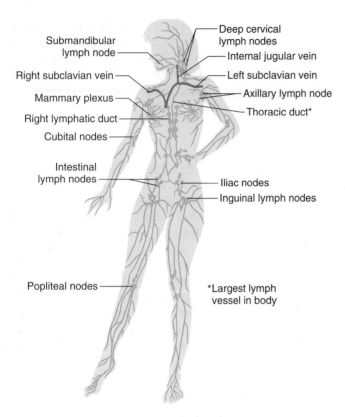

FIGURE 11–131 The lymphatic system

and removes and destroys worn-out red cells. The organ functions like a large lymph node. It is soft and elastic and varies in size according to the flow of blood through the organ. During an acute infection, it will become enlarged and tender. Patients with leukemia may have an enlarged, firm spleen that is palpable on examination. The spleen is filled with excess immature cells to be destroyed.

THE BLOOD

Blood is the life-giving fluid of the body. It flows through the blood vessels, transporting substances essential to the maintenance of life. The average adult has 8 to 10 pints of blood. A loss of two pints, or about 20%, is cause for concern. The blood carries oxygen from the lungs to the body's cells, nutrients from the digestive system to the cells, and cellular wastes from the cells to the appropriate organ for excretion. It picks up hormones excreted from endocrine glands and distributes them throughout the body to the appropriate receiving organ. Blood also delivers the minerals necessary for muscular contraction, heartbeat, stimulation of the respiratory system, and the homeostasis of cells. This vital substance is composed of only two main parts—the plasma and the cells—but each part has many essential components (Figure 11–132).

function purify the lymph by removing harmful substances, such as bacteria or malignant cells. The nodes increase and decrease in size in relation to the amount of material being filtered. In acute infections, they become swollen and tender because of the collection of cells gathered to destroy the invading substances. This condition is known as **adenitis**. With extensive involvement, the node may break down and an abscess will form.

Physicians palpate for nodes when patients have infectious conditions or when a malignancy is known or suspected. With malignancy, the cancer cells are abnormal and so are identified by the cells in the lymph node to be removed from the circulating fluid. As more cells accumulate, the node becomes enlarged and is therefore palpable. Early detection of lymph node involvement is critical to the prognosis of patients with cancer, for it is through the lymphatic system that a malignancy often **metastasizes** (spreads) to other sites. The extent of lymph node involvement is an important indicator of the ultimate prognosis of the patient.

The Spleen

The spleen is an organ composed of lymphatic tissue, lying just beneath the left side of the diaphragm, in back of the upper portion of the stomach. The spleen produces lymphocytes, stores red blood cells, keeps the appropriate balance between cells and plasma in the blood,

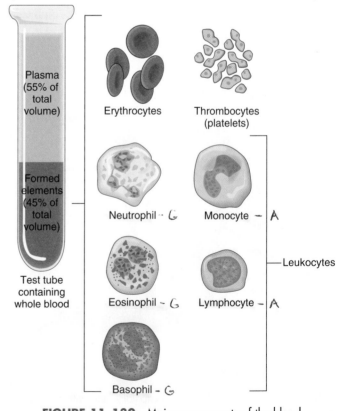

FIGURE 11–132 Major components of the blood

Plasma

Plasma is a straw-colored liquid that makes up a little over half the volume of blood. It is about 90% water, the remainder consisting of minerals, such as calcium, sodium, potassium, phosphorus, and bicarbonates. The minerals are commonly referred to as *electrolytes*. These elements are processed by the body from the foods that are eaten and play a major role in maintaining the acid–base balance of the blood.

Plasma contains other vital substances, such as vitamins, hormones, enzymes, and nutrients absorbed from the digestive system (i.e., glucose, fatty acids, and amino acids). Oxygen, carbon dioxide, and other waste products from the cells are also carried in the plasma.

In addition, three important proteins are found in plasma: fibrinogen, which is necessary to clot blood; serum albumin, which aids in maintaining blood pressure by regulating the exchange of water between the cells and the blood; and serum globulin, which assists in the formation of antibodies. A substance called prothrombin is a type of globulin formed by the liver with the aid of vitamin K. It plays an important role in the clotting of the blood.

Cells

The cellular portion of the blood can be divided into three types of cells: red, white, and platelets.

Red Blood Cells   Erythrocytes *(← no nucleus)* (red blood cells) are biconcave disks with very thin centers to enable them to fold over if necessary to pass through a narrow opening. Red cells number about 25 trillion in the body or about 5 million to a cubic millimeter of blood. It is the red cells which give blood its color. A red blood cell lasts about four months. They are produced in the bone marrow at a rate of about one million a second, the same rate at which they wear out.

Erythrocytes obtain their color from **hemoglobin,** which is a combination of a protein and an iron pigment. It is hemoglobin that attracts and carries the oxygen and carbon dioxide in the blood. When hemoglobin is carrying a lot of oxygen it is bright red in color. As the oxygen is given up to the cells and exchanged for carbon dioxide, the color changes to the dark reddish blue that is visible in surface veins.

White Blood Cells   White blood cells are called **leukocytes.** Leukocytes are present in the blood at approximately 5,000 to 9,000 per cubic millimeter, or about one white cell for every 600 to 700 red blood cells. White cells are about twice the size of red blood cells. Leukocytes play a vital role in defending the body against invasion, moving through capillary walls into the tissue fluid to chase down bacteria.

Leukocytes are divided into two major groups, granulocytes and agranulocytes, depending upon the presence of granules and certain staining characteristics.

Granulocytes are produced in red bone marrow and last for only a few days. There are three types. *Neutrophils* phagocytize (destroy) bacteria by surrounding, swallowing, and digesting them. *Eosinophils* are thought to consume the toxic substances in tissues because they are found in increasing numbers when the body has had a foreign protein injected, has an allergic reaction, or has been infected by a parasite. The third type, the *basophils,* are also thought to participate in phagocytosis because their numbers increase with chronic inflammation or during healing from an infection.

Agranulocytes are of two types: *lymphocytes,* which are produced by bone marrow and lymphoid tissues (such as the nodes and spleen), and *monocytes,* which are formed in the bone marrow. Lymphocytes primarily specialize in providing immunity for the body by attaching themselves to foreign bodies and destroying them and by developing antibodies. The monocyte assists with phagocytosis. Some enlarge greatly when they enter tissue and become fixed.

When an inflammation occurs, white cells can divide and proliferate into capsulelike structures around foreign objects that cannot be digested, such as silica dust and carbon particles, or causative organisms of infections, such as tuberculosis. This action effectively walls off involved tissue in an attempt to contain the foreign material or prevent the spread of disease. The evidence of a phagocytic reaction to invading bacteria or a foreign object is the presence of **exudate** (pus). Exudate is composed of lymph, bacteria, and dead white blood cells.

Platelets   *Thrombocyte* The third kind of cell is the **platelet.** These cells are the smallest of the three and are present in the blood at a rate of 200,000 to 400,000 per cubic millimeter. They are also formed in the bone marrow from cell fragments.

Platelets function in the life-saving process of clotting blood. When a blood vessel is cut or damaged, it is believed that the rough surface may catch and/or attract platelets to the area. This reaction occurs only when there is an incidence of bleeding; otherwise, the clotting process would stop circulation within the blood vessels. When there is a cut, platelets pile up at the site to form a small mass. Once attached firmly to the damaged area, they release the chemical, serotonin, which causes the blood vessel to spasm, resulting in a narrowing of the vessel and a decrease in blood loss until the clot can be formed (Figure 11–133). At the same time, platelets and injured tissues release thromboplastin, which triggers the clotting process to begin. The thromboplastin cooperates with calcium ions and other blood clotting factors in the blood to convert prothrombin (present in plasma) into thrombin. The thrombin acts on another protein in the plasma called fibrinogen. This reaction results in the formation of fibrin, tiny threads that form a network of fine mesh fibers over the cut. This net begins to catch the red blood cells, other platelets, and plasma, forming the clot.

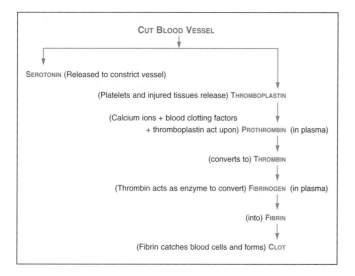

FIGURE 11–133 Process of blood clot formation

It should be remembered that unless the cut blood vessel is small, a clot may not be able to form. The force of the flow of blood will wash away the body's efforts to form fibrin nets and therefore will be unable to collect the ingredients of the clot. Clotting can be assisted by applying pressure over the area to stop the blood flow until a clot can form. When major vessels are cut, it may be necessary to surgically close the opening with sutures to control the bleeding. Fortunately, internal bleeding vessels can also undergo the clotting process. Complications can occur from the clotted mass, especially if the clot or its fragments break loose and enter the circulation before the body's natural "housekeeping" function can gradually remove it from the blood vessel.

Bleeding Time

The length of time required for blood to clot from an induced puncture wound is useful information when preparing a patient for a surgical procedure or evaluating the effects of certain disorders or medications. The normal range of bleeding time for the template puncture method is from two to eight minutes. The length of time varies with the method used.

Blood Types

There are four types of blood: A, B, AB, and O. The type of blood a person has depends on the presence of a protein factor called agglutinogen or antigen on the surface of the red blood cell. Type A blood has an A agglutinogen, type B has a B agglutinogen, type AB has both agglutinogens, and Type O has neither (Figure 11–134).

Similarly, a protein is present in blood plasma known as agglutinin or antibody. Type A blood has a b agglutinin, type B blood has an a agglutinin, type AB has no agglutinins, and type O has both a and b.

The term *agglutinate* refers to the process of clumping or sticking together. Blood clumps and forms clots in the blood vessels if agglutinins and agglutinogens of the same type are mixed together. This reaction can be fatal. Therefore, it is extremely important to determine the blood types of both the recipient and the donor when blood **transfusions** are required. A laboratory test known as type and **cross-match** is necessary to make this determination prior to the administration of either whole blood or packed cell transfusions. Not only is the blood typed, but it is also mixed and observed to assure that agglutination does not occur. Cross-matching will also detect the presence of subtypes and an agglutinogen known as H.

Figure 11–135 shows how the different types of blood would be distributed through 100 people as identified by the American Red Cross. The need for blood from donors is a constant concern for patients and their physicians. Information from the central area of a midwestern state indicates that 550 donors are needed each day. That translates to 16,775 per month or over 200,000 a year. A recent survey showed that 33% of Americans feel there is a great risk of getting AIDS or hepatitis from a transfusion. Currently, with the methods used to screen donors and the tests performed on the blood, it is highly unlikely. The risk of blood-borne AIDS is now only one in 420,000 units of blood; hepatitis is far smaller. A new form of hepatitis called hepatitis "G" has now been identified, so testing for it will be developed. To this point, six types have been found, and more are suspected. Scientists have been trying to develop an artificial blood as a substitute. One firm is now ready to test its product. Another research project has led to the creation of three pigs that carry

Blood Type	Percent of Population	Antigen/Agglutinogen on Red Blood Cells	Antibody/Agglutinin in Plasma	Can Receive	Can Donate To
A	41%	A	Anti-B	A or O only	A or AB only
B	12%	B	Anti-A	B or O only	B or AB only
A B	3%	A and B	None	A, B, AB, O Universal recipient	AB only
O	44%	None	Anti-A and B	O only	A, B, AB, O Universal donor

FIGURE 11–134 Blood types

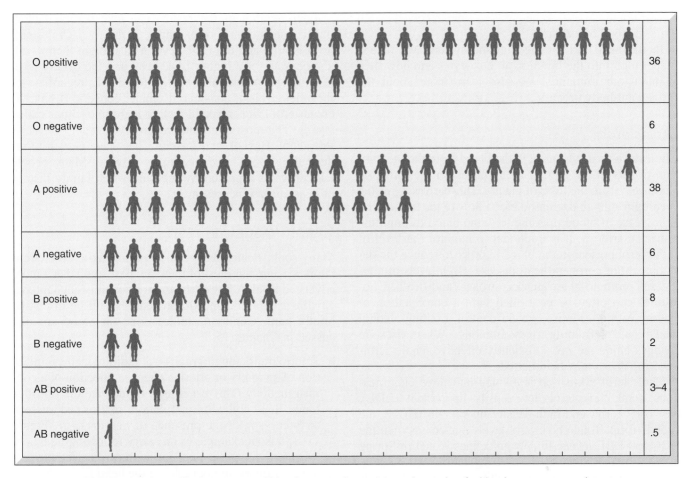

O positive		36
O negative		6
A positive		38
A negative		6
B positive		8
B negative		2
AB positive		3–4
AB negative		.5

FIGURE 11–135   The occurrence of blood types within 100 people as identified by the American Red Cross

genes that produce human hemoglobin that can be extracted, chemically modified, and then pasteurized for human use. It has a longer storage life, does not require refrigeration, avoids the risks of human viral diseases, and works in all blood types. At this point, it is in the testing stage.

Rh Factor

Red blood cells may have another factor known as the **Rh factor**. It is an antigen that was first detected in the blood of a Rhesus monkey, therefore it has the name Rh. If the red blood cell has the factor, it is said to be Rh positive or Rh+. If the factor is absent, then the blood is said to be Rh negative or Rh−. Blood must also be checked for the presence of this antigen when a transfusion is to be given. If an Rh negative person receives Rh positive blood, the antigen is "foreign" to the recipient's bloodstream. Within two weeks, the individual will produce antibodies in response to this invasion of a foreign substance. Usually no problems occur unless at a later date the person receives another Rh positive transfusion. This time the developed antibodies will react to the antigen being received and may cause serious complications.

It should be noted that persons who are Rh positive can receive either Rh positive or Rh negative blood, provided it is properly typed and cross-matched, because they already have the factor, and the Rh negative blood is without the antigen. When the two blood samples can mix without evidence of any clumping and the Rh factor is appropriate, the blood is said to be **compatible**.

The Rh factor is also of concern with pregnancy. If a female who is Rh negative becomes pregnant with an Rh positive baby, a few positive cells may enter the mother's blood at delivery and cause the production of antibodies. The firstborn will not be affected, but if later pregnancies are Rh positive, they may be affected by the antibodies that have been developed. These antibodies slowly filter into the fetal circulation and destroy the Rh positive red blood cells, making the newborn profoundly anemic and jaundiced. The situation must be treated vigorously with steps taken to alter the infant's blood.

This potentially fatal situation can be avoided by determining the Rh factor of the mother. If she is negative, then the father's factor must be determined before the first child is born. At the time of delivery, if the baby is positive, the Rh negative mother is given an injection of an Rh(D) immune human globulin, which prohibits the production of antibodies against the baby's Rh positive blood. Only when the mother is negative and the fetus positive is there cause for concern. If the father also happens to be negative, there is no need to treat for the antibodies unless the mother could have, at some previous time, received an Rh positive blood transfusion.

In the next unit on the immune system, we take a deeper look into the function of leukocytes and how they maintain our immunity. We also learn more about the antigen/antibody process.

Cholesterol

Cholesterol is a substance in the blood from the metabolism of fats in the diet. It accumulates on the lining of blood vessels in the form of plaque. This narrowing of the opening results in decreased blood flow to the tissues and an increase in blood pressure to pump blood through the restricted arteries. It is important to monitor the level of cholesterol present in the blood in order to reduce the development of coronary heart disease. High levels of cholesterol promote heart attacks, strokes, and death. Cholesterol can often be controlled with a combination of healthy eating, exercise, weight control, limiting alcohol intake, and refraining from smoking. When lifestyle changes alone are not sufficiently effective, cholesterol-lowering drugs may be required.

Cholesterol evaluation is divided into three classifications: total cholesterol; low-density lipoprotein (LDL), the "bad" form; and high-density lipoprotein (HDL), the "good" form. Total cholesterol levels matter less than the HDL and LDL levels. In new guidelines issued in Spring of 2001 by the National Heart, Lung, and Blood Institute of the National Institutes of Health, the acceptable levels were changed significantly because of continued high incidence of heart disease. A new emphasis was placed on the protective factor of high levels of HDL. There is also a lowering of acceptable levels of LDL in certain circumstances, such as having a previous heart attack, being a diabetic, and being at risk for attack because of age, smoking, high cholesterol, hypertension, family history, and obesity. Diabetes is now considered such a potent risk factor that it automatically places an individual in the lower level category.

The new general guidelines for cholesterol levels are as follows:

Total Cholesterol

Desirable	Less than 200 mg/dl
Borderline-high	200-239 mg/dl
High	240 mg/dl and above

LDL Cholesterol

Desirable	Less than 130 mg/dl
Borderline-high	130-159 mg/dl
High	160 mg/dl

HDL Cholesterol

Low (risk factor)	Less than 35 mg/dl
High (protective)	60 mg/dl

Interpretation of the results can take several factors into consideration. For example, if the total cholesterol level is high and the HDL level is also high, then it will compensate for a higher LDL level and the overall level may be acceptable. However, a low HDL, regardless of the other levels, is considered a major concern. High LDL cholesterol levels respond well to a group of drugs called statins. The most common are Lipitor, Zorcor, Mevacor, Pravachol, Baycol, and Lescor. They have proven to reduce the risk of coronary artery disease. Many people take drugs as a preventive measure when family history of heart disease is present.

CARDIOVASCULAR TESTS

Many sophisticated tests can be performed on the circulatory system, but most of them are best studied at a more advanced level. A few of the more frequently encountered **cardiovascular** diagnostic procedures will be discussed briefly here. Common studies done on blood are discussed in Chapter 15.

■ Arteriograph (angiograph)—a radiological examination of an artery or arteries after the injection of a contrast medium. The test is used to indicate the status of blood flow, collateral circulation, malformed vessels, an aneurysm, or the presence of **hemorrhage**. Figure 11–136 is an example of an artery following injection. It is often done in connection with cardiac catheterization. Coronary angiography of the heart is very helpful in diagnosis. It can reveal faulty motion of the heart wall, leakage of blood back through diseased valves, or a hole between the right and left sides. In the coronary arteries, angiography can help locate blockages, which can then be treated with an angioplasty procedure or identified for bypass surgery. About one million angioplasties are performed in the United States each year.

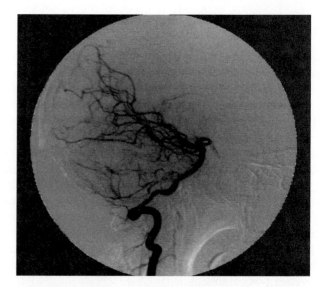

FIGURE 11–136 Example of angiogram (angiograph)

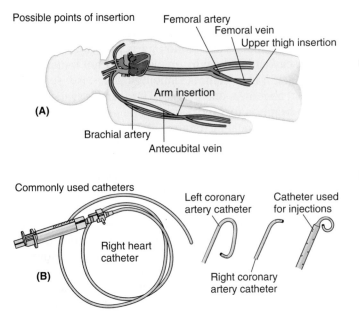

FIGURE 11-137 (A) Points of insertion for a cardiac catheter, (B) commonly used catheters

- Cardiac catherization—A catheter to the right side of the heart is inserted into a vein at the antecubital space of the right arm. A catheter to the left side of the heart is inserted into the brachial artery at the left antecubital space. The femoral artery or vein may also be used. The catheter is passed through the blood vessels until it reaches the heart. When it is determined by fluoroscopy that the catheter is properly positioned, a contrast medium is injected to permit visualization. The heart's chambers and valves and the coronary arteries or the pulmonary artery may be viewed, depending on the site being catheterized. The procedure can also be used to measure blood pressure within the pulmonary artery and some portions of the heart. It is used in connection with coronary angiography. Figure 11-137 illustrates the usual points of insertion of the cardiac catheter. Notice the different shapes of the catheter tips that help to guide the catheter into the desired position.

- Dobutamine stress test—Is a variation of the cardiac stress test that also combines the information from an echogram. A resting state echogram is performed first to evaluate the myocardium, the valves, the blood flow, and the action of the heart. Then, dobutamine is given intravenously in ever-increasing amounts to "stress" the heart chemically without the need for exercise. During the test, additional echogram findings are taken and the blood pressure is monitored. At peak stress, additional echogram pictures are taken. A continuous ECG records the activity of the heart throughout the examination. Upon completion, the effects of dobutamine gradually subside, and the patient's heart rate returns to normal. This combination of diagnostic tools gives the cardiologist a fairly complete picture of structural and functional aspects of the heart. Other

drugs, such as Persantine or Adenoscan, are used with a radioactive tracer (such as Cardiolite) and a special camera to produce similar studies of the heart.

- Doppler ultrasonography—Sound waves are transmitted through the skin and are reflected by the cells in the blood moving through the blood vessels (Figure 11-138). This diagnostic tool can evaluate the major blood vessels of the body to determine deep vein **thrombosis** (DVT), peripheral arterial **aneurysms**, and occluded carotid arteries.

- Echocardiograph—This is a non-invasive test that uses ultrasound (high-frequency sound waves) to make images of the internal structures of the heart. A special gel is applied to the chest wall, and a hand-held device called a transducer is maneuvered over the heart area. Sounds waves are transmitted through the skin and strike the structures of the heart, sending echoes back to the transducer. The machine converts the information into images that are displayed on the screen and produce an image or picture of the structures of the heart and its chambers. The test evaluates cardiac function and structure and can reveal valve irregularities, defects in the interior walls, and the presence of fluid between the layers of the pericardium.

- Electrocardiograph (ECG)—This test is also called EKG. It is perhaps the most common tool used to evaluate heart performance. The ECG is a graphic recording of the electrical activity of the heart. It identifies rhythm, abnormalities in conduction, and electrolyte imbalance. The graph is useful in documenting diagnosis and provides a method of measuring progression of cardiac disease conditions. The ECG also helps

How the Doppler probe works

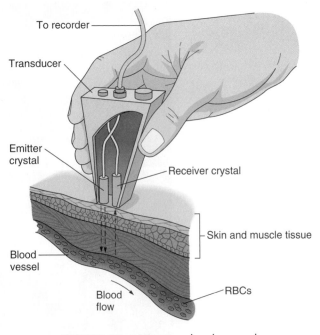

FIGURE 11-138 Doppler ultrasound

evaluate the effectiveness of an artificial pacemaker and cardiac medications.

The test may be taken while the patient is lying in a comfortable position or in an exercise mode, such as bicycling or walking a treadmill. The exercise mode measures the effects of controlled physical stress and is referred to as a *stress ECG*. Frequently, abnormalities of cardiac action are more evident upon exertion.

Another type of ECG is called the **Holter monitor** or **ambulatory** (walking) ECG. The ECG electrodes are attached to the patient's chest wall and a portable cassette recorder (monitor) is placed in a belt about the waist. For a 24 hour period, the patient's heart action is recorded, and a diary is kept of daily activities and any associated symptoms. At the end of the test, the recording is analyzed by computer, and a report is printed. This type of test is most beneficial for symptoms that occur irregularly or to evaluate the status of recovering cardiac patients. Another version permits the patient to activate the recording device only when experiencing symptoms. This patient-activated monitor can be worn for several days. (See Chapter 16.)

- Heart scan—A non-invasive test using a high speed scanner that takes accurate pictures of the heart in less than a second. The technology is known as ultra-fast CT scan and is done by an electron beam tomography scanner. (This same technology can also scan the chest, abdomen, and pelvis). The scanner sweeps electron beams across the patient so quickly that it actually freezes the beating motion of the heart. The scan is valuable in screening for calcified plaque in coronary arteries. Figure 11-139 illustrates the presence of calcified plaque. The amount of calcification is measured and given a score that is an indicator of the degree of coronary artery occlusion. Many physicians believe this scan is an excellent screening tool and provides a baseline assessment of coronary artery condition. It can identify coronary disease long before symptoms of artery blockage occur, thereby permitting lifestyle changes and treatment to prevent a heart attack. Typically, blockage must be about 50% before it can be detected by a stress test.
- **MUGA scan**—MUGA is an acronym for MUltiple Gated Acquisition; it is a test to evaluate the condition

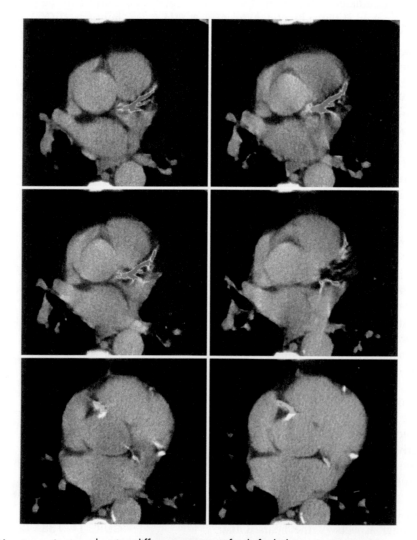

FIGURE 11-139 Heart scan images showing different amounts of calcified plaque in arteries (Courtesy of CAT SCAN 2000.)

of the myocardium of the heart. The test can be done in a resting or exercise mode. Isotopes are injected intravenously and are taken up by the myocardium. The scintillation camera records the motion of the heart. The test permits measurement of ventricular contractions to evaluate the strength of the heart wall. Patients who receive a chemotherapeutic drug that has cardiac toxicity side effects are monitored periodically by MUGA scans because of the drug's tendency to damage the myocardium.

- Myocardial perfusion imaging—This is a test to measure the passage of blood through the coronary arteries to the myocardium. The first part of the test involves "stressing" the heart by dilating the arteries with a special IV medication. This is done over a six-minute period. (Normal arteries will dilate more than partially or completely blocked arteries.) The heart is monitored during the test by ECG. After dilation, a radioactive imaging material is injected into the IV. The material concentrates in those parts of the myocardium that have the best blood flow. For about 45 minutes, the camera records images that identify any part of the heart that is not getting enough blood. Later, after the dilating drug has worn off, a series of images will be taken to show perfusion of the heart "at rest." The two series are compared to identify the differences in blood flow. A healthy heart will show little difference.

- Stress thallium ECG—A test to evaluate myocardial blood flow and the condition of the cells. The ECG electrodes are attached to the patient before performing the stress test on either a treadmill or a bicycle. The blood pressure and pulse rate are carefully monitored. When the patient reaches peak stress, the thallium is injected intravenously into the anticubital vein and the exercise continued for an additional minute to ensure circulation of the isotope to the heart. The ECG electrodes are removed, and within three to five minutes the patient is positioned under the scintillation camera. The scanner records the amount of thallium uptake by the heart over the next several minutes. Areas of the heart with normal blood supply and healthy cells rapidly take up the isotope. Areas of poor blood flow or damaged cells do not take up the material and appear as dark spots on the scan; these are known as cold spots.

  The test is indicated for assessing myocardial condition, demonstrating the location and extent of a **myocardial infarction (MI)**, diagnosing coronary artery disease, and determining the effectiveness of artery grafts and angioplasty procedures. Persantine Thallium is a new type of stress test. It is used for patients with arthritis or any other condition that prevents a patient from exercising. It determines the presence of coronary artery disease.

- Transthoracic echocardiography (TTE)—A procedure in which a transducer device is inserted into the esophagus behind the heart to more thoroughly view portions of the heart. In about 10% of patients, external echocardiography doesn't provide a clear enough pic-

ture. Chest deformities, chronic lung disease, and obesity are the main reasons for poor-quality imaging. TTE is particularly helpful when valve abnormalities, blood clots, tumors, growths, and aortic dissection (tearing open) are suspected. It may also be beneficial in detecting valve hardening, stenosis, and fungus-like vegetations that result from infections such as lupus.

- Venogram—A radiographic examination using a contrast medium to determine the condition of the deep veins of the legs. It is especially useful in determining the presence of deep vein thrombosis (DVT), which may occlude the vein systems and lead to pulmonary embolism, a potentially lethal situation. DVT may result from vein injury, prolonged bed rest, surgery, childbirth, irregularity in the coagulation process, and the use of oral contraceptives.

- Ultrasound—Cardiac—(See Echocardiograph.)

- Ultrasound—Carotid artery—A non-invasive test that measures the thickness of the carotid arteries of the neck using sound waves to create images. It was discovered that the risk of heart attack and stroke increased in direct proportion to the thickness of the artery walls. The thicker the walls, the greater the buildup of atheriosclerotic plaque. The people with the thickest walls had more than double the risk of stroke and heart attack as those with thin-walled arteries.

DISEASES AND DISORDERS

Anemia (Ah-ne-me-a)

Description—This term indicates that certain elements are lacking in the blood. There are various types of **anemias**.

Iron Deficiency Anemia is the most common form of anemia.

Description—This form is characterized by an inadequate supply of iron to form normal red blood cells. When the body's supply of iron decreases, so does the number of red blood cells and, as a result, the hemoglobin. This reduces the body's ability to carry oxygen to the cells.

Signs and symptoms—Symptoms include fatigue, listlessness, pallor, inability to concentrate, and difficulty in breathing on exertion.

Etiology—Iron deficiency anemia develops from an inadequate dietary intake of iron or inability of the body to absorb iron as the result of diarrhea, partial or total removal of the stomach, or certain diseases. It can also be caused by intestinal bleeding, heavy menstruation, colon cancer, or bleeding ulcers. It is most common among premature infants, children, adolescents (especially girls), and women before menopause.

Treatment—Iron deficiency is treated by first identifying the underlying cause. Once determined, iron replacement can begin. Oral preparations of iron or iron combined with ascorbic acid are given. Intramuscular injections are possible but not desirable because of the discomfort produced. Intravenous infusion is relatively painless and requires fewer injections.

Aplastic Anemia

Description and causes—It is a disease resulting from injury or destruction of the blood cell formation function of the bone marrow.

Signs and symptoms—This disease generally produces a fatal bleeding episode or a systemic infection, often as a result of infectious hepatitis.

Treatment—Treatment for aplastic anemia must first rule out any identifiable cause and follow with transfusions of pack cells. Recovery may take months. Bone marrow transplant is the treatment of choice in severe aplastic anemia and with those needing constant RBC transfusions. The use of corticosteroids and bone marrow stimulants is appropriate in some cases.

Acute Blood Loss Anemia

Description and causes—Describes conditions of low red blood cell count occurring over extended periods of time. However, low red blood cell count can also occur following an acute blood loss and is referred to by some as acute blood loss anemia.

Signs and symptoms—In this instance, there is a sudden loss of red blood cells and therefore hemoglobin and iron. The rapid loss of blood volume can be fatal.

Etiology—Acute blood loss can result from severe trauma, the inability to coagulate the blood, ruptured gastric or intestinal ulcers, postoperative bleeding, postpartum (after birth) hemorrhage, or a ruptured aneurysm. A loss of 20% to 30% of blood volume causes circulatory insufficiency with symptoms of shock, restlessness, low blood pressure, rapid pulse, perspiration, and cool, clammy skin. With a loss greater than 30%, the circulatory system may fail and be followed by shock and then coma. Blood loss beyond 40% is life-threatening, and the patient will die unless blood volume is immediately replaced.

Treatment—The treatment goal in acute blood loss anemia is to control the hemorrhage and restore blood volume. Prevention of shock is very important. Immediate infusion of IV fluids, electrolytes solutions, and plasma can increase the circulating volume while packed cells and/or whole blood are being typed and cross-matched for infusion.

Aneurysm (An-ur-ism)

Description—This is the ballooning out of the wall of an artery. Often an aneurysm is associated with **atherosclerosis** or **arteriosclerosis** and the resulting hypertension.

Etiology—A slight break or weakness in the muscular layer of an artery allows the pressure of the blood to push the walls of the blood vessel out (Figure 11–140). The larger the bulge, the thinner the arterial wall becomes. Eventually, the wall gives way and a hemorrhage occurs. The extent of the bleeding and its effects on the body depend to a great extent on the location of the aneurysm and the size of the involved blood vessel.

Aneurysms are found primarily in cerebral arteries, the thoracic or abdominal section of the aorta, and the femoral and popliteal arteries of the leg. Some aneurysms are without symptoms and are discovered by accident or an x-ray.

Cerebral Aneurysm occurs within the brain.

Description—Depending on its location, it may rupture and cause bleeding within the subarachnoid space, or an artery within the brain tissue itself may rupture. If the hemorrhage is not too massive, the blood clots. Later, the body will slowly reabsorb the blood clots, and function will return. Hemorrhage may be fatal, however, because of increased intracranial pressure from the blood, which compresses and damages brain tissue. Remember, the skull does not stretch; therefore,

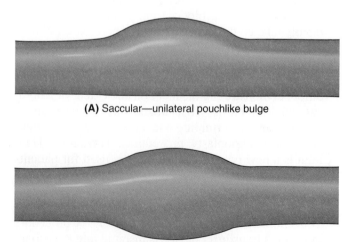

(A) Saccular—unilateral pouchlike bulge

(B) Fusiform—a spindle-shaped bulge of the entire artery wall

FIGURE 11–140 Types of aneyrysms

when bleeding occurs, the delicate tissues of the brain are displaced and damaged. Cerebral aneurysms are graded from I to V depending on the amount of bleeding. Rebleeding after 7 to 10 days is not uncommon. When the initial blood has clotted, the body resumes its normal function of removing clotted material, which may lead to a renewed and often fatal recurrence.

Signs and symptoms—Usually the onset is without warning, but headache, nuchal rigidity (back of neck), stiffness in the back and legs, and intermittent nausea may be present for several days preceding the rupture. Upon rupture, there is a sudden severe headache, nausea, vomiting, and maybe some altered level of consciousness, including coma. Following bleeding, there may be back and leg pain, restlessness, fever, irritability, and occasionally seizures and blurred vision. If there is bleeding into the tissues, there may be paralysis, sensory deficits, difficulty speaking, and visual defects.

Treatment—Treatment is directed toward reducing the risk of rebleeding by repairing the aneurysm surgically. When the patient's condition will not withstand the surgery, a conservative treatment is indicated. This involves bed rest for four to six weeks, avoidance of coffee, other stimulants, and aspirin; analgesics as needed; a hypotensive drug if there is hypertension; corticosteroids to reduce edema; a drug to delay blood clot destruction; and sedatives to reduce stress.

Thoracic Aortic Aneurysms

Description—Occur as a result of great pressure in the artery. Rupture of the aorta is usually fatal. If the thoracic aneurysm begins by "splitting" of the wall, the person may experience a tearing or ripping sensation accompanied by chest pain, pallow, rapid pulse, shortness of breath, loss of pulses below the neck, and other symptoms.

Treatment—Surgery can be accomplished to remove the damaged segment of the aorta and replace it with a Dacron or Teflon blood vessel graft.

Abdominal Aortic Aneurysms

Description—Usually without symptoms but detectable on palpation as a pulsating mass in an area around the umbilicus (navel). If it ruptures, the patient may experience pain similar to that of kidney spasms. About 20% of such patients die immediately; however, if the bleeding is in the retroperitoneal space (behind the peritoneal lining of the abdomen) the limited space puts pressure on the tear as it fills with blood, closing off the opening.

Treatment—An abdominal aneurysm is repaired like an aneurysm of the thoracic aorta. In addition, an external Dacron prosthesis (artificial part) may be applied around the aneurysm and sutured into place to support the weakened wall.

Aneurysms in the lower extremities may interfere with circulation and result in severe **ischemia** (lack of blood) and gangrene (tissue death), which may require amputation of the extremity.

Angina (An-jin-ah)

Description—This heart condition causes severe chest pain that radiates down the inner surface of the left arm, usually associated with emotional stress and/or physical exertion. The episode may last from a few seconds to several minutes.

Signs and symptoms—Symptoms, in addition to the pain, include irregular heart rate, lowered blood pressure, anxiety, and perspiration.

Etiology—The pain is believed to be caused by a spasm or blockage of one or more coronary arteries, which results in ischemia to a portion of the heart muscle.

Treatment—The treatment consists of nitroglycerin, in a tablet form, placed under the tongue. The nitroglycerin dilates the constricted artery or arteries to permit the flow of blood to the heart tissue. When **angina** pain persists after 10 minutes and the use of three sublingual tablets, the patient should go directly to the nearest hospital emergency room.

The patient must be instructed to have nitroglycerin available at all times. Tablets must be kept in a dark, tightly closed bottle, without cotton, and be protected from heat and sunlight. Tablets over three months old should be discarded. Nitroglycerin is also available as an oral spray or in the form of a paste that is applied to the skin to permit prolonged release of the drug in measurable doses. Other medications, such as calcium channel blockers, are also used to prevent angina.

A new little-known procedure is being used in specific centers in the United States. It is thought useful in about 5% to 15% of angina sufferers who are *not* candidates for established alternatives. It is called Enhanced External Counterpulsation. It involves the use of "cuffs" positioned around the legs, thighs, and hips. The apparatus is operated by a computer that synchronizes pulsations to the heartbeat and a compressor that inflates the cuffs, forcing blood to the arteries when the heart muscle is relaxed. This increases blood flow to the heart and decreases the workload. It requires daily one-hour treatments for 35 days. At present, the treatment is limited to patients with stable angina who are not candidates for other treatments. The patients treated have shown a decrease in the frequency and intensity of pain and an increase in exercise tolerance. Some have been able to resume work and even exercise. The treatment is non-invasive but does require a considerable investment in time. At present, insurance will not cover the costs because it is considered experimental.

Arrest (Cardiac)

Description—This is complete, sudden cessation of heart action. The condition is rapidly fatal, producing irreversible brain damage after five minutes.

Signs and symptoms—The major symptom is the sudden ending of heart function, hence the absence of heartbeat and pulse.

Etiology—It is believed to result from a failure in the body's ability to transport calcium, which interferes with its electrical and mechanical functions. It is associated with a severe lack of blood to the myocardium. Cardiac arrest can also be caused by heart failure, electrical shock, fibrillation, drowning, anesthetics, respiratory failure, and severe electrolyte imbalances.

Treatment—Arrest is treated initially by external cardiac massage (CPR or cardiopulmonary resuscitation technique), then supplemented by defibrillation, IV drug therapy, and ventilation procedures. Death is certain if function cannot be restored quickly.

Arrhythmia (A-rith-me-ah)

Description—This term is used to identify any abnormal changes in the heart rhythm. Arrhythmias vary in severity from mild to life-threatening, as with fibrillation. They are classified according to the origin of the irregularity (e.g., PVC or atrial flutter). The more the heart action is affected, the greater the consequences on the cardiac output and the blood pressure, which in turn determines the clinical significance.

Signs and symptoms—The presence of an irregular heart action pattern.

Etiology—Arrhythmias may be congenital or may result from myocardial anoxia, infarction, hypertrophy of muscle fiber from hypertension, or degeneration of conductive tissue required to maintain normal rhythm.

Treatment—Treatment varies in relation to the cause and severity of the irregularity from no treatment to medication, eliminating known causes, CPR, and the insertion of a pacemaker.

Arrhythmia that produces extra beats, delayed beats, or missed beats often results from caffeine, amphetamine or a medication reaction, and can usually be treated by removing the causative factor and taking a digitalis product, such as Lanoxin.

Arteriosclerosis (Ar-tear-e-o-sklur-o'-sis)

Description—A "hardening" of the arteries and arterioles. The muscular and elastic tissue is gradually replaced by fibrous tissue and calcification. Because the vessels are no longer capable of expanding and recoiling with each heartbeat, the heart must exert more pressure on the blood to pump it through the more rigid vessels. Arteriosclerosis results in high blood pressure and may lead to an aneurysm and cerebral hemorrhage.

Signs and symptoms—The major symptom is hypertension.

Etiology—The artery and arteriole walls become fibrous and contain calcium deposits.

Treatment—The prime focus of treatment is aimed at preventing the rupture of an aneurysm or a CVA (stroke) by reducing blood pressure.

Atherosclerosis (A-ther-o-sklur-o'-sis)

Description—This condition is characterized by the deposit of fatty material along the linings of the arteries (Figure 11–141). As the material builds up, the opening of the artery may become partially or totally closed, thereby reducing or eliminating the flow of blood to the area. Atherosclerosis can also result in elevated blood pressure, but the greatest danger is a blocked coronary artery and heart attack. There is also danger from the atherosclerotic plaque deposits that can break loose and circulate through the blood stream as emboli.

Signs and symptoms—The major symptom is hypertension. Examination of the interior of arteries would show plaque of lipids and fat deposits. Decreased circulation symptoms are particularly observable in the carotid, coronary, and lower extremity arteries.

Etiology—Atherosclerosis is linked to many risk factors: family history, hypertension, obesity, smoking, diabetes, stress, sedentary life-style, and high serum cholesterol and/or triglyceride levels.

Treatment—If there is coronary involvement, the goal of treatment is to prevent occlusion of the arteries and prevent myocardial infarction. Dietary restrictions to reduce intake of salt, fats, and cholesterol; abstaining

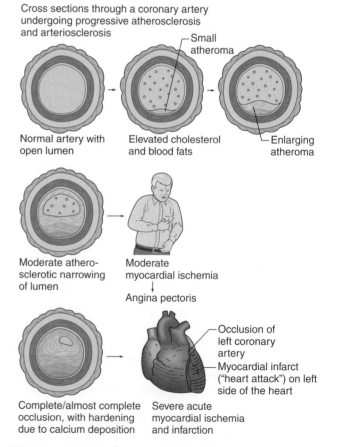

Cross sections through a coronary artery undergoing progressive atherosclerosis and arteriosclerosis

Small atheroma

Normal artery with open lumen

Elevated cholesterol and blood fats

Enlarging atheroma

Moderate atherosclerotic narrowing of lumen

Moderate myocardial ischemia
↓
Angina pectoris

Complete/almost complete occlusion, with hardening due to calcium deposition

Severe acute myocardial ischemia and infarction

Occlusion of left coronary artery

Myocardial infarct ("heart attack") on left side of the heart

FIGURE 11-141 The natural history of coronary heart disease

from smoking; and reducing stress are indicated. Angioplasty is used to compress, remove, or stent deposit areas. With complete obstruction, bypass surgery may be indicated.

Athletic Heart Syndrome

Description—This is a series of cardiac changes resulting from strenuous exercise. Primarily, the heart enlarges (cardiomegaly), particularly the ventricles, because of its adaptive ability to meet the body's need for increased output. Because the heart is a muscle, it reacts just as the biceps do to physical endurance training. This syndrome is increasing because of the emphasis on physical fitness.

Signs and symptoms—The athletic heart usually produces no symptoms except perhaps pounding or irregularity after strenuous activity. Bradycardia of 40 beats per minute is common and may be considered "normal" because of the heart's increased efficiency upon contraction.

Etiology—The syndrome is probably a physiological response to maintaining optimal cardiac performance during physical endurance training. The stress placed on the heart causes the left ventricle to enlarge in order to meet the demand for more oxygen and hence more blood flow.

Treatment—Nothing is required unless there is underlying cardiac disease, which will necessitate discontinuing training.

Carditis (Car-di-tis)

Description—Literally, it is inflammation of the heart. The term is usually used with one of three prefixes that define the portion of the heart that is involved. The inflammation results from an infectious process caused by a viral, fungal, or bacterial invasion. Other causes vary with the form of inflammation, as follows.

Pericarditis (Pear-e-car-di'-tis)

Description—An inflammation of the pericardium, the fibroserous tissue sac that covers the heart.

Signs and symptoms—It may result in a purulent or bloody exudate forming within the sac, or the tissue may become thickened and fibrous, constricting the filling action of the heart. Pericarditis can follow injury to the heart, an infarction, or cardiac surgery.

Acute pericarditis typically causes sharp, sudden pain that begins at the sternum and radiates across the back to the shoulders and arms. It is similar to pleurisy, becoming more intense on inspiration but decreasing when sitting upright and leaning forward. A very serious condition known as tamponade will occur if the collection of fluid within the pericardium is rapid. Pressure within the sac prevents ventricular filling during diastole, thereby severely decreasing cardiac output and resulting in pallor, hypotension, and eventually cardiovascular collapse and death.

Etiology—Acute pericarditis is caused by bacterial, fungal, or viral infections.

Treatment—With tamponade, emergency treatment to remove the fluid by needle aspiration or surgical incision will result in a dramatic improvement.

Pericarditis that causes a gradual fluid accumulation allows time for the pericardium to stretch, often to hold one to two liters of fluid. Chronic pericarditis that results in constriction or recurrent collection of fluid may necessitate partial removal of the pericardium to allow escape of the fluid or, if constriction, a total pericardectomy (removal of the pericardium).

Myocarditis (My-o-car-di'-tis)

Description—An inflammation of the myocardium (heart muscle). It can occur in both acute and chronic forms.

Signs and symptoms—Symptoms produced are generally nonspecific, such as fatigue, palpitations, fever, and dyspnea. It is usually an uncomplicated disease and is self-limiting in nature. Normally, it is associated with a recent upper respiratory infection (URI) and fever.

Myocarditis may produce mild chest soreness and a feeling of pressure but not the anginal type of pain. Occasionally, myocarditis may initiate a degenerative process of the tiny fibrils (small fibers) in the muscular tissue. This may result in heart failure, enlargement, and arrhythmia.

Etiology—Myocarditis is caused by a viral or bacterial infection, an immune reaction (rheumatic fever), radiation therapy to the chest, and effects of chemicals, such as in chronic alcoholism.

Treatment—Myocarditis is treated with antibiotics, bed rest, and appropriate measures for complications that may develop.

Endocarditis (En-do-car-di'-tis)

Description—This is infection of the endocardial lining, heart valves, tissue adjoining artificial valves, or the blood vessel linings. In the infectious process, fibrin and platelets collect where the invading circulating organisms have produced wartlike vegetations on the valves and often the surrounding structures. The vegetative growths may cause serious complications if they embolize to the spleen, kidneys, or lungs.

Etiology—The infecting organism in acute endocarditis is usually a streptococcus, staphylococcus, or pneumococcus. The gonococcus is also capable of causing endocarditis. Intravenous drug abuse may lead to infections from staph or fungi normally present on the skin surface. A subacute form may affect persons with valve or other cardiac lesions that may be acquired or congenital.

Treatment—If endocarditis is left untreated, it usually results in death. Recovery is improved to 70% with proper treatment. When severe valve damage occurs, resulting complications may include insufficient cardiac action and congestive failure caused by improper valve function. Damaged valves can be surgically removed with open heart surgery and replaced with artificial valves. If the infection involves an artificial valve, surgery to replace the prosthesis will be required. Often valves from pigs or cows are used to replace damaged human heart valves and function very effectively.

Cerebrovascular Accident (CVA) (Ce-re-bro-vas'-cu-lar)

Description—A condition commonly known as a stroke, CVA is the sudden impairment of the flow of blood to the brain, thereby diminishing or interrupting the supply of oxygen and causing serious damage or destruction of brain tissue. Because of the urgency for intervention and treatment, strokes are now being referred to as "brain attacks." The phrase "time is brain" also emphasizes the importance of immediate treatment. Strokes are the third leading cause of death and the leading cause of serious long-term disability in the United States. The risk of stroke doubles each succeeding decade of life, beginning at age 55. More men than women have strokes, but women are more likely to die. African Americans and Latinos have a higher rate than whites. Strokes are often referred to as the silent killer because usually no symptoms are noticed in advance.

CVAs are classified according to their cause and effect. **Transient ischemic attacks** (TIAs) are small, temporary interruptions of blood flow. These are referred to as "warning strokes" because they may happen before a major stroke. The symptoms usually last only a few minutes. The most common major stroke is an ischemic stroke, meaning a blood vessel is blocked by a clot and stops all flow of blood to a portion of the brain. A rarer but more dangerous type of stroke is called hemorrhagic, meaning a blood vessel has ruptured, and the escaping blood is damaging brain tissue either by pressure against it or from lack of circulation through the tissue.

Signs and symptoms—Symptoms vary with the area of the brain that is involved. CVAs involving posterior cerebral arteries affect the vision and often result in coma. Anterior artery involvement results in confusion, weakness, loss of coordination, personality changes, and numbness, especially in the legs. If the CVA occurs in the right hemisphere of the brain, symptoms are produced on the left side of the body, and if in the left hemisphere, on the right side. A CVA may leave the patient with many varied symptoms that may include: slurred speech, amnesia, dizziness, paralysis (one extremity, one side, or total), inability to speak, coma, double vision, incontinence (inability to control bladder and bowels), and rigidity. In addition, hemorrhagic stroke usually causes severe headache, difficulty breathing, nausea, and vomiting.

TABLE 11–5

THE WARNING SIGNS OF STROKE

- The development of difficulty in speaking or in understanding simple statements.
- Sudden blurred or decreased vision.
- Loss of balance or coordination when combined with another warning sign.
- Numbness, weakness, or paralysis of face, arm, or leg—especially on one side of the body.
- Loss of consciousness or severe drowsiness.
- A sudden, severe headache.

These signs could represent a stroke; call 911 or other emergency assistance immediately.

Etiology—A **cerebrovascular accident** is the result of high blood pressure, which ruptures an artery; atherosclerosis, which occludes an artery; or thrombosis (a blood clot), which interrupts the flow of blood. When a large enough area is involved, death will result.

All medical personnel should be familiar with the warning signs of stroke as listed in Table 11–5.

Treatment—Remember, with stroke every minute counts. Patients should go to the emergency room immediately either by EMS services, or, if it is quicker, by private car. The patient must NOT drive themselves. Upon arrival, a CT scan or MRI will be ordered to identify the type of stroke, the location, and the extent of the damage. With ischemic stroke, a clot buster called tissue plasminogen activator (tPA) is administered intravenously (IV) or directly into the brain by catheter for about one hour. It can dissolve about 60% to 80% of the clots and effectively prevent brain damage but ONLY if given within three hours of the onset of symptoms. A new clot-busting chemical called prourokinase is being tested and has shown to minimize brain damage up to six hours after a stroke. Also, a non-toxic form of snake venom was accidentally discovered that is effective up to six hours as well. There is always danger from any clot-buster because the blood rushes back in after the blockage is cleared, and the weakened arteries can result in life-threatening bleeding in about 6.5% of patients. An experimental device is being researched as an alternative treatment. It is a tiny pump called an AngioJet that vacuums up a clot almost instantly and without chemicals. It is hoped this proves to be a safer, more effective treatment.

A hemorrhagic stroke is treated differently. Administering tPA could cause life-threatening brain hemorrhage. These patients are treated with methods to control heart rhythm, stabilize blood pressure, and monitor brain function. Unfortunately, little can be done to quickly solve the effects of the hemorrhage.

Research has found that administering neuroprotective materials within 24 hours helps protect the damaged cells. Enzyme-blocking chemicals may be effective for more than a week to prevent damaged cells from dying. After approximately one year, little additional progress toward recovery is anticipated.

Scientists have developed many exciting devices to help maximize the patient's ability to function. A "Handmaster" uses voice activation to duplicate brain impulses to move extremities. A minute computer chip has been implanted in the brain to allow brain signals to form a readout on a computer screen so that a person who is paralyzed and mute can communicate. Also, encouraging results are being achieved from infusion of millions of fresh lab-grown neurons into the damaged brain. It was discovered that when cancerous cells in a lab were treated with retinoic acid, they transformed into healthy neurons. Initially, lab rats were induced to have strokes, and following neuron injection, they regained function. A few humans have received these neuron transplants and are showing improvements for the first time since their devastating strokes.

Perhaps the best treatment is prevention. The strongest predictors of stroke are hypertension, irregular heartbeat, diabetes, a sedentary lifestyle, and use of tobacco. Some protective measures may be beneficial. The use of vitamins B_6 and B_{12} and folic acid seems to help because they lower homocysteine levels. It appears that drinking up to two alcoholic drinks per day offers protection against ischemic stroke by increasing HDL cholesterol and tPA levels to keep clots from forming. Higher intake increases risk for hemorrhagic stroke. Figure 11–142 illustrates ischemic and hemorrhagic stroke effects.

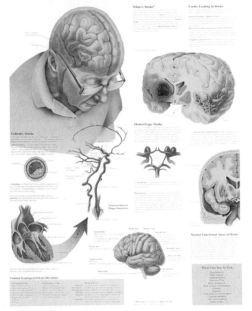

FIGURE 11–142 An illustration of ischemic and hemorrhagic stroke (Courtesy of Colwell, a Division of Patterson Dental Supply, Inc., 800-637-1140.)

Congestive Heart Failure (CHF)

Description—This group of cardiac dysfunctions results in poor performance of the heart with related congestion of the circulatory system. Usually the myocardium of the left ventricle is affected, often as a result of prolonged high blood pressure. **Congestive heart failure** can also be a complication of coronary artery disease or a result of a mechanical disorder involving the heart's valvular functions.

Left-sided Heart Failure

Description—Cardiac output is decreased; however, the left atrium continues to force blood into the ventricle, resulting in increased pressure and volume within the ventricle. As this backup continues, the left atrium becomes congested, backing up blood into the pulmonary veins and then the pulmonary capillary beds. The fluid in the capillaries fills the alveolar spaces, resulting in pulmonary edema. There is a lack of oxygen exchange, and a decrease in the emptying capability of the right ventricle.

Signs and symptoms—Symptoms of left-sided failure are shortness of breath, inability to breathe while lying down, periods of gasping for air, weak and rapid pulse, cool and clammy skin, and an ashen gray or cyanotic skin coloring. Often a cough produces pink, frothy sputum.

Etiology—Congestive heart failure is caused by the increased pressure of blood within the heart, primarily from the poor emptying of the ventricles, which causes fluid from the blood to collect in the tissues. With left-sided heart failure, blood backs up into the lungs, releasing fluid into the alveoli.

Right-sided Heart Failure

Description—Returning blood flow becomes congested in the systemic circulation, eventually causing fluid to enter the interstitial spaces.

Signs and symptoms—Initially, the fluid can be viewed as edema in the lower extremities, but as the failure continues, edema is present in the upper extremities and in various organs throughout the system. Right-sided failure symptoms include swelling of the extremities, enlarged liver and spleen, and ascites (fluid in the abdominal cavity) caused by filtration from portal circulation venous pressure.

Etiology—When the right ventricle fails to move blood forward into the lungs, the blood backs up into the atrium, which therefore cannot accept incoming blood, so congestion occurs in the lower extremities and abdomen.

Treatment—Heart failure is extremely serious. Treatment involves the use of drugs to quickly increase cardiac output and remove congested fluids. Arterial vasodilators increase the efficiency of heart action. Bed rest is enforced and antiembolism stockings are used to prevent thromboembolism resulting from venous stasis.

Continued treatment involves the use of cardiac drugs, frequent periods of rest, the use of elastic support stockings, skin care of the lower extremities, and dietary adjustments to reduce sodium intake and ensure proper nutrition.

Treating the underlying cause of congestive heart failure is the best first step. This may involve diseased heart valves, blocked coronary arteries, or toxins that directly damage heart muscle. Often there is no way to correct the cause, so doctors use medication to take some workload off the heart. An angiotensin-converting enzyme inhibitor (ACE inhibitor), such as Prinivil, Vasotec, or Zestril, works to decrease edema. These vasodialators work to relax stiffened blood vessels to make it easier for the weakened heart to push blood through the circulatory system. Diuretics or thiazide diuretics, such as Hydrodiuril, work to decrease edema in the lungs. A weak diuretic Spironolactone is given to some CHF patients because it helps the body hold on to potassium, whereas Lasix (a powerful diuretic) makes patient lose potassium, which then causes other problems. Doctors are now using beta blockers, such as Coreg, Lopressor and Toprol XL, that significantly reduce the risk of hospitalization and death in patients with mild to moderate heart failure. It is believed that this type of medication will become the standard of care for most patients with heart failure.

Coronary Artery Disease

Description—This is a disease of the arteries that surround the heart, carrying oxygen and nutrients to the myocardium.

Signs and symptoms—The lack of oxygen causes the typical symptoms of angina: tightness of the chest and crushing substernal chest pains radiating to the left arm, neck, and shoulder blades. Other symptoms may be nausea, vomiting, fainting, and perspiring. When angina pain persists, it suggests an infarction.

Coronary artery disease may be diagnosed by the ECG during an attack or during a treadmill or exercise bicycle test. An angiograph, also called an arteriograph, allows visualization by x-ray examination of the arteries following injection of a contrast medium into an artery.

Etiology—Characteristically it is caused by atherosclerosis that narrows the blood vessel opening, thereby reducing the volume of blood flow to that portion of the heart muscle served by the arterial branch resulting in angina symptoms.

Treatment—Narrowed, clogged arteries can be treated by three methods. First is the use of nitrates to dilate the vessel. Nitroglycerin in tablet form is placed under the tongue or can be applied in a paste form to the skin surface. When medication does not relieve symptoms and arterial openings are considerably narrowed, other treatments are required. Second, an **angioplasty** can be

performed during catheterization of the heart. A balloonlike device is inflated to compress the fatty deposits against the arterial walls, thereby opening the constricted vessel. This is called a balloon angioplasty (Figure 11–143A). About 54% of the vessels clog again within three years and require a second angioplasty or bypass surgery. Another similar procedure is known as directional coronary atherectomy. It is performed like the conventional balloon procedure except that one side of the tip has a metal cylinder with a cutting blade that is attached to an external motor that rotates the cutter, grinding up the deposits and sucking them out of the catheter (Figure 11–143B). This method is believed to better control the reformation of deposits. A third type of artery procedure is called a coronary stent (Figure 11–143C). A balloon catheter with a stent (stainless steel mesh tube) is inserted into the artery. The balloon is inflated, compressing the deposits toward the sides of the artery and opening up the stent, which expands and stretches the arterial wall. The balloon is deflated and the catheter removed, leaving the stent to keep the vessel open. So far it has produced the best results.

In total, about 700,000 angioplasties are performed each year, often on two or three vessels at a time. Stents are used about 60% to 70% of the time. Research has shown that six months after an angioplasty with a stent in place is performed, patients suffered less pain and less clogging and were less likely to need bypass surgery or additional angioplasty. However, there are some other results. The stent does not seem to decrease the risk of subsequent heart attacks or stroke primarily because the stents can become blocked with clots, scar tissue, or new fatty deposits. In an effort to improve the results with stents, intracoronary radiation at the time of insertion is being tried. The radiation technique called brachytherapy reduces the risk of new obstructions. Some researches feel that perhaps radiation alone might be the most effective because blood clots do not seem to appear later. Stents are also being coated to improve their effectiveness. Either heparin, an anticlotting agent, or rapamycin, an immune-suppressing drug, is used. The coated stents have remained open for eight months in all 30 patients studied, and none have had an additional heart attack, needed a repeat procedure, or died.

Another way to correct clogged arteries is coronary bypass surgery. This entails bypassing clogged arteries by redirecting blood through vein grafts surgically transplanted from the legs to the heart's surface. The replacement vessels, however, are subject to the same disease as the original vessels. Currently, 10% to 15% of bypass surgeries are repeat procedures. A new procedure uses the internal thoracic artery for the graft because it tends to remain free of atherosclerosis longer. Heart surgeons can now operate without opening the chest cavity. The method is called the daVinci Computer-Enhanced Surgical System. Basically, the

(A) Conventional balloon angioplasty

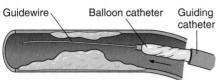

1. In conventional balloon angioplasty, a guiding catheter is positioned in the opening of the coronary artery. The physician then pushes a thin, flexible guidewire down the vessel and through the narrowing. The balloon catheter is then advanced over this guidewire.

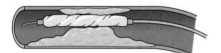

2. The balloon catheter is positioned next to the atherosclerotic plaque.

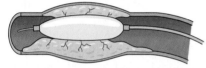

3. The balloon is inflated, stretching and cracking the plaque.

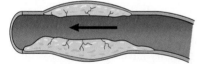

4. When the balloon is withdrawn, blood flow is re-established through the widened vessel.

(B) Coronary atherectomy

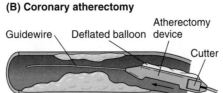

1. In coronary atherectomy procedures, a special cutting device with a deflated balloon on one side and an opening on the other is pushed over a wire down the coronary artery.

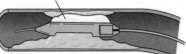

2. When the device is within a coronary artery narrowing, the balloon is inflated, so that part of the atherosclerotic plaque is "squeezed" into the opening of the device.

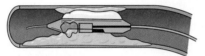

3. When the physician starts rotating the cutting blade, pieces of plaque are shaved off into the device.

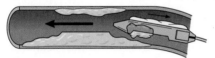

4. The catheter is withdrawn, leaving a larger opening for blood flow.

(C) Coronary stent

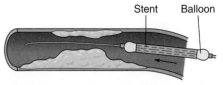

1. To place a coronary stent within a vessel narrowing, physicians use a special catheter with a deflated balloon and the stent at the tip.

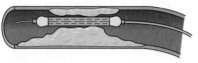

2. The catheter is positioned so that the stent is within the narrowed region of the coronary artery.

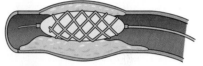

3. The balloon is then inflated, causing the stent to expand and stretch the coronary artery.

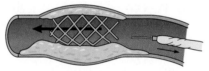

4. The balloon catheter is then withdrawn, leaving the stent behind to keep the vessel open.

FIGURE 11–143   Opening clogged arteries: (A) balloon angioplasty, (B) coronary atherectomy, and (C) coronary stent

surgeon sits at a computer keyboard with a monitor and joystick. The doctor controls robotic arms holding specially-designed surgical instruments and tiny cameras. The robot performs the surgery through tiny incisions in the chest. The vein graft is taken from the inside wall of the chest, thereby eliminating harvesting it from the leg. This new minimally-invasive procedure greatly reduces pain, post-operative scarring, and recovery time, which can be significant with the open-chest method.

Coronary artery disease is best treated by prevention. That includes weight control; a diet low in salt, fats, and cholesterol; regular active exercise; reduction of stress; and refraining from smoking.

Embolism (Em'-bow-lism)

Description—An embolus is defined as foreign matter that enters and circulates in the blood stream. Emboli (more than one) can be composed of blood, exudate, fat, or air.

Signs and symptoms—The symptoms vary according to the location of the **embolism**. Obstruction of a cerebral artery has already been described in CVA symptoms. Smaller emboli produce symptoms in relation to the location and size of the mass. The first symptom of pulmonary emboli is usually dyspnea and probably chest pain. Other symptoms include tachycardia, productive cough (often blood-tinged), low-grade fever, and pleural effusion. Signs may include leg edema, massive hemoptysis (coughing up blood), cyanosis, pleural friction, and signs of circulatory collapse, fainting, and coma. A fatty embolus is potentially fatal if it is in the brain or lung. It typically occurs within 24 to 72 hours following an extremity fracture or trauma. Signs are apprehension, sweating, fever, tachycardia, pallor, dyspnea, pulmonary effusion, cyanosis, convulsions, and coma. A distinctive sign is a petechial rash (small purplish hemorrhagic spots) on the chest and shoulders.

Etiology—A thrombus that forms within a blood vessel becomes an embolus when it breaks loose and begins to circulate. An embolus can also result from air introduced into a blood vessel. An infection may produce a circulating clump of exudate, as discussed under endocarditis. Skeletal fractures cause the formation of fat

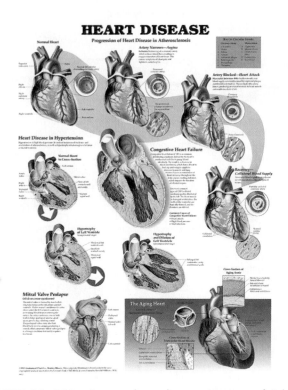

FIGURE 11–144 Common heart diseases (Courtesy of Colwell, a Division of Patterson Dental Supply, Inc., 800-637-1140.)

emboli. One theory holds that minute fat globules from the bone marrow enter the damaged blood vessels at the fracture site. The greatest danger of fat emboli is that they may circulate to the capillary beds in the lungs and block the alveolar exchange, resulting in an insufficient supply of oxygen.

An embolus of any type is potentially lethal if the circulating mass is of adequate size to obstruct the blood supply to a significant portion of an organ. The resulting **infarction** (interference with circulation) is especially rapid when it occurs within a major pulmonary artery or in one of the coronary arteries, and it can be fatal. Infarction of a kidney, the spleen, or the brain will produce symptoms related to the degree of tissue damage. If a nonvital organ is extensively destroyed, surgical removal may be indicated.

Treatment—Depending upon the location of the embolus, treatment can include administering oxygen, use of heparin, reduction of pulmonary edema, chest tubes and tracheotomy to restore and support breathing, medications to cause the mass to disintegrate, antibiotic with an exudate, and other supportive measures.

Figure 11–144 illustrates the most common heart diseases.

Heart Failure

Description—A condition, particularly with the aged, in which the heart pumps too weakly to supply the body

with blood. With severe failure, life expectancy is shortened. A transplant will correct the problem, but most patients with heart failure are too old or have additional medical conditions. Without the transplant, fewer than half survive for two years.

Symptoms—The prime symptoms are weakness, shortness of breath, and others resulting from poor circulation, such as edema.

Etiology—One cause of heart failure is dilated cardiomyopathy, a condition characterized by weakened walls of the left ventricle that allow it to expand outward. Eventually, the expanded walls pull the edges of the mitral valve apart, widening the opening. This results in the valve leaflets being unable to cover the opening, and blood flows backwards (regurgitates) into the left atrium when the ventricles contracts. This only complicates an already compromised circulation. A variety of conditions can contribute to the development of cardiomyopathy, such as viruses, heart attacks, and high blood pressure.

Treatment—Treatment of regurgitation and the loss of pumping strength involves specific medication, such as Aldactone, Coreg, or digoxin, and an ACE inhibitor, such as Vasotec, Prinivil, or Zestril. Diuretics are given to keep excess fluid from collecting in the lungs and extremities.

If drug therapy proves inadequate, then valve replacement or repair may be indicated. Artificial or animal heart valve replacements have been used for quite some time. Replacement procedures involve a temporary but substantial loss of pumping function because left ventricular tissue around the valve is lost when the valve is removed. This procedure is considered too risky for people with severe failure because their function is already critical. A new procedure called annuloplasty repairs the leaky valve by narrowing the expanded valve opening, which greatly reduces or eliminates regurgitation. The surgeon simply sews a plastic ring around the edge of the mitral valve opening, "cinching" it tighter so that the leaflets overlap. In one study of the procedure, only one patient out of 91 died as a result of the surgery. After two years, 80% were still alive, and 70% survived two years. Additional study is continuing, and the results are encouraging.

Heart Replacement

Perhaps the ultimate treatment for severe heart problems is heart transplant. This procedure involves an enormous amount of physical, financial, legal, emotional, and ethical preparation. Usually, the patient is not a good operative risk because of the extent of their disease. There is always an emotional rollercoaster of events while waiting to obtain a donor heart match. Many patients do not survive the wait. Even with the best odds possible, transplantation is not always successful. Some patients have transplant rejections and have been fortunate enough to receive and survive a second successfully. The ability to mentally and emotionally accept the placement of another person's heart into your body can be very difficult. The realization that someone had to die for you to get a chance to survive can be a life-changing experience. Fortunately, trained professionals provide support and counseling to assist in this ultimate procedure.

A new alternative has just been developed which may provide a solution to the transplant dilemma. In July 2001, a patient with only days to live received the first totally implantable, permanent, artificial heart. The Abio-Cor is the an experimental yo-yo–shaped mechanical heart, a plastic and titanium pump weighing less than two pounds. It is powered through the skin by an external battery pack. Earlier, in the mid 1980s, Robert Jarvik developed the Jarvik 7 heart that kept a man alive for more than 600 days. But it was a bulky external machine to which the patient was constantly connected. Jarvik described the new device as false hope, a sincere but misdirected effort. The heart is so large it would only fit in people weighing about 200 pounds. He believes many years of experience have proved cutting out the heart is unnecessary.

The new heart is being tested in at least five patients across the country. Little information has been given about their progress. The first patient appeared on television in late August 2001 with the main people involved in the experiment. He was very thin but was able to walk into the room and speak briefly. He obviously had a long way to go for complete recovery. The developing company has stated that every single patient involved in the experiment is going to die on AbioCor. The initial goal is only 60 days of survival. Only those patients who are ineligible for transplant and who have "end stage" heart disease with less than a month to live will be permitted to participate. If initial trials are successful, they will be expanded, and research will continue. For now, patients are just looking for the chance to interact with their families for a little while longer.

The first patient who had received the artificial heart in July, died November 30, 2001, from complications following a stroke and internal bleeding. He had survived for five full months, far exceeding the initial goal of 60 days. No information has been released about any of the other participating patients.

Hypertension (Hi·per·ten'·shun)

Description—In this condition, blood pressure is consistently elevated above 140/90 for persons under age 50 and 150/90 for those over 50. The severity can be gauged by the diastolic pressure, or the least amount of pressure present during the resting phase of the heartbeat. Mild **hypertension** diastole is about 100 mm Hg, moderate is 110, and severe is over 120 mm Hg.

Signs and symptoms—The presence of elevated blood pressure readings is the only observable sign of hypertension. Some people may sense that their blood pressure is high and experience headache or "feel" pressure.

Etiology—Hypertension may be classified as *essential* (unknown cause) or *secondary* (resulting from another disease or disorder). Essential hypertension is correlated with family history, race, obesity, stress, a diet high in saturated fats and salt, oral contraceptives, and aging.

Secondary hypertension may be the result of kidney disease; thyroid, pituitary, or parathyroid dysfunction; or neurological disorders that interfere with blood pressure regulation. Treatment of the primary cause will reduce the blood pressure.

Hypertension may also be classified as *benign* or *malignant.* In the benign form, the pressure rises moderately over a fairly long period. Malignant hypertension is characterized by an accelerated, rapid, and severe increase, which may not respond to treatment.

Hypertension is the foremost contributing factor to CVAs, kidney damage, and various cardiac conditions.

Treatment—Treatment of hypertension is directed at reducing the elevated pressure and maintaining an acceptable level of blood pressure. It is of great importance to prevent complications of the disease. Treatment focuses around diet, the control of sodium (currently being questioned), the use of diuretics to encourage elimination of retained body fluids, and antihypertensive drugs to reduce vasoconstriction and/or increase kidney filtration. It is of the utmost importance that the patient maintain the treatment regimen because hypertension is not curable, only treatable. Patients must be encouraged to continue with their medication even though they have no symptoms of hypertension. Compliance with dietary and drug therapy is the only means of preventing life-threatening complications.

Hypertrophic Cardiomyopathy (Hy·per·tro'·fick Car·de·o·my·op'·a·the)

Description—This is a disease in which the walls of the ventricles of the heart are markedly thickened, sometimes to three times their normal width. The "muscle-bound" heart is stiff and cannot fill with blood and pump efficiently. It affects an estimated one in every 2,000 people in the United States. It is recognized as an important cause of heart failure and sudden death. Some prominent victims have been young athletes who collapse and die during sports events. The enlargement is for no apparent reason and is not caused by increased workload as with hypertension or aortic narrowing. (Those problems result in left ventricular hypertrophy.) This disease is not to be confused with athletic heart syndrome.

Signs and symptoms—Some signs include lightheadedness, fainting, shortness of breath, heart palpitations, and occasionally chest discomfort like angina. Many patients have a heart murmur. There may also be arrhythmia of the atria and sometimes of the ventricular as well. Rapid ventricular arrhythmia or fibrillation can cause fainting and sudden death in about 2% of patients annually.

Etiology—In some cases the disease is caused by a defective gene located on the 14th chromosome. This form results in 50% of their offspring developing the condition. Other causes are unknown. Diagnosis is confirmed by echocardiogram.

Treatment—Most patients are placed on medication to slow the heart to encourage a relaxation phase using beta and calcium channel blockers. Some patients also require medication to control arrhythmia. Often, strenuous activity is to be avoided. A new experimental therapy involves the use of a permanent pacemaker to change the heart contraction and improve blood flow.

Hypotension (Hi-po-ten'-shun)

Description—It is defined as blood pressure below the normal range. **Hypotension** may become life-threatening when the circulation of blood becomes impaired and the exchange of gases is inadequate.

Etiology—Hypotension can result from an acute blood loss, heart failure, shock, kidney failure, thyroid disease, and other infectious conditions.

Treatment—The treatment of hypotension is determined by the underlying cause. Options include transfusion and intravenous fluid replacement, cardiac stimulants, thyroid medication, and other appropriate drugs.

Leukemia (Lu-keem'-e-ah)

Description—This is a malignant disease of the bone marrow (myelogenous) or lymphatic tissue (lymphocytic). **Leukemia** can be present in either an acute or chronic form. Leukemia will strike 94,200 Americans this year and will cause the death of 51,650.

Signs and symptoms—In the **acute phase**, a great number of immature white blood cells are produced in the bone marrow or lymph tissue. The excessive amount of white blood cells cause pressure and discomfort within the bones, swelling and pain in the lymph nodes, and greatly elevated white blood cell count in the blood. The earliest symptoms of the disease are fever, pallor, fatigue, swelling of lymphoid tissue (spleen, liver), and a tendency toward large bruises.

Even in the presence of great numbers of leukocytes and lymphocytes, the body has little defense against infection because of the immaturity of the cells. The major complication of leukemia is infection. The disease process may progress to produce bleeding within the brain and other vital organs. In acute leukemia, the onset is rapid, and death occurs within a few months unless treated aggressively with chemotherapy. Acute lymphocytic leukemia is the form common in children. Typically it is approximately 30% into its course before it is diagnosed. Acute myelogenous leukemia is more common in adults. Both acute forms are ultimately fatal, but long-term remissions in the childhood form and approximately 70% cures are now being reported.

Chronic leukemia differs from acute only in that its onset is more insidious (slow), and its course is more prolonged. The median survival rate is three to four years.

Signs and symptoms—Often the first symptoms are a general malaise (vague discomfort, feeling "bad") and weight loss. Anemia, fatigue, and greatly enlarged spleen and lymph nodes are typical symptoms. Chronic myelogenous leukemia is almost always associated with a chromosome irregularity known as the Philadelphia chromosome. Chronic myelogenous leukemia is characterized by two distinct phases: the chronic phase, which is insidious, lasting an average of three to four years, and the eventual acute phase, an immature cell crisis, lasting only a few weeks or months before death occurs.

Diagnosis can be confirmed initially by blood studies in addition to typical clinical findings. Differentiation of type and positive identification of acute or chronic forms is possible through cellular and chromosomal analysis of bone marrow aspirates. The bone marrow sample can be withdrawn through a large-gauge needle introduced into the sternum or preferably the posterior superior iliac spine.

Treatment—Treatment varies with the type and form of leukemia. Systemic chemotherapy is used to destroy abnormal white blood cells and induce a remission so that more normal function of the bone marrow will occur. The side effects of the drugs are loss of hair, nausea, vomiting, gouty arthritis, and a number of other complications. Some success has been achieved with bone marrow transplants among siblings, particularly twins. This procedure is especially indicated in treatment of children and younger adults. Before the marrow is given, the patient is medicated with large doses of drugs to completely suppress the body's ability to react to foreign material. Total bone radiation treatments are used to induce marrow aplasia (lack of function) and aid in lowering the body's resistance to the transplant. Approximately 1 liter (1,000 cc) of bone marrow is removed from the pelvic bones of the donor. The marrow is processed and then given to the recipient intravenously. To prevent contact with any microorganisms, the patient is placed in a reverse isolation unit. The patient is in an extremely vulnerable state, and a prolonged hospital stay is inevitable. Barring complications, which are numerous, chances for recovery are good.

Murmur

Description—The abnormal sound of blood flowing through a heart valve can be heard with a stethoscope and is known as a **murmur**. The murmur is named for the valve which is "leaking."

Signs and symptoms—The mitral valve is the one most frequently affected, and the gurgling or swishing sound is called a mitral murmur. Murmurs are further identified as systolic or diastolic. This classification specifies whether the sound is heard during the contraction or relaxation phase of the heartbeat.

Etiology—Valve damage that results in murmurs can be caused by rheumatic fever, an inflammatory disease which follows a streptococcal infection. The valves may become inflamed and in time thicken and develop scar tissue. Hence the valves lose their flexibility and no longer close completely.

Endocarditis is another condition that may lead to valve damage. As previously discussed, bacteria circulating through the heart collect on the valvular surfaces, causing the growth of vegetation and resulting in ulceration and death of some tissue. In its damaged state, the valve is no longer capable of normal function. Preexisting valve damage from rheumatic fever, especially of the mitral valve, is quite common in endocarditis.

Treatment—Artificial or pig valve replacement may be indicated to alleviate the problem if severe enough to interfere with circulation.

Myocardial Infarction (MI) (My-o-card'-e-al In-fark'-shun)

Description—MI is a complication of coronary artery disease that results from occlusion (partial or complete) of the artery, causing myocardial tissue destruction. MIs are one of the leading causes of death in the United States. Mortality is high when treatment is delayed; approximately 50% of patients will die within an hour after symptoms develop.

Signs and symptoms—It is characterized by severe, crushing pain, which radiates through the chest to the neck and jaw and down the left arm. It is not relieved by rest, as with angina, and is accompanied by nausea, perspiration, a change in blood pressure, hypo- or hypertension, and dyspnea.

Etiology—Predisposing factors include sedentary lifestyle, stressful occupation, obesity, cigarette smoking, hypertension, aging, positive family history, and elevated levels of cholesterol and triglycerides in the blood. An attack can often be precipitated by a heavy meal, physical exertion, or exposure to cold weather.

Treatment—Treatment of MI is directed at relieving the pain with strong analgesic drugs, such as demerol or morphine, and administering extra oxygen to maintain an adequate supply to the tissues. It is important to prevent complications. Heart rhythm must be stabilized to prevent arrhythmia, which can lead to congestive heart failure. Complete bed rest must be enforced to decrease cardiac workload and a possible additional infarction. **Anticoagulant** drugs are given to reduce the tendency to develop thromboembolism. The newest treatment includes the immediate use of a clot-busting drug to open the narrowed or blocked coronary artery in order to restore circulation to the myocardium. In about 20% of cases this fails to work, and if there are associated bleeding ulcers or a stroke, it is prohibited. An angioplasty is now being performed on these selective patients and is being evaluated for use with other MI patients. Immediate accessibility to qualified surgeons and angioplasty within one hour is a problem in many areas. In contrast, clot-busting drugs can be administered immediately almost anywhere, possibly even by specially-trained emergency vehicle personnel in the future.

Severe complications may occur in the damaged ventricular area in addition to the systemic threat of embolism and heart failure. Unusual and potentially-lethal conditions may develop. The ventricular septum may rupture, causing a circulatory defect in which blood flows between the ventricles. The ventricular wall may weaken because of necrosis following infarction. The wall may develop an aneurysm, leading to a ventricular rupture.

The patient who survives an MI will be faced with a lengthy recovery period. Lifestyles may need to be altered and dietary and smoking habits changed. An exercise rehabilitation program must be initiated and adhered to to promote optimum recovery and maintenance of a healthy state.

The following information was reported in Consumer Reports on Health in October, 1994.

HOW TO RECOGNIZE A HEART ATTACK

Any of the following symptoms lasting more than two minutes may signal the start of a heart attack.

- A sensation of uncomfortable pressure, fullness, squeezing, aching, or pain, usually located in the center of the chest.
- Pain, aching, or heaviness in the shoulders, neck, jaw, arms, or upper back or spreading to those areas from the chest.
- Pain accompanied by lightheadedness, fainting, sweating, nausea, vomiting, or shortness of breath.

Taking a 325 mg aspirin tablet while waiting for help will help prevent clots from getting any larger.

Clot-dissolving drugs, given intravenously within an hour of the first signs of a heart attack, could prevent about 90% of deaths. Unfortunately, half of all people wait more than two hours before getting to a hospital, often because they do not realize they are having a heart attack.

Phlebitis (Fle-bi'-tis)

Description—This localized inflammation of a vein causes an alteration in the epithelial lining, which is predisposing to the formation of a thrombus. **Phlebitis** can occur in deep or superficial veins (see thrombophlebitis for more information).

Sickle Cell Anemia

Description—This is a congenital anemia occurring primarily among blacks, about 1 in 10 of whom carry the abnormal gene. When two carriers have children, there is a 25% chance that each child will have the disease. When two persons with the disease **sickle cell anemia** have children, all children will have the disease. If only one has the disease and the other is normal, all children will be carriers of the trait.

Signs and symptoms—Sickle cell anemia is characterized by red blood cells with a hemoglobin defect in their molecular structure that causes the cells to become sickle shaped. Cells of this shape cannot pass easily through blood vessels and they tend to interfere with circulation.

Symptoms are tachycardia, cardiomegaly, cardiac murmurs, chronic fatigue, unexplained dyspnea, chest pain, enlarged liver, jaundice, pallor, swollen joints, aching bones, and leg ulcers. These symptoms begin after about six months of age when the protective excess amounts of hemoglobin present at birth are exhausted.

The most common feature of the disease is a painful crisis, which usually appears first at about age five. Sickled red blood cells become tangled, causing blood vessel obstruction and a lack of oxygen to the tissues, with possible destruction of the involved area. This tissue infarction causes severe pain to the affected area. Usual sites are the lungs, liver, bones, and spleen. The spleen, particularly, is affected so frequently that the resulting damage and scarring cause it to shrink and become useless. A crisis usually lasts from four days to several weeks and recurs cyclically.

Diagnosis can be made from a positive family history and the typical clinical features. It is confirmed by a blood smear that shows the sickled cell structure. At present, research has failed to discover a means to prevent the sickling alteration.

The disease produces long-term complications, such as delayed puberty and a tendency toward delayed growth. If the patient survives to adulthood, the body is described as spiderlike, with a narrow trunk and long extremities, curved spine, elongated skull, and barrel-shaped chest. Premature death may result from repeated infarctions within vital organs or from an infectious process.

Etiology—It is an inherited condition caused by a faulty gene.

Treatment—Treatment focuses on alleviating the symptoms of the disease and on transfusions with packed red blood cells when an aplastic crisis occurs (depression of the bone marrow activity and destruction of RBCs). The most successful treatment may be prevention through genetic counseling of persons known to

be carriers. Information is provided to allow individuals to arrive at informed decisions regarding the conception and birth of children.

There is no known cure for sickle cell anemia. However, recently, a cancer drug has been shown to help prevent the attacks. Hydroxyurea (Hydrea) can cut the rate of painful episodes and complication in half, but the drug poses risks, so only adults with the most severe form are advised to take it.

Stasis Ulcer (Stay'-sis All'-sir)

Description—This is a secondary condition resulting from chronic venous insufficiency. The most common site of **stasis ulcers** is the ankle at the internal malleous area.

Signs and symptoms—Varicosities and edema are common. Early signs are dusky red deposits in the skin with itching and dimpling of the tissue. Later, there is redness and scaling of large areas of the legs. Then, cracks develop with crusts and ulcers.

Etiology—Stasis ulcers develop following deep vein thrombophlebitis that destroys the valve structures. Communicating veins in the affected area fail to compensate for the damaged vein. The venous pressure increases, causing fluid to enter the interstitial tissues and produce edema. The tissue swelling leads to fibrosis and skin discoloration from blood entering the subcutaneous tissues. The poor condition of the skin and the inadequate circulation from the area lead to a breakdown of the surrounding tissues (Figure 11–145). They can also be caused by lower extremity trauma or a skin irritation.

Treatment—Treatment of small ulcers involves elevation of the affected extremity, warm soaks, bed rest, and the use of drugs to counteract infection. When the swelling subsides, pressure is applied by a sponge rubber dressing or an Unna's boot (zinc gelatin boot). Large stasis ulcers not responding to treatment may require removal of the ulcer site followed by a skin graft.

Thrombophlebitis (Throm-bo-fle-bite'-is)

Description—This is an acute condition in which the lining of the vein wall becomes inflamed and a thrombus forms. **Thrombophlebitis** can develop within small superficial veins and is usually self-limiting. Deep vein thrombosis (DVT) can affect small or large veins. When there is an alteration of the vein lining, platelets begin to collect at the area. The platelet fibrin catches red blood cells, white blood cells, and additional platelets, forming a blood clot. The thrombus enlarges rapidly, particularly if the blood flow is slow, causing an inflammation that becomes fibrotic. The enlarging clot may completely fill the vein opening, occluding the vessel, or it may break loose, becoming an embolus.

Signs and symptoms—Symptoms of deep thrombophlebitis include severe pain, fever, chills, and possibly edema,

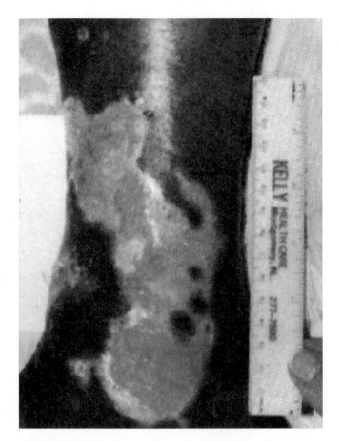

FIGURE 11–145 Venous stasis ulcer (Courtesy of Carrington Laboratories, Inc., Irving, TX.)

with discoloration of the affected extremity. When superficial veins are involved, visible and palpable signs may include heat, swelling, tenderness, redness and discoloration, and induration (hardening) along the affected portion of the vein.

Etiology—DVT usually results from lining damage, but it can also follow accelerated blood clotting and a slow, reduced flow of blood. Conditions that precipitate thrombophlebitis are prolonged bed rest, trauma, childbirth, surgery, and the use of oral contraceptives.

Treatment—Treatment is directed toward preventing complications, controlling the development of thrombi, and relieving the discomfort. The patient is maintained on bed rest, with the affected extremity elevated to aid circulation. Warm, moist soaks are applied to the affected area. Medication is given to relieve pain, and anticoagulants are frequently used to reduce the blood's clotting ability. Antiembolism stockings (tight-fitting, elastic, knee- or thigh-length hose) are indicated to assist the return of blood from the legs to the heart. Individuals who are prone to develop thrombophlebitis should avoid prolonged periods of sitting or standing, especially with little movement, to help eliminate pooling of blood in the lower extremities. When sitting, the legs should be resting on a support that does not cause pressure to interfere with return circulation.

Varicosities (Var-i-cos'-i-tees)

Description—Veins that become dilated, twisted, and inefficient are known as **varicose** veins. The condition usually results from weakness of the valves in the saphenous vein and its branches, which permits blood to leak backward as a result of incomplete closure. As the blood accumulates, the veins become dilated, the valve is no longer capable of reaching across the opening of the vein, and the situation becomes worse.

Signs and symptoms—Symptoms include a feeling of heaviness, night leg cramps, aching, and a feeling of fatigue. With deep vein involvement, edema may accumulate in the feet and ankles, often associated with the discoloration that precedes stasis ulcers. Superficial varicosed veins can often be seen or palpated behind the knees or on the medial surface of the calf. Varicosed veins are not to be confused with the tiny purplish red surface veins seen on the skin of most adults. These are commonly referred to as spider veins and are evidence of increased venous pressure. They are often associated with varicosities.

Etiology—This stasis (stagnation) of blood is often the result of occupations requiring long periods of standing or of other factors interfering with circulation, such as pressure against the veins during pregnancy.

Treatment—Treatment for mild to moderate varicosities includes an exercise program to improve circulation; use of antiembolism stockings; attention to sitting position; and the elimination of tight-fitting or constricting clothing, such as girdles, garters, elastic bands of clothing, and knee-high or thigh-high hose. More severe varicosities may require injection of a sclerosing agent into small venous areas to scar and harden the vein. Larger involvement will necessitate surgical ligation (tying off) of the involved vein from its branches and stripping the vein from the leg.

ACHIEVE UNIT OBJECTIVES

Complete Chapter 11, Unit 8, in the workbook to help you obtain competency of this subject matter.

UNIT 9

The Immune System

OBJECTIVES

Upon completion of the unit, meet the following performance objectives by verifying knowledge of the facts and principles presented through oral and written communication at a level deemed competent.

1. Spell and define, using the glossary at the back of the text, all the **Words to Know** in this unit.
2. List the body's three main lines of defense against antigens.

3. Define the function of the immune system.
4. Identify the three basic services of the immune system.
5. Describe the origin of blood cells.
6. List the organs of the immune system, and identify their locations.
7. Describe the purpose of MHC.
8. Explain the role of the B cell.
9. Identify the four types of T cells.
10. Tell how NK cell action differs from phagocytic action.
11. Explain what causes an inflammatory response.
12. Tell how immunizations and vaccines work.
13. Explain how the acquired immunodeficiency syndrome (AIDS) virus destroys the immune system.
14. Identify five ways to acquire the AIDS virus.
15. List four high-risk behaviors to avoid.
16. Name the three most common opportunistic diseases.
17. Define cancer.
18. Name the classifications of cancer.
19. Identify six characteristics of a cancerous cell.
20. Identify the basic cause of cancer.
21. Describe grading and staging of cancer.
22. List four types or categories of carcinogens.
23. Identify the three categories of diagnostic testing.
24. List the four major cancer treatment methods.
25. List five symptoms of chronic fatigue syndrome.
26. Explain how lupus affects the immune system and the major body organs it may affect.
27. Identify the symptoms of rheumatoid arthritis.

AREAS OF COMPETENCE (AAMA)

This unit addresses content within the specific competency areas of *Administrative procedures, Practice finances, Patient care, Communication skills*, and *Instruction*, as identified in the Medical Assistant Role Delineation Study. Refer to Appendix A for a detailed listing of the areas. (Note: Although *Anatomy and physiology* is not specifically identified in the study, a basic knowledge of the body's structure and function is an essential foundation to the competent performance of many roles.)

WORDS TO KNOW

abstinence	benign
acquired	biopsy
immunodeficiency	brachytherapy
syndrome (AIDS)	cancerous
allergens	carcinoembryonic
allergies	antigen (CEA)
anaphylaxis	carcinogens
antibody	carcinoma
antibody-mediated	cell-mediated
antigen	chemotherapy
autoimmune	clonal
basophils	complement

corticosteroids	monocyte
cytokine	monogamous
cytotoxic	monokine
debilitating	mutation
desensitization	neoplasm
discoid	neutrophils
eosinophils	oncogenes
extracellular	opportunistic
histamine	permeable
homosexual	phagocyte
humoral	prostaglandin
immune	psychoneuroimmunology
immunoglobulin	radiation
immunosuppressed	Raynaud's phenomenon
interferon	remission
interleukin	retrovirus
intracellular	sarcoma
lupus erythematosus	staging
lymphedema	suppressor
lymphocyte	surveillance
lymphokine	thymus
macrophage	transmission
malignant	vaccine
metastasis	virus
monoclonal	

Ⓐ Library

The **immune** system is not usually given the distinction of being identified as a body system. The function of immunity is primarily provided by specific cells and organs of the circulatory system, so it is usually included in that system's discussion. The role of immunity is essential to the health and well-being of humans. When the system misfires or is crippled, a whole host of diseases can develop, such as AIDS, allergy, arthritis, and cancer. Because its function is of such importance, it is being given significance equal to a body system in this text.

We live in an environment full of **antigens**, things that the immune system recognizes as non-self and responds to by destroying or rendering them ineffective. All antigens carry markers that identify them as foreign to the immune system. Foreign materials, bacteria, **viruses**, fungi, and parasites are antigens. Foreign material can be a cell, tissue, a protein, the food we eat, and even particles in the air. Blood from a transfusion or cells and tissue from a transplant are prime examples of foreign material. In abnormal situations, the immune system can mistake self for non-self and attack. This results in the development of an **autoimmune** disease, such as rheumatoid arthritis, diabetes, and lupus. Sometimes, the system responds inappropriately to harmless substances, such as ragweed pollen or cat hair. This kind of antigen is called an **allergen**, and the result is known as an allergy. When one's own cells become **malignant**, their structure changes, making them "different," and a response occurs. Many antigens can cause serious reactions, infections, diseases, and even death.

The body has three main lines of defense against antigens: barriers, the inflammation process, and **antibodies**. The first line of defense are the three types of barriers that prevent entry of antigens. (1) Anatomic barriers are the skin, which covers the body, and the mucous membranes, which line the respiratory, gastrointestinal, and genitourinary tracts. (2) Biochemical barriers are located within the anatomic barriers. Sebaceous glands in the skin secrete antibacterial and antifungal fatty acids and lactic acid. Tears, perspiration, and saliva contain enzymes that attack the cellular walls of gram positive bacteria. Secretions from certain glands make the skin acidic, which is hostile to bacteria. (3) Mechanical barriers work to eliminate substances. Skin sloughs off, and irritated membranes cause coughing. The acts of urinating and vomiting expel materials.

The second and third lines of defense involve cooperation of various components of the immune response that require additional specific explanation before the defense can be understood. For now, inflammation, the second line, occurs when the barriers have been penetrated. This response begins within seconds of an injury or invasion and results in the familiar warm, red, and swollen area that we recognize as an infection. The third line, antibody defense, is a dual-response system involving the actions of specific cells and other immune system components to attack the antigen. This is our immunity and is our last line of defense.

The function of the immune system is to create effective immune responses to continually defend the body against antigens. To do this, the immune system must be able to provide three basic services: (1) identify self and destroy non-self substances, (2) maintain homeostasis, and (3) conduct continual **surveillance**. To understand how these services work, it is necessary to learn about the way each part of the system contributes to the services. The system includes a variety of cells, the organs, the **complement** system, antibodies, cytokines, and the process of surveillance.

ORIGIN OF CELLS

In the last unit, it was stated that cells within the blood are of three types—red, white, and platelets. The leukocytes (white blood cells) were identified as playing a vital role in defending the body. It is these cells in cooperation with protein molecules that are responsible for immunity.

All blood cells originate in the bone marrow and initially develop from stem cells. They progress through different stages of maturation and differentiation until they become mature, functioning cells. Refer to Figure 11–146 as the origin and maturity of cells is explained. Erythrocytes (RBCs)

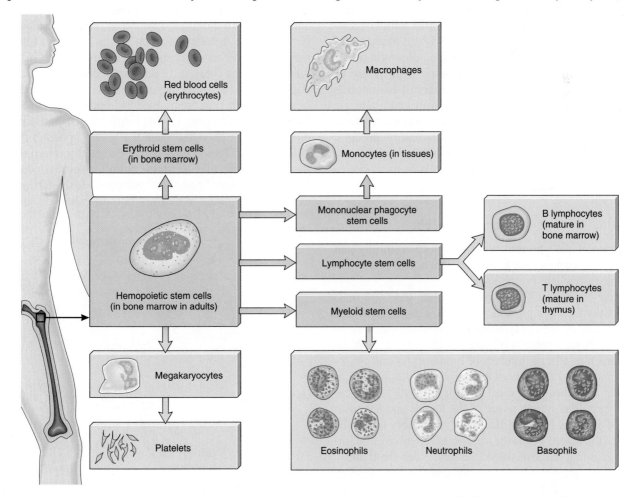

FIGURE 11–146 Origin of cells (From Starr and Taggart, *Biology: The Unity and Diversity of Life,* 5th ed., copyright 1989 by Wadsworth Publishing Company.)

develop from erythroid stem cells and mature in the bone marrow. White blood cells (WBCs), which become the granulated **eosinophils**, **neutrophils**, and **basophils**, develop from myeloid stem cells. One type of agranulocyte, the **lymphocyte**, develops from a lymphocyte stem cell into two major classes: B cells that mature in the bone marrow and T cells that mature in the **thymus**. A granulated cell means that it has granules within its cytoplasm. If no granules are present, the cell is agranulated. Mononuclear phagocyte stem cells become the **monocytes**.

Monocytes are immature cells that have little ability to fight infection. However, once they enter the tissue, they sometimes swell to as large as 80 micrometers, large enough to be seen by the naked eye. At this stage, they are called **macrophages** and are very effective at fighting infection. The most important function of macrophages is phagocytosis, the ability to engulf and destroy antigens. They can phagocytize as many as 100 bacteria and large organisms or cells, such as whole red blood cells and some parasites. Neutrophils are also phagocytic, but in addition, they carry granules of potent chemicals to destroy microorganisms. They can only engulf small particles, such as bacteria.

Neutrophils make up about 40% to 60% of all white blood cells. They are also known as segmentals (segs) and polymorphonuclear neutrophils (PMNs). They attack and destroy invading bacteria, viruses, and other antigens. Eosinophils make up about 2% to 3% of white blood cells. They are weak **phagocytes** when fighting common infections but are produced in large amounts in response to certain parasitic infections. A high number of eosinophils will be found when there is inflammation or an allergic reaction. Basophils release heparin and histamine, which are essential components of the inflammatory process. Eosinophils and basophils are also granulated cells. They release their chemicals onto harmful cells or microbes in their environment.

ORGANS OF THE IMMUNE SYSTEM

The organs of the immune system are located throughout the body and are generally known as lymphoidal organs because they are where lymphocytes develop, grow, and perform their functions. These organs include the bone marrow, the thymus, lymph nodes, spleen, tonsils, adenoids, appendix, and clumps of lymphoid tissue in the small intestine called Peyer's patches (Figure 11–147). The lymph tissue organs house large numbers of lymphocytes and are located strategically throughout the body. The lymph tissue in the Peyer's Patches is exposed to antigens invading the intestinal tract. The lymph tissue of the tonsils and adenoids intercept antigens invading the upper respiratory tract. The tissues in the spleen and bone marrow are involved in fighting antigens that reach the blood vessels. When the B and T lymphocytes leave the bone marrow and the thymus, they travel throughout the body in the blood. They exit the capillaries and enter the **extracellular** fluid surrounding the cells to patrol the environment. As the lymph flows around

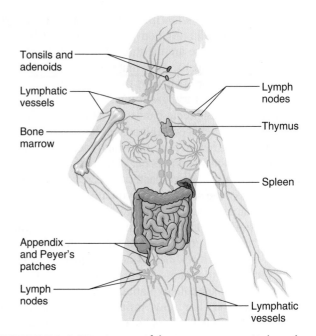

FIGURE 11–147 Organs of the immune system (Adapted from Schindler, *Understanding the Immune System,* United States Department of Health and Human Services.)

the cells and through the body, it carries the lymphocytes, macrophages, and the antigens into the lymph capillaries and vessels. All along the lymphatic vessels are clusters of lymph nodes. A node functions somewhat like a filter. Immune cells and antigens enter the nodes through incoming afferent lymph vessels. Each node contains specialized compartments that store large numbers of B and T cells and others. The antigens are trapped and presented to the T cells for destruction (Figure 11–148). After the response is completed, the lymphocytes leave the lymph nodes in the outgoing efferent lymph vessels that eventually return them to the blood where they begin the patrolling cycle once again.

Now that you know how lymph nodes function, it is easy to understand why they become swollen and ten-

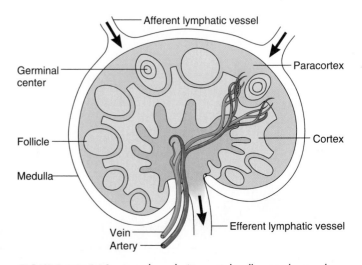

FIGURE 11–148 Lymph node (From Schindler, *Understanding the Immune System,* copyright 1990 by the United States Department of Health and Human Services.)

der during periods of infection. It is because of the increased amount of cellular activity within the nodes. In the same manner, when malignant cells break away from the primary tumor and begin to circulate in the lymph fluid, they become trapped in the nearest nodes. When the nodes cannot contain all the malignant cells, the cells are able to circulate to another body site and begin to produce another area of malignancy. This is known as metastasis. The amount of lymph node involvement is one of the criteria for determining the extent of the cancer. This assessment is called **staging** and is determined by the size of the tumor, the number of involved lymph nodes, and the metastatic progress. As an example, when a mastectomy is performed for breast cancer, the surgeon also removes the lymph nodes that drain from that area of the breast. The nodes are tested for cancer cells, and the results become one factor in determining the staging of the cancer and the plan of treatment.

CELL MARKERS

Basic to the immune system is the ability of immune cells to determine initially the self or non-self status of encountered cells and molecules. All body cells carry molecules that are encoded by a group of genes known as the *major histocompatibility complex* (MHC). This is like a biochemical "fingerprint" that serves as the "ID" for cells so that they are marked as "self." This allows immune cells to recognize and communicate with each other. The body's immune defenses do not normally attack cells carrying this "self" marker. In addition, the millions of lymphocytes have approximately 100 million different surface receptor molecules that can "read" the surface patterns of virtually all non-self molecules that might invade the body. When they meet molecules carrying foreign markers, they move quickly to destroy them. Any non-self substance capable of triggering an immune response is considered to be an antigen. An antigen announces its foreignness by carrying different kinds of characteristic shapes called *epitopes,* which stick out from its surface. The immune system is capable of recognizing millions of these non-self molecules, or it can produce matching molecules that can counteract and destroy the antigen.

The MHC markers enable the immune system to achieve its function of recognizing self from non-self. The second function, homeostasis, involves the maintenance of the steady state of the system. This is accomplished by destroying damaged or dead cells. An example is the function of the spleen when it destroys damaged and dead red blood cells. The third function, surveillance, involves the recognition and destruction of abnormal cells. It is estimated that 100 to 1,000 mutated cells are formed every day. If not held in check by the immune system, cancer might develop. This is demonstrated by statistics showing that individuals who are immunocompromised have an increased risk of cancer.

LYMPHOCYTES

Lymphocytes are the small white blood cells charged with immunity functions. Both T cells and B cells are able to recognize specific antigen targets.

T Lymphocytes

T lymphocytes make up about 80% of all circulating lymphocytes. They are capable of acting directly on their targets by a process called **cell-mediated** *immunity.* They are present in four identifiable types: helper T cells, suppressor T cells, memory T cells, and killer T cells.

- *Helper* T cells produce proteins called **lymphokines** that help other lymphocytes and phagocytes perform their functions. They also help B lymphocytes make antibodies. Helper T cells are identifiable by the CD4+ cell marker. The HIV virus affects the function of the helper T cells and the severity of the disease is measured by the CD4+ blood counts.
- *Suppressor* T cells stop or turn off the actions of the T cells when the "battle" is under control.
- *Killer* T cells can directly kill infected or malignant cells and those cells carrying a target antigen. They are also known as **cytotoxic** T cells and carry the CD8+ cell marker. One type of killer T cell can attach tightly to its target, secrete perforin and other chemicals, which make holes in the target cell's membrane, destroying it before it can reproduce. Unfortunately, killer T cells will also attack the non-self marker cells of transplant tissues and organs causing rejection.
- *Memory T* cells have a memory from a previous experience with specific antigens so are prepared to act immediately upon re-contact.

B Lymphocytes

B lymphocytes represent about 20% of the total lymphocytes. They act upon their targets by producing antibodies in a process called humoral immunity. When B cells are maturing, they go through two stages of development. The first begins with the cell inserting numerous molecules of one specific kind of antibody into its cytoplasmic membrane. Each type of B lymphocyte is capable of making only one type of antibody and only one specific antigen can activate it. There are about 100,000 antibodies on the cell membranes of B lymphocytes. These each have a "combining site" with specific characteristics that will match the same characteristic site on the surface of a specific antigen.

When B cells with their antibody molecules come into contact with antigens, they undergo a second change. When the combining site of a B cell's surface "fits" one of the variety of antigen's surface shapes, they join and are changed into an antigen–antibody complex, and the antibody begins to perform its duties. It causes the antigen to stick to other antigens forming clumps so the large macrophages can destroy large numbers of them at one time.

It also causes the B cell to begin to divide, rapidly producing many clone cells with the same antibody. Later the cells divide into memory or plasma cells (Figure 11–149). The memory cells go to the lymph nodes to stand by for the next same antigen invasion while the plasma cells continue to secrete millions of identical antibody molecules.

The immune system stockpiles a huge arsenal of cells, some for general defense, others for specific invaders. To be able to match millions of antigens, the system stores a few of each kind but can produce millions of the type to match the antigen within a very short period.

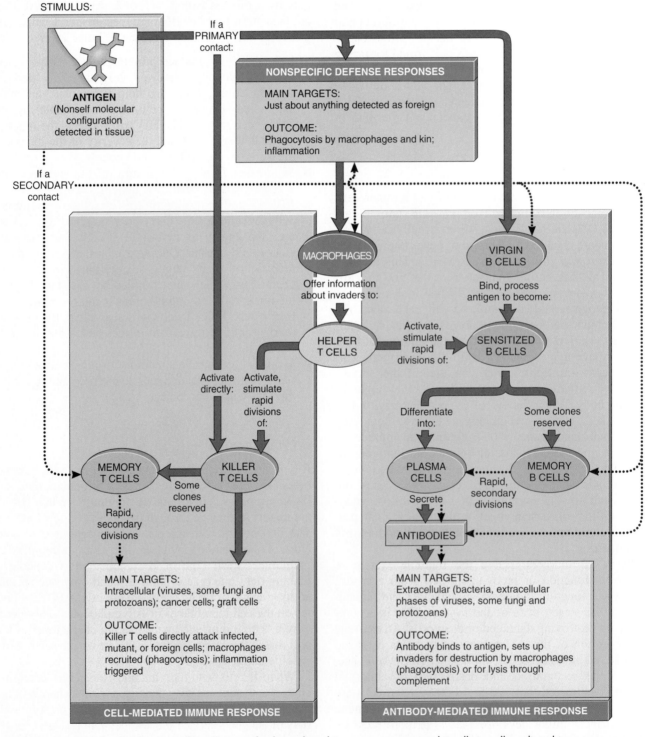

FIGURE 11–149 The development of B cells in antibody-mediated immune response and T cells in cell-mediated immune response (From Starr and Taggart, *Biology: The Unity and Diversity of Life*, 5th ed., copyright 1989 by Wadsworth Publishing Company.)

TABLE 11–6

ANTIBODY CLASS AND FUNCTION	
Class	**Function**
IgA	Concentrated in body fluids, such as tears, saliva, and respiratory and gastrointestinal secretions, to guard the entrances of the body
IgD	Located on B cell membranes. Believed to regulate B cell activity
IgE	Very effective against parasites but also involved in allergic responses, such as hayfever, asthma, and urticaria
IgG	Is the most plentiful antibody. It coats microorganisms in the tissues to speed up the uptake by other immune system cells. It carries out both antibacterial and antiviral activity. It can cross the placenta barrier
IgM	Is found in the bloodstream and is very effective in killing bacteria. It is responsible for initial formation of antibodies once exposed to an antigen

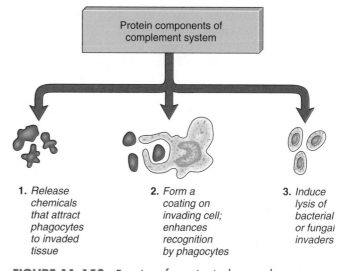

Protein components of complement system

1. *Release chemicals that attract phagocytes to invaded tissue*

2. *Form a coating on invading cell; enhances recognition by phagocytes*

3. *Induce lysis of bacterial or fungal invaders*

FIGURE 11–150 Function of proteins in the complement system (From Starr and Taggart, *Biology: The Unity and Diversity of Life*, 5th ed., copyright 1989 by Wadsworth Publishing Company.)

Antibodies

The antibodies from the B cells are protein substances belonging to a family of large molecules known as **immunoglobulins**. Five classes of human immunoglobulins have been identified and are classified by "Ig" for immunoglobin and a capital letter. The classes are: IgA, IgD, IgE, IgG, and IgM. Their presence in the body can be measured by a blood test called *serum protein electropheresis*. The role of antibodies is summarized in Table 11–6, which lists the antibody classes and key points of their function.

COMPLEMENT SYSTEM

Antibodies may change their shape slightly when they bind with antigens. This change will expose two regions called complement-binding sites. **Complement** is a group of about 20 *inactive* enzyme proteins normally present in the blood and involved in humoral immunity. When one complement protein meets an antibody–antigen complex, it will *activate* and begin a chain reaction of attracting the others to "complement" the activity of the antibodies in destroying bacteria. Complement proteins circulate in the blood in an inactive form. When the first of the complement substances is triggered—usually by an antibody interlocked with an antigen—it sets in motion a ripple effect. As each component is activated in turn, it acts upon the next in a precise sequence of carefully regulated steps known as the "complement cascade." This results in the creation of lethal chemicals to attract the phagocytes to the scene, coat the target cell to make it more recognizable, or destroy the antigen by puncturing its mem-

brane. In this way, antibodies and the complement system work together to destroy antigens by the **antibody-mediated** response also known as **humoral** immunity (Figure 11–150).

Inflammation

The events set off by antibody-mediated response and the other chemicals help to develop an inflammatory response. When complement proteins begin to act, basophils and mast cells are also activated. Both cells release the substance called **histamine**, which dilates blood vessels, slowing down the rate of flow. The vessel walls become more **permeable** which allows fluid to seep into the surrounding tissues. The result is localized warmth, redness, and swelling. The complement proteins and other factors in the fluid can easily leave the blood vessels and attract the phagocytes in the tissues to fight the intruders.

CYTOKINES

Cytokines are non-antibody proteins that regulate the immune response. These substances are diverse and potent chemical messengers. Cytokines produced by T cells are called *lymphokines*. Those produced by macrophages/monocytes are called **monokines**. Another group of cytokines are produced by both lymphocytes and macrophages/monocytes. Lymphokines bind to specific receptors on target cells and set off other actions, such as getting other cells and substances involved, encouraging cell growth, and stimulating macrophages. Two other cytokines are lymphotoxin from lymphocytes and tumor necrosis factor from macrophages. Both of these cytokines kill tumor cells. Many cytokines have been renamed as **interleukins** (IL), which means "messengers between leukocytes." IL-1 from macrophages helps to activate B and T cells. IL-2 is produced by antigen-activated T cells and promotes rapid growth of mature B and T cells and the development of different types of T cells. There are six types of interleukins identified at present.

Some of the first cytokines discovered were **interferons**. They are produced by T cells, macrophages, and some cells outside the immune system. Interferons are a family of proteins that can fight viruses. Interferon from immune cells activates macrophages. The cytokine called tumor necrosis factor, which also comes from macrophages, kills tumor cells and inhibits parasites and viruses. Scientists have genetically engineered genes with cytokines to attack cancer cells. The tumor necrosis factor is measured to determine the effects of chemotherapy on certain cancers.

A summary of the 14 groups of cytokines is included in the Components of the Immune System, a color-treated section of the text following the discussion on immune response.

Natural Killer (NK) Cells

Natural Killer (NK) cells are non-T and non-B lymphocytes. NK cells are numerous in the bloodstream and the reticuloendothelial system. (The tissue macrophages and phagocytes in the blood and lymph.) NK cells kill cancer cells and cells infected with viruses without using antibodies or having prior exposure to the antigen. Like the killer T cell, they contain granules filled with potent chemicals. They bind to their targets and deliver a lethal burst of their chemicals to produce holes in the target cell's membrane leading to its destruction. NK cells get the name "natural" because they do not need to recognize a specific antigen like other T cells in order to kill the invading antigen. The killing function of NK cells can be boosted by the administration of alpha interferon (a cytokine, non-antibody protein that is produced by T cells). Treatment with alpha interferon is used for many types of cancer, including chronic myelogenous leukemia and renal cell cancer, to increase the ability of NK cells to kill the cancer cells.

IMMUNE RESPONSES

The organs of the immune system, immune cells, cell markers, complement system, and related activities have been discussed. It is time to put it all together in an immune response as it would occur in the body.

The immune response system has two branches, one resulting from B cell activity, the humoral or antibody-mediated immune response, and one resulting from T cell activity, the cell-mediated immune response (review Figure 11–149). The response can also be primary when it is the first encounter with the antigen or a secondary response with subsequent encounters.

Primary Humoral (Antibody-Mediated) Response

In primary humoral response, an antigen enters the body and goes undetected past "virgin" desensitized B cells until it meets one with matching antibody sites. The B cell connects (becomes sensitized) and processes the antigen to attract helper T cells. When the sensitized B cell and the helper T combine, interleukins are released, which cause the cell to begin mitosis. At the same time, other similar antigens have been engulfed by the macrophages. Helper T cells bind with the macrophages, and interleukins are secreted. The secretion of interleukin stimulates the helper T cells to mature and secrete lymphokines to cause a rapid growth and division of the B cells. Some of the differentiated B cells become plasma cells and release identical antibodies in order to bind with more antigens for recognition and destruction. Some B cells convert to memory B cells. They do not produce antibodies at the time of the initial exposure, but they "remember" the encounter until the next exposure to the same antigen.

The immunoglobulins get other cells and substances involved. IgM and IgG activate macrophages and the complement system. IgE stimulates mast cells to release histamine. IgA causes secretions in the first line of defense in the saliva, tears, lungs, and intestines to protect the body's entrances. IgD works in the cell's membranes to regulate activity. A full primary immune response requires five to six days to develop.

Humoral antibody-mediated responses act against bacteria and extracellular viruses, fungi, and parasites. It *cannot* react to an invader already within a cell's cytoplasm, only those in circulation or attached to a cell's surface.

Secondary Response

In a secondary response, the reaction is much faster, taking only two to three days. This is possible because leftover **clonal** lymphocytes with memory are able to attack the antigen. Once one of the cells meets the same antigen, mitosis is immediate, and large numbers of appropriately-matched cells and antibodies are produced to destroy the antigen.

Primary Cell-Mediated Response

Primary response of T cells in cell-mediated response is both quick and direct. Some T cells are vital to the operation of other cells. The helper T cells assist B cells to produce antibodies. Helper T cells identify antigens trapped by macrophages. The processed antigen binds with helper T cells and with B lymphocytes. The helper T cells secrete interleukin and the B cell carries out humoral immunity. In cell-mediated immunity, the helper T cells' interleukin secretions activate the killer T cells to attack. Macrophages are recruited, and inflammation is triggered. The NK cells are also stimulated into action to directly destroy **cancerous** and virus-infected cells before they can divide and begin growing.

Some T cells will also develop memory and are held in reserve for subsequent invasions. Cell-mediated immune responses attack **intracellular** viruses, fungi and protozoans, cancer cells, and transplant tissue cells.

Killer cells that cause rejection of organ transplants do so because the MHC markers of the donor cells are not identical self-markers unless they are from an identical twin. Individuals who are to receive organs are given drugs to destroy the killer T cells to prevent rejection; however, that leaves the recipient without the ability to have a full immune response to other invaders and can lead to death from infections such as pneumonia.

Both antibody-mediated and cell-mediated immune responses are controlled reactions. When the "battle" is won, the binding sites are saturated with antibodies, and the **suppressor** T cells stop the attack. Without this feedback, immune reactions would go out of control.

The complexity of the immune system makes it very difficult to understand. The two features on the following pages provide summaries, one of the components and another of the surveillance process, to make the immune system a little clearer. This material is taken from a presentation by Elaine Glass, RN, MS, OCN; Clinical Nurse Specialist in Medical Oncology and Hematology. She explains the functions of the components of the immune system and relates them to the familiar roles of a police and military force (shown in italics). The cell-mediated responses are the duties of the police, whereas the antibody response is the job of the army. There is even one firefighter who is involved. Note that there are also statements in italics and parentheses concerning emotions, exercise, and personal interactions and their effect upon the immune system. This connection is now being recognized as important and as evidence of the impact of diet. Because these effects are often based on multiple and difficult to measure factors and usually cover long periods, studies require long-term commitments from participants and extended time to identify and validate apparent cause and effect relationships in the development of disease.

COMPONENTS OF THE IMMUNE SYSTEM

AGRANULOCYTES

A. Macrophages/Monocytes
The cop on the beat

Monocytes circulate in the blood; macrophages infiltrate the tissues. They engulf antigens and summon other cells to analyze them.

(Stress causes release of cortisol that renders the macrophage unresponsive.

Exercise increases endorphins [natural brain analgesic] which may increase macrophage activity.)

B. Lymphocytes
A collective label for T and B immune cells

1. T CELLS
Involved in the cellular immune system response. Mature in the thymus gland.

a. Helper T cell
The detective

Identifies the antigens trapped by macrophages or monocytes and stimulates other cells to destroy them. Does not attack or destroy by itself.

b. Activated helper T cell
Helps destroy identified antigens by producing interleukin-2, which stimulates other helper and killer T cells to multiply.

c. Killer T cell
SWAT team member

Destroys cells that have been invaded by antigens. They can trigger a process that punctures a cell membrane and destroys it before the invading virus inside has a chance to grow.

d. Natural killer T cell
Rambo or a vigilante

Attacks cancerous or virus-infected cells without previous exposure to the antigen. NKs are stimulated by interferon. They can recognize artificial antigens created in a lab to which humans have never come into contact.

(In one study, patients with a lot of support from their "significant others" and doctors had higher levels of NK cells.)

e. Suppressor T cell
The police chief

Slows down or stops other immune cell activity after antigens are destroyed.

2. B CELLS
Produces antibodies against antigens; involved in the humoral immune response.

a. Plasma cell
The army sergeant

Descends from B cells to produce antibodies. They make thousands of antibodies per second.

b. Antibodies
The foot soldiers

Proteins that neutralize antigens and destroy other cells where the antigen has invaded.

1) IgG

The most common protein antibody in the blood and tissue spaces, where it coats antigens speeding their uptake by other immune cells.

2) IgM

A protein antibody that circulates in the bloodstream in star-shaped clusters, very effective in killing bacteria.

3) IgA

A protein antibody in body fluids (tears, saliva, respiratory and digestive tracts) to guard body entrances.

(College students who watched a video of Mother Teresa had higher levels of IgG and IgA than students who watched a video that did not stimulate positive emotions.)

4) IgE

A protein antibody that attaches itself to mast cells and basophils. When it encounters its matching antigen, it stimulates the cell to pour out its contents. It provides protection by coating bacteria and viruses.

5) IgD

A protein antibody that inserts itself into the membrane of the B cell to regulate the activation of the cell.

c. Complement

Flying Aces

A series of 20 proteins that circulate in the blood in an inactive state until they are triggered by contact with antigen–antibody complexes or by contact with the cell membrane of an invading organism.

T cells = Police chief with a history on the force

B cells = Army sergeant with a history in the service

T and B cells that have been activated by an antigen and continue to circulate within the body, ready to attack an antigen if it reinvades. (These cells are the basis of how vaccines work.)

GRANULOCYTES

A group of immune cells filled with granules of toxic chemicals that enable them to digest microorganisms.

A. Neutrophil

Like cop on beat but more heavily armed

A circulating WBC that destroys foreign matter and cell debris by phagocytosis, by digesting cellular membranes, and by releasing chemotactants and pyrogenic substances that cause fever.

B. Basophil

A firefighter

A circulating WBC that is responsible for allergy symptoms by releasing heparin, histamine, bradykinin, and serotonin from its granules, to cause vasodilation and permeability.

C. Eosinophil

A circulating WBC that can digest microorganisms, especially parasites, and assists in allergic reactions by detoxifying some of the inflammation-inducing substances to prevent the spread of the local inflammatory process.

D. Mast cells

Special member of police force that is armed with chemicals.

Special cells found in tissues that contain granules of chemicals that produce redness, warmth, and swelling (allergy symptoms).

CYTOKINES

All non-antibody proteins that regulate the immune response. Cytokines produced by T cells are called *lymphokines*. Cytokines produced by macrophages/monocytes are called *monokines*.

A. Lymphokines

A number of proteins produced by T cells

1. Granulocyte-macrophage colony-stimulating factor (GM-CSF)

GM-CSF stimulates the growth of neutrophils, eosinophils, and macrophages. It increases the ingestion of bacteria and the killing of tumors coated with antibody. It activates mature granulocytes and macrophages.

2. **Interferons**

A class of lymphokines with important immunoregulatory functions, especially improving the activities of macrophages and NK cells. *Exercise may increase the production of interferon.*

a. Alpha (IFN-α)

Is produced by leukocytes in response to viral infections. It also increases NK activity and the numbers of cytotoxic T cells and starts the tumoricidal activity of macrophages.

b. Beta (IFN-β)

Its activity is similar to IFN-α.

c. Gamma (IFN-γ)

Is produced by T and NK cells. It (1) activates killer T cells; (2) increases the ability of B cells to produce antibodies; (3) keeps macrophages at the site; and (4) assists them in digesting bacteria and cancerous cells they engulf. IFN-γ also regulates other lymphokines, increases NK activity, and starts the production of T cell suppressor factor.

3. IL-2 (Interleukin-2)

Is produced by helper T cells and NK cells, which stimulates other helper, killer, and suppressor T cells to multiply. It starts cytokine production by T cells and monocytes. It improves NK cell activity.

4. IL-3

Is produced by activated T cells. It is a growth factor for mast cells and most bone marrow progenitor (after stem) cells.

5. IL-4

Is called B cell growth factor and causes B cells, mast cells, and resting T cells to multiply. It increases toxicity of killer T cells and macrophages. It is produced by helper T cells.

6. IL-5

Is produced by activated T cells. It is an important factor in the final differentiation of eosinophils and activated B cells. It increases IgA, IgM, and IgE development and secretion. It begins the appearance of IL-2 receptors on B cells.

7. Soluble immune response suppressor (SIRS)

SIRS is released by suppressor T cells and may slow down immune cell activity.

B. **Monokines**

Proteins produced primarily by monocytes

1. Granulocyte colony-stimulating factor (G-CSF)

G-CSF stimulates the growth and activity of neutrophils. It is produced by monocytes and some other nonblood cells.

2. Macrophage colony-stimulating factor (M-CSF)

M-CSF stimulates the growth and activity of macrophages. It is also produced by monocytes and other nonblood cells.

(GM-CSF, G-CSF, IL2, and Interferon are now produced synthetically and are being used as anticancer drugs. They have shown promise in the treatment of some types of malignancies.)

C. **Other cytokines**

(Produced by both lymphocytes and macrophages/monocytes)

1. IL-1

Is produced by macrophages, T cells, granulocytes, and NK cells. It activates helper T cells and raises the body's temperature. (Fever increases immune cell activity). It stimulates the production of lymphokines and activates macrophages to immobilize cancer cells. It starts the differentiation of stem cells and activated B cells and increases the number of activated B cells. Exercise may increase IL-1 production.

2. IL-6 (B cell differentiation factor)

Is called BCDF, which causes some B cells to stop dividing and to start making immunoglobin and antibodies. Improves the differentiation of killer T cells. Is produced by helper T cells, monocytes, and fibroblasts. It also stimulates the production of platelets.

3. Tumor growth factor-beta (TGF-β)

TGF-β is produced by T cells, macrophages, and tumor cells. It suppresses T and B cell growth and differentiation and antibody secretion.

4. Tumor necrosis factor-B (TNF-B)

TNF-B, also known as lymphotoxin, is produced by B cells, T cells, mast cells, and macrophages. It makes some cells more vulnerable to lysis by NK cells.

5. Tumor necrosis factor (TNF)

TNF is produced by monocytes, activated macrophages, NK cells, and mast cells. It can kill tumors or retard their growth. It causes some tumors to bleed and die. It stimulates the production of lymphokines and activates macrophages.

By now, you must be amazed at the complexity and function of the immune system. The previous outline of the duties of its components causes one to wonder how all that coordinated effort ever gets accomplished. And yet, so much more is not understood.

To give a brief overall picture of what happens when an immune system cell comes into contact with an antigen, consider the following box. In italics within parentheses are descriptions of the cartoon slides Elaine uses to summarize her discussion of the surveillance process of the immune system. She again uses the police and military roles in the scenarios. If you can visualize the scene, it may help you to get an understanding of the immune process.

IMMUNE SYSTEM SURVEILLANCE PROCESS

1. A macrophage (or complement protein, NK cell, or memory cell) recognizes an antigen.

   (A cop begins to struggle with an alien.)

2. Helper T cells bind to the macrophage and become activated by the cytokine, IL-1, which also causes fever.

   (The detective sees the cop and alien struggling and calls for help.)

3. Activated helper T cells produce a lymphokine, IL-2, which stimulates other helper and killer T cells to multiply.

   (Help arrives as detectives, SWAT team, and a few army sergeants.)

4. Helper T cells also secrete a lymphokine, IL-4, which causes B cells to multiply.

   (The detective decides more army personnel are needed and calls in the troops. The army comes marching in.)

5. Helper T cells also secrete a lymphokine, IL-6, which causes some B cells to stop dividing and start making antibodies.

   (The sergeant calls the foot soldiers into duty.)

6. Helper T cells also produce the lymphokine interferon, which activates killer T cells, increases the ability of B cells to produce antibodies, and keeps macrophages at the site and assists them in digesting the cells they engulf.

   (The detective calls out words of encouragement to the SWAT team, the sergeants, and the street cops.)

7. Killer T cells destroy the cells where antigens have invaded.

   (The SWAT team member nails an alien inside a phone booth.)

8. Antibodies neutralize the antigen and destroy other cells that have also been infected.

   (A foot soldier punches out an alien.)

9. Complement proteins, triggered by antigen–antibody complexes, or the cell membranes of some invading microorganisms:

   (The flying aces come into the action.)

   - Cause chemotaxis of macrophages and neutrophils to the area. *(An ace calls in the street cop.)*
   - Increase phagocytosis of macrophages and neutrophils. *(The street cops look mean and ugly.)*
   - Activate basophils and mast cells to release immobilizing chemicals and other products that increase inflammation. *(The firefighters and cops with chemicals soak the aliens.)*
   - Change the invader's cell surface, causing them to stick together. *(The aliens get stuck.)*
   - Attack the invader's structure and make it inactive. *(The aces crop-dust the aliens.)*
   - Rupture the invader's cell membrane. *(The ace's gunner blows a hole through the alien.)*

10. Suppressor T cells halt the immune response after the antigen is destroyed.

    (The police chief enters the scene and halts the action once the aliens are destroyed.)

11. Memory T and B cells are left in the blood and lymph system to defend against another attack.

    (The detectives and the army sergeants have the alien's ID in case future attacks occur.)

NOTE: Scientists have made great progress in understanding the functions of the many components of the immune system, but a great deal still remains a mystery. It is an unbelievably complicated interaction of cells, antibodies, and proteins against antigens and allergens. Recently, it has been recognized that the brain, nervous system, and hormones also have a relationship with the immune response. A new science called **psychoneuroimmunology** involves researching the connection between the brain, behavior, and immunity. Scientists have discovered that the brain produces over 50 neuropeptides that have receptors on WBCs and can affect the cell's activity. For example, people who feel hopeless have sluggish macrophages. Laughter increases NK activity, lymphocyte proliferation, migration of monocytes, and the production of IL-2 and IgA. It would seem we may have the power to influence our own immune system if we can learn how.

IMMUNIZATION

With the knowledge of immune reactions, it is easy to understand how immunizations (shots) and vaccinations provide protection against antigens. The smallpox **vaccine**, for instance, is the deliberate introduction of the smallpox antigen into the body in a state that causes only minor reaction, but it is sufficient for the body to produce an antigen–antibody complex and eventually memory cells against the disease. Other examples of purposeful antigen introduction are measles, mumps, diphtheria, hepatitis, pneumonia, pertussis, and tetanus toxoid (given routinely to infants and children).

Vaccines are given in initial and in "booster" doses to provide memory cells and antibodies for longer periods. These methods provide active immunity because the recipients make their own immunity. Another form is known as passive immunity and is given to people already exposed to a disease, such as tetanus. Antibodies from another source are injected into the person to provide a temporary immunity to counter the immediate attack of pathogens. This immunity is short lived. The tetanus antitoxin given after certain injuries or animal bites is an example of this type of vaccine.

DISEASES AND DISORDERS

Acquired Immunodeficiency Syndrome (AIDS) (A-qui'-erd Im-mu-no-de-fish'-en-see)

Description—**Acquired immunodeficiency syndrome** (AIDS) is a worldwide epidemic caused by the human immunodeficiency virus (HIV). The term AIDS refers to the most advanced stages of HIV infection. It is estimated that there are 36 million people in the world living with HIV infection. The AIDS epidemic is greatest in Sub-Saharan Africa. However, the largest increase in HIV/AIDS in 2000 was reported by the Russian Federation. Their incidence was larger than all previous years combined. In August 2001, China also revealed that HIV was rapidly increasing in part because of unscreened blood donations and medical practices of reusing needles. The beginning of AIDS in the United

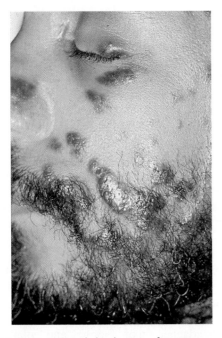

FIGURE 11–151 Typical skin lesions of Kaposi's sarcoma (Courtesy of Robert A. Silverman, M.D., Clinical Associate Professor, Department of Pediatrics, Georgetown University.)

TABLE 11–7

CUMULATIVE AIDS CASES BY AGE

Age	# of Cumulative AIDS Cases
Under 5:	6,812
Ages 5 to 12:	1,992
Ages 13 to 19:	3,865
Ages 20 to 24:	26,518
Ages 25 to 29:	99,587
Ages 30 to 34:	168,723
Ages 35 to 39:	168,778
Ages 40 to 44:	124,398
Ages 45 to 49:	72,128
Ages 50 to 54:	38,118
Ages 55 to 59:	20,971
Ages 60 to 64:	11,636
Ages 65 or older:	10,378

States is well documented. Between October 1980 and May 1981, five young, previously-healthy **homosexual** men were treated for a pneumonia caused by *Pneumocystis carinii*. They were treated at three different hospitals in Los Angeles. Doctors and health care professionals were curious because usually *P. carinii* pneumonia occurred only in **immunosuppressed** patients, especially those receiving cancer therapy. At the same time, a rare and unusual blood vessel malignancy called Kaposi's sarcoma was being diagnosed with increasing frequency in young homosexuals in California and New York (Figure 11–151). By July 1981, 26 cases of Kaposi's sarcoma had been diagnosed. Seven of these men also had serious infections; four had *P. carinii* pneumonia. These cases were an early indication of an epidemic of a previously-unknown disease. Later it was called the acquired immunodeficiency syndrome, or AIDS. As of June 2000, a total of 753,907 cases have been reported—745,103 adults and adolescents with 620,189 being male and 124,911 being female. Of these cases, the total number of reported deaths is 438,795, about 58% of the infected.

A PEDIATRIC PERSPECTIVE

There have been 8,804 AIDS cases reported in children under 13. During the same time, 5,086 children under age 15 died, also about 58% of the infected.

Table 11–7 lists the Cumulative AIDS cases by age. Observe that a very large number of patients, about 529,895 (approximately 70%), are less than 45 years old. This translates into a lifelong battle against the disease for a lot of people. This also translates into billions of dollars needed for their care.

The Centers for Disease Control and Prevention (CDC) in Atlanta, Georgia, reports that as many as 900,000 Americans may be currently infected with the virus. The CDC Surveillance Report (Vol. 12, 2000) indicates the epidemic is growing most rapidly in minority populations. AIDS affects seven times more African-American males that white males and three times more Hispanic males than white males.

Table 11-8 identifies the incidence of HIV/AIDS statistics as indicated in the CDC report.

TABLE 11–8

INCIDENCE OF HIV/AIDS

Estimated number of adults and children infected and living with HIV worldwide	36 million
Estimated number of adults and children who have died from AIDS worldwide	21.8 million Of these, 4.3 million are children
Estimated number of Americans currently living with HIV/AIDS	900,000
Estimated cases of AIDS in the US since 1981	753,907
Number of deaths from AIDS in the US since 1981	438,795

Etiology—AIDS is an infectious disease caused by the human immunodeficiency virus (HIV), which renders the body's immune system ineffective. The virus has been found in many body fluids but survives well only in those with numerous WBCs, such as blood, semen, and vaginal secretions. The virus invades the helper T cells and macrophages, hiding within their membranes. Because both stimulate one another at different times in the immune response, when the helper Ts are "disabled," they do not cause the macrophages to act, which results in the diversion of B cell antibody production and the absence of NK cell formation. HIV is a **retrovirus**: its genetic material is RNA instead of DNA. It wraps itself in components from the host helper T cell membrane. Once inside the host, an enzyme uses the viral RNA as a "pattern" for making DNA and inserts these new instructions into the host's chromosome.

The virus hides in the cells for months or even years. It is difficult to determine its average or maximum incubation period. The onset of AIDS following infection with the HIV virus has been observed from as little as six months to as many as 10 years or more. The average onset of symptoms of AIDS appears to be 10 years. At some time, the body makes a secondary response, and the infected cells are activated. They copy their new DNA with the viral RNA, and new virus particles are assembled. They form "buds" on the helper T cell membrane and separate. This process continues until the helper T cells are depleted and the immune system is destroyed, leaving the person vulnerable to opportunistic infections which may eventually cause death.

The HIV virus requires certain conditions to be able to transfer to a new host. Avoiding these situations will decrease the risk of becoming infected. The virus can be transmitted by the following methods:

- Unprotected sex with an infected partner. **Transmission** can occur through the vagina, vulva, rectum, penis, and mouth during sex.
- Sharing drug needles or syringes with a person infected with HIV.
- Women with HIV can transmit the virus to their babies during pregnancy, birth, and breast-feeding. Twenty-five to thirty-three percent of infected mothers will transmit the infection to their babies. (The medication AZT [zidovudine] and delivery by cesarean section can significantly reduce the transmission rate.)
- The risk of getting HIV from blood transfusions is extremely low. All blood in the United States is screened for HIV.
- The risk to health care professionals of obtaining HIV from accidental needle sticks and contact with blood and body fluids. These risks are eliminated by following protective Standard Precautions when providing care.

There are some people who fear that HIV can be transmitted in other ways, but it has not been proven by research. The most common misconceptions are:

- Casual contact with an infected person through sharing food utensils, towels, toilet, telephones, bedding, or swimming pools.
- Closed-mouth kissing. The CDC does recommend eliminating open-mouth kissing, although the risk is very low.
- Mosquitoes, bedbugs, or other biting insects.
- Tattooing and body piercing could theoretically transmit the virus if the open skin area comes into contact with the organism or if contaminated instruments are used. There have been no instances of HIV transmission in the United States from either activity.

Early signs and symptoms—Many people who are infected with the virus do not have any symptoms when first infected. Within a month or two after exposure, others, however, may have a flu-like illness that includes headache, fever, fatigue, and enlarged lymph nodes. The symptoms usually subside within a week. During this flu-like period, the HIV virus is present in high concentrations in genital fluids, and infected persons are highly contagious.

Later signs and symptoms—Severe symptoms of HIV infection may not appear for 10 or more years in adults and two or more years in children. However, during this asymptomatic period, the infected person is still capable of passing on the virus, and the T helper cells are being systematically destroyed. The numbers decline (as measured by the CD4 [T4] counts) and infections and other symptoms begin to occur, such as:

- Enlarged lymph nodes
- Fatigue
- Pelvic inflammatory disease
- Fever, sweats
- Weight loss
- Yeast infections
- Rashes, dry skin
- Short-term memory loss

Late signs and symptoms of AIDS—The signs and symptoms of AIDS are related to the effects of infections and cancer.

The presence of the opportunistic infections, such as *Pneumocystis Carinii Pneumonia,* are indicated by a fever, cough, and difficulty breathing; by *Kaposi's Sarcoma,* a form of cancer appearing as purplish blotches on the skin (Figure 11–151); by *Candidiasis,* a yeast infection that is sometimes present in the mouth, esophagus, and vagina; and by the usual infections. There are over 20 opportunistic infections that people with AIDS may experience, such as other forms of pneumonia, meningitis, encephalitis, esophagitis, persistent diarrhea, and skin inflammation. These are often resistant to treatment. About 60% of AIDS patients have neurological symptoms, including motor problems, inability to concentrate, memory loss, and progressive mental deterioration. They are believed to be caused by brain infection or cancer.

Diagnosis of HIV Infections Early HIV infection usually has no signs or symptoms, therefore it can only be detected by a blood test or by testing saliva. Blood tests detect antigens found on the virus or detect antibodies made against HIV. The antibodies may not be detectable for one to four months after infection and may be as long as six months before enough antibodies are present in the blood to test positive.

There are two different tests for HIV antibodies, the *ELISA* (enzyme-linked immunosorbent assay) and the *Western Blot*. A general guideline used is if the ELISA test is reactive, it is repeated two more times. If it is positive three times, a Western Blot test is performed. The Western Blot is used to confirm the diagnosis because a small number of ELISA tests may show a false positive. Another test called the Coulter HIV-p24 Antigen Assay can detect the presence of HIV antigens. In the clinical setting, it is used when patients are highly suspected to be positive but show negative tests on both the ELISA and Western Blot tests.

Home testing for HIV is available and is increasing the process of testing, primarily because it protects the patient's identity. Some tests use a blood sample, whereas another, called the Orasure, uses a treated cotton pad to collect an oral sample between the gum and cheek.

Physicians can now predict the risk of HIV progressing to AIDS by monitoring the HIV virus levels in the blood. The test is based on studies that have shown that higher levels of the virus in the blood correlate with an increased risk of the disease progressing to AIDS and AIDS-related infection or death.

Diagnosis of AIDS The CDC diagnosis for AIDS requires a positive confirmed test for HIV and at least one of the following:

- CD4 count less than 200 per cubic millimeter of blood or a CD4 count of less than 14% of the total number of lymphocytes. The CD4 count measures the number of helper T lymphocytes.
- The presence of an **opportunistic** infection, such as pneumocystis pneumonia.
- An AIDS-related cancer, a severe wasting, or dementia.

Table 11–9 lists the clinical conditions in patients which indicate AIDS.

AIDS Prevention AIDS can be prevented by practicing personal measures to protect oneself. The disease is contracted primarily through contact with an infected person's blood, semen, or vaginal secretions. The virus enters through the vagina, penis, rectum, or mouth (in oral sex). The safest lifestyle is sexual **abstinence** or a faith-

TABLE 11–9

CLINICAL CONDITIONS IN PATIENTS WITH AIDS

AIDS Indicator Diseases

OPPORTUNISTIC INFECTIONS

Candidiasis: bronchi, esophageal, trachea, lungs

Coccidioidomycosis

Cryptococcosis, extrapulmonary

Cryptosporidiosis, chronic intestinal greater than one month in duration

Cytomegalovirus, other than liver, spleen, or nodes

Cytomegalovirus retinitis with loss of vision

Disseminated histoplasmosis

Herpes simplex: chronic ulcers >one month in duration or bronchitis, pneumonitis, or esophagitis

Histoplasmosis, disseminated

HIV encephalopathy

Isosporiasis, chronic

Mycobacterium avium complex or *M. kansasii*, disseminated or extrapulmonary

Mycobacterium of other species

Pneumocystis carinii pneumonia

Pneumonia, recurrent in 12-month period

Progressive multifocal leukoencephalopathy

Salmonella septicemia

Toxoplasmosis of the brain

Tuberculosis, extrapulmonary

Tuberculosis, pulmonary

AIDS-RELATED CANCERS

Burkitt's lymphoma

Immunoblastic lymphoma

Lymphoma, primary brain

Invasive cervical cancer

Kaposi's sarcoma

OTHER

HIV wasting syndrome

ful **monogamous** relationship. If these conditions are not absolutely certain, then precautions must be taken.

1. Avoid high-risk sexual activities. Behaviors that may cause you to acquire the virus are clear:
   - Having unprotected sex, homosexual or heterosexual, with an HIV-infected person (oral, vaginal, or anal).

- Using IV drugs and sharing needles.
- Having many sexual partners; risk increases with number of partners.
- Having other sexually transmitted diseases, such as gonorrhea, syphilis, or genital herpes.
2. Use a latex condom *properly* to maintain a barrier to the transmission of the virus. It must stay intact and be in place from the beginning to the end of vaginal, anal, or oral sex. The use of a spermicide provides additional protection. The condom must be carefully removed and disposed of properly. Condoms must never be reused.

Treatment—Unfortunately, no vaccine, antitoxin, or drug "cures" AIDS. In 1981, when AIDS was first diagnosed in the United States, there were no effective medications to treat the disease. Over the past 10 years, researchers have developed drugs to fight the virus, the associated infections, and the cancers. A number of medications to treat HIV infection have been approved by the Food and Drug Administration (FDA). The virus can become resistant to any of these drugs; therefore, combinations of medications are used. All medications and combinations used to treat HIV have numerous side effects, including bone marrow suppression, nausea, and nerve damage. The side effects decrease the individual's compliance to taking the medications.

Medications to Treat HIV and AIDS

The following medications are used to treat HIV and AIDS.

- Nucleoside Reverse Transcriptase (RT) Inhibitors— These drugs interrupt an early stage of the virus from making copies of itself. They can slow the spread of HIV and delay the onset of opportunistic infections. Examples are AZT (zidovudine or ZDV), ddC (zalcitabine), ddI (didanosine), and d4T (stavudine).
- Protease Inhibitors—The inhibitors interrupt virus replication at a later stage in the lifecycle. Examples include ritonavir (Norvir), saquinivir (Invirase), and indinavir (Crixivan).
- Highly Antiretroviral Therapy (HAART)—HAART is a treatment regimen that combines reverse transcriptase inhibitors and protease inhibitors. It is considered highly effective and is believed to be responsible for reducing the number of deaths from AIDS by almost half in the United States. Patients who are newly infected with HIV and those with AIDS can take HAART. It has been found to decrease the amount of circulating virus to almost undetectable levels. However, it still cannot eliminate HIV from the body.

Treatment of Opportunistic Infections and Cancer

A variety of at least 22 FDA-approved medications are available to prevent and treat the many opportunistic infections and cancers experienced by patients with AIDS. Table 11–10 lists some of most common.

TABLE 11-10

MANAGEMENT OF OPPORTUNISTIC INFECTIONS IN AIDS	
Acyclovir	Herpes infection
Amphotericin B	Candida and aspergillus fungal infections
Fluconazole	Candida infections
Foscarnet	Cytomegalovirus infections of the eye
Gancyclovir	Cytomegalovirus infections of the eye
Interferon alfa-2a	Kaposi's sarcoma
Interferon alfa-2b	Kaposi's sarcoma
Pentamidine	Pneumocystis carinii pneumonia
Trimethoprim/ sulfamethoxazole	Pneumocystis carinii pneumonia

HIV Vaccines Research is being conducted in the United States and throughout the world to develop a safe and effective vaccination against HIV infection. The vaccines are designed to induce the development of antibodies to different strains of HIV.

Needless to say, AIDS must be prevented. To obtain a free brochure, materials, and confidential AIDS counseling, call the toll-free National AIDS Hotline (800–342–AIDS). Information is also abundant on the Internet. Search under various sites, such as CDC, AOL Health, and AIDS organizations.

Allergies (Al'-ler-gees)

Description—Sometimes the immune system can damage instead of protect the body. A secondary response to a normally harmless substance is seen in **allergies** and may actually damage tissues. About 15% of humans are predisposed to become sensitive. Allergies may affect different areas of the body.

In the nose—as hay fever or allergic rhinitis.

In the lungs—as asthma.

In the eyes—as conjunctivitis.

On the skin—as eczema, contact dermatitis, or hives.

In the digestive tract—as cramps, vomiting, and diarrhea.

When exposed to the sensitive allergens, the antibody IgE is produced, resulting in allergic symptoms. With each additional exposure to the allergen, IgE antibody is produced and becomes attached to the mast cells or basophils, which in turn release histamine and **prostaglandins** (Figure 11–152).

Signs and symptoms—The histamine causes the mucous membranes to secrete and capillaries to become more permeable. Prostaglandins constrict smooth muscle in

Allergy

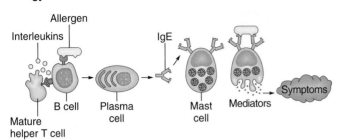

FIGURE 11–152   Response to allergens (From Schindler, *Understanding the Immune System,* copyright 1990 by the United States Department of Health and Human Services.)

some organs, such as the bronchioles of the lungs. The two initiate a local inflammatory response. With hay fever or asthma, for example, there is sneezing, runny nose, congestion, and difficult breathing.

Exaggerated reactions to allergens can be life-threatening. For instance, some people are very sensitive to bee stings and certain drugs. The histamine and prostaglandins cause extensive bronchial constriction, mucous production, and excessive capillary permeability. Breathing is difficult and extensive loss of blood plasma drastically lowers the blood pressure leading to circulatory collapse and death. This reaction is known as **anaphylaxis**, and the situation is called *anaphylactic shock.*

Etiology—The most common causative substances are dust, animal hair, certain foods, pollen, insect stings, and drugs. Other factors, such as emotional state, air pressure or temperature change, and infections, can either trigger or complicate allergic reactions.

Diagnostic procedures to confirm allergies consist of blood counts to determine eosinophil numbers (an increase denotes allergy), chest x-ray to determine congestion and perhaps focal atelectasis (mucous plugs with asthma), and pulmonary function test to evaluate lung condition. Often there is a family history of sensitivity. A series of skin tests can identify allergic substances (see Chapter 16).

Treatment—Treatment consists of eliminating contact with allergens and other causative factors as much as possible. **Desensitization** to specific allergens may be helpful. By injecting minute amounts of the allergen intradermally and gradually increasing the amount, the body can be caused to produce IgG antibodies that circulate and bind with the allergen, prohibiting its interaction with IgE. In addition, antihistamines, bronchodilators, antibiotics for secondary infection, and sometimes corticosteroids are helpful.

Cancer

Description—Cancer is a large group of diseases characterized by uncontrolled cell growth, tissue destruction, and spread of abnormal cells. It is the second leading cause of death in adults and the leading cause of death among children ages 1 through 14 in the United States. The American Cancer Society statistics for 2001 estimated that 1,268,000 Americans would be diagnosed with cancer and 553,400 would die during the year. One out of every four Americans is diagnosed with cancer. With proper treatment, 60% will survive five or more years after their diagnosis. Medical and surgical oncologists, physicians with specialized education in the management and treatment of cancer, are best suited to deal with this complicated disease. Figure 11–153 illustrates the leading sites of new cancer and deaths estimated for the year 2001 by the American Cancer Society.

A PEDIATRIC PERSPECTIVE

Childhood cancer, though rare, is the chief cause of death by disease in children between birth and age 14. An estimated 8,600 new cases and 1,500 deaths were expected to have occurred in 2001. Early detection of cancer in children is often difficult to recognize.

Characteristics of Cancer Cells

The word **neoplasm** is defined as new growth and can refer to both **benign** and malignant tumors. Both types of tumors contain growing tumor cells, connective tissue, and blood vessels. Benign tumors are usually slow growing, do not invade other tissues, and do not spread to other parts of the body. Usually they do not cause any problems unless they are growing in a confined space, such as in the brain. Malignant tumors are cancerous and differ from benign in several ways:

- Cancer cells have an altered cell structure that includes an increased nuclear size, irregular chromatin distribution, and prominent nucleoli.
- Cancer cells lack normal growth controlling mechanisms; growth is unorganized and disorderly.
- Cancer cells lack contact inhibition (normal cell growth stops when other cells are contacted). They continue to grow and invade into other tissue.
- Cancer cells do not respond to growth factors that stimulate or inhibit growth of normal cells. They have decreased requirements for growth and therefore grow rapidly with reduced growth factors.
- Cancer cells frequently escape immune surveillance. NK cells fail to recognize and therefore destroy them because they are capable of lowering their expression of being an antigen and abnormal.
- Cancer cells are invasive, causing destruction of normal tissue.
- Cancer cells can metastasize by invading other cells, traveling through the lymphatic or blood vessels, and then implanting into other body sites and creating additional tumors.
- Cancer cells have altered metabolism, often having an increased metabolic rate.

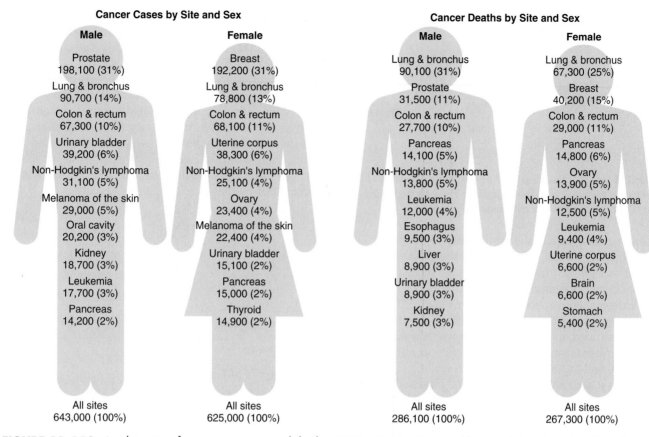

FIGURE 11–153 Leading sites of new cancer cases and deaths—2001 estimates (Reprinted by permission of the American Cancer Society, Inc.)

Classifications of Cancer

Cancer can be classified according to its cellular origin. Cancers arising from epithelial tissues are known as **carcinomas**, whereas those from connective tissues are called **sarcomas**. Cancers of the blood and blood-forming organs are called leukemias, and those from the lymph tissue are lymphomas. Table 11–11 lists benign and malignant tumors according to their cellular origins.

Cancers can also be described according to their degree of differentiation. This refers to how similar the cancer cell appears to the normal cell from which it was derived. A well-differentiated cancer cells looks similar to a normal cell, and a poorly or undifferentiated cancer cell appears very abnormal. Sometimes it is so poorly differentiated that it is difficult to tell from what type of cell it originated. This type of cell source is termed as "unknown primary." Grading refers to the degree of differentiation of the cancer cell. The grading system goes from Grade 1, which is a well-differentiated cell, to Grade IV, which is undifferentiated. The grading and staging findings allow for the determination of an anticipated prognosis.

Cancer Staging

Staging is a term used to identify the extent of the disease process. It is a system that is accepted worldwide for primary site evaluation. It provides a standardized description for planning treatments, exchanging information, evaluating outcomes and estimating progno-

sis. It is also a criterion for patient eligibility for individual clinical trials. The method is known as the TNM system and uses standardized measurement criteria:

(T)—the extent of the primary tumor

(N)—the presence or absence and extent of regional lymph node **metastasis**

(M)—the presence or absence of distant metastasis

Numbers are added to the three components to indicate the clinical extent of the disease to show an increase in tumor size, local involvement, regional lymph node spread, or distant metastasis:

Tumor size	T0	T1	T2	T3	T4
Nodal involvement	N0	N1	N2	N3	
Metastasis	M0	M1			

In addition to the letters and numbers, four staging classifications are also used:

c—Clinical based on acquired evidence from exams and studies

p—Pathologic based on information after a surgical procedure

r—Re-treatment based on disease-free interval with planned new treatment

a—Autopsy based on pathology after death

In the future, multiples biological factors, such as hormone receptors, genetic markers, cellular proliferation,

TABLE 11–11

CELLULAR ORIGINS OF BENIGN AND MALIGNANT DISEASES

Cell or Tissue of Origin	Benign	Malignant
TUMORS OF EPITHELIAL ORIGIN		
Squamous cells	Squamous cell papilloma	Squamous cell carcinoma
Basal cells	—	Basal cell carcinoma
Glandular or ductal epithelium	Adenoma	Adenocarcinoma
Transitional cells	Transitional cell papilloma	Transitional cell carcinoma
Melanocytes	Nevus	Malignant melanoma
Germ cells (testes/ovaries)	—	Seminoma (of testes), embryonal carcinoma, yolk sack carcinoma
TUMORS OF BLOOD AND BLOOD FORMING ORGANS/LYMPHOID TISSUE		
Bone marrow and blood	—	Leukemia
Lymph tissue and organs	—	Hodgkin's disease
Plasma blood cells (B lymphocytes)	—	Multiple myeloma
Lymph tissue and organs	—	Non-Hodgkin's lymphoma
TUMORS OF CONNECTIVE TISSUE		
Fibrous tissue	Fibromatosis (desmoid tumor)	Fibrosarcoma
Fat	Lipoma	Liposarcoma
Bone	Osteoma	Osteogenic sarcoma
Cartilage	Chondroma	Chondrosarcoma
Smooth muscle	Leiomyoma	Leiomyosarcoma
Striated (skeletal) muscle	Rhabdomyoma	Rhabdomyosarcoma
ENDOTHELIAL AND RELATED TISSUES		
Blood vessels	Hemangioma	Angiosarcoma
Lymph vessels	Lymphangioma	Lymphangiosarcoma
Synovium	—	Synovial sarcoma
Mesothelium	Meningioma	Malignant mesothelioma
Meninges	Meningioma	Malignant meningioma
NEURAL AND RETINAL TISSUE		
Nerve sheath	Neurilemoma Neurofibroma	Malignant peripheral sheath tumor
Nerve cells	Gangioneuroma	Neuroblastoma
Retinal cells (cones)	—	Retinoblastoma

and metastasis potential, will probably be used to further classify cancer.

Signs and symptoms—The signs and symptoms vary according to the type of cancer, its location, and the indi-vidual affected. The American Cancer Society has de-veloped the warning signals for cancer in adults and children (Tables 11–12 and 11–13). Unfortunately, these are often signs of fairly advanced disease. Many individuals have no symptoms, and the possibility of

TABLE 11–12

THE SEVEN WARNING SIGNALS OF CANCER
■ Change in bowel and bladder habits
■ A sore that does not heal
■ Unusual bleeding or discharge
■ Thickening or lump in a breast or elsewhere
■ Indigestion or difficulty swallowing
■ Obvious change in a wart or mole
■ Nagging cough or hoarseness

TABLE 11–13

WARNING SIGNALS OF CHILDHOOD CANCER
■ Unusual mass or swelling
■ Unexplained paleness and loss of energy
■ Sudden tendency to bruise
■ Persistent, localized pain or limping
■ Prolonged, unexplained fever or illness
■ Frequent headaches, often with vomiting
■ Sudden eye or vision changes
■ Excessive, rapid weight loss

cancer is detected through routine cancer screening tests. (Chapter 14, Units 3 and 4, discuss recommended screening tests.)

Etiology—Cancer is believed to be caused by cellular **mutation** or abnormal activation of cellular genes that control cell growth and division. These abnormal genes are called **oncogenes**. In normal cells, proto-oncogenes and tumor suppresser genes regulate the growth and repair of cells. If a proto-oncogene is mutated, it may be left permanently in the "on position," causing continuous cell proliferation. If the tumor suppresser gene is mutated, it may be left permanently in the "off" position, also allowing continued cell proliferation.

One of the most common known mutated genes in human cancers is the p53 tumor suppresser gene. This gene normally stops cell proliferation and promotes DNA repair of damaged cells. Some clinical trials using gene therapy are looking at ways to interact with the p53 tumor suppresser gene.

Only a small fraction of cells that mutate ever lead to cancer (remember it is estimated that 100 to 1,000 mutated cells are formed every day). Many of the mutated cells cannot survive because they are so defective. Others are destroyed by the immune system, particularly the NK cells. The probability of mutations is increased when a person is exposed to certain chemical, physical, or biologic factors called **carcinogens**. Carcinogens are usually categorized under chemical, viral, physical, and familial headings. Table 11–14 lists the types of known carcinogens and the resulting cancers.

TABLE 11–14

TYPES OF KNOWN CARCINOGENS AND THE RESULTING CANCERS	
Carcinogen	Type of Cancer
CHEMICAL CARCINOGENS	
Alkylating chemotherapy agents (e.g., nitrogen mustard, cyclophosphamide)	■ Leukemia
Arsenic	■ Liver ■ Lung ■ Skin
Benzene	■ Leukemia
Chewing tobacco	■ Oral cancer
Cigarette smoking	■ Oral cancer ■ Head and neck cancer ■ Lung cancer ■ Bladder cancer ■ Cervical cancer
Vinyl chloride	■ Liver cancer
VIRAL CARCINOGENS	
Epstein–Barr virus	■ Burkitt's lymphoma in Africa ■ Nasopharyngeal cancer
Hepatitis B virus	■ Hepatocellular liver cancer
Human T cell leukemia/lymphoma virus (HTLV-1)	■ T cell leukemias and lymphomas
Human papilloma virus (HPV 16 or HPV-18)	■ Found in at least 70% of cases of cervical cancer
PHYSICAL CARCINOGENS	
Asbestos	■ Bronchogenic lung cancer ■ Mesothelioma
Ionizing radiation	■ Leukemia ■ Lymphoma ■ Potentially all solid tumors
Ultraviolet radiation	■ Melanoma ■ Skin cancers
FAMILIAL CARCINOGENESIS	
Dysplastic nevus syndrome	■ Melanoma
Fanconi's anemia	■ Leukemia
Familial polyposis	■ Colorectal cancer
Gardner's syndrome	■ Colorectal cancer
Neurofibromatosis	■ Brain tumors ■ Endocrine cancers
Xeroderma pigmentosum	■ Melanoma ■ Skin cancer

A PEDIATRIC PERSPECTIVE

There is evidence that some tumor suppressor gene defects are inherited. Patients with inherited retinoblastoma, a rare pediatric tumor of the eye, are known to have a defective tumor suppressor gene.

Some other reasons for failure of the immune system to destroy mutated cells have been suggested:

- A decrease in antibodies and lymphocytes caused by cytotoxic drugs or steroids
- Stress, which stimulates production of *cortisol,* a lymphocyte destroyer
- Severe systemic infection, which depresses the immune system
- Cancer itself causes suppression of the immune system and eventual exhaustion of a response
- Increased infection caused by radiation, toxic drug therapy, and bone marrow depression, which interferes with leukocyte production

Some scientists believe that the mutated cell's surface markers either did not change (still say self), are disguised, or even are released and cause immune fighters to follow them instead of destroying the cell.

Diagnostic Tests Additional tests are indicated when a patient has a positive screening test or has symptoms of cancer. The diagnosis of cancer can only be considered 100% accurate if a sample of the cells are obtained and examined. The major goals of the diagnostic evaluation are to determine:

- The tissue type of the cancer (e.g. carcinoma, sarcoma)
- The primary site (e.g. breast)
- The grade of the cancer (the degree of differentiation)
- The extent of the disease in the body (stage)

Diagnostic tests for cancer can be categorized into biopsies, laboratory tests, and tumor imaging.

Biopsies A **biopsy** provides a piece of tissue for histologic examination to determine the type of cell. Treatment decisions for cancers arising from the same organ differ based upon the type of cell involved. For example, adenocarcinoma of the lung is treated very differently than a sarcoma of the lung. Common techniques for biopsies are: needle, incisional, excisional, and bone marrow aspiration. During a needle biopsy, a needle is inserted into the tumor and cells are withdrawn. Incisional biopsy involves removing a portion of the tumor for testing. The entire tumor is removed during an excisional biopsy. A bone marrow aspiration is used to test for leukemia and cancers that have invaded the bone marrow. A bone marrow aspiration requires the patient to lie prone. A local anesthetic is injected over the iliac crest, and a long needle is inserted through the bone and into the marrow where blood cells are made.

Sentinel lymph node biopsy is a newer technique used to remove and sample lymph nodes that may be cancerous. It is most commonly used for breast cancer and melanoma. The sentinel lymph node (SLN) is the first lymph node that drains the area of the cancerous tumor. The patient is injected with a radioactive material. SNLs will have a higher uptake of the material than other lymph nodes, identifying them for removal. The advantage of SLN biopsy is that fewer nodes are removed, resulting in fewer complications.

Stereotatic breast biopsy is used for breast tumors that are difficult to locate. The biopsy is done while the patient is having an x-ray or ultrasound, allowing the surgeon to see the location of the tumor in order to obtain the biopsy.

Laboratory Tests Different laboratory tests of the blood, serum, urine, and other body fluids help establish the diagnosis of cancer. In addition to standard tests, tumor markers and genetic testing can be done for different types of cancer.

Tumor markers are proteins, antigens, genes, hormones, or enzymes produced by the tumor and released into the blood. Tumor markers can help establish the diagnosis of cancer and its response to treatment. For example, if a patient has elevated tumor markers, then the numbers should decrease with cancer treatment. Tumor markers, however, are not always specific for cancer and can be effected by other factors. **Carcinoembryonic antigen (CEA)** is a tumor marker often elevated in patients with colon cancer; however, it can also be elevated in smokers.

Genetic Testing Conducting genetic testing is appropriate for some types of cancer and for individuals at high risk for developing inherited cancers. The ethical, social, and legal issues need to be considered. There are two examples of genetic testing, breast cancer genes BRAC 1 and BRAC 2. Defects in these genes are believed responsible for up to 80% of *inherited* breast cancers. (Note: fewer than 5% of all breast cancers have a direct genetic link.) BRAC 1 and 2 are present in everyone; however, when the genes mutate, the risk for breast and ovarian cancer increases. BRAC 1 mutations have also been linked to colon and prostate cancer. BRAC 2 genes have been linked to these and other cancers. Both men and women can inherit and pass on the genes. Women who inherit the BRAC 1 and BRAC 2 mutated gene have a 50% to 80% chance of developing breast cancer.

Tumor Imaging A variety of different radiology and imaging tests are used to aid in the diagnosis and staging of cancer, including x-rays, CT scans, MRIs, endoscopy, ultrasound, and nuclear medicine. X-rays include mammography used to screen for breast cancer. CT scans are commonly used to aid in the diagnosis of lung, liver, and head and neck cancers. MRIs are used to diagnose and stage cancers, such as brain and musculoskeletal cancers (e.g., sarcomas).

Endoscopy is used to visualize the interior of hollow organs. After a hollow tube is inserted into the organ, images may be taken, and tissue samples can be obtained through the scope. Bronchoscopy is used for diagnosis of lung cancers. Sigmoidoscopy and colonoscopy are used for the screening and diagnosis of colorectal cancer. Ultrasound is used to distinguish between a fluid-filled cyst and a solid tumor.

Nuclear medicine imaging involves the injection or ingestion of radioactive substances, followed by imagining of the organ or organs that concentrate the radioactive material. Common nuclear medicine scans include bone, liver, spleen, brain, thyroid, and kidney.

Positron emission tomography (PET) scan is a type of nuclear medicine test that has only recently been used to detect cancer. PET scans are computerized images of the metabolic activity of the body tissues that can detect the presence of cancer.

Radiolabeled monoclonal antibodies include Prosta-Scint scans used for the early detection of prostate cancer. With this technology, antibodies are made for specific tumor types and labeled with a radioactive substance. The radioactive antibody searches for the specific tumor antigen and is detectable by the scan. *Radiolabeled peptides* are most commonly used to detect neuroendocrine tumors.

Ductal Lavage

A new experimental diagnostic examination called ductal lavage is being tried on women at high risk for developing breast cancer. It is a way to detect early changes in the cells of the breast ducts before cancer would be evident on a mammogram or by breast examination. It is showing promise for early detection. In December 2000, Johns Hopkins Medical Center did a study on 500 high-risk women at 19 different breast centers in the United States. These women had a history of breast cancer, a positive BRCA 1/BRCA 2 gene mutation, or a first degree or two or more close relatives with breast cancer. Atypical or suspicious cells were detected in 15% of the participants, and cancerous cells were found in 5% of them. All had normal mammograms within the past year.

The procedure is minimally invasive. An anesthetic cream is applied to the nipple area. A nursing pump is attached to the breast to draw a small amount of fluid to the surface in order to locate the milk ducts. A hair-thin catheter is inserted into the duct, and a small amount of anesthetic mixed with sterile saline is injected into the duct. The breast is massaged to mix the saline with the fluid in the duct that contains ductal epithelial cells. The saline and the cells are withdrawn through the catheter and sent to a cytology lab for analysis. The procedure takes about 30 minutes to complete. The test may sound very uncomfortable, but the women who participated reported only mild discomfort

This type of test seems worthwhile because most breast cancers begin in the cells lining the milk ducts and have been growing for years before they were identifiable by mammogram or examination. Interpreting the results

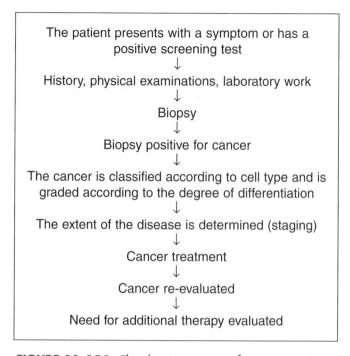

The patient presents with a symptom or has a
positive screening test
↓
History, physical examinations, laboratory work
↓
Biopsy
↓
Biopsy positive for cancer
↓
The cancer is classified according to cell type and is
graded according to the degree of differentiation
↓
The extent of the disease is determined (staging)
↓
Cancer treatment
↓
Cancer re-evaluated
↓
Need for additional therapy evaluated

FIGURE 11–154 The planning sequence for cancer treatment

of lavage studies is being evaluated. The presence of cells doesn't mean that cancer is inevitable. Most atypical cells do not progress to cancer. For the present, it presents the woman with a dilemma because the location within the breast where the cells came from is not known. Women at high risk have the option to watch and wait or to decide on preventive strategies, such as taking tomoxifen, having surgery to remove the ducts, or undergoing a preventative mastectomy.

Treatment—The treatment of cancer is based upon the type, grade, and stage of the cancer. In addition, treatment considerations include the risk or probability that the cancer will metastasize or recur after a "cure." The planning sequence for treatment is illustrated in Figure 11–154.

Goals of Cancer Therapy

The goals of therapy—cure, control, or palliation—are based on the patient's type and stage of cancer. Cure means that there will be no evidence of disease for a specified time. Control indicates that the disease cannot be cured but can be controlled for a period using the identified therapy. Palliation means that the disease cannot be cured or controlled, and palliative treatments will be used to control symptoms only.

Local Versus Systemic Treatment

The major treatment methods for cancer are surgery, **radiation**, **chemotherapy**, and biological response modifiers. Treatments can have local or systemic effects. A local treatment effects only the area of the therapy and any side effects that occur within that area. An example of local therapy is surgery. Systemic therapy travels throughout the

TABLE 11–15

TYPES OF CANCER TREATMENT

Type	Key Points
Surgery	■ Most common treatment ■ Local treatment ■ Diagnosis and staging ■ Treatment ■ Palliation of symptoms
Chemotherapy	■ Most routes: systemic treatment ■ Affects cell division in cancer and normal cells ■ Most effects seen in rapidly dividing normal and cancer cells ■ Side effects include: nausea, vomiting, bone marrow depression, hair loss, stomatitis (mouth sores)
Radiation: external beam therapy	■ Local treatment ■ Affects cell division of cancer and normal cells ■ Side effects: fatigue, skin reactions, other side effects dependent upon site treated
Radiation: brachytherapy	■ Local treatment ■ Radioactive isotope placed near site of cancer ■ Most common uses: cervical cancer, lung cancer, prostate cancer
Radiation: radiosurgery	■ Radiation used to "cut out" cancer ■ Most common uses: neurological tumors
Biological response modifiers	■ Also called immunotherapy ■ Examples: alpha interferon, interleukins, monoclonal antibodies, tumor necrosis factor, colony stimulating factors ■ Side effects: fatigue, fever, chills, muscle and joint aches, anaphylaxis
Gene therapy	■ Investigational ■ Affects growth-controlling factors of tumors
Complementary therapy	■ Complements standard therapies ■ Examples: massage therapy, biofeedback, music therapy, art therapy
Alternative therapy	■ Not approved by the Food and Drug Administration ■ Examples: shark cartilage, laetrile, megadoses of vitamins, herbs

body to treat cancer cells in different locations. Side effects will be systemic as well. An example of systemic therapy is chemotherapy. Most patients receive a combination of local and systemic therapies, especially if they already have or are at increased risk for metastasis. Table 11-15 lists the types of treatment and their key points.

Surgery is the oldest form of treatment for cancer. About 60% of all patients with cancer will have some type of surgery. It can be used for the purpose of diagnosis, treatment, or palliation of symptoms.

Radiation therapy is the use of high-energy particles or waves, such as x-rays or gamma rays, to destroy or damage the DNA or RNA of cancer cells. It is most effective on dividing cells. Radiation therapy can be delivered by external beam or brachytherapy. External beam therapy is delivered externally through the skin to the area. **Brachytherapy** uses radioactive isotopes that are placed directly on or very near the tumor. Brachytherapy can be delivered interstitially, using seeds "planted" into the tissues, or intracavitary, using a tube or catheter to instill the material. General side effects of radiation therapy include fatigue and weakness.

Chemotherapy involves the use of potent medications to treat cancer cells by altering cell division; therefore, it effects both rapidly dividing cancer cells and normal tissues. It can be administered orally, intravenously, subcutaneously, intramuscularly, intrarterially, topically, intraperitoneally, and into the central nervous system.

The route is dependent upon the type of chemotherapy and the type of cancer. Patients can receive one type of chemotherapy or combinations of chemotherapy. Although drug specific, common side effects of chemotherapy include hair loss, skin changes, mouth sores, and bone marrow depression. Bone marrow depression can lead to anemia, increased risk of infection, and increased risk for bleeding.

Biological response modifiers (BRM) are defined as any substance that is capable of altering the immune system by either stimulating or suppressing its action. BRMs are also referred to as immunotherapy or biotherapy. The action of BRMs can be divided into three categories:

1. Agents that restore, augment, or modulate the host's immune response
2. Agents that have direct antitumor activity
3. Agents that have other biologic effects, such as affecting tumor growth, differentiation, or the ability of the tumor to metastasize

There are numerous BRMs. Examples include colony-stimulating factors, interferons, interleukins, monoclonal antibodies, and tumor necrosis factor.

Colony stimulating factors (CSFs) are cytokines that regulate hematopoiesis, the growth and maturation of blood cells. The CSFs work on different blood cell lines. For example, granulocyte colony-stimulating factor works to promote the maturation of granulocytes, important white blood cells for fighting infection. Erythropoetin targets only red blood cell maturation. Other CSFs regulate stem cell growth and platelet growth. CSF is used to treat granulocytopenia (lack of granulocytes) and allow increased doses of chemotherapy to be given without the risk of long term granulocytopenia. It is administered subcutaneously or intravenously.

Interferons are naturally occurring cytokines that have antiviral, immunomodulatory, and antiproliferative effects. Interferon interacts with T cells to increase the activity of NK cells to have direct cytoxic affects on cancer cells. Alfa interferon is used to treat a variety of cancers, including renal cell cancer, hairy cell leukemia, melanoma, lymphomas, and Kaposi's sarcoma. It is administered intravenously or subcutaneously. Side effects include flu-like symptoms, such as fever, chills, fatigue, rigors, and headache.

Interleukins are important regulatory proteins produced naturally by lymphocytes and monocytes. The most commonly prescribed interleukin is interleukin-2 (IL-2). It is produced by helper T cells. An important function of IL-2 is to stimulate and activate NK cells, which have a cytoxic affect on cancer cells. IL-2 has been used to treat renal carcinoma, melanoma, and lymphoma. It is administered intravenously or subcutaneously. IL-2 has numerous side effects, including severe flu-like symptoms and third-spacing of fluids, which can lead to hypotension, ascites (fluid in the abdomen), and pleural effusion.

Monoclonal antibodies are antibodies directed at specific tumor antigens. They can be used alone to directly activate the host's immune system or can be attached to a chemotherapeutic agent for direct delivery to the cancer cell. Monoclonal antibodies are currently being used to treat a variety of cancers, including breast, B cell lymphoma, and melanomas.

Alternative Therapies

Alternative therapies are promoted as cancer cures; however, they have not been proven because they have not been scientifically tested or were tested and found to be statistically ineffective. Alternative therapies have not been approved by the Food and Drug Administration as treatments for cancer. Some examples include:

- Shark cartilage
- Laetrile
- Immunoaugmentive therapy
- Megadoses of vitamins

Complementary Therapies

Complementary therapies refer to supportive methods that are used to complement or add to recognized treatments, such as chemotherapy, radiation, and surgery. They are not given to cure cancer but to help control symptoms and improve well being. Examples of complementary therapies are:

- Art therapy
- Biofeedback
- Imagery
- Massage
- Meditation
- Music therapy
- Pet therapy
- Relaxation
- Yoga

Clinical Research Trials

Clinical trials are research studies that determine the effectiveness and safety of a cancer treatment regime. Before a treatment can be used for patients, it goes through many years of investigation—first through laboratory trials and then in animals. If the treatment is found effective and safe in animals, it is then tested on humans. Patients with specific criteria in their disease are permitted to participate in the trial treatment. After the studies are completed and there is evidence that the new therapy is more effective and safe, it is approved by the Food and Drug Administration to be used in mainstream therapy.

Chronic Fatigue Syndrome (CFS)

Description—This **debilitating** disorder was officially recognized and reported in 1984 by two doctors near Lake Tahoe, Nevada. It was officially declared a disease in 1988. The CDC started a surveillance program costing $1.5 million to track the frequency and impact of the disorder.

Signs and symptoms—The following guidelines have been established to help physicians diagnose the condition.

- Persistent overwhelming fatigue that lasts for at least six months and does not go away with rest
- Low grade fever

- Sore throat and/or swollen lymph nodes
- Headaches
- Lingering fatigue after levels of exercise that would normally be easily tolerated
- Unexplainable muscle weakness or pain
- Pain in joints without swelling
- Forgetfulness, irritability, confusion, inability to concentrate, depression, sensitivity to light, and impaired vision
- Sleep disturbances

Patients experience varying levels of ability to perform activity from profound fatigue to being completely bedridden. CFS affects twice as many women as men, particularly between 25 and 45 years old. However, children and senior citizens have also been diagnosed.

The disorder begins suddenly like the common flu, but the CFS symptoms last for three or four years. Only about 15% to 20% seem to recover fully; 5% are homebound or bedridden.

Etiology—The cause of the disorder appears to be genetically predisposed. About 79% to 80% of CFS patients have allergies. Current theories suggest that a virus, bacteria, allergen, or environment chemical enters the body but does not set off the normal immune response to fight the invasion. Instead, the system continues to make symptom-producing chemicals. A second theory suggests that some unidentified organism weakens the immune system, allowing normally-dormant viruses to become activated. This theory is supported by the presence of high levels of antibodies to Epstein–Barr virus and others.

Physicians still do not know much about the disorder; some deny its existence because it cannot be detected by a blood test. Diagnosis requires a thorough physical examination and laboratory tests to rule out other conditions with similar symptoms.

Treatment—Treatment consists of analgesics for pain, antihistamines for allergic symptoms, antidepressants to improve sleep and fatigue. Patients should avoid emotional and physical stress and have good nutrition. Exercise must be appropriate. Psychological counseling may be required to help a patient deal with the changes caused by CFS.

Lupus Erythematosus (Lu'-pus Er-ith-ema-toe'-sis)

Description—**Lupus erythematosus** is a chronic disease of unknown cause in which striking changes occur in the immune system. It causes inflammation of various parts of the body. It can involve only a few body organs or cause serious life-threatening problems. Lupus can affect the skin, joints, kidneys, lungs, heart, nervous system, and other body organs and systems.

In lupus, the usually-protective antibodies are produced in large quantities but react against the per-son's own normal tissue; therefore, it is called an **autoimmune** disease. There are three main types of lupus:

- **Discoid lupus erythematosus (DLE)**—Cutaneous or **discoid** lupus is confined to the skin and causes a persistent flush of the cheeks or disklike lesions on the face, neck, scalp, and other areas exposed to ultraviolet light. The lesions of the face are referred to as a butterfly rash. The rash is usually scaly and red but not itchy. If not treated, scarring may result, and if on the scalp, bald spots.
- Systemic lupus erythematosus (SLE) inflames the organs of the body. Some persons also have skin and joint involvement; in others, skin, lungs, kidneys, or blood may be affected. The disease is characterized by periods of **remission**, when few if any symptoms are evident, and other periods of active disease and symptoms.
- Drug-induced lupus can be caused by certain medications and is similar to SLE. The most common offenders are hydralazine for hypertension and procainamide for cardiac arrhythmia. The symptoms fade when the drugs are stopped.

The incidence of SLE in the United States is approximately 500,000 people. SLE affects women nine times more often than men, most frequently during the childbearing years. Lupus is more common in African, Asian, and Native Americans. About 16,000 new cases are diagnosed each year.

Signs and symptoms—**General symptoms** of beginning lupus are:

fever	loss of appetite
weight loss	nausea and vomiting
headache	easy bruising
fatigue	hair loss
swollen glands	edema
depression	

Suggestive symptoms of lupus include:

a rash over cheeks and bridge of nose	discoid lupus lesions
	ulcers inside mouth
rashes developing after being in the sun	pleurisy
	anemia
arthritis in two or more joints	**Raynaud's phenomenon** (fingers turn white or blue in the cold)
seizures	
bald spots	

Diagnosis is made on the strength of symptoms and blood tests showing low cell counts. Urine is checked for protein, RBCs and WBCs. A specific antibody test called ANA (antinuclear antibody) looks for antibodies to the nuclei of cells. Over 99% of people with lupus will have a positive test; however, only 33% of people with a positive ANA have SLE.

Etiology—Unknown immune system change.

Treatment—Treatment of SLE consists of assuring patients they can live near-normal lives. Limits on activities are dictated by the disease. Rest when needed, but otherwise engage in normal employment and exercise. Sun exposure should be avoided at peak hours (10:00 AM to 2:00 PM), otherwise, as tolerated. Sunscreens of at least SPF 15 are advisable. No medication has been developed to cure lupus. Joint and muscle pain is controlled with anti-inflammatory and analgesic drugs, such as aspirin, ibuprofen, Naprosyn, and Tylenol. During flareups or if major organs are involved, steroids, such as prednisone, are often used to suppress inflammation. The steroid also interferes with the proliferation and interaction of the cells in the immune system and causes T cells to gather in the lymph nodes, which removes them from concentrating at the inflammation sites. The drugs chloroquine and Plaquenil (antimalarials) are valuable in managing the skin lesions and also help control arthritis symptoms.

Many new treatments are being tested, several dealing with self-antigens, immunoreplacement therapy, and even plasmapheresis (the removal of blood plasma, and hence antibodies). It is believed with further understanding of the immune system, an effective treatment of lupus will be discovered.

Lymphedema (Limf–a-dee′-ma)

Description—**Lymphedema** is swelling in the tissues of the body caused by an accumulation of lymphatic fluid. Approximately 20% of women who have had breast cancer surgery develop the condition. It may begin as soon as a few months or as late as several years after surgery.

Signs and symptoms—A swelling within the fatty tissue just under the skin of the arm and hand. When it first begins, the arm may seem normal in the morning, but the hand or arm will swell during the day. If it occurs following overuse of the arm in the first year or year and one-half after surgery, it can often be reversed with aggressive treatment. If it occurs two or more years after surgery, complete reversal is unlikely, but the condition can be controlled. With chronic marked swelling in the arm, serious complications can arise, such as infection, loss of function, and skin breakdown.

Etiology—Normally lymph fluid circulates easily through the vessels and is filtered in the nodes. However, when the system is altered or damaged it cannot handle the amount of fluid. This is especially true when lymph nodes in the axilla are removed during surgery for breast cancer. Damage can also result from radiation therapy. The more extensive the damage, the greater the risk of developing lymphedema.

One way to reduce the risk from surgery is to perform the sentinel node biopsy procedure. A dye material is injected at the site of the tumor to identify the first node along the lymph vessel that drains the area. This node is biopsied to determine if cancer cells are present. If none are found, no lymph nodes are removed.

Treatment—The most comprehensive treatment for lymphedema is complete or complex decongestive physiotherapy (CDP). This involves massage, exercise, hygiene training, and compression bandages or clothing. A trained therapist is required to provide manual lymph drainage. This requires daily massage over a one to four week period. The message removes excess fluid by stimulating the lymph vessels to dilate to drain fluid and to open new passageways. After each massage, the affected limb is wound in compression bandages to prevent the build-up of fluid.

Exercise and skin care techniques are also used during the maintenance phase of CDP. Compression bandages may be required for 24 hours a day at the beginning, but once edema has decreased, a compression sleeve that is worn during periods of activity may be adequate. The sleeve is also necessary when exercising or traveling in a plane. CDP may not be appropriate for people under treatment for congestive heart disease. Diuretics are contraindicated because they contribute to protein build-up and may further affect the tissues.

Precautions—Physicians advise patients to take precautions to reduce the risk of lymphedema by observing the following advice:

- Avoid any injury to the arm or puncture to the skin. Avoid infection from cuts, burns, or insect bites by applying or taking antibiotics.
- Protect the affected arm from injections, vaccinations, blood withdrawal, or intravenous procedures. Avoidance of blood pressure readings may be advisable.
- Avoid constricting clothing or jewelry.
- Avoid an activity that might cause heat in the arm or chest, such as tanning, saunas, hot tubs or baths, and vigorous exercise.
- Wear compression bandages or garments when exercising or flying.

Rheumatoid Arthritis (Room′-a-toid Arth-ri′-tis)

Description—This chronic systemic inflammatory autoimmune disease affects the joints and surrounding muscles, tendons, ligaments, and blood vessels. It affects women three times more often than men. It occurs primarily between the ages of 20 and 60 with a peak onset period between 35 to 45.

Signs and symptoms—The symptoms develop insidiously, then become localized in joints, usually bilaterally. Following inactivity, the affected joints stiffen, swell, and may show beginning signs of deformity. They eventually become tender, painful, hot, and enlarged and have marked deformities and decreased function.

This disease was discussed in the unit on skeletal system; however, it is believed there is a connection to the immune system. Recent findings suggest a link to genetic defects, which cause the cells to display a specific cell marker. Patients may also have an autoantibody known as *rheumatoid factor,* which locks onto the body's own IgG molecule as if it were an antigen. These antigen–antibody complexes seem to be deposited on the synovial membranes of the joints and are the targets of the inflammatory response.

Etiology—This is a malfunction of the immune response. When the complement system is activated, the macrophages gather at the joint. The inflammatory response dilates the blood vessels, and fluid accumulates in the joint cavity. The cells of the membrane proliferate in response, thickening the joint membrane and causing more swelling. These events continue in cycles and result in the destruction of the joint.

Treatment—Treatment consists primarily of salicylates to reduce inflammation. **Corticosteroids** (prednisone)—anti-inflammatory agents, such as ibuprofen, gold salts, and antimalarial drugs—may prove helpful. Patients need periods of rest during the day and 8 to 10 hours of sleep every night. Activities that may be helpful are range of motion exercises, application of heat during chronic episodes, and ice packs with acute phases. Advanced disease may necessitate total joint replacement or joint fusion to relieve pain.

ACHIEVE UNIT OBJECTIVES

Complete Chapter 11, Unit 9, in the workbook to help you obtain competency of this subject matter.

A CAAHEP CONNECTION

This unit addresses multiple curriculum requirements of the CAAHEP Standards. The **Anatomy and physiology, Common pathologies, Diagnostic and treatment modalities,** A great amount of specific **Medical terminology,** discussions of **Radiological examinations and treatments,** and The types of **Medications** are included in this discussion of immune system–specific interventions. Even though much of this will not be encountered in a family practice setting, your knowledge of this content will allow you to explain procedures and assist your patients to understand the treatment they are undergoing.

UNIT 10

The Digestive System

OBJECTIVES

Upon completion of the unit, meet the following performance objectives by verifying knowledge of the facts and principles presented through oral and written communication at a level deemed competent.

1. Spell and define, using the glossary at the back of the text, all the **Words to Know** in this unit.
2. Name the four phases of the digestive process.
3. Define digestion.
4. Name the raw materials required for a healthy body.
5. Trace the pathway of food through the alimentary tract.
6. Describe the structures of the mouth and the digestive processes that occur there.
7. Explain the process of swallowing.
8. Describe how the esophagus propels food toward the stomach.
9. Describe the structure and function of the stomach.
10. Describe the structure and function of the small intestine.
11. Tell why the duodenum is a vital link in the digestive system.
12. List the functions of the liver, including the portal circulation connection.
13. Describe the role of the gallbladder and its association with the liver.
14. Describe the location and function of the pancreas.
15. Explain how and where nutrients are absorbed.
16. Name the sections of the colon, and describe its function.
17. Describe the function of the rectum.
18. Describe the structure and function of the anal canal.
19. Describe the diagnostic examinations of the digestive tract.
20. Describe the disorders of diseases of the digestive system.

AREAS OF COMPETENCE (AAMA)

This unit addresses content within the specific competency areas of *Administrative procedures, Practice finances, Patient care, Communication skills*, and *Instruction*, as identified in the Medical Assistant Role Delineation Study. Refer to Appendix A for a detailed listing of the areas. (Note: Although *Anatomy and physiology* is not specifically identified in the study, a basic knowledge of the body's structure and function is an essential foundation of many roles.)

■ WORDS TO KNOW

alimentary canal	hernia
anal	herniorrhaphy
anus	hiatus
appendectomy	hydrochloric acid
appendicitis	ileocecal
ascending	ileostomy
bile	ileum
bolus	impaction
bowel	incontinent
cardiac sphincter	insulin
cecum	intestine
cholecystectomy	jaundice
cholelithiasis	jejunum
chyme	liver
cirrhosis	mesentery
colitis	mouth
colon	nausea
colostomy	pancreas
common bile duct	pancreatitis
constipation	paralytic ileus
Crohn's disease	peptic
cystic	peristalsis
defecate	polyp
descending	proctoscope
diarrhea	pruritus ani
digestion	pyloric
digestive	rectum
diverticulitis	reflux
duodenum	saliva
emesis	salivary glands
enzyme	sigmoid
esophagus	sigmoidoscopy
fecal	spastic colon
fissure	stenosis
fistula	stomach
flatus	stool
gallbladder	tongue
gastric	transverse
gastrointestinal (GI)	ulcer
gastroscopy	varices
hemorrhoidectomy	vermiform appendix
hemorrhoids	villi
hepatic	villous adenoma
hepatitis	vomit

(A) **Library**

The **digestive** system is the group of organs that changes food that has been eaten into a form that can be used by the body's cells. The system is also known as the **gastrointestinal (GI)** tract or system, and the connecting chain of organs is sometimes referred to as the **alimentary canal**. The digestive process can be divided into four phases: *ingestion, digestion, absorption,* and *elimination.*

Food that is consumed is acted on by various mechanical and chemical means as it progresses through the body. Each organ, whether main or accessory, plays an important role in physically or chemically altering the composition of the food, selectively absorbing the elements, or eliminating the remains.

The main organs of the system are those through which the food passes. These organs form a continuous tube from the entrance to the exit of the body. They are the mouth, pharynx, esophagus, stomach, small intestine, and large intestine. As important as these organs are, it is the accessory organs that play a major role in the digestive process. In the mouth, there are the teeth, salivary glands, and tongue. The liver, gallbladder, and pancreas have access to the small intestine (Figure 11–155).

Digestion is the activity performed by the organs of the digestive system, and it is defined as the process by which food is broken down, mechanically and chemically, in the gastrointestinal tract and converted into an absorbable form that can be used by the cells of the body. This process cannot occur within the digestive system alone. As with all body functions, an interrelationship of systems is required to achieve the desired results. Digestion requires cooperation from the nervous system, the muscular system, the circulatory system, and the endocrine system.

The human body can be compared to an engine that needs appropriate fuel to operate. The energy we need to function must come from the foods we eat. The right fuel will not only supply the body with energy, but also provide the materials necessary to build and repair the body so that it can operate efficiently. If the wrong fuel is used too often, the machine will eventually break down.

The human body can manufacture the appropriate fuel if it receives an adequate supply of the right raw materials, mainly carbohydrates, proteins, fats, minerals, vitamins, water, and roughage. All these raw materials are available from the basic food groups and should be eaten daily.

Carbohydrates supply about two thirds of the energy calories needed each day. Fats are also an excellent source of energy; in fact, an ounce of fat yields about three times the calories of an ounce of carbohydrate. Unfortunately, the body does not waste excess energy-producing calories but stores them instead. Therefore, when all the calories eaten are not used for energy, they are stored as excess body tissue we may not desire.

Proteins are obtained primarily from plant and animal sources but are not stored by the body. It is especially important that they be eaten daily because they are the main ingredients needed to build and repair cells and tissue.

Other raw materials required for a healthy body are vitamins and minerals. Vitamins are regulating chemicals needed for growth and control of body activities. For instance, the chemical that becomes vitamin D must be absorbed by the body and then become activated in the skin by contact with the sun. The body needs vitamin D to ab-

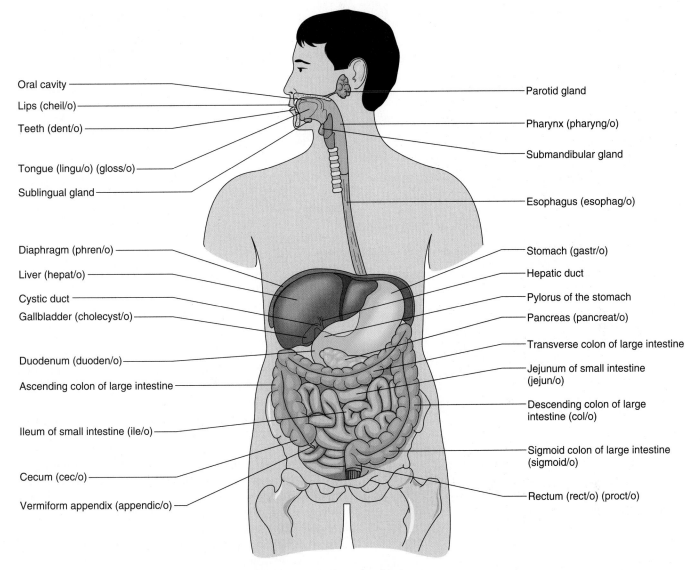

FIGURE 11-155 The digestive system

sorb and use calcium. Calcium and another mineral, phosphorus, are needed by the body for the muscles, nerves, blood, teeth, and bones. The formation of red blood cells requires iron and copper. We have already learned that the combination of an iron pigment and a protein forms the hemoglobin of the red blood cells, which enables them to attract O_2 and CO_2 as they move through the body.

All the raw materials the body needs are altered by the digestive system to provide the essential elements necessary for good health. The various stages in this process will become clearer by tracing the pathway of food through the alimentary canal.

THE MOUTH

Food enters the body through the **mouth**. It is held in the oral cavity while the initial digestive process is begun.

Teeth break up food into small pieces to make it easier to swallow and also to prepare it for more effective action by digestive enzymes. "Baby" teeth are called *deciduous* and begin to appear at about six months. They are gradually exchanged for permanent teeth beginning at about six years. Different teeth have specific duties to perform. The incisors bite food with their sharp edges. The canines or cuspids are pointed to puncture and tear. The premolars or bicuspids and the molars are for grinding and crushing (Figure 11–156). The **tongue** aids in the process by moving the food around within the mouth, bringing it into contact with the teeth. The tongue is a muscle and can alter its shape to reach all areas of the mouth. The surface of the tongue contains the taste buds, located within the papillae projections.

The **salivary glands** excrete the fluid known as **saliva**. It is released from three pairs of glands: the parotid, the submandibular, and the sublingual (Figure 11–157). Cer-

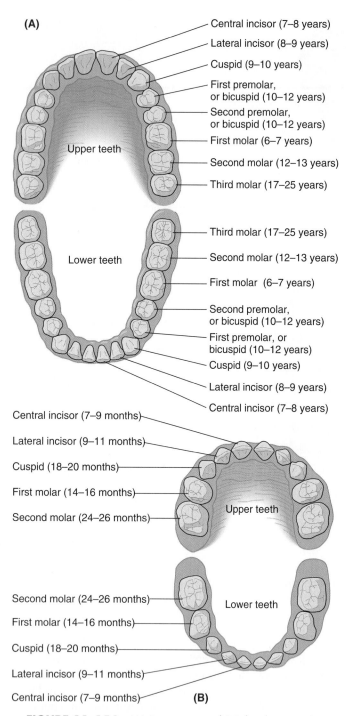

(A)

Central incisor (7–8 years)
Lateral incisor (8–9 years)
Cuspid (9–10 years)
First premolar, or bicuspid (10–12 years)
Second premolar, or bicuspid (10–12 years)
First molar (6–7 years)
Second molar (12–13 years)
Third molar (17–25 years)

Upper teeth

Third molar (17–25 years)
Second molar (12–13 years)
First molar (6–7 years)
Second premolar, or bicuspid (10–12 years)
First premolar, or bicuspid (10–12 years)
Cuspid (9–10 years)
Lateral incisor (8–9 years)
Central incisor (7–8 years)

Lower teeth

Central incisor (7–9 months)
Lateral incisor (9–11 months)
Cuspid (18–20 months)
First molar (14–16 months)
Second molar (24–26 months)

Upper teeth

Second molar (24–26 months)
First molar (14–16 months)
Cuspid (18–20 months)
Lateral incisor (9–11 months)
Central incisor (7–9 months)

Lower teeth

(B)

FIGURE 11–156 (A) Permanent and (B) deciduous teeth

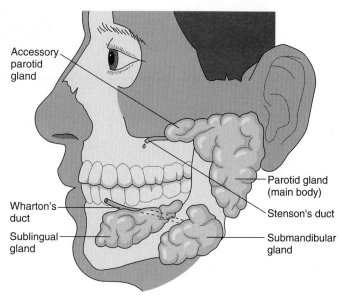

Accessory parotid gland

Parotid gland (main body)

Stenson's duct

Wharton's duct

Sublingual gland

Submandibular gland

FIGURE 11–157 Salivary glands

to perceive the sensations of sweet, sour, bitter, and salty. In addition, saliva aids in cleansing the teeth by washing away food particles that might allow bacteria to grow. The presence of saliva in the oral cavity keeps the surfaces moist and flexible, which aids in the production of speech.

The combination of mashed food substances and saliva is called a **bolus**. When it has been mixed well and contains sufficient moisture, it can be easily swallowed. For this to occur, several muscles must work together. The tongue presses upward and backward against the palate (roof of the mouth), while the muscles in the cheeks help in the formation of a chute to direct the bolus toward the back of the mouth and into the pharynx (Figure 11–158). At this point, the bolus could go in three different directions: into the nasal cavity, down and forward into the trachea, or down into the **esophagus**.

The directing of the bolus is accomplished by a complex combination of "lids" and muscles, which operate automatically. As the bolus is swallowed, it raises the soft palate, closing off the nasal cavity. At the same time, the epiglottis, a cartilage lid attached at the top of the larynx, moves across the opening into the larynx when the tongue pushes the bolus against the palate. At the moment of swallowing, the larynx moves upward against the epiglottis to close the opening. Usually, this reflex action works perfectly, but when the timing is slightly off, food may enter the larynx, triggering the cough reflex (to remove the material). We say, "It went down the wrong pipe."

THE ESOPHAGUS

Once food is swallowed, its movement through the body is maintained by the smooth, involuntary muscle action called **peristalsis**. The esophagus has two layers of invol-

tain foods cause the glands to excrete profusely, often producing some discomfort, as when eating something sour. The disease called mumps is the inflammation of the parotid glands. A virus causes the glands to enlarge and become painful. With mumps, mastication (chewing) causes great discomfort because the muscle action squeezes the swollen glands.

Saliva contains an **enzyme** called ptyalin. This chemical begins the breakdown of carbohydrates into sugar. Saliva also provides moisture that enables the taste buds

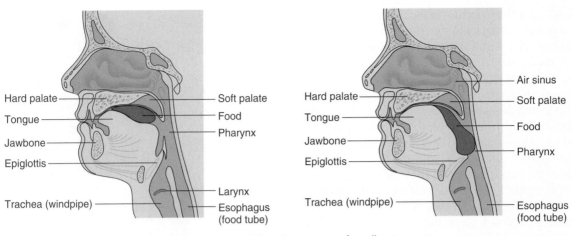

FIGURE 11-158 The process of swallowing

untary muscles. The inner layer forms circles around the esophagus, whereas the outer layer runs longitudinally along its approximately 10-inch length. When food enters the esophagus, the muscles alternately contract and relax, squeezing the bolus. Together they create the peristaltic "milking action," which moves the bolus to the **stomach**. The whole process only requires about five seconds. Because peristaltic action moves material in one direction only and this process does not depend on gravity, it is possible to drink a glass of water while standing on your head.

THE STOMACH

The upper opening to the stomach is controlled by a circular muscle called the **cardiac sphincter**. As the peristaltic wave approaches, the sphincter dilates, allowing the food to enter. Once the food is inside, this one-way "gate" closes to prevent its escape.

The stomach is a 10-inch-long, J-shaped organ constructed of three layers of strong muscle tissue (Figure 11-159). It lies just beneath the diaphragm. The inner lining of the stomach is thick and full of folds called *rugae*. Because muscle tissue is elastic and the folds in the lining can straighten out, the stomach is capable of expanding. It can hold about half a gallon of food and liquid.

Once the material has entered the stomach, the muscular layers begin to contract. A circular layer, a longitudinal layer, and an oblique layer work together in a strong rhythmic motion to break up the food into tiny particles. The stomach continues the digestive process that began in the mouth. The churning action is prolonged and made more difficult by poorly-chewed food.

The mechanical digestive process is assisted by a chemical process. The stomach lining is formed of mucous membrane, whose glands secrete mucus. The stomach lining also has about 35 million **gastric** glands, which secrete **hydrochloric acid** and several enzymes. As the stomach contents are being kneaded, acid and enzymes

are excreted by the gastric glands and thoroughly mixed into the bolus. One enzyme, rennin, curdles milk. Another enzyme, lipase, splits certain fats, while pepsin digests the milk curds from the rennin. The hydrochloric acid unites with protein to form another chemical, which in turn is split by the pepsin.

Because hydrochloric acid burns holes in most things it touches, you may wonder why it does not destroy the stomach. This is because the lining also secretes small amounts of ammonia, which is capable of counteracting normal amounts of the acid. However, when a sufficient amount of excess acid is present for a sufficient length of time, an **ulcer** (open sore) will develop, usually along the

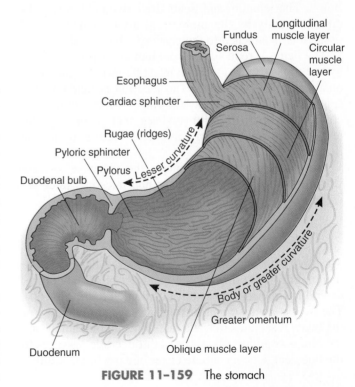

FIGURE 11-159 The stomach

posterior wall near the pylorus. An ulcer in the stomach is known as a gastric (stomach) or **peptic** ulcer.

The partially-digested food in the stomach is changed into a semiliquid state called **chyme** in three to five hours. Liquids, on the other hand, pass through the stomach in a matter of minutes. Of the solid foods, carbohydrates are digested first, proteins second, and fats last. When the consistency of the chyme is right, the **pyloric** sphincter, at the end of the stomach, allows the chyme to spurt through the sphincter into the small **intestine**.

Because of the two sphincters, food is held in the stomach until it is properly prepared to leave. But occasionally, when you suffer from **nausea** and **vomit**, it is obvious the material did not go in the right direction. This action is accomplished by the contraction of the abdominal muscles, forcefully squeezing the stomach as it is pushed downward by the diaphragm. With this pressure and reverse peristaltic waves, the contents of the stomach are forced out and **emesis** (vomiting) occurs.

THE SMALL INTESTINE

The small intestine is a tube about one inch in diameter and about 20 feet in length. It completes the digestive process and absorbs the nutrients from the chyme.

The small intestine is divided into three sections. The first is a C-shaped segment, about nine inches long, called the **duodenum** (see Figure 11–159). Because this area receives the highest concentration of acid from the stomach, it is especially prone to the development of ulcers. An ulcer in this area is called a duodenal ulcer.

The next segment, the **jejunum**, is about eight feet in length. The last segment, about 12 feet long, is called the **ileum**. The jejunum and ileum are suspended in the abdominal cavity by the **mesentery**, a fan-shaped fold of tissue that is attached to the posterior abdominal wall.

The ileum is reduced to about half an inch in diameter by the time it joins the large intestine in the right lower quadrant of the abdomen. The junction is marked by a sphincter called the **ileocecal** valve, which allows the chyme to enter the **cecum** (first segment of the large intestine) but prohibits anything from returning to the ileum.

The small intestine completes the digestive process with the aid of accessory organs and intestinal juice secreted by the glands of the small intestine.

The Liver and Gallbladder

The **liver** is the largest gland in the body. It lies below the diaphragm in the upper right quadrant of the abdomen, extending into the upper left quadrant (Figure 11–160). The liver is a vital organ performing several functions for the body. It secretes **bile** at a rate of over a pint a day, and the bile is continuously excreted through bile passages to the bile duct. Unconcentrated liver bile is a bitter, yellow-

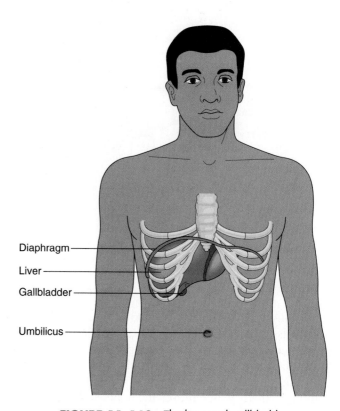

FIGURE 11–160 The liver and gallbladder

orange liquid that is required to digest fats. Bile is composed primarily of water and contains pigment from red blood cells that have been destroyed (carried to the liver from the spleen in the portal vein). The pigment is changed in the intestines and excreted in **fecal** material, giving it its yellow-brown color. The iron from the destroyed cells is reabsorbed into the body.

The liver also stores glycogen, a form of glucose (carbohydrate). When the body needs additional blood sugar, it changes the glycogen back to glucose and releases it. In addition, the liver processes proteins from amino acids and either burns fats as fuel or stores them. The liver performs the life-essential service of manufacturing fibrinogen, prothrombin, and other substances required for the process of clotting blood. Antibodies to counteract certain disease organisms are produced in the liver. Also, toxins (poisons) that have been absorbed from the intestine, inhaled, injected, or otherwise taken into the body are circulated in the blood to the liver, where for the most part they are rendered harmless. The liver is also an important storage area for blood and body fluid because of its large size.

The liver receives blood from two separate systems. It receives arterial blood for its own support and preservation from the hepatic artery. It also receives blood from the portal vein that conveys absorbed nutrients and other substances from all the abdominal organs for processing.

The **gallbladder** is a small sac attached to the underside of the liver (Figure 11–161). Its sole purpose is the

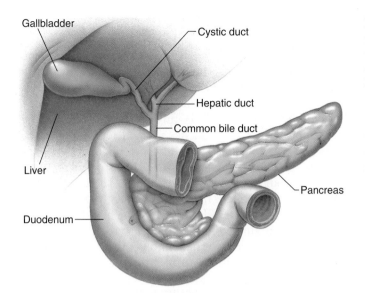

FIGURE 11-161 The gallbladder and cystic, hepatic, and common bile ducts on the undersurface of the liver

concentration and storage of bile. When the body needs bile to digest food, the gallbladder releases the concentrated bile to supplement that being currently produced by the liver. Concentrated bile is very bitter and is green-yellow in color. The gallbladder empties its contents via the **cystic** duct. The cystic duct from the gallbladder and the **hepatic** duct from the liver combine to form the **common bile duct**. This command duct empties the bile directly into the duodenum to be added to the chyme during the digestive process. The duodenum is a very vital segment of the digestive system. Not only does it receive chyme from the stomach and bile from the liver and gallbladder, but as we will soon see, it also receives pancreatic juices from the pancreas.

Obstruction of the bile ducts by **cholelithiasis** (gallstones) is not uncommon. Bile contains certain mineral salts that can become crystallized into "stones" in the gallbladder, perhaps from poor drainage or extended storage. Frequently the stones will be expelled into the cystic duct where they become lodged, causing pain and an inadequate supply of bile and frequently requiring surgical removal. If the stone reaches the common bile duct before becoming lodged, a much more serious situation results. Now neither the gallbladder nor the liver can empty its bile. The liver maintains its production, but now the bile is absorbed into the bloodstream, producing the yellow discoloration of the sclera, mucosa, and skin known as **jaundice**. The gallbladder itself may become infected or filled with stones and nonfunctional. Periodic "gallbladder attacks" will usually prompt a **cholecystectomy** (surgical removal). The hepatic duct and the common bile duct must remain for the liver to function, however.

A surgical procedure to remove cholelithiasis called endoscopic retrograde cholangiopancreatography (ERCP)

has revolutionized the way cholecystectomies are performed. The procedure is accomplished with the use of three laparoscopes inserted into the abdomen. One is placed in the RUQ, one at the umbilicus, and one mid-upper abdomen. One scope serves as the light source, another to supply air to manipulate tissues, and one through which the operation is performed. The gallbladder and its contents, if any, are excised and removed through the operative scope. Following surgery, only a few sutures are required to close the small abdominal openings. Previous surgery resulted in a long incision extending down the right side of the abdomen and a considerably uncomfortable postoperative period. The new laparoscopic surgery has shortened recovery to two weeks or less from about six weeks with the previous surgical method. In some instances, the surgery is even being done as an outpatient procedure.

The Pancreas

The **pancreas** lies behind the stomach, with its head in the curve of the duodenum (Figure 11–162). The pancreas, like the liver, is a gland, but it secretes substances in two different ways. Functioning as an *exocrine gland* (secreting through ducts), the pancreas secretes pancreatic juice via the pancreatic duct directly into the duodenum. The three powerful enzymes in pancreatic juice react chemically on all three types of nutrients to break them down for absorption into the bloodstream. Most of the chemical changes that occur in the intestinal tract are caused by pancreatic juices, which are probably sufficient to digest all foods by themselves. If pancreatic juice is absent, serious digestive problems occur.

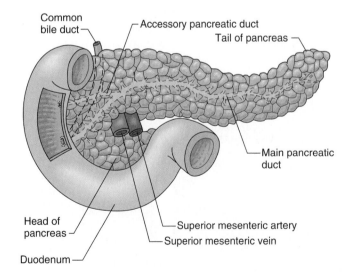

FIGURE 11-162 The duodenum and pancreas. A window has been cut into the anterior wall of the duodenum to show the openings of the common bile duct and the pancreatic ducts into the lumen of the duodenum.

Functioning as an *endocrine* (ductless) *gland,* the pancreas also secretes directly into the bloodstream a substance called **insulin**. This function will be covered in Unit 12, The Endocrine System.

It should be clear now why the duodenum is such a critical segment of the digestive tract. Because it receives products from four organs—stomach, liver, gallbladder, and pancreas—it is a vital connective link. When ulceration occurs or a tumor develops in this area, it may interfere drastically with the digestive process. Involvement of the duodenum is a cause for concern.

The Absorption Function

When all the digestive juices and enzymes have been added and the chyme passes into the jejunum, digestion has progressed to the point where absorption of some nutrients and other substances can begin. Absorption is a vital function of the small intestine, occurring primarily in the jejunum and gradually decreasing toward the end of the ileum.

Absorption is accomplished through millions of microscopic structures known as **villi** (Figure 11–163). The villi project from the lining of the major part of the small intestine. These fingerlike structures serve a dual purpose. First, they move continuously, swinging back and forth to keep the chyme thoroughly mixed with the digestive juices. Second, each projection is equipped with blood capillaries and a lacteal (intestinal lymphatic capillary) from the lymphatic system. The external cells of the villi absorb the nutrients, minerals, and water from the chyme. Some fats and all carbohydrates and proteins, in the form of sugar and amino acids, are absorbed into the capillaries of the villi, to be sent by way of the portal vein to the liver. Here, the products are processed and released into the body or stored in reserve. Many fats are absorbed into the lacteals of the lymphatic system to be processed through the lymph nodes and eventually returned to the circulatory system for distribution.

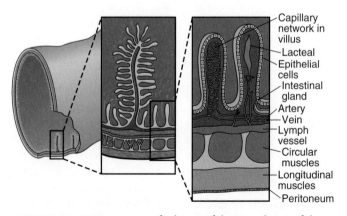

FIGURE 11-163 A magnified view of the inner lining of the small intestine, showing the villi with blood and lymphatic capillaries for the absorption of the products of digestion

THE LARGE INTESTINE

With digestion completed and the useful nutrients and other substances absorbed from the chyme, the waste products, any undigestible material, and the excess water are sent on to the large intestine through the ileocecal valve. The large intestine is only about five feet long, but it is approximately two inches in diameter. The **colon**, as it is also called, frames the abdomen (Figure 11–164).

The large intestine absorbs the excess liquid from the chyme through capillaries in the lining. There are no villi in the large intestine. The absorbed water, plus some salts and proteins, are later filtered out of the blood by the kidneys to be eliminated in the urine. The remaining fibrous waste materials are formed into semisolid feces to be eliminated through the **rectum**.

The Cecum and Appendix

When material leaves the ileum, it enters a small, pouch-like segment of the colon called the cecum. A small projection, the **vermiform appendix**, extends from the cecum. The appendix is a worm-shaped structure about the size of the little finger. It tends to become filled easily but drains rather slowly. Occasionally, a substance causes irritation to the lining, resulting in a painful, inflammatory process known as **appendicitis**. If it persists or progresses, a surgical procedure called an **appendectomy** is indicated.

The Ascending, Transverse, and Descending Colon

The large intestine is divided into **ascending**, **transverse**, and **descending** sections as a means of identification. The ascending section joins the cecum at the level of the ileocecal valve and continues upward along the right side of the abdomen to the hepatic flexure (bend at the liver). It is generally a little larger in diameter than the descending section. The upper right corner, the hepatic flexure, lies in front of the right kidney and behind the right lobe of the liver. The transverse section begins at the hepatic flexure and extends in a loop across the abdominal cavity to a point below the spleen, the splenic flexure (bend at the spleen). The center section is attached to the mesentery but can move freely. Both the hepatic and splenic flexures are firmly attached to the rear of the abdominal wall, with the splenic attachment being slightly higher.

The descending section begins at the splenic flexure and extends downward along the left side of the abdomen until it reaches the edge of the pelvic cavity. This section is somewhat smaller in diameter. It is firmly anchored to the abdominal posterior wall to maintain its position.

The Sigmoid, Rectum, and Anal Canal

After the large intestine enters the pelvic cavity, it makes two bends suggestive of an S and is therefore labeled the

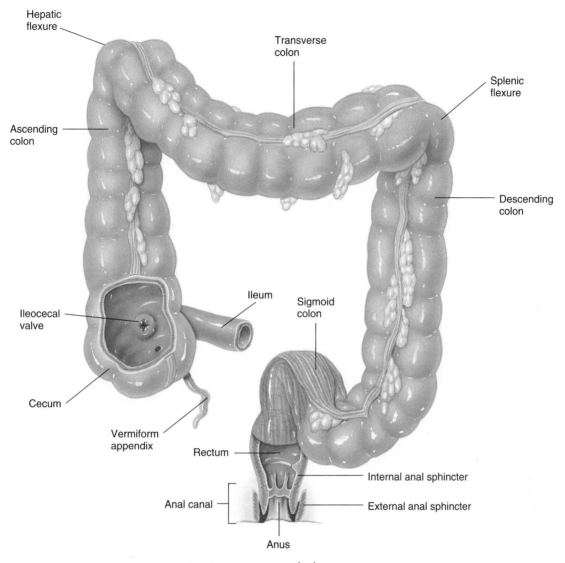

FIGURE 11-164   The large intestine

sigmoid section of the colon. The sigmoid section extends from the left iliac crest over and back to join the rectum. The rectum is six to eight inches long. It serves as a collecting area for the remains of digestion. When enough material is accumulated, sensors are activated, and the urge to **defecate** is felt.

The **anal** canal is a narrow passageway about an inch long, extending from the rectum to the **anus** (opening from the body). Both ends of the anal canal are controlled by sphincter muscles. The internal anal sphincter is an involuntary muscle. When defecation occurs, the nerve endings in the rectum are stimulated to contract, and the internal sphincter is relaxed, allowing the fecal material to enter the anal canal. The external anal sphincter is a voluntary muscle and can be consciously controlled to prevent the rectum from emptying when it is inappropriate. It is unwise to make a habit of delaying defecation unnecessarily, however, as this tends to lessening the urge, which can result in **constipation**.

When a patient's condition interferes with the ability to control the anus, as in a stroke with paralysis, and the rectum empties whenever the nerve impulse is triggered, the patient is said to be **incontinent** of feces. This situation can be extremely embarrassing to a patient who is still capable of being aware of this occurrence. The opposite problem is often the result of prolonged or serious illness causing a loss of muscle tone so that the patient is too weak to expel the contents of the rectum. This results in material becoming more and more solid as fluid content is lost and the mass becoming of such size that it cannot be expelled. This condition is known as a fecal **impaction**. The best solution is manual breakup of the mass followed by an enema to irrigate the rectum and remove the material. A patient may attempt to remove the impaction by taking a laxative. Laxatives work either by increasing the rate of passage through the tract, therefore reducing the water absorption time, or by stimulating the secretion of fluid into the tract. Regardless, the results will not help an impaction but only cause an uncontrollable flow of liquid **stool** around the mass.

The proper function of the digestive system is essential to health. If raw materials cannot be digested and absorbed, the patient will starve. If waste products are not adequately removed, toxins may accumulate and cause illness and even death. This vital function requires a total of about 36 hours from the mouth to the anus. Of course, this time period is influenced by the type of foods eaten and the rate of the peristaltic action.

DIAGNOSTIC EXAMINATIONS

A great many studies can be done on blood to determine the function of the digestive organs. Also, chemical analysis can be performed on secretions withdrawn by catheter from the stomach or small intestine. However, six other types of examinations will be discussed here because they are so frequently used in diagnosis.

- Cholecystography—An x-ray examination of the gallbladder following oral administration of a contrast medium. The patient is instructed to take the tablets, one at a time, five minutes apart, about two hours after dinner the evening before the examination is scheduled. After the tablets are taken, the patient must refrain from any food or drink. The medium is digested and absorbed by the small intestine and sent to the liver by the portal vein. The liver processes the blood, excreting the medium in the bile. The gallbladder concentrates the bile. X-rays taken 12 to 14 hours after ingestion of the pills will show the gallbladder filled with the medium. If a fatty substance is then given to the patient to eat or drink, the gallbladder should contract and empty bile into the duodenum. This study allows the physician to determine if the gallbladder is functioning properly. A nonfunctioning gallbladder will neither absorb nor empty the dye properly. The presence of cholelithiasis and obstruction of the bile ducts can be determined.

- Colonoscopy—An examination to view the entire large intestine using a flexible fiberoptic scope. It is indicated in patients with complaints of diarrhea, constipation, bleeding, or lower abdominal pain. It is usually indicated following negative or inconclusive results from barium enema studies or sigmoidoscopy examination. Preparation for the examination is like that for sigmoidoscopy. The patient is positioned on the left side, and the scope is guided and advanced through the large intestine. The physician may insert air to distend the walls of the intestine to facilitate passage. Manipulation of the abdomen also assists with insertion, and the repositioning of the patient facilitates passage through the splenic and hepatic flexures. It is possible to obtain tissue samples and secretions through the scope to provide cytology studies. Polyps can also be snared, and electrocautery can be performed through the instrument.

- Gastrointestinal series (x-rays)—Radiological studies of the GI tract are indicated for a wide variety of reasons and concentrated on various portions of the system.

Barium swallow—If the condition or function of the esophagus is in question, the patient may be asked to drink a radiopaque liquid called barium while the action of the esophagus is observed by fluoroscope. This test is known as a barium swallow. It aids in diagnosing conditions, such as hiatus hernia, diverticulosis, and varices. It also detects strictures, tumors, ulcers, and functional disorders. The barium swallow is usually included as part of the more complete GI series.

Upper GI series—A barium swallow is performed initially to evaluate the esophagus. Sixteen to twenty ounces of additional barium are drunk as the progress of the medium is observed by fluoroscope. X-ray films are taken at specific periods to permit further evaluation. The stomach is compressed to ensure that the barium coats the entire lining. As the barium enters the small intestine, the radiologist manipulates the abdomen to obtain distribution of the barium throughout the bowel loops. The patient is rotated to several positions to record pertinent areas. Spot films may be taken at 30- to 60-minute intervals until peristalsis carries the barium to the ileocecal valve.

An upper GI series is not painful, but the chalky taste and consistency of barium are unpleasant. Preparation for the test may require a two- to three-day diet of low-residue foods before the examination. All oral intake must stop at least eight hours before it is scheduled. The patient must also refrain from smoking. Both a laxative and a cleansing enema may be ordered the evening before the procedure to be certain the tract is empty.

An upper GI series aids in the diagnosis of gastric ulcers, tumors, strictures of the sphincters, inflammation of the lining, motility irregularities, duodenal ulcers, tumors, filling defects, and the like. Following the exam, another laxative may be ordered to aid in removal of the barium from the intestines. Retained barium may cause constipation, obstruction, or fecal impaction.

Lower GI series—To permit viewing of the entire large intestine, the barium mixture is administered as an enema. The medium outlines the interior wall of the colon for detection of mucosal changes, tumors, **polyps**, ulcerated sites, **diverticulitis**, and structural irregularities. The patient must be carefully prepared with a restrictive, low-residue diet for about two days, followed by a diet of liquids only the day before examination. A cathartic (strong laxative) is ordered the afternoon preceding the test and the colon is thoroughly emptied with tap water enemas until no more fecal material is expelled.

A barium enema of 1,000 to 1,500 cc is administered through a tube inserted into the rectum. This tube is often capable of being inflated with a balloonlike section to aid in retention of the medium until the examination is completed. As the medium is instilled, the filling is observed by fluoroscope. The patient is rotated on the x-ray table to assist the flow of the barium. The patient is placed on the left side to fill the descending, on the back to fill the transverse, and on the right side to fill the ascending colon. Periodic x-ray films are taken.

When the procedure is completed, the balloon is deflated and the tube is removed. The patient is instructed to expel as much barium as possible. An additional x-ray may be taken to record the ability of the colon to empty.

■ **Gastroscopy**/Esophagogastroduodenoscopy (EGD)—Viewing of the esophagus, stomach, and upper duodenum through a flexible scope that is lighted by fiberoptics. This permits observation of the inside of the organs without an exploratory operation. If an unusual area or growth is seen, a biopsy (small piece) can be removed through the scope. The procedure is also used to remove small foreign objects, obtain cells from the lining, and, with the attachment of a camera, to photograph suspicious areas for later study.

The patient is prepared by spraying the back of the throat with local anesthetic to block the gag reflex and given a sedative to produce drowsiness. The patient must be awake to swallow the scope. As it is passed into the patient, air is instilled to expand the pathway or flatten out folds. Water may also be instilled to wash off the lens and is removed, along with the air and any other secretions, by suction.

The examination is especially helpful in diagnosing tumors, ulcers, structural abnormalities, damage from ingested chemicals, and esophageal varices. Figure 11–165 shows a fairly large tumor attached to the wall of the stomach. It is clearly visible through the scope and easily accessible for biopsy.

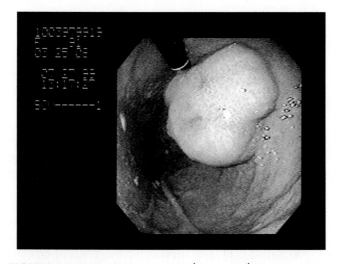

FIGURE 11–165 Tumor in stomach as seen during an esophagogastrosdenoscopy examination (Courtesy of Thomas Ransbottom, M.D.)

■ Nuclear medicine study—Scanning of structures, such as the liver or spleen, is made visible by radioactive materials. A special camera or scanning device may be used to screen the liver for disease processes, infarcts, cysts, tumors, and organ size. The patient is given an intravenous injection of a radioactive material that the body will absorb in the cells of the liver. The scanner is positioned above the patient and passes slowly back and forth in a descending pattern over the area being examined. The resulting pictures outline the organ and indicate irregularities in its composition. A gamma camera is capable of producing images instantly without the scanning procedure.

Similar studies are accomplished with different types of equipment. Computerized axial tomography studies (CT scans) are multiple x-ray beams passed into tissue to be interpreted and reconstructed by a computer into a three-dimensional picture on a screen. This type of study can be done on the liver, the ducts, and the pancreas.

■ Occult blood test—When bleeding from the intestinal tract is not visible because of the small quantity, it can be detected through analysis of the feces. Occult blood studies are frequently used to identify bleeding associated with colorectal malignancy.

Visible blood in the stool has a characteristic coloration that suggests the approximate location of the bleeding. Basically, the nearer the rectum, the brighter red the blood. Dark maroon stool is an indication of bleeding in the ileum or jejunum. Bleeding from the stomach or esophagus will be acted on by gastric juices, which cause it to turn black, resulting in a tarry-looking stool. A simple test involves the use of a Hemoccult slide upon which a thin smear of stool is placed. The Hemoccult Developer is applied to the smear, and results are read within a minute. A trace or change of color to blue is positive for occult blood. Refer to Chapter 15, Unit 4, for additional information.

■ Proctoscopy—An examination of the lower rectum and anal canal through a three-inch-long **proctoscope**. It is preceded by a digital examination to determine anal sphincter condition. The proctoscope permits detection of hemorrhoids, polyps, fissures, fistulas, and abscesses. The patient may need an enema if fecal material is obstructing the view.

■ **Sigmoidoscopy**—An examination to view the lower portion of the sigmoid and rectum through a 10- to 12-inch sigmoidoscope. A longer flexible fiberoptic scope is capable of manipulation into the descending colon. A digital examination to determine anal sphincter condition precedes insertion of the scope. The patient is examined, preferably on a special jackknife table, or otherwise in the less comfortable knee–chest position. Sigmoidoscopy aids in the diagnosis of inflammation, infection, or ulcerative conditions. It also permits viewing of tumors, polyps, and other disease processes. Biopsy through the scope permits confirmation of a diagnosis without surgery. The patient must be prepared for the examination with an enema administered a short time before. Soap or other irritants must not be added to the water because they may affect the appearance of the lining. (See Chapter 14, Unit 4.)

■ Ultrasound—Ultrasonography uses high-frequency sound waves directed toward the liver, gallbladder, or pancreas. The waves create echos of varying degrees, which are changed into patterns of dots on a screen. The patterns reveal the size, shape, and position of the organ being studied. Ultrasonography is especially useful when liver and gallbladder functions are impaired and the use of contrast media is ineffective.

DISORDERS AND DISEASES
Anorectal Abscess and Fistula (A-no-reck'-tal Ab'-cess Fis'-tu-la)

Definition—This localized infection is a collection of exudate in the soft tissue adjacent to the anus or rectum.

Signs and symptoms—It is characterized by a throbbing, painful lump, which makes sitting and coughing very uncomfortable.

Etiology—The abscess may be initiated from within the rectum because of a sharp object in the feces, such as a piece of seashell or bone, penetrating the surrounding tissue. Because the feces contain bacteria, an infection develops and an abscess results. The exudate may develop an escape route into the rectum, anal canal, or skin surface, which will periodically relieve the pain and excess pressure. Such a tract is known as a **fistula**.

Treatment—Surgical intervention is indicated to correct the condition by incision and drainage of both the abscess and the tract (Figure 11–166).

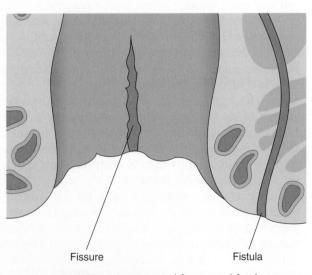

Fissure Fistula

FIGURE 11-166 Anal fissure and fistula

Occasionally, an abscess occurs without a fistula. It may appear on the surface of the perineum as a large, firm, red mass, with or without a yellow center. This abscess requires incision to promote drainage and eventual expression of the solid core of material. The application of heat by sitting in a tub of warm water aids in the drainage process and relieves discomfort.

Appendicitis (A-pen-di-ci'-tis)

Description—An acute inflammation of the appendix probably is caused by an obstruction of the intestinal lumen.

Signs and symptoms—Symptoms of appendicitis begin with generalized abdominal pain that later localizes in the lower right abdomen at a site known as McBurney's point. Increased tenderness, anorexia, nausea, vomiting, and rebound tenderness (produced by slowly compressing abdomen over site, then suddenly releasing the pressure) occur. A slight fever may be present. A moderately elevated white blood cell count (12,000 to 15,000) in addition to the physical findings supports the diagnosis. The sudden cessation of symptoms is an indication of infarction or rupture.

Etiology—When obstruction occurs, an inflammatory process begins and leads to infection, thrombosis, destruction of tissue, and eventually perforation of the appendix. On rupture, the infectious material spills into the abdominal cavity and initiates peritonitis, a serious complication. If left untreated, it is fatal.

Treatment—The only effective treatment for appendicitis is surgical removal, an appendectomy. When appendicitis is suspected, abdominal heat, enemas, or laxatives must never be administered because of the risk of causing perforation. Usually pain medication is avoided to prevent masking of the symptoms. Positioning patients on their right side with the knees flexed will usually help to reduce the discomfort.

Cirrhosis (Sear-o'-sis)

Description—This chronic disease of the liver causes destruction of the liver cells. The destruction leads to impaired blood and lymph circulation and interferes with the life-preserving functions of the liver.

Signs and symptoms—Early symptoms include a variety of GI tract signs, such as lack of appetite, indigestion, nausea, vomiting, constipation, and **diarrhea**. Later, nosebleeds, bleeding gums, and anemia may develop. The liver becomes enlarged, jaundice is present, and ascites (collection of fluid) occurs within the abdomen. Because the disease interferes with portal circulation, hypertension occurs in the portal system, causing esophageal varices that eventually rupture and bleed.

Various blood tests support the diagnosis of **cirrhosis**, but positive confirmation can be obtained through a liver biopsy. A liver scan will detect abnormal thickening and a mass.

Etiology—The most frequent cause of cirrhosis is malnutrition associated with alcoholism. Other causative factors are hepatitis or the suppression of bile flow resulting from a disease of the ducts.

Treatment—Treatment consists of taking measures to prevent further damage or complications and dealing with the underlying cause. Dietary changes, supplemental vitamins, rest, and appropriate exercise are indicated. Extra care is required when prescribing drugs because the damaged liver may not be able to process them. Alcohol must be prohibited. It is also important to avoid contact with infections. Mortality is high, with many patients dying within five years of diagnosis.

Colitis (Ko-li'-tis)

Description—This inflammation of the colon causes tenderness and discomfort. It may be acute, occurring as the result of a bacterial invasion, or chronic, associated with allergy, emotional stress, or other diseases. (See ulcerative **colitis**.)

Colorectal Cancer (Co-lo-reck'-tal)

Description—This is a malignancy of the colon or rectum. The American Cancer Society estimated 135,400 new cases of colorectal cancer in 2001. It is the third most common cancer in men and women. Incidence rates did decline 1.6% from 1985 to 1997, possibly because of increased screening and polyp removal. (Some polyps tend to become malignant over time.) The Society also estimated 56,700 deaths in 2001, which represented about 10% of all cancer deaths. The one-year survival rate is 82%, whereas the five-year rate is 61%. When detected early at the localized stage, the five-year survival rate increases to 90%; however, only 37% are detected this early. When there is distant metastases, the survival rate drops to only 8%. Figure 11–167 illustrates the percentage of incidence in the common sites and shows that 75% are within viewing distance of the flexible sigmoidoscope. This illustration emphasizes the importance of sigmoidoscopy screening on a regularly-scheduled basis as a way of identifying a large percentage of colorectal cancer in its early stage when intervention is most effective.

Signs and symptoms—Symptoms can vary in relation to the area involved. With right side colon involvement there may be black tarry stools, anemia, abdominal aching, pressure, and dull cramps in the beginning. As the disease progresses, weakness, fatigue, dyspnea, vertigo, and eventually diarrhea, anorexia, weight loss, vomiting, and other signs of intestinal obstruction will occur. (Because the wastes are liquid in the section, obstruction is delayed.) With left side involvement, obstruction signs occur earlier because of the formed consistency of the fecal material. There is rectal bleeding, abdominal fullness, cramping, and rectal pressure.

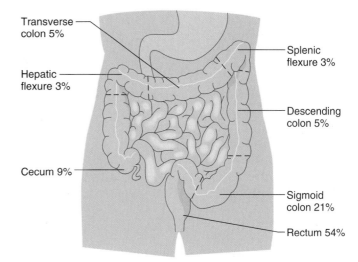

FIGURE 11–167 Percentages of incidence of colorectal cancer by sites

Later, there are diarrhea and "ribbon" or pencil-shaped stools. Bleeding in the form of bright red blood and mucous is in or on the stools. With rectal cancer, the first symptom is a change in bowel habits—often "morning diarrhea" may alternate with obstipation (constipation caused by obstruction). This will be followed by a feeling of incomplete evacuation and later pain and a feeling of rectal fullness.

Etiology—Basically the cause is unknown. However, certain risk factors have been identified.

- A personal or family history of colorectal cancer or polyps
- Inflammatory bowel disease
- Possible relationship to smoking, physical inactivity, high-fat and/or low fiber diet, alcohol consumption, and low intake of fruits and vegetables

Recent studies seem to suggest that estrogen replacement therapy and the use of NSAIDs, such as aspirin, may reduce the risk.

Treatment—The most effective treatment is surgery to remove the tumor, adjacent tissues, and any lymph nodes that may be involved. The type of tumor and extent of involvement determine the surgical procedure. It may involve only the removal of a section of the colon and its supporting structures, to total resectioning of the rectum and the construction of a permanent colostomy. Chemotherapy is indicated with metastasis, residual disease, or a recurring inoperable tumor. Radiation and chemotherapy may be used before surgery to reduce the tumor size and activity and also are given following surgery to treat any missed cells.

Colostomy (Ko-los'-toe-me)

Description—This is an artificial opening of the colon, allowing fecal material to be excreted from the body through the abdominal wall. **Colostomies** are classified

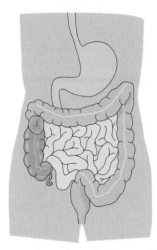
Ascending colostomy

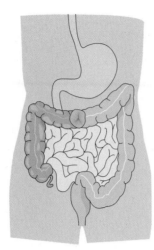
Transverse colostomy

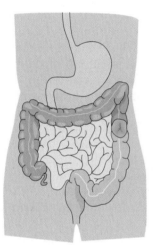
Descending colostomy

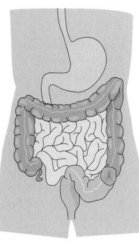
Sigmoid colostomy

Colostomy Sites

FIGURE 11–168 Colostomy sites

according to the portion of the colon involved (for example, transverse colostomy) (Figure 11–168). The terms *single* and *double barrel* tell whether only the proximal loop is involved or both the proximal and distal loop. A colostomy can also be temporary or permanent. If a disease process could improve if the colon were not constantly irritated by passing feces, then a temporary colostomy is indicated. By surgically providing for the fecal material to empty through an opening in the colon before reaching the affected area, the area is allowed to rest and heal. After an adequate period, surgery is performed to reattach the ends of the colon.

A colostomy is also indicated when an obstructive growth process, such as a tumor, prohibits the passage of feces. When the growth is close to the end of the rectum, there may not be enough healthy tissue remaining to which a segment of the colon can be attached. There may also be evidence that removal of the affected area, even if possible, would present no ad-

vantage. In these cases, a colostomy will be performed for elimination to occur until the disease process results in death.

The colostomy patient has a major emotional adjustment in addition to physical adjustment to make. The alteration in body image may be difficult to accept. The thought of fecal material being expelled into a pouch attached to the abdomen may be very unappealing. Consider also that there is no control over the expulsion of **flatus** (gas) or stool, and it is easy to understand the new patient's rejection. However, with time, diet control, and the use of irrigation, a colostomy can be regulated so that its emptying is at the patient's convenience. Support groups of colostomy patients provide emotional and physical assistance to help new colostomy patients adjust to their changed lifestyle.

Constipation (Con-sti-pa'-shun)

Description—This is a condition of sluggish bowel action.
Signs and symptoms—It is characterized by dry, hard, infrequent bowel movements.
Etiology—To have normal elimination of body wastes, three things are necessary: a proper diet including bulk, adequate fluid intake, and exercise. When one or more of these elements is missing, constipation is likely to occur. Other contributing factors are habitual disregard of the impulse to defecate and the chronic use of laxatives or enemas, which dull the impulse stimulation. Constipation is common among the elderly, persons with paralysis, and the chronically ill or bedridden, as a result of lack of activity.
Treatment—Treatment varies with the cause and condition of the patient. If possible, increasing the dietary bulk, fluid intake, and amount of exercise will usually solve the problem. Prompt response to the urge to defecate is necessary. Normally, a person's body will establish a routine schedule given the opportunity. The habitual use of laxatives and enemas must be stopped. The use of bulk-forming products and glycerin suppositories can be substituted until new bowel habits are learned.

A PEDIATRIC PERSPECTIVE

Constipation in an infant is commonly the result of early introduction of solid foods, such as cereal, or a switch from breast milk to formula. A history of fussiness, colic, or excessive gas is frequently described in addition to usual symptoms of difficulty and decreased frequency in passing stool. A second common time for constipation to occur is with toilet training because of the pressure the parent or caregiver places on the child to defecate or urinate in the toilet.

Treatment—For infants (less than one year of age), adding a fruit juice, such as pear or apple, may resolve the constipation. A glycerin suppository may be needed to soften the stool to reduce the discomfort with defecation. Constipation in infants that does not respond to juice or glycerin suppository needs to be thoroughly evaluated by a physician or gastrointestinal specialist. The parents of a child who is in the process of toilet training should be advised to stop the training until the child is interested in using the toilet or potty-chair.

Crohn's Disease (Kron's)

Description—This is an inflammation of any portion of the GI tract, most common in the terminal ileum. The inflammation involves all layers of the intestinal wall leading to edema, ulceration, narrowing, and the formation of abscesses and fistulas.

Signs and symptoms—Symptoms vary according to the location of the disease. An acute episode often causes appendicitis-type complaints of pain, cramping, and tenderness in the right lower quadrant with flatulence, nausea, fever, and diarrhea. Bloody stools are also possible. Chronic disease is characterized by diarrhea of four to six stools daily, marked weight loss, weakness, and difficulty in coping with everyday stress.

Etiology—The exact cause of **Crohn's disease** is unknown. Some feel it is caused by allergies or immune disorders, obstruction of the lymphatics, or infection.

Diagnosis is made after positive blood tests showing increased white blood cells, decreased hemoglobin, and other specific abnormalities. Barium enema studies showing segments of stricture separated by normal bowel, known as *string signs,* supports the diagnosis. Sigmoidoscopy, which reveals patchy areas of inflammation, helps to differentiate Crohn's disease from ulcerative colitis.

Treatment—Treatment is mainly symptomatic and may include dietary supplements, steroids to reduce the inflammation, and the use of antibacterial agents. Most important are changes in lifestyle to obtain more rest and dietary adjustments to eliminate contributing agents. The ingestion of fruits and vegetables must be restricted with intestinal stenosis (narrowing). Surgery may be necessary if certain conditions develop, such as a fistula, bowel perforation, hemorrhage, or obstruction. With extensive disease of the colon, a colectomy with **ileostomy** may be required (see Ileostomy).

Diarrhea (Di-a-re'-ah)

Description—This is a condition of repeated passage of unformed wastes.

Signs and symptoms—It is characterized by frequent, liquid stools, which can be very serious in infants and small children because of the excessive loss of body fluid.

Etiology—Diarrhea can be caused by a bacterial, viral, or amebic organism. It can also result from a poor diet, toxic substances, foods such as prunes that stimulate peristalsis, or an irritated colon. Basically, diarrhea occurs because the chyme is moved too rapidly through the colon without sufficient time for the water to be absorbed. When the lining is inflamed, as with colitis, rapid peristalsis occurs as soon as material reaches the affected area. In addition, the lining secretes excess mucus to counteract the irritating material. This response results in a liquid stool with shreds of mucus. Diarrhea can also result from nervousness or anxiety. Again, the peristaltic action is stimulated and the waves move rapidly.

Treatment—Diarrhea is best treated by providing an adequate intake of liquids and taking care of the underlying cause. Medication to slow down peristalsis is helpful, but it will not treat the underlying cause.

Diverticulosis (Di-ver-tick'-u-low-sis)

Description—This is the presence of bulging pouches in the wall of the GI tract where the lining has pushed into the surrounding muscle. The sigmoid colon is the most common site, but diverticuli can occur anywhere from the esophagus to the anus.

Signs and symptoms—Symptoms of diverticulitis include irregular bowel movements, lower left abdominal pain, nausea, flatus, low-grade fever, and an increase in WBCs. Chronic diverticulitis may result in fibrosis and adhesions (tissues growing together) that severely limit or obstruct the lumen. Symptoms progress from constipation to ribbon-like stools, diarrhea, distention (swelling up) of the abdomen, nausea, vomiting, pain, and abdominal rigidity.

Etiology—They are believed to be caused by a high degree of internal pressure and an area of weakness in the intestinal wall. There is a theory that lack of roughage in the diet permits the bowel lumen (opening) to narrow, resulting in higher pressure developing during defecation. The disease is much less common in nations where more natural food and fiber are eaten.

Diverticulitis develops when undigested food mixes with the bacteria normal to the tract and collects in a diverticular sac, forming a hard mass. The mass shuts off the blood supply to the thin-walled sac, followed by inflammation, infection, possibly perforation (a hole), abscess, or hemorrhage.

Treatment—Treatment initially consists of preventing constipation and combating infection. A liquid diet, antibiotics, one medication to soften the stool, and another medication to relieve pain and relax muscle spasms are called for. When conservative measures fail, the affected colon section may need to be removed.

Esophageal Varices (E-sof-o-ge'-al Var'-i-sees)

Description—Dilated, tortuous veins in the lower section of the esophagus are called esophageal **varices.**

Signs and symptoms—This results in fluid entering the abdominal cavity, causing ascites. With the veins dilated and therefore thinner and the number of platelets reduced, hemorrhage occurs readily and is often the first sign of the condition. Often massive hemorrhage occurs, producing bloody emesis and stools.

Etiology—They are the result of hypertension within the portal vein. The blood flowing through the portal system in the liver meets with resistance because of cirrhosis, a tumor, thrombosis, or occlusion of the veins. As a result, blood backs up to the spleen, causing it to enlarge, and the blood flows through other veins. The number of platelets decreases, and the other veins dilate.

Treatment—Treatment is limited. To control bleeding, a tube may be inserted into the esophagus to put pressure against the bleeding site. In addition, iced salt water may be instilled into the tube. A drug may be given to control bleeding temporarily. Surgical bypass procedures to correct venous flow may cause from 25% to 50% mortality, and the patient may still die eventually from liver complications instead of hemorrhage. Blood transfusions are also temporary measures. At best, the patient can be kept comfortable until the inevitable massive hemorrhage or coma from liver damage occurs.

Fissure of the Anus (Fish'-ur)

Description—An anal **fissure** is a crack or tear in the lining of the anus (Figure 11–166).

Signs and symptoms—Symptoms of acute fissure are a burning pain and a few drops of blood on the toilet tissue or underwear. The fissure may develop a swelling at the lower end known as a *sentinel pile*. This protrusion may ulcerate, resulting in painful anal sphincter spasms.

A fissure may heal completely or become chronic as a result of partial healing and retearing. Later, scar tissue develops in the area, narrowing the passageway. Because the anus must stretch each time stool is passed, healing is difficult.

Etiology—It is usually the result of passing large, hard stools that stretch the lining beyond its capacity.

Treatment—Treatment consists of digital dilation to prevent stricture, a low-residue diet, stool softeners, adequate liquid intake, hot sitz baths, and a local medication for pain. A chronic condition will require surgical excision of the scar tissue, providing two fresh surfaces that can heal by a gradual regrowth of tissue. Fissures can be prevented by drinking plenty of fluids (eight glasses of water a day), eating a proper diet, and passing stool promptly when indicated.

Gastroenteritis (Gas-tro-enter-i'-tis)

Description—This is an inflammation of the stomach and intestines. The term may be applied to such conditions

as intestinal flu, traveler's diarrhea, and food poisoning. The inflammation usually subsides within a couple of days and poses no threat to persons in good general health. However, people who are very young, elderly, and generally debilitated are at risk because of the loss of intracellular fluid.

Signs and symptoms—Gastroenteritis is characterized by fever, nausea, abdominal cramping, diarrhea, and vomiting. Other possible symptoms include fever, malaise, and a gurgling, splashing sound over the intestines.

Etiology—There are many possible causes, such as bacteria (associated with food poisoning), amoebas and parasites, viruses (usually with traveler's diarrhea), ingestion of toxic plants, drug reactions (perhaps to antibiotics), and food allergies.

Treatment—It is treated with bed rest, increased fluid intake, and diet. Antibiotics and intravenous fluids to combat dehydration may be indicated for the person at risk. Medication may be needed to control vomiting and diarrhea.

Gastroesophageal Reflux Disease (GERD) (Gas-tro-e-sof-o-ge'-all Re'-flux)

Description—This is a backflow of gastric and sometimes duodenal contents into the esophagus through the sphincter just above the stomach.

Signs and symptoms—The most common feature is heartburn, which becomes more severe with vigorous exercise, bending, or lying down. There may be esophageal spasms that mimic angina pain, radiating to the neck and arms. **Reflux** may be associated with hiatal hernia. If there is regurgitation of fluids, there may be pulmonary symptoms of aspiration, including nocturnal wheezing, bronchitis, asthma, morning hoarseness, and coughing.

Etiology—It is caused by a faulty lower esophageal sphincter (LES) that is supposed to prevent the backup of gastric contents by creating pressure, which closes the lower end of the esophagus. Normally, the sphincter relaxes after each swallow to allow food into the stomach. Reflux occurs when the pressure is insufficient or the pressure within the stomach exceeds that of the sphincter. Certain other factors may contribute to the condition, such as hiatal hernia, a position that increases intra-abdominal pressure, and any agent that lowers the LES pressure (such as food, alcohol, cigarettes, and certain drugs).

Treatment—Common treatment includes the use of common antacids, such as Alka-Seltzer, Maalox, Mylanta, Rolaids, Tums, and others. These work almost immediately after taken to suppress the symptoms and continue for about three to four hours. Another group of drugs, such as Pepsid AC are called H2-blockers. They suppress the secretion in the first place to prevent the heartburn. Their effects begin after about an hour but last for several. Perhaps the best treatment is prevention by:

- Avoid or cut back on foods that trigger heartburn (alcohol, chocolate, fat, peppermint, and spearmint); these tend to relax the sphincter.
- Avoid caffeine, it stimulates gastric acid (caffeine is found in coffee, strong tea, soda pop, and medication, such as Anacin, Excedrin, No Doz).
- Avoid carbonated drinks, which distend the stomach and increase the pressure.
- Lose weight if overweight.
- If a smoker, quit.
- Use gravity (Don't lie down after eating and raise head of bed on four- to six-inch blocks at night).

Hemorrhoids (Hem'-o-roids)

Description—The anal canal and the lower portion of the rectum contain vertical folds of mucous membrane called anal and rectal columns. The veins in the mucosa of the folds frequently become dilated, resulting in internal or external **hemorrhoids**.

Signs and symptoms—Hemorrhoids may be asymptomatic but characteristically cause painless, intermittent bleeding, which occurs with the passing of stool. There may also be some itching. As they worsen and prolapse, they are still painless as long as they return to the anal canal. With continued progression, constant discomfort may result because of prolapse, which must be corrected by manual reduction. If blood becomes trapped in prolapsed hemorrhoids, it causes thrombosis, which results in sudden rectal pain and a large firm lump that can be felt.

Etiology—Hemorrhoids can result from long periods of sitting or standing, diarrhea, constipation, vomiting, coughing, hepatitis, alcoholism, loss of muscle tone, pregnancy, or anorectal infections. Any condition that increases portal pressure, such as pregnancy or hepatitis, or that leads to a trapping of blood in the veins, as when stool is being expelled, interferes with the return flow of blood. As more blood enters the veins, it causes dilation, and the veins bulge into the anal canal or protrude to the outside, resulting in hemorrhoids. With protrusion comes the possibility of developing a thrombosis. The blood may become trapped externally, forming a painful, hard lump. Once this occurs, it will probably need to be incised to remove the clotted blood.

Treatment—Treatment of mild to moderate hemorrhoids involves regulating bowel habits; limiting sitting time on the toilet; increasing intake of water, raw vegetables, fruits, and fiber; and applying local heat. When swelling and discomfort persist with pain and bleeding on defecation, additional treatment is indicated. A sclerosis agent can be injected into internal hemorrhoids, which causes scar tissue to develop, thus reducing the

dilation. More severe involvement requires surgical removal of the dilated vein and the surrounding stretched mucosa in a procedure called a **hemorrhoidectomy**.

Hepatitis (Hep-a-ti'-tis)

Description—**Hepatitis** is an infection of the liver that can result in cell destruction and death. It is caused by a virus that has been identified in several different forms. Hepatitis B, serum hepatitis, was the first to be identified over 20 years ago. It is very contagious with a relatively high mortality rate. A vaccine was developed to control its spread. Next hepatitis A, infectious hepatitis, was identified. Type A is also highly contagious but seems to be self-limiting and rather benign. A vaccine also exists for type A hepatitis. For a while, all other types discovered were called non-A or non-B. After 15 years, a type C (HCV) was identified. It is the most worrisome form. It usually has a silent beginning but develops into a chronic form that causes the liver to scar; it requires powerful drug therapy and ultimately a liver transplant. Hepatitis B and C are transmitted only through blood and sexual contact with an infected person. Nearly four million Americans are infected with the virus, and many do not know it. About 10,000 people die each year, and the number is expected to triple by 2010.

Within the last five years, other strains have been identified. Because they do not meet the criteria for A, B, or C, they have been called D and E. D is like A but not highly prevalent in this country. E is like B. The latest strain, G, appears to be related to C and has been recently added to the family of viruses. There is no F; however, scientists do not believe this is the end of their discoveries.

Etiology—Type A is usually transmitted by the fecal-oral route, meaning organisms from sewage, human, or animal wastes get into the food chain. It is usually transmitted through ingestion of food, water, or milk that has been contaminated, and from seafood taken from contaminated water. Type B is usually transmitted parenterally (other than by mouth). Health care workers are especially prone to it because of contact with human secretions and feces. Universal precautions are indicated when caring for all patients to prevent acquiring or spreading the disease. Like AIDS, hepatitis B can also be acquired through sexual intercourse and contaminated needles, including ear piercing and tattooing. It can be passed from mother to newborn during delivery. But it can be spread by more casual contact through cuts in the skin and in saliva.

In most patients, involved cells will repair themselves, leaving little damage, and in the case of type A hepatitis only, confering a lifelong immunity. When other disorders are present, such as congestive heart failure, diabetes, severe anemia, cancer, and advanced age, complications are more likely and the prognosis is poor.

Type C hepatitis is acquired through blood and body fluids. It seldom causes illness when contracted, but about 75% of those afflicted develop a chronic form that goes undetected for years. Carriers never lose the virus or the ability to transmit it to others. No vaccine has been developed.

Signs and symptoms—Hepatitis produces a variety of symptoms, which appear suddenly with type A; type B symptoms are insidious. Clinical features of stage one include: fatigue, malaise, headache, anorexia (lack of appetite), sensitivity to light, sore throat, cough, nausea, vomiting, frequently a fever of 100° to 101°F (37° to 38°C), and possibly liver and lymph node enlargement. These symptoms occur during the preicteric (before jaundice) stage and disappear when jaundice begins. About 6% to 10% of adults and 25% to 50% of children become chronic carriers. These individuals are infectious and can develop potentially-fatal complications because of liver degeneration and cancer.

The second, icteric, stage has begun once the urine becomes dark, the stool is clay-colored, the sclera and skin is yellow, and a mild weight loss has occurred. The liver remains enlarged and tender, and the spleen and cervical nodes swell. The jaundice may continue for one to two weeks. Then, liver enlargement subsides, but the fatigue, flatulence (intestinal gas), abdominal tenderness, and indigestion continue. The third stage, posticteric, usually lasts for two to six weeks. Full recovery requires six months.

Complications may develop leading to a chronic hepatitis, which occurs in benign or active forms. The active form, known as chronic aggressive hepatitis, has about a 25% fatality rate because of liver failure from cell destruction.

Hepatitis C may be acquired completely without symptoms. Some people however, do experience nausea, vomiting, fever, and jaundice for a few days, but all symptoms disappear after a couple days of bed rest. These people are fortunate because early diagnosis may be made. Diagnosis is made based on history that reveals recent exposure to drugs, chemicals, a jaundiced person, or a blood transfusion and the presence of typical symptoms. Blood tests revealing hepatitis B antigens and the presence of B antibodies confirm type B hepatitis. Antigens are present only in the early phase of the disease, so a false negative result may occur if the blood is drawn too late.

Presence of the antibody (anti-HAV) indicates type A hepatitis. If these antigens and antibodies are absent but the patient still exhibits appropriate symptoms, then type C hepatitis is expected. There is a test to identify antibodies for HCV (type C). People testing positive should be treated before the disease progresses.

HCV can lay dormant for decades before symptoms appear. By then it may have destroyed the liver. It is a silent, deadly virus that infects an estimated four million Americans with 150,000–170,000 new cases diagnosed each year. In 1994, one third of all liver transplants in the United States were done because of this virus. The new organ will become infected but will not necessarily be seriously damaged. There is no vaccine, and only 10% to 25% become inactive with medical therapy. The carriers never lose the virus or the ability to transmit it to others. Most people discover they are infected when they undergo routine lab tests or when they donate blood. Fortunately, HCV is not highly infectious. The risk from blood transfusions is one in 3,300, but mother-to-child and needle-stick in health care workers is rare. Infection is possible from shared manicure tools, toothbrushes, and razors—things that can hold blood. The largest infected group is IV drug users. Sexual activity does not seem to be a very efficient means of transmission, although it increases with the number of partners. Hepatitis G is transmitted through blood but is very rare at this time. Currently, little is known about the strain.

Prevention—Vaccines have been developed to prevent hepatitis A and B and are recommended for the following groups of people:
- IV drug users
- Health workers
- Individuals living with an infected person
- Sexually active homosexuals
- Heterosexuals with multiple partners
- Recipients of certain blood products
- Children born to immigrants from regions where hepatitis B is common, such as Southeast Asia
- Infants born to infected women (Up to 90% of children born to infected mothers become infected and suffer a high death rate.)
- Travelers spending more than six months in an area with high incidence

The main problem with the vaccine is it requires three shots over a six-month period and is relatively expensive in the United States. Many of the targeted groups of people, except for health care workers and infected mothers, are difficult to reach. It is interesting to note several developing countries are immunizing newborns and others at a cost of about $1.

Treatment—There is no specific treatment nor cure for hepatitis B. Patients are expected to rest and eat small meals with high calorie and protein content. Medication to help relieve nausea and vomiting may be necessary. An effort is made to determine the source of infection or contagion. Hepatitis is one of several contagious diseases that are to be reported to the local public health department.

Health care workers should protect themselves from suspected or confirmed disease by wearing gloves to handle body secretions or draw blood. Hospitalized patients are isolated, with strict techniques used to prevent the spread of the disease.

Treatment of patients with HCV who develop progressive liver scarring usually require powerful drug treatments. Two antiviral agents are the only approved drug therapies of the disease. These are interferon alpha-2b and ribavirin. Interferon is one of the body's lymphokines. It helps boost the immune system and attack viruses. Ribavirin works by blocking the virus's ability to multiply. When they are used together, the drugs can destroy the virus to undetectable levels in about 40% of the patients. However, severe side effects of nausea, fatigue, seizures, and even heart or kidney failure make this option suitable only as a life-saving measure. The virus often comes back after treatment is discontinued. A vaccine is in the process of being developed but is not yet available.

Hernia (Hiatus) (Her'-ne-ah Hi-a'-tus)

Description—The protrusion of an internal organ through a natural opening in the body wall is known as a hernia or rupture. One form of hernia involves a defect in the diaphragm that allows a portion of the stomach to move up into the chest cavity through the opening for the esophagus. It is called a **hiatus** or hiatal **hernia**. There are three types of hiatal hernias: sliding, which is most common; rolling or paraesophageal (alongside the esophagus); and mixed, which is a combination of both. This condition is found in up to 50% of the population over 50 years old. If no symptoms occur, no treatment is required.

In all forms of hiatal hernia, some portion of the stomach, the end of the esophagus, or both slip(s) through the diaphragmatic opening (Figure 11–169).

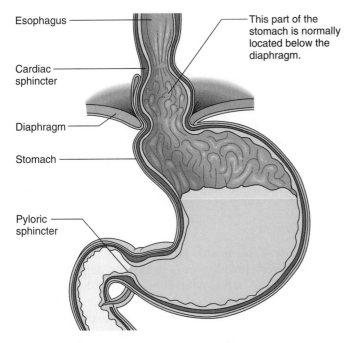

Esophagus

Cardiac sphincter

Diaphragm

Stomach

Pyloric sphincter

This part of the stomach is normally located below the diaphragm.

FIGURE 11-169 Hiatal hernia

Signs and symptoms—In paraesophageal, a portion of the stomach "rolls" through the opening into the chest but causes few symptoms except a feeling of fullness in the chest and angina-like pain. This type of hernia needs surgical repair. A sliding hernia may cause symptoms, such as heartburn from one to four hours after eating (which is often aggravated by reclining and occasionally results in regurgitation or vomiting), chest pain (caused by the reflux [return] of gastric juices), distention and spasms of the stomach, difficulty swallowing (caused by inflammation of the esophagus), or an ulcer. The most serious symptoms are severe pain and shock, which result from incarceration when a large portion of the stomach is trapped above the diaphragm, cutting off circulation to that part of the organ. Because strangulation leads to tissue death, immediate surgery is indicated.

Etiology—It is caused by a portion of the stomach and/or part of the esophagus protruding up through the diaphragm.

Treatment—Conservative treatment for uncomplicated hiatal hernia involves medication to strengthen the esophageal sphincter muscle, using gravity to decrease the reflux of gastric juices, and a diet of small, frequent, bland meals. Other helpful measures include waiting at least two hours after eating to lie down, eating slowly, and avoiding spicy foods, fruit juices, alcohol, and coffee. Smoking is discouraged because it stimulates the production of gastric acid.

Hernia (Inguinal) (Her'-ne-ah In'-gwin-al)

Description—The wall of the abdominal cavity has normal openings through which blood vessels or other body structures pass. For example, the male's spermatic cords pass through the inguinal rings of the lower abdominal wall to reach the testes, which are external to the body.

Signs and symptoms—Diagnosis of a smaller hernia can be made on manual examination of the inguinal ring while the patient is asked to cough. If the examiner feels something touch the examining finger, the patient has a hernia.

Etiology—When the surrounding structure of fibrous tissue, the fascia, becomes weak, it allows a loop of small intestine to protrude through the ring, following the path of the spermatic cord. This type of hernia is called an inguinal hernia, and it often extends into the scrotum when the patient stands.

Treatment—A protruding hernia is visible and can usually be reduced or pushed back into place. Some patients may wear a device called a truss, which exerts pressure directly over the herniated opening, to hold the protruding mass inside the cavity. Occasionally, the mass cannot be reduced and will remain in the hernial sac. It is then possible for additional intestine to enter the sac or the contents to become twisted or trapped,

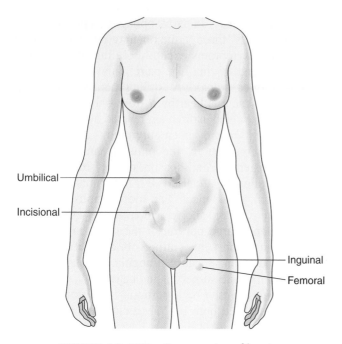

FIGURE 11–170   Common sites of hernias

interfering with the circulation of blood to the intestine. This condition is referred to as a *strangulated hernia* and requires a surgical procedure known as **herniorrhaphy** as quickly as possible. The procedure replaces the contents of the sac within the abdominal cavity and closes the opening.

Hernias can be the result of weak abdominal muscles caused by a congenital condition or the natural process of aging. Hernias can also develop from increased abdominal pressure caused by heavy lifting, pregnancy, obesity, or straining.

Other types of hernias are: femoral, which occurs where the femoral artery exits the abdomen to the legs; umbilical, involving the structure around the umbilicus; and incisional, in an area of previous surgery (Figure 11–170).

Ileostomy (Ill-e-os'-toe-me)

Description—This surgical opening of the ileum allows the chyme of the small intestine to empty through the abdominal wall. This is not a disease but rather a solution to a disease process. An ileostomy is similar to a colostomy except that the chyme is liquid and highly caustic to the skin because of the digestive juices. The patient with an ileostomy has no control over its function and must wear an ostomy appliance (collection bag) attached to a donut-like disk that perfectly surrounds the stoma (mouth or opening). A protective adhesive creates a watertight seal. A belt attached to the disk supports the device. A permanent type of bag may be attached, which must be emptied and cleaned period-

ically. Disposable plastic bags can also be used. Some disposable types incorporate a deodorizing material; the permanent type requires instillation of a deodorizer.

Etiology—The patient with an ileostomy must accept a great alteration in body image and function. The passing of flatus and the gurgling of liquid stool being expelled occurs without warning and cannot be controlled. Most patients who have had ileostomy surgery feel better off than before surgery. Many had extensive ulcerative colitis with much pain, bleeding, and excessive, sudden, and frequent diarrhea, and were in poor physical condition from the debilitating effects of the disease. The removal of the diseased colon necessitates the ileostomy. Other patients may have been affected by Crohn's disease, which causes inflammation, scarring, and near or complete obstruction of the bowel. These patients experienced pain, nausea, fever, cramping, bleeding, and diarrhea, occurring four to six times a day. The freedom from pain and relative increase in control over excretion are often considered to make an ileostomy worthwhile. Many times, these patients have been nearly confined to their homes because of their weakness and the characteristics of the disease. With an ileostomy they can regain fairly good health and live a nearly normal life.

Irritable Bowel Syndrome

Description—This is a common condition marked by chronic or periodic diarrhea and alternating constipation. Irritable **bowel** syndrome is also called spastic colon.

Signs and symptoms—The syndrome is characterized with lower abdominal pain that is relieved by passing flatus or defecation and diarrhea during the day. Stools are often small and contain mucus. There may be abdominal distention and digestion difficulties.

Etiology—It is generally associated with psychologic stress, but it may result from physical factors, such as ingestion of irritants (coffee, raw fruits and vegetables), an abuse of laxatives, food poisoning, a lactose intolerance, diverticular disease, or colon cancer.

Treatment—Treatment is aimed at relieving symptoms and teaching the patient to deal with stress. Elimination of known food irritants, rest, and heat to the abdomen are helpful. The use of sedatives and antispasmodics are recommended for a limited time.

Oral Cancer

Description—The mouth should be examined for oral cancer every time a visit is made to a dentist for routine cleaning and examination. It should also be inspected by the physician as part of a physical examination. People who do not visit a dentist or physician frequently should observe their own mouths for oral cancer.

Signs and symptoms—
- Swelling, lump, or growth anywhere in or about the mouth
- White scaly patches inside the mouth
- Any size sore that does not heal
- Numbness or pain anywhere in the mouth area
- Repeated bleeding in the mouth without cause
  Any of these signals should be examined by a physician or dentist.

*Etiology—*Oral cancer strikes about 30,300 per year with about 8,000 dying. About 90% of the cancers are squamous cell that develop in the tissue lining or covering of the mouth, lip, tongue, and throat. The single greatest risk factor is the use of tobacco, in the form of cigarettes, cigars, pipe, or chewing tobacco. The use of snuff is clearly linked with cancer of the cheek, tongue, and mouth structures. Abuse of alcohol is also a risk factor. Heavy drinkers who also smoke a pack of cigarettes per day have 24 times the amount of oral cancer risk. Overexposure to the sun is a factor in lip cancer.

*Treatment—*Oral cancer is usually treated with surgery or radiation or both. With advanced disease, chemotherapy in combination with surgery or radiation is being used. The choice of treatment depends upon the tumor size and location and the patient's willingness to undergo the side effects. Expected survival of five years is only 51%.

Oral cancer can result in a disabling and disfiguring condition when areas are excised. If the tongue is involved, speech and the process of eating become difficult.

Pancreatitis (Pan-cre-a-ti′-tis)

*Description—*This is inflammation of the pancreas, which occurs in both acute and chronic forms. **Pancreatitis** progresses in an unusual manner. The enzymes normally produced and excreted into the pancreatic duct remain and digest the pancreatic tissue. If the cells that produce insulin are destroyed, the condition will be complicated by diabetes.

*Signs and symptoms—*Mild pancreatitis is characterized by epigastric pain not relieved by vomiting. A severe attack causes extreme pain, persistent vomiting, a rigid abdomen, and rales (noisy, ausculated breath sounds) at the lung bases with pleural fluid on the left side. Tachycardia may occur, and a fever of from 100° to 102°F (38° to 39°C) with cold, perspiring extremities. Rapidly progressing pancreatitis can cause massive hemorrhage, which results in shock and coma. Mortality is as high as 60% when there is tissue destruction and hemorrhage.

*Etiology—*The most frequent predisposing factors are alcoholism, trauma to the pancreas, reaction to certain medications, and pancreatic carcinoma. It may also develop as the result of a duodenal ulcer.

*Treatment—*The complicated treatment consists of methods to decrease pancreatic secretions and relieve pain while maintaining adequate fluids. Shock is treated vigorously by replacing electrolytes and proteins intravenously (IV) to prevent death. After the emergency passes, IVs containing electrolytes and proteins that do not stimulate the pancreas are continued for five to seven days. This may be followed by tubal feeding if the patient is unable to take enough nutrients by mouth. In extreme cases, a pancreatectomy, the removal of the pancreas, may be indicated.

Paralytic Ileus (Pear-a-lit′-ick Ill′-e-us)

*Description—*A physiological intestinal obstruction, a **paralytic ileus** usually occurs in the small intestine. Peristalsis is either drastically reduced or totally absent.

*Signs and symptoms—*The condition causes severe abdominal distention and distress, frequently accompanied by vomiting.

*Etiology—*It is often precipitated by manipulation of the bowel during abdominal surgery or the paralyzing effects of the anesthesia. The ileus usually disappears after two to three days.

*Treatment—*If it continues for more than 48 hours, it may be necessary to insert a weighted tube into the small intestine to remove the accumulated fluids and gas. Medication to stimulate colon action may be given.

Peptic Ulcer (Pep′-tic All′-sir)

*Description—*This is an encircled lesion in the mucous membrane lining of the stomach, lower esophagus, duodenum, or jejunum.

Signs and symptoms—Duodenal peptic ulcers cause heartburn, epigastric pain that is relieved by food, a weight gain (caused by extra eating), and a strange feeling of bubbling hot water in the back of the pharynx. Attacks occur whenever the stomach is empty or after drinking alcohol, juice, or coffee. *Gastric* ulcers usually cause heartburn and indigestion, pain in the left epigastrium, and a feeling of fullness. There may be weight loss and repeated episodes of serious GI bleeding. Gastric ulcers tend to cause discomfort after eating because the stomach lining is "stretched," causing pain from the lesion in the membrane lining. Either type of ulcer may develop complications, such as perforation, hemorrhage, and pyloric obstruction.

*Etiology—*For years, physicians thought ulcers were caused by the overproduction of gastric juices from emotional stimulation. In 1982, an Australian physician drank a concoction with millions of bacteria to prove his theory that ulcers were caused by an organism. A few days later he developed an inflamed stomach lining—the beginnings of an ulcer—and proved that even though the stomach is full of acid, the *Helicobacter pylori* (H. pylori) bacteria could survive. The organism itself does not cause the ulcer, but the burrowing of the corkscrew bacteria into the membranes weakens the linings, allowing the stomach acid and the digestive enzymes to create an ulcer. Not everyone who has the organism develops an ulcer, and not every ulcer is the result of the bacteria. However, at least 80% of gastric and 95% of duodenal ulcers are associated with the bacteria, and the remainder are often caused by nonsteroidal anti-inflammatory drugs. Other contributing factors are smoking, drinking alcohol, aspirin taken over long periods, and an hereditary tendency.

Treatment—With the new discovery came a new treatment. If there is bacteria and the existence of an ulcer is confirmed with endoscopy, the infection can be permanently cured with drug therapy involving two antibiotics and a bismuth preparation, such as Pepto-Bismol. Most physicians also add a blocker to relieve symptoms and hasten the healing. A new blood test for H. pylori antibodies is probably adequate for people with confirmed ulcer history. Newly-diagnosed patients with mild to moderate symptoms may be placed on a couple of months of treatment with newer acid-suppressing drugs and blockers. They will usually heal, and one in three sufferers will not have a recurrence. If the ulcer returns, they are then treated with the antibiotic therapy.

Polyp (Pol'-ip)

Description—This is a mass of tissue that results from an overgrowth of upper epithelial cells of the mucosal membrane of the GI tract. There are five varieties, some hereditary, others of common adenoma structure. Most are benign, but **villous adenoma** and hereditary polyps show a tendency to become malignant. Most types develop in adults over 45 years old. Predisposing factors are age, heredity, diet, and infection.

Signs and symptoms—Polyps are difficult to diagnose because they are almost always asymptomatic. They are usually discovered accidentally during a rectosigmoidoscopy or lower GI series x-ray. The most common symptom is rectal bleeding. The structure of the polyps varies from small lesions covering the surface of the rectum or sigmoid to large lesions attached by long, thin stalks. The type of polyp determines its physical characteristics.

Etiology—Overgrowth of epithelial cells.

Treatment—Treatment consists of surgical removal often by electrocautery, especially if benign and pedunculated (on a stalk). If they are villous adenomas, which are invasive and therefore malignant, treatment usually involves abdominoperineal resection (removal of the colon and rectum, including the area around the anus), with a resulting permanent ileostomy. Each type of polyp is dealt with in relation to its current state or its tendency to become malignant.

Pruritus Ani (Prur-i'-tis A'-ni)

Description—This is itching of the area surrounding the anus, often associated with irritation and burning.

Signs and symptoms—Classical symptoms are itching after a bowel movement or at night. Scratching can cause reddened, weeping skin or thickened, leathery, darker tissue.

Etiology—The main contributing factors for **pruritus ani** are harsh, vigorous rubbing with soap and a washcloth; poor hygiene; spicy foods; anal skin tags (small pieces of suspended extra skin); excessive perspiration; a systemic disease, such as diabetes; the use of perfumed or colored toilet paper; coffee, alcohol, or food preservatives; a fungus or parasitic infection; an anorectal disease, such as fissure, fistula, or hemorrhoids; and certain skin cancers.

Treatment—Treatment consists of removing the underlying cause, such as a rectal tag, and eliminating irritants to the skin, such as soaps, powders, and colored tissue. The area should be kept clean and dry. Witch hazel applied on wiping pads or cotton balls is soothing. Steroid creams aid in reducing inflammation and controlling itching.

Pyloric Stenosis (Pie-lor'-ick Sten-o'-sis)

Description—This is a narrowing of the pyloric sphincter which interferes with the emptying of the stomach. The sphincter is enlarged and often cartilagenous, causing a narrowing of the opening, which results in the dilation of the stomach.

Signs and symptoms—Adults will experience symptoms when there is a delayed action of the stomach to empty its contents, which causes distention. Because of the thickening of the pylorus and the backup of contents, the most common symptom is projectile or forceful vomiting.

Etiology—**Stenosis** can be caused by scar tissue developed during healing of a gastric ulcer.

Treatment—In adult stenosis, the patient may be able to alter the diet and use medication for some time; however, surgical correction will probably be required eventually.

A PEDIATRIC PERSPECTIVE

Symptoms of pyloric stenosis usually begin before four weeks of age and are considered to be congenital. There is forceful vomiting that may lead to serious dehydration. This condition occurs almost exclusively in infant boys. If vomiting is not too intense, the condition will be observed and may self correct in time. Otherwise, surgical intervention to open the pyloric sphincter muscle is performed to correct the problem.

Spastic Colon (Spas'-tick Col'-on)

Description—This is a common condition of alternating periods of constipation and diarrhea.

Signs and symptoms—It is characterized by lower abdominal pain, which is relieved by expelling flatus or stool. There is frequently diarrhea during the daytime. This pattern alternates with constipation or normal function. Sometimes the stool contains mucous.

Etiology—A **spastic colon** is a functional disorder, often associated with stress. However, it can also be caused by physical conditions, such as diverticulitis, food poisoning, cancer of the colon, and eating certain irritants like raw fruits or vegetables.

Treatment—Treatment consists of therapy to relieve symptoms, such as counseling for stress, dietary restriction of known irritant foods, rest, heat to the abdomen, and the use of sedatives for a short time.

Ulcerative Colitis (All'-sir-a-tive Col-i'-tis)

Description—An inflammatory disease, often chronic, that affects the mucosa of the colon. It usually begins in the sigmoid and rectum, extending upward to involve the whole colon. The small intestine is seldom involved. The disease produces congestion followed by edema, which makes the mucosa fragile. As the lining breaks down, ulcers are formed, which eventually develop into abscesses. The disease can be confined to one area and be known as segmented colitis, or it can spread throughout the colon. Severe colitis may cause a perforation of the colon, which can result in a life-threatening infection called peritonitis and in toxemia (blood poisoning).

Ulcerative colitis primarily affects young adults, mostly female.

Signs and symptoms—The prime symptom of ulcerative colitis is recurrent bloody diarrhea, often containing exudate and mucus. The frequency and intensity will vary with the extent of the disease. Other symptoms include weight loss, weakness, anorexia, nausea, vomiting, irritability, and abdominal pain. The disease leads to other complicating conditions, such as anemia, coagulation defects, liver damage, arthritis, loss of muscle mass, hemorrhoids from frequent stools, and stricture resulting from no solid stool, perforated colon, and toxemia.

Etiology—Predisposing factors are a family history of colitis, a bacterial infection, overproduction of enzymes that damage the mucous membrane, emotional stress, an autoimmune reaction, and allergic reactions to some foods.

Treatment—Treatment consists of controlling inflammation, maintaining nutrition and blood volume, and preventing complications. Patients are usually placed on bed rest, IV fluid replacement, and a clear liquid diet. Drug therapy is used to control the inflammatory process and combat infection. Severe involvement may

DISEASES OF THE DIGESTIVE SYSTEM

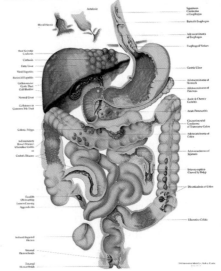

FIGURE 11–171 Diseases of the digestive system (Courtesy of Colwell, a division of Patterson Dental Supply Inc., 800-637-1140.)

A CAAHEP CONNECTION

This unit address *Anatomy and physiology, Diseases and their treatments, Medical terminology, Diagnostic testing* and *Principles of radiology*, and identifying developmental disorders associated with pediatric patients as they pertain to the digestive system. This type of information allows the medical assistant to more confidently communicate with patients and perform the necessary administrative and clinical procedures required with the related patient care.

necessitate antispasmotics and pain medication to relieve the cramping and discomfort. If the patient fails to respond to medical treatment and the symptoms become intolerable, surgical resection (removal) of the colon is indicated, with an ileostomy as previously described. Patients who develop colitis before age 15 and in whom the condition persists for at least 10 years are especially prone to colorectal cancer.

Figure 11–171 illustrates some of the disease conditions of the digestive system and may help in the visualization of their characteristics.

ACHIEVE UNIT OBJECTIVES

Complete Chapter 11, Unit 10, in the workbook to help you obtain competency of this subject matter.

UNIT 11

The Urinary System

■ OBJECTIVES

Upon completion of the unit, meet the following performance objectives by verifying knowledge of the facts and principles presented through oral and written communication at a level deemed competent.

1. Spell and define, using the glossary at the back of the text, all the **Words to Know** in this unit.
2. Explain the three main functions of the urinary system.
3. Identify the organs of the urinary system, and describe their physical characteristics.
4. Explain how the urinary system functions with other systems.
5. Describe the interior structure of the kidney.
6. Name the parts of a nephron, and explain how each part functions.
7. Describe the process of dialysis, and name two types.
8. Explain the likelihood of success with a kidney transplant.
9. List the two main categories of diagnostic examination, and give examples, explaining briefly how each test is performed and for what purpose.
10. Describe 10 diseases or disorders of the urinary system.

AREAS OF COMPETENCE (AAMA)

This unit addresses content within the specific competency areas of *Administrative procedures, Practice finances, Patient care, Communication skills*, and *Instruction*, as identified in the Medical Assistant Role Delineation Study. Refer to Appendix A for a detailed listing of the areas. (Note: Although *Anatomy and physiology* is not specifically identified in the study, a basic knowledge of the body's structure and function is an essential foundation of many roles.)

■ WORDS TO KNOW

acute glomerulonephritis	chronic
acute renal failure	glomerulonephritis
anuria	chronic renal failure
bladder	cortex
Bowman's capsule	cystitis
calculi	dialysis
calyces	dribbling
calyx	dysuria
catheterization	elimination

excretion	peritoneal
fistula	polycystic kidney disease
frequency	polyuria
glomerulus	ptosis
graft	pyelonephritis
hematuria	renal
hemodialysis	residual
hesitancy	retention
hilum	secretion
intravenous pyelography	stricture
invasive procedure	uremia
kidney	ureter
lithotripsy	urethra
medulla	urgency
nephron	urinary
nephrotic syndrome	urinary meatus
nocturia	urine
noninvasive procedure	void
oliguria	

 Library

The **urinary** system removes nitrogenous waste products, certain salts, and excess water from the blood and eliminates them from the body. At the same time, it evaluates the body's acid–base balance and selectively reabsorbs the elements needed to maintain the proper ratio.

The urinary system performs three main functions. The first is **excretion**, the process of removing waste products and other elements from the blood. The second is **secretion**, by which **urine** is produced. The third is **elimination**, the emptying of the urine from its bladder storage.

The major work of the system is performed by two organs called the **kidneys** (Figure 11–172). The well-being of the human body depends heavily on the function of the kidneys. When waste products are not removed from the blood, they build up, producing potentially-fatal toxicity. After the kidneys have performed their functions, the waste material, urine, is carried through the **ureters**, one for each kidney, to temporary storage in the **bladder**. When an adequate amount has been accumulated, the bladder expels the urine through the **urethra**, eliminating it from the body.

As we have said before, no system can function by itself. The urinary system is no exception. Waste products and other substances that are filtered out of the blood must first have been ingested, digested, and absorbed by the digestive system into the circulatory system, to be delivered in the blood to the kidneys. The peristalsis of the muscular system moves the urine through the ureters. The nervous system, in cooperation with a muscular sphincter, controls elimination. The respiratory system and the urinary system cooperate to control the body's acid–base balance and the amount of fluid retained. Pulmonary

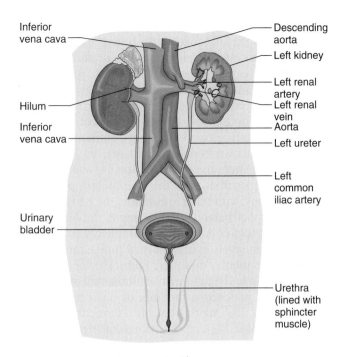

FIGURE 11–172   The urinary system

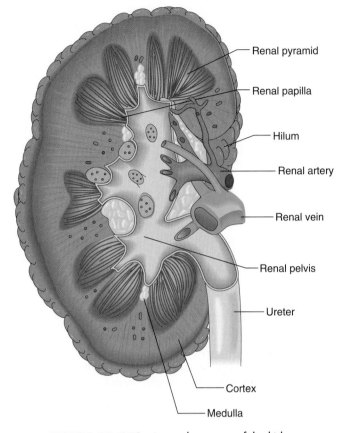

FIGURE 11–173   Internal structure of the kidney

action influences the amount of O_2–CO_2 exchange and the amount of fluid loss through respiration. Hormones from the endocrine system also influence the amount of urine excreted. And the integumentary system works in close relationship to the urinary system to remove or retain body fluid as required. Once again, it is apparent that the body is a complex, interdependent organism.

THE KIDNEYS

The kidneys are shaped like a lima or kidney bean. Each kidney is about $4\frac{1}{2}$ inches long, from two to three inches wide, and about an inch thick, and it weighs about $\frac{1}{4}$ pound. The kidneys are located on each side of the vertebral column, high up on the posterior wall of the abdominal cavity, between the muscles of the back and the parietal peritoneum that covers the abdominal organs. Because they are not within the area occupied by the organs, the kidneys are said to be retroperitoneal (behind the peritoneum). The left kidney is slightly higher than the right, which is displaced by the liver. Normally, a heavy cushion of fat helps keep the kidneys in their proper position. A condition known as **ptosis** (dropping) occurs in very thin persons as a result of an inadequate fatty cushion.

Externally, the kidney is covered with a tough, fibrous capsule. The concave border has a notch called the **hilum** through which the **renal** (kidney) artery enters and the renal vein and renal pelvis of the ureter exits. Internally, the kidney is divided into two sections: an outer layer, the **cortex**, and an inner layer, the **medulla** (Figure 11–173). The medulla is divided into triangular-shaped wedges

called renal pyramids with bases toward the cortex and "tops," or renal papillae, emptying into cavities called **calyces** (singular: **calyx**). The pyramids have a striated (striped) appearance; the cortex appears smooth. The cortex extends inward between the pyramids in sections called renal columns.

The Nephrons

The life-preserving service of the kidney is performed by microscopic units called **nephrons**. Each kidney has over one million of these units, which altogether contain roughly 140 miles of filters and tubes. Each minute, the kidneys filter over 1,000 cc of blood, producing about 60 cc of urine per hour. In an average day, a person takes in 2,500 cc of fluid ($2\frac{1}{2}$ quarts) and generates another 300 cc (10 ounces) of water, which is formed by the cells in the process of combining oxygen and other materials. About 1,500 cc ($1\frac{1}{2}$ quarts) is eliminated as urine each day. Additional fluid is lost through feces and respiration. Some moisture is also lost through the skin, especially when perspiring. Despite the amount of liquid consumed, the kidneys maintain a constant amount of fluid in the body's tissues, excreting the excess as urine. The concentration of the urine is in direct relationship to the amount of liquid consumed.

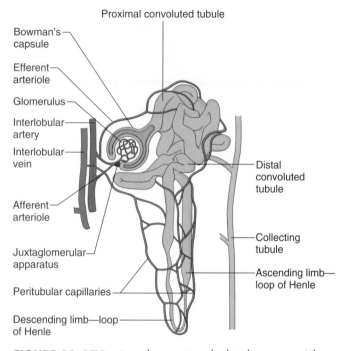

Proximal convoluted tubule
Bowman's capsule
Efferent arteriole
Glomerulus
Interlobular artery
Interlobular vein
Afferent arteriole
Juxtaglomerular apparatus
Peritubular capillaries
Descending limb—loop of Henle
Distal convoluted tubule
Collecting tubule
Ascending limb—loop of Henle

FIGURE 11–174 A nephron unit and related structures. (The collecting tubules, which are not microscopic, give the pyramids of the medullary portion of the kidney a striated appearance. As shown, there are some collecting tubules in the cortical portion of the kidney.)

The process by which the nephrons produce urine is complex. The nephron is a peculiarly-shaped structure, resembling a funnel with a long, twisted tail (Figure 11–174). The top of the funnel is a double-walled hollow capsule called the **Bowman's capsule**. Each capsule contains a cluster of about 50 capillaries called the **glomerulus**. The Bowman's capsule and the glomerulus together are known as the renal corpuscle.

Blood enters the glomerulus by way of an afferent arteriole, flows through the glomerular capillaries, and leaves through the efferent arteriole. The efferent arteriole branches into capillaries that surround the renal tubule. The capillaries come back together in tiny veins, which join a branch of the renal vein.

Beyond the Bowman's capsule is a twisted section of tubule called the *proximal convoluted tubule*. The capsule and this section of tubule descend into the medulla and are called the *loop of Henle*. This loop has a straight descending and ascending limb, but when it returns to the cortex, it changes into another twisted section called the *distal convoluted tubule*. Several distal tubules join into a straight collecting tubule, which empties into the calyx.

Filtration and Reabsorption Filtration is the first process in the formation of urine. Blood enters the capsule by way of the afferent arteriole, carrying waste products, water, salt, urea, and glucose. The arteriole divides, forming approximately 50 glomerular capillaries. Because so many capillaries are emptied by a single efferent arteri-

ole, blood pressure increases significantly. This higher pressure forces the fluid to leave the blood by filtration and enter the Bowman's capsule at the rate of about 125 mL a minute. This equals a rate of 60,000 mL (60 liters, or 56.8 quarts) in an eight-hour period.

By a reabsorption process, 99% of the filtrate is returned to the bloodstream. Not only fluid but also useful substances, such as glucose, vitamins, amino acids, electrolyte salts, and bicarbonate ions (base), are reabsorbed. As the filtrate enters the proximal tubule, about 80% of the water is reabsorbed into the surrounding peritubular capillaries along with other substances the body needs to maintain a proper balance. For example, the filtrate contains glucose, which is normally completely reabsorbed. However, when levels exceed normal limits, the selective cells lining the tubules no longer reabsorb glucose but allow it to remain in the tubule to be eliminated in the urine. The term used to describe the limit of sugar reabsorption is the *threshold*. Passing this level is referred to as *spilling over the threshold*. Patients who have diabetes spill sugar frequently and therefore test its presence in their urine to determine the need for additional insulin.

A final reabsorption takes place in the distal tubule. The remaining 10% to 15% of water may be reabsorbed, depending on the body's need. The process is controlled by a hormone that acts upon the nephron.

Secretion The secretion function of the nephron moves substances directly from the blood in the peritubular capillaries into the urine in the distal and collecting tubules. The substances secreted directly are ammonia, hydrogen ions, potassium ions, and drugs. The elements are selectively secreted to maintain the body's acid–base balance.

Urinary Output Anything that increases the volume of blood in the capillaries increases the output of urine; conversely, the urine output decreases with a lessening of blood volume. For example, a large fluid intake increases the volume of blood and the output of urine. Hemorrhage or dehydration decreases blood volume and urine output.

Another factor regulating secretion is the amount of solutes in the filtrate. Again considering the diabetic, when there is an increase in the amount of glucose, it spills over into the urine, increasing the urine volume eliminated that day because more liquid is allowed to pass through to dilute the glucose content.

The functional capacity of the healthy kidney is so great that removal of one kidney poses no problem to the body in removing liquid wastes.

The Ureters

The urine secreted by the nephrons drops out of the collecting tubules into the calyces, then enters the renal pelvis and continues down the ureters into the urinary bladder (Figure 11–175). The ureters begin with a widened upper portion, continuing as a long, slender, muscular tube ap-

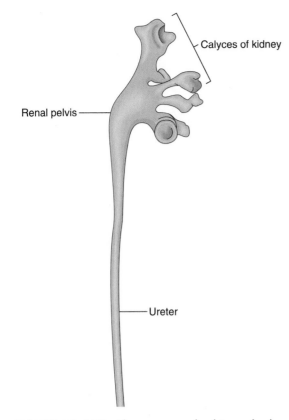

FIGURE 11–175 The ureter, renal pelvis, and calyces

proximately 10 to 12 inches in length. Peristaltic waves, at a rate of one to five a minute, move the urine down the ureter to enter the lower posterior wall of the bladder. Because of the solutes in urine, some persons tend to form renal **calculi** (stones). As the calculi form in the renal pelvis, they are washed into the ureter by the urine. When a stone is large enough to become lodged in the ureter, severe pain results. Frequently, removal of the stone may be required if it cannot be passed into the bladder. (See Renal Calculi in Diseases and Disorders.)

THE URINARY BLADDER

The bladder is a collapsible bag of muscular tissue lying behind the symphysis pubis. The lining has many folds, giving it the ability to expand. The bladder serves as a reservoir for urine, collecting approximately 250 cc before the urge to **void** (urinate) is felt. The capacity of the bladder is two to three times this amount, and in instances of **retention** (inability to empty bladder), may be in excess of 1,000 cc. In such instances, urine must be removed by inserting a catheter (a tube) through the urethra into the bladder to relieve the distention and discomfort. This procedure is known as **catheterization**.

THE URETHRA

The urethra is a tube leading from the bladder to an exit from the body. In the female, it is a straight tube about 1½

inches in length. It opens externally between the clitoris and the vagina within the folds of the labia minora. The opening is called the **urinary meatus**. Only urine passes through the female urethra. In the male, the urethra is about eight inches long, extending internally from the bladder down through the prostate gland and out through the penis to the meatus. The male urethra also serves as a passageway for semen.

A circular muscle sphincter within the urethra permits voluntary control of bladder function. This control, however, requires an intact nerve supply and motor area of the brain. Involuntary emptying of the bladder is known as *incontinence.*

Other medical terms commonly used to describe urinary output include: **anuria**, an absence of urine; **dysuria**, pain or discomfort associated with voiding; **hematuria**, blood in the urine; **nocturia**, having to urinate at night; **oliguria**, a scanty urinary output; and **polyuria**, excessive urination. Descriptive words used to clarify symptoms are: **dribbling**, the involuntary loss of drops of urine; **frequency**, the necessity to void often; **hesitancy**, difficulty in initiating urination; and **urgency**, the sudden need to void.

DIALYSIS

Dialysis is the mechanical process of removing waste products from the blood normally removed by the kidneys. Basically it is a process for purifying blood by passing it through thin membranes and exposing it to a solution that continually circulates around the membranes. The solution is called *dialysate.* Substances in the blood pass through the membrane into the lesser-concentrated dialysate in response to the laws of diffusion. This is called **hemodialysis**.

The term artificial kidney is often used to refer to the kidney dialysis unit. However, the part of the unit that actually substitutes for the kidney is a glass tube approximately eight inches long and about 1½ inches in diameter. The tube, called the dialyzer, is filled with thousands of minute hollow fibers attached firmly at both ends (Figure 11–176). Blood from the patient flows through the fibers, which are surrounded by circulating dialysate. The dialysate can be individualized for each patient to provide the appropriate levels of sodium, bicarbonate, and other substances. These cross the membrane and enter the blood. At the same time, extra water and waste products leave the blood to enter the dialysate.

The patient is connected to the dialysis unit by means of needles and tubing that take blood from the patient, circulate it through the machine and return it to the patient. New programmable dialysis management systems, as seen in Figure 11–177, can monitor blood pressure; allow variable control of solution substances; adjust temperature, flow, and filtration rate of the blood; preset the length of treatment time; and perform other functions, all automatically. (On the system pictured in Figure 11–177,

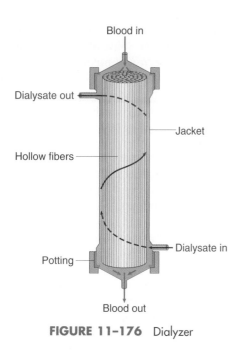

FIGURE 11–176 Dialyzer

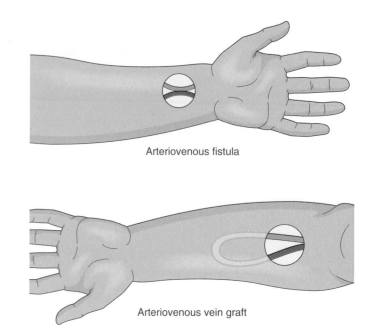

FIGURE 11–178 Hemodialysis sites

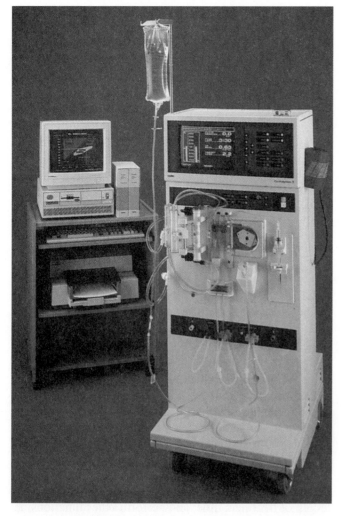

FIGURE 11–177 Hemodialysis unit

the dialyzer is located just left of center; it has black ends with tubing attached to both ends.)

A **fistula** (opening between an artery and vein), or a **graft** (vein inserted between an artery and a vein) is surgically constructed in the patient to provide a site for inserting the large needles required in dialysis (Figure 11–178). The fistulas and grafts are artificial veins that can withstand repeated needle insertions. They lie just under the skin surface and require two to four weeks for a graft and eight to twelve weeks for a fistula to completely heal before they can be used.

The initial site is the nondominant forearm, usually at the radial artery. When this begins to fail, sites are constructed at the brachial artery, then in the dominant arm, and finally grafts at the femoral artery in the groin area. Artificial veins last from three to five years. Some patients who have had a graft constructed from one of their own veins have had unusually successful sites for as long as 10 years, but this is not the norm. Because dialysis occurs so frequently, the multiple needle insertions not only affect the grafts or fistulas but the overlying skin as well. When too much damage has occurred, the site is no longer usable. The patient must learn to care for the site and protect it from damage. This is truly the lifeline for the patient with renal failure. Nothing, such as tight clothing or elastic cuffs, must constrict the site area. The patient is not allowed to sleep on the involved arm. Women cannot have purse straps across the forearm. Care must be taken when carrying any objects in the arms, such as grocery bags, boxes, firewood, books, and similar articles that could damage the site.

Another access to the bloodstream of patients is through a Permacath, a large double lumen (two open-

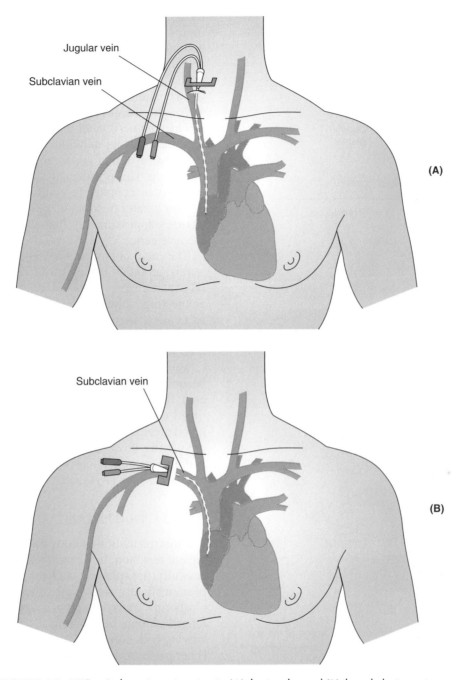

FIGURE 11-179 Catheter insertion sites in (A) the jugular and (B) the subclavian veins

ings) catheter. It can be surgically inserted into either the jugular or subclavian vein to provide temporary access for hemodialysis treatments. Figure 11–179 illustrates the catheter insertion sites in (A) the jugular and (B) the subclavian veins. The tubing from the hemodiaysis machine connects with the openings of catheter. The blood exits from the proximal opening on the catheter and goes to the machine for filtering. After being treated through the machine filters, the blood returns through the distal opening of the catheter to the body. The catheter is inserted to provide immediate use of a dialysis access to permit he-

modialysis. It is often used while waiting for a fistula or a graft to mature.

Because the rest of the patient's life depends on dialysis, access to a machine becomes critical. Most patients are assigned to dialysis centers for periodic treatment. However, equipment can be obtained for home dialysis if the patient and the family are willing to assume the responsibility. Patients usually require dialysis two to three times per week, for three to five hours each time.

An alternative to hemodialysis is continuous ambulatory **peritoneal** dialysis (Figure 11–180). Instead of an

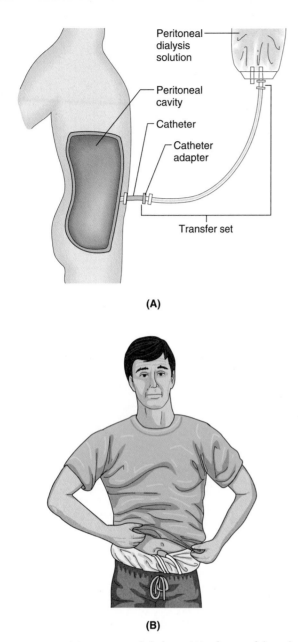

(A)

(B)

FIGURE 11–180 Peritoneal dialysis: (A) infusion of the solution, (B) rolled empty solution container hidden under clothing

artificial dialyzer to cleanse the blood, the patient's own peritoneal membrane is used (the peritoneum covers the abdominal organs and lines the abdominal cavity). The dialyzing solution is introduced into the peritoneal cavity where it comes into contact with blood vessels. The solution enters through a catheter permanently implanted into the abdomen. The solution tubing is aseptically attached and approximately two liters of dialyzing solution are infused by the process of gravity by suspending the bag at shoulder level. Then the empty bag is rolled up and placed around the waist under the clothing. The solution attracts the waste products and water from the blood, and they are suspended in the solution. After approximately four to six hours, the bag is unrolled, placed lower than

the abdomen, and the waste-bearing dialyzing solution is drained out. Another fresh bag is infused, and the dialysis continues. The exchange process of draining the solution and infusing fresh solution requires from 30 to 45 minutes. This is repeated about every four to six hours during the day and for an eight-hour period at night.

Another form of peritoneal dialysis is called *continuous cycling peritoneal dialysis* (CCPD). This is more acceptable to some individuals because the dialysis is accomplished during six to eight hours every night while they sleep. This is especially well-suited for children. The patient can completely control peritoneal dialysis, permitting greater freedom of activity; however, solution exchanges approximately four times daily do create some inconvenience.

The main complication of peritoneal dialysis is peritonitis, an inflammation of the peritonium from accidental contamination of the tubing when connecting and disconnecting solutions. Users of the method must be meticulous in performing the procedure. Peritonitis is painful and can cause scarring of the peritoneum, making it no longer useful for dialysis. Peritonitis can be fatal.

Many considerations must be weighed when dialysis becomes necessary. Routine procedures, must be considered: for example, when taking medications, they must be timed after dialysis to prevent removing them from the bloodstream. For additional information about this life-prolonging procedure, contact your local branch of the National Kidney Foundation, inquire at a dialysis center, or consult your physician.

KIDNEY TRANSPLANT

The transplantation of body organs is always at risk of recipient rejection; however the kidney can usually be successfully transplanted, and the survival of the graft has been markedly improved by the use of the drug cyclosporin. Transplantation is indicated in cases of prolonged chronic debilitating disease and renal failure involving both kidneys; unfortunately, transplantation often is not performed until patients have been on dialysis for a significant time because of a lack of organ donors.

The demand exceeds the supply for healthy organs. In addition, blood and other cellular structures must "match" to ensure the greatest probability for a functioning transplanted organ. There is an anticipated percentage of success within immediate family members. A twin provides the greatest likelihood, with a brother or sister, parent, or child providing decreasing percentages of success in that order. The surgical procedure itself is well established and presents virtually no concern as far as the success of the transplanted kidney. The patient, however, is almost always in a state of relatively poor physical condition because of the effects of the extended illness. This status and the tendency of the body to reject a "substance" that is foreign and not of the same cellular structure sometimes result in the organ not surviving in its new host. The use of drugs to control the body's natural defensive mechanism of rejection increases the rate of success. Neoral is the current commonly-used medication for kidney transplant patients. Research into new and more effective drugs is a continuing process.

DIAGNOSTIC EXAMINATIONS

Several procedures and tests are used to determine the physical characteristics of the urinary system and assess its function. Analysis of the blood can determine levels of uric acid and the amount of urea nitrogen present. Urinalysis (analysis of the urine) can determine the presence of blood cells and bacteria, acidity level, specific gravity (weight), and physical characteristics, such as color, clarity, and odor.

- **Noninvasive procedures**—Procedures that attempt to evaluate function deal with urinary output. An *intake–output measurement* involves keeping a record of all fluid, or food that melts to liquid, that is consumed, along with all urine or other fluid loss, be it measured or estimated. For example, emesis would be measured; perspiration estimated as slight, moderate, or profuse; diarrhea indicated as to frequency; and any other loss (such as bleeding, drainage through a stoma, or excessive respiratory activity) evaluated. Hence, intake is compared to output to evaluate fluid balance within the body.

A *24-hour urine test* collects all urinary output, from a specified hour one day until the same time the next day, in a special container under specific conditions (see Chapter 15). Urine can be collected by various methods, depending to some degree on the purpose for collection. A *routine specimen,* preferably the first of the morning, is simply voided into a clean container. A *clean catch specimen,* usually for culture purpose, pregnancy determination, or microscopic examination, involves specific cleaning of the meatal area and catching the specimen midstream in a sterile container.

An *x-ray* or *plain film* of the abdomen may be taken to determine size, shape, and position of the urinary organs. It may also indicate the presence of calculi. This is usually referred to as a KUB (kidney, ureters, and bladder) series.

The kidney may also be examined by *ultrasound* to detect abnormalities or to clarify findings from other tests. It is a safe, painless procedure that can be used especially in cases where sensitivity to the radiological opaque materials prohibits other tests. Examinations for kidney function that use a contrast medium are of little value when there is renal failure. Ultrasound, however, can be used to at least view the structure of the kidney in these instances.

Urine Analysis—A new urine test has been developed that can detect bladder cancer with 95% accuracy. It is capable of finding abnormal DNA material that is evidence of cancer. This makes diagnosis possible at a very early stage when the five-year survival rate is 91%. Previously, because no symptoms were present, cancer of the bladder was usually not detected until blood appeared in the urine, which was often too late. At this stage of advanced tumor, the five-year survival rate drops to only 9%. The current bladder tests detect only 20% to 30% of the patients with early disease because microscopic examination to distinguish malignant from normal cells is very difficult. In addition, early detection requires a cystoscopic examination to obtain the cells from a lesion. This test is invasive, painful, and expensive and is not suitable for bladder cancer screening. However, the new urine test could become a part of a routine physical examination. According to the American Cancer Society, estimates of new urinary bladder cancer cases for 2001 are 39,200 for males and 15,100 for females. The estimated death rate is 8,300 for males and 4,100 for females.

- **Invasive procedures**—Another means of collecting a urine specimen is to withdraw it directly from the bladder through a catheter into a sterile container by strict aseptic (sterile) technique.

One of the most common diagnostic procedures is an x-ray series called **intravenous pyelography (IVP)**. The patient is required to fast (no food or water) for approximately 10 hours beforehand. A laxative or cleansing enema removes from the colon any fecal material that might obscure the urinary organs. A contrast medium is injected into a vein, usually at the antecubital space of the arm. After a time, a film is taken to demonstrate the function, location, and position of the kidneys, as determined by the presence of the dye. Subsequent films outline the ureters and bladder as the dye is processed by the system. The film is taken at specific intervals to assess the efficiency of the kidney function. Because the contrast medium is iodine based, it is extremely important to determine if the patient has an allergic response to iodine or seafood before the injection.

Cystourethroscopy is an examination using a lighted instrument inserted into the urethra and bladder to view the interior surface (Figure 11–181). A local anesthetic (sometimes a general) is given. The scope is lubricated, and as it is inserted, the interior of the urethra is observed. The scope is then advanced into the bladder. A solution is instilled to distend the bladder for observation and to make the ureteral openings visible. At this point, based on findings, other procedures can be performed, such as *catheterization of the kidney(s)* by inserting a catheter up through the ureter(s), *biopsy of a tumor,* or *removal of calculi* in the bladder. It may be possible to crush larger calculi with an instrument and irrigate the pieces out through the scope. When examination of the bladder is completed, the scope is slowly withdrawn as the neck of the bladder and the interior of the urethra are examined.

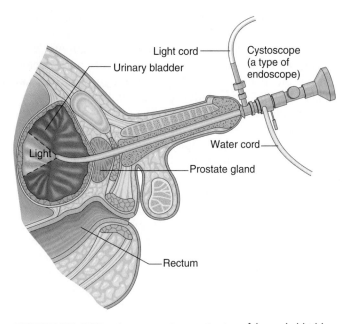

FIGURE 11–181   A cystoscopic examination of the male bladder

Other standard procedures performed initially during cystourethroscopy are obtaining a sterile specimen for culture, cytology (for cancer cells), and sensitivity testing. The *amount of residual urine* left in the bladder after the patient has voided (just prior to the examination) may be withdrawn and measured.

Other x-ray examinations can be performed in connection with endoscopic examinations. When a catheter is inserted into one of the ureters and passed into the pelvis of the kidney, a radiopaque medium can be instilled. This procedure, known as *retrograde ureteropyelography,* is especially useful for viewing the inside of the kidney when poor kidney function prohibits an IVP procedure. The structure of the ureters can be seen by an additional dye injection as the catheter is withdrawn.

Fluoroscopy and x-ray films aid in determining abnormalities. A delayed film, 15 to 20 minutes following instillation of the dye, can be taken to check for retention indicative of urinary stasis (stagnation). If an obstruction of the kidney is observed, it can be located by the film to be corrected. When an obstruction prohibits urine drainage, the catheter may be left in position temporarily to ensure adequate drainage. A kidney can be severely, if not permanently, damaged in a relatively short period if pressure from urine builds up because of the inability to drain.

DISEASES AND DISORDERS
Cystitis (Cys-ti'-tis)

Description—This inflammation of the bladder usually results from an ascending organism introduced through the meatus.

Signs and symptoms—Symptoms of cystitis are frequent urination, dysuria, spasms of the bladder, nocturia, and often fever and hematuria. Nausea, vomiting, chills, tenderness over the bladder area, and lower-back pain may occur. A frequent complaint is sharp, stabbing pain when voiding, especially at the end of the stream. This discomfort, together with the urge to void small amounts frequently, prompts the patient to seek medical help.

Diagnosis is confirmed by clinical characteristics and the presence of organisms in the urine.

Etiology—The most common cause in women is *E. coli* from the rectum, which may be carried to the meatus by improper cleansing following defecation. Women should be instructed to always cleanse from front to back when washing, wiping, or drying the perineal area. Cystitis can also be caused by organisms from the vagina. Women are far more prone to infection than men, presumably because the urethra is so short. Also in men, the prostatic fluid acts as an antibacterial shield, thereby providing protection.

Treatment—Cystitis is treated with antibiotics sufficient to sterilize the urine. Usually, medication is given for approximately five days. A culture of the urine after three days should show no organisms. If bacterial resistance to a certain medication has developed, the drug of choice will need to be changed. The sensitivity studies performed on the urine culture will identify appropriate alterations.

Urinary tract infections (UTI) are particularly common in patients with neurogenic bladders. The problem stems from the loss of innervation to the bladder, which can cause incontinence, residual retention, spasticity, or flaccidness. Bedfast patients or those confined to wheelchairs are especially susceptible. The use of indwelling catheters to deal with incontinence or the inability to void frequently results in UTI as a result of the direct entrance route for bacteria into the bladder.

Prevention—Women may be able to avoid cystitis by following some simple measures:

- Drink enough water to keep urine a light straw color; this washes out bacteria.
- Drinking 12 ounces of cranberry juice daily may also decrease bacteria.
- Don't use a diaphragm if you have recurrent UTIs; it boosts the risk for repeat infections.
- Urinate immediately after sex. Often, bacteria in the vagina may be introduced into the bladder, and urination expels the bacteria and decreases the likelihood of infection.

Glomerulonephritis (Glo-mer-u-low-nef-ri'-tis)

This inflammation of the glomerulus of the nephron occurs in both acute and chronic forms.

Acute glomerulonephritis (AGN)

Description—It can occur following bacterial infections of the respiratory tract, the urinary tract, or the bloodstream. It affects boys ages three to seven most frequently but can strike either sex at any age. Up to 95% of children and 70% of adults recover fully, with the remainder developing chronic renal failure.

Signs and symptoms—AGN usually begins from one to three weeks after an untreated throat infection. Symptoms include moderate edema, protein in the urine, hematuria, oliguria, and fatigue. Hypertension may develop because of retention of sodium or water from the decreased glomerular filtration rate. Diagnosis is made following a detailed history and clinical assessment. Laboratory findings confirm elevated electrolytes, BUN (blood urea nitrogen), creatinine in the blood, red and white blood cells, and protein in the urine. A throat culture may show a streptococcal organism.

Etiology—AGN results from a collection of antigen–antibodies from the streptococcal infections, which become entrapped in the glomeruli membranes. The entrapment causes interference in the glomerular function, damaging the membrane and resulting in the loss of its ability to selectively filter solutes. Red blood cells and protein molecules are allowed to filter out and the filtration rate drops. Uremic poisoning may result. (See Uremia.)

Treatment—Treatment consists of bed rest, fluid and salt restriction, and correction of the electrolyte imbalance. Diuretics (water pills) may be used to reduce the accumulation of cellular fluid. At this time, the use of antibiotics is controversial. The course of AGN usually resolves in about two weeks.

Chronic glomerulonephritis

Description—This is a slow, progressive disease. It causes scarring and sclerosing of the inflamed glomeruli, gradually leading to renal failure. Unfortunately, sufficient symptoms are not produced to cause early clinical investigation.

Signs and symptoms—The first symptoms are proteinuria (protein in the urine), hematuria, and a specific form of a urine cast. By the time it is diagnosed, chronic glomerulonephritis is usually irreversible.

The chronic stage can be asymptomatic for many years, suddenly becoming progressive and producing hypertension, proteinuria, and hematuria. In the later stages, uremic symptoms occur, such as nausea, vomiting, pruritus, dyspnea, fatigue, mild to severe edema, and anemia. Severe hypertension may cause enlargement of the heart, congestive heart failure (CHF), and eventually renal failure.

Etiology—Occasionally, the chronic form follows AGN, but most frequently it is an insidious disease precipitated by other primary renal disorders or systemic syndromes.

Treatment—Treatment consists of measures to treat the symptoms only, such as a diet to restrict sodium, antihypertensive drugs, correction of the electrolyte imbalance, reduction of edema, and prevention of cardiac failure.

Incontinence (In-con'-tin-ence)

Description—This is the uncontrollable loss of urine. It is estimated that at least 20 million people in the United States suffer from incontinence; 85% are women. It interferes with sleep, physical and sexual activity, travel, and daily activities. Many women avoid social activities and are home-bound because of the fear of an accident. Twenty-five percent of women ages 15 to 64 have incontinence. This increases to over 40% for those over 60. It occurs basically in three forms: stress, overflow, and urge. *Stress incontinence,* the most common, occurs when a person coughs, sneezes, or laughs. Urine may also leak from the stress on muscles when exercising or rising from bed or a chair. *Overflow incontinence* occurs because the bladder never empties completely and its fullness causes leakage. *Urge incontinence* occurs unexpectedly. There is a strong, uncontrollable urge to void requiring immediate emptying of the bladder to prevent wetting.

Males may also be affected by incontinence, but not as frequently as women. The rate among men is 1.5% to 5% but also increases with age. (It may be higher because so many prefer to be silent.) Nearly all older men have "dribbling" of urine when the prostate becomes enlarged and displaces the bladder. (The prostate, shaped somewhat like a donut, lies directly beneath the bladder with the urethra running through its center.) If the prostate is removed, the prostatic portion of the urethra is involved, and control of urine is affected.

Signs and symptoms—The primary symptom is the involuntary loss of urine.

Etiology—Age is not a cause. There are a number of reasons for incontinence; some are specific to one of the forms previously discussed. All involve the physical structure and function of the bladder and urethra. In the female, the bladder lies beneath and is somewhat supported by the uterus and its ligaments (Figure 11–182A). As the bladder fills, a message to void goes to the brain, but if it is not convenient, the external sphincter is contracted and the bladder neck stays closed. This signals the bladder to relax (Figure 11–182B). When it is time to void, the message goes to the external sphincter to relax and it opens; this signals the bladder neck to open and the bladder to contract (Figure 11–182C). With stress incontinence, coughing, sneezing, or laughing increases pressure on the bladder, thereby increasing pressure on the bladder neck, which is not able to stay closed. The external sphincter cannot control urine alone so it spurts out. With overflow incontinence, the urethra is narrowed, usually by scar tissue or a prolapsed pelvic organ preventing the bladder from emptying completely. The pressure builds up and overpowers the sphincter causing leakage. In women, the displacement of the bladder during pregnancy and the pressure during the process of

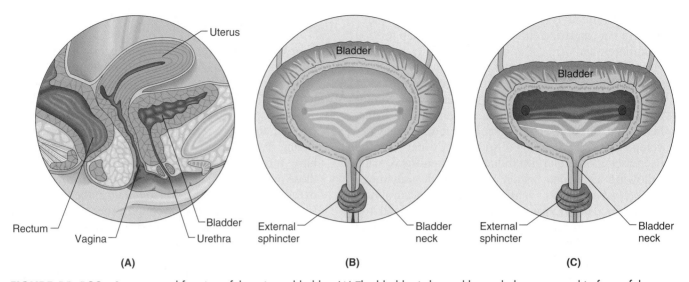

FIGURE 11–182 Structure and function of the urinary bladder: (A) The bladder is located beneath the uterus and in front of the vagina in a female, (B) the sphincter contracts to close the urethra and sends a message to the bladder to relax and the bladder neck to stay closed; (C) to void, the sphincter relaxes and a message goes to the bladder to contract and the bladder neck to open.

childbirth are definite factors in the development of incontinence. Often, following hysterectomy (removal of the uterus), the bladder will "drop" and protrude into the vagina causing a cystocele and resulting in improper positioning and the inability to empty completely. With urge incontinence, the urge to urinate is received even though there is little urine, the bladder continues to contract longer than the sphincter can prevent leakage, and urine is leaked. Menopause is often responsible because the drop in estrogen weakens the urethral sphincter causing an inability to keep it tightly closed, so a woman feels the urge to void small amounts several times an hour.

Treatment—A variety of things can be done. Many people find it necessary to wear sanitary napkins or specially designed incontinence pads in order to conceal their leakage. Others wear adult-style diapers or waterproof briefs. Some, especially men, wear an external appliance to catch the urine. For stress-related incontinence, exercises of the pelvic floor muscles may be helpful. These muscles act as a sling to keep the bladder and the bladder neck lifted and to control the external sphincter. These exercises are known as "Kegels." They involve contracting and briefly holding the muscles several times a day, which over time can tighten and strengthen the pelvic floor (Figure 11–183). The recommended "workout" is 25 to 40 repetitions of 5 to 10 seconds duration. For females, estrogen (female hormone) therapy is also helpful. The injection of collagen into the tissue surrounding the sphincter can be very effective in narrowing the urethra. Figure 11–184 illustrates the injection into the tissue from a needle within the cystoscope. This procedure may take several injections, which often cost up to $5,000 each. It has a 69% cure rate.

Overflow incontinence can be improved with medication that assists the bladder in emptying or with self catheterization to remove the urine. Surgery may be indicated if there is vaginal prolapse or if the bladder has partially descended through the muscles of the pelvic floor. Urge incontinence is best treated with drugs to relax the bladder contractions and estrogen to improve the sphincter tone. The Kegel exercises are also helpful. Drug therapy costs about $40 to $50 per month and must continue throughout life.

In males, exercises following prostate surgery are very important to regain urinary control. The surgical procedure weakens the related muscles and may injure the urethral sphincter. Occasionally, incontinence persists either because of increased bladder pressure or a sphincter problem, or both. If it persists, periurethral

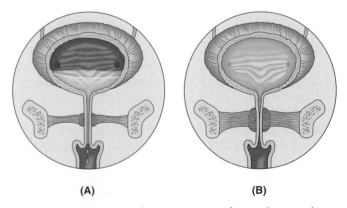

FIGURE 11–183 Kegel exercises: (A) Before, pelvic muscles are thin and the sphincter is weak, so the urethra cannot close; (B) after three months of exercise, the muscles are thicker and stronger, closing the sphincter.

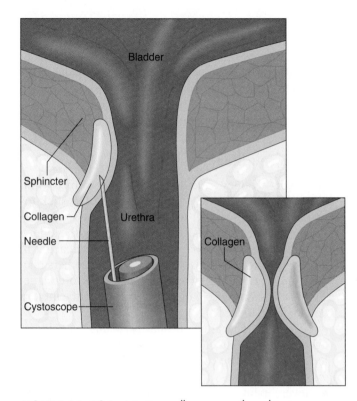

FIGURE 11–184 Injecting collagen near the sphincter narrows the urethra to control leakage.

collagen injections can be effective. A surgical procedure involving the insertion of an artificial sphincter can also be performed. This device has a valve mechanism that the person can activate to control and expel urine.

A change in behavior may be sufficient to control incontinence. With stress incontinence, a bathroom trip should be made every three hours. Urge incontinence requires bladder training by beginning bathroom trips every hour the first week, then every hour and a half, and eventually every three hours. Kegels are used to control the urge. The process is slow but rather successful, helping 54% to 75% but only curing 12% to 16%. Bladder surgery will achieve 85% success but will cost about $10,000.

There are other health problems that cause incontinence for both sexes. The effects of a stroke and Parkinson's disease, for instance, can damage the nerves, making control impossible. If leakage begins suddenly, it may signify a bladder infection or a medication side effect. High blood pressure drugs called alpha blockers weaken the sphincter. Antihistamines and sleeping pills may also cause problems.

Nephrotic Syndrome (Nephrosis) (Ne-frot'-ick)

Description—This noninflammatory disease involving the glomerular membrane allows a large number of protein molecules to leave the blood and enter the

urine. As a result, large amounts of water accumulate in the body, causing generalized dependent edema. This often leads to pleural effusion, swollen external sex organs, and ascites (fluid within the abdomen). **Nephrotic syndrome** occurs most often in children, but adults can contract the disease also.

Signs and symptoms—Symptoms range from the dominant clinical feature of edema to hypotension (especially on standing), lethargy, fatigue, lack of appetite, pallor, and depression.

Diagnosis can be confirmed with consistently-elevated proteinuria over a 24-hour period, the presence of characteristic fatty casts and oval fat bodies in the urine, and increased serum cholesterol levels with decreased albumin levels.

Etiology—The underlying cause of the disease is usually glomerulonephritis (75% of the cases). The remaining 25% are associated with diabetes; circulatory diseases, such as sickle cell anemia, CHF, and renal vein thrombosis; toxins that affect the nephrons, such as mercury, bismuth, or gold; allergic reactions; and systemic infections, such as tuberculosis.

Treatment—Treatment consists of correcting the underlying cause whenever possible. Supportive treatment involves a high-protein diet, restrictive sodium intake, diuretics for edema, and antibiotics to combat infection. Some favorable results have occurred with the use of corticosteroids, but they are limited to specific uses.

Polycystic Kidney Disease (Pol-le-cis'-tick)

Description—An inherited disorder, **polycystic kidney disease** is characterized by bilateral, grapelike clusters of fluid-filled cysts that replace normal renal tissue (Figure 11–185). The presence of the cysts greatly enlarges the size of the kidney externally and also compresses the nephrons inside, eventually replacing the functioning renal tissue. One form of the disease ap-

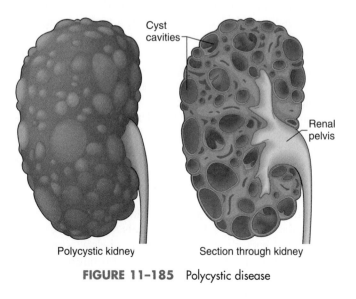

Polycystic kidney   Section through kidney

FIGURE 11–185 Polycystic disease

pears in infants and results in stillbirth or early newborn death. Occasionally, an infant will survive for about two years before developing renal failure. The adult form has an insidious onset, usually apparent between ages 30 to 50. The deterioration of the kidney is slower but is nevertheless fatal unless treated by dialysis or transplantation.

Signs and symptoms—Symptoms of the infantile form include a pointed nose, small chin, floppy low-set ears, and folds in the inner eyelids. The kidneys become huge bilateral masses between the bottom of the ribs and the top of the ileum and are symmetric, firm, and dense. Usually there is evidence of CHF and respiratory distress. Adult polycystic disease initially presents nonspecific symptoms, such as hypertension, polyuria, and UTI. Eventually additional symptoms appear relating to enlarged kidney masses, such as lumbar pain, widened body, and a swollen, tender abdomen. As the disease advances, the patient develops recurrent hematuria, life-threatening bleeding from cyst rupture, proteinuria, and pain caused by ureteral spasm from the passing of clots or calculi. Ultimately, the insufficiency of the kidney results in failure and uremia.

Etiology—This disease is an inherited disorder.

Treatment—Polycystic disease is not curable, but it can be managed, to a certain degree, by controlling hypertension and urinary infections. Treatment is like that for any chronic, destructive kidney disease.

Pyelonephritis (Pie-low-nef-ri'-tis)

Description—This is one of the most common kidney infections.

Signs and symptoms—Symptoms associated with pyelonephritis include fever, urgency, dysuria, back pain, burning during urination, nocturia, and hematuria. The urine may have an ammoniac or fishy odor and is usually cloudy in appearance. Other common symptoms include chills, lack of appetite, flank pain, and fatigue. The symptoms generally develop rapidly and may subside within a few days. However, a residual bacterial infection may recur at a later time.

Etiology—Acute pyelonephritis is caused by bacteria that normally inhabit the intestines. The bacteria typically spread from the bladder up the ureters and into the kidney pelvis, causing the development of colonies of bacteria within 24 to 48 hours. **Pyelonephritis** may also result from urinary stasis, the inability to empty the bladder completely, or urinary obstruction caused by strictures, tumors, or enlarged prostate in males.

Diagnosis is confirmed by urinalysis, which shows sediment containing bacteria leukocytes and possibly a few red blood cells. Culture reveals a significant population of bacteria. Specific gravity is below normal because of the temporary inability to concentrate urine.

Treatment—Treatment consists of antibiotics determined by culture and sensitivity tests. A course of treatment is usually 10 to 14 days even though urine becomes sterile after two to three days.

Reculturing is done one week after treatment and periodically for the next year to observe for residual infection. Mechanical problems causing urinary stasis, such as strictures, "dropped" bladder (positioned so that it cannot totally empty), or tumors, should be corrected.

Renal Calculi (Ree'-nal Cal'-q-lie)

Description—Kidney calculi (stones) are formed from chemicals in the urine, forming crystals that stick together. They may be as small as a grain of sand or as large as a golf ball. Small stones pass out of the kidney with the urine. Some that are larger become caught in a ureter where they cause severe pain. Still others may pass into the bladder where they continue to enlarge. They will again cause pain if they wash into the urethra and become lodged.

Kidney stones affect primarily young to middle-aged adults, with men being affected four times as often as women. The condition tends to recur.

Signs and symptoms—

- Severe pain, starting suddenly in the kidneys or lower abdomen and moving to the groin area. It may last for minutes or hours, alternating with periods of relief.
- Nausea and vomiting
- Burning and frequent urge to urinate
- Chills, fever, and weakness, probably from infection
- Cloudy or foul-smelling urine
- Blood in the urine
- Blocked urine flow

Diagnosis is made based on symptoms, x-rays (such as KUB or IVP), or ultrasound. Once size and location are determined, then an appropriate course of action can be selected. About 90% can be passed without requiring special treatment or surgery. Often, increasing fluids, being active, and a specific medication to dissolve the stone are sufficient. However, calcium-containing stones, the most common type, cannot be dissolved.

Etiology—The causes of calculi formation are not always clear; however, certain factors seem to contribute to their development.

- Drinking too little fluid
- Chronic UTIs
- Blockage of the urinary tract
- Prolonged limited activity
- Misuse of certain medications
- Certain genetic and metabolic diseases
- Specific foods in certain susceptible people

Treatment—The simplest treatment is chosen first. Many stones, if in the bladder or ureters, can be removed endoscopically either directly or following fracture of the stone with laser or shock waves. Stones in the kidney may be removed by a scope, inserted through the side of the body and directly into the kidney. This allows removal of the stone when it is visualized or fracture of the stone with instruments passed under direct vision.

Another new method of stone removal is called extracorporeal shock-wave **lithotripsy** (ESWL). Shock waves (high-energy pressure waves) similar to sonic booms generated by aircraft are produced outside the body by an electrical spark. The patient, in a disposable swimsuit, is positioned and strapped into a hydraulic chair. Intravenous sedation is given to make the patient comfortable. The chair is positioned, within a tank of warm water, so that the stone is in an area where the shock waves can be focused. The waves travel through the water and the body without damaging living tissue because all living tissue is about 80% water. Figure 11–186 illustrates the positioning of the patient for lithotripsy procedure.

It takes about 2,000 shock waves to break up the average stone and requires about 30 minutes to complete the treatment. Most describe the shock feeling as a slapping or tapping sensation. Patients are fitted with headphones to listen to music while the procedure is being done. About an hour after the treatment, most patients are allowed to leave. The small fragments of the fractured stone can easily be passed in the urine. It may take several weeks to completely pass all the fragments.

Most patients experience some abdominal discomfort with or without bruising on the abdomen or back. Frequent, bloody urination is common. Patients are instructed to collect passed stone fragments for analysis and to see their urologists as a follow-up to be certain there is no kidney blockage from the fragments.

Occasionally, people do not qualify for ESWL because of stone location or one of the following:
- Weight in excess of 295 pounds
- Height over six feet, six inches
- Involved kidney has little or no function
- Uncontrolled urinary infection
- It is the urologist's opinion that another form of treatment is more appropriate

If no other method can be used, the stone will be removed by surgical incision into the kidney. This is considered the final choice to solve the problem because of the risks involved with any major surgical procedure and the length of recovery time required.

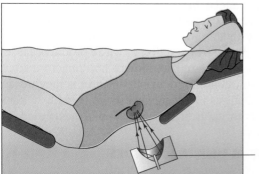

FIGURE 11-186   Lithotripsy procedure

Shock wave generator

Renal Failure

Acute renal failure

Description—A critical illness, **acute renal failure** results in the sudden cessation of kidney function. Effective medical treatment usually can overcome the problem. If not, however, it will progress to uremia and death.

Signs and symptoms—Symptoms initially apparent are oliguria and azotemia (nitrogenous products of protein metabolism in the blood). Without filtration, the waste products and excess solutes quickly collect in the blood, resulting in severe electrolyte imbalance, acidosis, and uremia, which interfere with the function of the other body systems. A vast number of other symptoms develop, listed here by body system and in ascending order within the system:
- Gastrointestinal: anorexia, nausea, vomiting, hematemesis (bloody vomitus)
- Nervous: headache, drowsiness, confusion, convulsion, coma
- Integumentary: dryness of the skin, pruritis, pallor, uremic frost (powdery white crystals of urea on the skin)
- Circulatory: hypotension initially, then hypertension, cardiac rhythm irregularities, CHF, edema, anemia, pulmonary edema
- Respiratory: Kussmaul's respirations (fast, deep respirations, over 20 per minute and usually sounding labored, resembling sighs)

Fever and chills, indicators of infection, are an expected complication.

Diagnosis of renal failure is confirmed by blood test findings of greatly-elevated quantities of urea, nitrogen, and creatinine and urine samples with casts, protein, and altered specific gravity. Additional verification with diagnostic examinations, such as KUB, IVP, ultrasound, and retrograde pyelography, may be indicated.

Etiology—Renal failure may be caused by an obstruction, inadequate circulation, or damage to the nephrons. Failure caused by bilateral obstruction is usually associated with calculi, blood clots, tumors, strictures, an enlarged prostate, or urethral edema. Inadequate blood flow results from low blood pressure and low volume in the arteries, which eliminates the force required for the kidney to filter water and solutes from the blood. This can result from shock, embolism, hemorrhage, loss of fluid caused by burns, congestive heart failure, and arrhythmias. Nephron damage, which may cause failure, can result from acute glomerulonephritis, sickle cell anemia, bilateral renal vein thrombosis, acute pyelonephritis, renal myeloma (tumor), or toxic substances.

Treatment—Treatment consists of a high-calorie diet that is low in protein, sodium, and potassium. Fluids are controlled. Dialysis may be required.

Chronic renal failure

Description—This is an end result of the progressive loss of kidney function.

Signs and symptoms—Symptoms do not develop significantly enough to warrant investigation until almost 75%

of glomerular function is gone. The remaining normal nephrons gradually deteriorate, causing symptoms of renal failure and other system involvement. Signs and symptoms initially are related to an imbalance of sodium and potassium and an accumulation of nitrogen from protein metabolism; these may include hypotension, dry mouth, listlessness, fatigue, and nausea. Later the patient will begin experiencing mental dullness and confusion. Symptoms increase as more nephrons fail.

Additional systems involvement is similar to that described with acute failure, but a few specific differences do occur with the slower progressive course.

A PEDIATRIC PERSPECTIVE

Children with chronic failure show stunted growth patterns because of endocrine abnormalities.

Infertility and amenorrhea (lack of menses) in women, impotence in men, and impaired carbohydrate metabolism also result from improper endocrine action. The skeletal system develops a mineral imbalance that results in bone pain because of parathyroid hormone imbalance. This in turn allows the minerals to be withdrawn from the bones, causing fractures. Calcifications develop in the brain, eyes, joints, myocardium, and blood vessels.

Diagnosis is made in the same manner as for acute renal failure.

Etiology—Chronic failure can be the result of many preexisting conditions, such as chronic glomerular disease, chronic infections, obstructions, stones, and endocrine diseases, such as diabetes, vascular diseases, hypertension, and chronic overdose of toxic agents.

Treatment—Treatment is almost exclusively dependent on dialysis to correct the chemical imbalance. Other treatment is required for the complications developed in the other body systems. Long-term dialysis requires specific physical and psychological therapy. Patients must be meticulous in their personal care. The skin must be clean and lotions should be applied to combat dryness and itching. Good oral hygiene is a must to alleviate bad breath and counteract excessive dryness and bad taste. Diet is extremely critical and requires individual adjustments in relation to dialysis. Daily records of intake and output aid in determining fluid status. If urine is not being excreted, fluid builds up within the body's tissues. Dialysis removes this fluid, causing the patient to express feelings of being "wrung out."

Stricture (Strick'-sure)

Description—This is a narrowing of a passageway that interferes with the movement of substances through its interior. For example, the **stricture** of a ureter interferes with the flow of urine to the bladder. A more common stricture occurs in the urethra, particularly in males.

A CAAHEP CONNECTION

Medical assisting curriculum standards must include content on **Communication** and **Common pathologies**. This content on renal failure and the important patient teaching information required to assist patients to cope with these life-changing conditions is very helpful. Understanding the progression of the disease, the importance of diet, skin care, fluid measurement, and the need for dialysis allows you to adapt your instruction and support for the individual needs of the patient.

Signs and symptoms—Symptoms of urethral stricture, such as a small urine stream and prolonged urination time, are indicative of a decreased passageway. Stricture of a ureter may not be evident until distention occurs because of the buildup of pressure or until kidney stones develop from urinary stasis. Complete stricture of a ureter will destroy the function of the affected kidney.

Etiology—It may be caused by a congenital abnormality or, in either sex, the result of scarring following infection.

Treatment—Urethral strictures can be readily treated by dilation to open up the narrowed passageway. Increasingly larger dilators are inserted into the urethra to stretch the constricted area. The procedure often needs to be repeated periodically to maintain patency (openness), especially with the growing child. If it is not successful, surgery to correct the problem will be necessary.

Uremia (Your-e-me-ah)

Description—Literally translated, this term means that the products normally found in the urine are instead in the blood.

Signs and Symtoms— Blood analysis shows excess protein byproducts because urinary disease prevents their excretion in the urine. It is a toxic condition, leading to coma and death if not treated. End-stage uremia may cause "uremic frost," the presence of crystals from the excretion of urine products through the skin.

Etiology—It can be the end result of many acute and chronic kidney diseases. Any condition, which renders the kidney unable to regulate the chemical composition of the blood by excretion of waste products causes the wastes to accumulate, slowly building to a toxic level. When renal failure exists, **uremia** is inevitable.

Treatment—Dialysis is the only substitute for kidney function, except for surgical transplantation of another kidney.

ACHIEVE UNIT OBJECTIVES

Complete Chapter 11, Unit 11, in the workbook to help you obtain competency of this subject matter.

UNIT 12

The Endocrine System

◼ OBJECTIVES

Upon completion of the unit, meet the following performance objectives by verifying knowledge of the facts and principles presented through oral and written communication at a level deemed competent.

1. Spell and define, using the glossary at the back of the text, all the **Words to Know** in this unit.
2. Differentiate between endocrine and exocrine glands, and give an example of each.
3. Give five examples of body functions affected by hormones.
4. Name and locate the nine glands discussed in the unit.
5. Describe the structure and function of the pituitary, thyroid, parathyroid, adrenal, pancreas, and thymus glands.
6. Describe the hormones and functions of the pineal body and the gonads.
7. Explain the hormone secretion abnormalities that cause: gigantism, dwarfism, acromegaly, goiter, tetany, diabetes, cretinism, Cushing's syndrome, and myxedema.
8. List the symptoms of diabetic coma and insulin shock.
9. Identify the diagnostic examinations used to confirm diabetes, thyroid function, pregnancy, and Cushing's syndrome.
10. Describe briefly the symptoms, characteristics, and the usual course of action of endocrine disorders presented in the unit.

AREAS OF COMPETENCE (AAMA)

This unit addresses content within the specific competency areas of *Administrative procedures, Practice finances, Patient care, Communication skills*, and *Instruction*, as identified in the Medical Assistant Role Delineation Study. Refer to Appendix A for a detailed listing of the areas. (Note: Although *Anatomy and physiology* is not specifically identified in the study, a basic understanding of the body's structure and function is an essential foundation to the competent performance of many roles.)

◼ WORDS TO KNOW

acromegaly	aldosterone
adrenal	cretinism
adrenaline	Cushing's syndrome
adrenocorticotropic	diabetes mellitus
hormone (ACTH)	dwarfism

endocrine	islets of Langerhans
epinephrine	luteinizing
estrogen	myxedema
exocrine	ovary
exophthalmia	parathyroid
gigantism	pineal body
glucohemoglobin	pituitary
glycosuria	progesterone
goiter	puberty
gonad	testes
gonadotropic	testosterone
hormone	tetany
hyperglycemia	thymus
hyperthyroidism	thyroid
hypoglycemia	thyroidectomy
hypothyroidism	

 Library

The **endocrine** system is a group of glands that secrete substances directly into the bloodstream. Endocrine glands are ductless; in other words, their secretions do not drain into the body by way of a duct but are secreted directly into the capillaries of the circulatory system (Figure 11–187). Glands secreting substances through ducts are **exocrine** glands. The liver secretes bile through the hepatic duct; therefore it is an exocrine gland. Similarly, the pancreas secretes pancreatic juices by way of a duct into the duodenum, so it is an exocrine gland. However, the pancreas also secretes insulin directly into the blood, which also makes it an endocrine gland.

The secretions from endocrine glands are called **hormones**. A hormone is a complex chemical that influences

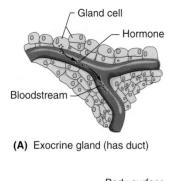

(A) Exocrine gland (has duct)

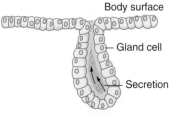

(B) Endocrine gland (ductless)

FIGURE 11-187 (A) Exocrine gland cells secrete substances directly into a duct; (B) endocrine gland cells secrete hormones into a capillary.

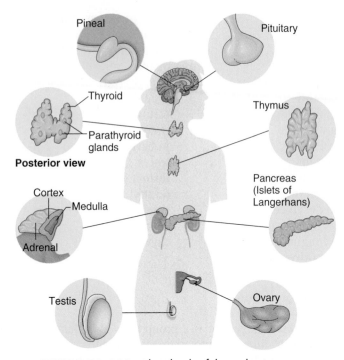

FIGURE 11-188   The glands of the endocrine system

and controls body functions. Hormones are chemical messengers that cause changes, which persist for a considerable time. Examples of body functions affected by hormones are growth and development, metabolism, the composition of the blood and bones, sexual maturity, and the function of all endocrine glands.

Nine glands or groups of glands will be discussed: the **pituitary**, **thyroid**, **parathyroids**, pancreas (introduced in Unit 10, The Digestive System), **adrenals**, **ovaries**, **testes**, **thymus**, and the **pineal body** (Figure 11–188). Each gland performs a specific function. The hyper- or hypoactivity of the gland causes changes in the body, often altering its appearance, always altering its function, even to the point of death in specific hormonal crises. Hormones either stimulate or inhibit glandular function to maintain homeostasis.

There are many diseases and disorders that develop from either too little or too much hormone influence. Some effects begin in early childhood, others after years of absence or excess of secretions. Fortunately, with appropriate health care, these abnormal conditions are discovered early, and the consequences are negligible. In developing nations or when there are religious beliefs that prohibit medical intervention, these conditions may still be observable.

PITUITARY GLAND

The pituitary gland is considered to be the "master" gland of the body, secreting a large number of hormones that affect other glands, growth, and development.

The gland is attached by a thin stalk to the undersurface of the brain. It is so vital to the body that it is protected

within a bony cradle deep within the skull. It sits in a bony depression of the spheroid bone of the skull, called the *sella turcica,* behind the bony orbits of the eyes at about the level of the bridge of the nose. This tiny gland, not much larger than a pea, secretes nine known hormones.

The pituitary is constructed of a large anterior and a small posterior lobe, each producing specific hormones. A thin sheet of tissue lies between the two lobes. The production of pituitary hormones is under the control of the hypothalamus of the brain by way of a feedback mechanism that senses the level of all hormones available to the body and the need for hormones to be released in response to stimuli.

Anterior Lobe

The hormones of the anterior lobe of the pituitary are as follows:

1. Growth hormone (GH)—Essential for normal growth of the body's tissues, affects the length of long bones and therefore height. Insufficient production during childhood results in **dwarfism**, whereas overproduction produces **gigantism** (Figure 11–189). Overproduction in adulthood will produce a condition known as **acromegaly**, which is characterized by overgrowth of cartilagenous and connective tissue resulting in a

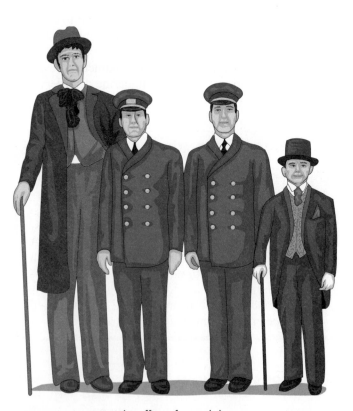

FIGURE 11-189   The effect of growth hormone: a giant, a dwarf, and two normal-sized people (Adapted from C.P. Anthony and G. Thibodeau, *Textbook of Anatomy and Physiology,* copyright by Mosby, reproduced with permission.)

bulky appearance, protrusion of the eyebrow area, enlargement of the hands and feet, and deformation of the features.

2. Thyrotropin, the thyroid-stimulating hormone (TSH)—Increases the growth and activity of thyroid cells to produce thyroid hormone.
3. **Adrenocorticotropic hormone (ACTH)**—Stimulates the cortex of the adrenal gland.
4. Melanocyte-stimulating hormone (MSH)—Increases skin pigmentation.

The following three **gonadotropic** hormones control the development of the reproductive system in both males and females, including the female menstrual cycle. If production fails before **puberty**, sexual maturity will not occur. If it fails after puberty, secondary sexual characteristics regress.

5. Follicle-stimulating hormone (FSH)—Enlarges the graafian follicle of the ovary to the point of rupture and stimulates the follicle to produce estrogen in the female. FSH stimulates the production of the sperm in the male.
6. **Luteinizing** hormone (LH)—In the female causes the ruptured ovarian follicle to become a corpus luteum that in turn secretes the hormone progesterone. Interstitial cell stimulating hormone (ICSH) in the male stimulates the interstitial cells in the testes to produce testosterone.
7. Prolactin (PR)—Responsible for breast development and the production of milk.

Posterior Lobe

The hormones of the posterior lobe of the pituitary are as follows:

1. Oxytocin—Stimulates the contractions of the uterus, especially during childbirth; it also is responsible for the flow of milk from the breast.
2. Vasopressin, or the antidiuretic hormone (ADH)—Acts on the kidney tubule cells to concentrate urine and conserve water within the body. It also stimulates the smooth muscles of blood vessels to constrict.

THYROID GLAND

The thyroid gland has two lobes, one on each side of the larynx, with a connecting central section called the isthmus (Figure 11–190). It is located in front of the upper portion of the trachea in the lower part of the neck. The gland is encased in a capsule of connective tissue.

The thyroid gland produces three hormones: thyroxine (T_4), triiodothyronine (T_3), and thyrocalcitonin. Thyrocalcitonin causes calcium to be stored in the bones to reduce the level of calcium in the blood. The other two hormones strongly affect metabolism, which influences both the physical and mental activity necessary for normal growth

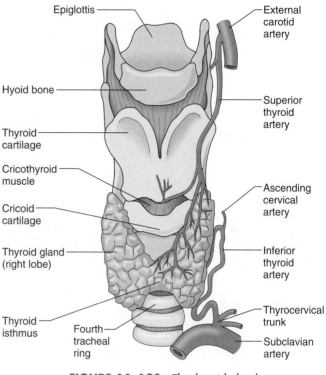

FIGURE 11-190 The thyroid gland

and development. When thyroid activity is below normal, it is called **hypothyroidism**, indicating a decrease in the basal metabolic rate. An overactive thyroid is called **hyperthyroidism** and indicates an increased metabolic rate.

The thyroid gland requires iodine to form the thyroid hormones. Iodine is obtained by eating vegetables grown in soil containing iodine or by eating seafood. Lack of the element causes the thyroid gland to enlarge because of the feedback mechanism. When the pituitary receives information that the level of thyroid hormones is too low, it sends out TSH to stimulate the thyroid cells. The cells in turn enlarge, trying to increase output, and eventually enlarge the entire gland. An enlarged thyroid gland is commonly known as a **goiter**.

A person who has hypothyroidism feels fatigued, has low blood pressure and pulse rate, often a subnormal temperature, and may be overweight due to decreased metabolism. The hyperthyroid patient is nervous, restless, and irritable, with heart rate above normal and elevated blood pressure. The patient may lose weight despite a good appetite. Occasionally the eyes protrude dramatically in a condition called **exophthalmia** (Figure 11–191).

Treatment of hypothyroidism is relatively simple: the thyroid hormone is taken orally as a supplement. Hyperthyroidism may initially be treated with supplemental iodine to prohibit or control gland enlargement. With progressive disease, it may be necessary to remove part or all of the gland or limit its function by radiation. The surgical removal of the thyroid is called a **thyroidectomy**.

A thyrotoxic crisis or thyroid storm is the extreme clinical development of hyperthyroidism. It produces a

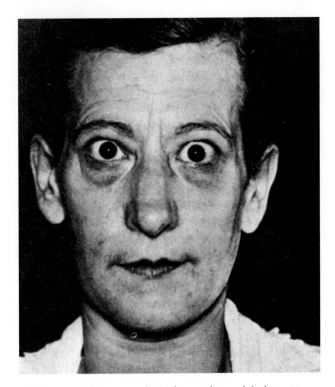

FIGURE 11–191 Hyperthyroidism with exophthalmia (From DeGroot, *The Thyroid and Its Diseases*, 4th. ed., copyright 1975 by John Willey & Sons.)

greatly accelerated metabolism, severe nervous system malfunction, overheating, and heart failure. The situation is precipitated by stress or a severe infection and is usually fatal. The vigorous use of antithyroid drugs can frequently prevent the complication from occurring.

PARATHYROID GLANDS

The parathyroid glands, usually two pairs, are embedded on the posterior surface of the thyroid gland. Their number and size vary greatly, but normally they resemble grains of wheat. The parathyroids are responsible for regulating the calcium content of the blood. The hormone parathromone cooperates with vitamin D to balance the level of calcium in the blood by stimulating the bones to release stored calcium and phosphate into the circulation.

Hyperparathyroidism results in increased levels of calcium in the blood, which causes lethargy and the excretion of large quantities of calcium salts in the urine, leading to the formation of kidney stones. The condition leads progressively to decalcification of the bones and is usually associated with a tumor of one of the glands. Decalcified bones are prone to pathological fracture.

Hypoparathyroidism is dramatically demonstrated by a condition known as **tetany**, an uncontrollable twitching of the muscles of the body. This results from hyperirritability of the nervous system in response to the lowered concentration of calcium throughout the body. The condition is easily treated by the addition of calcium. Hypoparathyroidism occurs following damage to or accidental removal of the parathyroids during a thyroidectomy.

ADRENAL GLANDS (SUPRARENAL)

The adrenal glands sit atop each kidney, hence the additional name of *suprarenal*. Each gland is contained in a fibrous capsule and is composed of two parts, each of which acts separately. The outer glandular tissue is called the *cortex,* whereas the inner tissue is referred to as the *medulla.*

The principal hormone of the medulla is **adrenaline**, also called **epinephrine**. Another hormone, norepinephrine, has a similar action on the body. Together they are considered to be the "flight or fight" hormones because of their effects in emergency situations. The hormones cause an increase in the heart rate, blood pressure, and flow of blood, and a decrease in intestinal activity. The adrenal medulla is considered to be nonessential to life.

The cortex of the adrenal gland, however, is essential to life. The cortex produces steroid hormones in three categories: mineral corticoids, glucocorticoids, and sex steroids. The mineral corticoids, of which **aldosterone** is the principal one, control electrolyte balances through regulating the reabsorption of sodium in the kidney tubules and the excretion of potassium. The glucocorticoids affect the metabolism of protein, fat, and glucose. They stimulate the liver to convert protein into glycogen and then break it down into glucose, thereby increasing blood sugar level. This change is seen when the body is subjected to stressful situations. The hormone level is increased, which in turn accelerates the conversion process to allow the body to cope.

The sex steroids govern certain sexual characteristics, especially those that are male oriented. These steroids are referred to as *androgens*. Excessive secretions cause the virilization and development of masculine secondary sex characteristics in the female and immature male (Figure 11–192). A mature female's voice will deepen, a growth of beard will appear, menstruation will become irregular, and sterility will result.

PANCREAS

The pancreas is a dual-function organ. It has an exocrine function, producing pancreatic juices excreted by way of the pancreatic duct into the duodenum to become part of the digestive juices. It is also an endocrine gland. The hormone *insulin* is secreted by the B cells of the **islets of Langerhans**, often called beta cells (Figure 11–193). They are one of four cell types, A, B, C, and D, located in the pancreas. It is known that the A cells secrete glucagon, but the exact function of this substance is uncertain. It may stimulate the liver to release glucogen, converting it to glucose to raise the blood sugar level.

Insulin is necessary for the metabolism of carbohydrates. With reduced islet function, the level of blood sugar rises to an abnormal amount and is referred to as **hyperglycemia**. Conversely, an abnormally low level of blood sugar is known as **hypoglycemia**. When excess glucose is present in the blood, it is excreted in the urine,

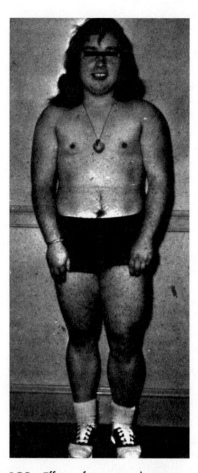

FIGURE 11-192   Effects of excess androgens on young female (Adapted from C.P. Anthony and G. Thilbodeau, *Textbook of Anatomy and Physiology*, 11th ed., copyright 1983 by Mosby; courtesy Dr. William McKendree Jefferies, Case Western Reserve University School of Medicine, Cleveland, Ohio.)

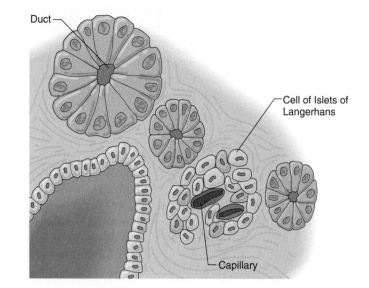

FIGURE 11-193   Pancreatic structure

a finding known as **glycosuria**. Hyperglycemia and glycosuria are the two outstanding characteristics of **diabetes mellitus**.

The exact function of insulin and its relationship to diabetes are not clearly understood. It is believed that insulin makes it possible for the cells to use the glucose present in the body tissues. Without the ability to burn glucose, it cannot be changed into energy and is therefore passed on to the kidneys for excretion. Insulin is also required for the metabolism of fat and protein.

THYMUS GLAND

The thymus gland is a two-lobed structure, located under the sternum. It is composed primarily of lymphoid tissue and enclosed in a fibrous capsule. The thymus is fairly large during childhood but begins to disappear with the onset of puberty, becoming a small mass of connective tissue and fat in adulthood. It appears to produce a hormone known as thymosin, which is believed to react on lymphoid tissue to mature T lymphocytes and develop immunity against certain diseases.

PINEAL BODY

The pineal body is a small mass of tissue attached by a slim stalk to the roof of the third ventricle in the brain. The pineal body is believed to produce a substance called melatonin. This substance combines with a hypothalamic substance to delay puberty until the normal time.

GONADS (TESTES AND OVARIES)

The ovaries in the female and the testes in the male are called the **gonads**, or sex glands. The ovaries are located in the pelvic cavity, one on each side of the uterus. The testes are located outside the body of the male, suspended in the scrotum. Both gonads secrete hormones that control the development of secondary sex characteristics.

In the female, the ovaries secrete **estrogen**, which reacts on the lining of the uterus, promotes growth and development of the primary and secondary sex organs, and maintains them throughout adult life. Estrogen also affects the release of other hormones from the pituitary. Another hormone, **progesterone**, is also secreted by the ovaries. It affects the uterine lining and the development of the secretory portion of the breasts. It aids in maintaining pregnancy.

In the male, the testes produce a hormone known as **testosterone**. This hormone develops the primary male sexual characteristics and the secondary characteristics of a deep voice, muscular development, and body hair distribution. It stimulates maturation of sperm cells.

The gonads are the organs of fertility and reproduction in both sexes. The maturity of the organs and the proper balance of hormonal secretions create the desire for and ability to engage in sexual activity.

See Table 11–16 for a summary of the glands and their functions.

TABLE 11–16

ENDOCRINE GLANDS			
Gland	**Location**	**Hormone**	**Principal Effects**
PITUITARY Anterior lobe	Undersurface of the brain in the sella turcica of the skull	Growth hormone (GH)	Normal growth of body tissues
		Thyroid stimulating hormone (TSH) (Thyrotropin)	Stimulates growth and activity of thyroid cells to produce thyroid hormone
		Adrenocorticotropic hormone (ACTH)	Stimulates the cortex of the adrenal gland
		Melanocyte-stimulating hormone (MSH)	Increases skin pigmentation
		Follicle-stimulating hormone (FSH)	Stimulates the maturity of the graafian follicle to rupture and to produce estrogen in the female. In the male, it stimulates the development of the testes and the production of sperm
		Luteinizing hormone (LH) Interstitial-cell stimulating hormone (ICSH)	Causes the development of the corpus luteum, which then secretes progesterone in the female. ICSH in the male stimulates the interstitial cells of the testes to produce testosterone.
		Prolactin (PR)	Develops breast tissue and stimulates secretion of milk from mammary glands
Posterior lobe		Oxytocin	Stimulates contraction of uterus, especially during childbirth; causes ejection of milk from mammary glands
		Vasopressin or Antidiuretic hormone (ADH)	Acts on cells of kidney tubules to concentrate urine and conserve fluid in the body. Also acts to constrict blood vessels
THYROID	Lower portion of the anterior neck	Thyroxine (T$_4$) and Triiodothyronine (T$_3$)	Increases metabolism; influences both physical and mental activity; promotes normal growth and development
		Thyrocalcitonin	Causes calcium to be stored in bones; reduces blood level of calcium
PARATHYROID	Posterior surface of thyroid gland	Parathormone	Regulates exchange of calcium between the bones and blood
ADRENAL Medulla	Superior surface of each kidney	Adrenaline (epinephrine)	Increases heart rate, blood pressure, and flow of blood; decreases intestinal activity
		Aldosterone (mineral corticoid)	Controls electrolyte balances by regulating the reabsorption of sodium and the excretion of potassium
Cortex		Glucocorticoids	Affect the metabolism of protein, fat, and glucose, thereby increasing blood sugar
		Sex hormones (androgens)	Govern sex characteristics, especially those that are masculine
PANCREAS	Behind the stomach	Insulin	Essential to the metabolism of carbohydrates; reduces the blood sugar level
		Glucagon	Stimulates the liver to release glycogen and convert it to glucose to increase blood sugar levels
THYMUS	Under the sternum	Thymosin	Reacts upon lymphoid tissue to produce T lymphocyte cells to develop immunity to certain diseases
PINEAL BODY	Third ventricle in the brain	Melatonin	Controls onset of puberty
OVARIES	Female pelvis	Estrogen	Promotes growth of primary and secondary sexual characteristics
		Progesterone	Develops excretory portion of mammary glands; aids in maintaining pregnancy
TESTES	Male scrotum	Testosterone	Develops primary and secondary sexual characteristics; stimulates maturation of sperm

INTERRELATIONSHIP OF THE GLANDS

As stated previously, hormonal secretion is regulated by a feedback mechanism. When the hormone is present or the substance produced by the effect of that hormone on another gland or organ is present, further secretion is affected. For example, the parathyroids increase secretion of parathormone to raise the serum calcium level to be withdrawn from the bones. When the serum level rises, a negative feedback message is signaled, and the secretion of parathormone is decreased. A more complicated feedback involves both positive and negative action. For example, the pituitary gland secretes TSH, which causes the thyroid gland to increase the production of hormones. When the appropriate level is reached, TSH secretion is inhibited, a negative feedback. The hypothalamus produces a thyrotropin-releasing hormone (TRH), which is stimulated by low levels of thyroid hormone. Therefore, when the level again drops, the hypothalamus secretes TRH, which stimulates the pituitary to release TSH, which in turn stimulates the production of the thyroid hormones, a positive feedback mechanism.

In the next unit, the interrelationship of the pituitary and the ovary will be discussed to explain how this complex balance prepares the female for pregnancy and then either sustains that hormonal state or allows it to alter, all in response to the feedback mechanism.

DIAGNOSTIC EXAMINATIONS

A great variety of diagnostic tests can be performed on blood and urine, which either measure the amount of specific hormones present in the body or measure the effectiveness of their function. A few of the more common tests are:

- Blood sugar, frequently measured after fasting (FBS)—To assess the function of the pancreas, including insulin production and use.
- T_3, TSH, and T_4—To measure the level of the thyroid hormones.
- Urine human chorionic gonadotropin (HCG) (pregnancy test)—To measure the presence of a hormone secreted by the placental cells
- Glucose tolerance—To measure the body's ability to process a large dose of glucose. Multiple blood and urine samples are taken at specific intervals following ingestion of the glucose mixture.
- **Glucohemoglobin** (GHB A1c)—Is a simple blood test that measures how well the glucose level has been controlled over the previous four to six weeks. The glucose collects in the hemoglobin of the red blood cells (RBC). A1c is the stable molecule formed when sugar and hemoglobin bind together in the RBC in a process called glycosylation. A1c can be measured. An elevated finding indicates poor glucose control. Measuring A1c reveals a truer picture of

blood sugar level control than conventional measurement. If the diabetic patient has not been conforming to diet, except in anticipation of an office visit, the cells will reveal that they have picked up excess sugar; conventional method shows only current day status, which can be manipulated with diet adherence in the recent past.

There are also specific tests measuring hormone levels in the blood to aid in confirming diagnoses, such as:

- ACTH, FSH, LH, and TSH—When acromegaly or dwarfism is suspected.
- FSH, LH, estrogen, and testosterone—When sex organs fail to develop properly.
- ACTH, cortisol—When Cushing's syndrome (chronic excessive glucocorticoids) is suspected.
- PTH—When hypo- or hyperparathyroidism is suspected.

Scanning Tests

The thyroid gland is probably the one most frequently scanned.

- Radioactive iodine uptake test—An oral dose of radioactive iodine is given to the patient. After intervals of 2, 6, and 24 hours, an external detector (scintillation counter) measures the amount of the original dose that is present in the gland. Thyroid function can be determined by the gland's ability to absorb and retain iodine.
- Thyroid scan—The thyroid gland is viewed by a scintiscanner camera following either an oral or IV dose of a radioactive iodine. The scan is indicated by discovery of a palpable nodule or mass, enlarged thyroid gland, or asymmetric goiter. The camera is capable of photographing the isotopes, which identify the size of the gland, position, and uniformity of absorption. A nodule with poor or no uptake capability shows as a "cold spot," suggesting a possible malignancy. A "hot spot" indicates a hyperfunctioning nodule, possibly a toxic nodular goiter. A total gland picture that shows little uptake is indicative of hypothyroidism; an enlarged gland showing uniformly increased uptake is indicative of hyperthyroidism.

DISEASES AND DISORDERS
Cretinism (Kree'-tin-ism)

Description—This is an endocrine disorder of the thyroid gland that has physical and mental ramifications.
Signs and symptoms—**Cretinism** is characterized by lack of mental and physical growth, resulting in mental retardation and a characteristic dwarflike appearance (Figure 11–194).
Etiology—This condition results from a serious lack of the thyroid hormone thyroxine beginning in the early stages of life.

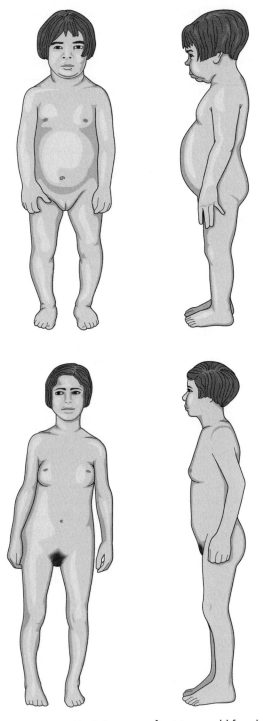

Cushing's Syndrome (Coo'-shings)

Description—This is an endocrine disorder of the adrenal glands which has physical and physiological effects.

Signs and symptoms—Symptoms include hypertension, obesity, weakness of the muscles, and a tendency to develop bruises. Typical characteristics result from the rapid deposit of body fat: a deposit of fat between the shoulders, referred to as "buffalo hump," and a rounded face referred to as "moon face" (Figure 11–195). Purple streaks develop in the skin, called striae (stretch marks). The trunk becomes obese, yet the arms and legs are slender.

The excess amount of glucocorticoids, which metabolize protein into glucogen and then into glucose,

FIGURE 11–194 (Top) Cretinism of a 16-year-old female caused by lack of thyroid hormone; (bottom) same female after two years of treatment with thyroid extract (From C.P. Anthony and G. Thilbodeau, *Textbook of Anatomy and Physiology*, 11th ed., copyright 1983 by Mosby; courtesy Dr. Edward E. Beard.)

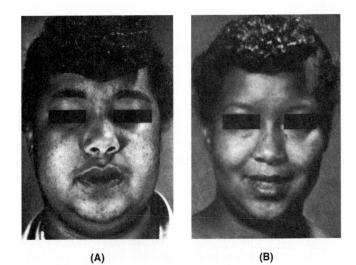

(A)   (B)

FIGURE 11–195 Cushing's syndrome from excessive glucocorticoids: (A) preoperatively, (B) six months postoperatively (Adapted from C.P. Anthony and G. Thilbodeau, *Textbook of Anatomy and Physiology*, 11th ed., copyright 1983 by Mosby; courtesy Dr. William McKendree Jefferies, Case Western Reserve University School of Medicine, Cleveland, Ohio.)

Treatment—If thyroid replacement is initiated early enough, a degree of normal development may be achieved, but once cretinism has developed, total normal development is not possible. An infant born without thyroid hormones of its own must be treated within a few weeks to prevent irreversible mental retardation.

results in a "steroid diabetes" with hyperglycemia and glucosuria. The urinary system is affected by the hormone imbalance and excretes excessive amounts of potassium, which results in hypokalemia. The lack of potassium results in muscular weakness. Muscle mass slowly wastes away. The decreasing amount of bone minerals results in pathological fractures.

Etiology—This disorder is characterized by a group of symptoms that result from the hypersecretion of glucocorticoids from the adrenal cortex caused by excess ACTH production. **Cushing's syndrome** may also be directly related to a tumor of the cortex of the adrenal gland.

Treatment—Treatment is related to the underlying cause. If there is an adrenal tumor, then the adrenal gland must be removed. If both adrenals are removed, replacement steroid therapy must be instituted. If the adrenals are being stimulated because of a pituitary tumor, then the pituitary gland must be irradiated or removed. Afterwards rigorous hormone therapy would be required to replace all the pituitary's secretions. Many drugs, some experimental, are used to suppress adrenal function and destroy adenocortical cells.

Diabetes Mellitus (Di-a-be'-tis Mell'-i-tus)

Description—A chronic disease of insulin deficiency or resistance, diabetes mellitus interferes with the metabolism of carbohydrates, proteins, and fats. Insulin in the blood "carries" glucose into the cell to be used for energy or stored as glycogen. It also stimulates the formation of proteins and free fatty acid storage. Without sufficient insulin being secreted by the pancreas, the body's tissues do not have access to essential nutrients for fuel or storage.

Diabetes mellitus affects an estimated 5% of the United States population or approximately 16 million people. About one half are unaware they have diabetes. Each year 625,000 people are newly diagnosed. The disease is three times as common today as it was in 1960. There are many long-term effects of diabetes. Diabetes is the leading cause of new cases of blindness, end-stage kidney disease, and lower limb amputation in the United States. It develops more often in people who are over 40, obese, sedentary, have a family history of diabetes, or are of African-American, Mexican, or Native-American descent. It more than doubles the risk for stroke and heart disease. Approximately 50% of patients who have had myocardial infarctions and 75% who have had cerebrovascular accidents are also diabetic. The disease also interferes with resistance to organisms, which may result in skin and bladder infections. Diabetic retinopathy results from circulatory changes in the retina of the eye in the poorly-controlled diabetic. In patients who have had diabetes for 20 or more years, 80% develop retinopathy. It is the leading cause of adult acquired blindness.

How Insulin Works   Insulin is the hormone made in the pancreas and released into the bloodstream when needed. It helps sugar to enter the body's cells, where it is used as fuel for the cell's activities (Figure 11–196). When the sugar level rises, the pancreas secretes more insulin so that the larger amount of sugar can move out of the blood and into the cells. When the sugar level falls too low, insulin secretion stops and the hormone glucagon is released. This causes the liver to release stored up energy into the blood. When this mechanism fails to work properly, the disease known as diabetes develops.

To completely understand the role of insulin, we need to consider a basic fact of life. All living organisms are programmed to withstand cycles of feast and famine and have developed ways of storing energy for the lean times. In humans and most animals, it is insulin that allows us to store glucose inside fat and muscle cells until it is needed. In most countries, life is a continual feast, but our bodies are programmed to store glucose that produces excess weight and obesity, which leads to diabetes and numerous other illness. In the United States, obesity is at alarming incidence rates not only for adults but also for children. There is much concern about the future health of our population.

There are two forms of diabetes: a Type 1 DM, or insulin-dependent diabetes mellitus (IDDM), and a Type 2 DM, noninsulin-dependent diabetes mellitus (NIDDM),

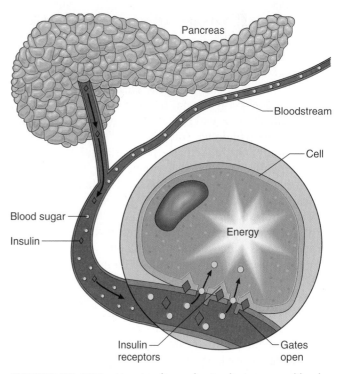

FIGURE 11–196 How insulin works. Insulin is excreted by the pancreas into the blood. It circulates to an insulin receptor on the membrane of a cell. When it binds to the receptor, a signal is sent and the gates in the cell wall open, allowing blood sugar to enter the cell to be converted to energy.

often called adult onset form. Type 1 DM tends to afflict children and young people.

A PEDIATRIC PERSPECTIVE

TYPE 1 DIABETES MELLITUS (TYPE 1 DM)

Etiology—Type 1 diabetes can be considered a genetic disease, but it is commonly considered an autoimmune disorder that affects primarily the pancreas. The immune disorder attacks the cells of the pancreas, known as the islets of Langerhans.

Signs and symptoms—The diagnosis of diabetes in childhood is usually straightforward. The parents report an increased thirst, increased urination, and weight loss. The child will appear to be dehydrated and may have a sweet odor to the breath from the ketones (a byproduct of fatty acids). A urinalysis will generally reveal a large amount of ketones and may be positive for glucose on the Clinitest test.

Treatment—A child with newly-diagnosed Type 1 DM will be admitted to the hospital for stabilization and treatment. Insulin injections or intravenous insulin are required for initial management. During hospitalization, the parents, caregivers, and the child (if of appropriate age) are taught to administer the insulin injections. Commonly, several types of insulin (short-acting, intermediate, and long-acting) will be used for the injections to control the elevated blood sugar and complications with childhood diabetes.

Signs and symptoms—Signs and symptoms of diabetes include fatigue, caused by the lack of energy production, and hyperglycemia, because the glucose cannot be used. The elevated glucose level in the blood causes fluid to be withdrawn from the body's tissues. The excess fluid in the blood causes polyuria and dehydration of the cells. The diabetic patient is frequently thirsty and has dry mucous membranes. The lens of the eye becomes affected by deposits of sugar and edema, which results in visual difficulties. Characteristically, glycosuria is present because the body tries to eliminate excess glucose from the blood. This wasting of sugar causes the weight loss and hunger of the Type 1 DM patient.

Etiology—Type 2 DM is the most common form, usually starting from insulin resistance. This is a complex problem where the cells resist both insulin and blood sugar that is trying to be delivered. The blood sugar level rises, and to add to the problem, the liver produces more sugar and releases lipoproteins full of triglycerides that increase LDL cholesterol and decrease HDL. Insulin resistance can also result from genetics, aging, and some medication, but being overweight and lack of exercise are the main non-ge-

netic factors. About 90% of all newly-diagnosed diabetics are overweight. There is a theory proposed that the fat cells secrete a hormone that is being called resistin, which interferes with insulin action. The role of fat cells is being studied specifically because being overweight is so often associated with the disease.

In addition to resistance, other factors are in effect. The pancreas will compensate resistance by pumping out more insulin for several months or years. Eventually, however, the insulin-producing cells can no longer keep up, and glucose builds up in the blood. Over time, this high level of sugar damages blood vessels, nerves, and other body parts. It also causes a vicious cycle of increasing resistance and further exhausts the pancreas.

Treatment—Treatment begins with a strict diet, planned to meet the nutritional needs of the individual patient and to control the blood sugar level. Diet can have a significant impact on controlling blood sugar and diabetes. Losing as little as 10 pounds will reduce blood sugar levels. A recent study determined that a high-fiber diet lowered blood sugar levels by 10%, a comparable figure to the effect of some medications. Exercise may be the most important activity. It not only uses up glucose in the blood, it also increases insulin sensitivity, which causes fat and muscle cells to respond to insulin and the sugar it is carrying. Diet and exercise can have a significant effect on preventing diabetes, but as a treatment, it can only go so far. In most people, the problem of insulin production and insulin resistance tend to worsen despite weight loss, diet, and exercise. When diet alone is inadequate, insulin injections or the use of an oral hypoglycemic drug are indicated. Injections may be necessary only once a day, using a long-acting insulin; when control is more difficult, a regular insulin, injected at specific times, may be used. Diabetic patients are taught to evaluate their glucose level by performing a urine test for sugar or a finger stick for blood analysis. The amount of the insulin injected is based on the findings. Hypoglycemic drugs are taken orally to aid in the metabolism of sugar. Oral therapy is usually adequate only for Type 2 DM patients.

The drugs used today address insulin resistance and secretion and blood sugar levels. Physicians are using more drugs and using them more aggressively. Drugs can be categorized according to their actions (see the following).

Increasing Insulin Supplies

1. *Sulfonylureas* work to stimulate beta cells to release more insulin. This works for a short period, and then the cells stop working. These drugs can work too well, causing hypoglycemia that can be dangerous for older patients because it causes fainting, falls, and fractures.

2. *Rapid-acting insulin stimulators* work like sulfony-lureas but faster. They are short-lived and less apt to cause hypoglycemia. Two drugs in this class are Prandin and Starlix.

3. *Injection of insulin* subcutaneously is the ultimate method of overriding pancreatic dysfunction. Type 1 diabetics who have complete shutdown of insulin production are dependent on injections. Patients with Type 2 diabetes often can control their disease with diet, exercise, and medications, but if that fails, insulin is the most potent and effective therapy. They usually require fewer injections but higher doses because of the need to overcome resistance. A form of insulin that can be inhaled is being developed. A February 2001 report indicated initial trials by 73 Type 1 diabetics have yielded positive results. This would be a great step forward in replacing the need for repeated injections.

Lowering Blood Sugar by Other Means

1. *Alpha-glucosidase inhibitors* block the action of a digestive enzyme that breaks down carbohydrates into smaller sugars. The effect is to moderate blood sugar surges after a meal. The drug is weaker than some others but very safe.

2. *Biguanides* work to lower sugar levels by blocking the release of glucose by the liver. The only drug currently approved is Glucophage, and it works well in overweight people because it does not cause weight gain or risk of hypoglycemia.

Overcoming Insulin Resistance

1. Thiazolidinediones (TZD) reduces insulin resistance, but how it works is unknown.

Multi-Drug Approach

More physicians are using a multi-drug approach to management. Previously, they would do one thing at a time: diet and exercise, then drug after drug until ineffective, and then insulin. However, this method of control only was successful in 25% of the patients. By using drug combinations, lower doses of each are effective, and therefore fewer side effects occur. This approach better addresses the new view of diabetes as a syndrome instead of a simple disease of high blood sugar.

The most common drug combination is metformin and sulfonylurea. A new clinical trial with metformin-rosiglitazone combination showed more effectiveness in control blood sugar, insulin sensitivity, and pancreatic function. When insulin becomes necessary, combining it with oral medications may mean a lower dose of insulin is needed.

Future Treatments

It is hoped that the human genome project will reveal new information on diabetes and its treatment, but researchers realize this will take some time to determine. Some researchers are focusing on preventing the complications associated with diabetes, such as atherosclerosis; others focus on therapies directed at fat cells.

A study also revealed that the simple action of taking an aspirin a day is a very effective health strategy for diabetics and would help those with cardiovascular involvements. Controlling blood pressure and lowering LDL are crucial even if there is no evidence of coronary disease.

Maintaining Health

The glucose level of the blood can be affected by circumstances other than food or insulin. For example, the diabetic will require either less insulin or more food when engaging in a high level of physical activity. Adjustments are also required with illness. A patient who has diarrhea and/or vomiting requires less insulin. Pregnancy, the use of contraceptives, a fever, and periods of stress all influence the diabetic's need for supplemental insulin or hypoglycemic therapy.

Specific symptoms indicate whether the blood sugar is too high or too low. A diabetic must be aware of their physical condition at all times. Should the blood sugar level become significantly low, they may enter into insulin shock; if it goes very high, there is a possibility of a diabetic coma. Both situations require urgent attention. When patients sense impending shock, they will drink orange juice or eat a piece of candy immediately. A patient going into coma needs an urgent blood sugar measurement and an injection of insulin. Figure 11–197 illustrates the contrasting symptoms of shock and coma. Become familiar with the signs and be prepared to act.

Diabetic patients must be encouraged to maintain their optimal level of health. They must guard against injury, especially to the lower extremities, because of difficulty healing. They must use extreme caution when cutting toenails and must never try to remove corns or calluses themselves. Diabetics frequently suffer amputations as a result of infection from an injury that would not heal or from the loss of peripheral circulation, which causes tissue death.

Patients should be encouraged to visit an ophthalmologist regularly to detect the possibility of retinal changes. Blindness will result from uncontrolled diabetes. The physician must be alert to signs of cardiovascular complications and urinary tract involvement. Cerebral vascular disease, coronary artery disease, and renal failure resulting from vascular deterioration in the kidney are not uncommon.

Graves' Disease

Description—This condition is the most common form of hyperthyroidism.

Signs and symptoms—The thyroid gland enlarges and the patient becomes nervous, has an intolerance to heat, loses weight, sweats, and may have diarrhea, tremors, and palpitations. The increased thyroxine may also cause difficulty in concentrating because of the acceler-

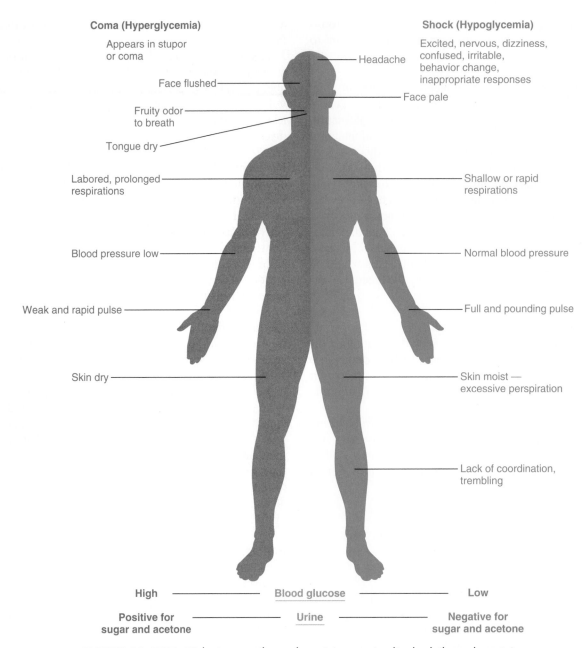

Coma (Hyperglycemia)

Appears in stupor or coma

Face flushed

Fruity odor to breath

Tongue dry

Labored, prolonged respirations

Blood pressure low

Weak and rapid pulse

Skin dry

Shock (Hypoglycemia)

Excited, nervous, dizziness, confused, irritable, behavior change, inappropriate responses

Headache

Face pale

Shallow or rapid respirations

Normal blood pressure

Full and pounding pulse

Skin moist — excessive perspiration

Lack of coordination, trembling

High —————— Blood glucose —————— Low

Positive for sugar and acetone —————— Urine —————— Negative for sugar and acetone

FIGURE 11–197 Diabetic coma (hyperglycemia) versus insulin shock (hypoglycemia)

ated cerebral functioning. Mood swings and emotional instability may occur. The cardiovascular system is also affected and results in tachycardia, increased cardiac output and blood volume, cardiomegaly, and possibly atrial fibrillation (especially in the elderly). The patient may experience dyspnea and an array of musculoskeletal symptoms ranging from weakness and fatigue to localized or generalized paralysis. The dominant feature of exophthalmus may also be present.

The patient can get into serious difficulty if the hyperthyroidism escalates into a thyroid storm. The symptoms persist and others develop, such as hypertension, extreme irritability, vomiting, high fever, delirium, and eventually coma.

Etiology—Graves' disease results from an increase in the production of thyroxine that may be caused by a genetic or immunological factor. It is also associated with the production of autoantibodies, which may be from a defect in suppressor T lymphocyte function that allows them to be formed.

Treatment—Primary treatment is the use of antithyroid drugs that block the formation of thyroid hormone. Some patients are candidates for a single oral dose of a radioactive element that concentrates in the thyroid, destroying some cells and reducing the size of the thyroid gland. In addition, a portion or all of the gland can be removed surgically to reduce or eliminate the hormone.

Myxedema (Mex'-e-de-ma)

Description—This is an endocrine disorder of the thyroid gland which affects adults.

Signs and symptoms—Clinically, **myxedema's** characteristics are in relation to the degree of hypothyroidism. If it is mild, the patient will probably complain of forgetfulness, dry skin, and an intolerance for cold. With more severe myxedema, the decreased metabolism and vital functions will become more evident. Decrease in heat production (because of decreased metabolism) causes a marked intolerance for cold. There is a noticeable weight gain. The motor function and reflex actions are slowed. The voice becomes low and husky. A characteristic yellowish discoloration of the skin, called *carotenemia,* results from reduction in the conversion of carotene to vitamin A. Levels of cholesterol are increased and may also produce atherosclerosis. Because cardiac function is depressed, the myocardium becomes flabby and weak. Protein and certain electrolytes accumulate in the tissue spaces, causing edema. Myxedema patients have a characteristic drowsy appearance, with puffiness about the eyes. There is a marked degree of fatigue and weakness. The temperature, pulse, respiration, and blood pressure are all below normal.

Etiology—This condition is caused by a hyposecretion of the thyroid gland. It varies in significance in relation to the amount of secretion.

Treatment—Treatment consists primarily of thyroid hormone replacement to a level necessary to maintain normal balance.

Hormonal Balance

Diagnosing, treating, and maintaining hormonal balance in patients with endocrine gland malfunctions is an involved and challenging endeavor because of the hormone interactions. What may appear to be a simple over-production by the thyroid may actually be a pituitary malfunction, a failed hypothalamus, or an inhibitor that did not cause the pituitary to stop secreting a thyroid stimulant. Many possibilities must be considered to explain the symptoms presented by a patient with endocrine dysfunction.

■ ACHIEVE UNIT OBJECTIVES

Complete Chapter 11, Unit 12, in the workbook to help you obtain competency of this subject matter.

UNIT 13

The Reproductive System

■ OBJECTIVES

Upon completion of the unit, meet the following performance objectives by verifying knowledge of the facts and principles presented through oral and written communication at a level deemed competent.

1. Spell and define, using the glossary at the back of the text, all the **Words to Know** in this unit.
2. Differentiate between sexual and asexual reproduction.
3. Describe the differentiation of reproductive organs.
4. Explain how sperm are able to fertilize an egg.
5. Describe male prenatal development.
6. Name the male sex organs, and describe their location and function.
7. Explain how pituitary hormones affect the functions of the testes.
8. Identify the male secondary sex characteristics.
9. Trace the pathway of sperm from production to expulsion.
10. Name the components of semen.
11. Describe four diseases and disorders of the male reproductive system.
12. Name the female sex organs, and describe their location and function.
13. Explain the interaction of pituitary hormones with the ovaries and other organs.
14. Identify the female secondary sex characteristics.
15. Describe the maturation and release of an ovum.
16. Compare the internal and external sexual organs of the male and female.
17. Describe the phases of the menstrual cycle and the purpose of menstruation.
18. Explain how fertilization occurs.
19. Describe the events occurring during each trimester of pregnancy as they relate to the woman and the embryo/fetus.
20. Describe the events that occur in the three stages of labor.
21. List the reasons for practicing contraception.
22. Identify the contraceptive methods, stating their relative effectiveness.
23. Describe the diagnostic tests of the female reproductive system.
24. Describe the diseases or disorders of the female reproductive system.
25. Identify the characteristics of the sexually transmitted diseases.

AREAS OF COMPETENCE (AAMA)

This unit addresses content within the specific competency areas of *Administrative procedures, Practice finances, Patient care, Communication skills*, and *Instruction*, as identified in the Medical Assistant Role Delineation Study. Refer to Appendix A for a detailed listing of the areas. (Note: Although *Anatomy and physiology* is not specifically identified in the study, a basic knowledge of the body's structure and function is an essential foundation to the competent performance of many roles.)

■ WORDS TO KNOW

ablation
abortion
alpha-fetoprotein
  screening (AFP)
amniocentesis
amniotic
anteflexed
anteverted
areola
Bartholin's glands
benign hypertrophy
bulbourethral glands
cervix
cesarean
chlamydia
circumcision
clitoris
coitus
colposcopy
conceive
conception
contraception
contraction
corpus luteum
cryptorchidism
dilation and
  curettage
dysmenorrhea
dysplasia
ectopic
effacement
ejaculation
ejaculatory duct
embryo
endometrium
epididymis
episiotomy
erectile
fallopian tubes
fertilization
fetus
fibroid
foreskin
gamete
genital herpes
genitalia
gonorrhea
graafian follicle
gynecology
hydrocele
hymen
hysterectomy
hysteroscopy
impotence

inguinal canal
inguinal hernia
interventional hysterosalpingography
labia majora
labia minora
ligation
mammary glands
mammogram
mastectomy
menarche
menopause
menorrhagia
menstruation
moniliasis
mons pubis
myometrium
nonspecific urethritis
os
ovulation
ovum
Papanicolaou (Pap)
  smear
penis
perineum
phimosis
placenta
pregnancy
prolapse
prostate
prostatectomy
rectocele
reproductive
retroflexed
retroverted
salpingo-
  oophorectomy
scrotum
semen
sperm
spermatozoan
syphilis
transurethral
trichomoniasis
trimester
uterus
vagina
vaginitis
vas deferens
vasectomy
vulva
womb
zygote

A Library

The **reproductive** system consists of the organs that are capable of accomplishing reproduction, the creation of a new individual. All living organisms reproduce, some very simply by an asexual method or without the need of sexual contact. An example of asexual reproduction is one of the simplest forms of life, a single cell. In binary fusion, a cell divides into two cells by simple cleavage. In mitosis, a single cell rearranges its chromatin into chromosomes and then divides into two cells (the method by which human cells reproduce). Both methods require that the "parent" become the "children"; therefore both parent and child cannot exist at the same time.

Sexual methods of reproduction are found in multicelled forms of life, including humans. The methods may vary but certain characteristics are common to all. In each species, there are sexes, namely a male and a female. Each sex has special sex glands, or gonads, which produce sex cells (**gametes**). In humans, the union of the male gamete (a **spermatozoan**) with the female gamete (an **ovum**) forms a new one-celled structure called a **zygote**. The zygote then undergoes mitosis repeatedly to form a new individual.

In Unit 1, the cell was described as having 46 chromosomes, or 23 pairs. Each chromosome has a partner of the same shape and size. One pair of chromosomes are the sex chromosomes. In the female, both chromosomes in the pair are X chromosomes, but in the male, one is an X and one is a Y. When the gonads produce the ovum and spermatozoan cells, the number of chromosomes is reduced to 23 (one half). When the two cells unite as fertilization occurs, the new cell, a zygote, will again have 46 chromosomes. If the spermatozoan carries an X chromosome, the embryo will develop female characteristics. If it carries a Y chromosome, the embryo will develop as a male.

The reproductive organs are the only organs in the human body that differ between the male and female, yet there is still a significant similarity. This likeness results from the fact that male and female organs develop from the same group of embryonic cells. For approximately two months, the embryo develops without sexual identity. Then the influence of the X or Y chromosome begins to make a differentiation.

DIFFERENTIATION OF REPRODUCTIVE ORGANS

The gonads of the embryo begin to evolve into the sexual organs of the female at about the 10th or 11th week of pregnancy. The ovaries of the embryo develop high in its abdomen from the same type of tissue as the testes. However, the testes evolve from the medulla of the gonad, whereas the ovaries develop from the cortex. Figure 11–198 illustrates how the undifferentiated external **genitalia** develop into fully-differentiated structures. In the male, the tubercle

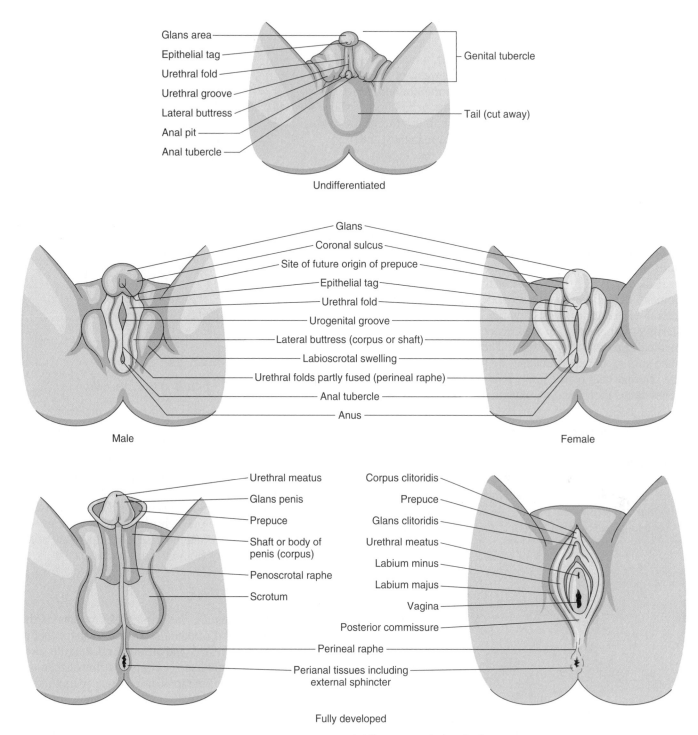

FIGURE 11-198 Sexual differentiation before birth

becomes the glans **penis**, the folds become the penile shaft, and the swelling develops into the **scrotum**. In the female, the tubercle becomes the **clitoris**, the folds the **labia minora**, and the swelling the **labia majora**.

Internally, there is also a similarity of structures. The embryonic müllerian ducts degenerate, and the wolffian ducts become the **epididymis, vas deferens**, and **ejaculatory duct** in the male. In the female, the wolffian ducts de-

generate, and the müllerian ducts develop into the **fallopian tubes**, the **uterus**, and the upper portion of the **vagina**. It is believed that the presence of the testes in the male is the differentiating factor in the development. Without the androgens (male hormones) from the testes, a female develops. With the androgens, a male develops. Another substance called the müllerian inhibitor works in partnership with the androgens to produce the sex differentiation.

MALE REPRODUCTIVE ORGANS

When the zygote contains a Y chromosome, a male child will develop. About the seventh or eighth week of pregnancy, the testes begin to develop within the abdominal cavity at about the level of the ileum of the pelvis bone. The sex of the fetus is evident by about the fourth month.

During the eighth and ninth months of pregnancy, the testes move from the abdomen through the **inguinal canal** into the external pouch called the scrotum (Figure 11–199). After the testes pass, the canal closes to prevent the descent of other structures into the scrotum or the return of the testes into the abdomen. When a loop of small intestine descends through the canal because of improper closure or later in life because of relaxed inguinal structures, it is known as an **inguinal hernia** (Figure 11–200).

If the testes fail to descend or if they return to the abdomen, a condition known as undescended testicle (unilateral or bilateral) exists, which must be corrected or sterility will result. An undescended testicle is known medically as **cryptorchidism**. The testes normally produce **sperm**, but sperm cannot be produced or survive in the internal heat of the body. It is this characteristic that necessitates their location outside the body.

A PEDIATRIC PERSPECTIVE

When testes do not descend spontaneously by age one, surgical correction is generally indicated and is performed before age six. An orchiopexy secures the testes within the scrotum to prevent sterility and the resulting harmful psychological effects.

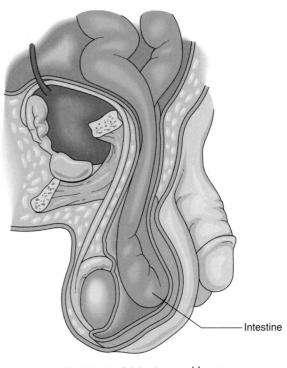

FIGURE 11–200 Inguinal hernia

The scrotum, which contains the testes, has another function, which is to regulate the temperature of the testes' environment. Sperm are most effectively produced at temperatures 1.5° to 2°C below body temperature. To maintain this difference, the scrotum contains many sweat glands that perspire profusely to dissipate heat. The scrotum also has cremasteric muscles, which can contract to draw the testes closer to the body and increase the temperature or relax to lower them away from the body and reduce it.

Testes

The testes or testicles are the primary sex organs of the male. They are almost of equal size, oval in shape, about $2 \times 1 \times 1\frac{1}{2}$ inches in size, and are suspended in the scrotum, with the left testis usually somewhat lower than the right. A testis has two functions: to produce sperm and to secrete testosterone, the male hormone. These functions begin to occur about age 10 when the hypothalamus releases a hormone that initiates puberty. The hormone stimulates the anterior pituitary gland, which releases the gonad-stimulating hormones to effect change in the testes.

Male gonadotropic hormones secreted by the pituitary are FSH (follicle-stimulating hormone) and ICSH (interstitial cell-stimulating hormones). FSH causes sperm to develop in the male and ova to mature in the female, a very similar function.

Sperm Production   Sperm develop and mature in microscopic tubes in the testes known as *seminiferous tubules* (Figure 11–201). FSH stimulates the production of sperm in the cells that line the tubules. There are about 300 sec-

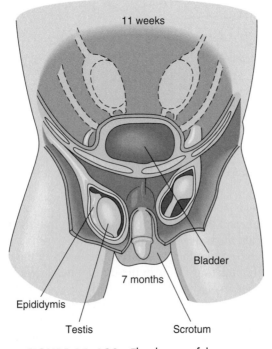

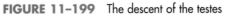

FIGURE 11–199 The descent of the testes

Seminiferous tubule

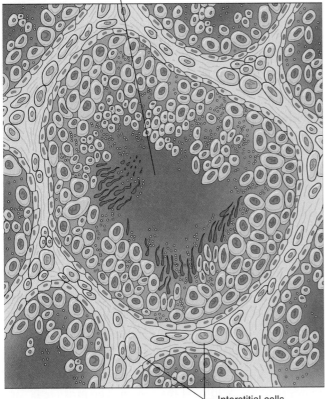

Interstitial cells

FIGURE 11–201 The production of sperm in the seminiferous tubules and the secretion of testosterone by the interstitial cells

tions of coiled tubules that, if uncoiled, it is estimated, they would extend over a mile. As the sperm develop, they are released into the tubules to start their journey from the testes. Sperm formation in an adult male requires about 74 days to maturity. The function normally begins to develop at about age 12, and the first mature sperm are ejaculated at about age 14.

Testosterone   As sperm are developing, ICSH is causing the interstitial cells in the network of structures around the tubules to secrete testosterone. Testosterone aids in the maturing of sperm and causes many changes in the male body as it circulates in the blood stream. These changes are referred to as the development of secondary sex characteristics (Figure 11–202).

In the male, secondary sex characteristics are:

1. Longer and heavier bone structure
2. Larger muscles
3. Deep voice
4. Growth of body hair
5. Development of the genitalia (external sex organs)
6. Increased metabolism
7. Sexual desire

Epididymis, Vas Deferens, and Seminal Vesicles

The epididymis is a coiled structure about 20 feet in length. It is shaped like a half-moon and sits with its head

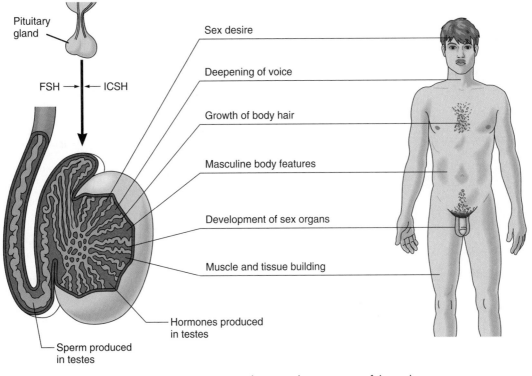

FIGURE 11–202 Secondary sex characteristics of the male

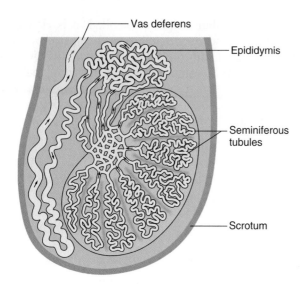

FIGURE 11–203 Seminferous tubules, epididymis, and vas deferens

on top of the testes with its tail extending down the side to join the vas deferens (Figure 11–203).

After sperm are produced in the tubules, they pass into the epididymis where a small number are stored. The sperm mature in the epididymis for about 18 hours. The fluid secreted by the epididymis adds to the volume of ejaculant.

The vas deferens serves as the passageway for sperm to exit the body from the epididymis. On each side, one vas deferens joins one epididymis extending upward for about 45 cm through an inguinal canal to the base of the urinary bladder. Each vas joins with a duct from a seminal vesicle to form a common ejaculatory duct (Figure 11–204).

The seminal vesicles are a pair of convoluted tubes lying posterior to the bladder. They also empty into the ejaculatory duct. The vesicles secrete a fluid that contains fructose, a simple sugar, which provides nutrition for the sperm. The fluid makes up a major portion of the ejaculant. The ejaculatory duct is a short straight tube that passes through the **prostate** gland to join the urethra.

Prostate Gland, Bulbourethral Glands, and Urethra

The prostate gland is a donut-like-pyramidal structure with the urethra extending through its center (Figure 11–204). The gland is positioned just beneath the bladder. It produces secretions that are drained through tiny tubules into the prostatic section of the urethra. The fluid secreted is alkaline in nature. Its addition to the ejaculant stimulates sperm motility and preserves sperm life by neutralizing the acidity of the vagina. The prostate is surrounded by muscular tissue that contracts during ejacula-

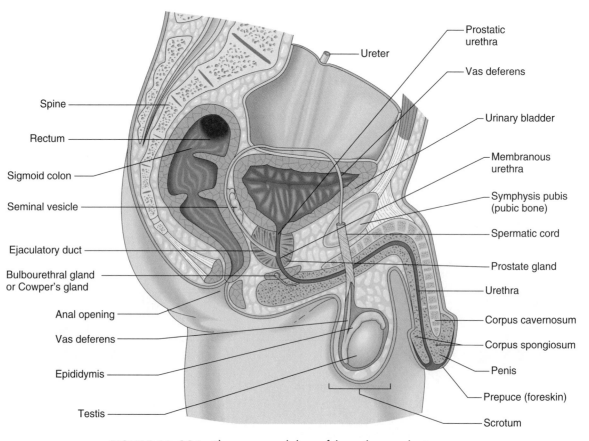

FIGURE 11–204 The organs and ducts of the male reproductive system

tion to empty the **semen** (ejaculant fluids and sperm) into the urethra to be propelled from the body.

The **bulbourethral glands** lie beneath the prostate and empty their contents into the urethra. The fluid the glands secrete aids in the movement of sperm and makes the normally acidic male urethra alkaline just prior to **ejaculation**. The secretions may serve as a lubricant for intercourse. Bulbourethral glands are sometimes called Cowper's glands.

Semen

The combined secretions from all the glands and ducts along with the sperm are called the seminal fluid or semen. Approximately 3.5 mL of total fluid are expelled per orgasm (series of rhythmic muscular contractions). Semen is composed of:

- Fluids from the testes and epididymis containing about 350 million sperm (5%).
- Fluid secreted by the seminal vesicles (30%).
- Fluid secreted by the prostate gland (60%).
- Fluid secreted by the bulbourethral glands (5%).

Penis

The penis is constructed of two columns of spongelike **erectile** tissue and the urethra, which are surrounded by a layer of subcutaneous tissue and covered with skin. The distal end of the penis enlarges to form the glans penis. A circular fold of skin that extends down over the glans is called the prepuce or **foreskin**. A number of small glands in the foreskin secrete a waxy, odoriferous substance called smegma onto the glans. A **circumcision** (surgical removal of the foreskin) may be performed on a male infant to prevent accumulation of the smegma, thereby avoiding bothersome infections later in life. It also has been observed that circumcised men have a lower incidence of cancer of the penis and that women married to circumcised men have a lower incidence of cancer of the cervix. Circumcision is indicated to correct **phimosis**, a narrowed opening of the foreskin, which prohibits its retraction over the glans. Phimosis contributes to the accumulation of smegma. Many men feel that sexual sensations are heightened when the glans is not covered or restricted by the foreskin. The urethra extends down the length of the penis, opening at the urinary meatus of the glans. The urethra serves two purposes, to empty urine from the urinary bladder and to expel semen.

Erection and Ejaculation

Successful intercourse is dependent on the two columns of erectile tissue in the penis. When a male is sexually aroused, nerve impulses cause the erectile tissue to engorge with blood, which makes the erectile tissue increase in size and become firm. Blood entering the dilated

arteries squeezes the veins against the penile structures prohibiting venous return.

After stimulation of the glans results in maximum stimulation of the seminal vesicles, impulses are sent to the ejaculatory center and orgasm occurs. Orgasm is the result of muscular contractions from the vas deferens, seminal vesicles, ejaculatory ducts, and prostate gland. Secretions produced and stored in these structures, along with the sperm, are forcefully expelled through the urethra after which the engorgement gradually subsides.

Vasectomy

Vasectomy is a simple surgical procedure to prohibit the ejaculation of sperm and effect sterilization of the male. It has become a popular means of birth control. The procedure involves making a small incision in each side of the scrotum. The vas deferens, on each side, is grasped and a loop is withdrawn through the incision. The physician ties the duct in two places and removes a piece of the duct between the ties. The ends are placed back into the scrotum, and the small incision is closed with sutures. The procedure can be performed in the physician's office under local anesthesia or in a hospital outpatient clinic. It is a much simpler means of sterilization than the surgery required to perform a similar procedure on a female.

A vasectomy neither interferes with the function of the testes nor with sexual ability. Sperm are still produced in the testes but, because their exit is blocked, they remain in the testes and epididymis until they die and are reabsorbed into the body. Testosterone, the male hormone produced by the testes, gains access to the body by way of the veins in the scrotum. Vasectomy will have no effect on testosterone levels. Most men report as much or more sexual activity after as before their vasectomy. The only negative aspect is that the procedure is likely to be irreversible. Recently, success at restoring fertility has been achieved by surgical reconnection in one out of five attempts. However, the patient may have developed autoantibodies toward his own sperm and may no longer be fertile.

Diagnostic Exams and Tests of the Male Reproductive System

Chromosomal analysis—Tests to determine genetic defects, such as Klinefelter's syndrome, that cause abnormal growth and development of sexual characteristics and chromosome basis for hypogonadism.

Digital rectal examination—A common manual examination involving insertion of a gloved finger into the rectum to palpate the prostate gland for size, density, and nodules or tumors.

Hormonal studies—Measurement of pituitary hormones, such as interstitial-cell stimulating hormone that causes development of testes and sperm production or adrenal cortex androgens that govern sex characteristics and testosterone levels of the testes, to diagnose conditions like hypogonadism, early or delayed sexual development, and infertility.

Prostatic specific antigen (PSA)—A blood test used to measure the amount of antigen present when there is prostate hypertrophy. An elevated amount may be indicative of cancer.

Semen analysis—Analysis of semen and the sperm to determine the volume of semen, the number, maturity and motility of sperm, the presence of abnormal or immature sperm, and other characteristics. Approximately 40% to 50% of fertility problems are attributed to the male when couples fail to achieve pregnancy.

Testicular biopsy—Examination of testicular tissue to determine unexplained oligospermia, the absence or great decrease in the amount of sperm, when diagnosing infertility.

Testicular self-examination—The American Cancer Society recommends that men perform routine testicular self-examination (TSE) as a means of early identification of testicular cancer. The testicle is the most common site of cancer in men from 29 to 35 years of age. It tends to occur primarily in men from 20 to 40 years of age. The society recommends monthly TSE beginning at 15 years of age (see Chapter 14).

DISEASES AND DISORDERS OF THE MALE REPRODUCTIVE SYSTEM

Epididymitis (Ep-eh-did-eh-mi'-tis)

Description—This is an infection of the epididymis and is an uncommon infection of the male reproductive tract. It may spread to the testicle, causing *orchitis* (inflammation of the testicle).

Signs and symptoms—The primary symptom is intense pain with swelling in the scrotum. Other symptoms include fever, malaise, and a characteristic waddle when walking.

Etiology—The causative organism is usually a coliform bacteria from the intestinal tract and generally follows urinary or prostatic infections. Other causes include trauma, gonorrhea, or syphilis.

Treatment—Treatment may consist of bed rest, elevation of the scrotum on towel rolls, and ice to relieve pain and swelling. A broad-spectrum (inclusive) antibiotic and pain medication are indicated. Therapy must be initiated immediately, especially if there is bilateral involvement, as a result of the threat of sterility.

Erectile Dysfunction (Impotence)

Description—This is an inability to have or sustain an erection to complete intercourse. Because of the negative connotation of the word "impotence," physicians and sex therapists use the term *erectile dysfunction* to identify the occurrence.

Signs and symptoms—Primary **impotence** refers to the patient who has never had an erection. Secondary impotence refers to the patient who is currently impotent but has had intercourse in the past. Transient periods of impotence are not considered a dysfunction and probably occur in half the adult male population. The incidence of impotence increases with age.

Etiology—Organic dysfunction causes most impotence and may result from a chronic illness such as diabetes, renal failure, or cardiopulmonary disease. Spinal cord trauma, the effects of alcohol, or the results of certain drug therapy may cause organic dysfunction. Impotence may be 30% psychogenic in origin. The usual causes are anxiety, fear of failure, depression, parental rejection, and previous traumatic sexual experiences. Impotence may result from stress. Interpersonal factors such as insufficient knowledge of sexual function or lack of communication with partner may cause impotence.

Treatment—Treatment of impotence may include sexual therapy to reduce the anxiety and usually involves both partners. The type of therapy chosen depends on the specific cause of the dysfunction. Most often it involves improving communication, reevaluating attitudes toward sex, restricting sexual activity, and encouraging attention to the physical sensations of touching. Many men may benefit from the use of the medication Viagra. It can be beneficial for men following prostatectomy where nerves involved in the erection process may be damaged or severed. It is also helpful for men with diabetes or those taking hypertensive medications. It is primarily a trial process to determine if it will be effective. The medication must be taken one hour prior to intercourse for it to be effective. The drug is contraindicated for patients with severe heart problems or those using nitroglycerine products. Additional methods of medicating may be developed, such as a nasal form to be inhaled or a topical ointment, and methods with a shortened period to effectiveness. Patients with organic impotence may need to develop alternative means of sexual expression. Some patients may benefit from learning to inject one or a combination of drugs into the spongy bodies of the penis. These drugs stimulate a normal erection. Some may use a vacuum device which pulls blood into the spongy bodies to effect a firm erection. Others may be candidates for the placement of a prosthesis, a device that is implanted into the spongy bodies. There are two basic types of prostheses: a semi-rigid and an inflatable style. The semi-rigid prosthesis will give a constant state of firmness with flexibility at the base so that the penis can be held against the body with underclothing. The inflatable prosthesis can be made erect for intercourse and can be deflated when not engaged in sexual activity.

Hydrocele (Hi'-dro-ceel)

Description—The presence of an excessive amount of fluid within structures around the testes is called a **hydrocele**.

Signs and symptoms—Enlargement of scrotum.

Etiology—It may occur following injury or inflammation or may develop as a result of the aging process. It usually is caused by excess production of normal body fluid, lack of reabsorption, or blockage of the circulatory process.

Treatment—Surgical correction is indicated with continued enlargement and discomfort.

Prostatic Hypertrophy (Pros-ta'-tic Hi-per'-tro-fe)

Description—This enlargement of the prostate gland is common in men over age 50. In **benign** (nonmalignant) **hypertrophy**, the prostate may enlarge sufficiently to constrict the urethra, making it difficult to empty the bladder. Surgery may be indicated to remove the obstructive tissue. A malignant prostate, one of the most common forms of cancer found in men, is a different disease.

Signs and symptoms—Symptoms of hypertrophy vary with the extent of involvement. Usually the initial symptoms are reduced force and size of urinary stream, difficulty in starting a stream, dribbling, a feeling of incomplete voiding, nocturia (having to void at night), and frequent urination. As the hypertrophy increases, symptoms become more pronounced, and eventually hematuria and retention may develop. Diagnosis of hypertrophy can be confirmed by a digital examination to palpate the prostate through the rectal wall (Figure 11–205).

Etiology—It may be caused by a change in hormonal activity.

Treatment—Treatment of benign hypertrophy of the prostate will be conservative until the gland squeezes the urethra and interferes with voiding. Sitz baths, prostatic massage, fluid restriction (for a short time), and several medications can be used, with the addition of antibiotics if an infection develops. Prostatic congestion may benefit from regular sexual intercourse. Conservative therapy is usually only temporary, with a more permanent surgical solution required to effectively relieve urinary retention and other symptoms.

A **prostatectomy** (removal of the prostate) can be performed by different methods. An open operation is indicated with a large prostate or with a contained malignancy. An incision is made in the skin above the pubic bone and below the umbilicus. The prostate is exposed as it lies below the bladder and above the penis. The benign tumor of the prostate is removed when no cancer is expected. When cancer is expected, the entire prostate gland and tumor is removed. Another common method is the **transurethral** prostatectomy (TURP). In this procedure, a resectoscope is inserted into the urethra, and the prostate is approached through an incision in the wall of the urethra (Figure 11–206). A wire loop with electric current removes a segment of the gland, thereby interrupting the integrity of the prostate and prohibiting its constricting action.

When there is a malignancy in the prostate, it may cause no symptoms or the patient may have urinary obstructive symptoms similar to those seen with benign hypertrophy. Cancer may be identified on a rectal examination as a hardened area and may be palpated, or the suspicion of a malignancy may be raised when the patient's Prostatic Specific Antigen (PSA) blood test is abnormal. PSA is a compound that is made only by cells in the prostate, and malignant cells cause this to

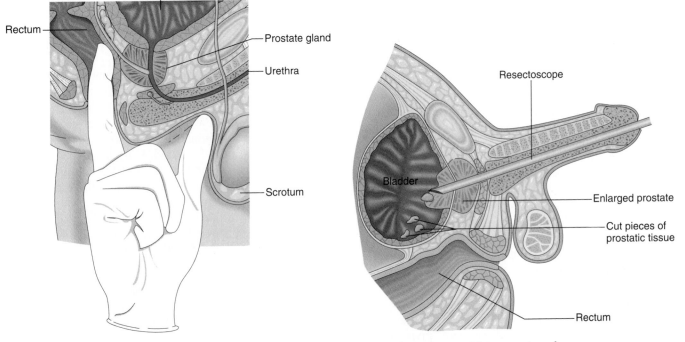

FIGURE 11–205 Digital examination of the prostate gland

FIGURE 11–206 Insertion of a resectoscope

rise more quickly than is normally seen with an enlarging prostate or with aging.

The incidence of prostate cancer appears to show a family tendency and to be more prevalent in the black race. All men over 50 years should have a rectal examination and a PSA blood test yearly, but those with a family history or who are black should begin annual testing at 40 years.

Treatment of prostatic cancer—Treatment is determined by clinical assessment, expected life span, the stage of the disease, and tolerance for the therapy. Radiation, a prostatectomy, an orchidectomy (removal of testes to stop hormone production), and oral doses of female estrogen are used alone or in combinations, according to the stage of the involvement, to arrest and control the malignancy. Favorable results are obtained from high doses of radiation. Not only does the cancer go into remission, but the associated metastatic skeletal pain, if present, is also relieved.

With the screening for prostate cancer that is now occurring, many younger, sexually active men are being found with prostate cancer, so treatment offers a chance to cure many individuals, and it is anticipated that survival rates will be greatly improved. Unfortunately, the curative treatments available—cryotherapy, radiotherapy, or radical prostatectomy—all have side effects that are disturbing but can be overcome. These include incontinence, impotence, cystitis, and proctitis (rectal inflammation). If the cancer has spread outside the prostate, making it incurable, it can be controlled by medications and/or orchidectomy. The cancer can be put into remission for a significant time.

New methods of prevention and treatment are being continuously developed. The National Cancer Institute is sponsoring a study called the Prostate Cancer Prevention Trial (PCPT) to test whether the drug finasteride can prevent prostate cancer. The study involves 18,000 men across the United States over seven years. To test the drug's effectiveness, only one half of the participants are receiving the actual medication; the other half receive a placebo (inactive pill). Not even their attending physicians know which medication their patients are receiving. Hopefully, this will prove beneficial. Prostate cancer currently strikes one out of every seven men age 55 and above and is the second most common cause of cancer deaths.

Two new treatments are being tested. Cryosurgery (freezing) using liquid nitrogen to kill cancer cells is showing promise for some men. It appears to be a good alternative to radiation and is less invasive than traditional surgery. But it still poses risks including impotence and often fails to remove all the cancer cells. It is not considered a good alternative for younger men or good candidates for traditional surgery.

Another treatment uses radioactive seeds, about the size of a grain of rice, implanted in the prostate. The pellets remain permanently in the body, giving off radiation within the prostate for approximately three months. It is believed to be more effective than traditional radiation because they deliver about two and a half times the dose without affecting neighboring organs. The seeds are planted through hollow needles that are positioned with the use of a transrectal ultrasound probe.

FEMALE REPRODUCTIVE ORGANS

Because the similarity in function of the male and female reproductive organs is another indication of their common origin, a comparison will be made, when appropriate, as each organ or structure is presented. The order of presentation will be, as with the male, from the formation of the sex cell to its exit from the body.

Ovaries

The embryonic gonadal tissue that is to become the ovaries begins to develop about the 10th or 11th week of pregnancy. The ovaries of the fetus develop high in the abdominal cavity near each kidney but descend to the pelvis as the time for delivery nears. Ovaries are small, almond-shaped glands measuring about $1\frac{1}{2} \times 1 \times \frac{1}{4}$ to $\frac{1}{2}$ inch (Figure 11–207). They are supported by the ligaments, which attach to the uterus and tubes to ensure their position near the fimbriated (fringelike projections) ends of the fallopian tubes. These two organs play a significant role in the life of every female. They have two main roles: to produce the sex cell and the ovum and to secrete hormones. These functions parallel the role of the testes in the male.

It is estimated that at birth the ovary has between 200,000 and 400,000 primary **graafian follicles** (podlike structures), which contain immature ova. Many follicles never mature and degenerate by puberty. During the reproductive life of a female, about 375 will develop and mature, releasing an ovum. By age 50, most of them have disappeared.

The ovaries are the primary sex organs of the female. When the female is about age eight, the pituitary gland begins to send hormonal messages that puberty is approaching. Within a few years, the messages get stronger, and the pituitary hormone causes the ovaries to begin releasing estrogen into the blood. Estrogen affects the development of the sex organs, such as the fallopian tubes, the uterus or **womb**, and the vagina, causing them to increase in size and maturity.

Estrogen also produces secondary sex characteristics, which alter the shape and appearance of the female body (Figure 11–208). In the female, secondary sex characteristics are:

1. Broadening of the pelvis, making the outlet broad and oval (to permit childbirth). (The male pelvic outlet is oblong and narrow.)
2. The epiphysis (growth plate) becomes bone and growth ceases. In the absence of estrogen, females

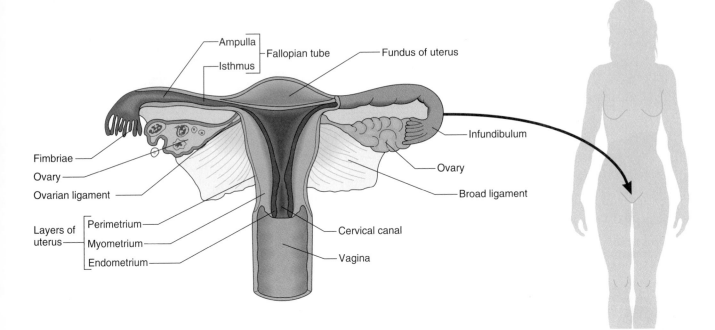

FIGURE 11–207   Female internal reproductive organs

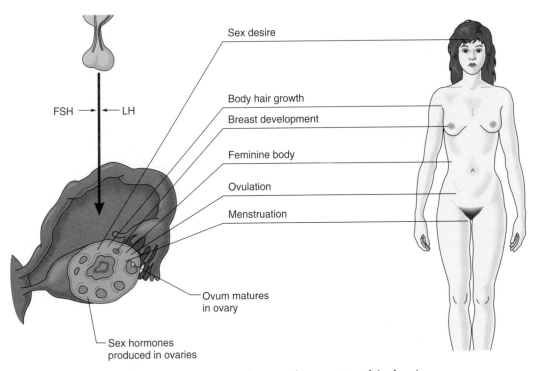

FIGURE 11–208   Secondary sex characteristics of the female

continue to grow, becoming several inches taller than normal.

3. Development of softer and smoother skin.
4. Development of pubic hair in a flat upper border pattern.
5. Deposits of fat in the breasts and development of the duct system.
6. Deposits of fat in the buttocks and thighs.
7. Sexual desire.

In addition to physical changes, two physiological functions begin to occur, namely **ovulation** and **menstruation**. Ova are produced in the germinal epithelium layer of the ovary (Figure 11–209). There, a "nest" of cells undergo change with some cells forming a wall around a liquid-filled cavity. Other cells join to thicken one area of the wall. This structure is known as a primary follicle. One of the inner cells will become the ovum.

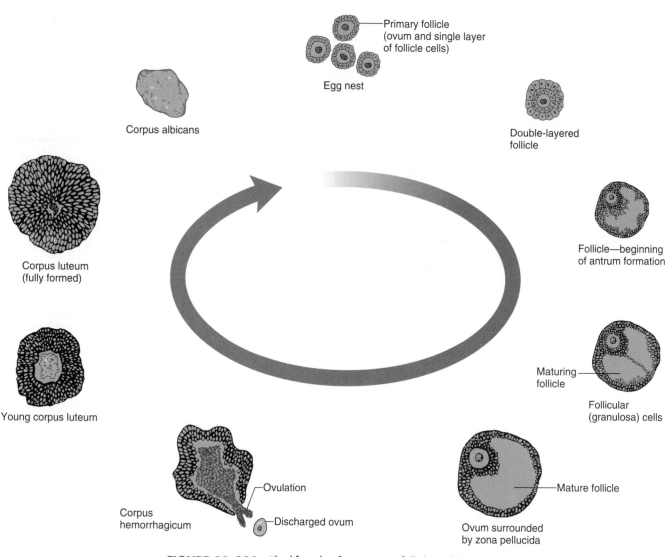

Primary follicle
(ovum and single layer
of follicle cells)

Egg nest

Corpus albicans

Double-layered
follicle

Corpus luteum
(fully formed)

Follicle—beginning
of antrum formation

Young corpus luteum

Maturing
follicle

Follicular
(granulosa) cells

Corpus
hemorrhagicum

Ovulation

Discharged ovum

Mature follicle

Ovum surrounded
by zona pellucida

FIGURE 11–209   The lifecycle of an ovarian follicle and the ovum

Under the continued influence of FSH and LH from the pituitary, the follicle and ovum mature. Additional fluid collects within the follicle, and it begins to resemble a blister. The follicle moves toward the surface of the ovary and develops a small protrusion called a stigma.

The maturing follicle, called a graafian follicle, produces estrogen, which in turn stimulates the pituitary to release increasing amounts of FSH and LH. When maturity has been achieved and the amount of LH is high, the stigma disintegrates, allowing the follicle to rupture and release the egg into the surrounding area. This action is known as ovulation. At this point, the follicle undergoes change to provide support to the ovum. Under the influence of LH, the follicle fills with a yellow material and begins to function as a temporary endocrine gland, secreting a hormone called progesterone. The follicle is now called a **corpus luteum** (yellowish body).

The high levels of FSH and LH act as a feedback mechanism to prevent the pituitary gland from secreting

FSH to mature an additional follicle. The corpus luteum continues to secrete estrogen and progesterone, which prepare the uterus for reception of a fertilized ovum. If fertilization does not occur, the ovum will pass from the body through the vagina, and the corpus luteum, after 10 or 12 days, degenerates and becomes inactive, causing a sharp decline in the hormonal level. This decline stimulates the pituitary to again begin releasing FSH and LH and the cycle starts again.

Fallopian Tubes

The fallopian tubes extend about four inches from the superior lateral surface of the uterus and are attached to the broad ligament (see Figure 11–207). The vas deferens and ejaculatory ducts of the male can be compared to the fallopian tubes of the female. The ducts provide a passageway for sperm, as the fallopian tubes provide a passageway for the ovum to reach the uterus.

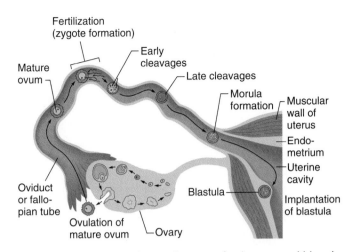

FIGURE 11–210 *Pathway of ovum to fertilization and blastula phase implantation in the uterus*

The fallopian tubes are constructed of four layers, including a muscle layer and ciliated mucosal layer. The distal ends of the tubes expand into funnel-shaped openings with many fingerlike projections (fimbriae). Upon ovulation, it is believed the fimbriae move the ovum toward the opening of the tube. At the same time, the muscular layer of the tube contracts to produce a vacuum within the tube, and the cilia beat to create a current moving toward the uterus.

The ovary and fallopian tubes lie close together but are not connected. An ovum may be lost within the surrounding abdominal space. Occasionally, sperm will locate and fertilize such an ovum, which will then attach itself to a nearby structure and develop into an abdominal pregnancy. At term, surgical removal of the baby is necessary because no outlet for delivery exists.

Normally, **conception (fertilization)** takes place in the outer third of the fallopian tube (Figure 11–210). Upon union, the two cells begin to multiply. The corpus luteum causes secretions to be released from glands within the mucosa of the tubes. The secretions provide nutrition for the new zygote, which must now move into the uterus within three to seven days for implantation and development. However, the opening of the tube narrows in the isthmus section to about 1 mm in diameter near the entrance to the uterus. If the zygote is unusually large or slow, or if there is any constriction of the tube, the zygote may not be able to pass through the opening, and an **ectopic** (abnormal location) tubal pregnancy develops. Because there is no space for growth, pain and discomfort will develop within a few weeks. Surgical removal of the embryo is imperative to prevent rupture of the tube.

Uterus

The uterus is a thick-walled, hollow, muscular organ lying within the pelvis, behind the urinary bladder, and in front of the rectum. It is shaped like an upside-down pear,

measuring, before pregnancy, about $3 \times 2 \times 1$ inch (Figure 11–211). The uterus is divided into three parts: the fundus, or rounded upper portion where the fallopian tubes are attached; the body, or middle and main portion; and the **cervix**, or narrowed section that opens into the vagina. The cervix has an internal and an external **os** (opening), with the cervical canal between them. The cavity within the uterus is a small triangular opening.

The uterus has three layers within its walls. The innermost is called the **endometrium**. The structure of the endometrium changes considerably in response to the influence of hormones, as will be discussed under menstruation. The **myometrium** is made up of three layers of muscle fibers running circularly, longitudinally, and diagonally. The outer layer consists of the serous membrane, which covers most of the body and fundus of the uterus.

The uterus has a great capacity for expansion. During pregnancy, its thick walls stretch and thin out until the fundus touches the diaphragm. Even at this great overextension, the powerful uterine muscles are still able to contract forcefully to produce labor and delivery. In addition, the uterus is flexible in its position, being easily moved in all directions. It is pressed posteriorly when the bladder fills and anteriorly when the rectum is full.

When the uterus is horizontal, at right angles to the vagina, it is in its normal position (Figure 11–212). There are five variances of normal positioning (from anterior to posterior): **anteflexed**, **anteverted**, mid position, **retroverted**, and **retroflexed**. The uterus may also **prolapse**, or drop downward into the vagina. If these positions cause discomfort or interfere with adjoining structures, a device called a pessary can be inserted into the vagina to support the uterus.

Vagina

The vagina is a collapsible muscular tube lined with mucous membrane, which is arranged in folds. The walls of the vagina lie in contact with each other. The posterior

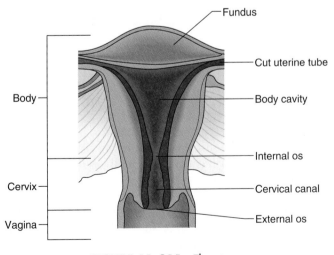

FIGURE 11–211 The uterus

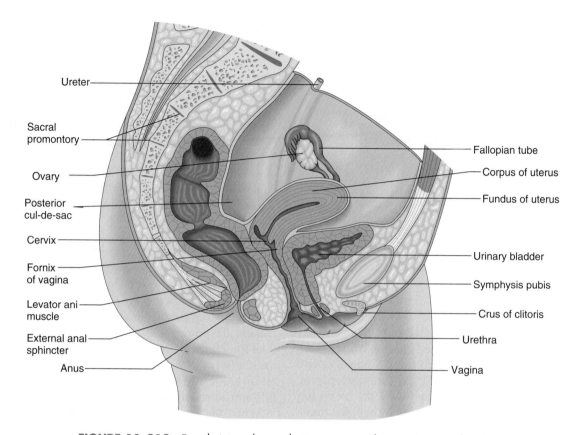

FIGURE 11–212 Female internal reproductive organs with uterus in normal position

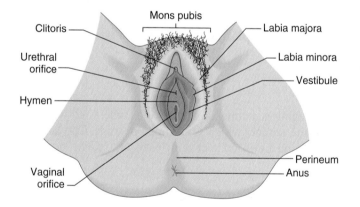

FIGURE 11–213 Female external genitalia

wall is three to four inches long. The anterior wall extends about two and one half or three inches to the cervix. The vagina is capable of great expansion. It serves as the passageway for menstruation, an organ of sexual intercourse, and the birth canal for the delivery of an infant.

Behind the vagina and anterior to the rectum is a rectouterine pouch, a space called the cul-de-sac or pouch of Douglas. Infection occasionally develops in this area and necessitates draining. A surgeon can make an incision through the vaginal wall, eliminating the need for abdominal surgery. This is also the area where abdominal ectopic pregnancies usually occur. Though rare, this type of ectopic pregnancy occurs because the fertilized ova goes out the open end of the fallopian tube instead of descending into the uterus. It falls naturally by gravity into the cul-de-sac.

Near the outlet of the vagina is a muscular sphincter that can be detected when inserting tampons or upon examination. The sphincter will maintain a tampon within the vagina and provides a "snugness" for sexual intercourse. The vaginal canal is kept moist by secretions from the uterus and by droplets of mucoid material from the vaginal walls.

Up to this point, all the structures discussed have been internal. Whereas the external genitalia of the male are quite visible, those of the female are practically hidden from sight. Many authorities recommend that women become familiar with their genitalia by making a thorough examination using a mirror and a good light.

The vagina opens onto the surface of the body at the **perineum**, posterior to the urinary meatus and anterior to the anus (Figure 11–213). The external opening is partially covered by folds of mucous membrane called the **hymen**, which border the edges prior to intercourse. Occasionally, the hymen is thicker than normal or covers the entire opening (imperforate hymen). The tissue must be removed prior to menstruation when imperforate. It occasionally requires surgical removal (hymenectomy) to permit intercourse when the narrowing tissue cannot be stretched naturally.

Vulva

The **vulva** is the area of the female external sexual structures. The large pad of fat that is covered with coarse hair on the mature female and overlies the symphysis pubis is known as the **mons pubis**. The labia majora (large lips) are a pair of rounded folds of skin on each side of the vulva and are continuous with the mons pubis. The labia are covered with hair on the exterior surface but with pigmented smooth skin on the inner surface. The labia are composed mainly of fat and numerous glands. The labia majora develop in the female from the same embryonic tissue that becomes the scrotum in the male.

The labia minora (small lips) lie within the labia majora and come together anteriorly in the midline continuous with the prepuce which covers the glans of the clitoris. The labia minora are covered with mucous membrane that is continuous with the lining of the vagina. The female labia minora develop from the same embryonic tissue as the male penile shaft.

The term vestibule is used to denote that portion of the vulva that lies inside the labia minora and posterior to the clitoris. It contains the opening to the urethra and the vagina. The ducts to the vestibular glands (**Bartholin's glands**) open at the base of the labia minora. They secrete a fluid which serves as a lubricant for **coitus** (intercourse). Posteriorly the labia minora are connected by a thin piece of tissue called the fourchette, which is just posterior to the vaginal opening. The fourchette is destroyed by the birth of the first child.

Clitoris

The clitoris is a rounded mass composed of two small columns of erectile tissue. The clitoris develops in the female similarly to the glans and penis of the male, except that the urethra does not descend through its interior. The clitoris and the glans penis are very sensitive and provide for heightening of sexual excitement. The clitoris becomes enlarged and engorged with blood and is involved in the orgasmic response to sexual arousal.

Perineum

The perineum is identified in two different manners. Some physicians consider the entire pelvic floor as the perineum and apply the term to both male and female. But in **gynecology** (the study of female diseases), the perineum refers to the area posterior to the vaginal introitus and anterior to the anus. In the male, the perineum in this sense is posterior to the scrotum and anterior to the anus. The perineal area is composed of muscles that form a sphincter for the vestibule. During childbirth, the perineum must stretch adequately to permit the delivery of the infant. If it appears the tissue might be torn, the physician will surgically cut the perineum to avoid a ragged tear. This procedure is known as an **episiotomy**. Following delivery, the straight, clean cut is sutured (sewn

closed). When the repair heals, the perineum is much smoother, with less scar tissue, than if torn tissue had healed.

Mammary Glands (Breasts)

The mammary glands are secondary sexual structures that develop and function only in the female. The breast consists of lobes separated into sections by connective tissue, somewhat like the structure of a grapefruit half. Each lobe has several lobules composed of connective tissue with grapelike clusters of secreting cells (alveoli) embedded in the tissue. The glandular clusters are drained by minute ducts that unite into a single duct for each lobe for a total of about 15 to 20 in each breast (Figure 11–214). The ducts are arranged like the spokes of a wheel, meeting at the nipple. Here they enlarge slightly to form small reservoirs. The main ducts exit on the surface of the nipple through tiny openings.

Fatty tissue is deposited around the surface of the gland, between the lobes and beneath the skin. A darkened area called the **areola** surrounds the nipple. The color of the areola varies from pink in light blonds and redheads to brown in brunettes. A pink areola will turn brown early in pregnancy and regress somewhat after delivery, but will not return to pink. About three days after delivery, the glands begin to secrete milk resulting from hormonal stimulation from the pituitary. The hormone prolactin stimulates the production of milk, whereas oxytocin causes it to be ejected in response to the infant's sucking.

Menstruation

When the ovum is not fertilized, and therefore the uterine structures prepared for reception of the embryo are not needed, the lining deteriorates and is discharged from the body in the process called menstruation. Menstruation begins at **menarche** (first cycle) and ends with **menopause** (last cycle). A complete cycle is approximately 28 days in length. If menarche occurs at age 13, the female will experience approximately 455 cycles over the following 35 years. A 28-day cycle is based on a lunar month, not a

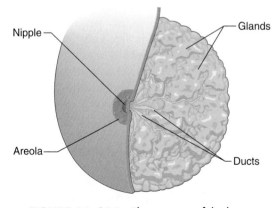

Nipple — Glands — Areola — Ducts

FIGURE 11–214 The structure of the breast

calendar month; therefore, there are 13 cycles (lunar months) per year.

The menstrual cycle is a result of the interaction of hormones and the endometrium of the uterus. Normally, menstruation is interrupted only by pregnancy or severe illness. The interrelated effects of the hormones and their effects on the sex organs are illustrated in Figure 11–215. The menstrual cycle can be divided into four phases, each characterized by hormonal, ovarian, and uterine changes.

Phase I—The Follicular Phase   Beginning about day five in the cycle (counting from the first day of menstruation), the pituitary secretes high levels of FSH to stimulate the ovarian follicles. One follicle ripens an egg and brings about ovulation, at the same time secreting estrogen. About day 10, the pituitary begins to secrete LH in large amounts to react on the follicle. As the estrogen increases, the FSH slows down. The follicle continues to move its maturing egg toward the ovarian surface. At the same time, the endometrium of the uterus has been stimulated by the high level of estrogen and grown a thick lining in preparation for receiving a fertilized egg. This change in the lining is known as *proliferation*.

Phase II—Ovulation   The follicle releases the matured ovum. Estrogen is at a high level; FSH is reduced just prior to ovulation. The high level of estrogen stimulates the release of LH by the pituitary, which causes the follicle to rupture about day 14 in the cycle. The endometrium has continued to grow a thick lining.

Phase III—The Luteal Phase   After the egg is released, the empty follicle undergoes a rapid change caused by the influence of LH. It becomes a glandular mass of cells called the corpus luteum and begins to release progesterone and estrogen. The progesterone reacts on the glands in the endometrium to begin secreting a nourishing substance for the egg. The corpus luteum continues to secrete progesterone for about 12 days until approximately day 26 of the cycle. As the level of progesterone rises, LH is inhibited and the LH level falls. When LH drops, the corpus luteum degenerates, causing the levels of progesterone and estrogen to decline sharply.

Phase IV—Menstruation   With hormonal support gone, the lining buildup in the uterus begins to slough off (shed), causing menstruation from day one to five. The excess endometrium and a small amount of blood pass out through the cervix. Estrogen and progesterone levels are low, but the FSH level is rising to start the next cycle, preparing the uterine lining and the next ovum for the opportunity of pregnancy.

FERTILIZATION

The miracle of reproduction begins with fertilization. In the process of sexual intercourse, sperm at the rate of about 360 million per ejaculation are deposited into the female vagina. From here the microscopic sperm begin an incredible journey toward a single female ovum, which will normally be in the outer one third of one of the fallopian tubes. The ovum must be fertilized within 24 hours after expulsion from the ovary, or fertilization will have to be postponed until the next ovum is ready in approximately one month.

The sperm travel at a rate of about 1 to 5 millimeters per minute; their course seems to be in a straight line but in a random direction. Studies on humans are difficult to do, but some research has been conducted. In one study, it was found that sperm deposited in the vagina of a woman just prior to surgery had migrated through the fallopian tubes 30 minutes later. This finding could not be explained based on sperm motility alone. It is hypothesized (suggested) that intercourse or artificial insemination causes the release of a hormonal substance that increases uterine contractions, propelling sperm toward their destination.

The ovum is considerably larger than the sperm, yet it is still only about $\frac{1}{125}$ of an inch in diameter (Figure 11–216). When the sperm reach the egg, they surround its outer surface attempting to enter. Only the strongest sperm are able to survive the acidity of the vaginal secretions to attack the protective corona radiata that surrounds the ovum. In repeated attacks, the sperm release an enzyme called hyaluronidase, which gradually breaks down the ovum's protection. Eventually, an exposed area of membrane will allow one spermatozoan to penetrate the ovum. The head and middle of the sperm enter the ovum while the tail drops off outside. Immediately, the membrane becomes sealed against additional sperm. The nucleus of the sperm moves to combine with the ovum nucleus, and a zygote is formed. At this time, the traits, which are inherited, and the sex of the new individual are determined and cannot be altered. The father has determined the sex, but the other characteristics are contributed by both parents. At this point, conception has occurred.

Following fertilization, the zygote begins the journey to the well-prepared uterus, arriving about six days after ovulation. There it implants itself in the thick wall, and a change in the menstrual cycle begins. At this point, phase III is at about day 20. The endometrium is at its peak. The levels of estrogen and progesterone are high. LH and FSH are low because of the feedback of adequate amounts of hormones; this is preventing stimulation of new follicle maturity. The secretions from the fallopian tubes and the uterine glands are providing nutrition for the embryo.

The high level of progesterone inhibits the myometrium from contracting; therefore, the embryo cannot be expelled. Progesterone also stimulates development of the ducts of the **mammary glands** (breasts). These effects must be continued to maintain the implantation. If the corpus luteum fails, so does the production of progesterone. Therefore, the developing **placenta** (afterbirth) secretes a hormone, human chorionic gonadotropin (HCG),

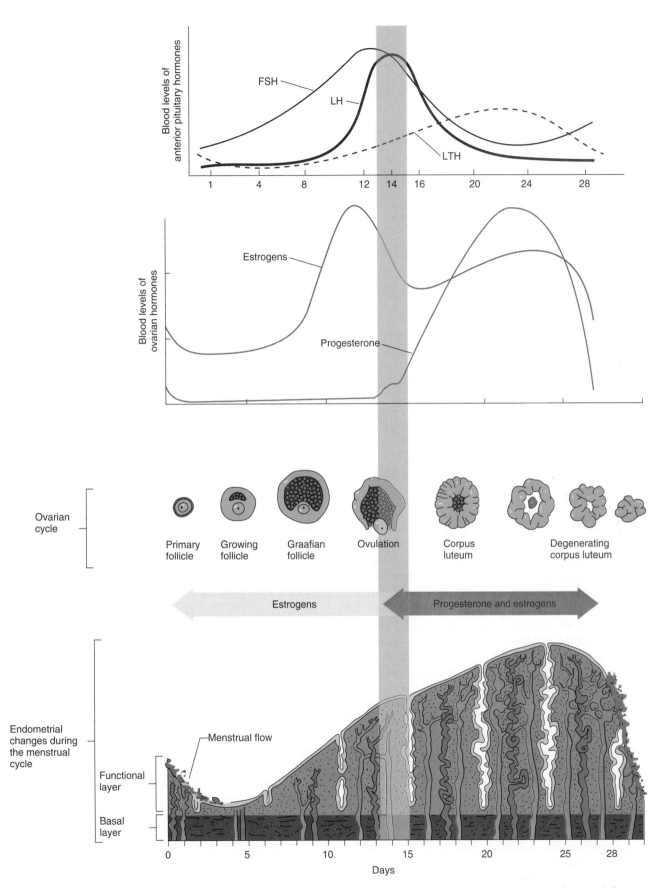

FIGURE 11–215 Menstrual cycle illustrating the levels of pituitary and ovarian hormones, ovarian cycle, and endometrial changes (Fig. 15–10, p. 351 from E.N. Marieb, *Essentials of Human Anatomy and Physiology,* 2nd ed. Copyright © 1988 by Benjamin/ Cummins Publishing Company, Inc. Reprinted by permission of Pearson Education, Inc.)

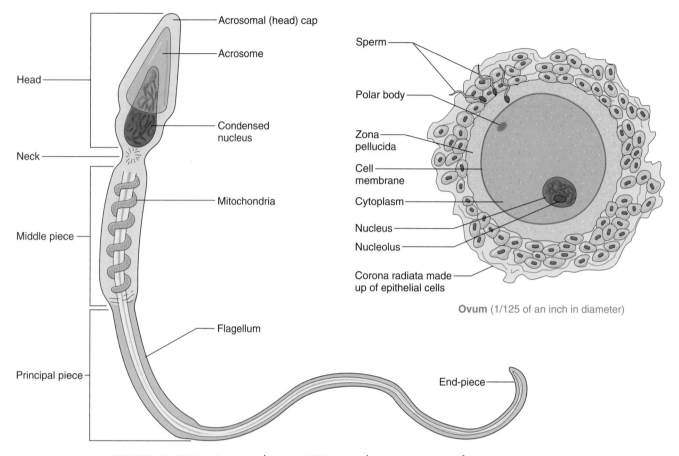

FIGURE 11–216 Sperm and ovum. NOTE: actual size comparison of sperm entering ovum

which maintains the corpus luteum during the early stages of pregnancy. This is the hormone that is detectable on urine pregnancy tests. As the embryo develops, the placenta begins to secrete progesterone and estrogen, and the corpus luteum degenerates and disappears.

The placenta maintains its high level of hormone output throughout pregnancy. When the time for delivery nears, the placenta decreases production of progesterone, which allows the myometrium to begin contracting, and labor begins. With progesterone diminished, the release of prolactin from the pituitary can occur. Prolactin stimulates the mammary glands to produce, for the first few days, *colostrum,* a thin nutritious liquid, and later, milk. The continued production of milk depends on stimulation from the regular sucking of the infant or the removal of milk by pumping.

PREGNANCY

About 36 hours after fertilization occurs, the zygote begins to grow from its one-cell beginning. It is almost beyond comprehension to realize that everything necessary to the formation of a new life, the bones, muscles, blood vessels, the brain, all the organs, and the skin and hair are all contained in one microscopic cell. In addition, the life-support system of the placenta and umbilical cord and the

protective membranes and **amniotic** fluid also develop from this single cell. By about day six, the small cluster of cells firmly implant within the uterine wall, and it enters the embryonic period (eight weeks) of development when most of the major organ systems are formed at an amazing speed. The group of cells arrange themselves into three layers from which the various organs are formed. One layer, the *ectoderm,* becomes the nervous system, skin, hair, and parts of the eye. The *endoderm* layer becomes the digestive and respiratory systems. The skeletal, muscular, connective tissue, reproductive, and circulatory systems develop from the *mesoderm* layer.

The **embryo** develops from the head down which explains why, in Figure 11–217, the head is so large when compared to the rest of the body. By the end of the 10th week of **pregnancy**, all systems are completed, even to nails on the fingers. Many of the organs begin limited function by the seventh week. After eight weeks, the embryo is called a **fetus**. By week 12, the sex can be determined, and the fetus is about four inches long and weighs about two thirds of an ounce. This marks the end of the first **trimester** or one third of the total pregnancy period.

It is obvious the fetus has a lot of growing to do, and it does so rapidly. By week 20, movement can be felt and the heartbeat is detectable with a fetascope. By now, the pregnancy is about half way through. A fetus must be car-

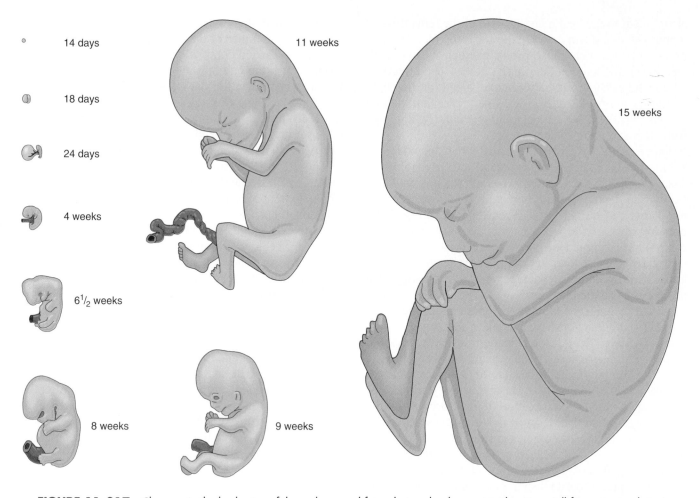

14 days

18 days

24 days

4 weeks

6½ weeks

8 weeks

9 weeks

11 weeks

15 weeks

FIGURE 11–217 Changes in the body size of the embryo and fetus during development in the uterus (all figures natural size)

ried past the next several weeks to survive. If born in week 23, a little past five months, it will weigh less than two pounds and has a one in 10,000 chance of surviving.

By the 20th week, the fetus opens its eyes, and by week 24, it can hear sounds from inside the uterus. The movements are very vigorous by now, and there are periods of sleep and wakefulness as the second trimester ends.

During the last trimester, the fetus adds greatly to its size. By the end of the seventh month, it has assumed a head-down position and if born would have over a 50% chance of survival. The odds increase to about 95% at eight months when weight reaches five pounds to 99% at full-term nine months with average weight being seven and one half pounds and a length of 20 inches.

The pregnant woman also undergoes body changes during pregnancy. Initially the first sign is a missed menstrual period. This is a time of joy for couples who have been trying to **conceive** but may be less than welcome to others. Another early sign is breast tenderness caused by the stimulation of hormones. Some women will experience "morning sickness," especially for the first six to eight weeks. Usually there is more frequent urination, fatigue, and the need for additional sleep. By the eighth to

tenth week, pregnancy can be detected by manual pelvic examination and the bluish hue of the formerly pale pink cervix. This change is called "Chadwick's Sign." Once pregnancy is confirmed, the woman is usually interested in the expected delivery date. It is calculated using Nagele's rule, which states: Take the first day of the last menstrual period, subtract three months, and add seven days, plus a year. For example, if the first day of the last period was September 1, 1996, the expected day of delivery would be June 7, 1997. Remember, this is only the "expected" date. Babies have a habit of being born when they are "ready." On a percentage basis, 39% are born within five days of the projected date and another 55% are within 10 days. The rest obviously are either early or late.

It is important to confirm pregnancy early so that good prenatal care is started. Proper nutrition, such as folic acid 1 mg, is recommended three months prior to conception to decrease the risk of neural tube defects of the fetus. If a woman has a history of a previous child with a neural tube defect, she should increase the dose to 4 mg prior to conception and continue throughout the pregnancy. Other vitamins and regular exercise are extremely important to promote a healthy baby and an uneventful pregnancy. It is also critical to the health and welfare of the fetus that the mother refrain from the use of tobacco, alcohol, and drugs, all of which cause problems such as low birth weight, drug addiction, and birth defects. The effects of AIDS, hepatitis, or genital herpes from an infected mother is a terrible inheritance. Every pregnant woman should consider it her responsibility to do everything possible to ensure the birth of a healthy baby.

Other symptoms experienced with pregnancy develop as the weeks pass. Usually there are psychological changes, such as the stereotypes of "being radiant," happy, and having "cravings" (e.g., for dill pickles at unusual times of the day). However, the symptoms of depression and fatigue are also common. In general, the symptoms are influenced by the attitude toward the pregnancy. If there are marriage conflicts or economic problems, or if it is an unwanted pregnancy, it can hardly be a time of joy and anticipation.

As the pregnancy continues, the morning sickness disappears and edema of the hands, face, feet, and legs appears. There may also be constipation caused by pressure on the rectum. Urinary frequency is universal because the bladder is limited in its expansion. As the third trimester progresses, the size of the uterus causes shortness of breath and indigestion because of pressure from displaced organs and the uterus against the lungs and stomach. Hemorrhoids are common resulting from constipation and pressure on the blood vessels of the rectum.

Weight gain continues throughout pregnancy. Most physicians prefer to establish a set amount of permissible gain. The total weight of the baby (seven and one half pounds), placenta (one pound), enlarged uterus (two pounds), enlarged breasts (one and one half pounds), and additional fat and water (about six pounds) add up to about 18 pounds, so 20 pounds is sometimes the recommended amount of gain. Excess weight causes complications such as hypertension, increased stress on the heart, and the problem of weight to be lost after delivery.

THE BIRTH PROCESS

The beginning of the birth process is usually signaled by a show of bloody mucous. This is from the mucous plug that was in the cervix to protect the fetus from organisms in the vagina. There may also be a slow leak or a gush of the amniotic fluid. Irregular **contractions** of the uterus will begin, and stimulation from prostaglandin may initiate labor.

Labor is divided into three stages. The first begins when uterine contractions become regular and proceeds through cervical dilation and **effacement** (thinning out). The cervix must dilate to about 10 centimeters (4 inches) in diameter before the baby can be delivered. Contractions increase in frequency and intensity until they become very strong, uncomfortable, and exhausting. First stage labor varies between as little as two to as long as 24 hours; 12 to 15 hours is average for a first pregnancy.

The second stage of labor begins with complete dilation and the entrance of the head (or another part) into the vagina. Continued contractions and bearing down by the woman push the baby through the vagina until it is visible at the entrance; this is known as *crowning* (if it is a head presentation). Strong contractions and pushing force the head through the vaginal opening, then the baby rotates to the side so the shoulders can be delivered. The rest is easily passed, and the second stage is completed.

The baby is suctioned to remove mucous from its mouth and nose, and crying begins to inflate the lungs. The baby's body function changes dramatically. For the first time it must breathe on its own to take in oxygen and begin to circulate its own blood. It changes from a bluish color to a healthy skin tone within a couple of minutes. As soon as the baby's condition is satisfactory, the umbilical cord is clamped, tied, and cut.

To help assess a newborn's condition, a universally-accepted evaluation technique called the Apgar scoring system is used. Observation of the newborn is made at one and five minutes following delivery. The ratings are entered on a chart and the scores totaled. A score of 10 is considered the best possible condition. A score of 7 to 9 is considered adequate, and no treatment is required. A score of 4 to 6 indicates close observation, and some intervention, such as suctioning, is necessary. A score below 4 requires immediate intervention and continued evaluation. Table 11–17 is an example of the Apgar scoring system.

TABLE 11–17

APGAR SCORING SYSTEM				Rating	
Sign	0	1	2	1 min	5 min
Heart rate	Not detectable	Below 100	Over 100		
Respiratory effort	Absent	Slow, irregular	Good, crying		
Muscle tone	Flaccid	Some flexion	Active motion of extremities		
Reflex irritability (response to flick on sole)	No response	Grimace, slow motion	Cry		
Color	Blue, pale	Body pink, extremities blue	Completely pink		
			TOTAL		

Scoring system developed by Dr. Virginia Apgar

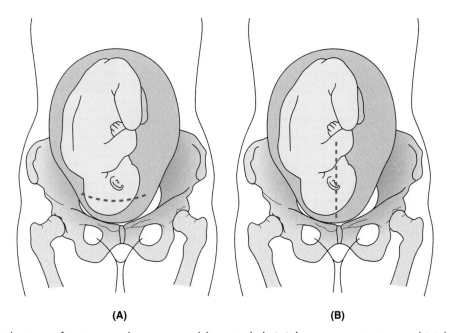

(A)   **(B)**

FIGURE 11–218   The types of incision used in cesarean delivery include (A) the transverse incision and (B) the low vertical incision

The third stage of labor begins with the detachment of the placenta from the uterine wall, and the *afterbirth* (placenta and its membranes) are expelled. Usually a few more contractions are required to accomplish this stage. After it has emptied, the muscles of the uterus maintain a level of contraction to close off open blood vessels and control bleeding.

In some cases, such as inadequate pelvic outlet, breech presentation (other than head), large baby, ineffective labor, or the development of a serious complication, the baby may need to be removed by **cesarean** section. This involves cutting through the abdomen and into the uterus to remove the baby and the afterbirth. About 10% of all deliveries are cesarean. Pregnancy following a cesarean section may undergo a trial of labor if certain factors are considered. It is commonly called vaginal birth after cesarean (VBAC) and is successful in 60% to 80% of the cases. One main concern is the type of *uterine* incision that was made. This may not be the same as that on the surface of the abdomen. If a transverse uterine incision has been made, across the lower, thinner part of the uterus (Figure 11–218), it is the least likely to result in complications in a subsequent vaginal delivery. The low vertical incision is an up and down cut in the lower, thinner area of the uterus, and risks are not well documented. The classical, a high vertical incision in the upper part of the uterus, is not as frequently done now because this type of incision requires that women have repeated cesareans because of the risk of uterine rupture during labor.

INFERTILITY

Infertility refers to the inability to become pregnant after one year of sexual intercourse without the use of birth control. It affects one in seven couples in the United States. One cause for infertility may be the delay in childbearing until after age 30. Infertility can be traced to the woman in about one third of the cases, to the man in another third, and to both in the last third. For the woman, the problem is usually a blocked fallopian tube, damaged ovaries, or abnormally-developed tubes. Many times, it is the absence or infrequency of ovulation. In the male, it is usually abnormally-developed testicles, a low sperm count, or low motility. Sexually transmitted diseases (STDs) account for a large percentage of infertility by silently damaging the fallopian tubes and ovaries. It is very important that young men and women understand the importance of practicing safe sex by using condoms and decreasing the number of sexual partners.

Treatment consists of medications to stimulate egg or sperm production or surgery to repair damaged organs or abnormalities. Other actions, such as determining ovulation, intercourse on alternating fertile days (to collect sperm), and the use of boxer shorts for men (this reduces the body heat transferred to the testicles by tight briefs), are indicated. When this is unsuccessful, other methods can be used, such as:

- *Artificial insemination*—the semen is spun down to concentrate the sperm, which are withdrawn and injected into the uterus through a catheter in the cervix. The specimen can be from the women's spouse or another male donor.
- *In vitro fertilization*—the eggs are retrieved through a needle inserted into the ovaries, fertilized with sperm in a laboratory, and placed into the uterus.
- *Gamete intra fallopian transfer (GIFT)*—this involves injection of egg(s) mixed with sperm directly into the fallopian tube(s) so that fertilization can occur.

■ *Intracytoplasmic sperm injection (ICSI)*—this is a microsurgical procedure involving the direct injection of a single sperm into an egg cell. This procedure is done in instances where only a very few sperm cells are produced or where those sperm cells are incapable of entering an egg on their own. ICSI is also used in those cases where sperm has to be recovered directly from the testes because of blockage of the normal route of sperm cells.

■ *Zygote intrafallopian transfer (ZIFT)*—this is a combination of in vitro fertilization and gamete intrafallopian transfer. Eggs are fertilized in the test tube, and the resulting embryos are transferred to the fallopian tube by laparoscopy. ZIFT is infrequently used.

Procedures to produce pregnancy are proceeded by medications that increase the maturation of eggs to increase the odds of fertilization. Often, when conception does occur, it results in multiple births—but the couple is usually more than happy to have multiple children.

CONTRACEPTION

The authors acknowledge that some religious and ethnic groups oppose birth control, and this text does not ignore that issue; however, this subject matter is presented factually, from a clinical viewpoint, as information required for practice as a medical assistant. As the word implies, **contraception** is literally "against" conception. Several reasons may be given to avoid pregnancy:

■ Avoid health risks to the woman. A woman in poor health may not survive a pregnancy.

■ Spacing pregnancies. Some women are very fertile and conceive every year or less. The infant death rate is reported to be 50% higher at one-year intervals than at two or more years.

■ Avoid having babies with birth defects. Some women have chromosome defects or are genetic disease carriers (or married to carriers) and choose not to risk pregnancy.

■ Delay pregnancy early in marriage to allow a time for adjustment to avoid additional stress in the new relationship and establish a strong marriage.

■ Limiting family size. It is sometimes a personal decision and other times a reality of limited resources.

■ Avoid pregnancy among unmarried couples. Single parenthood is difficult.

■ Permit the woman to develop a successful career with planned pregnancies to integrate motherhood. A career can be useful if the woman is left to raise the child alone.

■ Curbing population growth. The concern over worldwide food supply and supportive environment prompts some to promote contraception. It is expected that the population doubled between 1960 and the year 2000, only 40 years. Each successive doubling time becomes shorter.

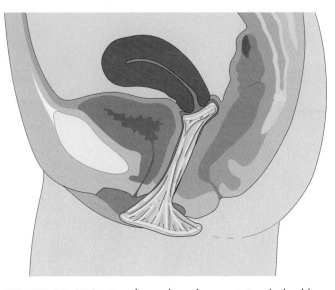

FIGURE 11–219 Female condom placement. Pouch should not be twisted. Outer ring must be outside the vagina.

Several methods to prevent conception and their relative percentage of effectiveness are listed in Table 11–18. Selection is usually made by the woman in consultation with her doctor. The cost, ease of use, degree of effectiveness, and likelihood of side effects must be taken into consideration when selecting a method. A relatively new product has been introduced into the United States market. It is the female condom. This gives women another method of birth control and protection from sexually transmitted diseases. The device is constructed with a ring at one end similar to a diaphragm, which is fitted internally over the cervix. A latex "tube" extends from the ring to another ring which hangs outside the vagina (Figure 11–219). Intercourse is accomplished within the lubricated latex tube. It is relatively effective, providing that the ring remains outside the vagina and the insertion is within the tube.

Pregnancy Termination

Abortion (Miscarriage) (A-bore'-shun)

Description—This is the spontaneous (unforced) or induced (therapeutic) loss of a pregnancy of less than 20 weeks' gestation.

Signs and symptoms—Symptoms of spontaneous abortion are a pink or brownish discharge for several days followed by uterine cramping and increasing vaginal bleeding. When contractions are sufficient, the cervix dilates and the fetus is expelled. A complete abortion includes expulsion of the fetus, placenta, and membranes, resulting in the end of cramping and minimal bleeding because the uterus contracts to close off the blood vessels. An incomplete abortion results from the retention of some or all of the placenta.

TABLE 11–18

DIFFERENT METHODS OF PREVENTING CONCEPTION

% Effective	Method	Description/Comments
100%	Abstinence	Refraining from sexual intercourse; absolutely most effective.
100%	Sterilization	Tubal ligation (cutting of the fallopian tubes) is done in the female. The cut ends can be sewn back in opposite directions or cauterized. The surgical procedure is done through a laparoscope inserted into the abdomen. The procedure is considered permanent. A vasectomy is done in the male, with the ends being sewn in opposite directions. The surgery is performed through a small incision at the base of the scrotum. Vasectomies are usually not reversible; however, in some instances, reconstructive surgery has been successful, especially in cases of shorter duration; sperm production is usually significantly decreased in time. Usually a second marriage and the desire for another child prompt the attempt. The method is relatively expensive initially.
99%	Depo medroxyprogesterone acetate (DMPA) suspension	This is an intramuscular injection that is given quarterly and provides protection for three months. The injection is given during the first five days of a normal menstrual period and provides contraceptive effects immediately. It is contraindicated if there is a possibility of being pregnant, a history of blood clots in the legs or lungs, known or suspected breast cancer, a liver tumor, or unexplained vaginal bleeding. Some side effects may occur, such as nervousness, dizziness, stomach discomfort, headaches, or fatigue. It may reduce the amount of minerals stored in bones, which could contribute to the development of osteoporosis. The most common side effect is irregular or unpredictable menstrual periods. Some women will stop having periods until six to eighteen months after stopping the injections.
99%	Lunelle	Lunelle is a hormonal birth control that is injected once a month into the arm, thigh, or buttocks. It contains hormones that work like natural estrogen and progesterone. It is given within the first five days of the menstrual period and every 28 to 30 days, but no later than 33 days, after the last injection. It is contraindicated if there is a possibility of pregnancy, blood clots, chest pain, certain cancers, or unexplained vaginal bleeding or a history of liver disease, stroke, or heart disease. Women over 35 and who smoke 15 or more cigarettes a day should not take Lunelle. The most common side effects are change in periods, such as irregular or no bleeding, spotting, and possible weight gain.
95%–99%	Birth control pills	Many different kinds are available. They are a combination of hormones that prevent ovulation; no ovum means no pregnancy. Failure occurs when pills are not taken as prescribed. Side effects can be prohibitive for some women. Available only by prescription and requires regular visits to a physician. Cost is a factor to consider.
93%–99%	Intrauterine device (IUD)	The intrauterine device is a small piece of plastic or coiled material inserted into the uterus to prevent implantation of a fertilized egg, presumably by providing irritation to the endometrium. Failure can occur if the device is expelled and during the first few months after being inserted. Initial insertion costs and the cost of removal are involved. IUDs are only recommended for women who have had children and who are in monogamous relationships because there is an increase risk of uterine infection with this device. Side effects include increase in menstrual cramping and possible increase in vaginal discharge throughout the month. IUDs are available in two types: one is copper and is effective for up to 10 years. Another contains progesterone and comes in a one-year or five-year form.
90%–99%	Diaphragm	A thin piece of dome-shaped rubber with a firm ring, which is inserted into the vagina to cover the cervix and provide a barrier to sperm. It is most effective when used in combination with a contraceptive cream placed into the dome before inserting. Failure usually results from improper insertion; a defect in the rubber, such as a hole; failure to insert before any penile penetration; or failure to maintain in place at least six hours following intercourse. There is an initial cost to examine and fit and purchase. No side effects. Requires cleaning and inspection after each use.

(continues)

TABLE 11–18 (continued)

DIFFERENT METHODS OF PREVENTING CONCEPTION—CONT'D

% Effective	Method	Description/Comments
85%–97%	Condom	A thin sheath of rubber or latex that fits over an erect penis to catch the semen. A properly used condom is very effective. It must be unrolled onto an erect penis *before* any penetration occurs. It is important to leave about one-half inch of free air space at the tip (unless the condom is constructed with a tip) to catch the semen; otherwise, the force of the ejaculant may burst the condom. It must also remain in place throughout intercourse. After ejaculation has occurred, care must be taken to withdraw with the condom in place. It may require grasping with the fingers. This is the only contraceptive that also provides a level of protection against sexually transmitted diseases. It is relatively inexpensive, easy to use, and readily available. Remember, only a latex condom is also effective against the AIDS virus.
80%–90%	Cervical cap	This is a small thimble-shaped latex cup device very similar to a diaphragm except that it is much smaller. It must be inserted from one-half hour to 48 hours before intercourse. It must remain in place for at least eight hours afterwards. This is considered a barrier method because it provides a physical "wall" over the cervix. Cervical caps come in various sizes and require fitting by a physician.
75%–97%	Female condom	This is a latex pouch suspended from an inner ring which fits over the cervix. The pouch extends to the outside and has an external ring which holds the opening outside the vagina. The condom provides a barrier for protection against sexually transmitted diseases and contraception. A new condom must be used with each intercourse. Care must be taken to ensure that the penis enters inside the pouch and that the pouch remains in the proper position throughout intercourse.
70%–75%	Spermicides	Contraceptive foams, jellies, and creams with *sperm-killing* ingredients, inserted by applicator, deep into the vagina before intercourse. It must remain for at least six to eight hours afterward. Each application is good for only one act of intercourse. They should not be relied on alone as an effective contraceptive. Combined with a diaphragm or condom, they are effective. Few side effects (some report allergic reactions), easily used, and readily available. Must not be confused with lubricants such as KY jelly or Lubafax, which contain *NO* spermicide.
?%	Douching	Absolutely not reliable. It only takes a couple of minutes for sperm to enter the cervix. In all reality, douching cannot be accomplished quickly enough. In fact, it may even assist sperm toward the cervix.
70%–80%	Withdrawal	This method has been practiced since Biblical times. It simply requires that the penis be withdrawn and ejaculation occur outside the vagina. It is not very effective because some sperm are deposited in the vagina before ejaculation occurs. In addition, the man may not be able to withdraw in time. It requires a lot of concentration to control. It is also not advised because it may lead to a sexual dysfunction if practiced for a prolonged time.
65%–85%	Rhythm	Is the practice of abstinence during an eight day period from day 10 to 17 of the menstrual cycle when conception is theoretically possible. The method works fairly well for women who are extremely regular in their cycles and couples who can practice strong self-control. However, it requires a careful assessment of at least six months of cycles to establish ovulation days. If cycles vary in length, the period of abstinence must be increased to cover the longest possible time.

Etiology—A spontaneous **abortion** usually results from one of three factors: (1) *fetal:* defective implantation or development of the embryo (most common cause); (2) *placental:* premature separation or abnormal implantation of the placenta; or (3) *maternal:* endometrial rejection, infection, malnutrition, trauma, drug reaction, endocrine difficulties, or blood group incompatibility. Spontaneous abortions occur in about 30% of all first pregnancies and up to 15% of all pregnancies.

Treatment—If the placenta (or a portion) adheres to the uterine wall, bleeding will persist, necessitating a D & C (**dilation and curettage**) to scrape out the retained placenta and permit the uterus to close off the blood vessels.

A therapeutic abortion is one performed to preserve the mother's mental or physical health in such instances as rape, unplanned pregnancy, or an existing medical condition, such as cardiac or kidney disease.

Diagnostic and Screening Tests in Pregnancy

- **Alpha-fetoprotein screening (AFP)**—This is a blood test taken at about the 15th to 18th week of pregnancy to aid in the detection of birth defects. It can also indicate the presence of multiple births. If the blood level is too high, additional tests will be performed to rule out neural tube defects. These are instances when there is a failure of the brain and skull to develop or there is an opening in the spine, exposing the spinal cord—a condition known as spina bifida. When the blood level is too low, Down syndrome is suspected. The tests are not 100% accurate but serve as a screening device detecting about 85% of open neural tube defects and about 75% of fetuses with Down syndrome in women under 35 years of age. When positive results are obtained, another blood sample, an ultrasound, and an amniocentesis are indicated. Remember that a negative test does NOT guarantee a baby free of birth defects but only that it is unlikely that there is neural tube defect or Down syndrome.
- Amniocentesis—Down Syndrome is caused by a chromosomal error (see Unit 1). This occurs in one of every 1,000 live births. A test known as an amniocentesis can be done on women who apparently are at risk. Amniotic fluid is withdrawn from the amniotic sac in which the fetus is growing (Figure 11–220). Cells from

DOWN SYNDROME AND MATERNAL AGE	
Maternal Age	**Frequency of Down Syndrome**
30	1 in 885 births
31	1 in 826 births
32	1 in 725 births
33	1 in 592 births
34	1 in 465 births
35	1 in 365 births
36	1 in 287 births
37	1 in 225 births
38	1 in 176 births
39	1 in 139 births
40	1 in 109 births
41	1 in 85 births
42	1 in 67 births
43	1 in 53 births
44	1 in 41 births
45	1 in 32 births
46	1 in 25 births
47	1 in 20 births
48	1 in 16 births
49	1 in 12 births

FIGURE 11–221 Risk of giving birth to a Down syndrome infant by maternal age

the skin of the fetus can be grown in a culture and examined for chromosomal abnormalities and neural tube defects. The test is usually done between 13 and 16 weeks, and ultrasound is used to visualize the fetus and amniotic fluid. Amniocentesis is 100% accurate in findings, but it is not without risk. A miscarriage rate of 1 in 200 to 1 in 300 is associated with the procedure. The incidence of Down Syndrome correlates to the age of the mother. In her 20s, a woman has only a one in 2,500 chance of having a Down Syndrome child. That incidence increases dramatically as the woman ages. By age 45, the risk increases to one in every 40 births. Figure 11–221 shows the frequency of Down Syndrome in relationship to age from 30 to 49 years old.

- Chorionic villi sampling (CVS)—A procedure similar to the amniocentesis but done by removing cells from the chorionic villi. This procedure is not as common as amnio and is associated with more complications. Like amniocentesis, this is 100% accurate for chromosomal testing.
- Gestational diabetes screening—This test is done between 24 and 28 weeks of pregnancy by drawing a blood sample after drinking a loading dose of glucose. Gestational diabetes only affects pregnant women. It is absent after delivery.
- Group B streptococcus (GBS)—GBS is one of the many bacteria that do not usually cause serious illness. It may be in the digestive, urinary, or reproductive tract, but it is most common in the vagina and rectum. Infected persons who show no symptoms are said to be

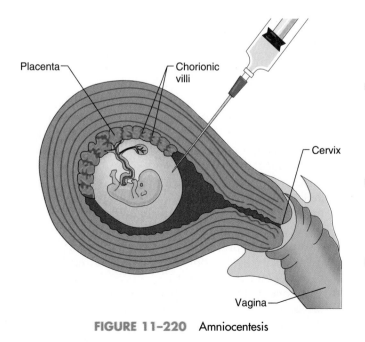

Placenta

Chorionic villi

Cervix

Vagina

FIGURE 11–220 Amniocentesis

colonized and usually do not pose any danger to their own health and may not be treated. However, when there is a pregnancy, one to two out of every 100 babies will be infected. Vaginal cultures are used to test during 35 to 37 weeks of pregnancy. This type of bacteria is found in up to 40% of pregnant women. It can be passed on to the fetus during pregnancy, to the baby during delivery, or to the baby after birth. Most babies who get GBS do not have any problems; however, a few will become sick. It can cause them major health problems and may even become life threatening. Antibiotics are given during labor to the women who test positive for GBS.

■ Routine pregnancy screening tests—There are several routine tests that are taken for routine information, such as blood typing, antibody screenings, sexual transmitted disease screening, and urine cultures.

Diagnostic Tests of the Female Reproductive System

■ **Colposcopy**—An examination and biopsy of the cervix using a colposcope. It is done to rule out cancer when there are abnormal PAP smear results. Often cell structure may be temporarily altered by antibiotics, yeast infections and other reasons, which might give a false positive pap smear. The cervix is cleansed with a solution of acetic acid and the scope introduced. The cervix can then be viewed through the colposcope, which magnifies the mucosa and makes cellular structure visible. In most cases, biopsies are taken from the abnormal sites. A PAP smear is a screening test, whereas colposcopy is used to obtain a definitive diagnosis.

■ **Hysteroscopy**—A hysteroscope is inserted vaginally into the uterus. It is connected to a monitor that permits viewing of the endometrium. By using instruments through the scope, it is possible to biopsy suspicious areas and remove polyps and fibroid. It is possible to take photographs or make a videotape for documentation of findings (Figure 11–222). When the hysteroscope is used with a laparoscope, it is possible to increase the visual field and facilitate the performance of surgical procedures. In the Figure 11–222, the use of both scopes permits visualizing both the inside and outside of the uterus at the same time.

■ **Interventional hysterosalpingography** (HSG)—This is a procedure used to evaluate fallopian tubes in cases of infertility. It is an alternative to laparoscopy or laparotomy with tubal resection. It is performed on women with tubal obstruction, which has been confirmed with regular HSG. A catheter is placed through the cervix into the uterus while x-ray dye is being injected. The catheter is then pushed into the opening of a blocked tube. Additional dye is injected into the tube. A small, soft wire is pushed into the fallopian tube through the catheter until the tube is reopened and the dye fills the entire fallopian tube. The success rate for

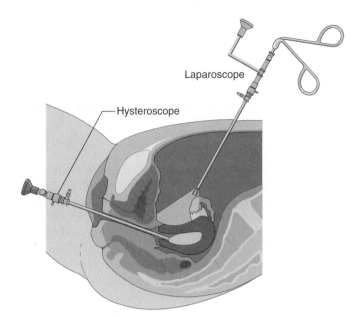

FIGURE 11–222 Laparoscopy performed with hysteroscopy

opening an obstruction is 75% to 95%. Pregnancy is greater than 50% within one year following the procedure. If unsuccessful, a second procedure may result in pregnancy.

The main benefits of the IHSG procedure are that it is relatively inexpensive, and it is a non-surgical approach to restoring tubal patency.

■ **Mammogram**—An x-ray of the breast for the detection of malignancy. A mammogram is indicated whenever there are palpable breast masses, breast pain, or nipple discharge. The film can also help differentiate between benign breast disease or breast malignancy. The American College of Radiologists recommends a single baseline mammogram for all women between ages 35 and 40. All women over 40 should have an annual mammogram. Women at risk require earlier and more frequent examinations. Risk-related factors are fibrocystic disease; history of breast, uterine, ovarian, colorectal, or salivary gland cancer; and a family history of breast malignancy.

■ Maturation index—A means of determining hormonal level by examining the percentage of certain types of cells in scrapings taken from the lateral vaginal walls.

■ **Papanicolaou (Pap) smear** (test)—A routine examination done on secretions removed from the cervix and upper vagina to determine the presence of cancerous cells.

■ Pregnancy test—Conducted on a first voided morning urine specimen to determine presence of the hormone human chorionic gonadotropin (HCG), which is produced by the developing placenta at the onset of pregnancy.

■ Ultrasonography—A test for malignancy. A transducer is used to focus a beam of high-frequency sound waves through the skin into the breast. Sound waves bounce back echos, which are displayed on a computer screen for diagnosis. Ultrasound can detect tumors less than one-fourth inch in diameter and can distinguish between cysts and solid tumors. It is anticipated that ultrasonography will eventually replace mammography in breast cancer screening programs.

■ Ultrasonography is also used to observe the fetus in utero. It can help determine the status of pregnancy, confirm the expected date of delivery, and identify the gender, if desired.

DISEASES AND DISORDERS OF THE FEMALE REPRODUCTIVE SYSTEM

Cervical Erosion (Serv'-i-cal E-ro'-zhun)

Description—This is an ulceration of the epithelium on a portion of the cervix.

Signs and symptoms—The area bleeds easily when touched during examination and may cause intermenstrual bleeding.

Etiology—It results from chronic cervicitis.

Treatment—Erosion is treated locally by cauterization (burning) to destroy the abnormal tissue growth. Cauterizing agents used can be chemical, such as silver nitrate sticks, or electrical, such as the electrocautery. The treatment is administered through a vaginal speculum and produces immediate cramping, which subsides quickly. Vaginal discharge will increase for a few days as the tissue sloughs off.

Cervicitis (Serve-eh-ci'-tis)

Description—This is the inflammation of the cervix.

Signs and symptoms—Often, the only symptoms are a purulent, foul-smelling vaginal discharge and a tenderness of the cervix.

Etiology—It is caused by an invading organism which is usually a staphylococcus or streptococcus. Herpes simplex II is a possible cause. A large percentage of patients are infected with the gonorrhea bacteria when the cervicitis is associated with pelvic inflammatory disease.

Treatment—Treatment is usually an antibiotic appropriate for the causative organism.

Cystic (Fibrocystic) Breast Disease (Fi'-bro-sis-tick)

Description—This is the presence of multiple lumps within the breast tissue. The lumps may be fibrous tumors that have degenerated or cysts (sacs) containing fluid.

Signs and symptoms—They may occur singularly or in multiple clusters. Fibrous tumors are either round or lobular. They are usually firm, well-defined (with definite borders), freely moveable, and painless. Cysts are also round, soft to firm, elastic, well-defined, moveable, and often tender. Neither type is attached to underlying tissues or to the skin to cause signs of retraction.

Etiology—There is probably no specific "cause" of this disorder. It is not a "disease" as such but rather a condition of normal breast tissue that has just "developed." It tends to occur with aging.

Treatment—Treatment may include needle aspiration of cystic fluid. Often, the cyst will not refill. Women with fibrocystic disease are believed to be at greater risk of developing a malignancy in one of the masses.

Many women naturally have "lumpy" breasts and should not be classified as having a "disease." Young women often have dense breast tissue that feels lumpy all over. This is just a condition of being fibrocystic. Often breasts become fibrocystic as a woman ages. Only professional examination and mammography can accurately diagnose a fibrocystic condition.

Cystocele (Sis'-toe-ceel)

Description—This is the bulging of the anterior wall of the vagina and the bladder into the vaginal canal, sometimes into the introitus.

Signs and symptoms—It can be demonstrated by asking the patient to bear down or strain as the vaginal opening is observed.

Etiology—Cystocele appears in older women because of poor musculature from aging and the effects of childbearing. Other predisposing factors are obesity, lifting of heavy objects, instrument deliveries, and chronic coughing. The displacement of the bladder contributes to improper emptying, which results in cystitis, frequency (because some urine is always in the bladder), urgency, and incontinence, particularly stress incontinence as a result of coughing, sneezing, or laughing.

Treatment—If it causes discomfort or continual urinary problems, it may be necessary to surgically reposition the bladder and repair the vaginal wall.

Dysmenorrhea (Dis-men-or-re'-ah)

Description—This is the lower abdominal and pelvic pain associated with menstruation common among young females and tends to decrease with maturity, particularly after pregnancy. **Dysmenorrhea** in women in their late 20s or early 30s may be a symptom of an organic disease, such as cervical stenosis, pelvic congestion, or endometriosis.

Signs and symptoms—Dysmenorrhea typically begins 12 to 14 hours before the onset of the menses and lasts between 24 to 48 hours. It may be associated with headache, nausea, vomiting, fatigue, and diarrhea. Occasionally, pain may be felt in the back and upper legs.

Etiology—It is unrelated to any identifiable cause. However, certain contributing factors are known, such as hormonal imbalances and psychogenic factors. The discomfort probably results from increased secretion of the hormone prostaglandin, which intensifies uterine contractions. Dysmenorrhea is also present with other conditions, such as endometriosis, cervical stenosis, uterine leiomyomas (tumor in the muscle tissue), incorrect uterine positioning, and PID (pelvic inflammatory disease).

Treatment—Treatment consists of analgesics, heat, drugs to decrease uterine contractions, and the use of hormonal therapy, such as oral contraceptives, to suppress ovulation. When discomfort has an organic cause, the underlying condition must be corrected.

Endometriosis (En-do-me'-tree-o-sis)

Description—The presence of endometrial tissue outside the uterus is most commonly found in the pelvic area, affecting the ovaries, ligaments, and peritoneal tissues.

Signs and symptoms—The condition is characterized by dysmenorrhea, with constant pain in the lower abdomen, pelvis, vagina, and back beginning about a week before menses and lasting two to three days after onset. The degree of pain depends on the location of the endometrial tissue. Other symptoms include excessive, profuse menses when ovarian; hematuria when located in the bladder; rectal bleeding when located in the colon; and nausea, vomiting, and abdominal cramps when located in the small intestine.

Etiology—The cause of endometriosis is unknown, but it is believed to be the result of the following:

- Recent surgery that opened the uterus.
- Endometrial fragments expelled through the fallopian tubes at menstruation.
- Alteration in the epithelium by inflammation or hormones that changes it to endometrium.

Treatment—Treatment consists of conservative methods in younger women, such as analgesics, non-steroidals, and oral contraceptives. Oral contraceptives are the current treatment of choice for long term therapy because of the action of ovulation suppression. Other injectable medications such as Lupron Depot is used for six-month therapy. It works by decreasing estrogen and progesterone normally produced by the ovaries. This is mainly used after the diagnosis of endometriosis has been determined, although some physicians are now using Lupron Depot prior to surgery for treatment. After the six-month month therapy, menstrual cycles will return to normal. When ovarian masses exist, they may be surgically removed. In women who no longer desire children, the treatment of choice is **hysterectomy** (removal of the uterus) and bilateral **salpingo-oophorectomy** (removal of both fallopian tubes and ovaries). The condition is not life-threatening, but pain and anemia must be controlled. Because the disease may cause sterility, childbearing should be accomplished as soon as convenient. Endometriosis generally subsides with menopause if surgery is ruled out.

Fibroids (Fi'-broid)

Description—**Fibroids** are known technically as uterine leiomyomas or myomas, they are a common benign, smooth tumor formed of muscle cells, not fibrous tissue as suggested by the name. Usually fibroids do not occur singly and are located most often in the body of the uterus.

Signs and symptoms—The primary symptom associated with leiomyomas is **menorrhagia** (excessive menstruation). Other characteristics are pain, a feeling of heaviness in the abdomen if the mass is large, discomfort from pressure against other organs, possible urinary frequency or constipation, and an irregular enlargement of the uterus. When a leiomyoma is attached to the lining by a stalk and is suspended within the uterine cavity, pain is caused by the uterus contracting in an attempt to expel the mass. The patient is frequently anemic because of excessive bleeding. The diagnosis is usually confirmed by a D & C, showing cells from leiomyoma in the scrapings from the endometrium.

Etiology—The cause of leiomyomas is unknown, but it is believed they are cells that have grown into a tumor, probably stimulated by estrogen and the growth hormone, because following menopause they usually shrink in size and disappear.

Treatment—Treatment depends on several factors, such as the patient's age, general health, and desire for children; the size of the tumors; and the severity of the symptoms. Lupron Depot is used to treat uterine fibroids for one to three months prior to surgery. The medication shrinks the fibroids, therefore minimizing bleeding with surgery. Small masses can be surgically removed, but a complete hysterectomy is indicated with greater involvement. The ovaries are left intact if possible to maintain hormone levels naturally. Uterine leiomyomas occur in about 20% of all women over age 35, with leiomyosarcoma (malignancy) developing in only about 0.1% of the patients.

Hysterectomy (His-ter-ec'-tomy)

Description—This is the surgical removal of the uterus. It is one of the most common procedures performed on female patients. It is not usually done on an elective or request basis but as a solution to a problem, such as endometriosis, leiomyomas, uterine rupture, or malignancy. A hysterectomy can be performed in different ways, depending on the situation. Figure 11–223 illustrates the extent of surgery. Removing the uterus through an abdominal incision is called an abdominal hysterectomy. When the uterus is positioned appropriately, it can be removed through the vagina, called a vaginal hysterectomy.

Endometrial **ablation** is used in cases of excessive bleeding from the buildup of endometrium or benign fibroid. A pen-sized instrument called a resectoscope is

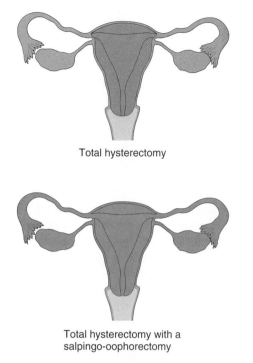

Total hysterectomy

Total hysterectomy with a
salpingo-oophorectomy

FIGURE 11-223 Types of hysterectomies

inserted into the uterus through the cervix. The procedure removes the lining by electrical cautery, using a loop or rollerball attached to the end of the scope. It requires about 20 minutes to perform, is relatively painless, avoids surgery, takes only a few days' recovery time, and is a fraction of the cost of a hysterectomy. In contrast, a hysterectomy is major surgery, requiring well over an hour to perform, approximately six weeks to recover, and costing between $4,000 and $7,000. The ablation is probably an alternative for 20% to 50% of the annual 600,000 hysterectomies done mainly to stop uncontrollable bleeding. The procedure almost always results in sterilization, which of course would also happen with a hysterectomy. There is a slight chance of perforating the uterine wall, which may then lead to a hysterectomy.

Ovarian Cyst

Description—This is a sac of fluid or semisolid material on an ovary; it is usually nonmalignant, small, and produces no symptoms. Common cysts include follicular and lutein types that occur in the follicle or the corpus luteum. They can occur any time between puberty and menopause, including during pregnancy.

Signs and symptoms—An ovarian cyst may cause an acute abdomen (a sudden condition, probably requiring surgical treatment) if the ovary is twisted by the cystic mass or the cyst ruptures. Large or multiple cysts may cause pelvic discomfort, lower-back pain, and abnormal uterine bleeding. Symptoms vary according to the type of cyst. Other possible symptoms

are acute abdominal pain similar to appendicitis, massive intraperitoneal hemorrhage, and delayed menses followed by prolonged or irregular bleeding.

Etiology—Follicular cysts develop as a result of an overdistended follicle that fails to close off properly. They secrete excessive amounts of estrogen in response to the FSH hormone. Granular lutein cysts are enlargements of the ovaries caused by excessive accumulation of blood during the bleeding phase of the menstrual cycle. Another form of lutein cyst is usually found bilaterally and contains clear, straw-colored liquid.

Treatment—Follicular cysts generally require no treatment because they spontaneously disappear within 60 days. Oral contraceptives or progesterone for five days reestablishes the hormonal cycle and induces ovulation. Treatment may also include drugs to induce ovulation or surgery to remove a portion of the ovary if drug therapy fails. Treatment generally consists of observation if the cyst is known to be nonmalignant. Signs of cyst rupture, such as increasing abdominal pain, distention, rigidity, fever, tachypnea, hypotension, and symptoms of intraperitoneal hemorrhage, are carefully watched. Occasionally, a cyst becomes so large that it causes discomfort and surgical removal becomes necessary.

PMS (Premenstrual Syndrome)

Description—This combination of characteristics appears from 7 to 14 days before menstruation and usually subsides with the onset. It is estimated that the syndrome occurs in 30% to 50% of women, particularly between the ages of 25 and 40.

Signs and symptoms—Symptoms include any or a combination of the following:

- Behavioral changes, such as nervousness, irritability, fatigue, and depression.
- Neurological changes, including headache, dizziness, numbness of extremities, and fainting.
- Respiratory changes, including increase in colds, exacerbation (aggravation or increase) of allergic rhinitis, and asthma.
- Gastrointestinal changes, such as constipation, diarrhea, abdominal bloating, and change in appetite.
- General symptoms of backache, palpitations, temporary weight gain, increase in acne, or breast tenderness and enlargement.

Etiology—The cause of premenstrual tension is unknown. For whatever reason, intravascular fluid enters the body tissues and results in secretion of an antidiuretic hormone. This causes fluid retention with characteristic bloating. The tissue edema results in headaches and alterations in mood because of central nervous system changes.

Treatment—Treatment basically is symptomatic. Medication can be used to help relieve emotional symptoms and the physical manifestations.

Polyp (Pol'-lip)

Description—This is a growth with a slender stem attachment usually arising from the mucous membranes.

Signs and symptoms—Polyps of the cervix can often be visualized protruding from the external cervical os. They are red, soft, and rather fragile. If only the tip can be seen, it cannot be differentiated from a polyp of the endometrium.

Etiology—Probably result from the unrestrained cell growth of the epithelium.

Treatment—Depending on the location, size, and attachment, removal may be a simple office procedure or an outpatient surgical procedure. Protruding polyps can be chemically cauterized in the office. The procedure causes some immediate discomfort, primarily cramping, but soon subsides.

Rectocele (Rec'-toe-seal)

Description—This is bulging of the posterior vaginal wall, by the rectum, into the vagina.

Signs and symptoms—Inspection of the introitus may disclose a posterior mass, or it may be demonstrable on requesting the patient to bear down. It is most common in postmenopausal women.

Etiology—Contributing factors are believed to be pregnancies, prolonged labor, instrument deliveries, obesity, chronic coughing, and lifting of heavy objects. A **rectocele** of advanced degree may cause difficulty in emptying the rectum.

Treatment—If severe, surgical intervention to repair the vaginal wall and support the rectum can be performed.

Vaginitis (Va-gin-i'-tis)

Description—This is an inflammation of the vaginal mucosa. There are several causes of **vaginitis**, with varying symptoms and treatment.

1. Allergic reaction—this usually happens as a result of douche solutions (especially those that are scented), spermicidal materials, deodorant-treated tampons, or other materials inserted into the vagina. This can be treated easily by discontinuing the causative agent.

2. Bacterial vaginitis—this was formerly called Garnerella or non-specific vaginitis. It is a complex condition that is not understood well at present. The cause of this infection is thought to be an overgrowth of several different types of organisms. The predominant symptom is an increase in vaginal discharge, often with an unpleasant "fishy" odor. Redness and itching are rare, however, because bacterial vaginitis can occur with other types of infections, and other symptoms may be present. Treatment involves oral antibiotics or an antibiotic vaginal cream therapy.

3. Candidiasis—also called fungus, yeast infection, or **moniliasis**, is the most common type of vaginal infection that causes irritation symptoms.

   Etiology—It is caused by a fungus like yeast that requires glucose for growth. It can effect any woman but is more frequent amount women who are pregnant, diabetic, or obese. These conditions alter the metabolic balance of the body and the acidity of the vagina, thereby promoting growth of the fungus. The use of antibiotics and birth control pills also increase the risk of the infection.

   Signs and symptoms—Many women do not notice a discharge, but if present, it is usually described as odorless with a "cheesy" appearance. The main symptom is intense itching, burning, and redness of the vaginal tissues.

   Treatment—With confirmation by exam and lab tests, medication will be prescribed to destroy the fungus. This may include vaginal suppositories or tablets or the insertion of an applicator of cream into the vagina.

4. Vaginal mucosa atrophy—this occurs in menopausal women because of decreased levels of estrogen. This can be treated with estrogen cream inserted into the vagina or by estrogen replacement therapy.

MALIGNANCY OF THE FEMALE REPRODUCTIVE ORGANS

Breast

Description—This is the most common malignancy among females and the number two cause of death. It occurs most often in women over age 35.

Breast cancer is more common in the upper outer quadrant and in the left breast. It spreads through the lymphatic and circulatory system to the lungs, liver, bone, adrenal glands, kidneys, and brain. Cancer may be classified according to its location and cellular type as adenocarcinoma (from the epithelium) or Paget's disease (cancer of the nipple). In addition, most cancers are classified according to stages to identify the amount of tumor, node, and extent of metastasis.

Signs and symptoms—Specific warning signals that may indicate breast cancer are:

- A lump or mass in the breast tissue.
- Change in breast size or shape.
- Change in appearance of the skin.
- Change in skin temperature (a warm, hot, or pink area).
- Drainage or discharge from a non-nursing woman or discharge produced by manipulation.
- Change in the nipple, such as itching, burning, erosion, or retraction.

Pain should be investigated but is not usually an early symptom.

Diagnosis is most often made by mammography, ultrasonography, and surgical biopsy. The best and most reliable means of detecting breast cancer early is mommography. Numerous studies have shown that early detection saves lives and increases treatment options. Estimates of new invasive cases of breast cancer in women for the year 2001 were 192,200 with an additional 1,500 in men. New cases of *in situ* cancer are expected to be 46,400, with 88% being ductal. A total of 40,600 death were estimated for 2001.

Etiology—The cause is not known, but estrogen is believed to be in some way responsible. Predisposing factors include: a family history of breast cancer, long menstrual cycles, early menarche or late menopause, first pregnancy after age 30, obesity, and drinking alcoholic beverages. There is also a correlation with diet, especially fat intake.

Treatment—The type of surgical treatment selected for breast cancer takes into consideration, first of all, the stage, the woman's age, the medical circumstances, and the patient's preferences. Physicians have become more aware of the woman's fears, attitudes, and feelings about the disfigurement of her body and will, if possible, choose the least radical method of surgery.

A lumpectomy (removal of the tumor only) can be done on a small mass when there is no evidence of lymph node involvement. The next step would be a lumpectomy and removal of axillary lymph nodes but not the breast itself. With additional breast involvement but no node enlargement, a simple **mastectomy** would remove just the breast and no underlying muscles. A modified radical mastectomy removes the breast and axillary nodes. A radical mastectomy removes the breast, axillary lymph node, and muscles from the chest wall. Radical mastectomies are seldom performed because of the lack of statistical data to verify their additional survival benefit. Treatment of ductal carcinoma in situ includes local excision, radiation, and tomoxifen.

Recent advances have been achieved in mastectomy surgery. Reconstruction of a breast mound can be provided for most patients. A prosthesis may be implanted after underlying tissues are excised with the skin and breast surface structures being maintained. The approach is determined by the extent of involvement. A mastectomy is disfiguring surgery that may alter the patient's body image drastically. Because it can affect a woman's opinion of her sexuality and her relationship with her sexual partner, numerous volunteer support groups and other services are available to assist with the problems of adjustment.

Surgical treatment is usually combined with chemotherapy and/or radiation in an attempt to destroy cells within other structures of the body. Hormone therapy involves the use of androgens, progesterone, or an antiestrogen, depending on the hormone-receptive nature of the tumor.

The five-year survival rate for localized breast cancer is 97% today. If it has spread regionally, the rate drops to 77%, and with distant metastases, the rate is only 21%. After five years, the rate of survival continues to decline, with the best survival being among women with early stage disease.

Cervical

Description—This is a cancer of the cervix of the uterus. An estimated 12,900 cases of invasive cervical cancer were expected in 2001 with a death rate of 4,400. The Pap screening has reduced the incidence steadily over the past decades. The Pap test is a simple procedure involving a sampling of cells from the cervix that are easily obtained and examined under a microscope.

Signs and symptoms—It produces no symptoms until the cancer cells penetrate through the membranes and begin to travel through the lymphatic vessels or spread directly to nearby structures. The earliest symptoms are abnormal vaginal bleeding, persistent discharge, and pain and bleeding after intercourse. Cervical cancer can be detected very early by a Pap smear before any clinical evidence is observable. For this reason, the American Cancer Society recommends that all adult women under 40 (and sexually active teens) have Pap smears done at least every three years, and women over 40 should be checked annually. The Pap test is not a reliable diagnostic tool for uterine cancer, only cervical. Women at risk require more frequent evaluation.

Etiology—Specific causes are unknown, but certain factors are contributory, such as: early age intercourse, multiple sexual partners, multiple pregnancies, herpes simplex virus II, and other bacterial or viral venereal diseases.

Treatment—A variety of treatments, surgery, radiation and chemotherapy, are used depending upon the stage of cancer. More common, especially in younger women, are pre-cancerous cells called **dysplasia**, which are detected by Pap smear or **colposcopy**. For these pre-invasive lesions, cryotherapy is used to freeze the area, or a procedure called LEEP (loop electrical excision procedure) uses electric current to destroy tissue with intense heat. Other methods use laser ablation or localized surgery.

With invasive cancers, surgery, radiation, or both and chemotherapy may be used. Survival rate for patients with pre-invasive lesions is nearly 100%. Eighty-eight percent survive for one year, and 70% survive five years. Even invasive cervical cancer survival is at 92% for five years when discovered early.

Ovarian

Description—Ovarian cancer is one of the most common causes of cancer deaths among American women. It accounts for 4% of all cancers among women and ranks second among gynecologic cancers. An estimated 23,400 new cases were expected in 2001 with an estimated 13,900 deaths—more than from any other cancer of the female reproductive system. Prognosis varies with the stage and type of tumor, but only about 25% of patients survive for five years. One type, primary epithelial, accounts for about 90% of the cases. Another form strikes children. It is more prevalent in higher socioeconomic women between 40 and 65 and in single women. Ovarian cancer spreads rapidly by local extension and occasionally through the blood or lymphatics. The most common metastasis is through the diaphragm into the chest cavity. Because of its location, early diagnosis is difficult.

Signs and symptoms—Symptoms are confined to vague abdominal discomfort and mild gastrointestinal disturbances. With progression, urinary frequency, constipation, pelvic discomfort, and distention develop. Symptoms may be confused with appendicitis. Diagnosis requires careful evaluation, complete history, surgical exploration, and lab studies on tissue samples.

Etiology—Risk factors for ovarian cancer increase with age and peak during the 80s. Women who have never had children, who have had breast cancer, or who have a family history of breast or ovarian cancer are at increased risk. Other genetic factors like BRCA1 and BRCA2, a type of hereditary colon cancer, and living in an industrialized country increase the incidence.

Treatment—Treatment generally involves aggressive surgery to remove all reproductive organs, affected lymph nodes, the omentum (the apron of tissue covering the organs), and the appendix. Chemotherapy may be beneficial in early stages, to extend the survival time. Recent therapy is resulting in prolonged remissions in some patients.

Uterine

Description—Uterine cancer is the most common gynecologic malignancy, usually affecting postmenopausal women between ages 50 and 60. Estimates for 2001 were 38,000 cases of uterine body cancer, usually of the endometrium, with an expected death rate of 6,600. The incidence is higher among white women, but the death rate is higher among black women.

Signs and symptoms—The first signs of uterine cancer are uterine enlargement and unusual premenopausal or any postmenopausal bleeding. It may begin as blood-streaked watery discharge but changes gradually to more bloody drainage. The only reliable diagnostic test is biopsy, with a follow-up D & C if the biopsy is negative.

Etiology—The prime risk factor that may lead to the most common form of uterine cancer is a high cumulative exposure to estrogen. This can be from hormone replacement therapy, tamoxifen, early menarche, late menopause, never having children, or a history of failure to ovulate. Other factors include infertility, diabetes, gallbladder disease, hypertension, and obesity. A familial tendency, a history of uterine polyps or hyperplasia of the endometrium, and the normal process of aging are also factors.

Treatment—Surgery is the treatment of choice, removing all reproductive organs. Radiation, either by an implanted internal device or externally administered, is indicated before surgery if the tumor is poorly defined. Chemotherapy and hormonal therapy with progesterone may be used. Both cervical and uterine cancers are rated by stages from 0 to IV with 0 being suspicious and IV-b indicating metastasis to distant organs. The one-year survival rate for endometrial cancer is 92%, and the five-year rate is between 64% and 69%, depending on whether it is discovered early or in a regional stage.

Vaginal

Description—Pertains to the vagina. Vaginal cancer is far less common, occurring primarily in women in their early to mid 50s. It occurs most often in the upper third of the vagina and, like cervical cancer, begins in the epithelial layer, then deepens. It spreads very slowly.

Signs and symptoms—Symptoms include vaginal discharge and bleeding, with an ulcerated, usually firm, lesion of the vagina. Diagnosis is made by the presence of abnormal vaginal cells on a Pap smear. Any visible lesion is biopsied. Involvement of the cervix must be ruled out. Lesions of the vagina are often difficult to visualize because of its physical structure and the presence of the vaginal speculum blades, which obstruct the view.

Etiology—Vaginal cancer appears to be caused by the same factors that contribute to uterine malignancy.

Treatment—Treatment of early stages may be confined to the area alone. Surgery or radiation varies according to the involvement. With extensive disease, surgical exenteration (removal of all pelvic organs) may be required, with construction of a colostomy and an ileal conduit (ureter emptying into the ileum). Radiation is the preferred treatment for vaginal cancer.

Vulva

Description—Pertains to the area of the external genitalia. Cancer of the vulva accounts for 5% of gynecologic malignancies. It occurs usually among older women, most often in their mid 60s, but can occur at any age, even in infancy. Early diagnosis and treatment greatly enhance survival. A five-year survival rate is possible in 85% of patients without lymph node involvement and 75% when removed nodes are positive.

Signs and symptoms—Symptoms often begin with pruritis, bleeding, and a small surface ulcer that becomes infected and painful. Diagnosis is tentatively made from abnormal cells on a Pap smear and the typical clinical findings. Firm diagnosis requires biopsy of the suspected lesion.

Etiology—Risk factors related to vulvular cancer are chronic pruritis of the vulva with friction, swelling, and dryness and the presence of vulval diseases, including venereal diseases. Also, pigmented moles that are constantly irritated by clothing and perineal pads tend to be predisposing. Other systemic conditions, such as obesity, hypertension, diabetes, and absence of childbirth, present risks.

Treatment—Treatment consists of surgery, which varies with the extent of involvement. Small, confined lesions without lymph node involvement are treated by simple vulvectomy, perhaps on only one side. With node involvement in advanced stages a radical vulvectomy is required. This involves the vulva and superficial and deep inguinal lymph nodes. With adjoining tissue metastasis, it may be necessary to excise the urethra, vagina, and rectum, leaving an open perineal wound requiring two to three months to fill in and heal. If surgery is prohibited, radiation may be used to make the patient more comfortable.

SEXUALLY TRANSMITTED DISEASES (STD)
AIDS—Acquired Immune Deficiency Syndrome

Refer to Unit 9, The Immune System, for an in-depth look at this disease.

Chlamydia (Klah-mid'-e-ah)

Description—This is one of the most frequent sexually transmitted diseases in North America, affecting between 3 and 10 million people each year. Approximately 10% of all college students are infected. It is probably present in half the patients with pelvic inflammatory disease (PID).

Signs and symptoms—Symptoms do not easily lead to diagnosis. Men may experience burning on urination and have a mucoid discharge from the penis. They are often misdiagnosed as having gonorrhea. Women experience a vaginal discharge mimicking gonorrhea and have frequent painful urination associated with urinary tract infections. Sometimes **chlamydia** does not cause any visible signs. If there are visible signs, they will be noticeable within one to three weeks after having sexual contact with an infected person.

Etiology—This disease is caused by a specialized bacterium that lives as an intracellular parasite. There are two types of bacteria, both of which are pathogenic to humans. One strain causes a type of pneumonia. The other, *Chlamydia trachomatis,* lives in the conjunctiva of the eye and the epithelium of the urethra and cervix.

Treatment—If misdiagnosed, penicillin (for gonorrhea) or a medication for urinary infection may be given, and the chlamydia remains unaffected. Proper treatment requires repeated doses of tetracycline or erythromycin for at least a week to destroy the organism. If left untreated, or mistreated, men usually have no lasting effect but carry the organism and infect their sexual partners. In women, the bacteria will travel up the reproductive tract, causing inflammation of the fallopian tubes and eventual scarring. The scarring can interfere with pregnancy by causing tubal implantation of the fertilized ova because of the narrowed opening. Complete blockage may also occur, which prevents conception.

The disease, if contracted during pregnancy, will be transmitted to the baby during birth. The infant may develop conjunctivitis or pneumonia. Some evidence suggests that the infection may cause an increase in premature and still births. Two recently developed tests, which are inexpensive and quick to perform, accurately diagnose the disease. Because of its widespread incidence, many physicians routinely treat patients with symptoms and evidence of PID or gonorrhea even without positive chlamydia test results because of the risk of sterility.

Gonorrhea (Gon-oh-re'-ah)

Description—This is a common venereal disease. The usual sites are the vagina, penis, rectum, mouth, and throat. Because the organism dies almost immediately on exposure to air, it can be spread only by direct sexual contact.

Signs and symptoms—Symptoms vary between the male and female. Men notice burning, itching, or pain on urination; a sore throat with gland involvement; discharge from the anus; or penile drainage that begins as a clear, watery fluid but changes to a thick, milky consistency. Women are usually asymptomatic, but they often develop an inflammation with a greenish-yellow discharge from the cervix. Other common symptoms are similar to those experienced by men, including sore throat, anal discharge, and swollen glands. Women may also develop lower abdominal pain, especially if fallopian tubes and other structures become involved (see PID). Diagnosis can usually be made on visual inspection, but confirmation depends on a microscopic examination of the discharge or a positive culture of the gonococcus organism from the discharge. Treatment is necessary; gonorrhea will not go away by itself.

Etiology—An infection caused by the gonococcus bacteria is known as **gonorrhea**. The organism is fragile and can survive only in a moist, dark, and warm area within the body.

Treatment—Large doses of penicillin or tetracycline are required to destroy the organism. A follow-up examination after treatment is important because strains of the gonococcus organism have become so resistant to the drugs that one course may not be sufficient.

Untreated or undertreated gonorrhea can continue to spread, causing much damage. Men may develop chronic urethritis, long-term urinary tract inflammation, and sterility. Women may develop PID, which damages the reproductive organs and results in sterility.

Women who are infected with gonorrhea when giving birth pose a grave danger to the newborn. The gonococcus organism can infect the delicate tissues of the newborn's eyes and cause permanent blindness. Because of this possibly happening, all newborns routinely receive silver nitrate solution in their eyes as part of immediate after-birth care.

Gonorrhea can be controlled and prevented with proper education, treatment, and common sense. Knowledge of a partner's sexual frequency and use of protection with others—*before* engaging in sexual activity—can prevent a person from becoming infected in the first place. Since the advent of the contraceptive pill and the IUD, the use of condoms, diaphragms, and foams has diminished. These chemical and mechanical barriers, especially the condom, deterred the spread of the disease. The condom is encouraged as a deterrent to the spread of all sexually transmitted diseases.

Herpes (Her'-pees)

Description—Genital herpes is an acute, inflammatory disease of the genitalia. It is one of the most common recurring disorders of the genitalia. Prognosis varies according to the age of the patient, the strength of the immune system, and the infection site. Primary genital herpes is usually self-limiting but may cause painful local or systemic disease. For people with weak immune systems, newborns, and others with widespread disease, genital herpes is often severe, with complications and a high mortality rate. Herpes is passed by direct skin-to-skin contact with your own or someone else's lesions, even 24 hours before they erupt. It is possible to spread your own herpes without being aware of its presence.

Signs and symptoms—Herpes takes from three to seven days to erupt. With **genital herpes**, fluid-filled vesicles appear on the cervix (primary site), labia, vulva, vagina, or perianal skin of the female. The male lesions appear on the glans, foreskin, or penile shaft. Nongenital lesions may cause complications, such as herpetic keratitis of the eye, which may lead to blindness. Vesicles are usually painless at first but may rupture and develop into shallow, painful ulcers with edema, redness, and tender inguinal lymph nodes.

Diagnosis is made by observation and from patient history. Confirmation of herpes simplex II is possible from a culture of the vesicle fluid.

Etiology—The virus causing herpes has two strains: type I and type II. Type I is the typical cold sore on the lip or at the edge of the nose. Type II is the form that appears on the external genitalia, mouth, or anus.

Treatment—Treatment with the usual antiviral medications helps reduce edema and ease discomfort. Antibacterial agents help combat secondary infections. Neither medication will treat the virus, but they will help to speed the healing process of the lesions.

After lesions heal, the virus becomes dormant. It may never recur, but about two thirds of herpes sufferers have additional attacks, some within a few months. Future recurrences decrease in frequency and severity. The best defense is a healthy, well-rested body that can fight the disease organism with its natural defense mechanisms.

Other complications demand attention. Newborns can be infected with herpes during vaginal delivery. Some infants survive, but others develop a brain infection that rapidly leads to death. If a woman has active herpes type II lesions at the time of birth, a cesarean section delivery is indicated. Women with herpes genitalis also have a higher-than-usual rate of spontaneous abortion. One major long-term risk associated with the disease is cervical cancer; therefore, women infected with or exposed to herpes type II should have a Pap smear every six months.

Human Papillomavirus (HPV) Infection

Description—Human papillomarvirus is the common name given to a group of related viruses. HPV is one of the most common sexually transmitted diseases (STDs). One form, genital warts, has been around for centuries. Today, its increase may result from women having more sexual partners and being less likely to rely on condoms for birth control—hence, there is no physical barrier.

Signs and symptoms—There are different types of HPV. One causes the common warts that appear on the fingers and hands and rarely spread to the genitalia. These are unsightly but do not cause any health problems. Other types of HPV found on the genitalia cause condylomas or genital warts. These are usually found in clusters growing on the external structures and inside the vagina and on the cervix. However, HPV can be present without the visible warts because the virus can cause changes that cannot be seen by the naked eye. Often the virus is discovered by the Pap test. When the Pap is positive, a visual examination and sometimes a colposcope, a magnifying instrument, may be used to examine the vagina, cervix, and vulva. Suspicious areas are usually biopsied for diagnosis and signs of precancerous changes.

Etiology—HPV is a very small virus that needs to infect cells in order to survive. Once inside a cell, the virus directs the cell to make copies of itself and to infect other healthy cells. The infected cells eventually die and are shed with the virus from the body. When shed, the virus can be passed to another person who then becomes infected. It often takes several months and maybe even years for the person to show signs of infection. The virus can be passed during sex and is therefore considered to be a STD.

Treatment—Some signs of infection may go away, but the following treatments may still be adviseable:

- Trichloroacetic acid (TCA) and bichloroacetic acid (BCA) are strong chemicals that can be applied to destroy genital warts.
- Podophyllin is an old treatment that can also be applied with care to warts because it can burn surrounding tissue. It should not be used during pregnancy.
- Interferon is a new drug to treat genital warts. It can be injected into the warts or into muscle. It must also be avoided during pregnancy.
- Cryotherapy destroys the lesions by freezing.
- Laser treatment destroys the warts with a high-intensity beam of light.
- Electrosurgery uses electric current to burn away the lesion or shave it with a loop.
- Excisional biopsy cuts away the tissue.
- TCA, cryotherapy, or a laser are used to treat pregnant patients.

Genital warts are difficult to remove, and repeated treatment may be necessary for several weeks or months. Even after visibly gone, they may return at a later time. The major concern with HPV is the increased risk of other major health problems, such as cancer.

Nongonococcal Urethritis (NGU, NSU) (Non-gon-o-cock'-al Ur-reth-ri-'tis)

Description—This is a group of infections with similar manifestations that are not linked to a single organism. Sometimes it is also called NSU or **nonspecific urethritis**. In men, it causes urethral inflammation; in women, vaginitis. NGU is transmitted by sexual intercourse. Men can also develop inflammation or allergic reactions from vaginal creams, contraceptive foams, soaps, douching solutions, and deodorants used by their sexual partners.

Signs and symptoms—Symptoms are similar to cystitis: burning on urination, frequency, itching (penile or vaginal), and possibly a thin discharge (penile or vaginal).

Differential diagnosis between NGU and gonorrhea must be made because the symptoms are similar, but the treatment is different. Confirmation is made by absence of the gonococcus from the culture of the discharge.

Etiology—It is usually the result of a bacterial infection. In males, it often results from *Chlamydia trachomatis* infection or from bacteria such as staphylococci, diphtheroids, coliform organism, and *Hemophilus vaginalis*. In females, less is known about non-specific genitourinary infection. The chlamydia or corynebacterial organisms may also be the cause of infection. The disease often has no obvious cause, but sometimes bacteria or bacteria-like organisms are found in the urethral discharge.

Treatment—Treatment is normally with tetracycline or a similar antibiotic because NGU does not respond to penicillin therapy. If untreated, it may lead to complications like those associated with gonorrhea. The most serious complication is a scarred urethra, which results in problems with urination. In addition, some strains can cause birth defects in newborns whose mothers have the disease.

Pelvic Inflammatory Disease (PID)

Description—This is any acute or chronic infection of the reproductive tract, including the cervix (cervicitis), uterus (endometritis), fallopian tubes (salpingitis), and ovaries (oophoritis). It can also involve the surrounding tissues. Early treatment is important to prevent reproductive damage, infertility, pulmonary emboli, septicemia (blood poisoning), and death.

Signs and symptoms—Symptoms include purulent vaginal discharge, fever, and malaise (especially if gonorrhea-related). There is lower abdominal pain, with severe pain on manipulation of the cervix and adjoining structures.

Etiology—PID is caused by an infection from aerobic or anaerobic organisms. The *Gonorrhea coccus* is the most common aerobic organism. It can rapidly destroy the bacterial barrier of the cervical mucus. With the barrier gone, the bacteria present in the vagina can ascend into the uterus and cause infection. Uterine infection can also develop following insertion of an IUD (intrauterine device), which accidentally introduces contaminated cervical mucus into the uterus. Other factors causing PID are abortion, tubal examinations that test patency by inserting air, pelvic surgery, and infection associated with pregnancy. Organisms can enter from the bloodstream, an abscess, an infected tube, or a ruptured appendix.

Treatment—PID can be treated with antibiotics to prevent progressive involvement. Culture of the drainage to identify the organism is important to be certain the appropriate drug is being used. Improper treatment will result in a chronic disease state. If the causative organism is gonorrhea, syphilis may also be present and require treatment. Bed rest, analgesics, and IV therapy may be indicated. Pelvic abscesses may develop, which require drainage. If permitted to rupture, they may cause a life-threatening situation.

Pediculosis Pubis (Pubic Lice) (Pe-dick-u-low'-sis Pu'-bis)

Description—These are little yellowish-gray insects, about the size of a pinhead. They attach themselves to the moist hair roots in the pubic area of humans and feed on the blood of their host, hopping from person to person during sexual contact. It is possible, however, to get lice from contaminated towels, upholstery, clothing, or bedding, because they can survive for about a day without a supporting host.

Signs and symptoms—The prime symptom is an intense itching which can not be ignored. They are visible on close inspection.

Etiology—Pediculosis is caused by parasitic forms of lice.

Treatment—Treatment is quite simple with a product called Kwell, which is applied to the infected area. All clothing, bedding, and linens must be washed in very hot water and detergent to destroy the nits (eggs) and lice. Nonwashable items can be dry-cleaned or ironed with a hot iron. Lice eggs can survive for a week, so uncleaned items must be avoided.

Syphilis (Sif'-uh-lus)

Description—This is a venereal disease that inhabits the warm, moist areas of the genitals and rectum. The organism can be viewed by dark-field microscope examination. **Syphilis** is spread by direct sexual contact during either the primary, secondary, or early latent stages of infection. Prenatal transmission to the fetus across the placental barrier is possible, resulting in an infant with congenital syphilis. If the mother is in the primary or secondary stage, the infant will probably die before or shortly after birth. If syphilis is diagnosed and treated before the fourth month of pregnancy, the fetus will not develop the disease. Therefore, a blood analysis for syphilis is routinely performed as part of early prenatal care.

Signs and symptoms—Symptoms vary according to the stage of involvement. Primary stage syphilis begins with entrance of the organism through the mucous membrane of the genitals as the result of contact with an infected person. After three to four weeks, a lesion called a *chancre* appears at the point of entrance. It is an ulcerlike area with a raised, hard edge, which looks painful but is not. In the female, it often appears on the cervix and is therefore hidden from sight, going undetected. It may also develop on the vulva and be visible on examination. In the male, the usual site is the glans or corona (ridge) of the penis. It may develop on the penile shaft or scrotum. The bacteria can also enter the mucous membranes of the mouth or rectum during nongenital intercourse, causing chancres to develop on the lip, tongue, tonsils, or around the anus.

The disease progresses through four stages. The primary stage, chancre, even if untreated, disappears within one to five weeks, giving the infected person a false sense of having healed. Actually, the disease enters an asymptomatic period during which the bacteria circulate through the body in the blood. About one to six months later a secondary stage begins. This stage is characterized by a generalized painless, nonitching rash. It is particularly distinctive because of its appearance on the soles of the feet and palms of the hands. During this stage, the following may occur: hair loss, a sore throat, headache, loss of appetite, nausea, constipation, persistent fever, and pain in the bones, muscles, or joints. These symptoms could be indicative of any number of illnesses. If the disease is diagnosed accurately and treated, it can be cured without permanent effects. Without treatment, the disease again "goes away" in two to six weeks, leading to the belief that nothing is wrong, while, on the contrary, a dangerous stage is approaching.

The third stage is the latent stage, which may last for years. There are no symptoms during this stage, but the organism is at work, burrowing into blood vessels, the spinal cord, the brain, and the bones. After the first year, the disease is no longer infectious except to a fetus. About 50% of those who contract syphilis move into the dangerous late or tertiary stage. This stage is further categorized according to the type of involvement: benign late (affecting internal organs); cardiovascular late (affecting the heart and major blood vessels); or neurosyphilis (affecting the brain and spinal cord). Cardiovascular forms can lead to death; neurosyphilis is almost always fatal.

Diagnosis is difficult by history alone, and physical examination at certain periods would be negative. However, a definitive blood test has been developed and is used routinely for suspected infection and as a mass screening test by some states for persons seeking a marriage license. The test is known as a VDRL, named for the Venereal Disease Research Laboratory of the United States Public Health Service. The blood test is fairly accurate, cheap, and easy to perform; however, it does not give accurate results until four to six weeks after initial infection. About 25% of the tests will be false negatives during the primary stage, but they are completely accurate in the secondary phase.

Etiology—Syphilis is caused by the spirochete *Treponema pallidum*.

Treatment—Penicillin is the treatment of choice for syphilis, which is relatively easily destroyed. Because some of the spirochetes may survive, a large initial dose of long-acting penicillin (1.2 million units) is divided into two injections, one in each buttock. Much greater doses are required for latent, late, or congenital syphilis. A follow-up exam should be done to confirm freedom from organisms.

Trichomoniasis (Trick-oh-moh-ni'-a-sis)

Description—This is a protozoal infection of the lower genitourinary tract. It occurs in 15% of sexually-active females and 10% of sexually-active males. **Trichomoniasis** can be passed back and forth between sexual partners; therefore, treatment must involve both persons.

Signs and symptoms—The prime and discriminating symptom is abundant, frothy, white or yellow vaginal discharge, which irritates the vulva and has a characteristic foul odor. There are usually no symptoms in the male, except for urethral itching. Diagnosis is made by placing a drop of the secretion on a slide and identifying the organism by microscope. This confirmation rules out ordinary vaginitis from female hygiene products or the presence of rectal *Escherichia coli* in the vagina.

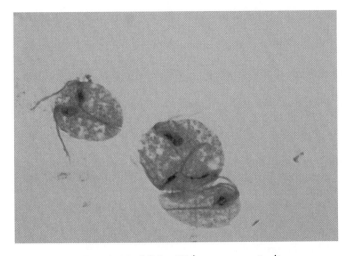

FIGURE 11–224   *Trichomonas vaginalis*

Etiology—It is caused by the single-celled parasitic organism called *Trichomonas vaginalis* (Figure 11–224). It is oval in shape with four hairlike strands protruding from it, which whip back and forth to propel the organism.

Treatment—Treatment of choice is a product called Flagyl, which is taken orally. If left untreated, the female may develop an inflamed cervix and urethra and exhibit abnormal Pap smears. Damaged cells of the cervix may make it more susceptible to cancer. Men develop an infected prostate, testicle, or bladder.

ACHIEVE UNIT OBJECTIVES

Complete Chapter 11, Unit 13, in the workbook to help you obtain competency of this subject matter.

A CAAHEP CONNECTION

This unit covers many **Diseases, disorders, diagnostic tests, and treatments** and introduces **Medical terminology**. It has discussed and illustrated **Anatomy and physiology** as it pertains to the reproductive systems of both males and females. This content addresses the requirement of the standards to cover these topics.

RELATING TO ABHES

Chapter 11 discusses the 11 systems of the body, fundamental body structure, and the senses. It also introduces a large amount of medical terminology, discusses appropriate diagnostic examinations, tests for each system, and has a structured discussion of many diseases and disorders with the usual treatment modalities as they are associated with each system. This content relates to the ABHES accreditation requirements of **Anatomy and physiology** and **Study of diseases and etiology** within the content area of **Anatomy and Physiology** and **Medications prescribed for the treatment of illness and disease based on a systems method** within the content area of **Pharmacology**.

RESOURCES

American Academy of Otolaryngology, Head and Neck Surgery, Inc. (1995). Snoring: Not funny, not hopeless [Pamphlet]. Alexandria, VA: Author.

American Cancer Society (2001). Cancer facts & figures [Booklet]. Altanta: Author.

Bartlett, J. S. (2001, June). Possible solution found for replacing defective C F genes. In *Infectious diseases in children*, (p. 67). American Academy of Allergy, Asthma, and Immunology.

Brody, J. E. (2001, May). Better choices in heart bypass surgery. *Bottom Line Health*.

Cable News Network Health (2001, February 12). Landmark gene studies released [Online]. Available: www. cnn.com

Congestive heart failure and beta blockers (2001, August). *Harvard Health Letter*.

Diabetes treatment: The tried and true and what's new (2001, April). *Harvard Health Letter, 26*(6), 1–3.

Ductal Lavage (2001, September). *Women's Health Watch*, p. 647.

Ehrlich, A. (2000). Medical terminology for health professions (4th ed.). Clifton Park, NY: Delmar Learning.

Eight ways to avoid Alzheimer's disease (2001, August). *Dr. Andrew Weil's Self Healing*, p. 6.

Floria, B. (2001, Spring). Assessing your osteoporosis risk. *Perspective*, p. 7.

Gugliotta, G. (2001, July 1). Doctors implant new heart pump. *The Washington Post*.

Hepatitis C: How to protect yourself against the new blood plague (2001, September). *Bottom Line Health*, pp. 11–12.

Lifesaving asthma secrets. (2001, May). *Bottom Line Health*, pp. 7–9.

Mitral valve repair for severe heart failure (2000, November). *HeartWatch, 4*(10), 1–2.

More iron overload screening recommended (2001, January). *Health and Nutrition Letter 18*(11), 7.

New solutions to those too, too embarrassing skin problems (2001, June). *Bottom Line Personal*, p. 11–12.

New treatment for osteoarthritis (2001, January). *Health and Nutrition Letter 18*(11), 4–5.

Pfeifer, J. D., and Wick, M. R. (1995). The pathologic evaluation of neoplastic diseases. In G. Murphy, W. Lawrence, and R. E. Lenhard, (eds.), American Cancer Society textbook on clinical oncology (2nd ed., 75–95). Atlanta: American Cancer Society.

Robb-Nicholson, C. (1999, March). Essential tremor. *Harvard Health Letter*, p. 6.

Robotic arms aid those of physician in heart surgery (2000, Winter). *The OSU Medical Center Health Connection*, p. 10.

Scott, A., & Fong, E. (1998). Body structures and functions. (9th ed.). Clifton Park, NY: Delmar Learning.

Seven out of 10 stroke patients suffer disability or death—How to beat the odds (2001, August). *Bottom Line Health*, pp. 3–4.

Wade, N. (2000, May 9). Another chromosome is decoded. *The New York Times*.

What is Bell's Palsy? (2001, June). *Women's Health Watch*, p. 8.

WEB LINKS

http://www.aaaai.org **(American Academy of Allergy, Asthma, and Immunology)**

Provides information on allergic diseases.

http://arthritis.org **(Arthritis Foundation)**

Provides information on arthritis.

http://cancer.org **(American Cancer Society)**

Provides information on cancer.

http://www.lymphnet.org **(National Lymphedema Network)**

Provides information on lymphedema.

http://www.nof.org **(National Osteoporosis Foundation)**

Provides information on osteoporosis.

http://www.mayoclinic.com **(Mayo Clinic)**

Affiliated with the Mayo Clinic, this site offers an index of diseases listed A-Z, 11 Condition Centers, and 8 Healthy Living Centers.

SECTION 4

The Clinical Medical Assistant

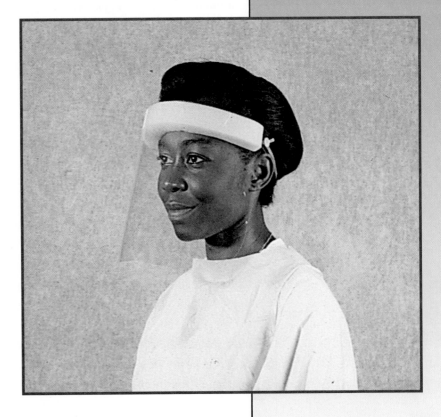

CHAPTER 12

Preparing for Clinical Duties

To be a valuable employee, the clinical assistant must be proficient in many skills. Patients will ask questions regarding their illnesses and treatments. You should be able to reply with correct and understandable information. You are also expected to be knowledgeable about office policies. You must perform tasks in a minimal amount of time while also conserving supplies because health care costs are high. It is up to each medical assistant to practice the necessary skills. Patience and perseverance are necessary to reach the goal of proficiency.

You will be assisting in many procedures that are extremely personal in nature. Considering the patient's feelings and emotions will help in dealing with these delicate matters. The procedures patients must experience are sometimes painful, often discomforting, and may be embarrassing for them. You must try to ease the patient's fears and anxieties. Ask patients if they have any questions concerning the examination or procedure for which they are scheduled. Procedures that have become routine to you and other medical personnel may be new or at least unfamiliar to patients. Patients may be apprehensive not only about the procedure itself, but about what the physician may find. Finally, patients usually do not feel well and are not themselves. Try to exhibit a caring attitude with all patients at all times. You should also be careful not to rush patients even though it can be tempting when the schedule is backed up and there are many others waiting to see the physician. Empathy and understanding in handling patients will make tasks more pleasant.

Patients who are intellectually impaired, developmentally disabled, hearing impaired, deaf, vision impaired, blind, elderly, senile, or non-English speaking may need the undivided attention of the medical assistant during their visit and may take considerably more time than the average patient. Some of your patients may have an assistance dog (or other animal) to help them get around. These animals are "working" and are on duty. Even though most owners are patient with both children and adults wanting to pet the dog, it is best to leave the animal alone so that they do not feel threatened or distracted from doing what they have been trained to do. Kindness and patience are important qualities to use especially with these patients. Assistance should be offered but not imposed.

Being friendly is a sure way to gain a good rapport with patients (Figure 12–1). Even the blind will hear a smile in your voice. Everyone smiles in the same language.

For a vision-impaired or blind patient, it is appropriate to offer to take his arm to guide him. You must also explain what is going on and describe floor plans and furniture arrangements to help the patient feel more comfortable, especially during times when you are not present.

In communicating with the deaf or hearing-impaired patient, speak clearly in a normal tone of voice while facing the patient so that your lips can be read. If the patient does not read lips, you can write notes to explain procedures and other important information. For a patient who is deaf or hard of hearing, it is important to show her around the facility, pointing out the restroom, insurance office, where the examination room is, and so on. If you need to leave the person alone, it is not only common courtesy but a necessity to let her know where you will be in case of further questions or problems.

Patients who have physical disabilities are usually self sufficient and will need little if any assistance in getting around. Try to make them feel comfortable and do not dwell on their disabilities.

All of us can learn a great deal from patients who have a disability, no matter what it may be, for they have learned to accept life and make the best of it.

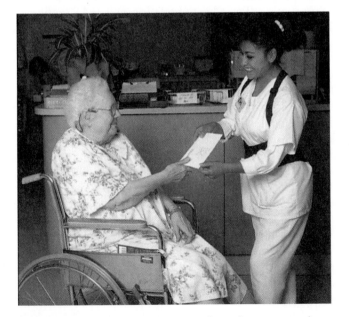

FIGURE 12–1 The medical assistant faces the patient and speaks to her in a pleasant manner.

A CAAHEP CONNECTION

Keep in mind that you will be dealing with patients from literally all parts of the world. They will be from different cultures and ethnic groups and have different religious beliefs. One who speaks no English must have an interpreter scheduled for the time of the patient's appointment. If an interpreter is not with the patient, you must do your best to relay information in an emergency situation. A family member usually accompanies the patient to translate what you and other health care professionals need to say regarding procedures and patient education.

In addition to the service of an interpreter, printed materials and signs should be provided in appropriate languages for the patients who come to your office who do not speak English.

UNIT 1

Guidelines for the Personal Safety and Well-being of Staff and Patients

▮ OBJECTIVES

Upon completion of the unit, meet the following performance objectives by verifying knowledge of the facts and principles presented through oral and written communication at a level deemed competent by the instructor or employer. Demonstrate the specific behaviors as identified in the performance objectives of the procedures, observing all aseptic and safety precautions in accordance with health care standards.

1. Spell and define, using the glossary in the back of the text, all the **Words to Know** in this unit.
2. Explain the medical assistant's role and responsibility in maintaining personal safety and well-being of staff and patients.
3. List potential hazards and problems in a medical facility and the action that should be taken for each.
4. List and name the location of housekeeping items and supplies that should be on hand for use as necessary.
5. Describe daily routine care of the medical facility.
6. Explain the importance of proper hand washing.
7. Demonstrate the proper procedure for hand washing.
8. State the purpose of wearing latex or vinyl gloves.
9. Explain how to prevent disease transmission to a patient with a cold.
10. List the admirable habits a medical assistant should practice to reduce disease transmission.
11. List general guidelines for lab safety.
12. Explain the importance of posting informative signs and diagrams for patients and visitors in a medical facility.

AREAS OF COMPETENCE (AAMA)

This unit addresses content within the areas of *Fundamental principles, Patient care, Legal concepts, Instruction*, and *Operational functions* in the Medical Assistant Role Delineation Study. Refer to Appendix A for a detailed listing of the areas.

▮ WORDS TO KNOW

asepsis	microbes
biohazard	microorganism
emesis	✳pathogens
esthetic	vigilance
harbor	warranted

✳vector - insects, rats etc
spread of disease

Fomite - inanimate object - nails, doorknobs

In the course of routine daily activities in a medical facility, there should be a scheduled time for inspection of the entire facility. Established guidelines should be followed to maintain a safe and comfortable environment for the safety and well-being of all patients and staff. Establishing and adhering to these standards will help to avoid problem situations regarding potential hazards and possible disease transmission. Foremost in protection for all is cleanliness, which is the best way to prevent the transmission of disease. Because a medical facility is a place where many people, both well and sick, convene, it is a prime target for pathogenic organisms to grow and multiply. Constant and consistent **vigilance** must be upheld to help ensure environmental control and safety. The schedule of duties to perform this important function should be outlined and regulated by the supervisor or office manager on a daily basis.

KEEPING THE ENTIRE MEDICAL FACILITY CLEAN

In the performance of clinical procedures, the medical assistant must be mindful of the necessity of **asepsis**, which is a state of being free from all pathogenic **microorganisms**. Even though there cannot be a completely sterile environment throughout the entire general medical facility, it must be clean and safe for all who enter. Although there is generally a contracted commercial cleaning service (this service is usually referred to as environmental or custodial service) established to do the heavy cleaning and scrubbing of the office walls, windows, furniture, carpets, and so on, it is the staff's job to check dust, debris, and clutter to keep a clean and **esthetic** appearance of the entire facility. Periodic remodeling and redecorating of the facility should be done before furniture and carpets become a safety hazard or an eyesore.

The reception area and the rest of the facility should be a pleasant and comfortable place for those who enter. Therefore, all those who are employed in a medical facility have a responsibility to observe, report, and assist in keeping the appearance and safety of the facility assured. It is your duty to take a good look around to inspect the facility daily before patients arrive.

All surfaces, doorknobs and plates should be dusted or washed appropriately as necessary and repeated as often as necessary throughout the day, especially in areas where there may be close quarters and where heavily populated. Attention should also be given to water fountains, public restrooms, trash cans, telephones (clean mouthpiece often), and the areas around them where either periodic restocking of supplies or cleanup is indicated. Occasionally, a considerate person may report that more toilet tissue or paper towels are needed in the restroom, but this should be the exception and not the rule. The conscientious medical assistant should already have matters under control in keeping a well cared-for facility. Trash containers are to be lined with disposable trash bags, and this is generally done by the custodial staff. However, there may be times when the container becomes too full, must be disposed of in the appropriate location for trash pick-up, and a new trash bag is placed in the container. The trash containers in the patient restrooms and in the reception area sometimes contain contents that may be unpleasant and should be changed. It is much more attractive in the reception area to have a receptacle with a lid to conceal unsightly trash. In the event that a general cleanup would become necessary (some cleaning services are only contracted on a weekly basis), a standard list of cleaning equipment and supplies should be kept in a convenient place. The following housekeeping list contains standard items that should be kept on the premises:

- broom and dust pan
- vacuum cleaner
- mop and bucket
- sponges
- cleaning solutions
- bleach (including a 10% bleach solution)
- dust cloths
- disposable trash bags
- disposable latex or vinyl gloves
- **biohazardous** puncture-proof containers and bags
- disposable **emesis** basins
- glass cleaner
- disposable paper towels
- disinfectant spray

Note: A solution of one-fourth cup bleach per gallon of tap water (a 10% dilution of common household bleach) should be made fresh daily and kept readily available for cleanup of accidental spills of blood or body fluids. A disinfectant spray is a good idea to disinfect small areas and to help eliminate odors (a fresh citrus fragrance is very effective against unpleasant odors). In an allergist's practice and for patients' comfort in general, an odorless disinfectant spray should be used.

A good way to add a nice touch to the decor in a reception room is to place some healthy, live, leafy plants in corners and on end tables. This is an attractive and inexpensive way to decorate and increase the oxygen content in the room as well. These plants must be cared for regularly (tended and watered as needed), or they will begin to look neglected and unattractive. If silk flowers or artificial plants are a part of the decor, they should be dusted or cleaned when necessary to be kept attractive. The same applies to an aquarium. Most of the time, a medical facility has made a commercial business contract for services, such as plants and sea life aquariums. However, it is up to the staff to contact the company regarding any problems that occur between scheduled service visits. You must pay attention to these needs and report them so that they can be remedied.

Proper ventilation and maintaining an ideal temperature of 72°F is necessary. Seating should not be placed directly under, over, or beside blowers or heating or cooling vents. Placing a plant, table, or lamp in an area of the room where there may be a draft is a good idea so that patients will not be sitting in an uncomfortable spot. You should also watch for any throw rugs or mats near doorways and keep them from buckling so that patients and staff do not trip over them and fall. Absorbent floor mats should be used on rainy days if the floor of the entrance is not carpeted. All furniture, lamps, wires, carpet, and so forth should be periodically inspected and cleaned as necessary. Any repairs or replacements should be made immediately as **warranted**. Keeping all reception room furniture and decor in a neat and clean manner will provide a pleasant and comfortable atmosphere for all patients, helping to make them feel safe, secure, and well cared for as they wait for their appointments.

Maintaining Cleanliness and Order in the Waiting Areas

Many facilities that provide medical care to children have a play area for the children to occupy while they wait to see the doctor. Even though the babies and children who are very ill will most likely not be playing with anything, it is important to remember to routinely clean and disinfect all items that children play with in the children's area. Remember that the health status of any child cannot be assessed before the physician examines them. This section where toys and games are kept for the entertainment of the young patients is a potential source of disease transmission and should be monitored closely. The most efficient way to control this is to have the child bring into the exam room whatever toy he or she played with in the reception area. Then you can clean it before it is placed back out with the other toys and need not worry that other little patients will become infected with whatever the child before them may have had. These toys should be made of a washable plastic or smooth non-pointed (no sharp edges) metal for children's safety and well-being. Any malfunctioning toys or toys with loose parts should be discarded immediately. Very small toys, such as beads or miniblocks, are not recommended because babies and toddlers tend to put everything into their mouths and small toys could choke them. The furniture that is used for young patients should also be made of a washable material and be cleaned routinely with a disinfectant solution. Remember to bring in those patients who are feeling very sick or who are in obvious pain or distress as soon as they arrive because it may be possible to help eliminate further problems and save the patient further stress or embarrassment.

For adult patients, there should be an appropriate assorted supply of printed materials, such as magazines, newspapers, patient education pamphlets, and booklets. These should be displayed in an orderly fashion for patients to read while they wait. Be sure to straighten up printed material as needed. Periodic checks of these materials should be done, and old or tattered ones should be discarded as necessary. Also, replace light bulbs as necessary so that there is adequate lighting for patients to read easily without eye strain. Patients should be discouraged from eating and drinking in the reception area. Spills and crumbs attract pests (such as ants, cockroaches, and mice). Used tissues, paper cups, and other assorted waste items are sometimes left behind, often unintentionally, by patients. As you pick up these trash items, wear disposable gloves or pick them up with a disposable paper towel or tissue so that you do not come in direct contact with the object as you throw it away in the appropriate waste container. Clutter and trash should be removed properly as soon as possible, not only to maintain an attractive environment, but also to eliminate potential insects and other pests. If pests do become a problem, a professional pest control company should be contacted immediately to deal with the elimination of this situation.

Wearing Gloves

C **Skills Menu:**
- Sterile Gloves and Gown
- Gloves and Gown

Wearing gloves is necessary when cleaning up blood or bodily fluid in the reception area and in the examination or treatment room. There are three very important reasons why latex or vinyl gloves are worn:

1. to provide protection as a barrier and prevent contamination of the hands when touching any blood or body fluid
2. to reduce the possibility that any **pathogens** present on your hands will be transferred to another
3. to diminish the chance of any pathogens being transmitted from you to patients as you go from one patient to another.

Wearing gloves is no substitute for hand washing. Because there is the possibility of gloves having imperfections, such as small holes or tears, or if gloves are ill-fitting, hand washing is a must before and after wearing them. There is also the risk of becoming contaminated during the removal of soiled gloves. Always remember to protect yourself and follow proper procedure (later in this chapter) when it comes to hand washing and gloving.

Avoiding Accidents

In addition to the reception area and examination and treatment rooms, the entire facility should be inspected daily and as you bring patients in to prepare them to see the physician. Even though this may seem like an obvious task, a problem situation could occur at any time; for example, someone could trip and fall over something (a toy, for instance) that was left in the usual walking path of the room. Accidents can and do happen from time to time even in the most cared for facilities. You must be alert to these potential situations and handle them with care and tact. Figure

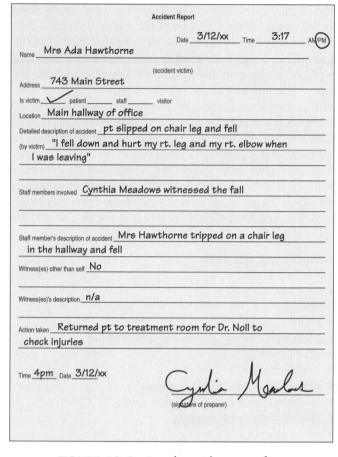

FIGURE 12-2 Sample accident report form

12–2 provides an example of an accident report form that should be used in case of any accident on the premises. If you are not aware of a problem because of neglect and a patient is injured or becomes ill because of a previously known problem that was never taken care of (such as a natural gas leak or a frayed wire), your facility can be held liable for any injury or illness caused to a patient.

Any and all repairs or replacements should be made or arranged for immediately for safety reasons and to keep the office schedule flowing as smoothly as possible. Because the administrative assistant stays primarily in the business office area and generally sees patients only at the reception window, many of the potential problems are not observed as readily as when the clinical medical assistant opens the door to the reception room to bring patients into the clinical area. This is a prime time to quickly observe the entire area, make a note of the situation, and then report it to the receptionist or whomever the appropriate person is to see to the need. If you do see a faulty chair or a frayed wire, for example, it is your responsibility to do something about it *before* someone gets hurt. Your initiative and follow-through is necessary to maintain surroundings that are as safe as possible for all concerned.

Additionally, it is a good idea to post a sign in the reception area to alert patients who are waiting about what to do in certain situations. Emergency exits should be clearly posted with easy-to-follow paths for evacuation

For Your Safety and Health

Please:

1. Report any safety hazard or emergency to the receptionist immediately.

2. Use tissues provided to cover your mouth and nose to catch your coughs and sneezes.

3. Dispose of all waste in the plastic-lined waste can.

4. Tell the receptionist if you feel nausea or need to use the restroom.

5. If you are feeling faint, weak, dizzy, nausea, chest pain, shortness of breath, or see another in similar distress, please notify the receptionist immediately.

Thank you.

FIGURE 12–3 A sign that conveys important information such as this one should be displayed in the reception area in clear view for patients and the general public in case of need.

and security in each of the rooms in the facility where you are employed. There should also be signs clearly posted for public restrooms, water fountains, telephones, and other facilities, such as the lab or pharmacy where patients may need to be sent from your office. Figure 12–3 gives an example of a concise list of advice for patients to follow if there is a problem. This will also give patients clear instructions to follow if they need attention while waiting for their appointment or in case of an emergency.

GUIDELINES FOR PREVENTING THE TRANSFER OF DISEASE

How you can be useful in preventing disease transmission and helpful in providing a safe and comfortable environment for staff and patients have been discussed. Yet there are more ways that you can be of help to ensure the health and safety of others. In this unit, you will find important regulations regarding how you can avoid the risks of contracting disease and help in preventing the transfer of disease-causing pathogens to others. Microorganisms (microscopic organisms) that are the cause of disease are called pathogens. They have certain requirements for growth and multiplication. If steps are taken to interrupt and prevent their growth, disease transmission can be reduced. Breaking the infection cycle helps prevent the spread of disease. The requirements of microbial growth are covered in Unit 2 of this chapter.

General guidelines for lab safety follow for your information. These are steps which can be taken to keep yourself and others from coming into contact with contaminated items. Further guidelines are discussed in Unit 2 regarding mandatory Occupational Safety and Health Administration (OSHA) and Clinical Laboratory

A CAAHEP CONNECTION

Because other staff members and patients observe your work and learn from your example, it is important that you follow Standard Precautions and proper hand washing procedure. Patients will appreciate the care and responsibility you take on their behalf.

Improvement Amendments (CLIA) regulations. Once you realize the seriousness of these matters, you will become conscientious about compliance. It is up to each health care provider to be honest and credible about following guidelines. Remember: Some diseases are dangerous and can be fatal. You also have a legal, moral, and ethical responsibility to protect yourself and others from such preventable problems. Obviously, the best way to do this is to establish a routine and stick to it. It is far better and easier to learn good habits than to break bad ones.

Never put your hands in your mouth (no nail biting) or any other objects (such as pens or pencils) that could transfer your germs to others who come into contact with these objects. After using tissues, wash your hands to avoid possible spread of pathogens from yourself to others. Promote a good patient education tip by demonstrating to patients how to use tissues when coughing and sneezing to help diminish the transfer of germs. Refer to Figure 12–13 to see how a patient uses tissues to catch the germs of coughing and sneezing and discards the used tissues properly. If you or a co-worker has the sniffles or a cold, it is wise to keep from being in contact with patients lest you (or they) contaminate someone. If and when you are sick and feverish, stay home and take care of yourself until you are well, and return to work only after you have been fever-free for at least 24 hours. Being in the health field, your employer should be understanding and appreciate your situation. Working as a cooperative team helps to solve these types of problems that can and do happen from time to time. Also remember that the multi-skilled medical assistant is a well-prepared team member who can fill in when other staff members are absent.

HAND WASHING GUIDELINES

C **Skills Menu:**
■ Hand Washing

The very first way to prevent the transfer of microorganisms is by washing your hands. This is the responsibility of all health care providers and all people in general to arrest the spread of pathogens. This one task alone could help to eliminate many diseases before they even begin. You must develop the routine of hand washing before you begin your daily work schedule by performing Procedure

PROCEDURE

12-1 Hand Washing

PERFORMANCE OBJECTIVE: Provided with liquid hand soap in a dispenser, nail brush, paper towels, waste receptacle, and lotion, the student will stand at a sink with hot and cold faucets and demonstrate each step in the hand washing procedure as specified in the procedure sheet.

EQUIPMENT: A liquid soap dispenser is desirable. It eliminates the possibility of dropping a bar of soap in the sink or on the floor during the procedure. It is also more economical and more attractive. Bar soap is often wasted because it becomes soft and starts to separate. The water that collects in the soap dish is also a good environment for microorganisms and therefore cancels the effort made in removing them from the hands.

Standard Precautions recommend that proper hand washing is performed to avoid the transfer of microorganisms to other patients, yourself, or the environment.

1. Remove all jewelry, including bracelets and rings (wedding rings may be left on but must be scrubbed). **RATIONALE: Jewelry harbors microorganisms.**

2. Stand at the sink and turn faucets on using a paper towel to avoid direct contact with faucets (Figure 12–4A). Adjust water temperature to moderately warm and discard paper towel. Leave water running at desired temperature. **RATIONALE: The sink and faucets are considered contaminated; water temperature must be properly adjusted because once the procedure is begun, the faucets cannot be touched.**

3. Wet hands and press soap dispenser with the heel of your hand to obtain approximately one teaspoon of soap in palm of one hand. Work soap into lather, and distribute soap over both palms and backs of hands in circular motions constantly and vigorously for two to three minutes. Keep hands lower than forearms. **RATIONALE: Circular motion and friction is more effective. Removed soil and water flows into sink, not onto arms (Figures 12–4B and C).**

4. Use nail brush to dislodge microorganisms around cuticles and under nails (Figure 12–4D).

5. Rinse well, being careful not to touch inside of sink or faucets during procedure (Figure 12–4E).

6. Rinse hands thoroughly. Leave water running, and reach for sufficient paper towels to dry hands completely.

7. Turn off faucet with paper towel and discard in waste container. **RATIONALE: Touching faucet would contaminate clean hands (Figure 12–4F).**

8. Hand lotion may be applied to prevent skin from becoming dry and chafed.

Refer to the patient education section for guidelines that all health care professionals should also follow.

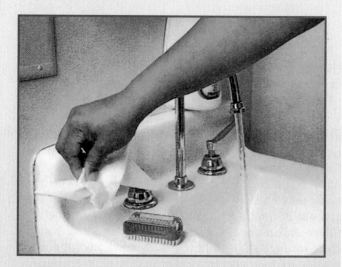

(A)

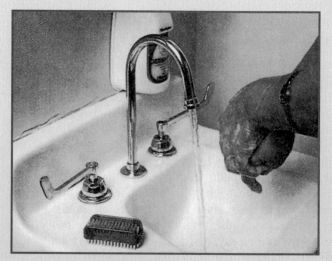

(B)

(Continued)

PROCEDURE

12-1 Hand Washing (continued)

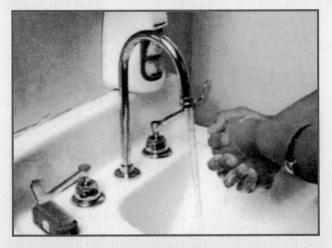
(C)

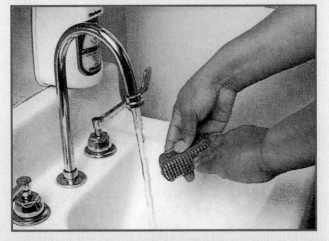
(D)

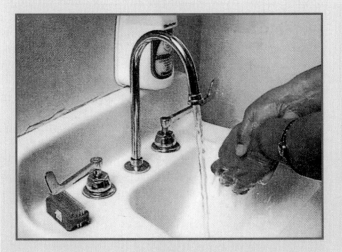
(E)

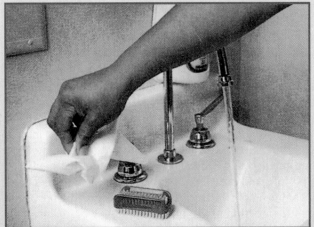
(F)

FIGURE 12–4
(A) A dry paper towel should be used to turn the faucet on.
(B) Fingertips should be pointed down while washing hands. Use the palm of one hand to clean the back of the other hand.
(C) Interlace the fingers to clean between them.
(D) Clean under the fingernails using a hand brush.
(E) Rinse the hands thoroughly with the fingertips down.
(F) Use paper towels to dry the hands and to turn off the faucets.

12–1 for two minutes. Hand washing thereafter should be done for approximately 20 seconds before and after seeing each patient and before and after handling specimens or any soiled or contaminated materials. A five- to six-minute hand washing and scrub should be performed before gloving for a surgical procedure. After removing gloves, you should wash your hands for at least 30 seconds. Lotion may be applied to the hands to prevent dry skin. It is important to avoid using lotions that have a petroleum or mineral oil content before putting latex gloves on because it can break down the latex and could intensify a latex allergic reaction. Those who are allergic to latex should use vinyl gloves. To be safe, it is a good practice to use a water-based lotion without perfume. To protect yourself from the transfer of **microbes**, remember to wash your hands both before and after using the restroom and before and after eating. Proper basic hand washing helps to remove microorganisms from the skin and from under fingernails. Minimal jewelry should be worn because it is impossible to eliminate all pathogens from the crevices of jewelry items unless they are sterilized by autoclaving. Autoclaving is not recommended because it is damaging to most jewelry, and it is highly impractical and timeconsuming. It is better to wear minimal jewelry or, better yet, none at all.

In places where a sink is not readily available for hand washing between patients, such as in an area designated for allergy injections or blood pressure readings, a practical way to cleanse the hands is by using a commercial foam cleaner preparation. This is a foamed alcohol preparation that is applied and spread over the hands in the same manner as you would use soap and water. It dries in approximately one minute. For those who have problems with dry skin, this foam seems to be less drying and irritating than some products used in washing the hands. A supply of hand cream should be readily available. Treating chapped skin with soothing lotions can help prevent a possible infection of the hands.

Carefully adhere to each hand washing step to prevent disease transmission. Even though the hand washing procedure may seem extensive, it takes only a couple of minutes to complete it, and it is done to prevent the spread of disease. Repeated hand washing between your many duties should take 20 seconds and is well worth the time. In Chapter 17, which deals with assisting in surgical procedures, you will learn how to perform a surgical handwashing, which takes considerably longer to complete (approximately 5 to 6 minutes). Learning the correct way to properly wash the hands is outlined in Procedure 12–1. Acquiring this extremely important habit is necessary for your well-being and that of others.

BASIC GUIDELINES FOR LAB SAFETY

1. Proper hand washing before and after every procedure and before and after gloving must become a habit for all health workers for self-protection from disease transmission. (Immediately washing *any* skin surface thoroughly that has been contaminated with any blood or body fluids is vital.)

2. Gloving is always a must when handling *any* blood or body fluid specimens. (If you find that you are allergic to latex gloves, disposable gloves made from materials other than latex, such as vinyl, are available. Disposable gloves are also available with or without powder.)

3. Cover all scratches, paper cuts, or any breaks in the skin with a bandage after hand washing and before gloving for self-protection against possible contamination.

4. Never eat, drink, chew gum, smoke, place hands or fingers to mouth, or place any item in your mouth (such as a pen or pencil) while working.

5. Wear protective gloves, a mask, a gown (or apron), and goggles when splashing of any blood or body fluids is possible while you are working (Figure 12–5).

6. Always recap or close bottles, jars, and tubes immediately after desired amounts are obtained to avoid spills, waste, and accidents.

7. Clean up spills immediately to avoid accidents (Figure 12–6). Spilled blood or any body fluids should be flooded with a liquid germicide or bleach solution (a 1:10 ratio) before cleaning up with paper towels (wear latex or vinyl gloves). Commercial preparations may also be used to solidify liquids, which makes cleanup easier.

8. Record lab test results immediately on charts or in logs to ensure accuracy.

9. Work in a well-lighted, properly ventilated, uncluttered, and quiet area for better concentration.

10. Discard all disposable sharp instruments, lancets, syringes, and needles (intact) in proper biohazard puncture-proof containers (Figure 12–7). (*Never*

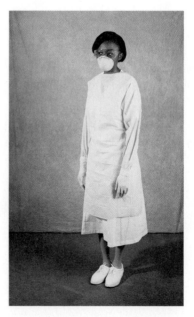

FIGURE 12–5 This medical assistant is wearing personal protective equipment (PPE): goggles, mask, gown, and latex or vinyl gloves. PPE prevents possible splashing of blood or other body fluids from coming into contact with skin or with mucous membranes of the eyes, nose, and mouth.

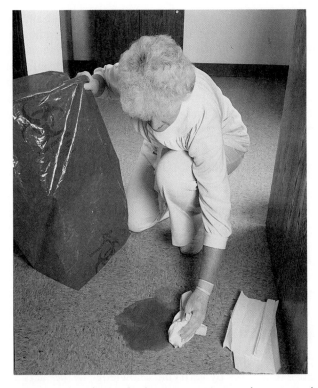

FIGURE 12–6 This medical assistant is wearing latex or vinyl gloves to clean up a specimen spill. The biohazard waste bag is used to dispose of the contaminated materials.

break needles off, handle after use, or reuse.) One should never put the needle cover between the teeth to remove it when giving an injection. Place reusable metal instruments in a disinfectant solution after rinsing in cold water in preparation for proper cleaning and sterilization.

Package broken glass or any sharp unusable items in a sturdy cardboard box or puncture-proof container

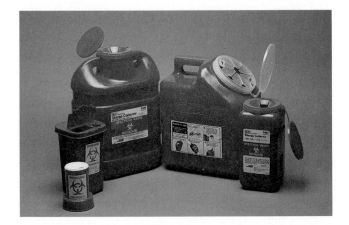

FIGURE 12–7 A few of the various sizes of biohazard puncture-proof (sharps) containers are displayed (they are generally bright red or yellow to alert caution). Notice the biohazardous material symbol that also alerts you to caution. These containers should be autoclaved when they are three-fourths full and returned to the biohazard agency for proper disposal.

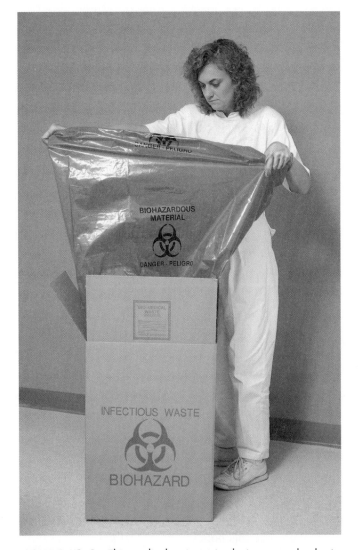

FIGURE 12–8 This medical assistant is placing a sturdy plastic bag marked with the biohazardous waste symbol into a durable cardboard box marked the same for collection of infectious waste material. When three-fourths full, these boxes are picked up by an agency for incineration or for autoclaving before being taken to a public landfill.

marked "caution—broken glass" to discard in the proper waste receptacle. (This will protect unsuspecting custodial personnel from injury.)

11. Discard *all* hazardous waste in proper containers (Figure 12–8).

12. Make periodic checks of all electrical appliances and equipment for frayed wires or faulty operation, and tag for repair if needed.

13. Make sure that your hands are dry before using any electrical appliances or equipment.

14. Report all accidents to your supervisor or instructor immediately.

15. Clearly post emergency phone numbers near the telephone in the lab (i.e., local fire, police, emergency medical unit, and poison control center) (Figure 12–9).

EMERGENCY PHONE NUMBERS

EMS	911
Police	555-1111
Emergency Squad	555-1010
Fire Dept.	555-0000
Rescue Squad	555-5050
Hospital	555-7171
ICU	ext. 210
CCU	ext. 250
ER	ext. 265
Admitting	ext. 200
Ambulance	555-1818
Poison Control Center	555-6101
Coroner	555-9914
Taxi	555-2222

FIGURE 12–9 Example of recommended phone numbers to post near each phone for emergency assistance.

16. Have available (nearby or in the lab) first aid items (i.e., sterile gauze, bandages, tape, and so on) for emergency use.
17. Post clearly the sign over the functional emergency eye wash station in the lab (Figure 12–10).
18. Do not wear loose-fitting or bulky clothing or jewelry that could contribute to accidents while working with machines or equipment in the lab or any area in the office or clinic.
19. Use gas or air valves and Bunsen burners with caution. Keep flammable chemicals away from them.
20. Use only paper disposable cups for drinking.
21. Designate a "dirty" and a "clean" area in your lab, and enforce this policy.
22. Never lean into work area when working with flame or chemicals (pour at arm's length) to avoid self-injury or accident.

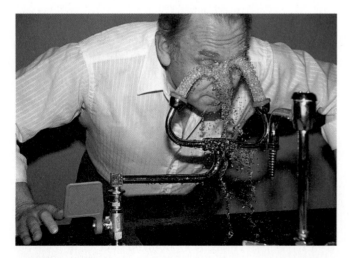

FIGURE 12–10 The emergency eye wash fountain connects to existing plumbing. The two streams of water wash both eyes simultaneously and continuously.

Another sensible practice is to avoid leaning into sinks or onto equipment or counters that could **harbor** pathogenic microorganisms. Routine housekeeping duties should be performed faithfully, such as scouring and disinfecting sinks and counters. Even if surfaces do not look dirty, you must remember that microorganisms cannot be seen with the naked eye and that preventing the disease is much smarter than taking a chance in getting it.

ACHIEVE UNIT OBJECTIVES

Complete Chapter 12, Unit 1, in the workbook to help you obtain competency of this subject matter.

UNIT 2

Infection Control

OBJECTIVES

Upon completion of the unit, meet the following performance objectives by verifying knowledge of the facts and principles presented through oral and written communication at a level deemed competent by the instructor or employer. Demonstrate the specific behaviors as identified in the performance objectives of the procedures, observing all aseptic and safety precautions in accordance with health care standards.

1. Spell and define, using the glossary in the back of the text, all the **Words to Know** in this unit.
2. List patient education suggestions to prevent transmitting disease to others.
3. Describe the recommended universal and standard precautions in regard to human tissue, blood, and body fluids.
4. Explain the purpose of the regulatory bodies (OSHA, CLIA) regarding disease transmission in the medical facility.
5. Explain the recommended written statement (and the reason for it) concerning universal precautions that should be posted in the physician's office laboratory.
6. Describe methods of controlling the growth of microorganisms.
7. List the growth requirements of microorganisms.
8. Describe the infection process cycle.
9. Explain what direct and indirect contact is.
10. Describe the body's defense against disease.
11. Explain the difference between sanitization, disinfection, and sterilization.
12. Explain the purpose of sterilization.
13. Explain the purpose of sterilizing all contaminated items before you can safely reuse them (including disposables before discarding).
14. Explain the function of the autoclave.
15. Explain the importance of safety when using the autoclave.

AREAS OF COMPETENCE (AAMA)

This unit addresses content within the specific competency areas of *Fundamental principles, Patient care, Legal concepts, Instruction,* and *Operational functions* in the Medical Assistant Role Delineation Study. Refer to Appendix A for a detailed listing of coverage.

A CAAHEP CONNECTION

Knowledge of common pathology, asepsis and infection control, risk management, and basic medical office functions included in this unit are important components in the medical assisting curriculum.

16. Demonstrate the proper procedure for preparing and wrapping instruments to be autoclaved. (Note: Many different types of autoclaves/sterilizers are on the market—pay strict attention to the operating instructions displayed by the manufacturer.)
17. Explain the purpose of using sterilization indicators for autoclaving.
18. Explain the preventative measures for health care professionals against the hepatitis B virus.
19. Locate and interpret from the communicable disease chart the means of transmission, incubation time, symptoms, and treatment for a given disease.

■ WORDS TO KNOW

aerobe	fungi
anaerobes	heterotrophs
autoclave	hygiene
autotrophs	incineration
bacteria	incubation ✳
Clinical Laboratory	inorganic
Improvement	invasive
Amendments (CLIA)	malaise
coma	morphology ✳
communicable	nits
confinement	obligate
contaminate	Occupational Safety and
debilitated	Health Administration
disinfection ✳ (unit not	(OSHA)
gloss)	organic
droplet infection	parasite
exudative	pH
fecal	perinatal
flora	

personal protective	seizures
equipment (PPE)	shelf life
petechial	spores
protozoa	sterilization ✳ book
pruritic	susceptible
pustular	vulnerable
resuscitation	virulent
sanitization ✳ book	virus
	permeable

In addition to giving special regard to patients, health care workers have the responsibility of self-protection. It is recommended that standard blood and body fluid precautions be used for all patients, especially when the infection status of the patient is unknown. Appropriate protection against exposure to blood and body fluids should be routine practice for all health care workers. Gloves should be worn when in contact (direct or indirect) with blood or any body fluids, mucous membranes, or nonintact skin; in handling items or surfaces soiled with blood or body fluid; and when performing venipuncture or any other surgical procedure. After each patient contact, gloves should be changed and hands washed. If procedures could possibly generate droplets of blood or other body fluids, the health care worker should wear shields to protect the eyes or face in addition to gloves and gown. This will protect the mucous membranes of the eyes, mouth, and nose.

After gloves are removed, hands should be thoroughly washed. If hands and other skin surfaces have been in contact with blood or other body fluids, they should be washed immediately.

At all times, extreme caution must be used by health care workers in handling needles, scalpels, and other sharp instruments to avoid self-injury. To prevent possible self-injury, it is recommended that needles should never be recapped, broken off, or removed from disposable syringes by hand after use. They should be carefully placed in puncture-proof containers after engaging the safety guard over the needle.

All infectious waste must be disposed of by placing each contaminated item in its appropriate hazardous waste container provided by your employer. Any disposable material that has even a trace of human tissue, blood, or other body fluid on it must be considered as infectious and must be treated with extreme caution. Latex or vinyl gloves must be worn when handling any contaminated item to reduce the possibility of disease transmission, especially the human immunodeficiency virus (HIV) and the hepatitis B virus (HBV). The precautions are recommended for all health care professionals by the Centers for Disease Control (CDC) and the United States Public Health Service.

Note that many of the patients you will serve and possibly some of your coworkers may be highly allergic to latex. A practical way to care for the patients with this sensitivity to latex is to make one of the examination rooms free of all latex products. When latex-allergic patients are treated in this way, they may be less likely to have an allergic episode when visiting your office.

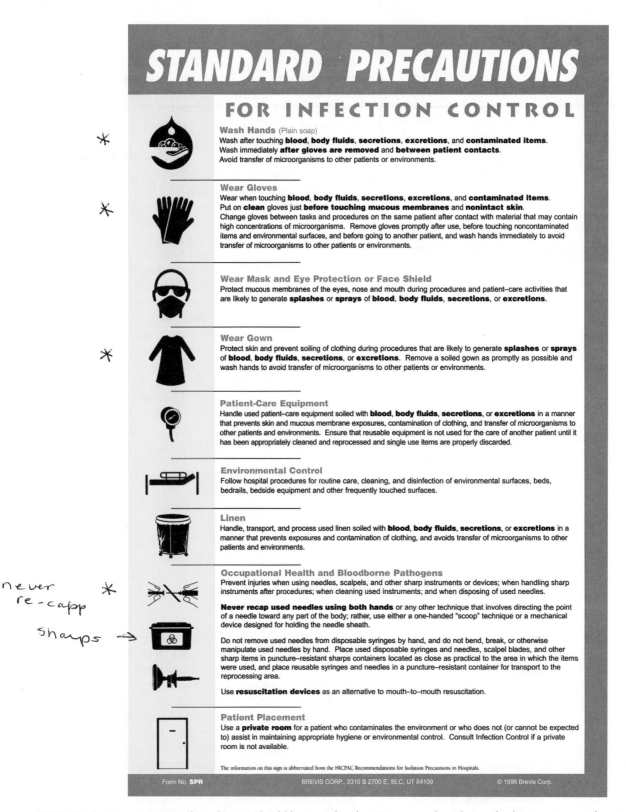

FIGURE 12–11 A poster such as this one should be posted in the POL to comply with Standard Precautions and to remind employees of safety precautions. (Courtesy of Brevis Corp.)

DISEASE PREVENTION

Beginning in the mid 1980s, following the frightening reality of the acquired immunodeficiency syndrome (AIDS) epidemic, the ways that health care professionals practice caring for patients has changed dramatically. Regulatory bodies have been established to provide standards for all who are employed with managed care of the public to ensure quality care. Two of the most prominent are the **Occupational Health and Safety Administration (OSHA)** established long before the epidemic, and the **Clinical Laboratory Improvement Amendments (CLIA)** in 1988. These guidelines have become federal regulations and must be followed not only because of lawful mandate, but foremost to protect both health care professionals and the patients whom they serve. These standards, called Standard Precautions (Figure 12–11), have been recommended by the Centers for Disease Control since 1987 and pay attention to the welfare of both health care providers and the public regarding health care standards. In each physician's office laboratory (POL) there must be posted a statement in writing that agrees with compliance of the OSHA regulations. Those who do not follow these regulations will be fined. Having this in clear view provides a constant reminder to all who work in the area of health care. Figure 12–12 shows this type of document. This statement must be signed and dated by the employer as well. Knowing that following these regulations can save the lives of so many makes it easier to cooperate. Employees quickly realize the importance of the guidelines and soon respect and appreciate their intent. This reminder helps to keep the health care provider alert and reminds them to safeguard against carelessness in the performance of their duties because they may be exposed to blood or other hazardous body fluids or infectious waste in the course of their duties. Each employee must have this statement explained when he is hired and have evidence of this in writing with his signature in a permanent file.

All items, such as mouthpieces, **resuscitation** bags, or any other ventilation supplies necessary for emergency use in mouth-to-mouth resuscitation, should be disposable to eliminate any risk of disease transmission—especially in an emergency situation where the health status of the afflicted is unknown. This practice protects both patient and health care provider.

A health care provider who has a skin condition or a laceration that is either seeping or bleeding should refrain from direct patient care until the condition clears up to avoid any possibility of transmitting microorganisms to another. An appropriate bandage that is adequate in covering the affected area should be worn, and the affected provider should follow proper gloving procedures to keep the condition contained. Caution should also be taken in handling all equipment and supplies.

Any female health care provider who is pregnant (or could possibly be pregnant) and works directly with patients whose health care status is unknown should be especially cautious. If a female contracts HIV while pregnant, the unborn fetus is at risk of contracting the fatal disease through **perinatal** transmission.

Employees must also be protected from HBV, which is a highly contagious and potentially fatal disease. Preventative immunization involves a series of three injections. Employers must offer this immunization to new employees within their first 14 days of employment, with no cost to the employee; then, documentation of the immunization offer must be filed in the employee's record. If the person has already had the vaccine or refuses to be given the vac-

---

Standard Precautions

All employees in this medical practice must follow standard precautions at all times in performing procedures that may expose them to **bloodborne pathogens** possibly contained in the blood and body fluids from any patient regardless of the patient's health status. All employees must wear protective barriers that are appropriate for the procedure being performed to prevent possible infection. Employees who work with direct patient contact must have HBV vaccine. Any accidental needle sticks, other injuries, or contacts with a potentially infectious body fluid must be reported to the physician at once for treatment and **documentation.**

FIGURE 12–12 This statement should be posted in clear view regarding Standard Precautions.

---

cine, documentation must be filed in her employee record. Human nature is imperfect, and the reality is that many serious diseases can be spread by careless acts. Needlestick injuries are unfortunately common because of human error. Safeguard yourself against this accident by never recapping needles. Always dispose of the entire used needle intact with the syringe to prevent injury. If you ever need to re-cap prior to performing an injection, a needle resheather should be used. Further information can be found regarding this procedure in Chapter 18, Unit 3. Because there are diseases that do carry a fatal risk and there are measures one can take to prevent such a risk, it is obvious that safeguarding from contracting the disease is wise. There are many ways for health care professionals to practice safety in regard to the prevention of disease. Use of barriers, such as gowns and masks, are recommended to avoid possible contamination by splash or spill of blood or blood-containing fluids. Where appropriate, protection should be made with goggles, face shields, or any other protective disposable clothing articles according to the circumstances. These protective barriers are referred to as **personal protective equipment (PPE)** and have been recommended by the Centers for Disease Control.

Following is a summary list of the basic recommended precautions:

- Routine use of appropriate barriers to prevent contact with mucous membranes, blood, or any other body fluid of a patient (any person)
- Proper routine, thorough hand washing
- Immediate placement of used sharps and needles (intact with syringe) in biohazard puncture-proof containers
- Use of disposables in resuscitation procedures
- Refraining from direct patient care if you have an **exudative** skin condition (or other contagious disease)
- Especially strict adherence to precautions during pregnancy

If all health care workers would follow Standard Precautions to help in the control of contagious diseases, it would set a good example for the public. We all must realize that actions speak louder than words.

Indirect and Direct Contact — means of transmission

The posted guidelines will be a constant reminder to pay special attention to safety. Because diseases can be transmitted in different ways, a brief discussion regarding direct and indirect contact is necessary for you to realize and understand the potential danger that an infected person can have. When a person is sick or infected with a disease, that person is the host of the microorganisms causing the illness. When the person coughs, sneezes, or whistles, the vapor that is projected from the mouth carries the microbes of the disease with it into the air. This is called **droplet infection** because the vapor contains tiny drops of vapor (moisture) from the person's breath. Depending on the force of the breath, laughing and shouting carry droplets quite far, possibly projecting them up to 20 feet or more. This force is determined by the size and strength of the person and also determines the potential radius of the spread of the microbes. The same is true for sneezing. This is the reason that patient education is so important. When a patient in the reception area is waiting to see the doctor for a routine checkup and another comes in with a terrible coughing and sneezing problem, the entire area is infected with the sick person's germs. It is your responsibility to remove the infected individual immediately to prevent others from being **contaminated** with an unwanted disease. Offer the patient instruction on catching the coughs and sneezes in the tissues you provide (Figure 12–13) and show the person where to deposit the waste. Make sure you follow the person's steps with a spray disinfectant to help contain the germs to protect those who will be in that place after the sick patient leaves. If you do not clean up after the person carefully (by gloving to pick up used tissues, for example), there is a risk that you and others may come down with the same illness. You and others may catch it by indirect contact. This means that you may contract the disease from having handled soiled tissues, by touching the door knob that the infected patient touched, or that you possibly inhaled the contaminated air following a cough or sneeze of the patient. When you are around a person who is sick, you should not deeply inhale when you breathe, or you may subject yourself to an even greater risk of contracting the disease. In some infectious disease cases, it is wise to wear a face mask that covers the mouth and nose. The physician usually suggests this for protection against disease. These are examples of indirect contact. A direct contact is actual contact with the patient or his body fluids. Direct contact includes eating, drinking, smoking after another, touching, kissing, and sexual intimacy.

DISEASE TRANSMISSION

It is suggested that you become familiar with the **communicable** diseases listed in Table 12–1. A description of the disease, the means of transmission, **incubation** time, symptoms, and treatment will inform you about the diseases so that you can be of better service to patients. The incubation time refers to the time between the initial exposure to the disease-causing microbes and the appearance of the first symptoms or signs of the disease. If a person is **susceptible** to a disease, it means that she is receptive, or **vulnerable**, to catching it. Generally, when one is susceptible, she is weakened because of a pre-existing illness or

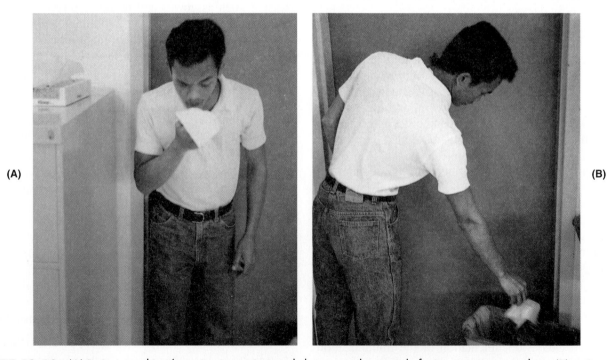

(A)

(B)

FIGURE 12–13 (A) Patient coughing/sneezing into a tissue to help prevent the spread of microorganisms to others; (B) patient properly discarding the used tissue into a waste receptacle

condition; is overall run down and worn out; or has poor **hygiene** and health habits. All of these points are considered to be factors in one's poor resistance to disease. Study the infection cycle in Figure 12–14. Follow the cycle to see how easily diseases are transferred from one to another un-

less the cycle is broken. You can be instrumental in the interruption of the cycle by being vigilant in your efforts against the transmission of disease. As you can see, taking care of yourself is extremely important in the scope of disease prevention and protection.

TABLE 12–1

COMMUNICABLE DISEASES				
Disease	Means of Transmission	Incubation	Symptoms	Treatment
AIDS (acquired immunodeficiency syndrome)*	Direct contact: sexual, anal, or vaginal intercourse, sharing IV drug needles, infected mother to child (childbirth), blood to blood (from cuts, scrapes, punctures of skin). Indirect contact: blood transfusions	Onset of AIDS following infection with human immunodeficiency virus (HIV) from 6 months to 10+ years	Early—loss of appetite, weight loss, fever, night sweats, skin rashes, diarrhea, fatigue, poor resistance to infections, swollen lymph nodes. Later—cough, fever, shortness of breath, dyspnea, purple blotches on the skin	Research and new developments continue in the search for a cure and/or a vaccine. Current treatment most commonly used is zidovudine (AZT).
Chickenpox* (*Varicella zoster* virus)	Direct or indirect contact, droplet, or airborne secretion of infected person	2–3 weeks, usually 13–17 days	Crops of **pruritic** vesicular eruptions on the skin, slight fever and headache, **malaise**	Bed rest, topical antipruritics
Common cold (upper respiratory infection— URI)	Direct or indirect contact with infected person	12–72 hours (some viruses 2–7 days), usually 24 hours	Slight sore throat, watery eyes, runny nose, sneezing, chills, malaise, low-grade fever	Rest, decongestant, mild analgesics, increased fluid intake
Conjunctivitis* (pink eye)	Direct or indirect contact with discharge from eyes or upper respiratory tract of infected person	Viral: 24 hours to days; bacterial: 24–72 hours	Redness of eyes, itching, burning of eyes, matted eyelashes	Antibacterial agents, antibiotics, corticosteroids depending on causative agent
Head lice* (pediculosis)	Direct contact with infected person; indirect contact is rare	1 week (**nits**, or eggs, hatch in 1 week, mature in 2 weeks)	Itching of scalp, presence of small light gray lice and nits (eggs) at the base of hairs	Topical use of 1% lindane: shampoo, lotion, or cream (7–10 days); comb nits from hair; launder washable items in hot water with hottest drying cycle, dry-clean or seal in plastic bags nonwashable items (2 weeks); thoroughly vacuum the environment
Haemophilus influenzae type b Hib (H-flu)*	Direct and indirect contact and droplet infection from respiratory tract	3+ days	URI symptoms, fever, aches, sleepiness, no appetite; as disease progresses, child is irritable and fussy	Antibiotics, increased fluid intake, antipyretics, rest, analgesics
Hepatitis A* (acute infective hepatitis)	Direct contact or by **fecal**-contaminated food or water	14–50 days, avg. 25–30 days	Slow onset, fever, malaise, loss of appetite, nausea, vomiting, jaundice, weakness, dark urine, whitish stool	Bed rest, increased fluid intake, proper nourishment (no fats or alcohol)
Hepatitis B* (serum hepatitis)	Contaminated serum in blood transfusion or by use of contaminated needles or instruments	14–50 days	Same as hepatitis A, of rapid onset, of acute symptoms	Same as hepatitis A

(Continued)

TABLE 12-1

| COMMUNICABLE DISEASES—CONTINUED | | | | |

Disease	Means of Transmission	Incubation	Symptoms	Treatment
Hepatitis C* (formerly non-A, non-B or NANB)	Direct contact with blood, contaminated needles	14–50 days acute onset	Same as above	Same as above
Herpes simplex virus (HSV) (cold sores, fever blisters)	Direct contact with infected person	2–14 days, usually 4–6 days	Painful blisters on lips, which turn **pustular** and then form crusted scabs; oral lesions are small ulcerated areas	Topical applications of drying medications; antibiotics for secondary infections.
Impetigo	Direct contact with draining sores	2–10 days	Blisterlike lesions (later become crusted), itching	Cleansing of areas with antibacterial soap and water, topical and/or oral antibiotics
Influenza*	Direct and indirect contact and by airborne secretions	1–3 days	Sudden onset of fever, chills, headache, sore muscles, malaise, (commonly runny nose, sore throat, and cough)	Bed rest, increased fluid intake, antipyretics
Meningitis* (aseptic)	Direct contact, fecal–oral route, and respiratory secretions	2–21 days	Sudden or gradual fever, intense headache, nausea, vomiting, stiff neck, irritability, sluggishness	Hospitalization, bed rest, increased fluid intake, antipyretics, analgesics
Meningitis* (bacterial) haemophilus and meningococcal	Direct contact and droplet infection from respiratory tract	1–10 days, usually 3–4 days	Sudden onset of fever, intense headache, nausea, vomiting; sometimes **petechial** rash, irritability, sluggishness (possible **seizures** and/or **coma**)	Same as above plus antibiotics, by intravenous and/or oral administration
Pinworms (*Enterobius vermicularis*)	Direct transfer of eggs from anus to mouth; indirect contact with eggs in clothing, bedding	3 weeks–3 months	Anal itching, insomnia, irritability.	Anthelmintics, initiate scrupulous personal hygiene, shorten fingernails; launder washable items in hottest or boiled water
Pneumonia	Direct and indirect contact	Abrupt onset	High fever, shaking, chills, productive cough	Antibiotics, liquids, rest, antipyretics
Scabies*	Direct contact or indirect contact with infected clothing/bedding	2–6 weeks	Intense itching of small raised areas of skin that contain fluid or tiny burrows under the skin, resembling a line—may be anywhere on the body	Topical scabicide, oral antihistamines, and sabicylates to reduce itching
Strep throat	Direct contact	1–3 days	Fever, red and sore throat, pus spots on back of throat, tender and swollen glands of neck	Antibiotics, analgesics, antipyretics, increase fluid intake
Scarlet fever* (scarlatina) (streptococcal)	Direct or indirect contact	1–7 days	Same as above, plus strawberry tongue, rash of skin and inside mouth, high fever, nausea, and vomiting	Same as above, plus bed rest

*Report these diseases to local health department. Refer also to sexually transmitted diseases in Chapter 11, Unit 13.

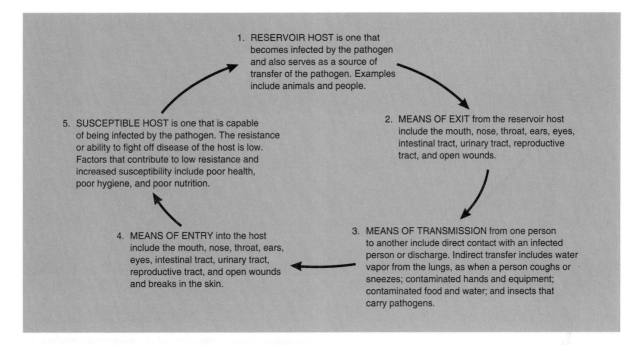

1. RESERVOIR HOST is one that becomes infected by the pathogen and also serves as a source of transfer of the pathogen. Examples include animals and people.

2. MEANS OF EXIT from the reservoir host include the mouth, nose, throat, ears, eyes, intestinal tract, urinary tract, reproductive tract, and open wounds.

3. MEANS OF TRANSMISSION from one person to another include direct contact with an infected person or discharge. Indirect transfer includes water vapor from the lungs, as when a person coughs or sneezes; contaminated hands and equipment; contaminated food and water; and insects that carry pathogens.

4. MEANS OF ENTRY into the host include the mouth, nose, throat, ears, eyes, intestinal tract, urinary tract, reproductive tract, and open wounds and breaks in the skin.

5. SUSCEPTIBLE HOST is one that is capable of being infected by the pathogen. The resistance or ability to fight off disease of the host is low. Factors that contribute to low resistance and increased susceptibility include poor health, poor hygiene, and poor nutrition.

FIGURE 12–14   The infection cycle can be broken if one is aware of the process. It is important to include this in patient education to help prevent disease transmission.

As you learned in Chapter 11, Unit 9, the body's immune system has amazing abilities. Immunity is best when the body is in a state of good physical, emotional, and mental condition. Essentially, this means that defense against disease can be maintained most efficiently by practicing the good health habits of proper exercise, adequate rest, good nutrition, and proper hygiene. Exercise is most helpful in resisting disease because it promotes circulation, encourages nutrition, and reduces stress. Good eating habits that provide a variety of nutrition following the food pyramid guidelines help keep energy levels at a maximum. Getting enough rest according to individual needs gives the body time to restore strength and vitality.

The body also has specialized defense mechanisms. The respiratory tract contains hairlike cilia that filter out invading pathogens. Coughing and sneezing are reflexes to rid the body of invaders. Body secretions, such as tears, sweat, urine, and mucous, also wash pathogens from the body. These body secretions have a low *pH*, which discourages bacterial growth. Hydrochloric acid with its low *pH* discourages the growth of pathogens in the digestive tract.

In the effort to prevent disease transmission, it is helpful to have an idea of what you are trying to prevent. All living organisms have requirements to sustain life and for growth and development. These requirements are oxygen, proper *pH* and temperature (98.6°F), nutrients, water, and a host to inhabit. Because microorganisms cannot be seen with the naked eye, a brief description follows of the disease-producing microbes, which are **viruses, bacteria, protozoa, fungi,** and **parasites**.

■ Bacteria are microorganisms that vary in their **morphology**. These single-celled microorganisms are differ-

ent from all other organisms because they lack a nucleus and organelles (mitrochondria, chloroplasts, and lysosomes). Bacteria reproduce by cell division approximately every 20 minutes. Figure 12–15 shows the various forms of bacteria. Many different species of bacteria are pathogenic to humans and animals. Some examples: *Escherichia coli* causes urinary tract infections (among other illnesses) in humans; *Bordetella pertussis* causes whooping cough, which is transmitted by droplet infection; and *Vibrio cholerae* causes cholera in humans who ingest contaminated food and water.

■ Viruses, which are the smallest of the microorganisms, may be viewed only by an electron microscope. Figure 12–16 shows a magnified view of a virus. Viruses can only reproduce themselves within a host. Commonly known viruses cause herpes, most childhood diseases, the common cold, and influenza.

■ Protozoa are complex single-celled microorganisms that attach themselves to other organisms (Figure 12–17). Amebic dysentery, malaria, and *Trichomonas vaginalis* are diseases caused by protozoa.

■ Fungi are simple parasitic plants (molds) that depend on other life forms for a nutritional source. They reproduce by budding. Multicellular fungi reproduce by spore formation. Approximately one hundred different types of fungi are common in humans; however, only 10 of these are pathogenic. Some examples of pathogenic fungus conditions are histoplasmosis, caused by *Histoplasma capsulatum,* and tinea pedis (athlete's foot) (Figure 12–18).

■ Parasites are organisms that depend on another living organism for nourishment. An **obligate** parasite is one that depends completely on its host for survival. Fac-

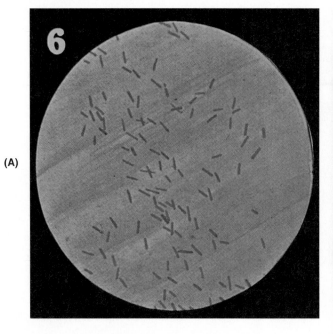

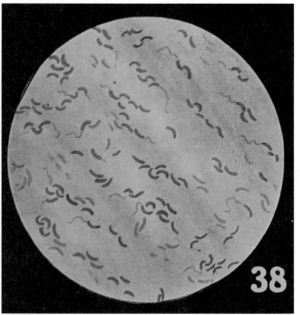

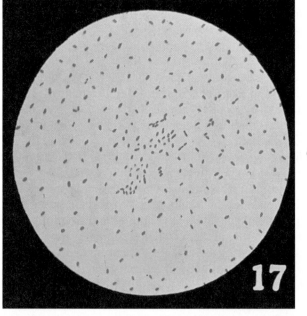

FIGURE 12–15   Bacterial forms: (A) *Escherichia coli;* (B) *Hemophilus pertussis;* (C) *Vibrio cholerae* (Courtesy of the Centers for Disease Control, Atlanta GA.)

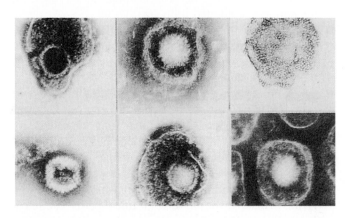

FIGURE 12–16   Electron micrographs of the various types of herpes simplex virus (Courtesy of the Centers for Disease Control, Atlanta GA.)

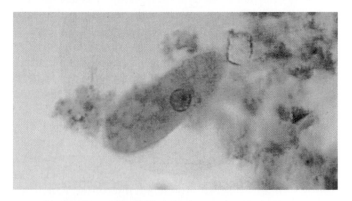

FIGURE 12–17   Intestinal protozoa *Entamoeba coli* (Courtesy of the Centers for Disease Control, Atlanta GA.)

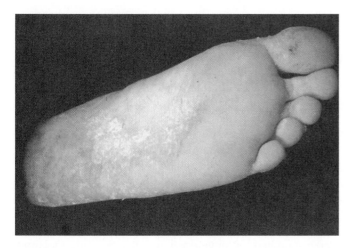

FIGURE 12–18   Ringworm of the foot (tinea pedis) (Courtesy of the Centers for Disease Control, Atlanta GA.)

ulative parasites are able to live independently from their hosts at times. Protozoa, mentioned earlier, are internal parasites because they live within the body of a human or an animal. *External parasites* are those that attach themselves on the outside of the body, such as fleas and ticks on animals. Humans are sometimes troubled with the itch mite (scabies), pinworms *(Enterobius vermicularis)* and hookworms *(ancylostomiasis)* (Figure 12–19). Other microorganisms are helpful and necessary to normal **flora** in humans and animals because they provide a balance in the body and destroy pathogens. Normal flora is the cohabitation of microorganisms (non-pathogenic and pathogenic in balance) that live in or within an organism to provide a natural immunity against certain infections. Infection occurs when this balance is disturbed.

Microorganisms that feed on **organic** matter are called **heterotrophs**; those that feed on **inorganic** matter are called **autotrophs**. Those that need oxygen to grow are

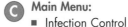

FIGURE 12–19   Strongyloides—filariform larvae of hookworm and strongyloides (Courtesy of the Centers for Disease Control, Atlanta GA.)

called **aerobes**, and those that grow best in the absence of oxygen are called **anaerobes**. Microorganisms grow best at the average body temperature (98.6°F or 37°C). The human body has not only a desirable temperature for microbial growth, but also furnishes darkness and moisture, other growth requirements. In addition, the body has a 6.0 average *p*H, which is an acidic level high enough to protect the body from microorganism invasion. If the *p*H level is higher, it indicates that microbial growth is present. As bacteria grow and multiply, the *p*H level becomes higher in alkalinity. A low *p*H reading, one less than 6, can be the result of not eating for a long period or ketosis. An environment that is too acidic will not support microbial growth.

Disease begins when a pathogen finds a body (a host) that offers it the conditions necessary for growth. Microorganisms, in the proper growth environment, can be extremely **virulent**, particularly for **debilitated**, aged, or young vulnerable patients. When the microorganism has reached the stage of causing an infection, the patient should take precautions against transmitting it to another. **Confinement** is the best way, but many patients insist on taking their colds and flu to work or play, thereby infecting others. The next step in the cycle, then, is transmission to another person by way of body openings. The microorganisms leave the host through the discharge of body secretions and make either direct or indirect contact with another host. When a patient with a cold coughs or sneezes, the vapor contains the microorganism that is causing the infection. The vapor may be projected through the air as far as 20 feet, and someone else may breathe in that microorganism. The growth requirement is then met by a susceptible host, one whose body resistance is low because of poor nutritional habits or poor hygiene.

INFECTION CONTROL

Ⓒ   Main Menu:
  ■ Infection Control
  Skills Menu:
  ■ Removing Contaminated Items

To diminish the spread of pathogens in the medical facility, there are three methods that are recommended in addition to the Standard Precautions. They are **sanitization**, **disinfection**, and **sterilization**.

Sanitization is the process of washing and scrubbing to remove materials such as body tissue, blood, or other body fluids. Again, hand washing is the number one step for sanitizing the hands. You should wear latex or vinyl gloves (double-glove as necessary). It is an additional recommendation that utility gloves be worn during the process of sanitization of items and equipment to protect your hands from any possibility of contamination and injury from the articles that you handle. Items should be rinsed in cool water, soaked in a warm detergent solution for generally 20 minutes, washed and scrubbed thoroughly with a brush, rinsed in warm to hot water to remove the detergent, and dried completely. During this process, the gloves also serve to protect your hands from the harshness of repeated contact with soap and water, which may result in chafing and cracking of the skin and possibly lead to infection. Remember to wash your hands before and after gloving. You should use a soothing hand lotion routinely to help prevent dryness caused from excessive hand washing.

Disinfection is a process by which disease-producing microorganisms, or pathogens, are killed. The term *disinfect* pertains to a chemical or physical means of destroying bacteria. It is sometimes referred to as a germicide or bactericide. There are many disinfectant solutions used in medical facilities. Common ones are zephrin chloride and chlorophenyl. Remember that disinfectants are used on objects, not on people. They are chemical solutions that must be changed often (depending on the frequency of use of the container) to ensure the effect intended. Always follow manufacturer's directions for time of exposure and how often to change the solution. Antiseptics are used in preparing the patient's skin for injection or a surgical or invasive procedure. The most commonly used antiseptics are alcohol and Betadine (povidone-iodine). The physical means of destroying pathogens is by intense heat. This is accomplished in a variety of ways which will be discussed later in this unit.

Sterilization is the process that destroys all forms of living organisms. Disinfectants and antiseptics do not always kill **spores**. Spores are thick-walled hard capsules formed by some bacteria when conditions for growth are good (Figure 12–20). When the proper growth conditions are present the bacteria break out of the capsule, grow, and multiply, starting infection. An example of bacteria that produce spores is *Clostridum tetani*, the cause of tetanus, or lock jaw. The only way to be sure that spores are eliminated is to sterilize them. Following the sterilization procedure, generally performed by **autoclaving**, the item remains sterile for 30 days if its packaging is kept dry and

intact. This period is referred to as **shelf life**. You should pay attention to the expiration date on all packages to ensure that the contents are sterile. Do not use any sterile package if it is beyond the expiration date (or more than 30 days from the time it was sterilized). If the package is labeled with just the date, it denotes when it was autoclaved. These sterile packages will remain sterile up to 30 days if they are still intact and have not been dampened. Autoclaved packages can also be labeled with "expiration date, 3-10-XX," which is the last date you could use the contents and be assured that they are sterile. If the packaging is torn or punctured, has signs of having been wet (water marks), or is wet, this is an indication that the sterility of the contents has been lost. Microorganisms can enter wrapped or enveloped articles through moisture. Give careful study and practice to the procedure of wrapping items for autoclaving within this unit.

CARE OF INSTRUMENTS

Processing items and instruments for use in procedures that are **invasive** is a vitally important responsibility. When handling any of the instruments or articles that need to be sanitized, disinfected, or prepared for sterilization, you should always wear gloves. This will protect you from becoming contaminated with any possible lingering microorganisms on the item. It will also protect the item from any possible contamination from your hands. Whenever you have a cold or the sniffles, you should glove and mask to avoid disease transmission. Never sneeze or cough on or over any items you are preparing for any procedure. Always follow Standard Precautions in performing procedures with patient contact.

Because there are microorganisms everywhere, the medical assistant should be ever mindful that pathogens could be present. Practicing proper handwashing and developing good habits is essential in disease control and eliminating the fear of contracting disease.

Many types of sterilization techniques are used in medical practice. The most common method is autoclaving. However, sharp instruments become dull from sterilizing by this method. Rubber or vinyl articles are damaged by intense heat of autoclaving. An alternative method for these items is to place them in a chemical disinfectant for at least 20 minutes. Sterilization requires that instruments remain in the disinfectant solution for 10 hours. All instruments must be thoroughly cleaned in a detergent (specifically for this purpose) before placing them into the disinfectant. A way to help prevent injury while cleaning instruments is to wear utility gloves. All instruments, including those with hinges and handles, should be cleaned with a brush and thoroughly dried to prevent diluting the disinfectant. The hinges and handles should be kept open to allow all parts to be exposed to the solution. A cover over the disinfectant container prevents the evaporation of the solution and keeps the vapor from being inhaled by members of the health care team. This disinfectant solution

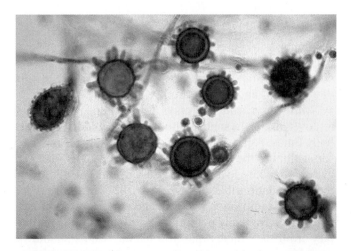

FIGURE 12–20 This picture shows the tough outer wall of spores, which explains their resistance to disinfectants. (Courtesy of the Centers for Disease Control, Atlanta GA.)

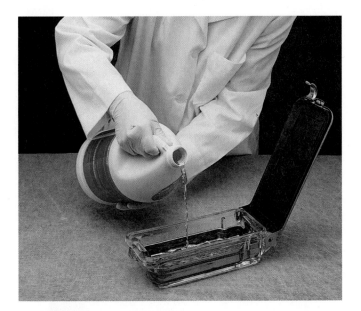

FIGURE 12-21 Chemical disinfectant solutions are used for aseptic control of sharp instruments (dulled by autoclaving) and other articles that can be damaged by the intense heat of autoclaving.

TABLE 12-2

STERILIZATION TIMES AND TEMPERATURES	
Articles	Time At 250° to 270°F (121° to 123°C)
Glassware: empty; inverted	15 minutes
Instruments: metal in covered or open tray; padded or unpadded	
Metal syringe cartridges	
Instruments: metal combined with other materials in covered and/or padded tray	20 minutes
Instruments wrapped in double-thickness muslin	
Dressings: wrapped in paper or muslin—small packs only	30 minutes
Silk, cotton, or nylon: wrapped in paper or muslin	
Treatment trays: wrapped in muslin or paper	

must completely cover the instruments to be effective. Follow the manufacturer's recommendations regarding disinfectant strength and proper disposal. The number of articles placed in this solution will determine how frequently it must be changed. Obviously, the more you use the solution for sterilizing items, the more often it needs to be changed. If this means of sterilizing instruments is only occasional, changing the solution once a week should be sufficient (Figure 12–21).

Autoclaving

Every medical practice should have an autoclave for sterilization of instruments by steam under pressure, which is a method that guarantees the destruction of spores. The manufacturer's instructions should be followed for the operation and care of the equipment. Instructions are usually printed either on top of the machine or on a tray that pulls out underneath it. It is important that the desired temperature of the sterilizer be maintained for the proper time. Table 12–2 lists the most commonly used articles and the desired times and temperatures for sterilization.

In the process of sterilization, the autoclave exerts approximately 15 pounds of steam pressure per square inch at a temperature between 250° and 270°F. The steam flows through the items and destroys all microorganisms and spores (Figure 12–22).

Articles to be autoclaved must be sanitized and then wrapped in a double thickness of paper or muslin. Envelope packaging is manufactured for some instruments, such as scissors (Figure 12–23). Figure 12–24 shows a medical assistant inserting an instrument into an envelope

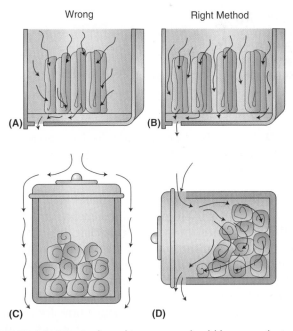

FIGURE 12-22 Packaged instruments should be properly spaced within the autoclave so that the steam can adequately penetrate each pack from all sides: (A) incorrect method of loading packages in autoclave and (B) correct method of loading packages in autoclave. When placing jars of dressings in the sterilizer, the jar should lay on its side with the cover loosely in place. This will allow the steam to flow freely through the jar and properly sterilize the dressings: (C) incorrect way and (D) correct way to place jar of dressings in the autoclave. (Courtesy of STERIS Corporation.)

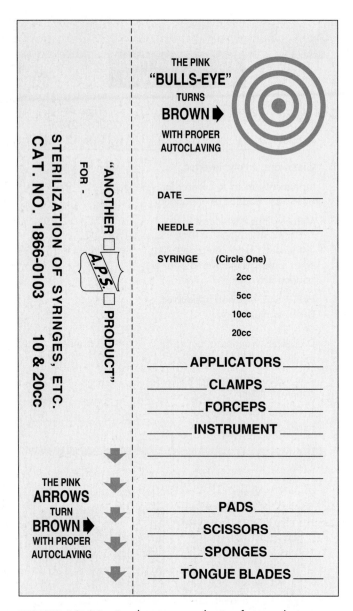

THE PINK
"BULLS-EYE"
TURNS
BROWN ➡
WITH PROPER
AUTOCLAVING

DATE _____

NEEDLE _____

SYRINGE   (Circle One)
2cc
5cc
10cc
20cc

_____ APPLICATORS _____
_____ CLAMPS _____
_____ FORCEPS _____
_____ INSTRUMENT _____

_____

_____ PADS _____
_____ SCISSORS _____
_____ SPONGES _____
_____ TONGUE BLADES _____

THE PINK
ARROWS
TURN
BROWN ➡
WITH PROPER
AUTOCLAVING

STERILIZATION OF SYRINGES, ETC.
CAT. NO. 1866-0103   10 & 20cc

FOR -   "ANOTHER ☐ A.P.S. ☐ PRODUCT"

FIGURE 12–23 Envelope-type packaging for autoclaving small or single items. Note the message about the color change to indicate that sterilization has taken place.

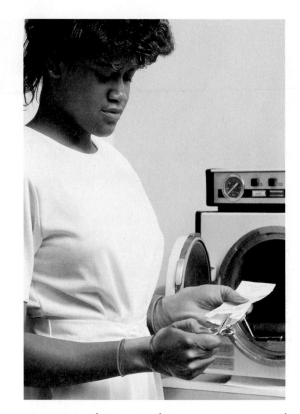

FIGURE 12–24 Placing a single instrument into an envelope package for autoclaving

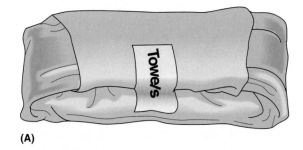

(A)

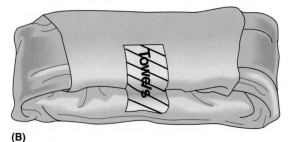

(B)

FIGURE 12–25 Package of towels: (A) before and (B) after autoclaving. Note the sterilized package has diagonal lines on the pressure-sensitive tape indicating that sterilization of contents was done correctly.

type of packaging in preparation for autoclaving. A section on the paper envelope permits recording the instrument name, the date, and the initials of the person who sterilized it. Sterilization indicators register proper and complete sterilization (Figure 12–25). Autoclave tape has an indicator stripe that changes color when the proper temperature has been maintained for a long enough time for sterilization to have taken place. The same principle applies to indicators placed inside the wrapped package. You should be aware that gas sterilizers and steam autoclaves require different indicator tapes. There are also envelopes for both types of sterilizers. The manufacturer can inform you of the proper indicator tape to use when you purchase a sterilizer or can tell you which one(s) to use with your present equipment. You should also clean the sterilizer routinely according to the manufacturer's recommendations.

Study the steps in Procedure 12–2 to learn how to properly wrap items for sterilization by autoclaving. Make sure that you do not put several items together unless they are separated by a gauze square. Items that are up against oth-

P R O C E D U R E

12-2 Wrap Items for Autoclave

PURPOSE: To wrap items to be autoclaved so that they will be protected from contamination after the sterilization process is completed for storage and handling.

EQUIPMENT: Muslin, autoclave paper, disposable paper bags, envelopes, autoclave tape, items to be sterilized or autoclaved, sterilization indicator, pen.

PERFORMANCE OBJECTIVE: Provided with several items, to be autoclaved or sterilized, the student will wrap each in autoclave paper or muslin, in preparation for the sterilization process. Each item must be wrapped neatly and snugly but not too tightly; the instructor and student will jointly determine if each wrapped item is suitable for autoclaving.

After the paper-wrapping procedure is demonstrated and checked, the paper should be removed from each item and discarded. The above-stated procedure will be repeated using muslin cloth. **(NOTE: When the muslin cloth wrapping procedure is completed, the muslin cloth is retained.)**

1. Wash hands and assemble all necessary items. **NOTE: Work in a clean area where there is sufficient work space.**

2. Check items for flaws and to make sure that they function properly. **NOTE: Items must be sanitized before wrapping for autoclave process. RATIONALE: Instruments must be working properly and materials must be in usable condition.**

3. Wrap item(s) in desired wrap so that there is a double thickness of protection. Make sure that there is no opening and seal with autoclave tape. Wrap item(s) snugly but not too tightly (Figure 12–26). **RATIONALE: Double thickness and complete enclosure prevent pathogenic entry as illustrated below.**

   NOTE: For envelope wrap, place item into envelope, seal, and label. Items suitable for envelope wrap include but are not limited to forceps, hemostats, needle holders, and towel clamps. All hinged instruments must be autoclaved open. RATIONALE: Sterilizing process must reach all parts of the instruments.

   Place spinal needles (small items) in glass test tube with cotton or gauze padding at bottom. Wrap autoclave tape around top to seal, with a pull tab for ease in opening. Label contents on a piece of tape secured to glass.

4. Make a tab for ease in opening wrapped packages after autoclaving by taping one to two inches of tape to itself at edge of package.

5. Label contents, write date and your initials on tape. **NOTE: Refer to Table 12–2 for proper time and temperature for items to be autoclaved.**

6. Return all items to proper storage area when finished.

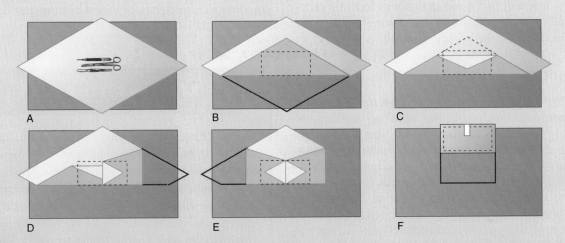

FIGURE 12–26 To wrap instruments or other items for autoclaving: (A) Place item(s) in center of wrap, (B) fold the material up from the bottom, (C) double back a small corner, (D) fold the right and then (E) left edges in again leaving corners doubled back, (F) fold the pack up from the bottom, and secure with pressure-sensitive tape.

ers during sterilization do not permit the steam to flow properly, and the items do not become sterile. Wrap each package snugly, but not too tight or too loose. If the package is too tight, the steam flow will not be able to get through the package or around each item sufficiently. Packages that are too loose or leave gaps could threaten the sterility of the contents, and they may even come apart. Allow adequate time for the packaging and contents to cool and dry before handling. Special care should be taken to avoid touching the autoclave while sterilization is in progress to avoid an accidental burn. It is a good practice to alert the staff when the sterilizer is operating so that they will also be cautious. When opening the autoclave door after the temperature and pressure are lowered, step to the side to avoid the possibility of a steam burn to the face and upper body. Being careless results in unfortunate injuries. Use caution with any type of sterilizer. You should leave the items in the autoclave with the door partially opened so that the packages can dry. If packs are touched before they are thoroughly dry, they are subject to become contaminated because microorganisms may enter through the wrap by the moisture.

Some offices or medical centers use the autoclaving service of a hospital. In this case, minimum cleaning is all that is necessary, for all items are properly sanitized before autoclaving.

All items, whether disposable or reusable, must be properly autoclaved. The sterilized disposables may then be discarded in proper receptacles without fear of transmitting disease. Blood and other body fluid specimens must also be sterilized before discarding.

Incineration

Another type of sterilization is by flame. This is a method for completely destroying disposable items by **incineration**. Items that will be treated in this way must be properly bagged for the procedure so that anyone handling the contaminated articles will not be affected.

Dry Heat Oven

Still another method of sterilization is the *dry heat oven.* Instruments with sharp blades, such as scissors or scalpels, are sometimes sterilized in this way. It is not the most desirable sterilization method because it is time-consuming. The process takes one to two hours at a temperature of 350°F, depending on the article. It is *not* a way to sterilize items made of rubber. For rubber articles, thorough washing and rinsing is the first step in preparing them for reuse. They must be completely dry before being placed in a disinfectant for chemical sterilization. Spores may still be a threat with this method. Finally, in every medical practice the policy of the establishment must be followed.

Many companies provide this service for medical facilities with large volumes. They supply containers in various sizes for disposables and schedule periodic pickup of these biohazardous items to take back to the

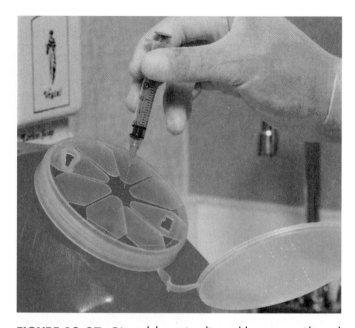

FIGURE 12–27 Discard the entire disposable syringe with used needle intact into the biohazard sharps container. The lid should be tightly affixed only when the container is three-fourths full.

company for sterilization before discarding in general city trash dumps.

Any disposable items, such as needles (never recap), scalpels, suture removal forceps, and scissors, must be placed in the sharps container for company sterilization (Figure 12–27) or wrapped and sterilized before discarding in a general trash receptacle.

ACHIEVE UNIT OBJECTIVES

Complete Chapter 12, Unit 2, in the workbook to help you obtain competency of this subject matter.

RELATING TO ABHES

Chapter 12 discussed the general considerations necessary to provide a clean, orderly, and safe office environment and the procedures known as Standard Precautions to prevent transmission of organisms. This content is related to the ABHES accreditation requirements of *Study of diseases and etiology* within the content area of **Anatomy and Physiology;** *Medical asepsis/sterilization and minor office surgery* and *Universal precautions in the medical office* within the content area of **Medical Office Clinical Procedures;** and *HIV/AIDS and blood borne pathogens* and *OSHA compliance rules and regulations* within the content area of **Medical Laboratory Procedures.**

Medical-Legal-Ethical Scenario

Ella was in a hurry when she took care of the last patient. She was trying to help catch up because they were so far behind schedule. The patient presented herself with a very sore throat and had a fever of 102°F. Ella prepared her to see the doctor. The doctor ordered a CBC (Complete Blood Count) and a nasopharyngeal culture because strep is suspected. Ella was rushing, so she did not wear gloves when she took the culture. Immediately after Ella withdrew the sterile swab from the patient's throat, the patient sneezed on Ella's hand. She hurried and only rinsed her hands to remove the discharge from her hand so that she could clean up the room and bring another patient back. Her nose was itching, and she rubbed it with the back of her contaminated hand. Ella then wrote out the CBC order and handed it to the patient who then handed it to the phlebotomist.

CRITICAL THINKING CHALLENGE

1. What is being jeopardized here?
2. What gain is there in rushing through your work?
3. Is Ella likely to contract what the patient has?
4. Who else is being subjected to becoming sick?
5. What should she have done?
6. Should Ella be reprimanded?
7. How do you think the patient felt?
8. Would you like to have Ella as your medical assistant if you get sick? Why or why not?

RESOURCES

Garza, D., and Becan-McBride (1989). Phlebotomy handbook (2nd ed.). East Norwalk, CT: Appleton and Lange.

Groust-Lakomia, L., and Fong, E. (1999). Microbiology for health careers (6th ed.). Clifton Park, NY: Delmar Learning.

Guidelines for prevention of transmission of human immunodeficiency virus and hepatitis B virus to health-care and public-safety workers (1989). *Morbidity and Mortality Weekly Report, 38*(S-6).

Miller, B.F., and Keane, C.B. (1992). Encyclopedia and dictionary medicine and allied health (5th ed.). Philadelphia: W.B. Saunders.

Mosby's medical & nursing dictionary (4th ed.). (1994). St. Louis: Mosby.

Nurse's ready reference diagnostic tests (1991). Springhouse, PA: Springhouse.

Raphael, S.S. (1983). Lynch's medical laboratory technology (4th ed.). Windsor, Ontario: W.B. Saunders.

Taber, C.W. (1997). Taber's cyclopedic medical dictionary (18th ed.). Philadelphia: F.A. Davis.

Ware, B.E. (June 1991). CLIA '88 physicians office laboratory, are you ready?

WEB LINKS   http://www.cdc.gov (Centers for Disease Control and Prevention)
Provides information on disease control and prevention.

13

Beginning the Patient's Record

Establishing an accurate database is a most important duty. When you assist the physician in collection of vital information about patients, you must keep in mind that patients have feelings and empathy is essential in your communication with them. Realize that some patients may be seeing a physician for the first time or may have fear and anxiety about what the outcome of their visit might be. Even though you must be efficient and use your time well to help patient flow run smoothly, patient care should not be rushed. Every effort should be made to treat each patient as an individual. Gaining the patient's trust will yield better compliance in treatment.

Accuracy is extremely important in recording information and in establishing the patient's record. You will learn to assist with beginning the database in the following text. You will also gain a better understanding of how valuable you can be to both physician and patient as a medical assistant, a most versatile health care team member.

UNIT 1

Medical History

OBJECTIVES

Upon completion of the unit, meet the following performance objectives by verifying knowledge of the facts and principles presented through oral and written communication at a level deemed competent. Demonstrate the specific behaviors as identified in the performance objectives of the procedures, observing all aseptic and safety precautions in accordance with health care standards.

1. Spell and define, using the glossary at the back of the text, all the **Words to Know** in this unit.
2. Complete a medical history form.
3. Describe the parts of a medical history form.
4. List the guidelines in regard to patient education.
5. Measure and record height of patients accurately.
6. Weigh patients and record accurately.

WORDS TO KNOW

abnormalities *persm, thg or cond ≠ norman*
adequate - *sufficient.*
elicit - *draw out, derive*
irrelevant *not imp to matter @ hand*
over the counter (OTC) *av. aid s Rx*

patronize - *"Honey" etc.*
remedy - *relieves/cures diseas*
stature - *height*
symptoms - *perceptible Δ that indicates disease*

AREAS OF COMPETENCE (AAMA)

This unit addresses content within the areas of *Administrative procedures, Fundamental principles, Patient care, Professionalism, Communication skills, Legal concepts, Instruction,* and *Operational functions*, as identified in the Medical Assistant Role Delineation Study. Refer to Appendix A for a detailed listing of the areas.

PATIENT'S MEDICAL HISTORY

Information needed for administrative purposes is obtained from the patient by the medical assistant in the receptionist's role. If the patient has a hearing or visual impairment or any other type of disability, be sure to address the patient and not the person providing assistance to the patient. This is also true when an interpreter (for those who are hearing impaired or who speak a different language) is relating to the patient instructions and all general information. The clinical medical assistant then escorts the patient to a private area away from distractions to assist the patient in completing the medical history form. Keeping the patient out of earshot of others will allow the patient to answer personal questions without stress. It is up to you to reassure and put the patient at ease.

It is a common practice to ask the patient to fill out this form, but most patients will appreciate help because of terminology they may not understand or the manner in which questions are asked. In some cases, the patient may be too ill or lacking in basic reading skills and will obviously need assistance. Assistance should always be offered but not insisted on. In some practices, the medical history and patient information forms are mailed to a new patient before the initial visit. This is a most convenient practice because it not only gives patients **adequate** time to gather all the necessary information about their health history, it helps with keeping the medical office on schedule by eliminating unnecessary time in completing the sometimes lengthy form during the appointment.

This completed medical history provides the physician with vital information to assist in making decisions about the diagnosis and course of treatment for the patient. Thereafter, when the patient comes in for an appointment, this data may be used again as an essential reference in that patient's health care plan (see Procedure 13–1).

The following terms are found on most medical history forms.

- Chief Complaint (CC)—Gives a description of why the patient has come to seek medical attention. Asking an open-ended question (e.g., "What brings you here to see the doctor today?") will **elicit** an answer that will furnish you with the main reason for the office/clinic visit. The response to your question from the patient should be in quotation marks. The following are examples (you should ask the length of time that the patient has had the complaint, and it should then be added if the patient does not include it when responding to your question).
  CC—*"I think I have the flu."* (past 3 days)
  CC—*"I have pain when I urinate."* (2 days' duration)
  CC—*"I fell and twisted my left ankle this morning."*
  It is recommended that you write exactly what the patient complains of in the patient's own words. If there are several chief complaints, you should make a list of the **symptoms**.

  If the patient has no complaints or symptoms to list and has an appointment to see the physician for a checkup or a report of a physical examination or consultation, that should be noted on the chart as well. Examples of charting other reasons for appointments are as follows:
  Patient states he is here for a physical examination, no complaints.
  Patient says she is here for annual Pap test, no physical complaints.
  Patient said this visit is for routine checkup; feels fine.
- Present Illness (PI)—A detailed description of the patient's chief complaint, including what the patient has

PATIENT EDUCATION

Patient education is a primary function of the medical assistant. Most patients are not trained health professionals and are somewhat confused by medical terminology, tests, procedures, and medications they encounter. Therefore, patient education becomes an important part of their medical care.

Whenever possible, the patient should be involved in making decisions about treatment or care. This will encourage the patient to participate more fully in the procedure. Patients will be more willing to cooperate if they understand the necessity for a particular procedure or treatment. Your careful and clear explanations of these procedures will encourage the patient to be more cooperative. If patients sense that you are truly concerned about their well-being, this will motivate them to comply. Always offer encouragement and praise where appropriate, even for the smallest accomplishment.

To properly instruct a patient, the medical assistant must know the material. Be prepared to answer any questions from the patient. If you cannot answer one of the patient's questions, tell the patient that you do not know the answer but will ask the physician. Never try to answer a question that you are not prepared to discuss. You could give incorrect information that could harm the patient's well-being. Never give information that is beyond your scope of practice.

In teaching a patient about health care and all that is involved in medical well-being, the primary goal of the medical assistant should be good communication. This means that each patient must be treated as an individual with particular needs. As the patient educator, you will have to meet these needs. You must communicate in the most efficient and effective manner for each individual. Listening is vital to this education. Patients may be shy or embarrassed by their problems or questions and may not ask direct questions. Therefore, you must listen carefully to the patient's comments and questions. Be familiar with information about the patient before proceeding with an explanation. This will help determine how to communicate best with each individual.

Never assume that a patient already knows the information you are conveying. Sometimes a patient will state that he understands something to keep from being embarrassed. If you sense that this is the situation, you should briefly repeat the information and provide printed material for the patient to take home to read. Printed materials, such as one-page handouts, brochures, pamphlets, and booklets on various procedures, examinations, diseases, conditions, and treatment plans, should be clear and concise in content. These informative materials should be appropriately distributed routinely to patients.

One very important aspect of patient teaching is your attitude toward the patient. The medical assistant must be open when approaching patients. This means that you must accept each patient as an individual who needs your help. There is no room in the medical office for prejudice. All patients should be treated with respect regardless of their financial status, race, religion, age, or station in life. Remember, your job is to provide assistance. Calling patients by pet names (e.g., Honey, Hon, and Dear) may be taken as **patronizing**, especially if your attitude is questionable. It is more respectful to patients if you call them by their titles (i.e., Mr. or Ms.) or their full names as you call them in for the appointment. The patient will let you know if a first-name basis is all right with her. If the patients sense any negative feelings on your part, then they will be less likely to pay attention to your instructions and suggestions.

Most patients are interested in getting better and staying healthy. Patient education involves not only instructing those who are sick but helping healthy patients stay well. By following current trends in wellness and prevention of medical problems, you can help patients help themselves to a healthier life.

The following are some general guidelines for patient education: _Know !_

1. Become familiar with your office's or clinic's policy concerning patient care.
2. Thoroughly read all handout information given to patients to explain procedures, examinations, or treatment plans so that you can intelligently answer patients' questions.
3. Make yourself available to patients for answering questions. Always remember to ask patients if they have any questions about their treatment or diagnosis.
4. Always take the opportunity to explain procedures to patients and offer additional information, when appropriate, at the time of their visits. For example, be sure to explain warmup and stretching exercises to the weekend athlete with a sprained ankle.
5. Attend continuing education programs to keep abreast of the latest medical information to pass on to patients.
6. Post charts, posters, and other information that will benefit the patient. Be sure that this information is kept current and is posted in areas where patients may spend time waiting.
7. Have current health-conscious magazines available in the reception area.
8. Post meeting times and information for patient support groups (weight control groups, stop smoking groups, tough love meetings) and encourage their participation. Keep this information current.

P R O C E D U R E

13-1   Interview Patient to Complete Medical History Form

PURPOSE: To obtain important information about the patient in assessment and plan of the treatment and total care of the patient.

EQUIPMENT: Medical history form, clipboard, pen (black and red ink).

PERFORMANCE OBJECTIVE: Using copies of the medical history forms included in this text and a pen (blue/black ink), obtain and record a medical history from another student within a set time as specified by the instructor. *All* items should be appropriately marked. **(NOTE: the only exception to this is in items the instructor has specified that only the physician should complete.)**

1. Assemble clipboard, medical history form, and pen.

2. Escort patient to private area where you can both sit comfortably.

3. Sit opposite patient. **RATIONALE: Facing the patient allows you to establish eye contact.**

4. Ask patient necessary questions, and record answers neatly and accurately.
   NOTE:
   - Speak in a clear and distinct voice so that the patient can easily understand you.
   - Give the patient time to answer before going on to the next question.
   - Explain any terms that the patient may not understand. **RATIONALE: Patients cannot give correct answers to inquiries they do not understand.**
   - Avoid getting off the subject. **RATIONALE: This is inappropriate, nonprofessional, and wastes time unless it is obvious that the patient needs to vent feelings.**

   - Because the AIDS and hepatitis B viruses and other dangerous diseases have been made apparent as a serious threat to health, additional questions must be asked concerning any history of IV drug use and the patient's sexual activity to determine if further investigation should be made about the health status of that patient. This is a delicate subject and must be handled with the greatest degree of tact and diplomacy.

5. Forms have spaces to make check marks or write in answers. If further explanation is needed, use section for comments. If there is not an appropriate space to enter information, write a note on a separate sheet of paper to alert physician. For example, a recent death in the family or loss of a job are stress-inducing situations that could influence care and treatment of patient. Patients do not always mention these types of problems to the physician because the patient may think they are irrelevant.

6. You may be instructed to make certain notations about a patient's medical history in red ink to alert physician. **RATIONALE: The patient's chief complaint should be obvious to the physician before entering the examination room.**

7. When finished with the form, thank the patient and explain the next step in examination. Ask if the patient needs to use the restroom, and if a urinalysis is to be performed as a part of the physical examination, obtain a urine specimen at this time. **RATIONALE: Having the patient empty the bladder helps to make the examination more successful and more comfortable for the patient.** Make the patient comfortable and explain if there will be a wait.

8. Gather all necessary forms into the patient's permanent chart, and give it to the physician to use during the examination.

---

done for the symptoms, if it has helped or not, how long it has been since the symptoms first occurred, and if the patient has ever experienced the symptoms before. Any medications the patient is taking to relieve the symptoms should be listed, whether prescription, **over the counter (OTC)**, or home **remedy**.

- Review of Systems (ROS)—A systematic review of all body systems to detect any problems the patient may not yet be aware of.
- Past History (PH) or Past Medical History (PMH)— Includes Usual Childhood Diseases (UCHD), major

illnesses (including mental health), surgeries, allergies, injuries, immunizations, and medications that the patient has taken, past and present.

- Family History (FH)—Past and present health of the patient's biological mother, father, and siblings; if they are deceased, the cause and their age at the time.
- Personal/Sociocultural History (PSH)—Refers to a profile of the patient's personal life history. It includes the patient's self-concept, role relationships, coping patterns, and life-style. Risk factors are also identified. This is most helpful to the physician in planning treat-

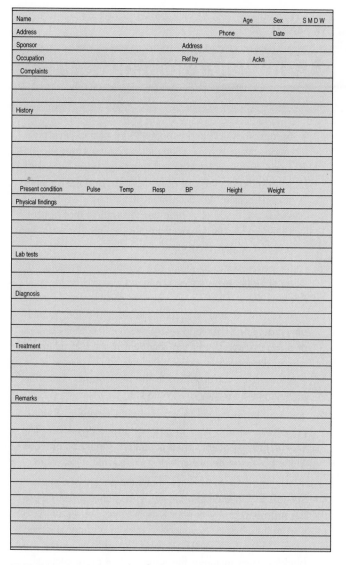

Name							Age	Sex	S M D W
Address						Phone		Date	
Sponsor					Address				
Occupation					Ref by		Ackn		
Complaints									
History									
Present condition	Pulse	Temp	Resp	BP		Height	Weight		
Physical findings									
Lab tests									
Diagnosis									
Treatment									
Remarks									

FIGURE 13–1 Example of a basic (general) medical history form

ment programs for patients. (Confidentiality must be practiced in regard to the information disclosed by patients to all health care professionals.)

Medical history forms vary with the type of practice. Some forms are short; others are quite extensive and time-consuming (Figures 13–1 and 13–2). Another concept of recording a family health history is by using the genogram (Figure 13–3). This method shows a diagram of the family's medical history over several generations. Most genograms include at least three generations. This is most helpful to the physician in reviewing the patient's chances of developing particular hereditary diseases. The diagram makes it easy to check the family history at a glance to detect genetic tendencies. Specialized printing companies can assist in designing a form for a particular practice. Forms may be color coded for easy identification.

A CAAHEP CONNECTION

Throughout this unit, discussion and instruction is provided in gathering information regarding patients to provide quality care. **Communication skills** and **Patient care** are included in instruction. Accuracy in obtaining and recording patient measurements is an important part of assessment of patients.

HEIGHT AND WEIGHT

Skills Menu:
- Weighing a Patient

The patient's height and weight must be recorded at the initial visit to serve as a reference point. Accuracy is important both in measuring and in recording this information (Procedures 13–2 and 13–3). Infants and small children should have height and weight measured and recorded routinely for growth and development patterns to be established. See Procedures in Chapter 14.

Because either the gaining or the losing of weight can change the course of a patient's diagnosis and treatment, proper balancing of the scales should be a routine practice to ensure accuracy.

Most physicians require that patients are weighed routinely at each visit. Measuring the height of patients should be done periodically after age 18 because of certain degenerative conditions and anatomical changes of the body from aging. Patients are often weight conscious, so the remarks of the medical assistant should be positive ones, if any. A chart of desirable weight of men and women may be posted above the scale for patient education (Figure 13–4).

ACHIEVE UNIT OBJECTIVES

Complete Chapter 13, Unit 1, in the workbook to help you obtain competency of this subject matter.

UNIT 2
Triage

OBJECTIVES

Upon completion of the unit, meet the following performance objectives by verifying knowledge of the facts and principles presented through written and oral communication at a level deemed competent. Demonstrate the specific behaviors as identified in the performance objectives of the procedures, observing all aseptic and safety precautions in accordance with health care standards.

MEDICAL HISTORY FORM

Date _____

Patient's name _____

Age	Date of birth	Sex

Address	City	State	Zip code

Phone ( ) _____   E-Mail _____

Insurance company	Policy number

Place of employment	Address

Phone ( ) _____   Job responsibilities _____

Parent/Guardian if minor _____

Address	City	State	Zip code

Phone ( ) _____   E-Mail _____

Family History:

List family members: (mother, father, brothers, sisters, grandparents, etc.)—ages and health status (if deceased write their age at the time of their death and the cause). List allergies and/or any conditions or diseases they may have or have had, such as asthma, arthritis, tuberculosis, diabetes, cancer, heart disease, hypertension, kidney disease, mental illness, depression, or any other health problems that you know of in your family.

_____

_____

_____

Patient's Past History: Mark the boxes to the right either "yes" or "no" for the following questions:*

Do you ever have or have you ever had any of the following: **(yes) (no)**

SKIN

	(yes)	(no)
Rashes, hives, itching or other skin irritations	( )	( )

EYES, EARS, NOSE, THROAT

Headaches, dizziness, fainting	( )	( )
Blurred or impaired vision	( )	( )
Hearing loss or ringing in the ears	( )	( )
Discharge from eyes or ears	( )	( )
Sinus trouble/colds/allergies	( )	( )
Asthma or hay fever	( )	( )
Sore throats/hoarseness	( )	( )

CARDIOPULMONARY

Shortness of breath	( )	( )
Persistent cough or coughing up blood or other secretions	( )	( )
Chills and/or fever	( )	( )
Night sweats	( )	( )
Tuberculosis or exposed to TB	( )	( )
Scarlet fever or rheumatic fever	( )	( )

Chest pain	( )	( )
Heart palpitations or rapid heart-beat or pulse	( )	( )
High blood pressure	( )	( )
Swelling of hands and/or feet	( )	( )

GASTROINTESTINAL

Heartburn or indigestion	( )	( )
Nausea and/or vomiting	( )	( )
Loss of appetite	( )	( )
Belching or gas	( )	( )
Peptic ulcer, gallbladder, or liver disease	( )	( )
Yellow jaundice or hepatitis	( )	( )
Diarrhea or constipation	( )	( )
Dysentery	( )	( )
Rectal bleeding, hemorrhoids (piles)	( )	( )
Tarry or clay-colored stools	( )	( )

GLANDS

Weight gain or loss	( )	( )
Diabetes	( )	( )

Thyroid or goiter	( )	( )
Swollen glands	( )	( )

GENITOURINARY

Kidney disease or stones or Bright's disease	( )	( )
Painful, frequent, or urgent urination	( )	( )
Blood or pus in urine	( )	( )
Sexually transmitted disease (venereal disease)	( )	( )
Been sexually active with anyone who has AIDS or HIV or hepatitis	( )	( )

NEUROMUSCULAR

Problems with becoming tired and/or upset easily	( )	( )
Nervous breakdown/depression	( )	( )
Poliomyelitis (infantile paralysis)	( )	( )
Convulsions	( )	( )
Joint and/or muscular pain	( )	( )
Back pain or injury/osteomyelitis/rheumatism	( )	( )

Are you currently taking any medications?	Yes ( )	No ( )
If yes, please list them _____		
Have you ever had or been treated for cancer or any tumors?	( )	( )
Are you anemic or have you ever had to take iron medication?	( )	( )
Do you use tobacco?	( )	( )
What type? _____		
Do you use IV drugs or alcohol?	( )	( )

WOMEN ONLY

Painful menstrual periods	( )	( )
Pregnancy/abortion/miscarriage	( )	( )
Vaginal infection or discharge/abnormal bleeding	( )	( )

Last menstrual period _____

Birth control _____

List dates of all operations/surgeries, injuries, and illnesses that required hospitalization:

_____

_____

Did you ever receive benefits from a medical insurance claim due to illness or injury?	Yes ( )	No ( )
Were you ever rejected from the military or for employment?	( )	( )
Were you absent from school/work in the past 10 years because of illness or injury?	( )	( )
Did you ever file a workers' compensation claim?	( )	( )
Did you ever seek psychological or psychiatric treatment?	( )	( )

*Please use the back of this form to explain any "yes" answers. Thank you.

FIGURE 13–2   Example of a complex, in-depth medical history form

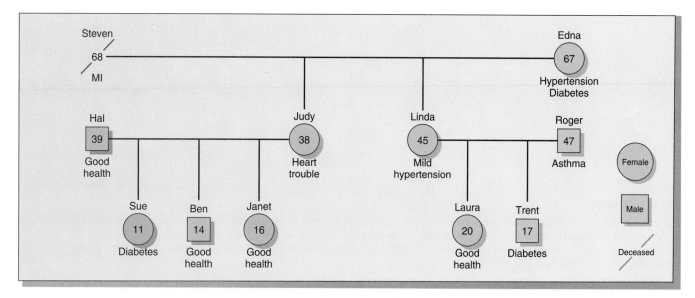

FIGURE 13–3   Example of a genogram tracing a family's medical history

PROCEDURE

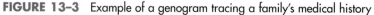

13-2   Measure Height

PURPOSE: To obtain an accurate measurement of a patient's height.

EQUIPMENT: Upright scale with extension measuring bar, patient's chart, pen (a measuring scale may be fixed to the wall).

PERFORMANCE OBJECTIVE: After the instructor has measured and recorded the height of all students, each student will, in turn, select five other students. Demonstrate on five other students each step in the height measurement procedure to determine the precise height of each of the other five students. The height measurements obtained should not be one-eighth of an inch more or less than the heights for those five students as measured and recorded by the instructor.

1. Raise measuring bar and extension higher than apparent height of patient. **RATIONALE: Avoids the possibility of striking the patient with the extension when it is raised.**

2. Ask patient to remove shoes. (Patients ready for physical exams will not have on shoes.) Place a paper towel on platform of scale. **RATIONALE: Accurate measurement cannot be obtained if shoes are worn. The paper towel provides a clean surface for the shoeless foot.**

3. Help patient onto scale facing you with his back to measuring device. Advise patient to stand erect (Figure 13–5).

4. Slide measuring bar down slowly and carefully to rest on top of patient's head, gently compressing hair. **NOTE: Measurement of height is from the top of the head, not the hair.**

5. Read measurement in inches or centimeters, and tell patient what it is.

6. Help patient down from scale. Tell patient to put shoes back on unless ready for physical exam.

7. Place measuring extension bar back in place, and discard paper towel.

8. Record height measurement on patient's chart.

CHARTING EXAMPLE:
5-12-XX
Ht. 5'8"

B. Hale, CMA (CL)

Note: Because there are insurance companies that require health care team members to sign after each order is performed as "B. Hale," the physician checks off the chart by writing his initials in parentheses to indicate that orders were completed as directed: (CL).

---

1. Spell and define, using the glossary at the back of this text, all the **Words to Know** in this unit.
2. Explain the origin of triage.
3. Explain the purpose of triage in today's medical office.

4. Name and describe the forms used to document patient information during return office visits.
5. Describe the types of questions that can be used during the interview to obtain pertinent information regarding a patient's condition.

PROCEDURE

13-3 Weigh Patient on Upright Scale

PURPOSE: To obtain an accurate measure of the patient's weight.

EQUIPMENT: Upright balance scales (Figure 13–6), patient's chart, pen.

PERFORMANCE OBJECTIVE: After the instructor has measured and recorded the weight of all students, each student will, in turn select five other students. Demonstrate on five other students each step in the weight measurement procedure to determine the accurate weight of each of the five students. The weight measurements obtained should one-fourth pound more or less than the weights for those five students as measured and recorded by the instructor.

1. Wash hands and balance scales.
2. Ask patient to remove shoes. *Some patients prefer to be weighed in a paper gown to give lowest weight.*
3. Place a paper towel on base of scale. **RATIONALE: Provides a clean surface for the shoeless foot.**
4. Help patient onto scale.
5. Make sure patient is in center of platform. Ask patient to stand still while you adjust balance and read weight (Fig-

ure 13–7). If you are to obtain both the height and weight of a patient, it is best to have the patient remain on the scales. Raise the bar by pushing it up with one hand and holding the extension of the bar with the other hand, protecting the patient from possible injury (the patient is still facing the measuring device). Refer to Step 4 of the Procedure 13–2 to complete.

6. Help patient from scale and discard paper towel.
7. Return scale to balance at zero.
8. Record weight on patient's chart. Be sure to record whether patient was wearing street clothing or gown.

CHARTING EXAMPLE:
5-12-XX
Wt. 147# (147 lbs) without shoes

B. Hale, CMA (CL)

NOTE: If patients are weighed with their clothes on, it is common to allow at least three pounds for women's clothing and five pounds for men's (according to office policy).

---

6. List the topics that should be covered each time a patient visits the office to see the physician.
7. List and explain the categories for determining the urgency of a patient's condition.
8. Discuss appropriate patient education during triage of patients.

◼ WORDS TO KNOW

carrel   prioritize
dispatch   triage

AREAS OF COMPETENCE (AAMA)

This unit addresses content within the specific competency areas of *Patient care, Professionalism, Communication skills,* and *Legal concepts,* as identified in the Medical Assistant Role Delineation Study. Refer to Appendix A for a detailed listing of the areas.

Triage is one of the most critical and significant of all the responsibilities you will perform as a medical assistant.

The term *triage* originated during war time. It referred to the sorting and assessment of soldiers' injuries. The French word *triage* means to sort. After the medics made a decision regarding the seriousness of the wounds, the soldier was **dispatched** as soon as possible for treatment. Those in charge of treatment had a clear description of the nature of the wounds from the initial triage. In addition, triage is a term also used in **prioritizing** the conditions of the injured following a disaster. The injured were separated into groups according to the seriousness of their needs. Usually they were tagged with a particular color-coded tape or cloth so that the other members of the emergency medical team would know which victims required immediate attention. The rules of first aid are that those who have difficulty with breathing are always taken first. Chest pain, severe bleeding, head injury, poisoning, open wounds of the chest and abdomen, shock, and second and third degree burns also should be given first priority. The conditions that should be considered next are major (and multiple) fractures, second degree burns (other than of the neck and face), back injury, and severe eye injuries. Conditions that are not life threatening, such as fractures, sprains, and minor injuries, can wait a short time.

MEN			
Height	Small	Medium	Large
5' 2"	128–134	131–141	138–150
5' 3"	130–136	133–143	140–153
5' 4"	132–138	135–145	142–156
5' 5"	134–140	137–148	144–160
5' 6"	136–142	139–151	146–164
5' 7"	138–146	142–154	149–168
5' 8"	140–148	145–157	152–172
5' 9"	142–151	148–160	155–176
5'10"	144–154	151–163	158–180
5'11"	146–157	154–166	161–184
6' 0"	149–160	157–170	164–188
6' 1"	152–164	160–174	168–192
6' 2"	155–168	164–178	172–197
6' 3"	158–172	167–182	176–202
6' 4"	162–176	171–187	181–207

WOMEN			
Height	Small	Medium	Large
4'10"	102–111	109–121	118–131
4'11"	103–113	111–123	120–134
5' 0"	104–115	113–126	122–137
5' 1"	106–118	115–129	125–140
5' 2"	108–121	118–132	128–143
5' 3"	111–124	121–135	131–147
5' 4"	114–127	124–138	134–151
5' 5"	117–130	127–141	137–155
5' 6"	120–133	130–144	140–159
5' 7"	123–136	133–147	143–163
5' 8"	128–139	138–150	146–167
5' 9"	129–142	139–153	149–170
5'10"	132–146	142–156	152–173
5'11"	135–148	145–159	155–176
6' 0"	138–151	148–162	158–179

FIGURE 13–4 Chart of desirable weights for men and women

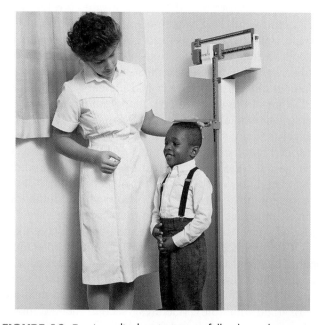

FIGURE 13–5 A medical assistant carefully places the measuring bar at the vertex of the head to obtain an accurate height of the child.

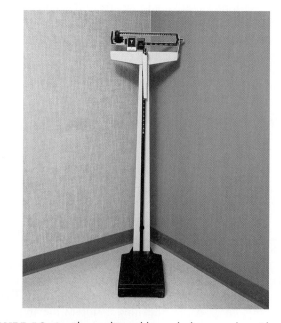

FIGURE 13–6 The traditional beam balance scales with measuring bar

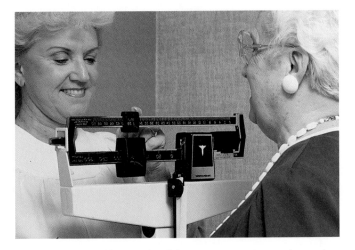

FIGURE 13-7 The weight of the patient may be read on either side of the scales.

It is during triage that one's symptoms are appraised and a judgment is made regarding the nature of the patient's complaints. Even though this is not the last word concerning her managed care, it is vital that the patient's immediate needs are met. All other problems should be listed in the order of their importance and severity.

The term has become common in medical facilities across the country. There are triage areas in emergency rooms, offices, and clinics. These areas are often set up as small **carrels** (Figure 13–8), to give some privacy to the patient during the interview. Why the patient is there to see the physician is determined by the medical assistant (or another qualified member of the health care team) who performs the triage interview. Initially, a decision is

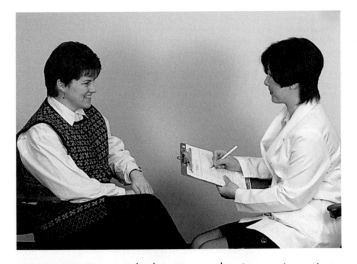

FIGURE 13-8 A medical assistant and patient are in a private area discussing symptoms and assessing the patient's condition. This is known as triage.

made and an appointment is given as the direct result of the information received by the medical assistant.

PHONE TRIAGE

Phone triage is assessing the patient's symptoms over the phone and responding in an appropriate manner. The assistant who speaks to patients over the phone must have knowledge of medical terminology, anatomy and physiology, diseases and disorders, emergency procedures, and medications; communication skills (especially listening); problem-solving and decision-making skills; compassion; self-control; patience; and understanding. Taking information regarding a patient's condition by phone requires careful listening and thorough questioning to ascertain the nature and the extent of the problem. In a medical office/clinic, the person who handles the phone and screens the calls is essentially at the heart of the practice. This person is usually the one who controls the schedule. Efficient patient flow and appointment schedules in the medical office are the result of the ability of the medical assistant's skill in phone triage. The anticipation of what examinations and/or procedures may have to be performed, how long it will most likely take, and the seriousness of the patient's condition are all vital. Timely communication with the rest of the health care team is essential in meeting the needs of the patients who must be worked into the schedule. If the nature of the patient's condition is too serious or complicated to be dealt with in your facility, this can and should be determined before the patient is advised to come in to be seen by the physician. A true life-threatening emergency should be referred to an emergency medical service (i.e., 911 where applicable) or to an emergency room for treatment.

The physician (and all office personnel) should have a written plan of action developed regarding telephone and face-to-face triage. The guidelines for prioritizing should follow those of first aid. All office personnel must be familiar with standard first aid procedures and cardiopulmonary resuscitation (CPR). Any changes in office policy should be communicated at the regularly scheduled weekly staff in-service meeting. Employees also need to have a printed copy of the revision noting any changes in policy with their initials by each one to show that they have been made aware of the changes.

FACE-TO-FACE TRIAGE

As patients come in for their appointments, information that pertains to their condition needs to be reviewed, confirmed, and documented. This data should be written in the patient's record on the progress notes sheet. Even if a notation is brief, but states how the patient is getting along, it is better than nothing at all. Their initial visit contains their medical history and any reports that were the result of the first visit. Each time the patient returns,

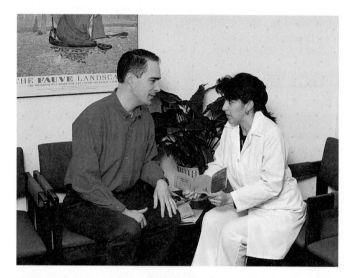

FIGURE 13-9 Patients comply with the instructions from the physician when they are given both orally and in written form.

additional information should be recorded. To obtain this information, the assistant should ask the patient open-ended questions, such as, "Tell me how you have been feeling since you were in last time to see the doctor," or "What brings you in to see the doctor today?" Open-ended questions need to be answered with a statement and cannot be answered with just a "yes" or "no."

While you are talking to the patient is a prime time to give patient education appropriate to his needs. For example, give those who complain of cold symptoms printed material about the respiratory system and advise them how to stay healthy by not smoking, eating sensibly, drinking plenty of fluids, getting enough rest, and exercising regularly. It is also a good time to ask patients if they have any further questions and encourage them to ask if and when they do have concerns. Advising patients to write down questions and subjects they wish to discuss with their doctor is especially helpful to patients who may be forgetful (Figure 13-9). Remember to include the companion (husband, wife, daughter, son, and so on) who accompanies the patient in the plan for the patient's treatment and follow-up care. Because the patient will have a caregiver, or someone who will look in on her, it is a standard practice to give printed instructions for care to help avoid any confusion. Supply the phone number where the physician (or other service provider the patient may need) can be reached at any time of the day or night. This reassurance will give the patient, caregiver, and family a more confident and secure feeling when in a time of stress and worry.

ACHIEVE UNIT OBJECTIVES

Complete Chapter 13, Unit 2, in the workbook to help you obtain competency of this subject matter.

A CAAHEP CONNECTION

This unit provides instruction in obtaining information from patients and prioritizing their needs. **Communication, Anatomy and physiology, Medical terminology, Medical law and ethics, Psychology,** and **Clinical procedures** are included in this information. Listening and accurate recording of information is vital to quality patient care.

UNIT 3
Vital Signs

OBJECTIVES

Upon completion of the unit, meet the following performance objectives by verifying knowledge of the facts and principles presented through oral and written communication at a level deemed competent. Demonstrate the specific behaviors as identified in the performance objectives of the procedures, observing all aseptic and safety precautions in accordance with health care standards.

1. Spell and define, using the glossary at the back of the text, all the **Words to Know** in this unit.
2. Identify the four vital signs and the body functions they measure.
3. Explain how the body controls temperature.
4. Describe the different designs of glass clinical thermometers and their appropriate uses.
5. Demonstrate the cleaning and storing of mercury thermometers.
6. Accurately measure oral, rectal, and axillary temperature with disposable, electronic, and infrared thermometers, identifying the normal temperature value and relative accuracy of each.
7. Explain situations when oral measurement is contraindicated.
8. Describe what causes pulse and why it can be felt; name and locate five pulse points.
9. Identify normal pulse rates and describe five factors that affect the rate.
10. Measure radial and apical pulse, and describe the quality characteristics to be observed.
11. Define pulse deficit, explaining its significance and how it is measured.
12. Measure respiration, identifying the normal rate and describing the quality characteristics to be observed.
13. Describe normal respiration, and explain four abnormal breathing patterns.

14. List the five circulatory factors reflected by the measurement of blood pressure.

15. Explain how the body maintains blood pressure.

16. Identify the phases of blood pressure, comparing them to the action of the heart.

17. Measure blood pressure by palpation and auscultation, explaining pulse pressure and normal findings.

18. Explain an auscultatory gap.

AREAS OF COMPETENCE (AAMA)

This unit addresses content within the specific competency areas of *Fundamental principles, Patient care, Legal concepts,* and *Communication skills,* as identified in the Medical Assistant Role Delineation Study. Refer to Appendix A for a detailed listing of the areas.

■ WORDS TO KNOW

afebrile	infrared
aneroid	inhale
antecubital	mercury
apex	oral
apical	orthostatic
apnea	palpate
arrhythmia	popliteal
aural	pulse
auscultate	pulse deficit
axillary	pulse pressure
blood pressure	pyrogen
brachial ← brady- .	radial
cardinal signs cardia	râles
carotid	rectal
Cheyne–Stokes	respiration
dorsalis pedis	rhythm
dyspnea	sphygmomanometer
essential	stethoscope
exhale	sublingual
fatal	temperature
febrile	thermometer
femoral	thready
groin	vital
hyperventilation	volume
idiopathic	

The term **cardinal signs** or **vital** signs is used by health care personnel to identify the measurement of body functions that are essential to life. The four vital indicators are **temperature, pulse, respiration,** and **blood pressure,** commonly referred to as TPR and B/P. They indicate the body's ability to control heat; the rate, volume, and rhythm of the heart; the rate and quality of breathing; and the force of the heart and condition of the blood vessels. The vital signs give the physician an assessment of the status of the brain, the autonomic nervous system, the heart, and the lungs.

The correct measurement of vital signs is extremely important. Proper technique and attention to details are essential. Findings should be recorded immediately following measurement to avoid a memory error. Always repeat the procedure if you think you may have made a mistake in measuring or recording. Occasionally, you may have a problem measuring a vital sign because of a patient's unusual physical condition that makes measurement difficult. Inform the physician of your problem and follow the course of action advised. Avoid alarming the patient. *Never* estimate the measurement. The physician's choice of treatment and medication is often based on the findings; therefore, they must be accurate.

TEMPERATURE

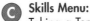
Skills Menu:
Taking a Temperature

The temperature of the body indicates the amount of heat produced by the activity of changing food into energy. The body loses heat through perspiration, breathing, and the elimination of body wastes. The balance between heat production and heat loss determines the body's temperature.

Conditions affecting body heat include metabolic rate, time of day, and amount of activity. Body temperature is usually lower in the morning following a period of rest. In the afternoon and evening, body temperature rises because of the heat produced by activity and the metabolism of food. These activities warm the blood that circulates through the body. "Normal" body temperature for an individual is that temperature at which his body systems function most effectively. Not all people have the same normal oral temperature. Refer to Table 13–1. An *average* normal oral temperature is 98.6°F (Fahrenheit) or 37°C (centigrade) (Figure 13–10). Normal oral temperature of patients may vary from 97.6° to 99.6°F. A person with a temperature above normal is said to be **febrile** or to have a temperature elevation. A person with a temperature which is normal or subnormal is said to be **afebrile**.

TABLE 13–1

TEMPERATURE VARIATIONS CONSIDERED "NORMAL"			
	Oral	Axillary	Rectal
Average Normal Temperature	98.6°F (37°C)	97.6°F (36.5°C)	99.6°F (37.5°C)
Range	97.6–99.6°F (36.5–37.5°C)	96.6–98.6°F (36–37°C)	98.6–100.6°F (37–38.1°C)

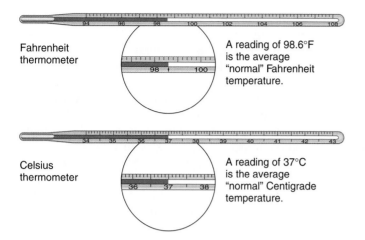

Fahrenheit thermometer

A reading of 98.6°F is the average "normal" Fahrenheit temperature.

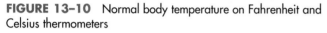

Celsius thermometer

A reading of 37°C is the average "normal" Centigrade temperature.

FIGURE 13–10 Normal body temperature on Fahrenheit and Celsius thermometers

Controlling Body Temperature

The temperature-regulating center in the body is located in the hypothalamus of the brain. The action of the hypothalamus can be compared to a thermostat that turns the furnace in your home off and on to keep the room temperature at the set number of degrees. As discussed previously, the brain, autonomic nervous system, blood vessels, and skin cooperate to regulate temperature. This is achieved through a feedback mechanism from temperature receptors. In the body, the hot and cold peripheral receptors in the skin send messages to the hypothalamus about the environment surrounding the body. Temperature receptors in the spinal cord, abdomen, and other internal structures send messages about the internal body temperature. One section of the hypothalamus also has many heat-sensitive neurons, which increase their output of impulses when temperature rises and decrease their output when it drops. The signals from this section of the hypothalamus merge with those received in another section, along with the internal and skin receptors, to evaluate the situation and send signals to control heat loss or heat production. Therefore, this central center is referred to as the *hypothalamic thermostat.*

The hypothalamic thermostat is very effective. When receptors sense the body is too warm, they send a message to the brain, which in turn acts on the sweat glands of the skin to produce moisture. The moisture evaporates from the skin's surface and cools the body. At the same time, nerve impulses are sent to the surface blood vessels to dilate, which brings more blood in contact with the surface of the skin. The blood gives up heat, which cools the blood within the vessels and therefore cools the body.

When the body senses coolness, the opposite activities occur. Surface blood vessels constrict to keep the blood away from the surface of the skin and prevent the loss of heat. Impulses to the sweat glands are stopped when temperature falls below normal. The small papillary muscles around the hair follicles contract, causing gooseflesh. Heat is produced by the activity of the papillary muscles, thereby helping to warm the body. In addition, a portion of

the hypothalamus becomes active when cold signals are received. Now hypothalamic messages are sent to skeletal muscles throughout the body, causing increased muscle tone that produces heat. When the muscle tone rises above a certain level, shivering results and heat production is raised dramatically. This is evident with an infectious process, such as influenza. Microorganisms cause the patient to experience chills and shivering until the temperature rises to warm the body and a fever develops.

During an infectious process, the presence of microorganisms cause **pyrogens** to be secreted, which raise the "set point" of the hypothalamic thermostat. Pyrogens are toxins from bacteria or a by-product of degenerating tissues. When the set point is higher than normal, the body's heat production and conservation processes are activated. Surface blood vessels constrict, causing the person to feel cold even though the temperature is above normal. No sweat is secreted. Increased white blood cell activity from fighting bacterial invasion also produces heat. Chills and shivering begin and continue until the temperature reaches the higher set point where the hypothalamus will continue to operate until the infectious process is reversed. Once this occurs, the hypothalamic thermostat is reset to a lower or normal value, and the body's temperature reduction process results in profuse sweating and a hot, red skin from general vasodilation. After this onset reaction, the temperature will begin to fall.

The extent of the infection determines the amount of heat (fever) generated. A mild infection may cause the temperature to rise to 100°F. A moderate infection may elevate the temperature to 102°F. Fevers are categorized by the degree of body heat as slight, moderate, severe,

TABLE 13-2

	CLASSIFICATION OF FEVERS	
	Fahrenheit	Celsius
Slight	99.6°–101.0°	37.5°–38.3°
Moderate	101.0°–102.0°	38.3°–38.8°
Severe	102.0°–104.0°	38.8°–40.0°
Dangerous	104.0°–105.0°	40.0°–40.5
Fatal	over 106.0°	41.1°

dangerous, or **fatal** (Table 13–2). Fatality-associated elevated temperature depends on the extent of time the fever is present. Fevers of short duration well above 106.0°F have not proved fatal, but immediate measures to reduce body temperature must be administered. Temperatures below normal are called subnormal. Collapse will occur at about 96.0°F, and death follows if temperature goes below 93.0°F except briefly.

Thermometer Types and Designs

Body temperature is measured by means of a **thermometer** in scales of Fahrenheit or the metric system equivalent, Celsius. Thermometers are of the following main types: glass **mercury**, also called clinical; disposable, in the form of plastic strips; self-contained digital; battery-operated electronic; and the most recent, a tympanic **infrared** thermometer. The mouth (**oral**), underarm (**axillary**), rectum (**rectal**), and ear (**aural** or tympanic membrane) may be

used to measure body temperature. The large variety of thermometers, each with its own advantages and disadvantages, allow for personal preference in equipment selection for the physician's office. Table 13–3 briefly outlines the main features for each type.

Glass mercury thermometers are of three designs to measure the temperature by oral, rectal, and axillary method (Figure 13–11). An oral thermometer has a long slender bulb to fit under the tongue. A rectal thermometer has a fat, rounded bulb that is stronger and safer to insert into the anus. An oral thermometer that is constructed with a rounded bulb is known as a stubby or security thermometer and is suitable for oral or axillary measurement. Many thermometers are further identifiable by a color-coded dot at the stem end. Blue indicates oral; red indicates rectal. Usually the word *oral* or *rectal* is inscribed on the stem.

It is extremely important that thermometers be used for their intended purpose. It is not safe to insert an oral thermometer into the rectum. The slender bulb may perforate

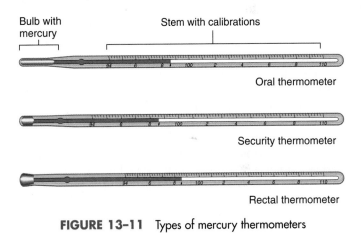

FIGURE 13-11 Types of mercury thermometers

TABLE 13-3

	COMPARISON OF THERMOMETER TYPES	
Type	Advantage	Disadvantage
Glass mercury	Accurate, inexpensive, familiar.	Slow, somewhat difficult to read, easily broken, requires cleaning and plastic cover.
Plastic disposable	Single use avoids cross-contamination, no cleaning, relatively fast.	Must protect from heat, somewhat unpleasant for patient, storage and inventory costs.
Digital	Quick, signals when registered, easily read, self-contained.	Moderate initial cost, plastic cover, and battery expenses.
Electronic probe	Quick, signals when registered, easily read, self-contained.	Fairly expensive, cumbersome cord, requires recharging, probe cover costs, may cause inaccurate readings if patient bites too hard on probe.
Tympanic infrared	Instant results, easily read, core temperature, individualized probe cover, eliminates mucous membrane concerns.	Expensive, probe cover costs, replacement battery costs. An improper seal in the ear canal, the presence of cerumen, or an infection of the middle ear, may cause inaccurate readings.

(puncture) the tissues, and it is more easily broken. Be equally careful that a rectal thermometer is *never* used to measure an oral temperature.

Reading a Mercury Thermometer and Recording Measurements

Clinical thermometers are slender glass rods with a hollow central cavity, extending from a bulb reservoir of mercury. The stem of the Fahrenheit thermometer is calibrated in even tenths (.2, .4, .6, .8) (Figure 13–12). The whole degrees are marked with long lines, but only the even-numbered degrees are printed on the thermometer. There is also a long line at 98.6°F with an arrow because this is the average normal body temperature when it is measured orally.

To view the numbers, lines, and column of mercury, hold the thermometer at eye level, between the thumb and index finger of the right hand, by the stem end only. Look directly at the edge of the glass triangle with the lines at the top and the numbers at the bottom. Rotate the stem slightly back and forth until you see the silver mercury column in the middle (Figure 13–13). The point where the mercury stops is read and recorded as the body temperature. When the mercury is between tenth markings, it is read to the next highest two tenths of a degree (Figure 13–14). Many thermometers have markings printed in blue below the normal arrow and in red above to make temperature identification easier.

It is extremely important that you not only read the thermometer accurately but that you also record the findings accurately. Remember that every line on a Fahrenheit thermometer represents two tenths of a degree. Note the difference between 100.2°F and 102.0°F, for example (Figure 13–15). When reporting verbally, 100.2° is referred to as "one hundred and two tenths" or "one hundred point two." A temperature of 102.0° is reported as "one hundred two" or "one hundred two point zero." It is good practice to read the thermometer and record the

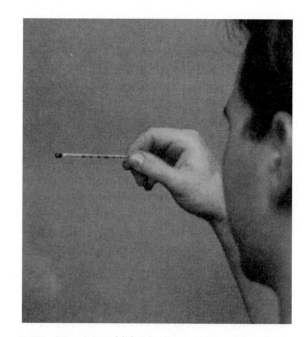

FIGURE 13–13 Hold the thermometer at eye level to read.

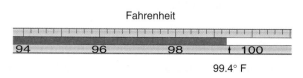

FIGURE 13–14 A temperature reading of 99.4°F. When the mercury is between the tenth markings, it is read to the next highest tenth.

temperature as soon as possible after measuring. After you have written it down, read the thermometer again and check what you wrote to be certain you are accurate. The implications of an error in reporting should be obvious.

CAUTION: Taking temperatures requires contact with mucous membranes in the mouth or rectum. Discussion and procedure descriptions will reflect Standard Precautions. In any clinical setting, it is advisable to eliminate cross-contamination to prevent the spread of disease-producing organisms that cause hepatitis, AIDS, and

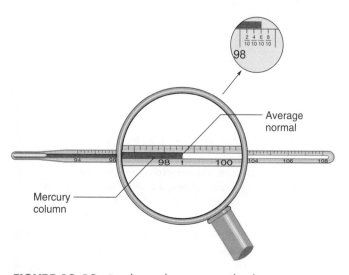

FIGURE 13–12 Reading a thermometer. This thermometer reads 98.6°F.

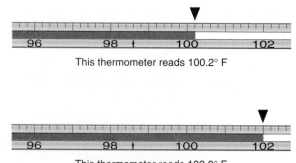

This thermometer reads 100.2° F

This thermometer reads 102.0° F

FIGURE 13–15 It is important to read and record temperature accurately.

many other transmittable diseases. Until a method of prevention or effective treatment is discovered, <u>EVERYONE</u> should be considered to be infected.

Care of Thermometers

Each time a temperature is taken, the thermometer must be cleaned and soaked in disinfectant. Even when covered with a plastic sheath, it is possible to accidentally contaminate the thermometer, depositing organisms on the bulb or stem. Glass mercury thermometers are extremely fragile, and care must be taken to prevent breakage.

When many thermometers are used daily, they will be processed in quantity. Each thermometer is cleaned and rinsed after use, then placed in a gauze-lined basin filled with disinfectant. Timing must begin after the last ther-

mometer is added. All thermometers must be completely covered by the disinfectant. The thermometers are then removed from the solution, rinsed, and inspected. They may be stored in a container, in individual dry storage, or placed in individual clean envelopes and stored in a drawer. Solution used in quantity disinfection is discarded after soaking time has elapsed.

A common container filled with disinfectant solution is not recommended. It is no longer considered safe to use an unsheathed thermometer even when it is cleaned after each use and returned to a solution-filled container. If such a common storage method is used, wipe the solution from the thermometer with a cotton ball, from the bulb to the stem, and discard cotton in a biohazardous container. Slip a sheath over the thermometer and continue as indicated in Procedure 13–4. Stop and think: Would *you* like

---

PROCEDURE

13-4 Clean and Store Mercury Thermometers

PURPOSE: To properly clean soiled clinical thermometers and store them for reuse. **NOTE: Oral and rectal thermometers are cleaned and disinfected separately.**

OSHA GUIDELINES: Standard Precautions require gloves to be worn if there is any possibility of coming into contact with blood, body fluids, or wound drainage. Biohazardous waste containers are required for disposal of soiled cotton balls and damaged mercury thermometers.

EQUIPMENT: Soiled clinical thermometers, cotton balls, soap or other cleanser, water, gloves, disinfectant, biohazardous waste container, soaking container, and storage equipment.

PERFORMANCE OBJECTIVE: Given soiled mercury thermometers and access to all necessary equipment and supplies, clean, inspect, disinfect, and store the thermometers aseptically in accordance with procedure technique and observing aseptic and safety precautions.

1. Wash hands and put on gloves.
2. Take soiled thermometers to sink.
3. Apply soap or other cleanser to cotton ball.
4. While holding thermometer by stem, rotate and wipe it from stem to bulb with soapy solution. **RATIONALE: Cleansing action forces soap into calibrations while working from clean to soiled area.**
5. Discard cotton ball in biohazardous waste container.
6. While holding by stem with bulb pointed downward, rinse thermometer in cool running water. **RATIONALE: Hot water will overexpand mercury and either damage or break thermometer.**

7. Inspect for cleanliness and condition. If still soiled, repeat steps 3 to 6. Discard a chipped or cracked thermometer in a sharps biohazardous waste container. **RATIONALE: A damaged thermometer is unsafe and may be inaccurate.**
8. Grasp stem firmly between thumb and index finger.
9. Shake mercury down to 95.0°F or below. **NOTE: Use a wrist-snapping action. Avoid striking faucet, sink, or counter. Remember, the mercury will not go down unless forced. RATIONALE: The next patient's temperature will not be measured accurately if it is LESS than the previously measured temperature.**
10. Place thermometers in gauze-lined container filled with disinfectant. **RATIONALE: Gauze aids in preventing breakage. NOTE: Thermometers must be completely covered and allowed to remain in solution for at least 20 minutes. If additional thermometers are added, timing must begin after last one is placed in the container.**
11. Using correct procedure, remove and discard gloves.
12. Wash hands.
13. Set timer or note time.
14. Following adequate time for disinfection, wash hands. Rinse, inspect, and place clean thermometers in individual envelopes, individual dry holders, or storage container. Remember that, if thermometers are stored in individual holders, place a cotton ball in the bottom to prevent breakage of the bulb.
15. Clean area and equipment. Return thermometers to appropriate locations.

to be your next patient? Remember your responsibility to others in stopping the threat of disease transmission. AIDS and hepatitis are very dangerous communicable diseases. Follow correct procedure each time you measure the temperature of any patient.

Slip-on Thermometer Sheaths

Clear plastic slip-on sheaths must be used when taking oral or rectal temperature with a glass thermometer. This narrow plastic cover slides over the thermometer like a loose skin. The covers come packaged in individualized narrow paper envelopes (Figure 13–16). The clean thermometer is inserted into the open end marked "insert." The opposite end is separated and peeled back, revealing the plastic cover. Peel back the envelope to the stem end, and snap off the tear tab. Check the cover to be certain it has remained intact before using. The thermometer is used exactly as if it were not covered. The covering is somewhat undesirable from the patient's viewpoint as it

is a rather strange feeling to have a "minibaggie" under one's tongue.

When the temperature has been measured, the cover is simply held by the tear tab, pulled off, and discarded in the biohazardous waste container. The design is such that the sheath inverts itself, thereby reducing the chance of contamination of the thermometer. The temperature is then read and recorded, and the thermometer cleaned, ready for use with the application of another sheath. A rectal thermometer *must* always be covered with a sheath and used only for rectal temperatures. It will require lubrication for ease of insertion. Some manufacturers of sheaths for rectal thermometers will package them prelubricated, however, you will need to inspect to be certain there is an adequate amount.

Measuring Oral Temperature

Measuring temperature orally is the method of choice because it is relatively convenient, quick, and accurate. The oral clinical thermometer is placed **sublingually** (under the tongue) and for a *minimum* of three minutes (Figure 13–17 and Procedure 13–5). (A study indicated that eight minutes are necessary to obtain the most accurate oral measurement.) Remember that a reading of 98.6°F or 37°C is considered normal.

A CAAHEP CONNECTION

Curriculum standards specify that program content in psychology be included in the program. Apply psychology techniques to assure the patient that covers are used for all mercury thermometers to be certain there is no chance of transferring any organisms so that he doesn't feel that you think he has a disease or is somehow not clean. The additional content in this chapter on asepsis and infection control is also a curriculum requirement.

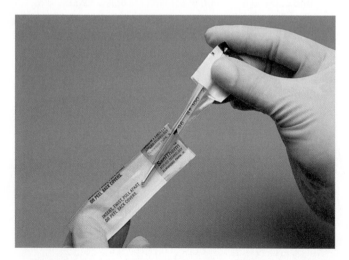

FIGURE 13–16 Slip-on disposable thermometer sheaths

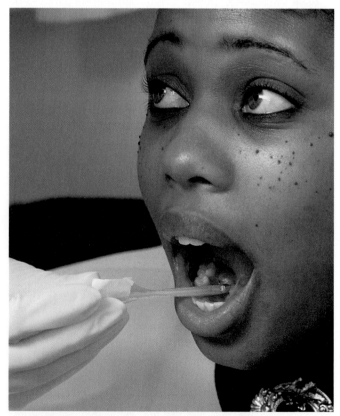

FIGURE 13–17 Place oral thermometer sublingually into a heat pocket.

PROCEDURE

13-5 Measure Oral Temperature with Mercury Thermometer

PURPOSE: To determine a patient's oral temperature using a clinical thermometer.

OSHA GUIDELINES: Standard Precautions require gloves to be worn if there is any possibility of coming into contact with blood, body fluids, or wound drainage. Biohazardous waste containers are required for discarding gloves, sheaths, and damaged mercury thermometers.

EQUIPMENT: Oral clinical/mercury thermometer, thermometer sheath, latex or vinyl gloves, biohazardous waste container, soiled thermometer container, watch or timer, paper, and pen or pencil.

PERFORMANCE OBJECTIVE: In a simulated or actual situation and given access to all necessary equipment and supplies, measure and record a patient's oral temperature. The procedure will be done within six minutes, following correct procedural technique and observing aseptic and safety precautions. The recorded findings must agree with the instructor's reading.

1. Wash hands; put on gloves.
2. Identify patient. **RATIONALE: Speaking to the patient by name and checking chart ensures that you are performing the procedure on the correct patient.**
3. Explain procedure.
4. Determine if patient has recently had a hot or cold drink or smoked. **NOTE: If so, allow 10 minutes before measuring. RATIONALE: Hot or cold substanes in the mouth prevent accurate temperature measurement.**
5. Remove thermometer from holder or envelope. Avoid touching bulb end with fingers. **RATIONALE: Bulb must be untouched because it is inserted into the patient's mouth.**
6. Inspect thermometer. Discard a chipped or cracked thermometer in a sharps biohazardous waste container. **RATIONALE: A damaged thermometer is unsafe and may be inaccurate.**

7. Read thermometer and shake down to 95°F or below. **RATIONALE: Temperature will not be measured accurately if LESS than the previously measured temperature.**
8. Put plastic sheath on thermometer. **NOTE: Check that sheath is intact. RATIONALE: Plastic sheaths protect against cross-contamination.**
9. Place bulb sublingually in patient's mouth. **NOTE: Take care not to probe sensitive sublingual tissues. Rationale: Heat pockets in the mouth are located sublingually (see Figure 13–18).**
10. Tell patient how to maintain proper position of thermometer: to keep lips closed, breathe through nose, and avoid biting.
11. Leave thermometer in position a minimum of three minutes. **NOTE: Time by watch or timer.**
12. Remove and read thermometer. **NOTE: Reinsert for additional minute if reading is less than 97.0°F.**
13. Reread thermometer.
14. Holding by stem end, pull off plastic sheath and discard in biohazardous waste container.
15. Follow procedure for soiled thermometers.
16. Remove gloves and discard in biohazardous waste container.
17. Wash hands.
18. Record temperature.
19. Follow procedure to clean thermometer, returning to storage when completed. **(NOTE: If greater accuracy is desired, adjust time and performance objective.)**

CHARTING EXAMPLE:
3-6-XX
T. 98.2

B. Davis (SEM)

Temperature readings will be inaccurate if the patient has smoked or had either a hot or cold drink within the previous 10 minutes. Always ask patients about this before placing the thermometer in their mouth. Tell them to keep the thermometer under their tongue with their lips closed around the stem. Readings will also be inaccurate if the patient breathes through the mouth. Caution the patient against biting down on the glass stem. It is possible to break the thermometer with the force of the teeth, cutting the tongue, gums, or inside of the mouth. The possible ingestion of glass fragments and poisonous mercury presents a real hazard.

Note: In temperature procedures, recording of findings is delayed until after gloves have been removed and hands washed. This is necessary to avoid contamination of pens/pencils, charts, and in turn yourself.

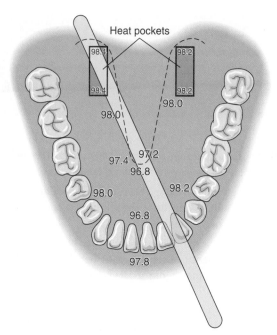

Heat pockets

FIGURE 13–18 Dot matrix portion of disposable thermometer must be placed sublingually into a heat pocket. (Courtesy 3M Health Care.)

FIGURE 13–19 Measuring rectal temperature of an infant.

Contraindications to Oral Measurement

Oral temperature measurement is not always the method of choice. Temperature must be measured by an axillary, a rectal, or a tympanic method in the following situations:

- infants and children under age six
- patients with respiratory complications that result in mouth breathing or use of supplemental oxygen
- confused, disoriented, or emotionally unstable patients
- patients with oral injuries
- patients with recent oral surgery
- patients with facial paralysis
- patients with nasal obstruction

Measuring Rectal Temperature

Rectal temperature is a very accurate measurement, simply because it is taken internally. Rectal measurement is appropriate with babies and young children who have not yet learned how to keep an oral thermometer in place or who might break it by biting down. Often children complain bitterly about having a rectal temperature taken when they think they are "too big." The physician usually has a policy concerning the age limit for rectal temperatures, which you will follow.

When measuring the temperature of infants, they may be positioned on the stomach or the back. If positioning on back, unfasten the diaper to expose the anus. Grasp the ankles securely with one hand, flexing the knees to the abdomen. With the other hand insert the lubricated sheathed thermometer about one inch through the anal

canal into the rectum. Hold the thermometer securely in place. Maintain your grasp on the ankles so the infant cannot turn over. Be prepared for the procedure to initiate urination or expelling of stool. It would be wise to cover the male infant's penis with a diaper to absorb the urine stream. When positioning prone across a person's lap or on a table, be certain to maintain control of the infant or child's position to prevent turning over and causing injury to the rectum from the inserted thermometer (Figure 13–19). In either position, the thermometer position can be maintained by holding it securely between the index and middle finger with the palm of the hand against the buttocks.

Older children can be positioned either on their abdomen or side, whichever is preferred. Adults would be positioned on their side and draped with a sheet for privacy.

Temperatures measured rectally require a minimum of three minutes insertion time (five minutes for greater accuracy). When recording a rectal measurement, place the letter *R* in parentheses following the reading. Normal rectal temperature is 99.6°F or 37.5°C, one full degree above normal oral temperature. Temperature must never be measured rectally if the patient has had recent rectal surgery. It is possible to damage the operative site or perforate newly sutured lines. See Procedure 13–6.

Measuring Axillary Temperature

Temperature can also be measured by placing the mercury thermometer in the axilla (armpit) (Figure 13–20). This method is the least accurate and requires a full 10 minutes. Axillary measurement is appropriate only when oral is contraindicated and rectal is inconvenient, undesirable, or contraindicated. An oral stubby or security design thermometer is best suited for axillary measurement. Normal axillary temperature is 97.6°F or 36.4°C, one full degree *below* normal oral temperature. When recording axillary findings, place the letters *Ax* in parentheses following the reading. See Procedure 13–7.

PROCEDURE

13-6 Measure Rectal Temperature with Mercury Thermometer

PURPOSE: To determine a patient's rectal temperature using a clinical thermometer. **NOTE: Rectal measurement may be indicated for an older child or adult when oral measurement is contraindicated.**

OSHA GUIDELINES: Standard Precautions require gloves to be worn if there is any possibility of coming into contact with blood, body fluids, or wound drainage. Biohazardous waste containers are required for discarding gloves, sheaths, and damaged mercury thermometers.

EQUIPMENT: Mannequin (if simulated), rectal clinical/mercury thermometer, thermometer sheath, drape (if adult), latex or vinyl gloves, lubricant, tissues, biohazardous waste container, soiled thermometer container, watch or timer, paper, and pen or pencil.

PERFORMANCE OBJECTIVE: In a simulated or actual situation and given access to all necessary equipment and supplies, measure and record a patient's rectal temperature. The procedure will be done within eight minutes, following correct procedural technique, and observing aseptic and safety precautions. The recorded findings must agree with the instructor's reading.

1. Wash hands and put on gloves.

2. Identify patient. **RATIONALE: Speaking to the patient by name and checking chart ensures that you are performing the procedure on the correct patient.**

3. Explain procedure and what you are going to do to child and parent or to adult patient.

4. Place a small amount of lubricant on a tissue. **NOTE: Lubricant should be water-soluble.**

5. Remove thermometer from holder or envelope. **NOTE: Hold by stem end only.**

6. Inspect thermometer. Discard a chipped or cracked thermometer in a sharps biohazardous waste container. **RATIONALE: A damaged thermometer is unsafe and may be inaccurate.**

7. Read thermometer and shake down to 95°F or below. **RATIONALE: Temperature will not be measured accurately if LESS than the previously measured temperature.**

8. Place thermometer in plastic sheath. Check that sheath is intact. **RATIONALE: Plastic sheaths protect against cross-contamination.**

9. Rotate thermometer bulb in lubricant on tissue and place in convenient location. **RATIONALE: A lubricated thermometer inserts with less discomfort and reduces chance of injury. NOTE: When performing this procedure on an adult patient, proceed with the following steps:**

   - Instruct patient to remove appropriate clothing, assisting as needed. **Note: Provide privacy.**

   - Assist adult patient onto examining table and cover with drape. Avoid overexposure.
   - Position patient on side. Ensure patient's comfort and safety.
   - Arrange drape to expose buttocks.
   - With one hand, raise upper buttock to expose anus.
   - With other hand, carefully insert lubricated thermometer into anal canal approximately one and one half inches. **NOTE:**
      - Do not force thermometer. Rotating will often facilitate insertion.
      - If opening is not apparent, request patient to bear down slightly; this will usually expose opening.

   NOTE: When performing the procedure on infants or small children, ask the parent or accompanying adult to prepare the child while you prepare the thermometer.

   - Position infant as to parent's or physician's preference.
   - Ensure safety during procedure by maintaining control of the infant's or child's position. (A parent can be instructed to assist you, as in Figure 13–19, especially if it comforts the child.)
   - Expose anus.
   - Carefully insert well-lubricated thermometer one inch into anal canal. (See Note in Step 9 for adults.)

10. Hold thermometer in place for a minimum of three minutes (five minutes for greater accuracy). **NOTE: Time by watch.**

11. Withdraw thermometer. Carefully remove plastic sheath and discard it in biohazardous waste container.

12. Read thermometer.

13. Reread to check temperature.

14. Place thermometer on tissue. **RATIONALE: A soiled thermometer must never be placed on an unprotected surface.**

15. Remove any excess lubricant from anal area with tissue. Wipe from front to back.

16. Ask parent or accompanying adult to dress infant or child.

17. Assist adult patient from examining table and instruct to redress. **NOTE: Provide privacy as appropriate.**

18. Follow procedure for soiled thermometer.

19. Remove and discard gloves in biohazardous waste container.

20. Record temperature, placing (R) after the finding.

21. Return thermometer to storage after cleaning.

CHARTING EXAMPLE:

3-6-XX

T. 100.2 (R)

B. Davis (SEM)

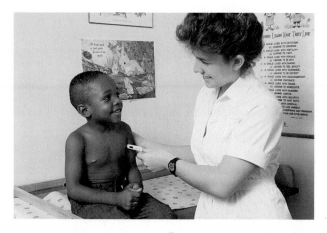

FIGURE 13–20 Measuring axillary temperature with a digital thermometer.

Disposable Thermometers

Disposable plastic oral thermometers may be used in some offices, urgent care centers, and hospital emergency rooms. Because they are used only once and discarded, they are free from cross-contamination, and no time or equipment is required for cleaning. One disadvantage is the cost factor. The patient's reaction may also be less than enthusiastic. The plastic is thin and almost sharp. Also, care must be taken to avoid touching the dot matrix portion, which is placed in the patient's mouth. The dots can be placed up or down. The thermometer must be held under the tongue as far back as possible in the heat pocket with the tongue pressed against the end and the mouth closed on the stem. Wait 60 seconds, then remove the thermometer. Allow 10 seconds for the dots to stabilize, then read and record

PROCEDURE

13-7 Measure Axillary Temperature with Mercury Thermometer

PURPOSE: To determine a patient's axillary temperature using a clinical thermometer.

EQUIPMENT: Oral security clinical/mercury thermometer, tissues, watch or timer, paper, pen or pencil, and soiled thermometer container.

PERFORMANCE OBJECTIVE: In a simulated or actual situation and given access to all necessary equipment and supplies, measure and record axillary temperature within 14 minutes, following correct procedural technique and observing aseptic and safety precautions. Recorded findings must agree with the instructor's reading.

1. Wash hands.
2. Identify patient. **RATIONALE: Speaking to the patient by name and checking chart ensures that you are performing the procedure on the correct patient.**
3. Explain procedure and what you are going to do.
4. Remove thermometer from holder or envelope.
5. Inspect thermometer. Discard a chipped or cracked thermometer in a sharps biohazardous waste container. **RATIONALE: A damaged thermometer is unsafe and may be inaccurate.**
6. Read thermometer and shake down to 95°F or below. **RATIONALE: Temperature will not be measured accurately if LESS than the previously measured temperature.**
7. Place thermometer on tissue or in envelope in convenient location.
8. Assist patient, as necessary, to expose axilla. **NOTE: Provide privacy.**
9. Pat axillary space with tissue to remove perspiration. **RATIONALE: Perspiration prevents thermometer from com-**

ing into direct contact with skin. It also makes it more difficult to keep thermometer in place.

10. Place thermometer deep in the axillary space. Position so that the bulb is in direct contact with the top of the axillary space with the stem projecting anteriorly. **NOTE: The thermometer may be placed with the stem extending posteriorly if desired.**
11. Hold arm tightly against body. Have patient maintain position for a minimum of 10 minutes.
    NOTE:
    - Time by watch or timer.
    - Help weak or confused patient maintain position.
    - Be certain thermometer remains deep in axillary space. Children will require close attention and assistance.
12. Remove thermometer and wipe with tissue from stem to bulb. **RATIONALE: Removes perspiration to facilitate reading. Action is from clean to soiled area.**
13. Read and record findings. **NOTE: Place (Ax) after the reading.**
14. Reread and check recording.
15. Help patient replace clothing.
16. Follow procedure for soiled thermometer.
17. Wash hands.
18. Return thermometer to storage after cleaning.

CHARTING EXAMPLE:
3-6-XX
T. 97.2 (Ax)

B. Davis (SEM)

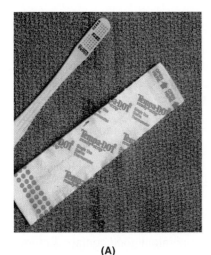

(A)

FIGURE 13–21 (A) Disposable plastic thermometer. (B) The matrix reads 101°F. (Courtesy 3M Health Care.)

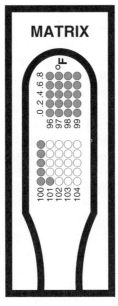

(B)

the temperature. The heat in the mouth causes a reaction on the heat-sensitive dots printed on the surface of the plastic strip. Readings are calculated by counting the number of dots that change color within a degree grouping (Figure 13–21). The last changed dot on the matrix indicates the correct temperature. Then discard the thermometer in a biohazardous waste container. Plastic thermometers are not considered to be precisely accurate; however, for usual temperature determination, their single use and freedom from cross-contamination concerns may outweigh any minor disadvantages. See Procedure 13–8.

The disposable plastic thermometer can also be used to measure axillary temperature. The dot matrix portion is placed next to the body, deep in the axillary space, with the handle extending straight down the patient's side. The arm must be held tightly at the side. After three minutes, remove the thermometer; wait 10 seconds, then read and record the temperature.

A variation of the disposable thermometer is available for rectal use. It is packaged with a plastic sheath and is

---

PROCEDURE

13-8 Measure Oral Temperature with Disposable Plastic Thermometer

PURPOSE: To determine a patient's oral temperature using a disposable plastic thermometer.

OSHA GUIDELINES: Standard Precautions require gloves to be worn if there is any possibility of coming into contact with blood, body fluids, or wound drainage. Biohazardous waste containers are required for discarding gloves and plastic thermometers.

EQUIPMENT: Disposable plastic thermometer, watch or timer, latex or vinyl gloves, biohazardous waste container, paper, pen or pencil.

PERFORMANCE OBJECTIVE: In a simulated or actual situation and given access to all necessary equipment and supplies, measure and record oral temperature within four minutes, following correct procedural technique and observing aseptic and safety precautions. Recorded findings must agree with the instructor's reading.

1. Wash hands and put on gloves.

2. Identify patient. **RATIONALE: Speaking to the patient by name and checking chart ensures that you are performing the procedure on the correct patient.**

3. Explain procedure and what you are going to do.

4. Determine if the patient has recently had a hot or cold drink or smoked. **NOTE: If so, allow 10 minutes before measuring. RATIONALE: Hot or cold substances in the mouth prevent accurate temperature measurement.**

5. Open package by peeling back top of wrapper to expose handle end of thermometer.

6. Grasp handle and remove from wrapper. **NOTE: Do NOT touch dot matrix portion, which will be placed in the patient's mouth. RATIONALE: Your hands would contaminate the thermometer and may interfere with the chemical reaction of the dots.**

7. Insert thermometer into patient's mouth as far back as possible into one of the heat pockets (see Figure 13–18).

8. Instruct patient to press tongue down on thermometer and keep mouth closed. **RATIONALE: Firm direct contact is necessary for accurate measurement. Breathing through the mouth admits air which may affect accuracy.**

9. Maintain position for 60 seconds. **NOTE: Time by watch.**

10. Remove thermometer and wait 10 seconds for dots to stabilize. **NOTE: Take special care to avoid touching the portion that has been in the patient's mouth.**

11. Read thermometer. Discard in biohazardous waste container.

12. Remove gloves and discard in biohazardous waste container.

13. Wash hands.

14. Record temperature.

CHARTING EXAMPLE:

3-6-XX
T. 97.8

B. Davis (SEM)

not recommended for infants or toddlers. The thermometer must be well lubricated and inserted until the dot matrix is completely covered. After three minutes, it is withdrawn and the sheath discarded. After 10 seconds, the temperature may be read and recorded.

When disposable thermometers are exposed to high temperatures in their environment, the matrix dots will turn blue. If this should occur, place them in a freezer for one hour for each box of 100 thermometers. Rectal thermometers will require two hours per 100 thermometers. Then let them stand at room temperature for one day. The thermometers will then be ready for use, and their accuracy should not be affected.

Electronic Thermometers

The use of electronic thermometers is becoming more common. They are quick, sanitary, easily read, and do not require cleaning. A small, battery-operated unit with a digital read-out window is very accurate and capable of measuring a temperature within a few seconds (Figure 13–22). A metal probe, blue for oral, red for rectal, is used like a mercury thermometer. It is attached by a cord to the battery unit. A disposable cover slips over the probe to provide each patient with an individual thermometer. The covered probe is inserted in the patient's mouth like a mercury thermometer. It is usually held in place by the medical assistant because the time involved is short, and the probe, with its cord, is heavy and somewhat cumbersome. As soon as the temperature level has been reached, the unit will sound a signal and the final reading will appear in the window of the unit (Procedure 13–9).

Electronic thermometers are time-saving and convenient, but they are somewhat expensive. Care must also be taken to adjust the unit frequently and correctly. It is critical that the dial be observed from a direct view at eye level while making adjustments. The unit must be returned to its charging stand after use to maintain the battery.

Electronic thermometers may also be used to measure axillary and rectal temperature. Use the rectal (red) probe to take a rectal temperature. Remove the rectal probe from its holder and attach a probe cover. The probe is inserted into the rectum one-half inch for adults and one-fourth inch for children. The use of lubricant is optional. The probe should be angled slightly to ensure contact with the rectal mucosa. After the reading is registered, remove the probe, and discard the cover in a biohazardous waste container.

When taking axillary temperature, some manufacturers recommend using the rectal probe; others recommend the oral probe. Consult the instructional booklet with your equipment to determine which to use. Apply a probe cover, and insert the tip well into the axillary space with the probe extending down and slightly forward along the patient's side. Press gently into the space to establish good tissue contact. Have patient lower arm over probe. Hold probe in position to maintain good contact. Remove and read after unit signals completion.

Some units have built-in operator prompts to signal when technique or problems exist. If the phrase OPER ERR 9 (or something similar) shows on the readout window, it means the probe is not in contact with tissue. A readjustment of the thermometer will erase the message and allow the continued measurement of the temperature. A BAT LO (or similar) message indicates the unit's batteries do not have enough charge to take a temperature. The unit must be returned to the charger base for six to eight hours to be fully charged or 45 minutes to permit a limited number of measurements. A PROB BAD (or similar) message indicates the probe is damaged and will not sense temperature properly. This can be corrected only by installing a new probe.

Another electronic thermometer is simple and self-contained. It is also a digital thermometer and is excellent for home use (Figure 13–23). The thermometer will register the temperature in about 60 seconds on an easy-to-read LCD panel that shows the temperature in tenths of degrees. The thermometer can be cleaned with soap and water and sanitized with a disinfectant. Probe covers are available for clinic or office use. It may be used for oral, axillary, or rectal measurement. Some models have a beeper that sounds when the maximum temperature is reached. This feature is especially appealing to children.

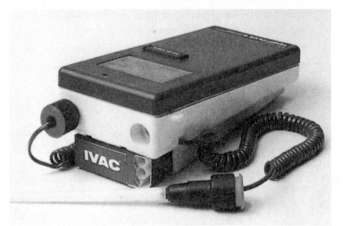

FIGURE 13–22 Electronic thermometer

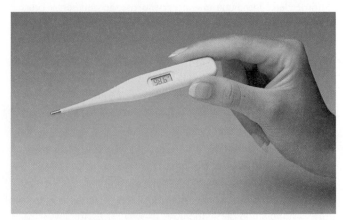

FIGURE 13–23 Electronic digital thermometer (Courtesy of Omron Healthcare, Inc.)

PROCEDURE

13-9 Measure Oral Temperature Electronically

PURPOSE: To determine a patient's oral temperature using an electronic thermometer.

OSHA GUIDELINES: Standard Precautions require a biohazardous waste container for discarding probe covers.

EQUIPMENT: Electronic thermometer unit, oral probe, probe cover, biohazardous waste container, paper, pen or pencil.

PERFORMANCE OBJECTIVE: In a simulated or actual situation and given access to all necessary equipment and supplies, measure the patient's temperature electronically. The temperature will be read and recorded in two minutes, following correct procedural technique and observing aseptic and safety precautions. Recorded findings must agree with instructor's reading.

1. Wash hands; assemble equipment.

2. Identify patient. **RATIONALE: Speaking to the patient by name and checking the chart ensures that you are performing the procedure on the correct patient.**

3. Explain procedure and what you are going to do.

4. Place probe connector in receptacle of unit base and check to make sure it is properly seated.

5. Holding it by the collar, remove appropriate probe from stored position.

6. Insert probe firmly into probe cover to ensure that it is properly seated.

7. Insert covered probe into mouth. **NOTE: The probe and connecting cord is rather heavy and cumbersome. It may be necessary to hold the thermometer steady in place.**

8. Maintain covered probe in position until unit signals, approximately 10 to 15 seconds. **RATIONALE: Early removal results in inaccurate measurement.**

9. Remove probe from patient. Do not touch probe cover. **RATIONALE: Probe is contaminated with patient's saliva.**

10. Read and record temperature measurement. **NOTE: Temperature is displayed digitally in window of unit.**

11. Recheck your reading and recording.

12. Press the eject button to discard used probe cover into biohazardous waste container. **RATIONALE: All materials coming into contact with bodily secretions are deposited in biohazardous waste container.**

13. Return probe to stored position in unit. Thermometer display will read zero and shut off.

14. Store unit in charging stand. **NOTE: A red light in the upper left hand area of the display indicates that the thermometer is charging. RATIONALE: The unit should remain in the stand so it is fully charged and ready for use.**

CHARTING EXAMPLE:
5/10/XX
T. 99.8

B. Davis (SEM)

Tympanic Membrane Thermometers

A newer concept in temperature measurement is the instantaneous tympanic membrane (aural) thermometer. The thermometer operates by the principle of measuring the strength of the infrared heat waves generated by the tympanic membrane and digitally displays that temperature in less than two seconds. Because the tympanic membrane shares the same blood supply as the hypothalamus, it is believed the auditory canal is an ideal site for obtaining an accurate assessment of the body's core temperature. Studies conducted with temperature-sensing devices placed internally in a large blood vessel have shown strong correlation in results.

Although its greatest asset is the instant result, it has become a real benefit to health care professionals in hospital emergency rooms, labor and delivery rooms, and pediatric units because it does not involve contact with mucous membranes and the site is so easily accessible. Another advantage is the readings are not affected by hot or cold liquids or smoking as are oral methods. In addition, the patient does not even need to be conscious. There are a few instances, however, when inaccurate readings may be obtained, for instance: if the probe is not properly sealed in the ear canal; if the beam is not directed toward the eardrum; if there is ceramen present; or if there is an infection of the middle ear.

The thermometer is extremely easy to use. You simply position the covered plastic tip properly inside the auditory canal, press the scan button, and an infrared beam measures the heat waves (Figure 13–24). The results are displayed digitally on the screen. A release button ejects the probe cover and in 10 seconds another temperature can be taken. The method is acceptable to patients and a time saver to the health care worker. The units operate on three AAA alkaline batteries and will measure at least 10,000 temperatures before needing to be replaced. As the aural thermometer becomes more acceptable and less expensive, many clinics, urgent care centers, and group

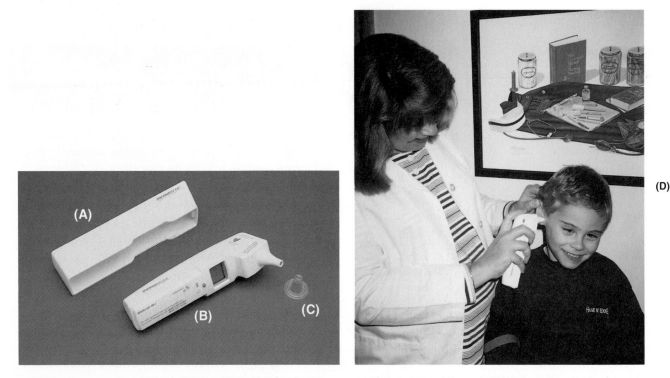

FIGURE 13–24 Tympanic (aural) thermometer: (A) holder (B) tympanic thermometer, (C) cover. (D) Measuring core body temperature with an aural thermometer

---

PROCEDURE

13-10 Measure Core Body Temperature with an Infrared Tympanic Thermometer

PURPOSE: To determine a patient's core body temperature using an infrared tympanic thermometer.

EQUIPMENT: Tympanic thermometer unit, probe cover, waste container, paper, and pen or pencil.

PERFORMANCE OBJECTIVE: In a simulated or actual situation and given access to all necessary equipment and supplies, measure and record core body temperature within three minutes, following correct procedural technique and observing aseptic and safety precautions. Recorded findings must agree with instructor's reading.

1. Wash hands.
2. Identify patient. **RATIONALE: Speaking to the patient by name and checking the chart ensures that you are performing the procedure on the correct patient.**
3. Explain procedure and what you are going to do.
4. Remove thermometer from base.
5. Attach a disposable probe cover to the ear piece. **NOTE: The display should read "ready."**

6. Insert covered probe into ear canal, sealing opening.
7. Press the scan button to activate the thermometer.
8. Withdraw the thermometer.
9. Observe the display window, noting the temperature.
10. Press the release button on the thermometer to eject the probe cover into a waste container.
11. Record the temperature using (T) or (Tc) to indicate tympanic or tympanic core temperature.
12. Return thermometer to base.
    NOTE: Thermometers can be set to correlate with an oral or rectal reading. Usually, the oral mode is used, and a reading of 98.6°F is considered "normal."

CHARTING EXAMPLE:
5-10-XX
T. 100.3 (Tc)

B. Davis (SEM)

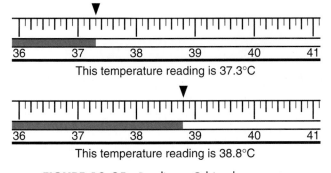

This temperature reading is 37.3°C

This temperature reading is 38.8°C

FIGURE 13–25   Reading a Celsius thermometer

practices may use the new technology. See Procedure 13–10.

Celsius Thermometers

The only difference between Celsius and Fahrenheit thermometers is the calibration. On a Celsius thermometer, each long line represents a degree. They are numbered consecutively, with the nine lines that are between each number representing one tenth of a degree (Figure 13–25).

Temperature can be converted from one scale to another by a mathematical calculation. To convert Celsius to Fahrenheit, multiply the degrees by $\frac{9}{5}$ and add 32. To change Fahrenheit to Celsius, subtract 32 and multiply by $\frac{5}{9}$. Another way to convert temperature uses a different mathematical calculation. Some people find this easier to do. Centigrade equals Fahrenheit minus 32 with the remainder divided by 1.8.

$$C = \frac{F - 32}{1.8}$$

To convert Fahrenheit to Centigrade the math is:

$$F = (C \times 1.8) + 32.$$

Table 13–4 shows examples of temperature conversions and compares some common temperatures.

PULSE

C   Skills Menu:
  ■ Taking a Pulse

Each time the heart beats, blood is forced into the aorta, temporarily expanding its walls and initiating a wavelike effect. This wave continues through all the body's arteries, causing the alternating expansion and recoil of the arterial walls (Figure 13–26). This effect can be **palpated** (felt) in the arteries that are close to the body surface and that lie over bone or firm structures. When the artery is pressed against the underlying structure, it is possible to feel the rhythmic pulsation, known as the pulse.

Pulse Points

The pulse can be felt in several locations on the body (Figure 13–27). The **radial** pulse point is on the thumb

TABLE 13–4

TEMPERATURE CONVERSION AND COMPARISON

To convert Celsius to Fahrenheit:

$$37°C \times \frac{9}{5}\left(\frac{333}{5}\right) = 66.6 + 32 = 98.6°F$$

$$C = \frac{F - 32}{1.8} \quad (C = 98.6 - 32 = \frac{66.6}{1.8} = 37)$$

To convert Fahrenheit to Celsius:

$$98.6°F - 32 = 66.6 \times \frac{5}{9}\left(\frac{333}{9}\right) = 37°C$$

$$F = (C \times 1.8) + 32 \quad (F = 37 \times 1.8 = 66.6 + 32 = 98.6)$$

Comparison	Celsius (C)	Fahrenheit (F)
Freezing	0°	32°
Body Temperature	37°	98.6°
Pasteurization	63°	145°
Boiling	100°	212°
Sterilizing (Autoclave)	121°	250.0°

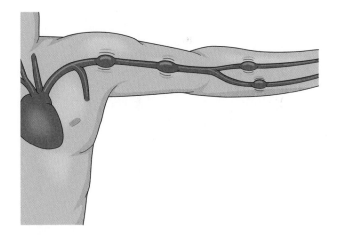

FIGURE 13–26   Blood pumped from the heart causes a wave-like effect in the arteries.

side of the inner surface of the wrist, lying over the radius bone. The radial pulse point is used most frequently when measuring pulse rate.

The **brachial** artery pulse point is on the inner medial surface of the elbow, at the **antecubital** space (crease of elbow). This point is used to palpate and **auscultate** (listen to) blood pressure.

The **carotid** pulse can be felt in the carotid artery of the neck when pressure is applied to the area at either side of the trachea. It is the carotid pulse that is palpated during the cardiopulmonary resuscitation (CPR) life-saving maneuver.

The **femoral point**, located midway in the **groin** where the artery begins its descent down the femur, the **dorsalis**

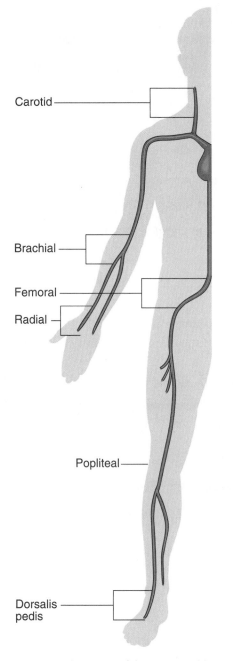

Carotid

Brachial

Femoral

Radial

Popliteal

Dorsalis
pedis

FIGURE 13–27 Pulse points of the upper and lower extremities and the neck

TABLE 13–5

PULSE–AGE RELATIONSHIP	
Age	Pulse Rate
Less than 1 year	100–170
2–6 years	90–115
6–10 years	80–110
11–16 years	70–95
Midlife adult	65–80
Aged adult	50–65

tivity, the heartbeat increases 20 to 30 beats per minute to meet the body's needs. It should return to normal within three minutes after activity has stopped. Of course, the rate of increase will be in proportion to the level of activity.

Age is directly related to pulse rate. The younger the person, the faster the heartbeat. A sample of age-related average pulse rates is shown in Table 13–5.

Pulse rate is also related to the sex of the patient. A female's pulse is approximately 10 beats per minute more rapid than a male's of the same age. Pulse rate is also related to size; therefore a larger person will have a slower rate than a smaller person. The relationship of size is particularly evident in animals. The heart rate of a bird may be well over 200 beats per minute while an elephant has a rate of about 30.

The physical condition of the body is another factor. Athletes, especially those who run or engage in strenuous sports, have a considerably slower pulse rate as a result of a more efficient circulatory system.

In general, the heart rate increases when the sympathetic nervous system is stimulated by feelings such as fear, anxiety, pain, or anger. The rate also increases with certain other conditions, such as thyroid disease, anemia, shock, or fever. A consistent rate of over 100 beats per minute is known as *tachycardia.*

When the parasympathetic nervous system affects the heart, it causes the rate to be much slower. A consistent rate below 60 beats per minute is known as *bradycardia.* This may also occur with the use of certain medications, heart disease, emotional depression, and drugs. A rate below 60 beats per minute is also normal for many athletes.

pedis, on the instep of the foot, and the **popliteal**, at the back of the knee, are other points palpated to evaluate circulation in the lower extremities.

Pulse Rate

The number of times the heart beats per minute is typically measured by counting the pulse in the radial artery. The average adult pulse rate is 72 beats per minute. The pulse rate is recorded as beats per minute preceded by a capital *P* (i.e., P. 72).

The rate of the pulse is influenced by several factors. The most obvious is exercise or activity. With increased ac-

Pulse Characteristics

When measuring pulse rate, two other characteristics must also be observed and recorded. The force or strength of the pulse is referred to as its **volume**. Words used to describe this quality are normal, full or bounding, weak, and **thready** (scarcely perceivable).

The quality of **rhythm** of the pulse refers to its regularity, or the equal spacing of the beats. The term **ar-**

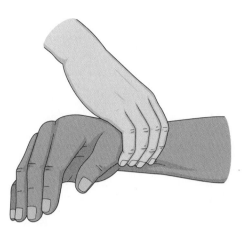

FIGURE 13–28   Measuring radial pulse

occasionally skip or insert beats. Often caffeine or nicotine react on the heart to cause irregularity and increased rate.

Measuring Radial Pulse

The patient should be completely relaxed and sitting comfortably or lying down when the pulse is measured and evaluated. Ideally the arm should be well supported, with the wrist near the level of the heart. Place the tips of your first three fingers at the wrist area, about an inch above the base of the thumb (Figure 13–28). Never use your thumb to measure pulse rate; there is a chance you may feel and record your own heart rate in your thumb's artery.

An appropriate amount of pressure applied to the artery will permit the pulsations to be felt. Too much pressure will shut off the circulation and therefore eliminate the pulse beat. Too little pressure will not compress the artery sufficiently against the radius. With practice, applying the correct amount of pressure will become routine. See Procedure 13–11.

rhythmia refers to a pulse that lacks a regular rhythm. The pulse can be irregular (without a consistent pattern) or regularly irregular (unequally spaced but consistently the same beating pattern). A pulse can also be intermittent and

P R O C E D U R E

13-11   Measure Radial Pulse

PURPOSE: To determine the rate, rhythm, and quality of a patient's radial pulse.

EQUIPMENT: Watch with sweep second hand, paper, and pen or pencil.

PERFORMANCE OBJECTIVE: In a simulated or actual situation and given access to all necessary equipment and supplies, within four minutes, assess and record the quality, and measure and record the rate of a patient's radial pulse following correct procedural technique. Recorded rate findings must be within two beats per minute of instructor's measurement and agree as to rhythm and quality characteristics.

1. Wash hands; assemble equipment.
2. Identify patient. **RATIONALE: Speaking to the patient by name and checking the chart ensures that you are performing the procedure on the correct patient.**
3. Explain procedure. Identify what you are going to do.
4. Determine patient's recent activity. **RATIONALE: Exertion within the past three to five minutes will cause temporary increase in pulse rate.**
5. Have patient assume a comfortable position with arm supported, palm of hand down, wrist near level of heart or placed across upper abdomen if lying down.
6. Locate radial artery on thumb side of wrist. **NOTE: Do not use your thumb. Place tips of fingers lightly over artery.**

7. Observe quality of pulse before beginning to count. Determine if regular, strong, weak, or thready. **RATIONALE: Concentration on the quality prior to measurement assists in accurate evaluation.**
8. Check watch. Begin counting beats when second hand is at 3, 6, 9, or 12. **(NOTE: Makes 30 seconds easier to observe).**
9. Count a *regular* pulse for 30 seconds and multiply results by 2. This will always be an even number. If *irregular*, count for full minute. Do not multiply by 2. **RATIONALE: The pulse rate is recorded in beats per minute, you have already determined the total beats per minute.**
10. Record pulse in beats per minute. **NOTE: Immediate recording helps eliminate errors.**
11. Describe quality characteristics. **RATIONALE: In certain disease conditions the presence or absence of quality characteristics is a significant finding.**
12. Wash hands.

CHARTING EXAMPLE:
5-10-XX
P. 96, weak but regular

B. Davis (SEM)

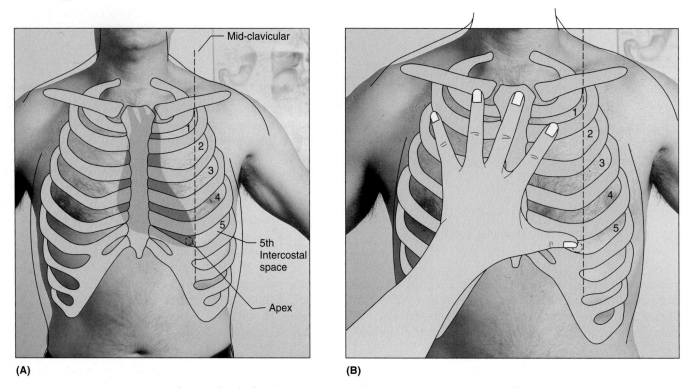

Mid-clavicular

5th
Intercostal
space

Apex

(A)

(B)

FIGURE 13–29 (A) Locating the apical pulse by counting intercostal spaces; (B) alternative method for locating the apex of the heart

Measuring Apical Pulse

In instances when measuring heart rate by the radial pulse is not appropriate, it is necessary to listen to the heart at its **apex** with a **stethoscope**. This is a very accurate method of measuring pulse rate. The contraction of the atria and the ventricles will be heard as two closely occurring sounds, known as the "lubb dupp;" however, both contraction phases are counted as only one beat. Whenever a pulse rate is measured at a point other than radial, that fact should be noted when recording the rate (e.g., P. 97 [Ap]). Note that an **apical** pulse is counted for a full minute, so it is possible to record an uneven number.

Locating the Apex The bottom or lower edge of the heart is known as the apex. This is the point of maximum impulse of the heart against the chest wall. It can be palpated at the left fifth intercostal space in line with the middle of the left clavicle. This spot may be located by pressing the fingertips between the ribs and counting down five spaces on the left chest wall (Figure 13–29A). Often the beat at the apex can be felt with the fingertips.

Another, quicker method for estimating the location of the apex is to place the outstretched LEFT hand on the chest wall with the tip of the middle finger in the suprasternal notch and the thumb at a 45° angle (Figure 13–29B). The end of the thumb will be approximately over the apex. This is only an approximate measurement because the size of the chest and the hand will vary. For a

ready reference point, the apex should be just below the left breast. Again, this is a variable, particularly in the female, because of the size and placement of the breast. Refer to Procedure 13–12.

Apical Indications Apical pulse measurement is indicated for infants and small children because of their normally rapid rate, which is easier to hear and count than to palpate. Patients with heart conditions, especially if being medicated with cardiac drugs, will require apical measurement for greater accuracy. Apical measurement is always indicated if you have difficulty feeling a radial pulse and believe you may be missing beats. Other indications are an excessively rapid or slow rate, a thready or irregular quality, or with an existing or suspected pulse deficit.

Measuring Apical-Radial Pulse

Certain heart conditions cause a symptom known as **pulse deficit**. A patient with a pulse deficit will have a higher apical than radial pulse rate. This difference indicates that some heart contractions are not strong enough to produce a palpable radial pulse. It is important to determine the extent of the deficit by measuring the apical and radial rate at the same time.

A procedure called *apical-radial pulse* requires one person to measure the pulse rate radially while another auscultates the apical rate with a stethoscope (Figure 13–30). The radial rate is then subtracted from the apical,

PROCEDURE

13-12 Measure Apical Pulse

PURPOSE: To determine the rate, rhythm, and quality of a patient's apical pulse.

EQUIPMENT: Watch with sweep second hand, stethoscope, alcohol wipe, paper, and pen or pencil.

PERFORMANCE OBJECTIVE: In a simulated or actual situation and given access to all necessary equipment and supplies, within five minutes, locate the apex of the heart, assess and record the quality and measure and record the rate of a patient's apical pulse, following correct technique and observing aseptic precautions. Recorded rate findings must be within one beat per minute of instructor's measurement and agree as to rhythm and quality characteristics.

1. Wash hands.
2. Prepare stethoscope by wiping earpieces and chestpiece with germicidal solution to prevent transfer of organisms.
3. Identify patient. **RATIONALE: Speaking to the patient by name and checking the chart ensures that you are performing the procedure on the correct patient.**
4. Tell patient what you are going to do. If patient is an infant or small child, explain the procedure to parent.
5. Provide privacy and a gown or drape if indicated.
6. Uncover left side of chest. **RATIONALE: Auscultation must be done directly against the skin surface.**
7. Place earpieces in ears. Openings in tips should be forward, entering auditory canal.
8. Locate apex by palpating to left fifth intercostal space at midclavicular line. **NOTE: If chestpiece does not have a chill ring, warm it in palm of one hand while locating apex. This also prevents accidental striking against hard surface and resulting noise in ears.**

9. Place chestpiece of stethoscope at apex.
10. Determine quality of heart sounds. **NOTE: Concentrate on rhythm and volume. RATIONALE: The quality of the beat is significant in evaluation of the heart action.**
11. Concentrate on rate of beats. **Note: Be certain of sounds and pattern.**
12. Observe watch and begin counting rate when second hand is at 3, 6, 9, or 12. **RATIONALE: It is easier to measure one minute when beginning at one of these four numbers.**
13. Count beats for a full minute. **NOTE: Both pulse phases count as one beat. RATIONALE: Apical rates are indicated when quality or rhythm irregularities are present or possible; therefore, full-minute measurement is essential.**
14. Remove earpieces from ears.
15. Record rate and quality of heart sounds.
    NOTE:
    ▪ Immediate recording aids in eliminating errors.
    ▪ Indicate it is apical measurement.
16. Assist or instruct patient to dress unless physician also wishes to assess heart action. Determine this by asking physician prior to measurement of if your findings indicate the need.
17. Wipe earpieces and chestpiece of stethoscope with disinfectant. Return to storage.
18. Wash hands.

CHARTING EXAMPLE:
5-10-XX
P. 103 (Ap), full but irregular with an extra beat every four beats

B. Davis (SEM)

---

the difference being the pulse deficit. Ideally, two people measure the rate at the same time. If this is not possible, then the apical rate is measured and recorded, followed immediately by the radial. Apical-radial rates are always measured for one full minute. The physician may have a preferred method for recording this procedure. It will probably include both apical and radial pulse rates and the deficit. Examples of a format that can be used are:

P. 97 (Ap) 75 (R), 22 deficit

or written as a fraction: P. $\dfrac{97\ (Ap)}{75(R)} = 22$ deficit

RESPIRATION

Skills Menu:
▪ Counting Respirations

The third vital sign to be measured is respiration. One respiration is the combination of total inspiration (breathing in) and total expiration (breathing out). Other frequently used terms are **inhale** and **exhale**.

Respirations are usually measured as one part of total vital signs assessment. Because patients can voluntarily control the depth, rate, and regularity of their breathing to some extent, it is important that they not be aware the

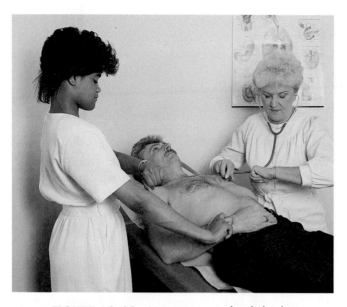

FIGURE 13–30 Measuring apical-radial pulse

procedure is being done. To accomplish this, it is common practice to observe and measure respiration immediately after assessing the pulse, while maintaining your fingers at the radial pulse or auscultating the apex. Using this method, the patient assumes you are still measuring pulse rate.

Quality of Respiration

Respirations should be quiet, effortless, and regularly spaced. Breathing should be through the nose with the mouth closed. Excessively fast and deep breathing, commonly associated with hysteria, is called **hyperventilation**. Difficult or labored breathing is called **dyspnea**. Frequently dyspnea is accompanied by discomfort and an anxious expression, caused by the fear of being unable to breathe. This patient will use the accessory respiratory muscles of the rib cage, neck, shoulders, and back to assist the breathing process.

The presence of **râles** (noisy breathing) usually indicates constricted bronchial passageways or the collection of fluid or exudate. Râles may be present with pneumonia, bronchitis, asthma, and other pulmonary diseases.

Respirations should be observed for the depth of inhalation. Three words are used to describe this quality: normal, shallow, or deep. Depth of inhalation can be de-

termined by watching the rise and fall of the chest. The rhythm of the respirations must also be assessed. This quality can be described as regular or irregular. Absence of breathing is known as **apnea**. A breathing pattern called **Cheyne–Stokes** occurs with acute brain, heart, or lung damage or disease and with intoxicants. It is characterized by slow, shallow breaths that increase in depth and frequency to be followed by a few shallow breaths, and then a period of apnea for 10 to 20 seconds and often more (Figure 13–31). This type of breathing pattern frequently precedes death.

Respiration Rate

Normal respiration rate for adults is from 16 to 20 times per minute. The respiration rate in infants and children has a greater range and fluctuates more during illness, exercise, and emotion than adult rates do. In the newborn, the rate per minute may range from 30 to 80; in early childhood, from 20 to 40; and during late childhood from 16 to 26. The rate will reach an adult normal range of 16 to 20 by age 15. An abnormally slow rate of respiration is known as *bradypnea*. A faster than normal rate of respiration is known as *tachypnea*.

Counting Respirations

It is necessary to observe the patient carefully while measuring respiration rate. If the patient is lying on the examination table, position the patient's arm across the upper abdominal area, placing your fingers over the radial pulse point. In this position you can visualize and feel respiration. With the patient in a sitting position, you will need to observe more carefully as you count the respirations (Figure 13–32). Remember, it is also necessary to keep your watch in view as you observe. With a little practice, you will be able to manage both at the same time.

When counting respirations as part of the TPR assessment, it is very important that you remember the number of heartbeats you have just counted. It may help you to use the following method:

1. Assume the pulse measuring position.
2. Observe, determine the characteristics, and describe to yourself the qualities of both the pulse and the respirations.
3. Count the number of heartbeats during the first 30 seconds of the minute.

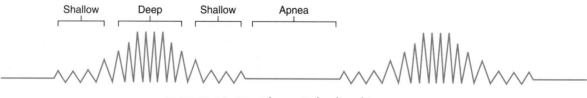

FIGURE 13–31 Cheyne-Stokes breathing pattern

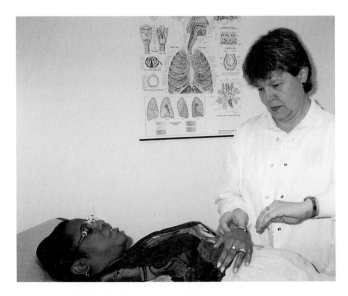

FIGURE 13-32 Measuring respirations

4. Repeat the pulse rate to yourself as you count the number of respirations during the second 30 seconds. (Note: You MUST use the word "and" between each respiration so you do not accidentally add counts to the pulse rate.)

For example, if your patient's pulse rate after 30 seconds is 40, repeat this number as you count the respirations: "40 and 1, 40 and 2, 40 and 3," and so on, until the second 30-second period is past. At the end of a minute, you will have both rates counted. Multiply the rates by 2 and record. Refer to Procedure 13–13.

TEMPERATURE–PULSE–RESPIRATION RATIO

Respiration rate, like pulse, will increase with activity, excitement, fear, other strong emotions, and certain disease conditions. Whenever a patient, either child or adult, has been upset and crying, a time must pass before an ac-

---

P R O C E D U R E

13-13 Measure Respirations

PURPOSE: To determine the rate, rhythm, sound, and depth of a patient's respirations.

EQUIPMENT: Watch with sweep second hand, paper, and pen or pencil.

PERFORMANCE OBJECTIVE: In a simulated or actual situation and given access to all necessary equipment and supplies, assess and record the quality and rate of a patient's respirations within three minutes, following the correct procedural technique. Recorded rate findings must be within two breaths per minute of instructor's measurement and agree as to rhythm, sound, and depth quality characteristics.

1. Wash hands.
2. Identify patient. **RATIONALE: Speaking to the patient by name and checking the chart ensures that you are performing the procedure on the correct patient.**
   NOTE: In this procedure, it is preferable *not* to explain to the patient what you are about to do. If the patient knows that you will be counting respirations, control of breathing is possible, resulting in an inaccurate measurement.
3. Ask about recent activity level. **RATIONALE: Patient should have been relatively quiet for the past two to five minutes to obtain accurate assessment.**
4. Place patient in comfortable position, sitting or lying down.

5. Assume pulse measurement position. **RATIONALE: Respirations are more easily counted if patient's arm is across upper abdomen.**
6. Assess respiration quality. **NOTE: Determine depth, rhythm, and sound.**
7. Count respirations for thirty seconds.
   NOTE: One rise and fall of the chest equals one respiration. Maintain radial pulse position. RATIONALE: Patients must be unaware you are measuring respirations so they do not unintentionally or purposely alter the rate or rhythm.
8. Multiply results by 2 and record. **NOTE: If respirations are irregular, count for a full minute and do *not* multiply results by 2. RATIONALE: The rate per minute has already been determined.**
9. Record quality characteristics. **RATIONALE: In certain disease conditions, the presence or absence of quality characteristics is a significant finding.**
10. Wash hands.

CHARTING EXAMPLE:
5-10-XX
R. 24, shallow, regular, and somewhat noisy

B. Davis (SEM)

TABLE 13–6

TEMPERATURE-PULSE-RESPIRATION RATIO		
Respiration	Pulse	Temperature (F°)
18	80	99
19 (plus)	88	100
21	96	101
23	104	102
25 (minus)	112	103
27	120	104
28 (minus)	128	105
30	136	106

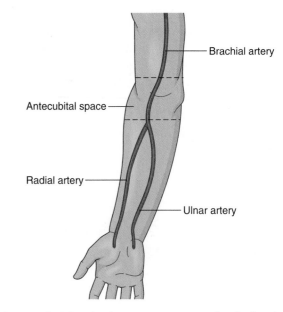

FIGURE 13–33 Blood pressure is measured in the brachial artery at the antecubital space.

curate measurement of either pulse or respirations can be made. Strong emotions elevate the vital signs and may make a true measurement impossible. Respirations and the pulse are also affected by the degree of fever present. Table 13–6 demonstrates the relationship of the three vital signs.

BLOOD PRESSURE

C Skills Menu:
- Taking Blood Pressure

The fourth vital sign is blood pressure. Learning to assess blood pressure accurately requires attention to details, careful listening, and correct technique. The term *blood pressure* means the fluctuating pressure that the blood exerts against the arterial walls as the heart alternately contracts and relaxes. The blood pressure reflects the condition of the heart, the amount of blood forced from the heart at contraction, the condition of the arteries, and to some extent the volume and viscosity (stickiness) of the blood.

Blood pressure is measured in the brachial artery of the arm at the antecubital space (Figure 13–33). It should be measured in both arms, at least initially. There is normally a 5- to 10-mm difference. Subsequent readings should be made on the arm with the higher pressure.

Maintaining Blood Pressure

Two main factors cooperate to maintain a fairly constant blood pressure. The first is the heart or pump, which exerts pressure on the blood. About 100,000 times a day the heart contracts, forcing blood into the aorta and throughout the blood vessels of the body. Without a strong, effective pump, the blood will not flow and the pressure will drop.

The second factor is the brain, which controls, through the autonomic nervous system, the rate of the heart and the size of the opening or caliber of the arteries. When sensors in the arteries detect an increase in arterial pressure, a message is sent to the brain, which in turn directs the arteries to dilate slightly (reducing resistance to the flow of blood) and directs the heart to slow down (reducing the amount of blood being forced out). When the pressure drops too far, the message to the brain results in slightly increased heart action and constriction of the arteries, which cause the pressure to rise. Both actions are needed to maintain homeostasis.

Blood Pressure Phases

The phases of blood pressure are identical to those of the pulse. A contraction phase, known as *systole,* corresponds to the beat phase of the heart, and is the period of greatest pressure. The relaxation phase, known as *diastole,* corresponds to the resting or filling action of the heart, and is the period of least pressure.

Normal Blood Pressure

Blood pressure is measured in millimeters of mercury (mm Hg) using a stethoscope and a **sphygmomanometer**, which may have either a calibrated column of mercury or an **aneroid** dial (Figure 13–34). Blood pressure readings are measurements of systolic and diastolic pressure written as a fraction; for example, B/P 120/80, where 120 is systolic and 80 is diastolic pressure.

A normal adult should have a systolic pressure less than 140 mm Hg, and a diastolic pressure less than 90. Blood pressure readings persistently above 140/90 indicate *hypertension* (high blood pressure).

Hypertension can result from things such as stress, obesity, high salt intake, sedentary lifestyle, and aging. Physical conditions that cause hypertension are kidney disease,

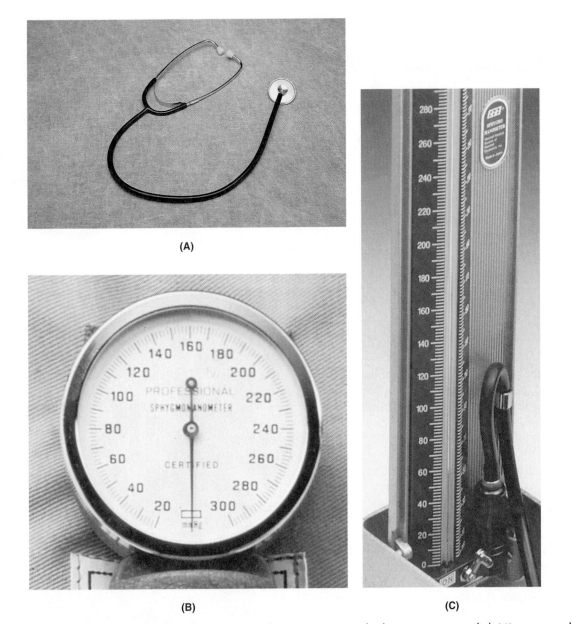

(A)

(B)

(C)

FIGURE 13–34 Blood pressure measuring equipment: (A) stethoscope, (B) aneroid sphygmomanometer dial, (C) mercury sphygmomanometer scale

thyroid dysfunction, neurological disorders, and vascular conditions (such as atherosclerosis and arteriosclerosis), which make circulation more difficult, therefore requiring a greater pressure to circulate the blood. An elevated pressure without apparent cause is said to be **idiopathic** or **essential** hypertension. Other terms used to identify types of hypertension include:

- Primary—without another identifiable cause
- Secondary—results from renal disease or another identifiable cause
- **Orthostatic**—occurs when in an erect or standing position
- Malignant—severe, difficult, or impossible to control

Hypertension can also be defined by stages as they relate to blood pressure findings. Table 13-7 contains information from the Fifth Report of the Joint National Com-

mittee on Detection, Evaluation, and Treatment of High Blood Pressure.

A blood pressure consistently below 90/60 indicates *hypotension* (low blood pressure), which may be normal for some persons. Hypotension will be present with heart failure, severe burns, dehydration, deep depression, hemorrhage, and shock.

Pulse Pressure

Pulse pressure refers to the difference between the systolic and diastolic reading and is an indicator of the tone of the arterial walls. For example, when the pressure is 120/80, the pulse pressure is 40, which is a normal finding. A pulse pressure over 50 or less than 30 mm Hg may be considered abnormal. A general rule of thumb is that the pulse pressure should be approximately a third of the systolic measure-

TABLE 13-7

HOW BLOOD PRESSURE IS DEFINED		
Category	Systolic/ Diastolic	Recommendations
Stage 1	140-159/90-99	Confirm in two months; begin lifestyle modifications
Stage 2	160-179/100-119	Medical evaluation; begin treatment within one month
Stage 3	180-209/110-119	Medical evaluation; begin treatment within one week
Stage 4	210/120 and over	Immediate medical evaluation and treatment

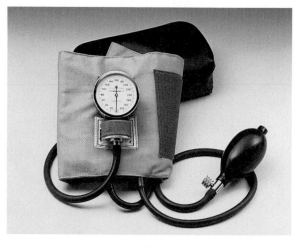

(A)

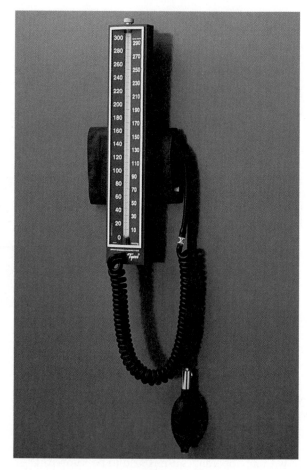

(B)

FIGURE 13–35 Types of sphygmomanometers: (A) aneroid (Courtesy Omron Healthcare, Inc.); (B) wall-mounted (Courtesy Welch Allyn, Inc.)

ment. If less, the patient may have an auscultatory gap (absence of sound) and the pressure may have been incorrectly measured. This disorder will be described later.

Equipment Factors

It is important that sphygmomanometers be in proper working order and correctly calibrated. A mercury manometer that leaks mercury or has bubbles rising in the mercury column when used may not measure accurately. If correctly calibrated, the meniscus of the mercury is at 0 when viewed at eye level. The desktop manometer must always be placed on a flat, level surface. Wall-mounted units should be at a height permitting eye-level viewing. The medical assistant must view a mercury manometer at eye level. Figure 13–35 shows two types of sphygmomanometers.

The aneroid dial should be calibrated occasionally by attaching it to a calibrated mercury manometer with a Y connector (Figure 13–36). Elevate the manometers to 250 mm Hg together, then let the pressure fall, noting the reading at four different points. There should be no more than a 3-mm Hg difference according to the National Bureau of Standards. Mercury sphygmomanometers are much more accurate than aneroid models; however, they still need to be checked for faults every 6 to 12 months, depending on use. They should be serviced and calibrated to ensure accuracy in measurement. Aneroid models must be checked every three to six months over the entire pressure range against an accurate mercury manometer. Figure 13–36 illustrates how the manometers are connected together by a "Y" tube and measured simultaneously.

Studies have shown many sphygmomanometers used in family practice to be faulty. There are two primary areas of failure in both models. The control valves of the cuffs often result in leakage. The mercury monometers also have unsatisfactory conditions of the mercury columns either because of inadequate mercury in the reservoir or dirt from oxidation in the glass calibrated tube, which makes reading more difficult. The aneroid models showed a

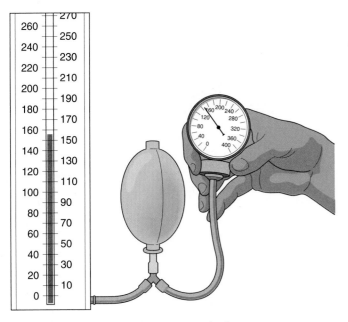

FIGURE 13-36 Testing an aneroid sphygomomanometer

greater problem with accuracy resulting from dial errors because they are rarely calibrated.

It is important that sphygmomanometers be serviced regularly. Faults in aneroid models have to be corrected by service technicians or the manufacturer. A mercury manometer can be maintained by the owner if desired. The common sources of error—the mercury level, the glass tube, and the air vent—can be solved by topping off the mercury in the reservoir, cleaning the glass tube to permit better viewing and mercury flow, or replacing the chamois leather in the air vent. Because mercury is a harmful substance, it is probably best to use trained technicians to service the equipment.

Blood pressure cuffs are critical to correct measurement. They are available in different sizes to measure blood pressure in neonates (infants), children, adults, obese adults, and adult thighs (Figure 13–37). If the reading is to be accurate, the cuff must be the appropriate size. If it is too

small for the upper arm, the reading will be falsely high; if too large, falsely low. To determine the proper size, compare the cuff width to the width of the upper arm. The cuff should be about 20% wider than the arm. When a cuff is too small and you do not have access to a wide adult cuff, measure to the width of the forearm. If the cuff is of adequate size, take the blood pressure reading in the forearm by placing the stethoscope over the radial artery.

Measuring Techniques

Because blood pressure readings are so critical to the determination of hypertension and consequently to the medication given for managing it, strict procedure techniques must be followed. Several factors affect the accuracy of results.

1. The cuff must be completely deflated when applied.
2. The patient must be comfortable, with the arm slightly flexed at the elbow and the brachial artery on a level with the heart. The arm must be free of a constricting sleeve (Figure 13–38). Note: A study at Duke University, reported in the Harvard's Medical School *Heart Letter,* stated that researchers had taken blood pressure measurements through clothing on 36 volunteers to determine if readings would be inaccurate. One arm was bare whereas the other was covered with clothing, either a shirt or a shirt with a light sweater. Simultaneous automated blood pressure measurements revealed that findings through light

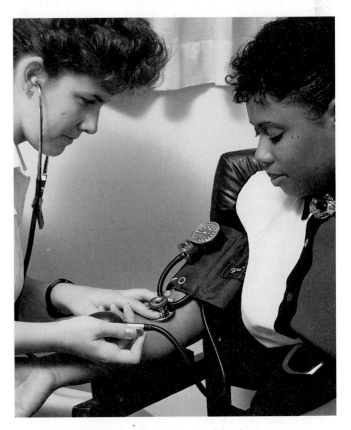

FIGURE 13-38 Measuring blood pressure

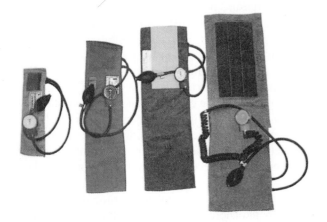

FIGURE 13-37 Blood pressure cuffs in different sizes to fit the arm of a small child to an adult thigh

P R O C E D U R E

13-14 Measure Blood Pressure

PURPOSE: To determine a patient's palpatory and auscultatory blood pressure measurements.

EQUIPMENT: Stethoscope, mercury or aneroid manometer, alcohol wipe, paper, and pen or pencil.

PERFORMANCE OBJECTIVE: In a simulated or actual situation and given access to all equipment and supplies, within a four minute period of time, measure palpatory and auscultatory blood pressure and record findings, following correct procedural technique and observing safety and aseptic precautions. Recorded findings must be within four mm Hg of instructor's measurement. (**NOTE: Accurate procedure evaluation requires the use of a dual teaching stethoscope.**)

1. Wash hands.

2. Assemble equipment.

3. Clean earpieces and head of stethoscope with antiseptic. **RATIONALE: This prevents the transference of microorganisms.**

4. Identify patient. **RATIONALE: Speaking to the patient by name and checking the chart ensures that you are performing the procedure on the correct patient.**

5. Explain procedure. **RATIONALE: If it is new to a patient, especially if a child, explain that the cuff will squeeze but that they must not move.**

6. Place a mercury manometer on a flat, level surface near patient. Put aneroid type within easy reach.

7. Place a patient in a relaxed and comfortable sitting or lying position.

8. Expose patient's upper arm well above elbow, extending arm with palm up. The arm may be either bare or covered with light clothing. (See note regarding clothing on page 587.) Remove arm from a constricting sleeve. **NOTE: Arm must be relaxed, on a supporting surface, slightly flexed at elbow, with brachial artery approximately at level of heart.**

9. With valve of inflation bulb open, squeeze all air from bladder, fold to identify center, placing bottom edge of cuff one to two inches above elbow. Wrap cuff smoothly and snugly around arm, with deflated bladder centered over brachial artery. If using mercury manometer, cuff and tubing may be disconnected for easier application. Reattach tubing after cuff applied. If using aneroid, be certain dial can be easily viewed and end of cuff does not interfere. (**CAUTION: Be alert to patient's movements, which could pull attached desk-type mercury manometer off table.**)

10. Take position with mercury manometer or aneroid dial in view or in a direct line at eye level.

11. With *one hand*, close valve on bulb, clockwise. **NOTE: Do not overtighten, or it will be hard to open.**

12. Position other hand to palpate radial pulse.

13. Observing manometer, rapidly inflate cuff to 30 mm above level where radial pulse disappears.

---

clothing were within 2 mm Hg of the results on bare skin. It was felt that based on this data, patients visiting a physician for a simple blood pressure reading may not need to change into a gown if the clothing covering the arm is light. This decision, however, needs to be made by the employing physician.

3. The center of the bladder in the cuff must be placed over the brachial artery. Fold the bladder area of the cuff in half to locate the center. Many cuffs have improper artery markings.

4. The manometer must be viewed directly from a distance of not more than three feet.

5. A palpatory reading should be taken first to determine proper inflation. Afterward, deflate cuff completely by compressing with hands before reinflation.

6. A minimum of 15 seconds should elapse between inflations (30 is better) to allow blood pressure to normalize.

7. The cuff should be inflated rapidly to 30 mm Hg above the palpatory reading.

To obtain a baseline reading for new patients it may be desirable to measure the pressure twice in each arm, once while the patient is sitting and once while lying down.

Blood pressure has two phases, both of which must be determined. When the cuff is properly inflated, the valve must be opened carefully to allow deflation at a rate of two to three mm per beat. Listen for the first sounds of heartbeat, and note the reading as the systolic pressure once you have heard at least two consecutive beats. Continue to listen and observe as the cuff is deflated until you hear a sudden change in sound to a softer, muffled tone. Note this reading as the diastolic pressure. Continue to observe the manometer until the sound disappears. Note this reading also, even if 0. To record, for example, you would write: B/P 140/90/70. You should ask the physician which sound, the change or the absence, you are to record as the diastolic measurement. There are reasons to support either method.

Probably the mistake made most often in measuring blood pressure is reinflating the cuff after only partial deflation or too soon after complete deflation. Either error

PROCEDURE

13-14 Measure Blood Pressure—continued

14. Open valve, slowly releasing air until radial pulse is detected. (NOTE: **Provides information for auscultatory measurement.**)

15. Observe mercury or dial reading. NOTE: **This is palpatory systolic pressure, which may be recorded, for example, as B/P 120 (P).**

16. Deflate cuff rapidly and completely. Squeeze cuff with hands to empty all. RATIONALE: **All the air must be expressed between inflations to obtain accurate results.** Adjust position if necessary.

17. Position earpieces of stethoscope in ears with openings entering ear canal.

18. Palpate brachial artery at medial antecubital space with fingertips.

19. Place head of stethoscope directly over palpated pulse. NOTE: **Stethoscope head should not touch cuff (creates static).**

20. Close valve on bulb and rapidly inflate cuff to 30 mm above palpated systolic pressure. NOTE: **A minimum of 15 seconds must have elapsed since the previous inflation. RATIONALE: This is the minimum time required for the normalizing of blood flow through the artery.**

21. Open valve, slowly deflating cuff. NOTE: **Pressure should drop two to three mm Hg per second.**

22. With eyes at level of descending meniscus or directly in line or over dial, note reading at which you hear systolic pressure. NOTE: **Must be at least two consecutive beats. Remember systolic measurement.**

23. Allow pressure to lower steadily until you note a change in sound to a softer, more muffled sound. Note this as diastolic pressure (if so instructed).

24. Continue to release pressure until all sound disappears. Note point as diastolic pressure (if so instructed).

25. Release remaining air. Squeeze cuff between hands. RATIONALE: **This removes all the remaining air to make the patient more comfortable and ensures accurate results if reevaluation is necessary.**

26. Record systolic and whichever diastolic the physician prefers.

27. Reevaluate if indicated after a minimum of 15 seconds.

28. Remove stethoscope from ears.

29. Remove cuff from patient's arm.

30. Assist patient with clothing, if necessary.

31. Clean tips and head of stethoscope with alcohol to disinfect. Fold cuff properly, and place with manometer and stethoscope in storage.

32. Wash hands.

CHARTING EXAMPLE:
6-30-XX
B/P 186/94/56

B. Davis (SEM)

---

may cause a false reading and will also cause difficulty in hearing the sound changes because of venous congestion in the forearm. Refer to Procedure 13–14.

Augmenting Sound   To augment heartbeat sounds when they are difficult to hear, use the following technique.

1. With the cuff properly applied and deflated, have the patient elevate the arm above the shoulder and make and release a fist a few times to aid in emptying forearm veins (Figure 13–39).
2. With the patient's arm still raised, rapidly inflate the cuff to 30 mm Hg above palpated pulse.
3. Have patient lower arm.
4. Begin deflation, listening for initial beats. The sounds will be intensified because the blood spurting through the cuff tourniquet is striking against the walls of a near empty artery.

Auscultatory Gap   In some patients, usually those who are hypertensive, there is a silent interval between systolic and diastolic pressure, called an *auscultatory gap* (Figure 13–40). If this is not detected, it may lead to serious undermeasurement of the systolic pressure. For example, the patient's actual systolic pressure is 200, with a gap from 170 to 140 and a diastolic of 120/110. You inflate the cuff to 170 and hear nothing until the manometer reaches 140, which you presume is the systolic pressure. You would continue deflation and record 120/110 as the diastolic; therefore, you would have a pulse pressure of only 20 or 30 mm Hg. Keeping in mind the normal range for pulse pressure; however, you would view 20/30 as suspicious. Taking one third of 140 would give you about 47. To be certain you had not missed a portion of the pressure, you would remeasure, palpating the systolic and then inflating the cuff 30 mm above. If sounds were still audible at that point, you would reinflate it higher *after complete deflation* until you hear the first sounds of systolic pressure.

When recording a blood pressure with an auscultatory gap, list your complete findings (e.g., B/P 200/120/110 with the auscultatory gap from 170 to 140).

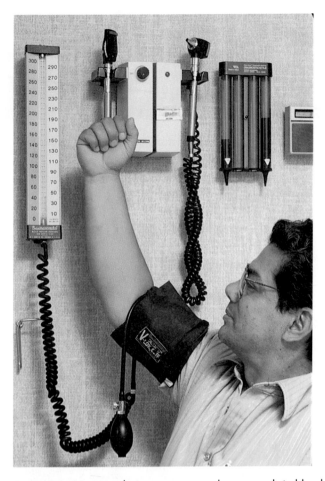

FIGURE 13–39   A technique to augment heart sounds in blood pressure measurement

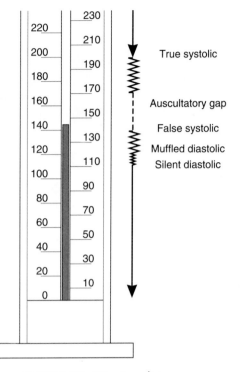

FIGURE 13–40   Auscultatory gap

Blood Pressure in Children

The blood pressure of infants and children is often omitted from the physical examination because it is so difficult to obtain. Variation in blood pressure caused by anxiety and emotional upset make accurate readings very challenging. Basically, the procedure is the same as with adults. Often physicians prefer to do the measurement last after having established some rapport with the child.

The cuff size is important in measuring a child's pressure. It should be appropriate to the size of the arm. The inflatable bag must entirely encircle the extremity.

The level of systolic pressure gradually rises throughout childhood. Normal pressure for a six-month-old is 70; at one year it is 95, and it rises to 100 at six years. By age 16, the systolic pressure will be 120, the adult average. The diastolic pressure reaches 65 by age one and does not change appreciably during childhood.

ACHIEVE UNIT OBJECTIVES

Complete Chapter 13, Unit 3, in the workbook to help you obtain competency in this subject matter.

A CAAHEP CONNECTION

This unit has discussed the physiology and measurement of vital signs, critical skills performed by the medical assistant on a daily basis. The curriculum standards require that instruction be given in **Diagnostic testing** and **Patient care**. Obtaining accurate vital signs is one element in the evaluation of the patient.

RELATING TO ABHES

Chapter 13 discussed the beginning of the database for the patient consisting of the personal and health history, the determination of the chief complaint, the current health status, and a measurement of basic features, such as height, weight, and vital signs. This content is related to the ABHES accreditation requirements of **Manual and computerized records management** within the content area of **Medical Office Business Procedures/Management** and **Basic clinical skills (e.g., vital signs)** and **Patient examination** within the content area of **Medical Office Clinical Procedures**.

Medical-Legal-Ethical Scenario

Susan had been in to see Dr. Morrison a week ago. She had been experiencing a lot of fatigue, a loss of appetite and consequently weight, and elevated temperature along with night sweats. For some time her lifestyle had been rather carefree, and she had not been very responsible with her sexual behavior. She was frightened and felt she needed to rule out any chance of an HIV infection. Her work outlook was very promising. She was being considered for a new position with her company and would gain a nice salary increase if she was chosen. She would also be eligible for a higher level package of health and life insurance benefits.

The appropriate blood tests were done, and when the results were available, Mr. Smith called her office. Because she did not answer, he left a message on her voice mail that her HIV test was positive, and that she needed to make an appointment to begin treatment and counseling.

Susan returned to her office late in the day after a sales appointment. She thought she would finish up a few details before she went home. It seemed like everyone else had gone. While she was cleaning off her desk, she activated her speaker phone to listen to see if there were any messages. She was shocked when she heard Mr. Smith's message and sat there stunned. It was then that she realized her boss had just gone past her cubicle to retrieve his forgotten briefcase. She wondered if he too had heard this very personal message. As she sat there, she became very angry. Early the next morning she phoned the physician's office and demanded to talk with the doctor. She wanted to know how this type of call could have happened and why would anyone be so inconsiderate and unprofessional to leave such a message.

CRITICAL THINKING CHALLENGE

1. What areas of the Role Delineation Study were ignored? (Refer to Appendix A.)
2. How might this incident effect Susan's employment opportunities?
3. What effect could this have on her current and future insurance coverage?
4. How might the medical assistant and the physician be affected?

RESOURCES

Harvard Medical School (1993, November). *Harvard Heart Letter 4* (3).

Hegner, B., Caldwell, E., and Needham, J. (1999). Nursing assistant: A nursing process approach (8th ed.). Clifton Park, NY: Delmar Learning.

Scott, A., and Fong, E. (1998). Body structures and functions (9th ed.). Clifton Park, NY: Delmar Learning.

WEB LINKS

http://www.lifeclinic.com/focus/blood/whatisit.asp (LifeClinic)

Maintained by physicians and educators, this site provides information about several medical conditions that can be positively affected by lifestyle and the close monitoring of changes in vital signs.

CHAPTER 14

Preparing Patients for Examinations

The medical assistant is a significant **liaison** between the patient and the physician. You should be **discreet** and courteous at all times with all patients. Listen carefully and observe closely as patients disclose their complaints and symptoms to you and while you are performing the many procedures dealing with their care. Some patients (themselves) may not even be aware of a condition or symptom that you could bring to their attention. Often a patient becomes so used to a problem that it may be overlooked, such as clearing the throat, a change in weight, or a skin discoloration. When changes like these happen gradually, sometimes the patient is really not aware of them. You can then alert the physician to initiate treatment for a problem that may have otherwise gone undetected.

The medical assistant's responsibility is for the overall preparation of patients for examinations and procedures performed by the physician. To gain full cooperation, patients need to be fully informed about what to expect. Keep in mind that just because these procedures and exams are routine for the health care team, they are not for the patient. Patients come to see the physician for many health concerns. The reason for the patient's office visit is generally established at the time the appointment was made. When a patient is brought in for her visit, a brief assessment is made to make sure you prepare the patient for the appropriate exam. Part of your duties is to answer any questions of the patient. Patients commonly ask:

- what exactly is the exam or procedure (brief definition)
- why it has to be done
- if it hurts
- how long it lasts
- if there will be additional exams/procedures
- when results/reports will be available

Even if the physician has already explained all this to the patient by phone or during the previous appointment, you may have to review it and answer questions. As you are getting patients ready for their exams/procedures, it is an ideal time to provide them with **pertinent** information regarding the maintenance of their overall health. The patient education boxes offer many suggestions you may find helpful. The units that follow provide valuable information in preparing for and assisting with simple to complex preparations and examinations for patients from infancy through adulthood.

UNIT 1

Procedures of the Eye and Ear

OBJECTIVES

Upon completion of the unit, meet the following performance objectives by verifying knowledge of the facts and principles presented through oral and written communication at a level deemed competent. Demonstrate the specific behaviors as identified in the performance objectives or procedures, observing all aseptic and safety precautions in accordance with health care standards.

1. Spell and define, using the glossary at the back of the text, all the **Words to Know** in this unit.
2. Describe patient education concerning the eye and the ear.
3. Assist with examinations of the eye and the ear.
4. Describe and administer screening tests of visual acuity.
5. List and describe screening tests of auditory acuity.
6. Demonstrate the procedure for eye irrigation.
7. Demonstrate the procedure for eyedrop instillation.
8. Demonstrate the procedure for eardrop instillation.
9. Demonstrate the procedure for ear irrigation.
10. Explain the purpose of the Pelli–Robson and Vectorvision visual screening chart.
11. Describe the Ishihara color vision acuity method.
12. Explain the various types of color vision disorders.
13. Identify common behaviors of patients who have vision or hearing problems.

AREAS OF COMPETENCE (AAMA)

This unit addresses content within the specific competency areas of *Fundamental principles, Patient care, Professionalism, Communication skills, Legal concepts,* and *Instruction,* as identified in the Medical Assistant Role Delineation Study, Refer to Appendix A for a detailed listing of the areas.

■ WORDS TO KNOW

achromatic	lavage
acuity	liaison
anesthetize	occluder
audiometer	OD
auditory	ophthalmic
cerumen	OS
daltonism	otic
decibel	OU
discreet	pertinent
deuteranopia	protanopia
funduscopy	Snellen chart
instill	tonometry
irrigate	tritanopia
Ishihara	vertex
Jaeger	wick

(handwritten) AD A S A u

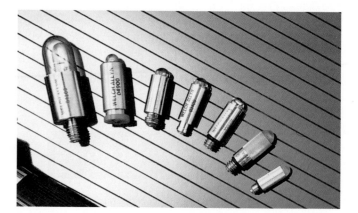

FIGURE 14–2 These tiny lamps are used in instruments requiring a light source and should be checked regularly for power availability. (Courtesy of Welch Allyn, Inc.)

EYE AND EAR EXAMINATION

In assisting with eye and ear examinations, you are expected to hand instruments to the physician as needed. Assembling the instruments in the order of use will be most helpful. You will be responsible for making sure that the instruments are clean and in working order. Otoscopes and ophthalmoscopes should be checked to be sure that the light bulbs are providing strong enough light (Figure 14–1).

These tiny light bulbs (shown in Figure 14–2) must be changed from time to time because they eventually burn out, as do any other kind of bulbs. If these instruments are the hand-held portable type, the batteries must also be changed periodically. The medical assistant is usually responsible for these minor but important tasks. More popularly used in most medical offices are the wall-mounted units with both otoscope and ophthalmoscope instruments (Figure 14–3), which give an electrically powered light source.

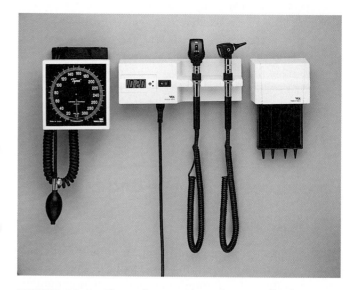

FIGURE 14–3 This wall-mounted set of scopes affords an attractive and efficient access. (Courtesy of Welch Allyn, Inc.)

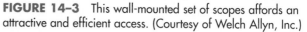

(A)   (B)

FIGURE 14–1 These illustrations show power sources and recharging methods for hand-held ophthalmoscopes and otoscopes: (A) for C-cell conversion, remove the recharging module and rechargeable battery, and replace with two C-cell batteries and converter; (B) for rechargeable batteries, place transformer on handle, and plug in outlet for easy overnight recharging. (Courtesy of Welch Allyn, Inc.)

Most physicians use the disposable plastic ear speculum, which eliminates the worry of disease transmission. The reusable ones must be washed after every use with a mild detergent and placed in a disinfectant solution for at least 20 minutes before they can safely be reused to examine another patient. If the patient has an infected ear that has a discharge containing blood, a disposable ear speculum must be used, and protective gloves must be worn.

The clinical medical assistant should check all exam and procedure rooms daily to make sure there is adequate lighting. A large part of the examination by the physician is of the sensory system by visual inspection. Lighting is also important to you and patients. You are constantly reading and recording information every day.

Some patients will need reassurance during the examination because of apprehension caused by an earlier experience or for other reasons. Usually a kind word and a reassuring smile will help them feel at ease, and their cooperation will follow. Remembering their comfort is vital.

Patients with discharge of the ear or the eye may require **irrigation** (also known as **lavage**) to remove the matter. The physician will then examine the ear or eye to make certain that no damage was done. See Procedures 14–1 and 14–2.

PROCEDURE

14-1 Irrigate the Eye

PURPOSE: To irrigate the patient's eye(s) to soothe tissues, relieve inflammation, remove foreign objects, and aid the eye in draining.

OSHA GUIDELINES: To comply with Standard Precautions, gloves must be worn if there is any possibility of coming into contact with blood or any body fluids.

EQUIPMENT: Latex or vinyl gloves, small basin for irrigation solution, towel, emesis basin to catch the solution, bulb syringe or bottle of solution, patient's chart, and a pen.

PERFORMANCE OBJECTIVE: Provided with a mannequin and all equipment required for the eye irrigation procedure, irrigate the eyes of the mannequin; each step of the procedure must be accurately demonstrated in proper order.

1. Wash hands and put on gloves.

2. Assemble items needed for procedure; prepare solution.

3. Identify patient. **RATIONALE: Speaking to the patient by name and checking the chart ensures that you are performing the procedure on the correct patient.**

4. Explain to patient reason for procedure and how it will be done.

5. Ask patient which position would be more comfortable, sitting or lying down, and assist in draping with towel to protect clothing.

6. Ask patient to tilt head back and to side. Place emesis basin against head for patient to hold to catch solution during irrigation. **NOTE: Placing a couple of tissues, gauze squares, or a towel between the face and the basin will help prevent the patient from getting wet during the procedure. You may have to hold the basin yourself (Figure 14–4).**

7. Wipe eye with gauze square from bridge of nose to outer corner to remove any particles before proceeding with irrigation.

8. Fill bulb or metal syringe with ordered solution.

9. Hold affected eye open with thumb and index finger of one hand or with the little finger of the hand in which you are holding the bottle of solution and slowly release the solution over the eye gently and steadily. **RATIONALE: This must be done from inner canthus to outer canthus to prevent any solution from entering other eye, which may not be affected, and for comfort of patient in catching solution at side instead of near nose.**

10. When irrigation is completed, use sterile gauze squares or tissues to blot area dry and make patient comfortable.

11. Record procedure in patient's chart and initial. **NOTE: Be sure to record type of solution that was used, which eye was irrigated, results, and any other important information you may have observed while performing procedure.**

12. Wash items and return them to proper storage area.

13. Remove gloves and wash hands. **NOTE: Deposit gloves in an appropriate container based upon the conditions under which irrigation was performed.**

CHARTING EXAMPLE:
3-30-XX
Rt eye or OD irrig w/ H$_2$O to remove sand, tolerated well.

T. Edwards (CL)

NOTE: Because there are insurance companies that require health care team members to sign after each order is performed as "T. Edwards," the physician checks off the chart by writing his initials in parentheses to indicate that orders were completed as directed: (CL).

PROCEDURE

14-2 Irrigate the Ear

PURPOSE: To irrigate the ear canal to remove foreign objects, impacted cerumen, or to relieve inflammation and swelling.

OSHA GUIDELINES: To comply with standard precautions, gloves must be worn if there is any possibility of coming into contact with blood or any body fluids.

EQUIPMENT: Latex or vinyl gloves, small basin for ordered irrigation solution, towel, ear basin to catch solution, Pomeroy or bulb syringe, gauze squares, otoscope, ear speculum, and tissues.

PERFORMANCE OBJECTIVE: Provided with an anatomical model of the ear or a mannequin and all equipment required for the ear irrigation procedure, first irrigate the anatomical ear, then the ears of the mannequin; in each process, the steps of the procedure must be demonstrated in proper order.

1. Wash hands and put on gloves.

2. Prepare solution as ordered, and assemble necessary items for procedure. **NOTE: Solution is usually between 100°F and 105°F for patient comfort. Remember to check the expiration dates of all medications before administering to patients.**

3. Identify patient. **RATIONALE: Speaking to the patient by name and checking the chart ensures that you are performing the procedure on the correct patient.**

4. Explain procedure.

5. View affected ear with otoscope to see where cerumen or foreign object is located so that the flow of solution can be directed properly. **RATIONALE: The flow should be directed upward and to one side (as you would rinse out a bucket with a hose).** To use the otoscope for viewing the ear canal, place one hand gently against the patient's head, and grasp the auricle with your thumb and index finger, pulling up and back for adults and down and back for babies up to 36 months. Hold the otoscope with the thumb, index, and great finger of your other hand to avoid using too much pressure as you insert the speculum into the ear canal (Figure 14–5).

6. Ask patient to turn head to affected side and back. Position ear basin under ear for patient to hold to catch solution as it returns during procedure. Place a towel over patient's shoulder to protect clothing (Figure 14–6). For pediatric patients, ask parent to hold the child on lap and assist you during procedure.

7. Use gauze square to wipe away any particles from outer ear before proceeding.

8. Fill syringe with ordered solution.

9. With one hand, gently pull auricle up and back for an adult (down and back for an infant or small child). **RATIONALE: To straighten ear canal.** With other hand, place tip of syringe into canal, and aim flow of solution upward so entire ear canal will be irrigated. DO NOT direct the flow of the solution straight into the ear or use force, or the result will be quite painful for the patient and may damage the tympanic membrane.

10. Use gauze square to wipe excess solution from outside of patient's ear.

11. Give patient several gauze squares or tissues and have patient hold head tilted to side to allow drainage of excess solution from canal.

12. Inspect ear canal with otoscope to determine if desired results have been obtained. **RATIONALE: All material must be removed to adequately inspect the outer ear and tympanic membrane. Patients sometimes feel a little dizzy following this procedure. Allow the patient time to gain balance; assist patient from the examination table.**

13. Record procedure on patient's chart and initial, including which ear was irrigated, solution used, the results of the procedure, and any other important observations.

14. Wash equipment and return to proper storage area.

15. Remove gloves and wash hands.

CHARTING EXAMPLE:

5-20-XX

Irrigated pt's L ear with ordered solution @ 102°F, which returned three large pieces of cerumen (1.25 cm each). Pt states, "I can hear again!"—eardrum is shiny with a pearl-gray color.

T. Edwards (CL)

Be sure to check exp. date & appearance of meds

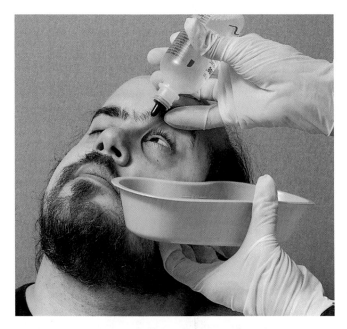

FIGURE 14–4 Direct the flow of irrigation from the inner canthus to the outer canthus.

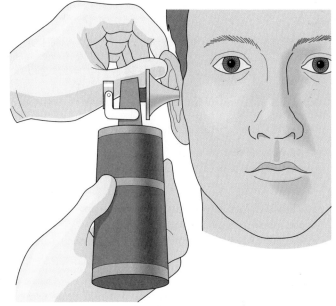

FIGURE 14–5 The examiner is using the otoscope to view the ear canal. This instrument has a light source and a magnifying lens that assists with inspection.

You may also have the responsibility of **instilling** drops into a patient's eye or ear. This simply means dropping a solution into the patient's eye or ear to medicate the tissue or to soothe an irritation. Sterile technique should be used. Recording the amount of medication and the organ to which it is administered is a must.

Instillation of the ear is also performed to soften cerumen (ear wax). **Cerumen** is a protective secretion of the ear, produced to ward off invading microorganisms. Patients sometimes try to remove it by using a cotton-tipped swab, but this often pushes it farther into the ear canal, where it becomes lodged and hardens. This buildup can be very uncomfortable and eventually impair hearing.

Sometimes it is necessary to instill medication into the ear to soften ear wax before an irrigation procedure can be performed. Irrigation of the eye and the ear may be ordered before a successful examination can be conducted by the physician. See Procedures 14–3 and 14–4 for eye and ear instillation.

Patients should have impacted cerumen removed by a member of the health care team to avoid further discomfort or possible injury to the ear. Many offices and clinics have adopted the water pic for this purpose because of the gentle flow it produces and its convenience for irrigation procedures. A bulb, metal, or plastic syringe is also used to perform the ear irrigation procedure. Some patients will need both irrigation and instillation procedures. A softening solution may be instilled into a severely impacted ear, followed by irrigation to remove the excess ear wax.

After having irrigation procedures performed, even with gentle care, many patients feel a little dizziness. You

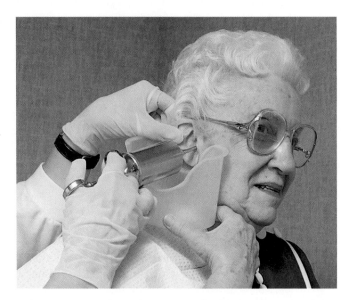

FIGURE 14–6 Drape the patient's shoulder, and position the basin under the ear. Ask the patient to hold the basin as you straighten the ear canal and position the syringe for irrigation.

must be sure that patients are completely stable before permitting them to leave.

A simple method of medicating the eye is by placing a small amount of ointment just inside the lower eyelid. The tip of the ointment tube must not touch the eyelid, where its contents would become contaminated by the secretions of the eye. Care must also be taken when instilling eyedrops so that the tip of the dropper does not come in contact with eye tissue.

PROCEDURE

14-3 Instill Eardrops

PURPOSE: To treat infections, relieve pain, and soften ear wax.

OSHA GUIDELINES: To comply with Standard Precautions, gloves must be worn if there is any possibility of coming into contact with blood or any body fluids.

EQUIPMENT: Latex or vinyl gloves, gauze squares, sterile cotton-tipped applicators and cotton balls, sterile dropper, ordered medication (may be in the form of drops or ointment), tissues.

PERFORMANCE OBJECTIVE: Provided with an anatomical model of the ear or a mannequin and all equipment required to perform the ear instillation procedure, first instill drops into the anatomical ear model, and then into the ears of the mannequin; in each process, the steps of the procedure must be demonstrated in proper order.

1. Verify medication ordered by physician (and check expiration date) in the patient's chart, and assemble necessary items for procedure. Otic medications are often kept in the refrigerator after they have been opened, so it is necessary to bring them to room temperature by letting container sit out for a while or by running warm water over the bottle before using. This is for the comfort of the patient.

2. Wash hands and put on gloves.

3. Identify patient. **RATIONALE: Speaking to the patient by name and checking the chart ensures that you are performing the procedure on the correct patient.**

4. Explain procedure to patient.

5. a. Open the bottle of otic medication and draw into the dropper the ordered amount of drops for instillation. **NOTE: Many prepared ear medications have their own dropper. It is vital that this dropper be used very carefully so as to keep it sterile. DO NOT touch the tip of the dropper to the ear! It is a good practice to place the lid inside up or on side on a gauze square. RATIONALE: If the dropper touches anything OTHER THAN the solution INSIDE the bottle, it is considered contaminated.**

   b. If the medication ordered is an ointment, you should open the tube by removing the cap, being very careful not to touch the tip. **RATIONALE: If the tip of the tube or inside of the cap is touched, it is considered contaminated.** Medication should be instilled by placing a small amount on the tip of a sterile cotton applicator stick and applying it gently into the ear canal. Use extreme caution to avoid puncturing the tympanic membrane.

6. Ask the patient to sit up straight and tilt the head slightly to the left for instilling the right ear; and to the right for the left ear (some patients may prefer to lie down). If the patient is very young or uncooperative, you may need to have another's help with holding the patient during the procedure.

7. Hand a couple of tissues to the patient before you begin. Hold the auricle of the ear *gently* with one hand while you hold the dropper in the other. To straighten the ear canal to allow the medication to enter, pull up and back for adults, and down and back for infants and children up to 36 months.

8. Position the dropper with the medication into (but not touching) the ear canal (Figure 14–7). Depress the bulb to release the prescribed amount of drops into the ear. **NOTE: Advise the patient to remain in this position for a minute or so to allow the medication to settle. Any excess may be wiped away with the tissues or gauze squares.** (This is an ideal time to go over patient education material concerning the ears.) Repeat for the other ear if ordered. Sometimes physicians will request that sterile cotton be inserted into the ear canal to hold the medication in. Simply place a small portion of the sterile cotton ball gently into the canal after instilling the medication; this is sometimes referred to as a wick. It is often saturated with the medication before being placed in the ear canal.

9. Close the bottle or tube of medication. Avoid touching the dropper to the outside of the bottle. **NOTE: If you have touched the patient's ear or anything else, the dropper must be either sterilized or replaced before any other doses of medication can be taken from the bottle.**

10. Remove gloves and wash hands.

11. Record procedure on patient's chart and initial. Be sure to note any complaints of the patient while performing the procedure (e.g., stinging or other discomfort).

12. Return items to proper storage area.

CHARTING EXAMPLE:

6-13-XX
Instilled 3 gtt (drops) of ordered medication into L ear

T. Edwards (CL)

PROCEDURE

14-4 Instill Eyedrops

PURPOSE: To instill medication (in the form of drops or ointment) into the eye(s) to relieve irritation; treat infection; dilate the pupil; or anesthetize the eye in preparation for an examination or for a surgical procedure.

OSHA GUIDELINES: To comply with Standard Precautions, gloves must be worn if there is any possibility of coming into contact with blood or any body fluids.

EQUIPMENT: Latex or vinyl gloves, ordered medication, sterile eye-dropper, sterile gauze squares, tissues.

PERFORMANCE OBJECTIVES: Provided with an anatomical model of the eye or a mannequin and all equipment necessary to perform instillation of the eye, instill drops into the eyes of the anatomical model or of the mannequin; in each process, the steps of the procedure must be demonstrated in proper order.

1. Verify medication ordered by physician in the patient's chart (check the expiration date), and assemble necessary items for procedure. Ophthalmic medications are often kept in the refrigerator after they have been opened, so it is necessary to bring them to room temperature by allowing the drops to sit out for a while or by running warm water over the bottle before using. This is for the comfort of the patient.

2. Wash hands and put on gloves.

3. Identify patient. **RATIONALE: Speaking to the patient by name and checking the chart ensures that you are performing the procedure on the correct patient.**

4. Explain procedure to patient.

5. a. Open the bottle of ophthalmic medication and draw into the dropper the ordered amount of drops for instillation. (Many prepared eye medications have their own dropper. It is vital that this dropper be used very carefully to keep it sterile. DO NOT touch the tip of the dropper to the eye!) **RATIONALE: If the dropper touches anything OTHER THAN the solution INSIDE the bottle, it is considered contaminated.**

   b. If the medication ordered is an ointment, you should open the tube by removing the cap, being very careful not to touch the tip or it will become contaminated. Medication should be placed carefully and sparingly just inside the lower eye lid without touching the eye tissue. **RATIONALE: The tip can be contaminated if it is touched or touches any surface.**

6. Ask the patient to sit up straight and tilt the head back slightly (some patients may prefer to lie down). If the patient is very young or uncooperative, you may need to have another's help with holding the patient during the procedure.

7. Hand a couple of tissues to the patient before you begin. With one hand, use a sterile gauze square to touch the patient's skin just under the eye and gently pull down. This will expose a small pocket (a recessed area between the eye just inside the lower lid) (Figure 14–8).

8. Hold the dropper steadily approximately one-fourth inch from the area, being careful NOT to touch the tissue. Tell the patient to look up while you gently drop the prescribed amount of drops into the pocket of the patient's eye. Ask the patient to blink to further distribute the medication. **NOTE: Advise the patient NOT to rub the eye and not to squeeze out the medications from the eyes. Remind the patient to use the tissues to gently blot excess medication from eyes and not to touch the eyes with bare hands.** (This is an ideal time to go over patient education material concerning the eyes.) Repeat for the other eye if ordered.

9. Close the bottle or tube of medication. Avoid touching the dropper to the outside of the bottle. **NOTE: If you have touched the patient's eye or anything else with the dropper, it must either be sterilized or replaced before any other doses of medication can be taken from the bottle, otherwise the contents will become contaminated.**

10. Remove gloves and wash hands.

11. Record procedure on patient's chart and initial. Be sure to note any complaints of the patient while performing the procedure (e.g., burning or other eye discomfort).

12. Return items to proper storage area.

CHARTING EXAMPLE:
3-06-XX
2 gtt of ordered medication instilled in OU, c/o stinging sensation OS (L eye) only

T. Edwards (CL)

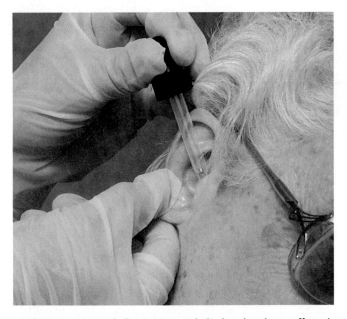

FIGURE 14–7 Ask the patient to tilt the head to the unaffected side as you instill the medication drops carefully into the affected ear canal.

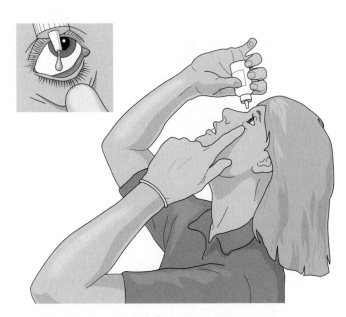

FIGURE 14–8 When instructing patients to use eye drops at home, tell them to tilt the head back slightly and look up. Then instruct the patient to gently pull the skin down just under the eye. This forms a small pocket where the drops should be instilled.

VISUAL ACUITY

Measuring visual **acuity** is a diagnostic screening procedure most often done by the medical assistant on the patient's initial visit prior to the physical examination. It should be performed in a well-lighted room with no interruptions. Observation of the patient for any conditions or behaviors that may indicate visual disturbances is an essential part of the overall examination.

The most common screening device for distance vision is a **Snellen chart**, which shows at what distance a patient can read (Procedure 14–5). The regular chart has letters arranged in rows from largest to smallest.

Those who may have difficulty with reading, such as preschool children or non-English speakers, should be tested with the chart or cards of the letter *E* arranged in different directions. Figures 14–9 and 14–10 show the various Snellen vision screening charts, which are made to standard specifications. These charts are hung on the wall with a mark 20 feet away to show where the patient should stand or sit to read the chart. The chart should be at the patient's eye level. Charts are available on a lighted view box to increase the visibility of the letters.

Most preschoolers have a short attention span. You may need some assistance in screening them for visual acuity, either by having a parent or guardian help to interpret your instructions to them or in the positioning and covering of their eyes during the screening process. It is best to familiarize the child with either chart (Big E or Kindergarten) at a short distance before you begin to screen them for visual acuity. This will help you determine whether or not the child is actually having trouble seeing, or if the child simply does not know what to call the letter or symbol you are pointing to on the chart. You can make it fun for the child by taking your turn first to read the chart and then letting the child have a turn to read it to you. Remembering to praise the child will encourage good behavior. Usually it is not recommended to screen three-year-olds below the 30-foot line. Make sure that you pay close attention to the patient (child or adult) during the procedure. The following are suggestions of what to look for in performing visual acuity tests:

- tilting the head to the side or forward
- blinking or watering of the eyes
- frowning or puckering of the face
- closing of one eye when testing both eyes
- any sign of straining to see

Often while you are preparing a child for this procedure, the parent may offer one or more reasons why the child was brought in for the examination. For instance, the child may hold story books too close to the face or rub the eyes frequently. You should record the symptoms and the results of the visual screening on the patient's chart. A list of common complaints that may indicate vision problems are in Table 14–1. These complaints pertain to both children and adults.

Patients should be screened with and without their corrective lenses and the results recorded as such on their charts. Note that if visual acuity does not exceed 20/200 in the better eye with corrective lenses, the patient is considered legally blind.

The **Jaeger** system is a common method of screening for near vision acuity. The chart used for this procedure is small compared to the wall-mounted charts for distance visual acuity. The card is held by the patient between 14 inches and 16 inches from the eye. You should measure with a yardstick, a meterstick, or a tape measure for accu-

PROCEDURE

14-5 Screen Visual Acuity with Snellen Chart

PURPOSE: To measure the visual acuity of a patient.

EQUIPMENT: Patient's chart, pen, Snellen chart (Figures 14–9 and 14–10), pointer, occular eye **occluder**, card or paper cup.

PERFORMANCE OBJECTIVE: Provided with the necessary vision-screening equipment, measure the visual acuity of at least two other students or visitors by demonstrating each step of the vision-screening procedure; the results of each test will be accurately recorded on the individual patient's chart.

1. Identify patient. **RATIONALE: Speaking to the patient by name and checking the chart ensures that you are performing the procedure on the correct patient.**

2. Explain procedure to patient—that patient is to read each line from the chart as you point to it with pointer.

3. Ask the patient to read the chart with both eyes (**OU**) first, standing 20 feet from the chart.

4. Have patient cover left eye (**OS**) with a card or paper cup. If patient wears corrective lenses, procedure should be performed first wearing lenses and then without and recorded as such.
   NOTE:
   - Chart should be at patient's eye level.
   - Tell patient to keep both eyes open but to cover one eye. This prevents squinting and blurring.

   - Record any observations of individual accommodations made to read chart, such as squinting or turning head.
   - Follow office policy in giving test. Asking patients to read only certain lines of chart is sometimes less time-consuming and less tiring for patient. Covering part of chart that is not being read keeps patients from "studying" for their eye test.

5. Record smallest line that patient can read without making a mistake.

6. Have patient cover right eye (**OD**), and test acuity of left, following same procedure.

7. Record the number of the lowest line that the patient can see. Distant visual acuity is written as a fraction, 20/20, which is average. The numerator is the number of feet, or the distance from the chart; the denominator is the numbered line the patient read. If one's distant visual acuity results are 20/100, it means that the person stood 20 feet from the chart and read the line that should be read at 100 feet. One who has 20/10 acuity can see at 20 feet what should be seen at a distance of 10 feet.

CHARTING EXAMPLE:
2-14-XX
Snellen findings: OD 25/30; OS 20/40 OU 25/30, no squinting observed

T. Edwards (CL)

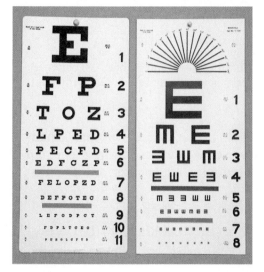

FIGURE 14–9 Snellen visual acuity screening charts. On the left, the letters appear in descending sizes; on the right, the letter E appears in various directions and in descending sizes.

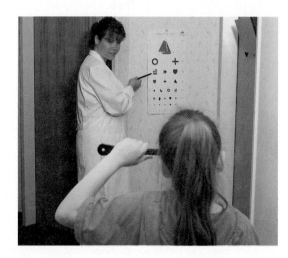

FIGURE 14–10 This photo shows the Kindergarten vision screening chart with pictures in descending sizes. For accurate results, the pictures should be reviewed with the child at a short distance prior to testing to be sure the child knows what the picture is when you ask them during the screening procedure.

TABLE 14-1

POSSIBLE INDICATIONS OF VISUAL DISTURBANCE

During Activities That Require Reading Shows	Illness	Condition	Behaviors	Complaints
1. Difficulty with near or distant vision 2. Avoids reading, writing, and other related activities.	1. Childhood 2. Current infection/ condition	1. Redness of the eye(s) or eyelid(s) 2. Crusting/swelling of eyelid(s) or styes 3. Poor eye coordination 4. Watering and/or discharge 5. Accident/injury to the eye	1. Looks cross-eyed 2. Rubbing eyes frequently 3. Confuses letters (e.g., *a* and *c*, *f* and *t*, *m* and *n*) 4. Turns head or leans forward to see better 5. Blinks continually 6. Irritable at attempting close work	1. Blurriness of vision 2. Nausea 3. Headaches often 4. Dizziness 5. Eyes sensitive to light 6. Feels like something in the eye(s)

If a patient has a past history or a current complaint of any of the areas listed above, a visual disturbance is suggested.

racy. This is the distance at which one with normal vision is able to read printed material (a newspaper) or work on something that requires close attention (sewing). The Jaeger screening test consists of reading material that has ascending sizes of type ranging from .37 mm to 2.5 mm (Figure 14–11). The test contains excerpts from a manuscript sectioned into short paragraphs, none of which are the same. The medical assistant should pay attention to

No. 1.
.37M

In the second century of the Christian era, the empire of Rome comprehended the fairest part of the earth, and the most civilized portion of mankind. The frontiers of that extensive monarchy were guarded by ancient renown and disciplined valor. The gentle but powerful influence of laws and manners had gradually cemented the union of the provinces. Their peaceful inhabitants enjoyed and abused the advantages of wealth.

No. 2.
.50M

fourscore years, the public administration was conducted by the virtue and abilities of Nerva, Trajan, Hadrian, and the two Antonines. It is the design of this, and of the two succeeding chapters, to describe the prosperous condition of their empire; and afterwards, from the death of Marcus Antoninus, to deduce the most important circumstances of its decline and fall; a revolution which will ever be remembered, and is still felt by

No. 3.
.62M

the nations of the earth. The principal conquests of the Romans were achieved under the republic; and the emperors, for the most part, were satisfied with preserving those dominions which had been acquired by the policy of the senate, the active emulations of the consuls, and the martial enthusiasm of the people. The seven first centuries were filled with a rapid succession of triumphs; but it was

No. 4.
.75M

reserved for Augustus to relinquish the ambitious design of subduing the whole earth, and to introduce a spirit of moderation into the public councils. Inclined to peace by his temper and situation, it was very easy for him to discover that Rome, in her present exalted situation, had much less to hope than to fear from the chance of arms; and that, in the prosecution of

No. 5.
1.00M

the undertaking became every day more difficult, the event more doubtful, and the possession more precarious, and less beneficial. The experience of Augustus added weight to these salutary reflections, and effectually convinced him that, by the prudent vigor of

No. 6.
1.25M

his counsels, it would be easy to secure every concession which the safety or the dignity of Rome might require from the most formidable barbarians. Instead of exposing his person or his legions to the arrows of the Parthinians, he obtained, by an honor-

No. 7.
1.50M

able treaty, the restitution of the standards and prisoners which had been taken in the defeat of Crassus. His generals, in the early part of his reign, attempted the reduction of Ethiopia and Arabia Felix. They marched near a thou-

No. 8.
1.75M

sand miles to the south of the tropic; but the heat of the climate soon repelled the invaders, and protected the unwarlike natives of those sequestered regions

No. 9.
2.00M

The northern countries of Europe scarcely deserved the expense and labor of conquest. The forests and morasses of Germany were

No. 10.
2.25M

filled with a hardy race of barbarians who despised life when it was separated from freedom; and though, on the first

No. 11.
2.50M

attack, they seemed to yield to the weight of the Roman power, they soon, by a signal

FIGURE 14–11 This shows the near distance visual acuity screening chart, which is to be held by the patient at arm's length (approximately 14 to 16 inches) for screening.

PROCEDURE

14-6 Screen Visual Acuity with Jaeger System

PURPOSE: To determine near distance visual acuity of a patient using the Jaeger system.

EQUIPMENT: Jaeger near vision acuity chart, pen, patient's chart.

PERFORMANCE OBJECTIVES: Using the Jaeger near vision acuity chart, in a well-lighted area, determine the near distance visual acuity of at least two other students or visitors by demonstrating each step of the visual acuity procedure; the results of each test will be accurately recorded on the individual patient's chart.

1. After identifying the patient, explain the procedure. **RATIONALE: Speaking to the patient by name and checking the chart ensures that you are performing the procedure on the correct patient.**

2. Have the patient sit up straight but comfortably in a well-lighted area.

3. Hand the Jaeger chart to the patient to hold, between 14 inches and 16 inches from the eyes. Figure 14–12 shows proper positioning of the card.

4. Instruct the patient to read (out loud to you) the various paragraphs of the card with both eyes open, first without wearing corrective lenses and then with. **NOTE: Each eye should be tested individually having the person cover the left eye first while reading the card and then the right. Observe carefully for any difficulty the patient has in reading any of the lines on the card. Listen also to any remarks made by the patient and note on chart.**

5. Record the results and problems, if any, on the patient's chart to assist the physician in determining the visual acuity of the patient. The smallest line of print that the patient can read should be recorded and initialed.

6. Thank the patient for cooperation and answer any questions.

7. Return Jaeger chart to proper storage.

CHARTING EXAMPLE:
8-17-XX
read No 3 (62M) OU w/corrective lenses; No 11 (2.5) OD (squinting); No 10 (2.2) OS

T. Edwards (CL)

---

observe any difficulty the person exhibits (e.g., holding the chart right in front of the face, squinting, or blinking) while the patient reads this card. The medical assistant records the results on the chart. Record the line number that the patient can read easily. The screening procedure should be conducted in a well-lighted room without interruptions. The patient ought to be tested with and without wearing corrective lenses, and each eye is tested separately for a complete assessment to be made by the physician. Refer to Procedure 14–6. note c̄/s̄ correction

Many devices for screening visual acuity are available besides the methods already discussed in this unit. One compact instrument is the Titmus Vision Tester (Figure 14–13). In this system of screening, the patient looks into the instrument to view eight different specialized fields designed to detect all common vision problems. While administering this test, the medical assistant sits or stands next to the patient to operate the selection of visual fields. A vision occluder is within the device for testing each eye individually as the patient reads the various lines. Again, the medical assistant must be alert in observing and listening while the patient completes this test. All complaints or observations should be recorded on the patient's chart along with the results of the test. The

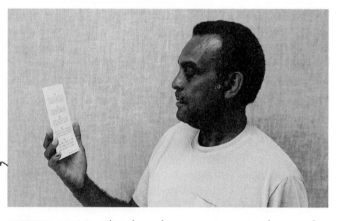

FIGURE 14–12 This photo shows a patient using the near distance vision acuity chart being held at the proper distance (14 to 16 inches) from the eyes.

instrument comes with forms for recording the results of the test.

Color vision acuity means that one can accurately recognize colors. Deficiency in this ability to perceive colors of the spectrum distinctly is commonly termed *color blindness.* This is caused by changes that happen in the

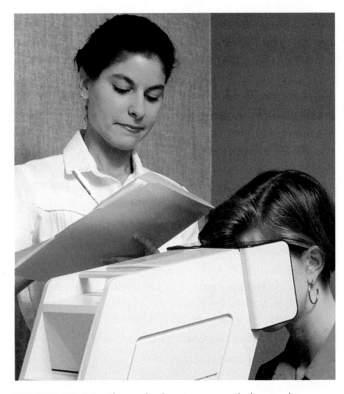

FIGURE 14–13 The medical assistant records the visual acuity as the patient is being tested by looking into the Titmus Vision Tester.

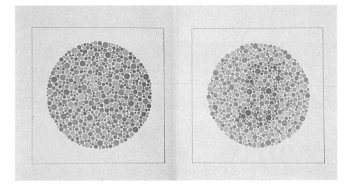

FIGURE 14–14 Sample color plates from the Ishihara's Test for color deficiency (Reproduced with permission from the Isshinkai Foundation.)

pigments of the cones in the retina of the eyes as they react to colored lights of red, green, and blue.

There are two primary types of color blindness: **Daltonism**, which is the most common, is a visual disorder in which the person cannot tell the difference between red and green. It is an hereditary disorder. **Achromatic** vision is total color blindness and very rare, where the person cannot recognize any color at all. These people see everything in white, gray, and black. The probable cause for this condition is that the cones in the retina are defective, or there may be none at all.

Several other conditions involve one's inability or weakness in distinguishing certain colors. In **deuteranopia**, the person has trouble telling any difference between varying shades of green and also of bluish reds and neutral shades. **Protanopia** is partial color blindness. These people have trouble with the perception of reds, and sometimes yellows and greens are confused. This condition is often referred to as red blindness. **Tritanopia**, which is the rarest, means that the person cannot distinguish blue color.

A method for screening patients for defects in distinguishing color vision acuity is with the **Ishihara** color plates book. A sample of the series of multicolored charts in the test book is shown in Figure 14–14. In these pictures of the color plates, one with normal color vision acuity can see a blue-green number 5 against a pink-red background and a pink-red number 8 against a blue-green background.

Patients are asked to trace the patterns of color with their finger as you observe them. There are letters and numbers (and curved lines and shapes for nonreaders) that are one color within another. When administering this procedure, make sure that the room is well-lighted, preferably with natural daylight (not direct sunlight), so that the patient is able to follow your instructions without straining to see. Whatever method of color vision assessment is used where you are employed, it is vital that you are accurate in reporting the results. Medical assistants should first be tested to determine if they have normal color vision to administer the test to patients. Refer to Procedure 14–7.

All patients with thyroid conditions should routinely be screened for color vision acuity during their scheduled visits. The procedure should include testing with both eyes first and then each eye separately to see if there is any difference in the perception of color in either eye. The eye not used should be covered and not held shut. Grave's disease patients especially need frequent assessment of their color vision acuity changes to detect possible damage to the optic nerve. In conditions such as this where swelling occurs behind the eye, pressure builds up and hypertrophy of the tissues results. This interferes with the patient's ability to distinguish colors because the optic nerve is being compressed. The color vision test results may lead to earlier diagnosis and treatment of Grave's ophthalmopathy.

PELLI–ROBSON CONTRAST SENSITIVITY CHART

A recent advance in the measurement of visual acuity is the development of the Pelli–Robson contrast sensitivity chart (Figure 14–15). This chart measures contrast sensitivity by determining the faintest contrast that an observer can see. Recent clinical evidence shows that contrast sensitivity is affected by all of the major eye diseases—diabetic retinopathy, macular degeneration, glaucoma, and cataract. Therefore, measuring contrast sensitivity provides a sensitive screening test for eye disease to provide earlier diagnosis and treatment.

PROCEDURE

14-7 Determine Color Vision Acuity by Ishihara Method

PURPOSE: To determine color vision acuity of a patient using the Ishihara method.

EQUIPMENT: Ishihara book, pen, patient's chart, proper lighting.

PERFORMANCE OBJECTIVE: Using the Ishihara book in a well-lighted area, determine the color vision acuity of at least two other students or visitors by demonstrating each step of the color vision screening procedure; the results of each test will be accurately recorded on the individual patient's chart.

1. Obtain chart from back of book. **NOTE: Before administering this screening test, you should first be tested.**

2. Explain procedure to patient.

3. Conduct the test by asking the patient first to read the plates with both eyes (if the patient wears corrective lenses, with them on). A common practice is to ask the patient to trace with the index finger the letters, numbers, or patterns of color printed in the various plates. Continue testing by having the patient cover the left eye to test the right eye, and then cover the right to test the left. Make sure to note any difficulty or complaint of the patient during the screening process.

4. Compare answers with those given on chart. Record frames patient misses and write down what patient reports so that degree of color impairment may be determined by physician.

CHARTING EXAMPLE:
9-24-XX
Ishihara color plates—no abnormalities

J. Baker (CL)

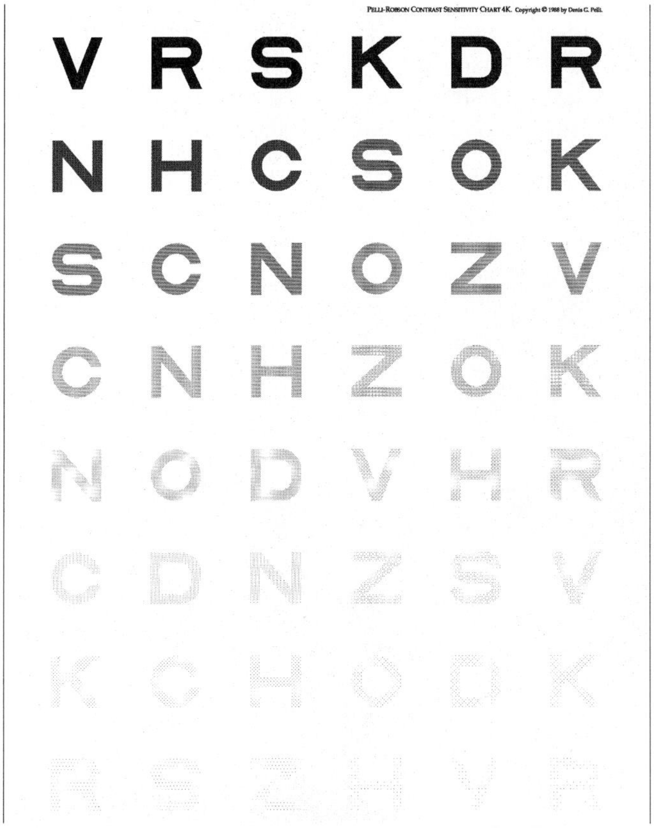

FIGURE 14–15 The Pelli-Robson contrast sensitivity chart is pictured here. The faintest letters that can be read on this chart determine an individual's contrast sensitivity. The use of this chart is an aid to earlier diagnosis of certain eye diseases. (Courtesy Dr. Denis Pelli, NYU.)

Another contrast sensitivity screening method has been developed by Vectorvision. Even though all patients can be tested in this way, it is especially useful in screening small children, internationals, and people who are illiterate. This test has a series of four groups of circles. In these rows of circles, some are solid gray colored and some have vertical lines with them. The patient is instructed to look at the first group and tell you which circles have lines within them. The last correctly identified circle in each group is charted on a graph. The results of this test are interpreted by the physician.

AUDITORY ACUITY

The function of the ear is to enable sound to be perceived. If this process is impaired, hearing loss results. Diseases or conditions of the ear, if not treated, can cause damage to nerves and tissues, which may result in mild to complete deafness. Often patients try to hide a problem such as hearing loss because it is an embarrassment to them. They are sometimes afraid they may have to wear a hearing aid or worry that they may need surgery. Often the patient will try to compensate for the hearing loss by:

- learning to read lips
- always turning the best ear toward the sound source
- pretending that they heard
- increasingly turning up the volume on audio equipment
- standing very close during conversation
- sometimes withdrawing *Avoid social situations*

The family members of the patient may relate this information to you. You should advise the person to have the patient schedule a time to have a doctor examine the ears and have a hearing test. You should note the information on the patient's chart and bring it to the physician's attention. The physician will discuss the problem with the patient during the scheduled appointment.

Sometimes the problem may be as simple as the patient having impacted cerumen, and after an irrigation, the person's hearing usually returns to normal. Sometimes it is not that simple, and further measures are necessary. The medical assistant is in contact with the patient usually more than the physician. It is the assistant's responsibility to act in the best interest of the patient in conveying important information observed. You can watch for any behaviors as you are getting patients ready for their scheduled appointments or when you talk to them over the phone. Often, it is a family member who makes the appointment for the one who has the obvious hearing problem. One of your most important duties is relaying information to the physician about patients.

Common behaviors of patients that indicate the loss of hearing ability are:

1. frequently asking someone to repeat what was said during conversation
2. talking in an inappropriately loud voice
3. not responding at all when spoken to if out of sight range
4. not pronouncing words well
5. responding only when you speak very loudly

Certain complaints may suggest hearing loss or **auditory** nerve damage. When patients disclose any of the following symptoms you should bring it to the attention of the physician for further assessment:

■ ringing in the ears
■ decreased hearing in one ear (or both), sometimes caused by impacted cerumen
■ infection or injury to the ear
■ bleeding or discharge from the ear(s)
■ any unusual noise or feeling inside the ears

These signs, or any others, which patients tell you should be written on the chart during triage. Further examination by the physician is necessary to determine the extent of the problem and its treatment.

HEARING TESTS

An **audiometer** is an instrument used to measure one's hearing. The audiometer determines the hearing thresholds of pure tones of frequencies that are normally audible by an individual. Some also measure bone and air conduction. The threshold of hearing is the point where a sound can barely be heard. A person with normal hearing should hear all frequencies up to 15 **decibels**, depending on the surrounding noise levels (Figure 14–16).

Audiometric devices are powered either by batteries or electricity. Whatever type is used in the facility where you are employed should be checked periodically for proper performance and accuracy. If the batteries need to be

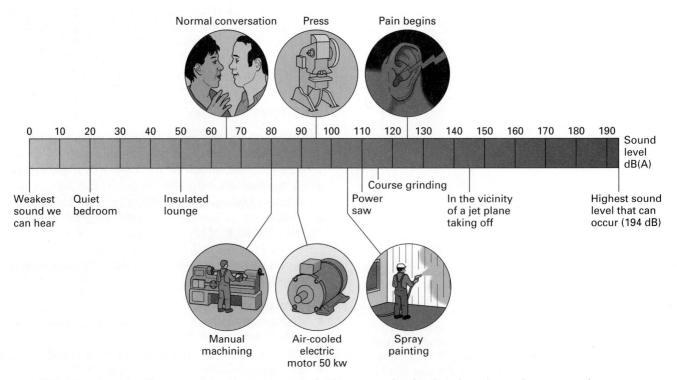

FIGURE 14–16 This illustration shows the various noise levels associated with selected conditions, locations, and operations.

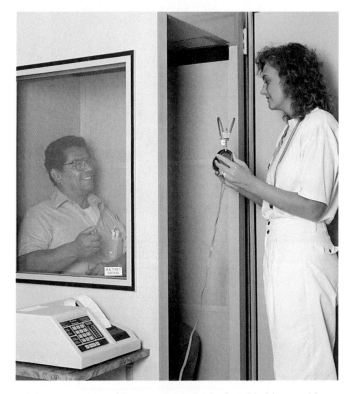

FIGURE 14–17 The patient presses the hand-held control button each time he hears a sound while in the soundproof booth. The signals are transmitted to the computer outside the booth and printed as an audiogram.

changed or if a wire is frayed, it should be taken care of before being used with patients, not only for their safety, but to make sure that it works efficiently. Several types of audiometers are available for use in determining hearing acuity. Many are still used, requiring that the operator manually turn a dial to emit the various frequencies for the patient to hear during the test. Companies that manufacture audiometers offer in-service demonstrations to make sure their equipment is used properly. Operations manuals should be kept with the instrument for handy reference.

The procedure for most audiometers is basically the same. The patient is instructed to place the earphones (marked red for the right ear and blue for the left ear) over the ears. The medical assistant tells the patient in the soundproof booth how the earphones are to be placed and how to work the control signal (Figure 14–17). The printer on the table next to the booth records the results of the hearing test. The printout is called an audiogram, which is filed in the patient's chart after the physician reads the results of the test and makes an evaluation.

During the procedure in whichever ear that is not being tested, the sound is automatically blocked by the machine. In the ear which is being tested, the machine provides a series of tones. The patient listens and signals (either by raising a finger or by using a hand-held control) to the medical assistant as the various sounds are heard. The tones range in frequencies from very low to very high with a varied level of decibel intensity. After the right ear

has been tested, the machine switches automatically to test the left ear. The medical assistant should report any complaints that the patient may have had before or during the hearing test and any unusual behavior to the physician. You should make a note of this information on the patient's chart along with the results of the test and place your initials indicating that you have completed the test.

Physicians use several audiometric assessment procedures to determine the cause of the patient's hearing loss, some of which are a part of the complete or routine physical examination.

During the physical examination, the physician will use a tuning fork to test the patient's hearing. A two-pronged metal tuning fork is used, its frequency varying with the size of the instrument. The common tests done are the Rinne and the Weber.

In the Rinne test, the examiner strikes the fork and then holds the shank (stem) against the patient's mastoid bone until the patient no longer hears the sound. The prongs of the tuning fork are then placed about one inch from the auditory meatus (opening to the ear) and then next to it. In a normal ear, the sound is heard about twice as long by air conduction as by bone conduction. If hearing by bone conduction is greater, the result is spoken of as a negative Rinne.

In the Weber test, the vibrating tuning fork is held against the **vertex** (crown of the head) or against the skull or forehead in the midline (Figure 14–18). The sound is heard best by the unaffected ear if deafness is caused by disease of the auditory apparatus or by the affected ear if deafness is caused by obstruction of the air passages.

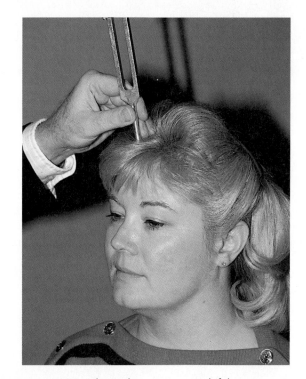

FIGURE 14–18 The Weber test is normal if the patient can hear the sound made in both ears equally well as the end of the tuning fork is placed against the skull.

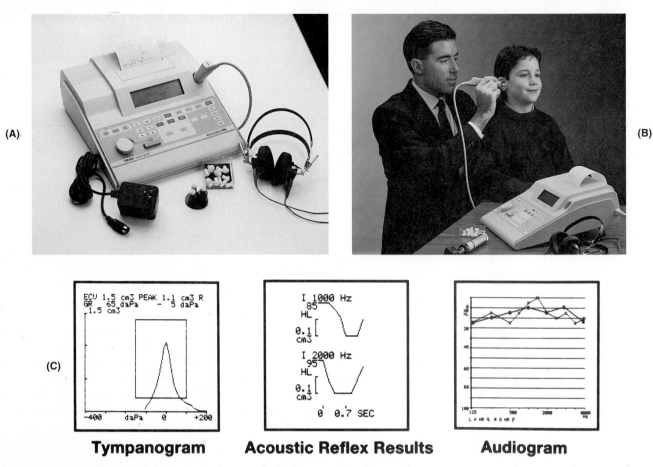

Tympanogram   **Acoustic Reflex Results**   **Audiogram**

FIGURE 14–19 This type of diagnostic tool is easy for both operator and patient because it requires only a minimal amount of time to complete: (A) the Auto Tymp with transformer, eartips, and headset; (B) Auto Tymp being used; (C) printed results of the test. (Courtesy of Welch Allyn, Inc.)

 # Medical-Legal-Ethical Scenario

Tonya had been designated as the clinical medical assistant for the day because the other clinical assistant was on vacation. Tonya had a headache and didn't feel like working at all. She brought patients back and tried to be pleasant but was not herself. Mrs. Agnew reported to the doctor that Tonya was patronizing and rude to her when she got her ready for her exam. She was working as fast as she could to get patients ready for the physician but kept making mistakes and forgetting things. Darlene was at the front desk and realized that the schedule was getting backed up. In attempting to help Tonya, Darlene brought patients in as much as she could in between answering the phone and greeting patients as they came into the reception room. Darlene finally pulled Tonya aside and asked her to try to speed it up, or she would involve the office manager, who was at another location. Darlene knew that they were already short staffed and tried to help as much as possible, but doing two jobs was beginning to wear her down.

CRITICAL THINKING CHALLENGE

1. What should Tonya have done to begin with to eliminate the problem?
2. What do you think the physician thought was going on?
3. Should the physician be involved? Why or why not?
4. Discuss whether Darlene was helping or adding to the problem?
5. What should have been done? When?
6. Should Darlene be thanked for what she did? By whom?
7. Should the office manager have been notified?
8. What would you have done in this situation?

A simple means of screening the hearing of an infant or a small child is to place a ticking watch behind her shoulder, without her seeing it, and see how quickly they become aware of the noise.

A small amount of hearing loss may be temporary because of a patient's physical condition, and a recheck in one or two weeks may be advisable.

A most useful diagnostic instrument that affords both audiogram and tympanogram, as well as acoustic reflex results, is shown in Figure 14-19A, B, and C. This device, the TM 262 Auto Tymp, is useful in providing objective data in determining complete diagnoses and documentation of diseases and disorders of the ear. It is additionally helpful in evaluation of follow-up treatment.

ACHIEVE UNIT OBJECTIVES

Complete Chapter 14, Unit 1, in the workbook to help you obtain competency of this subject matter.

PATIENT EDUCATION

1. Advise patients not to put anything into their ears to avoid damaging the tympanic membrane. The ear wax produced by the body has a purpose. It is to protect and moisten the membrane of the ear canal. Many people feel that they must completely remove this daily with a swab, which often results in being packed down into the ear canal where it hardens. This impacted ear wax (cerumen) must be removed by a qualified medical team member.

2. Instruct patients that eardrops and other ear medications should be used only with the advice of their physician. Earache, pain, or discharge should be reported to and examined by the physician as soon as possible.

3. Discuss the possibility of permanent hearing loss with patients who work around extremely loud noise or who have gotten into a habit of turning the volume way up when listening to audio systems, radios, or TVs. Explain to these patients that protective ear coverings should be worn while on the job (it is a safety requirement) and advise those who listen to loud music to turn down the volume before their hearing is lost from damage to nerves.

4. Urge patients to have regular hearing tests to detect loss of hearing or other related problems. It is recommended that this be done annually unless otherwise instructed by the physician or if there is a noticeable difference or problem with hearing. Patients who have a history of ear infections should have periodic hearing tests.

UNIT 2

Positioning and Draping for Examinations

OBJECTIVES

Upon completion of the unit, meet the following performance objectives by verifying knowledge of the facts and principles presented through oral and written communication at a level deemed competent. Demonstrate the specific behaviors as identified in the performance objectives of the procedures, observing all aseptic and safety precautions in accordance with health care standards.

1. Spell and define, using the glossary at the back of the text, all the **Words to Know** in this unit.
2. Describe and explain the purpose of each of the examination positions.
3. Demonstrate the proper method of positioning and draping patients for the various examinations.
4. Explain safety precautions regarding both the medical assistant and patient in positioning for examinations.

AREAS OF COMPETENCE (AAMA)

This unit addresses content within the specific competency areas of *Fundamental principles, Patient care, Professionalism, Communication skills, Legal concepts, Instruction,* and *Operational functions,* as identified in the Medical Assistant Role Delineation Study. Refer to Appendix A for a detailed listing of the areas.

WORDS TO KNOW

anterior	incompetent
body mechanics	lithotomy
dorsal	postpartum
dowel	prolapsed
dyspneic	prone
fenestrated	recumbent
flexed	shock
genucubital	supine
genupectoral	Trendelenburg
horizontal	

POSITIONING AND DRAPING PATIENT

Positioning the patient for examination is an important function of the medical assistant. There are a number of standard positions for specific examinations and treatments that you should know. If a power table is used, you should learn how to operate it. The power table illustrated in Figure 14–20 is considered to be an advanced power examination table in America. It is possible to program

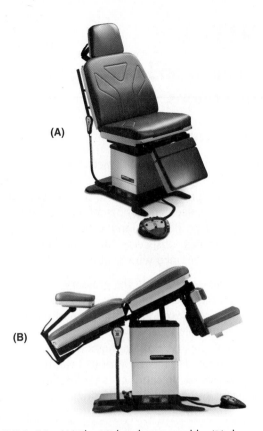

FIGURE 14-20 (A) The Midmark power table; (B) shows table in position for specialty exam. (Courtesy of Midmark Corp.)

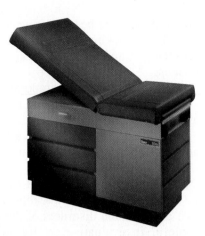

FIGURE 14-21 A medical examination table that is commonly used in medical offices. (Courtesy of Midmark Corp.)

this table to the best height for the physicians who will use it and to the positions desired. The desired position is then achieved by the press of a button. This table has an optional plug-in foot control that could be used in the event of a failure in the computer circuit. This table also has two rolls of paper under the frame at the head of the table. The paper supply should be checked periodically and replenished as necessary.

Most examination tables (Figure 14–21) are vinyl covered and easily cleaned with antiseptic soap and a sponge or cloth if any body fluids are noted after a patient has been examined. The table needs to be cleaned regularly. The table is covered with a roll of paper, which needs to be the proper width to cover the table. The paper roll is

usually inserted on a **dowel** under the head of the table and is secured at the bottom of the table with a strap. The strap is useful in your practice of tearing off the paper when you pull down a clean paper for the next patient. The paper that you pulled down to the edge of the exam table can be folded under about an inch so that it has a neat appearance (to hide the jagged paper edge). You should pull the new paper down in the presence of patients, so they will know it is clean for them.

A female medical assistant should remain in the room when a female patient is being examined by a male physician. The patient should feel more relaxed, and the physician is protected from lawsuits that could result from patients claiming the physician acted improperly during the examination. Patient gowns and drapes are made of cloth or disposable paper. The patient is instructed on the use of the gown to avoid unnecessary exposure. If the examination table is too high for the patient to sit on it comfortably, a foot stool should be provided. A very ill patient or a small child should never be left alone on a table; a member of the family may be asked to sit with them if you must leave the room.

gown is for privacy & warmth

BODY MECHANICS

Body mechanics are important. Never try to lift a patient who obviously weighs more than you can safely handle; have someone help you. If a patient needs help in moving on the table, reach under the arm at the shoulder and help the person move up. You should move with the patient. If it is necessary to help a patient out of a wheelchair, position the chair and lock the wheels before trying to help the patient move from the chair to the table. A procedure for this will be given later. The standing erect or anatomical position may be used, especially for neurological examination, range of motion, and flexibility while the patient is being instructed by the physician in bending and walking. This position begins with the patient standing upright with arms at sides and palms facing forward (see Chapter 11, Unit 1). If the patient is well enough to sit on the edge or end of the table with feet hanging down and

---

PATIENT EDUCATION

Instruct the patient about the need for a specific position for the examination to be performed. This information should be included with the instructions on preparing for the examination. The patient must understand that the physician needs to examine certain parts of the body or perform certain procedures and tests, and the patient must be positioned in the most accessible manner.

no back support, this position may be used to begin the examination.

EXAMINATION POSITIONS

The **horizontal recumbent** or **supine** position is used for examination and treatment of the **anterior** surface of the body and for x-rays (Procedure 14–8 and Figure 14–22). The term **dorsal** *recumbent* is used to indicate that the legs are **flexed**. This position allows for relaxation of the abdominal muscles and thus easier examination of the abdominal area. This position may also be used for vaginal or rectal examination. This position may also be used to test reflexes. The gown is open in the front, and a drape sheet of

---

PROCEDURE

14-8 Assist Patient to Horizontal Recumbent Position

PURPOSE: To position the patient into a comfortable and appropriate position for a specific exam.

OSHA GUIDELINES: Standard Precautions recommend that proper hand washing and gloving is performed to avoid the transfer of microorganisms to other patients, yourself, and the environment.

EQUIPMENT: Table, table paper, drape sheet, pillow, disposable pillow cover or towel.

PERFORMANCE OBJECTIVE: In a simulated situation, using an appropriately prepared examining table and drape, assist the patient to assume the horizontal recumbent position while providing for safety and privacy according to the standards identified in the procedure sheet.

1. Check examination room for cleanliness. **NOTE: Always have clean paper on table and a clean pillow cover or clean towel over pillow. RATIONALE: Every precaution must be maintained to prevent any possible cross-contamination of disease.**

2. Identify the patient. **RATIONALE: Speaking to the patient by name and checking the chart ensures that you are performing the procedure on the correct patient.**

3. Give clear instructions to the patient regarding amount of clothing to be removed and where it is to be placed.

4. Instruct patient on use of gown. **RATIONALE: The procedure to be performed dictates whether the front or back should be open.**

5. Assist patient if help is needed. Otherwise respect privacy and modesty of patient by leaving room while patient changes.

6. Instruct patient to sit on side of table.

7. Instruct patient to lie flat on table with legs together.

8. Pull out end extension on table for leg support if needed.

9. Patient may rest head on small pillow if desired.

10. Instruct patient to cross arms on chest or put them at sides of body. To position for dorsal recumbent, ask patient to put bottoms of both feet flat on table with knees flexed.

11. Drape sheet evenly over patient but leave loose on all sides. For vaginal or rectal examination, drape patient with one corner of sheet over chest, a corner wrapped around each leg, and fourth corner over pubic area. Physician will turn back sheet at pubic area.

12. Assist physician as necessary with examination.

13. Assist patient from table if help is needed when examination is completed. Patients may be dizzy from an abrupt change in position.

14. Clean room and replace supplies. **NOTE: Examination table surface and base must be thoroughly cleaned with disinfecting cleanser at regular intervals and following any contact with body fluids which may contain bloodborne pathogens.**

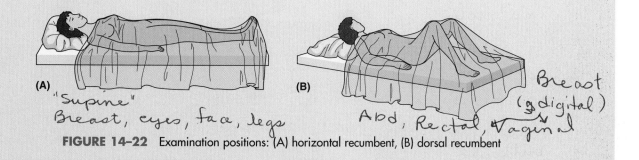

(A) "Supine" Breast, eyes, face, legs

(B) Abd, Rectal, Vaginal   Breast (g digital)

FIGURE 14–22 Examination positions: (A) horizontal recumbent, (B) dorsal recumbent

cloth or paper is used to cover the patient. The **prone** position is used for examination of the back or spine, with the gown open in the back (Procedure 14–9 and Figure 14–23).

The Sims' position is used in examination and treatment of the rectal area and for enemas, rectal temperature, and sigmoidoscopy (Procedure 14–10 and Figure 14–24). This position may also be used for pelvic examinations. This is also called the lateral recumbent position.

The knee-chest position is used for rectal examination and specifically for sigmoidoscopy examination (Procedure 14–11 and Figure 14–25). When properly done, this position helps straighten out the sharp curve in the sigmoid

---

PROCEDURE

14-9 Assist Patient to Prone Position

PURPOSE: To position patient into a comfortable and appropriate position for a specific exam.

OSHA GUIDELINES: Standard Precautions recommend that proper hand washing and gloving is performed to avoid the transfer of microorganisms to other patients, yourself, and the environment

EQUIPMENT: Table, protective gloves, table paper, drape sheet, pillow, disposable pillow cover or towel.

PERFORMANCE OBJECTIVE: In a simulated situation, using an appropriately prepared examining table and drape, assist the patient to assume the position while providing for safety and privacy according to standards identified in the procedure sheet.

1. Check examination room for cleanliness. **NOTE: Always have clean paper on table and a clean cover or clean towel over pillow.**

2. Identify the patient. **RATIONALE: Speaking to the patient by name ensures that you are performing the procedure on the correct patient.**

3. Give clear instructions to patient regarding amount of clothing to remove and where it is to be placed.

4. Instruct patient on use of gown—to be open in back. Some offices furnish a modesty gown with a rectangular piece of material to be put on diaper fashion and tied on sides. If so, instruct in use.

5. Assist patient if necessary. Otherwise respect privacy of patient by leaving room while patient undresses.

6. Instruct patient to sit on side of table.

7. Instruct patient to lie flat on table with legs together.

8. Pull out end extension on table for leg support if needed.

9. Cover patient with drape sheet and instruct patient to turn toward you onto stomach, being careful to stay in center of table to avoid a fall. **NOTE: Always instruct patient to turn toward your body to prevent a fall. You can grasp cover drape and keep it smoothly in place as patient turns over.**

10. Instruct patient to turn head to side.

11. Instruct patient to flex arms at elbows with hands at side of head.

12. Drape sheet evenly and loosely on all sides.

13. Assist physician as necessary with examination.

14. Instruct patient to turn on back, being careful to stay in middle of table to avoid fall.

15. Instruct patient to sit up for a moment to regain balance before trying to leave table.

16. Clean room and replace supplies. **NOTE: The examination table surface and base must be thoroughly cleaned with disinfecting cleanser at regular intervals and following any contact with body fluids which may contain bloodborne pathogens.**

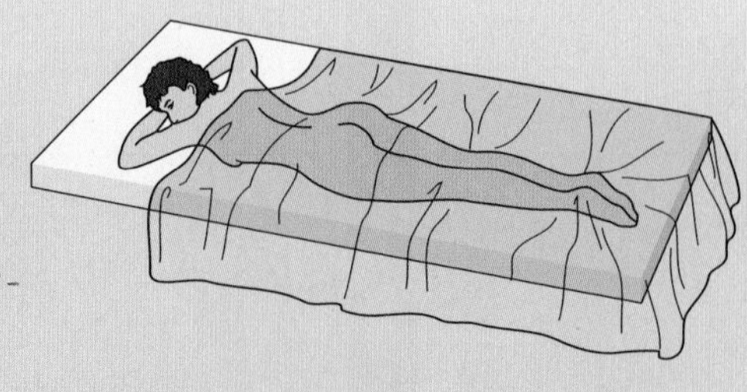

FIGURE 14-23 Prone position

PROCEDURE

14-10 Assist Patient to Sims' Position

PURPOSE: To position the patient into a comfortable and appropriate position for a specific exam.

OSHA GUIDELINES: Standard Precautions recommend that proper hand washing and gloving is performed to avoid the transfer of microorganisms to other patients, yourself, and the environment

EQUIPMENT: Table, table paper, drape sheet, pillow, disposable pillow cover or towel.

PERFORMANCE OBJECTIVE: In a simulated situation, using an appropriately prepared examining table and drape, assist the patient to assume the horizontal recumbent position while providing for safety and privacy according to standards identified in the procedure sheet.

1. Check examination room for cleanliness. **NOTE: Always have clean paper on table and a clean cover or clean towel over pillow.**

2. Identify the patient. **RATIONALE: Speaking to the patient by name ensures that you are performing the procedure on the correct patient.**

3. Give clear instructions to patient regarding amount of clothing to remove and where it is to be placed.

4. Instruct patient on use of gown. **RATIONALE: The procedure to be performed dictates whether the front or back should be open.**

5. Assist patient if needed. Otherwise respect privacy and modesty of patient by leaving room while patient undresses.

6. Instruct patient to sit on side of table.

7. Instruct patient to lie on left side. A pillow may be placed under head.

8. Instruct patient to place left arm and shoulder behind body. This places weight of body on chest.

9. Instruct patient to flex right arm with hand toward head in front of body.

10. Instruct patient to flex left leg slightly with buttocks near edge of table, being sure patient does not fall.

11. Instruct patient to flex right leg sharply toward chest.

12. Cover patient with a fenestrated drape. If a regular sheet is used, hang drape free from under arms to below knees. Edge will be turned back for procedure.

13. Assist physician as necessary with examination.

14. Instruct patient to turn to back, sit up, and then move from table. Assist patient as necessary.

15. Clean room and replace supplies. **NOTE: The examination table surface and base must be thoroughly cleaned with disinfecting cleanser at regular intervals and following any contact with body fluids that may contain bloodborne pathogens.**

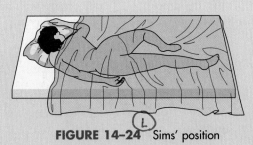

FIGURE 14-24 Sims' position

digital rectal, vag.
enemas (small -fleets
sigmoidoscopy
colonoscopy
suppository
Adult Rectal T

colon and makes it safer and easier to pass the sigmoidoscope. This position is sometimes called the **genupectoral** and is used as therapy for **postpartum prolapsed** uterus. The position is difficult to assume and to maintain for a long time. Special care must be taken to keep the patient from falling.

The Fowler's position is used for patients with respiratory or cardiovascular problems (Procedure 14–12 and Figure 14–26). The patient who is **dyspneic** must be in a sitting or semisitting position to breathe comfortably. This position may be used to examine the trunk of the body (head, neck, and chest area). The position may be

PROCEDURE

14-11 Assist Patient to Knee-Chest Position

PURPOSE: To position the patient into a comfortable and appropriate position for a specific exam.

OSHA GUIDELINES: Standard Precautions recommend that proper hand washing and gloving is performed to avoid the transfer of microorganisms to other patients, yourself, and the environment

EQUIPMENT: Table, table paper, drape sheet, pillow, disposable pillow cover or towel.

PERFORMANCE OBJECTIVE: In a simulated situation, using an appropriately prepared examining table and drape, assist the patient to assume the knee-chest position while providing for safety and privacy, according to standards identified in the procedure sheet.

1. Check examination room for cleanliness. **NOTE: Always have clean paper on table and a clean pillow cover or clean towel over pillow.**

2. Prepare examination equipment on tray with cover over instruments. Each office will have special equipment, which physician will want you to have ready. Check office procedure manual or make up your own card for each procedure.

3. Identify the patient. **RATIONALE: Speaking to the patient by name ensures that you are performing the procedure on the correct patient.**

4. Give clear instructions to patient regarding which clothing to remove and where it is to be placed.

5. Instruct patient on use of gown. **RATIONALE: The procedure to be performed dictates whether the front or back should be open.**

6. Assist patient if needed. Otherwise respect privacy and modesty of patient by leaving room while patient undresses.

7. Instruct patient to sit on side of table.

8. Instruct patient to lie down on table.

9. Cover patient with drape.

10. Instruct patient to turn toward you onto stomach, being careful to stay in middle of table.

11. Instruct patient to get on hands and knees.

12. Instruct patient to flex arms and fold under head, bringing chest down to table. If this is too difficult, have patient rest on elbows (**genucubital** position).

13. Instruct patient to separate knees slightly and keep thighs at right angle to table.

14. A fenestrated drape is usually used, but two small sheets may be draped to meet at rectal area. Diamond drape may also be used.

15. Call physician immediately to complete examination.

16. Assist physician as necessary with examination.

17. Instruct patient to lie flat on stomach and then turn over on back (while lying in middle of table) and sit up before moving from table.

18. Clean room and replace supplies. **NOTE: The examination table surface and base must be thoroughly cleaned with disinfecting cleanser at regular intervals and following any contact with body fluids which may contain blood-borne pathogens.**

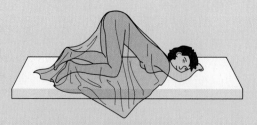

FIGURE 14–25 Knee-chest position

semi-Fowler's (partially sitting) or Fowler's (sitting upright). A female patient would be more comfortable in an examination gown opened in front if the sheet covers the chest area on down to the feet.

The **lithotomy** position is used for vaginal or rectal examination (Procedure 14–13 and Figure 14–27). This position can also be used for examination of the male genital area and for catheterization of a patient.

In the **Trendelenburg** or **shock** position, the patient is supine with feet elevated slightly (Figure 14–28). This position may easily be accomplished with a power table. This position may be used for postural drainage

P R O C E D U R E

14-12 Assist Patient to Semi-Fowler's Position

PURPOSE: To position the patient into a comfortable and appropriate position for a specific exam.

OSHA GUIDELINES: Standard Precautions recommend that proper hand washing and gloving be performed to avoid the transfer of microorganisms to other patients, yourself, and the environment

EQUIPMENT: Table, table paper, drape sheet, pillow, disposable pillow cover or towel.

PERFORMANCE OBJECTIVE: In a simulated situation, using an appropriately prepared examining table and drape, assist the patient to assume the semi-Fowler's position while providing for safety and privacy according to standards identified in the procedure sheet.

1. Check examination room for cleanliness. **NOTE: Always have clean paper on the table and a clean pillow cover or clean towel over the pillow.**

2. Identify the patient. **RATIONALE: Speaking to the patient by name and checking the chart ensures that you are performing the procedure on the correct patient.**

3. Give clear instructions to patient if clothing is to be removed.

4. Instruct patient on use of gown. **RATIONALE: The procedure to be performed dictates whether the front or back should be open.**

5. Assist patient if needed or leave room while patient undresses.

6. Ask patient to sit at end of table and move back toward the center.

7. Raise head of table to desired height for comfort of patient, usually 45° angle for semi-Fowler's and completely upright for Fowler's.

8. Ask patient to lean back on rest.

9. Support legs with extension rest at end of table.

10. Drape patient from underarms to below knees.

11. Assist patient as necessary.

12. Ask patient to sit up before lowering head of table. Be sure you understand how to lower head of table. **RATIONALE: Some tables have a release lever, and it is necessary to support head of table with one hand while releasing lever so that head of table will not fall with a crash.**

13. Assist patient from table.

14. Clean room and replace supplies. **NOTE: The examination table surface and base must be thoroughly cleaned with disinfecting cleanser at regular intervals and following any contact with body fluids which may contain bloodborne pathogens.**

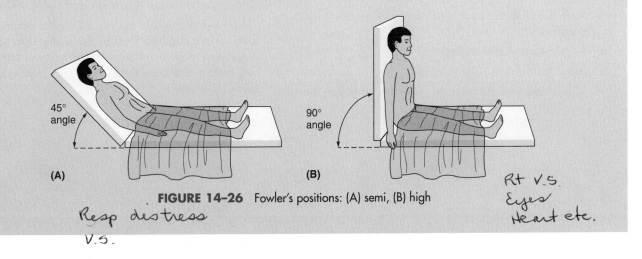

FIGURE 14–26 Fowler's positions: (A) semi, (B) high

(handwritten notes) Resp distress V.S. · Rt V.S. Eyes Heart etc.

with the patient turning into various positions. It can be used for a patient with low blood pressure and to displace organs for some abdominal surgical procedures. This position is also useful as a simple test for **incompetent** valves in persons with varicose veins. After being placed in this position, the patient is asked to stand, and the physician observes whether the veins fill from above or below.

A special table would be needed for the jackknife position to be comfortable (Figure 14–29). The patient is in a semisitting position with the shoulders elevated and the thighs flexed at right angles to the abdomen. This position

PROCEDURE

14-13 Assist Patient to Lithotomy Position

PURPOSE: To position the patient into a comfortable and appropriate position for a specific exam.

OSHA GUIDELINES: Standard Precautions recommend that proper hand washing and gloving is performed to avoid the transfer of microorganisms to other patients, yourself, and the environment

EQUIPMENT: Table, table paper, drape sheet, pillow, disposable pillow cover or towel.

PERFORMANCE OBJECTIVE: In a simulated situation, using an appropriately prepared examining table and drape, assist the patient to assume the lithotomy position while providing for safety and privacy according to standards identified in the procedure sheet.

1. Check examination room for cleanliness. **NOTE: Always have clean paper on the table and a clean pillow cover or clean towel over the pillow.**

2. Assemble necessary equipment.

3. Identify the patient. **RATIONALE: Speaking to the patient by name and checking the chart ensures that you are performing the procedure on the correct patient.**

4. Give clear instructions to patient to remove clothing from waist down. If breast examination is also to be performed, ask patient to put on a gown.

5. Assist patient if needed or leave room while patient is undressing.

6. Ask patient to sit at end of table.

7. Instruct patient to lie back on table.

8. Support legs with extension on table. (If no extension, be sure patient moves back on table before lying down.) **NOTE: Newer examination tables allow patient to sit while table is tilted back, leg supports come up under legs, and end of table is lowered, all by use of a foot pedal.**

9. Position stirrups as far away from table as possible and adjust height if necessary. If heels are too close to table and buttocks, patient may get leg cramps.

10. Stabilize stirrups so they will remain in position during examination. **NOTE: Some tables are designed so that you must turn a knob at side of table. Some tables have several locking positions for stirrups as they swing outward.**

11. Ask patient to move toward end of table while you guide feet into stirrups. **NOTE: Place the back of your hand against the drape sheet at the end of the table. Request the patient to move until she touches your hand.**

12. Instruct patient to move down so that buttocks are at end of table.

13. Push in table extension, position stool for physician, and position light.

14. Assist physician with examination.

15. Ask patient to slide back up on table.

16. Instruct patient to sit up before moving from table.

17. Offer tissues to remove excess lubricant before dressing.

18. Clean room and replace supplies. **NOTE: The examination table surface and base must be thoroughly cleaned with disinfecting cleanser at regular intervals and following any contact with body fluids which may contain bloodborne pathogens.**

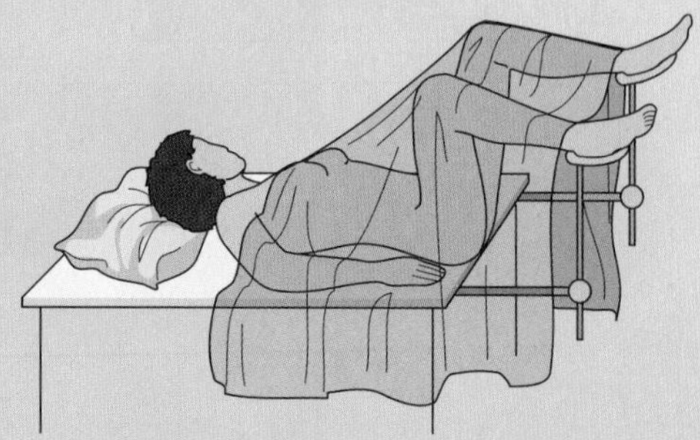

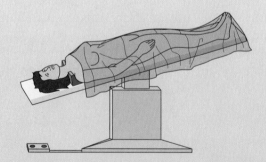

FIGURE 14–27 Lithotomy position

pelvic/pap
digital rectal
vag

FIGURE 14–28 Trendelenburg or shock position

(Face pale – raise the tail)

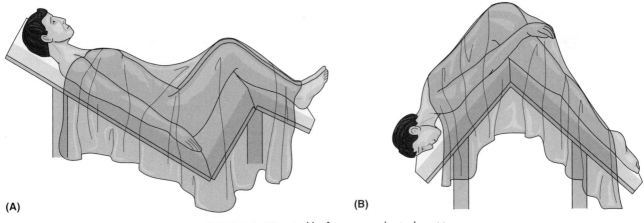

(A)   **(B)**

FIGURE 14–29   Jackknife or proctological position

A CAAHEP CONNECTION

In this unit procedures for positioning and draping patients is discussed. The medical assistant should continue to develop good communication skills in caring for patients. The importance of treating patients with empathy and respect cannot be stressed too often. Give clear instructions for procedures according to their age or level of education. Curriculum standards require instruction in *Anatomy and physiology, Medical terminology, Clinical procedures, Communication, Professionalism,* and *Psychology.*

---

is especially useful for examination and instrumentation of the male urethra.

ACHIEVE UNIT OBJECTIVES

Complete Chapter 14, Unit 2, in the workbook to help you obtain competency in this subject matter.

UNIT 3

Preparing Patients for Examinations

OBJECTIVES

Upon completion of the unit, meet the following performance objectives by verifying knowledge of the facts and principles presented through oral and written communication at a level deemed competent. Demonstrate the specific behaviors as identified in the performance objectives of the procedures, observing all aseptic and safety precautions in accordance with health care standards.

1. Spell and define, using the glossary at the back of the text, all the **Words to Know** in this unit.
2. List the duties that involve the medical assistant in preparing for the complete physical examination (CPE) of a patient.
3. Name the instruments, equipment, and supplies used in the CPE, and state the function of each.
4. Identify each section of the CPE, and describe how the physician conducts each part of the examination.
5. Explain the role of the medical assistant in the examination process.
6. List and discuss appropriate patient education for the various parts of the examination.
7. Identify the nine sections of the abdominal cavity, and name the visceral organs therein.
8. Define the POMR and SOAP methods of charting patient information.
9. List reasons for progress reports.
10. Explain subjective and objective symptoms, and give five examples of each.
11. Describe the seven warning signs of cancer in adults and children.
12. Describe the physical examination schedules for adults and children.
13. Refer to the following CDs to further your knowledge in this subject matter. V Weighing a client; X Hand washing; XI Safe lifting; XIII Gloves and gowns; XIV Removing contaminated items.

AREAS OF COMPETENCE (AAMA)

This unit addresses content within the specific competency areas of *Fundamental principles, Patient care, Communication skills, Professionalism, Legal concepts, Instructions,* and *Operational functions,* as identified in the Medical Assistant Role Delineation Study. Refer to Appendix A for a detailed listing of areas.

■ WORDS TO KNOW:

acute	manipulation
alcohol-saturated gauze	mensuration
square	nasal speculum
anxiety	objective
asymmetry	occult
audibility	otoscope
auscultation	palpation
bimanual	penlight
bold	percussion
bruit	percussion hammer
caustic	peripheral
chronic	physical
coordination	pitch
cytological	progress report
detection	prolapse
dimpling	resonance
douche	R/O (rule/out)
duration	sphincter
enema	sphygmomanometer
evacuate	sterile gauze square
explicit	stethoscope
exudate	subjective
fast	subsequent
fistula	symmetry
gait	tape measure
glaucoma	tentative
gooseneck lamp	tissues
guaiac test paper	tonometer
heart murmur	tongue depressor
hernia	tuning fork
initial	vaginal speculum
inspection	visceral
laryngeal mirror	void
latex gloves	warrant
laxative	water-soluble lubricant
light and accommodation	writer
(L & A)	

ASSISTING WITH THE EXAMINATION

Assisting with the complete physical examination (CPE), the general physical exam, history and physical (H & P), physical exam (PE), or just plain **physical** (as it is often termed) is not difficult but is complex in that it is a *set* of procedures. The responsibilities of the medical assistant are to prepare the room for the physician and patient and then prepare the patient for the physician to examine. You may also assist with the exam or write the findings. In the following pages, you will be shown this process.

In many facilities, the medical assistant accompanies the physician in the examination room and records the findings while the physician dictates the information as the examination proceeds. The term **writer** is given to the medical assistant who writes what the physician dictates

PATIENT EDUCATION

The patient needs to know why the physical examination must be performed accurately. Explain that the data collected form a database against which all future examinations and observations will be compared. The patient must understand what is taking place and why. It is very important for the patient to be relaxed while being examined. Some examinations can be embarrassing to a patient, but a clear explanation of each procedure can help relax the patient. You can assist the patient greatly by giving empathy and support. Never assume that a patient knows what clothing to remove or what position to assume simply because that patient has visited the office before. Be sure to answer all questions the patient has about the procedure to be performed.

during the exam. One who performs this duty must have sound knowledge in medical terminology, anatomy, and physiology, and of course, good spelling and writing skills. Because the physician bases the diagnosis on these findings, accuracy is vital. Many physicians prefer to write their own findings on plain sheets of lined paper (a common practice is to use a rubber stamp that outlines a particular exam format), or on specially printed forms in the outlined order of their choice. Still other physicians prefer to dictate the findings of an examination into a recorder for transcription later by the medical assistant.

There is no absolute pattern of examination to follow as long as the examiner is consistent and forms a personal habit so as to be thorough and complete with each patient. The complete examination should include the whole body, from the head to the toes, front to back, and inside and out. In your career as a medical assistant, you will work with many physicians who may be quite different in their systematic approach to patient care.

EVALUATION TECHNIQUES

Physicians are skilled in a variety of techniques used in evaluating patients in the examination process. In assisting with H & P, the medical assistant is expected to have a basic knowledge of these procedural terms.

The **initial** part of the exam is the **inspection**, in which the physician looks for any abnormalities of speech, skin condition, color, posture, **gait**, awareness, sensitivity, **anxiety**, grooming, or general appearance.

Whenever patients come in to the office/clinic for an appointment, whether it is for a checkup or a visit for an illness or injury, it is a perfect opportunity for you to motivate them to practice better health habits. The medical assistant usually has more time than the physician to talk with the patients because many procedures do take time to perform. While you are conducting these matters, you can suggest many different ideas to patients. Often, for various reasons, the patient must wait for the physician. Making use of this time for patient education is wise. Sometimes a beginning medical assistant may be at a loss for words with patients and does not know what to talk about with them except for the weather. This may help you learn some appropriate topics to speak about with patients to benefit them. Refer back to Chapter 11, Unit 9, The Immune System, which contains the warning signs of cancer. It is a good practice to have printed information for patients and posters to assist you with patient education. A few other suggestions for topics to discuss with patients follow.

Palpation is a means of examination by touching with the fingers or hands. Digital (one-finger) palpation is used to examine the anus. **Bimanual** (two-handed) palpation is used in vaginal examinations. Palpation of the breasts is done with the flat of the fingers, palmar side, of both hands.

Percussion is a means of producing sounds by tapping various parts of the body. The physician listens to the sounds to determine the size, density, and location of underlying **visceral** organs. **Pitch**, quality, **duration**, and **resonance** are terms used by physicians when referring to percussion. Direct percussion is termed *immediate* and is done by striking the finger against the patient's body. The type of percussion most often used is *indirect* or *mediate.* With indirect percussion, the examiner's finger is placed on the area and struck with a finger of the other hand.

Auscultation is listening to sounds made by the patient's body. Indirect auscultation is done with the stethoscope to amplify sounds that arise from the lungs, heart, and visceral organs. Sounds heard by this method of examination include **bruits**, murmurs, and rhythms. Direct auscultation is done by placing the ear directly over the area.

Mensuration means measurement. In this part of the examination, the patient's chest and extremities are measured and recorded in centimeters. Usually a standard flexible tape measure is used. Mensuration includes all of the following measurements: height, weight, head, chest, other parts of the body as appropriate, temperature, pulse, respirations, and blood pressure. All measurements should be recorded in inches, feet, and pounds, or kilograms and centimeters. Being consistent is necessary in

---

PATIENT EDUCATION

A. To prevent injuries of the face and head:
   1. In work and recreational environments, wear protective head gear: hard hat at work (construction sites), helmet for sports (motorcycle riding, football).
      a. Wear protective face mask/goggles for sports, such as football/basketball/wrestling, to prevent possible eye injuries.
      b. Use ear plugs to protect ears from exposure to loud noises that can lead to possible damage to auditory nerves resulting in hearing loss (machinery, band concerts); water when swimming.
B. To protect the skin:
   1. Keep skin clean and soft by using mild soap and water for bathing and a moisturizing lotion as necessary.
      a. Discourage sun worship. Encourage keeping covered in the sun or the use of a sun blocker to prevent damage of ultraviolet rays if one must be in the sun for prolonged periods. Limit time in tanning beds.
      b. Wash hands of (chemical) irritants immediately to prevent **caustic** burns.
C. To prevent diseases of the respiratory system and other contagious diseases:
   1. Discourage eating or drinking after others to keep from transmitting viruses and diseases to others.

   2. Wash hands after handling items in or from public places, which probably have been handled by multitudes of others (money, doorknobs, etc.).
   3. Discourage smoking or tobacco use of any kind (post anti-smoking pamphlets or meetings for patients to read).
   4. Remind patients of the dangers of drug and alcohol use/abuse (display information about Alcoholics Anonymous meetings).
   5. Encourage exercise/physical fitness programs with the advice of the physician.
   6. Promote proper nutrition and weight control by reminding patients to eat well-balanced meals regularly, and help them plan their diets.
   7. Encourage *safe sex* by providing **explicit** information to teach patients about the dangers of sexually transmitted diseases and AIDS.
   8. Discourage patients from using **laxatives** and **enemas** unless specifically ordered by the physician.
   9. Remind patients about immunizations and encourage their compliance.
   10. Encourage patients to read labels for contents of the products they buy and use for their safety.
   11. Remind patients to use seat belts.
   12. Promote regular medical and dental checkups.

keeping track of the patients growth and development or in assessment and evaluation of a change in readings that may contribute to a diagnosis.

Manipulation is the passive movement of a joint to determine the range of extension and flexion. Range of motion (ROM) exercises are an excellent patient education tool that you can show patients how to do properly. If patients do these exercises regularly, they will be able to move more freely and strengthen muscles besides increasing muscle tone. An illustration may be found in Chapter 20, Unit 4. Advise patients not to force themselves in this exercise; they should proceed only until it begins to be uncomfortable and stop.

DOCUMENTATION OF THE EXAM

In documenting the physical examination, many physicians use the Problem Oriented Medical Record (POMR) method described previously (see Chapter 7, Unit 1). It is sometimes referred to as POS, or problem-oriented system. This system is used for a new patient workup and for patients with serious or **chronic** illnesses. It is also used to document specific multiple complaints of patients. For **acute** or single minor complaints (such as a sore throat or a splinter), this system may not be used, for the chief complaint would not **warrant** such detail. Using this system ensures that pertinent data is recorded in logical order on the patient's chart with each return visit to the physician. Data is recorded under the following headings:

S   Subjective findings
O   Objective findings
A   Assessment of problems
P   Plan for treatment

Under **subjective** findings are those symptoms that the patient feels but that cannot be seen by another. Nausea, joint pain, headache, and abdominal pain are examples of subjective findings. **Objective** findings are those symptoms that can be seen by another and by the patient, such as redness, rash, swelling, watery discharge, or bleeding. It can also include the patient's past health history and any information concerning the patient that a family member or friend has conveyed to either you or the doctor. Assessment documents measurement of the symptoms. This includes laboratory reports, x-rays, vital sign recordings, and other aids to diagnosis.

The **tentative** diagnosis is made in this section of the patient's chart. The final section of the system outlines the plan of treatment for the patient to follow. This includes referrals, medication, surgery, therapy, exercise, and any further orders to return the patient to better health. Patient education is obviously a great part of this systematic method of record keeping. All action taken in the course of the patient's treatment generates additional information that continually modifies the original data base. **Subsequent** visits of the patient are recorded in the same manner (SOAP) as was the initial visit on sheets termed *progress notes,* sometimes referred to as *progress reports* or chart notes. Following each entry on the patient's chart should be the signature or initials of the health care provider or the person who performed the procedure.

PREPARATION OF THE EXAMINATION ROOM

Getting the examination room ready consists of making sure that the temperature in the room is comfortable, it is clean and tidy, the examination table has a clean covering (either disposable table paper or a cloth sheet), and all appropriate instruments, equipment, and supplies are arranged conveniently for use during the examination.

The medical assistant should routinely clean and restock the examination room. Carefully checking the room for necessary items will ensure efficient, expedient patient care. Make sure all equipment is in proper working order and that the room is cleaned following each patient.

These items are displayed and labeled in Figure 14–30 in the order in which they are commonly used for a complete physical examination. You should learn the name and function of each item.

PREPARATION OF THE PATIENT

It is a usual practice to schedule the CPE early in the morning because patients are normally required to **fast** (have nothing by mouth [NOP]) from midnight on for blood chemistry tests, which are based on a fasting normal range. Other procedures within the examination process are more comfortable if the patient has not eaten before the physical.

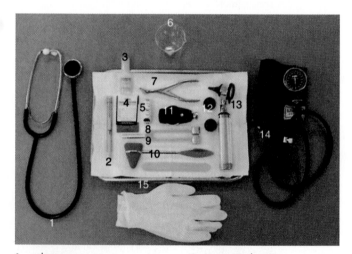

1. stethoscope	9. percussion hammer
2. penlight	10. tongue depressor
3. guaiac/occult blood test developer	11. ophthalmoscope (head)
4. guaiac/occult blood test	12. ear and nose speculum
5. flexible tape measure	13. otoscope head attached to base
6. urine specimen container	handle
7. metal nasal speculum	14. sphygmomanometer
8. tuning fork	15. latex or vinyl gloves

FIGURE 14–30 Example of instruments and supplies used in the physical examination

When these preliminary tasks have been completed, the medical assistant escorts the patient into the examination room and explains the proceedings, answers any questions, and may begin patient education where appropriate. Triage will have already determined what chief complaints the patient has. You may want to verify what the patient feels is the problem at this point. Make sure that you allow the patient time to use the restroom for comfort during the exam. You should ask the patient to urinate in a specimen cup if he did not bring a first morning specimen for you to test (complete instructions for specimen collection are in Chapter 15). Sometimes the physician must delay the examination of the abdominal area because the patient has to **void** or **evacuate** the bowel. Occasionally this is obviously unavoidable even if the patient has already made an elimination. Unnecessary interruptions are annoying and hinder the patient flow schedule. The success of the physical examination is attributed largely to the preparation of the patient. Until you are sure of yourself in remembering details, it is helpful to keep a checklist in your uniform pocket for handy reference.

The next duty of the medical assistant is to ask the patient to disrobe and put on the examination gown. Explain how by showing the patient, for instance, whether the gown should be open in the front or the back. You should offer assistance with this and show the patient where to store belongings. Pull out the step at the end of the exam table (or provide a portable one) and help the patient up to the exam table. Cover the top of the patient's legs with a drape sheet, which provides both privacy and warmth.

General instructions about the physical may be offered at this point. You may want to tell the patient that some parts of the examination may be uncomfortable but usually not painful. The patient should be urged to let the physician know of any pain or unusual discomfort during any part of the procedure and to offer any complaint that has not previously been made known.

PHYSICAL EXAMINATION FORMAT

In reviewing the medical history form in the previous chapter (see Figure 13–2), you will notice that the section immediately following "present illness" has all of the areas outlined for recording the findings of the complete physical examination.

The format of the examination section of this form has been extracted and completed in the following text with an explanation of each of the body areas examined. Hopefully this will help you become familiar with what the doctor does in each section of the physical examination. Even though H & P forms vary in appearance, the contents will basically be the same. In the spaces that say general appearance, skin, and mucous membranes, a brief written description by the examiner is far more helpful for future reference than just writing "normal," or its

equivalent N (negative or normal), or simply drawing a straight line that means "no comment."

(taken from the "in depth" medical history form)
Patient _____ Date _____

PHYSICAL EXAMINATION:
Ht.— recorded in: _____ cm (centimeters) or _____"
        (inches) or _____' (feet) and _____" (inches)
Wt.— recorded in _____ kg (kilograms) or _____ lbs
        (pounds)
Temp.—recorded in degrees of _____ Fahrenheit or
        _____ Centigrade
Pulse—recorded _____ per minute
Respirations—recorded _____ per minute

Notice that the very first part of the physical includes measurement, vital signs, and vision screening, which the medical assistant normally completes. You may want to refer to appropriate units to review these procedures.

The instruments and equipment to be used in examining each area of the body are in **bold** print at the beginning of each section where necessary or appropriate. The patient's chart, pens (one with black ink, and one with red for alerting allergies), and any forms (laboratory request or others) necessary for completion should be at the disposal of the physician and the medical assistant to begin the examination.

Blood pressure—**stethoscope, sphygmomanometer**— Readings should be taken and recorded from both right and left arms and marked appropriately. It is generally advised that two or more readings be taken, preferably from two different positions (i.e., sitting and standing), and recorded.

GENERAL APPEARANCE OF THE PATIENT

General Appearance—This generally describes the patient and the state of health, such as "Mr. G. is a spirited, energetic, medium-built, well-groomed, 34-year-old His-

---

A CAAHEP CONNECTION

Preparing patients for examinations is discussed in this unit. Good communication skills in caring for patients and giving empathy and respect is necessary. Giving patients instructions for procedures according to their age or level of education will return better cooperation from them. Curriculum standards require instruction in *Anatomy and physiology, Medical terminology, Clinical procedures, Communication, Professionalism,* and *Psychology.*

panic male who has a history of allergies. He has no speech or hearing defects."

Skin—Includes inspection of color (or discoloration) and texture; temperature; assessment of the condition of the hair and nails, lesions, rashes, masses, swollen areas, scars, wounds, warts, moles, and bruises; and any other significant changes the patient reports.

Eyes—Vision: OD 20/30 OS 20/25 OU 20/30

Ishihara—Record plate numbers that are both seen and not seen by the patient for evaluation or physician may write that patient's color vision is intact for red and green or normal or abnormal after interpreting the results of the test.

Near Vision—Record the number of the line that the patient can read most easily on the Jaeger card. Physician will determine if the patient's near-distance acuity is normal or abnormal from test results.

Pupil—Fundus—ophthalmoscope, **tonometer**—The physician uses the ophthalmoscope to look deep into the center of the eye to check the condition of the tiny capillaries behind the retina; if there are no abnormalities, there will be what is called a *red reflex,* or a red reflection that fills the pupil as the examiner views the eye (Figure 14–31). Then, testing the pupils for reaction to light is done. During this part of the exam, the overhead light is temporarily turned off (by the medical assistant) so that the doctor can watch for pupillary constriction, which, if normal, will happen right away. The patient is instructed to keep looking straight ahead while this is done in both eyes. The examiner looks to see if the patient has eye-lashes and brows (or not) and checks ocular tension, if the patient exhibits a stare or any ocular protrusion, if the sclera is white, if there is any defect of the cornea or iris, if the pupils are round and equal in size, and if they react to **light and accommodation (L & A)**. At some point during this part of the exam, the examiner will test the patient's **peripheral** vision and the horizontal and vertical fields. These tests are several hand/finger movements made by the doctor, which the patient is instructed to follow while the doctor observes.

A test with the tonometer may be done next to detect **glaucoma**. There are several different types of tonometers. A tonometer measures the intraocular pressure by determining the resistance of the eyeball to an indentation made from an applied force. Assistance with this procedure consists of preparation (by instilling drops to anesthetize the eyes), instruction regarding the procedure, positioning the patient, and handing the instrument to the physician.

Ears—otoscope, **tuning fork**—The examiner inspects the ears for size and for any abnormalities, such as lesions or nodules, or diagonal creasing of the lobe. The otoscope is used to examine the inner ear. Refer to Figure 14–5 for use of the otoscope. The physician traditionally assesses the hearing during examination of the ear with the tuning fork.

Nose—**nasal speculum, penlight** (otoscope), **alcohol-saturated gauze square**—The physician checks for any outward signs of abnormalities and then uses a nasal speculum to view the right and left nostril for any lesions,

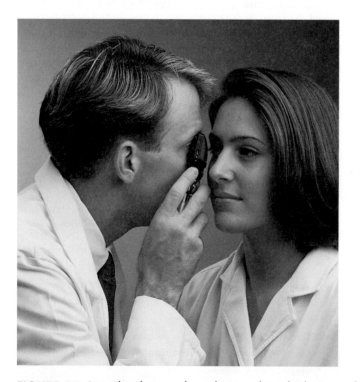

Normal Fundus—structures are defined clearly: a normal red-orange color distinguishes the retina from the darker area which is the fundus; arteries are red, veins are light purple.

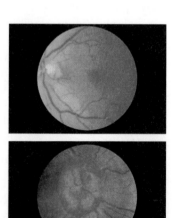

Papilledema—shows swelling of the vessels with a small hemorrhage close to the optic papilla (optic disc) caused from head injury.

Giant Papillary Conjunctivitis (GPC)—an inflammation of the conjunctiva may occur as a reaction to contact lenses. A fluorescein dye is used to help in the identification of the microorganism.

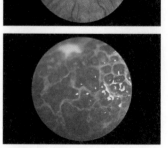

FIGURE 14–31 The photographs and text on the right show samples of what the examiner may see during the examination of a patient's eye using the ophthalmoscope. (Courtesy of Welch Allyn, Inc.)

obstructions, **exudate**, tenderness, or swelling. A test to check the sense of smell often is done at this point by having the patient close the eyes and identify a common substance, such as alcohol.

Oral Mucous Membranes—penlight, **tongue depressor, sterile gauze square, laryngeal mirror,** stethoscope—The physician looks into the oral cavity with a penlight or by using the light of the otoscope (without the ear speculum attached), to check for any unusual condition of the teeth, tongue, throat, etc. The patient is asked to tilt the head back, hold the mouth open, stick out the tongue, and say, "ahh," while the physician uses the tongue depressor and/or a gauze square to hold the tongue to the side during the exam of the floor of the mouth. A laryngeal mirror may be used here to check areas difficult to view in the mouth, besides looking down the throat of the patient. It is a good opportunity to remind patients at this point to brush their teeth and use dental floss after eating and to have regular dental checkups (especially if there is a noticeable need for dental care). The pharynx and neck are generally examined next by palpation. By auscultation, the physician listens to the carotid artery bloodflow for any abnormal sounds. The sound made by the blockage of the carotid artery is referred to as bruit (Figure 14–32).

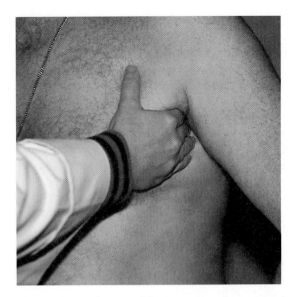

FIGURE 14–33 Palpation of the patient's axillary region by the examiner

Chest—stethoscope—During this portion of the exam, the patient's gown must be removed to the waist so the physician can inspect the chest for visual signs of abnormality, such as lesions, tumors, swelling, or skin disorders, and to observe the patient's breathing. The back is also checked in this manner. The chest is normally examined next by the physician palpating several areas, including the neck and axillary region, by using the hands placed against the skin (Figure 14–33). This allows the examiner to feel any nodules, lumps, swelling, or any other abnormal condition of the patient. Percussion is the next means of examination where the doctor taps the fingers over several areas of the chest to evaluate the condition of the underlying structures. Figure 14–34 shows the examiner using blunt percussion to examine the kidney.

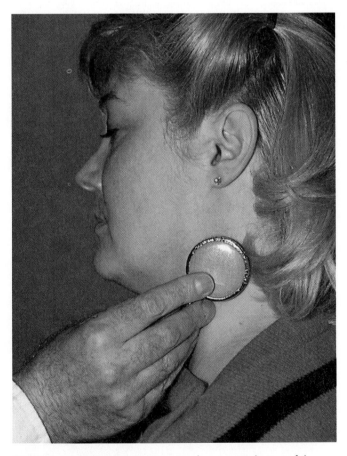

FIGURE 14–32 The physician performs auscultation of the neck to listen for the sounds normally made by blood flowing through the carotid artery.

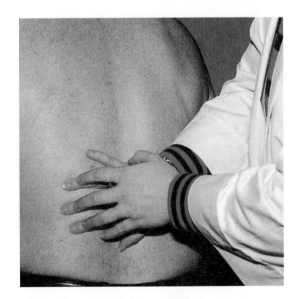

FIGURE 14–34 The examiner uses blunt percussion to examine the kidney.

The stethoscope is used finally to auscultate the chest and allow the physician to hear the sounds within the chest cavity, including breath sounds in the lungs and the heartbeat. The doctor will ask the patient to breathe through the mouth to make the sounds easier to hear while using the stethoscope.

Breasts—The inspection of the size, shape, **symmetry**, and position of the breasts and nipples is done first, then palpation while the patient is sitting and then lying down. The examiner looks for abnormalities, such as tenderness, discharge from the nipples, swelling or masses, lumps or nodules, **dimpling**, skin disorders, and any other signs of disease. Routine patient education should be done at this point in urging breast self-examination after her monthly menstrual period and in scheduling mammograms. An instruction booklet should be provided for the patient to take home (Figure 14–35). Men are also examined for abnormalities of the breasts.

Heart—stethoscope—Evidence of heart disease is indicated by many other areas of the body besides the findings from examination of the heart. The examiner visually inspects the chest and then palpates the chest wall to determine the cardiac border. The stethoscope is used to listen to the chambers of the heart to detect different characteristic heart sounds. The physician has the patient move into several positions to achieve maximum **audibility** (i.e., lying down, sitting up, leaning forward, etc.) while the doctor listens for any abnormal sounds, such as a **heart murmur**.

Lungs—spirometer—The physician may use the spirometer to measure the patient's lung capacity. The spirometer measures the amount of air that goes into the lungs and measures the amount of return air. Generally the physician, or whoever administers the spirometry, will give the patient instructions about what to do and allow the patient to practice once or twice what is expected.

HOW TO DO BREAST SELF-EXAMINATION (BSE)

1. Lie down and put a pillow under your right shoulder. Place your right arm behind your head.
2. Use the finger pads of the three middle fingers on your left hand to feel for lumps or thickening. Your finger pads are the top third of each finger.

4. Move around the breast in a set way. You can choose the circle (A), the up and down (B), or the wedge (C). Do it the same way every time. It will help you to make sure that you have gone over the entire breast area, and to remember how your breast feels each month.

5. Now, examine your left breast using right hand finger pads.
   You might want to check your breasts while standing in front of a mirror right after you do your BSE each month. You might also want to do an extra BSE while you are in the shower. Your soapy hands will glide over the wet skin, making it easy to check how your breasts feel.

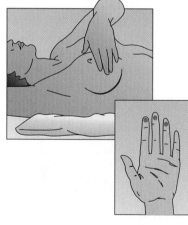

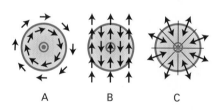

A B C

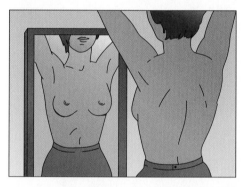

3. Press hard enough to know how your breast feels. If you are not sure how hard to press, ask your health care provider. Or try to copy the way your health care provider uses the finger pads during a breast exam. Learn what your breast feels like most of the time. A firm ridge in the lower curve of each breast is normal.

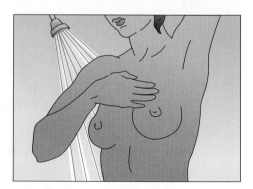

FIGURE 14–35 Breast self-examination (Reprinted by permission of the American Cancer Society Inc.)

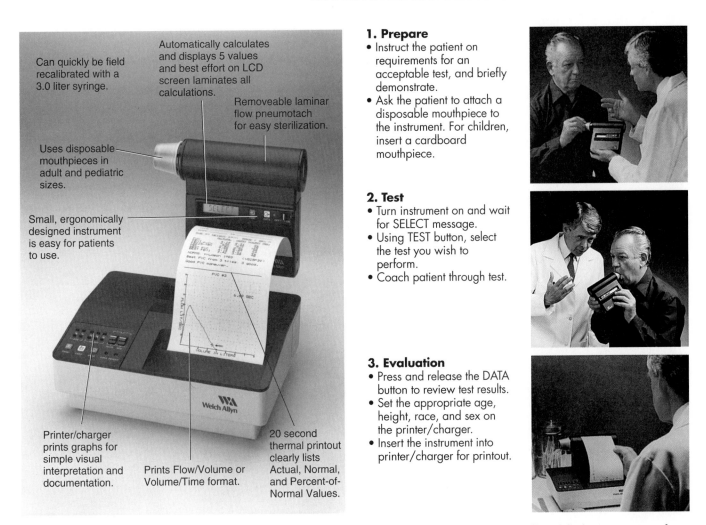

1. Prepare
- Instruct the patient on requirements for an acceptable test, and briefly demonstrate.
- Ask the patient to attach a disposable mouthpiece to the instrument. For children, insert a cardboard mouthpiece.

2. Test
- Turn instrument on and wait for SELECT message.
- Using TEST button, select the test you wish to perform.
- Coach patient through test.

3. Evaluation
- Press and release the DATA button to review test results.
- Set the appropriate age, height, race, and sex on the printer/charger.
- Insert the instrument into printer/charger for printout.

Can quickly be field recalibrated with a 3.0 liter syringe.

Automatically calculates and displays 5 values and best effort on LCD screen laminates all calculations.

Removeable laminar flow pneumotach for easy sterilization.

Uses disposable mouthpieces in adult and pediatric sizes.

Small, ergonomically designed instrument is easy for patients to use.

Printer/charger prints graphs for simple visual interpretation and documentation.

Prints Flow/Volume or Volume/Time format.

20 second thermal printout clearly lists Actual, Normal, and Percent-of-Normal Values.

FIGURE 14–36 The PneumoCheck™ Spirometer provides ease with use and printed data for patient files. (All photos Courtesy of Welch Allyn, Inc.)

This encourages the patient to do the best he can and give a better test result. Refer to Figure 14–36, which shows the physician and patient and the steps in using this instrument for aid in the diagnosis of lung diseases and disorders.

Abdomen—stethoscope—Refer to Figure 14–37 for an outlined description of the organs within the same areas of the abdominal cavity and the position of abdominal organs. This will help you to understand the use of the various techniques used by the physician during the examination. For successful examination of the abdominal cavity, the patient should be lying in the supine position with the head supported by a pillow. The arms should be to the side or folded across the chest. The medical assistant should help the patient into position. You should place a drape sheet over the patient to provide privacy. The physician will inspect the skin (refer to discussion of skin previously) and proceed with the exam usually in this order: inspection, auscultation, palpation, and percussion. The examiner looks for any abnormalities, some of which may include **hernias**, masses, tenderness, or en-

largement of organs. In males, the inguinal hernia is the most common. It is caused by a loop of the intestine entering the inguinal canal and sometimes filling the entire scrotal sac.

Genitalia—Note: For both male and female patients, this is an ideal time to stress the importance of using condoms during sexual intercourse (vaginal and anal) each and every time.

Males—**latex** or vinyl **gloves, water-soluble lubricant**—(The physician wears latex or vinyl gloves for this exam.) In general, the doctor inspects the external genitalia for gross **asymmetry**, comparing one side to the other; checks for any deformities, lesions, swelling or masses, or varicosities; and checks whether the patient has pubic hair or not. Skin temperature is also noted to determine circulation. The penis is examined for lesions, scars, masses, tumors, edema, and discharge. The scrotum is palpated for content and then each side is pressed upward (palpated) while the patient holds his arms over the head and pushes downward with abdominal muscles while the examiner observes for hernias (the patient is in-

Right Hypochondriac	Epigastric	Left Hypochondriac
Right lobe of liver	Pyloric end of stomach	Stomach
Gallbladder	Duodenum	Spleen
Part of duodenum	Pancreas	Tail of pancreas
Hepatic flexure of colon	Aorta	Splenic flexure of colon
Part of right kidney	Portion of liver	Upper pole of left kidney
Suprarenal gland		
Right lumbar	**Umbilical**	**Left Lumbar**
Ascending colon	Omentum	Descending colon
Lower half of right kidney	Mesentery	Lower half of left kidney
Part of duodenum and jejunum	Transverse colon	Parts of jejunum and ileum
	Lower part of duodenum	
	Jejunum and ileum	
Right Inguinal	**Hypogastric**	**Left Inguinal**
Cecum	Ileum	Sigmoid colon
Appendix	Bladder	Left ureter
Lower end of ileum	Pregnant uterus	Left spermatic cord in male
Right ureter		Left ovary in female
Right spermatic cord in male		
Right ovary in female		

(A)

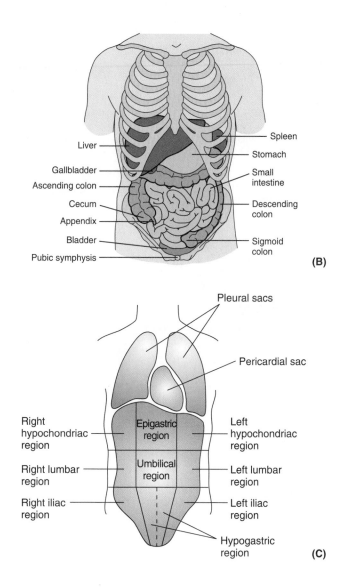

(B)

(C)

FIGURE 14–37 (A) The nine sections of the abdominal cavity with underlying visceral organs, (B) position of abdominal organs in the nine abdominal regions, (C) position of the nine abdominal regions

structed to cough during the exam to detect any discomfort with abdominal straining). The physician places a gloved index finger (with water-soluble lubricant) into the rectum to examine the prostate gland. The patient usually stands for the exam; the examiner is seated. Patient education in testicular self-examination (TSE) to **detect** tumors of the testes is appropriate during this portion of the exam (Figure 14–38). Distributing pamphlets is recommended because of the increasing numbers of cases of testicular cancer being reported in young men aged 20 to 35. Early detection may save lives!

Females—latex or vinyl gloves, **vaginal speculum**, water-soluble lubricant, **gooseneck lamp**, **tissues**—Refer to Unit 4 of this chapter for in-depth information regarding the gynecological (GYN) exam. At the time the patient schedules the CPE, she should receive instructions regarding this section of the exam. In general, female patients are advised not to **douche** or engage in sexual intercourse for 24 to 48 hours before the appointment. It is

preferred that she make the appointment either before or after the menstrual period. (Findings may be masked or misinterpreted during this time. Also remind her that routine vaginal douching should be done only by the direction of the physician.)

This part of the exam is often referred to as a pelvic exam. In general, you may help the patient lie down and then into the lithotomy position by placing your hand at the edge of the exam table and asking the patient to scoot down until she can feel the back of your hand (the buttocks should be just at the edge of the table). Assist the patient in placing the feet in the stirrups, and provide a drape for privacy. (The physician wears latex or vinyl gloves for this exam.) The gooseneck lamp should be placed at the end of the examining table to aid in visual inspection. The physician first inspects the external genitalia for lesions or ulcers, reddening, scratches, edema, inflammation, tumors, cysts or masses, scarring, varicosities, bleeding, or discharge.

These symptoms may be evident with testicular cancer:
— a heavy feeling
— a dragging sensation
— the accumulation of fluid
— breast tenderness

The American Cancer Society recommends that men:
1. begin monthly TSE at 15 years of age
2. perform careful 3 minute exam following a warm shower or bath when scrotal skin is relaxed
3. observe for any changes in appearance
4. manually examine each testis by gently rolling it between fingers and thumbs of both hands to check for any hard lumps or nodules

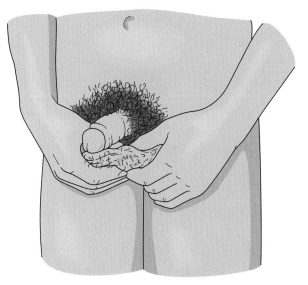

FIGURE 14–38 Testicular self-examination. Men should be advised to be examined by a physician as soon as possible if there are any abnormal findings (such as lumps or masses) with TSE.

During this exam, the patient should be instructed to try to relax and breathe slowly and deeply through the mouth. The vaginal speculum is warmed with water before being inserted into the vagina. This part of the exam is for internal inspection and to access vaginal and cervical scrapings, cultures, and **cytological** specimens. Using a water-soluble lubricant, a bimanual exam is performed to determine any abnormalities in the female reproductive organs. Offer tissues to the patient following this procedure to remove excess lubricant. Help patient out of stirrups and to a sitting position. Your role in assisting is to hand items to the physician as needed and to offer the patient your support.

Rectum—Male—latex or vinyl gloves, water-soluble lubricant, **guaiac test paper**, tissues—The patient stands with feet apart and bends over the examination table or is placed in the knee-chest position. The physician, wearing gloves and using a water-soluble lubricant, spreads the buttocks and inspects the patient for lesions, **fistulas**, external hemorrhoids, prolapse, or any other abnormalities. The internal exam determines **sphincter** control and other abnormalities and is performed as part of the exam-

ination of the genitalia (see above). It is followed by a guaiac test for **occult** blood by the placing of a small amount of stool from the gloved finger on the test paper.

Female—latex or vinyl gloves, water soluble lubricant, guaiac test paper, tissues—The physician wears gloves for this exam. A water-soluble lubricant is used to insert the index finger into the rectum to palpate sphincter control, any fistulas, tumors, hemorrhoids, **prolapse**, or any other abnormalities. A guaiac test for occult blood is performed by placing a small amount of stool on the test paper from the gloved finger.

Vagina—see above, female genitalia.

Extremities—**tape measure**—This is a general overall examination of inspection that the physician does during the course of the examination. It begins with the head and neck, and includes evaluation of the patient's gait and posture, the appearance of the back, arms, and legs. The examiner also looks for muscle strength, the condition of the patient's circulation, and the range of motion (ROM) of the joints. Sometimes measurements of the chest, arms, and legs are done at this point in the examination with a flexible tape measure and recorded in the patient's chart.

Reflexes—**percussion hammer**—The patient sits on the exam table with the legs dangling at the side. The patient must be relaxed during these procedures to elicit an involuntary reaction or response (as the absence of such response could mean neuropathy) as the physician strikes the tendon of each extremity. The examiner watches the response of the limb as contraction of the stretched muscle causes the sudden movement. The reflexes tested are biceps, triceps, patellar, Achilles, and plantar (Figure 14–39).

Lymph nodes—The physician palpates the lymph nodes of the neck, axilla, inguinal, and abdominal areas of the body during the course of the examination to determine if infection is present. Enlargement of these nodes may indicate infection; clustering of nodes may indicate pathology (refer back to Figure 14–32).

In addition to the many examinations already discussed, the physician normally includes many others, such as:

1. *Romberg balance test*—Performed to detect any muscle abnormality. The patient stands with feet together and eyes open; if the balance seems all right, the examiner asks the patient to close the eyes. If there is any muscle abnormality, the patient possibly will fall. You should assist by standing close to help prevent this from happening.
2. Other tests involve checking for **coordination** and may include:
   a. The patient sits up, spreads the arms out wide, and touches the fingertip to the nose, first the right and then the left quickly, with eyes open and then closed (Figure 14–40).
   b. The heel-to-shin test is performed by the patient while lying in the supine position: first the right

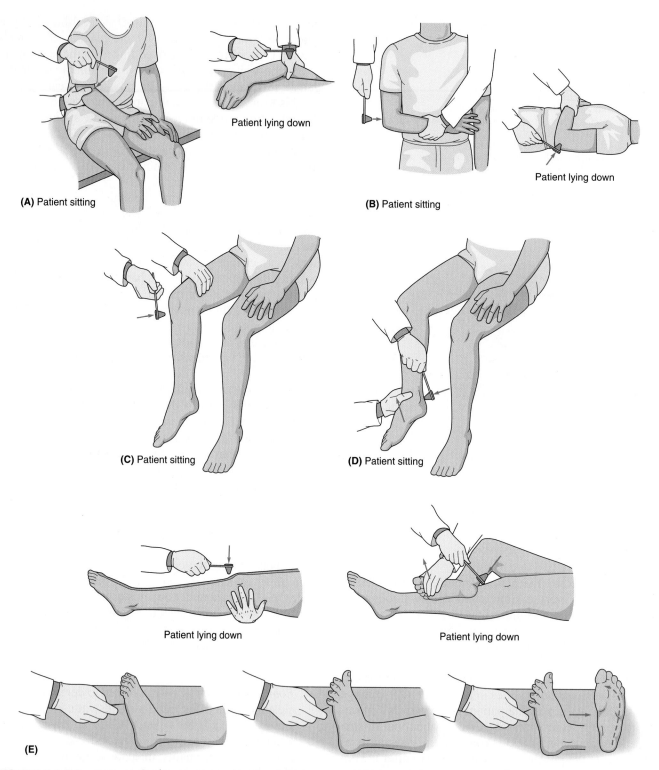

(A) Patient sitting

Patient lying down

(B) Patient sitting

Patient lying down

(C) Patient sitting

(D) Patient sitting

Patient lying down

Patient lying down

(E)

FIGURE 14–39 A percussion hammer is used by the physician to test (A) biceps, (B) triceps, (C) patellar, (D) Achilles, and (E) plantar reflexes.

heel traces the left leg down from the knee, and then the left heel down right leg; may also be done while patient stands.

c. Alternating motion is a test that may involve tapping the foot or clapping.

d. The heel-to-toe test of coordination is having the patient touch the right heel to the left great toe and

then the left heel to the right great toe; it can be done while the patient is standing or lying down. The patient is observed and evaluated by the examiner.

Remarks—Physicians note additional observations of important information concerning the patient in this section of the form (i.e., birth mark or scar is noted).

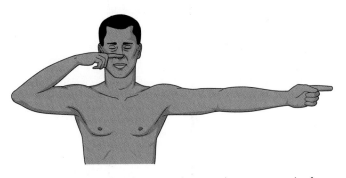

FIGURE 14–40 The physician observes the patient as the finger is touched to the nose to determine normal coordination.

From the desk of Dr. H. N. Finklestein
(Today's date)

Dear Mr. G.:

We are pleased to inform you that the results of your physical examination, lab tests, EKG, and chest x-ray were normal. Your next physical exam should be scheduled within the next two to three years unless you experience any medical problems. Please feel free to call if you have any further questions or concerns or if we can be of service to you.

Sincerely,

H N Finklestein MD

H.N. Finklestein, M.D.

FIGURE 14–41 Example of a brief letter as a report of the physical exam

The Diagnosis

Diagnosis (Diagnoses)—Here the physician makes a decision about the patient's condition based on the health history, symptoms, examination findings, and any other procedures and laboratory tests thought necessary to confirm the decision. The term **R/O**, or **rule/out**, may be used to indicate that there is not yet conclusive evidence in the decision concerning a patient's condition or in confirming a diagnosis (i.e., R/O gallbladder disease—awaiting diagnostic x-ray studies).

Treatment—This section of the form is where *all* measures for management of the care of the patient are listed, including diet, exercise, physical therapy, medication, surgery, and any others.

Following the completion of the physical examination, the physician will usually leave the patient's chart in the chart holder on the door or in some other designated area for the medical assistant. You should then check the chart for orders to perform any additional procedures for the patient, such as ECG, lab tests, scheduling x-rays, or an appointment with a specialist. After you have finished the procedures, you should write your initials after each one, signifying that you completed the orders.

Patient Care

Always be sure to help the patient down from the examination table. Often after sitting there for some time, especially if the (elderly) patient has been lying down, one can become dizzy or lightheaded, and there is the possibility of a fall, which you could prevent. You may also offer the courtesy of assisting her in getting dressed when appropriate, possibly with the elderly. Answer any questions she may have about the follow-up appointment or further studies. Always let the patient know how long to expect to wait for reports from lab, radiology, or other diagnostic procedures. Tell her when to call and with whom to speak when they phone for the report. It is a common practice to give the patient an appointment one week to 10 days after the physical for a report of the findings; others mail a report (Figure 14–41). Still others phone the

patient or have the patient phone the office at a specific day and time. Whatever the policy where you are employed, you must realize that the patient is usually very concerned about what the physician will find, and waiting makes the anxiety far worse. Letting patients know about their health status as soon as possible in a professional manner will be appreciated.

Patients may ask how often they need to have a physical or a checkup as they call it. You may use Table 14–2 as a guide in giving advice to adult patients about examination and specialty procedures routinely performed on patients. Some physicians recommend annual physicals for their patients, others every two to three years unless a specific or chronic medical problem exists. The age of the patient has some consideration in this matter. Pediatric patients should be examined more often than adults and monitored very closely because their growth and development, especially the first year, is so rapid. Initially, infants are examined by the physician in the office or clinic at age three or four weeks. In addition to the physical exam, diet and nutritional concerns are discussed, and any laboratory tests or procedures are performed during each of these appointments. At two months the baby has a checkup and begins the immunization schedule (you will learn about this in detail in Chapter 18). At four and six months the baby has checkups and continues with the initial series of immunizations. Additional exams and/or immunizations are generally scheduled for the child at 9, 12, 15, and 18 months. Even though there are no immunizations needed again until between four and six years old, children should have annual examinations to detect any diseases or abnormal condition. You will, however,

TABLE 14–2

PHYSICAL EXAMINATION TABLE

Procedure/Screening	Age
Hearing	65 years+ or as necessitated by symptoms
Vision	65 years+ or as necessitated by symptoms
	tonometry/fundoscopy at 40, then q4yrs
Urinalysis	65 years+ or as necessitated by symptoms
Skin/melanoma	Begin at 40, then annually
Fecal occult blood test	Begin at 40, then annually
Digital rectal exam	Begin at 40, then annually
Sigmoidoscopy (flexible fiberoptic)	Begin at 50, then annually
Double contrast barium enema	every 5 years as directed by physician
Colonoscopy	q10yrs or as directed by physician
Pulmonary function tests	PRN for high-risk pts (COPD/smokers)
Total blood cholesterol	19–65+ as directed by physician
Thyroid testing	PRN symptoms; baseline for females at menopause, then q2yrs
H & P	20–39 q3yrs, then annually after 40
Height/weight	13–65+, then as directed by physician
Blood pressure	13–65+, then as directed by physician
Counseling	13–65+, then as directed by physician
Males: self-testicular exam	monthly (by physician, 13–65+ PRN symptoms)
Females: mammogram	baseline at 35, q1–2yrs, then annually at 50
Breast self-exam	monthly (by physician), 35 annually
Pap test and pelvic exam	annually beginning at 18 or when sexually active

This physical exam schedule is meant to serve as a guide. The medical needs of patients will vary, as will physicians' recommendations.

Medical-Legal-Ethical Scenario

Martina and Sylvia (clinical assistants) are having a discussion over lunch in the employee's lounge at the office talking about the overweight patient (weighing 278 pounds) who was in earlier that morning for a CPE. They were both embarrassed for her at how tight her clothes were. The new administrative assistant, Cassie, entered the lounge, said hello to Martina and Sylvia, and put her lunch in the microwave. The two of them waved to Cassie as they continued to say that she could at least wear clothes that fit. While Cassie was waiting, she couldn't help but hear them talking. She took her lunch and quickly ran out of the room. Since Cassie was apparently quite upset about something, Sylvia followed her to see what was wrong. She learned that they had been talking about Cassie's mother's dear friend (and Cassie's friend, too). Cassie explained that their friend had been without employment for almost a year and was having a hard time. Cassie's feelings were hurt.

CRITICAL THINKING CHALLENGE

1. What are Martina and Sylvia guilty of doing?
2. Should they apologize to Cassie?
3. Should the office manager or physician be informed of this behavior?
4. Do you think Sylvia and Martina meant any malice?
5. Is there any legal action that should be initiated in this situation?
6. Should Cassie have responded immediately to what she overheard?
7. What would you do in this situation?

have to check with the physician who employs you because office policies may vary.

The examinations discussed in this unit are by no means the only ones performed in medical offices and clinics. You will learn many others as you gain experience and knowledge in assisting. To learn other instruments used in medical offices or clinics, refer to the appendix of this text.

ACHIEVE UNIT OBJECTIVES

Complete Chapter 14, Unit 3, in the workbook to help you obtain competency in this subject matter.

UNIT 4
Assisting with Special Examinations

OBJECTIVES

Upon completion of the unit, meet the following performance objectives by verifying knowledge of the facts and principles presented through oral and written communication at a level deemed competent. Demonstrate the specific behaviors as identified in the performance objectives of the procedures, observing all aseptic and safety precautions in accordance with health care standards.

1. Spell and define, using the glossary at the back of the text, all the **Words to Know** in this unit.
2. Instruct a female patient for a Pap test appointment, and explain why it is necessary.
3. List and describe the necessary instruments and supplies for a pelvic exam and Pap test.
4. Prepare a female patient for a pelvic exam and Pap test.
5. Demonstrate the proper way to assist with a pelvic exam and Pap test.
6. Prepare the Pap test specimen for laboratory analysis.
7. Explain breast self-examination to a patient and the best time of the month to do it.
8. Describe patient education appropriate for females having a pelvic exam and Pap test.
9. List and describe the way to obtain a complete prenatal evaluation of a patient.
10. Explain the appointment schedule for prenatal and obstetric patients.
11. List and describe three sections of prenatal patient evaluations that should be given careful attention.
12. List and describe the nine questions/diagnostic tests that should be a part of each prenatal visit.
13. Demonstrate obtaining height, weight, and head and chest measurements of infants/children.
14. Demonstrate the correct way to plot measurements on a pediatric growth graph.
15. Explain the importance of accepted normal growth patterns of infants/children.
16. Describe ways to gain compliance of pediatric patients and make them feel at ease.
17. List topics that may be of concern to parents/caregivers during the office visits.
18. List the responsibilities of the medical assistant regarding obstetric and pediatric patients.
19. Demonstrate how to administer an enema.
20. Instruct a patient to prepare for a sigmoidoscopy and explain why it is necessary.
21. List and describe the necessary instruments and equipment for a sigmoidoscopy.
22. Explain how to assist with a sigmoidoscopy.
23. Describe appropriate patient education for patients having a sigmoidoscopy.

AREAS OF COMPETENCE (AAMA)

This unit addresses content within the specific competency areas of *Administrative procedures, Fundamental principles, Diagnostic orders, Patient care, Professionalism, Communication skills, Legal concepts,* and *Instruction,* as identified in the Medical Assistant Role Delineation Study. Refer to Appendix A for a detailed listing of areas.

WORDS TO KNOW

atypical	Lamaze
cervical	lumen
constipation	Maturation Index (MI)
cytology	mucosa
diagnostic	obturator
disclose	occult
douche	Papanicolaou
endocervical	percentile
endoscope	pregnancy
enema	prenatal
evacuants	proctology
evacuate	risk
exfoliated	sigmoidoscopy
fecal	stool
fetal monitor	suction
flatulence	tarry
flexible	trimester
formaldehyde	trivial
gestation	tumor
Healthcheck	ulceration
heartburn	vaginitis
hormonal	warranted
intercede	

Many special examinations are performed on patients in various medical practices. Specialties often require additional staff training in assisting with particular procedures.

It is important to stay within your boundaries until you have been properly instructed and evaluated in specific areas.

This unit addresses examinations that are specialized and/or specific. In assisting with the CPE (Unit 3), the examination of the vagina and genitalia was described as a part of the total exam; the Pap test is not necessarily done at that time. Frequently women schedule appointments with their general/family practitioners for the Pap test alone, definitely in the specialty of gynecology. One must make the distinction between a *physical* and a *Pap test.* The CPE is a review of systems (ROS) of the total body. The gynecological exam is that of the female reproductive organs only. In Procedure 14–14, you will learn about assisting with this exam. As a rule, the specialists refer other symptoms or conditions of their patients back to the "family doctor" or general practice physician for treatment.

PROCEDURE

14-14 Assist with a Gynecological Examination and Pap Test

PURPOSE: To assist in evaluation of the patient's gynecological condition.

OSHA GUIDELINES: To comply with Standard Precautions, gloves must be worn if there is any possibility of coming into contact with blood or any body fluids.

EQUIPMENT: Two (or more) frosted-end glass slides, Mayo tray, cloth or paper towel, pen and pencil, fixative spray and container to hold slides (or jar with alcohol–ether solution), disposable latex or vinyl gloves, water-soluble lubricant, vaginal speculum, endocervical brush, vaginal/cervical spatula (Ayer blade), sterile cotton-tipped applicators, tissues, lab request form, rubber band, (cultures and uterine dressing forceps as requested by physician).

PERFORMANCE OBJECTIVE: With all equipment and supplies provided, demonstrate (insofar as feasible) each of the steps required in assisting with the GYN examination and Pap test.

1. Wash hands; place gown or drape sheet on exam table; cover Mayo tray with towel; assemble all necessary items on tray.

2. Take the patient into the examining room. Request her urine specimen if brought or ask the patient to go to the bathroom to void if one is needed. Determine if the patient needs to empty her bladder before the examination is performed.

3. Obtain the necessary information and complete cytology request form, label slides.

4. Explain procedure, disrobing, and gowning to patient (assist if needed). Ask her to leave door unlocked when ready.

5. Assist patient onto the exam table and drape.

6. Accompany physician into exam room to assist both the doctor and the patient during the exam.

7. Assist patient into lithotomy position, helping her place her feet in the stirrups (adjust accordingly), and place drape sheet over the knees. **NOTE: Place the back of your hand against the drape sheet at the end of the table. Request the patient to move until she touches your hand.** Place a pillow under her head for comfort.

8. Physician will sit at the end of the exam table on exam stool and adjust the lamp for inspection of vaginal and anal tissues. Hand gloves to the physician. You should also put on gloves. Run warm water over the vaginal speculum, and hand it and the vaginal spatula to the doctor to obtain Pap smear as you carefully hold the slide by the frosted end. The endocervical brush is used next to obtain a smear from the interior of the cervix. Slides for these specific areas must be marked appropriately: V–vaginal; E–endocervical; and C–cervical for proper analysis to be done at the lab.

9. Immediately apply fixative spray and place into container, or place in alcohol–ether solution, for transport to lab.

10. The physician performs the bimanual exam after smears have been taken. Assist by placing a small amount of lubricant on the doctor's gloved finger and handing a fresh glove to the examiner for the rectal exam. Further assistance in obtaining cultures, a biopsy, or any other GYN procedures may be performed at this time. Refer to Figure 14–42 for other instruments that may be used in these procedures that you will assist in handing the physician.

11. Hand tissues to the patient for removal of any residual lubricant. Discard all disposables in biohazardous waste container. If metal speculum was used, place in cool water to soak until it can be properly washed, wrapped, and autoclaved; remove gloves and wash hands.

12. Help patient sit up, push table extension and stirrups in, and help her down from table when her sense of balance has returned.

13. Instruct patient to dress (give assistance if needed).

14. Advise patient when results will be available and schedule follow-up appointment if indicated.

15. Place specimen(s) in lab pick-up area.

16. Clean and restock exam room to make ready for next patient.

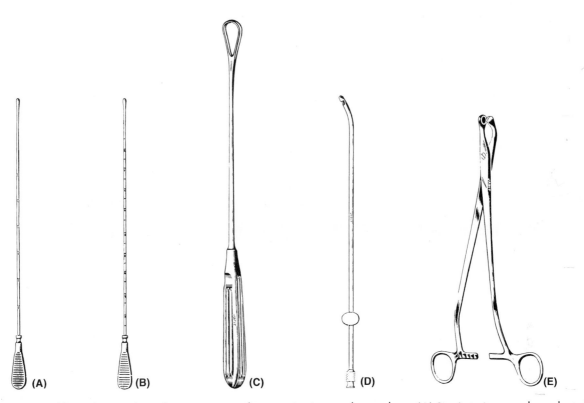

FIGURE 14-42 Additional gynecological instruments used in examinations and procedures: (A) Sims' uterine sound, graduated in inches; (B) Sims' uterine sound, graduated in centimeters; (C) Sims' uterine curette; (D) Randall uterine curette; (E) Toms-Gaylor uterine punch biopsy forceps (Courtesy of JARIT® Surgical Instruments.)

The sigmoidoscopy is another special diagnostic examination performed in most general or family practices, besides in the specialty practice of internal medicine. Assisting with this procedure requires that you are familiar with the instruments and equipment used by the physician, that you have a sound understanding of the process in giving support to the patient, and that you are an efficient assistant to the physician.

With both of these exams, it is essential that the patient receive proper preparation before the procedures can be successfully performed. Because the medical assistant is usually responsible for instructing patients, it is important that both verbal and written information is given. In consideration of the patient, the nature of both of these procedures can be embarrassing; having to go through the process only once will be appreciated.

THE PAP TEST AND HORMONAL SMEARS

The **Papanicolaou** technique is a cytologic screening test to detect cancer of the cervix. This method of detection was developed by an American physician, George N. Papanicolaou, in 1883. This simple smear technique can also be used to screen tissue from other parts of the body for **atypical cytology** as the form in Figure 14–43 shows ("special cytology"). The "thin prep" is the technique now used to read the smear; it has a single layer of cells for a more accurate study. Female patients usually have

the Pap test done routinely either as a part of the CPE with their family doctor or by their gynecologist. Patients who have complaints of severe menstrual pain or discomfort, unusual vaginal discharge, or lower abdominal pain (or any other problems) may have a Pap smear taken during the pelvic examination to rule out gynecological problems. Women should be especially conscientious in scheduling annual Pap tests if they have a family history of uterine or **cervical** cancer.

Some physicians recommend that females over age 35 have a Pap smear done every six months. Others feel that in healthy women one test every one to three years is sufficient. The American Cancer Society recommends that females have a Pap test done at least every three years, beginning when they become sexually active, or at age 20 if there have been two initial negative Pap test results one year apart. You should check with your employer and advise patients accordingly.

Patients should not **douche** for 24 to 48 hours prior to the Pap test, or the smear may be reported as negative because sloughed-off (**exfoliated**) cells would have been washed away. The Pap test should not be done during the menstrual flow because red blood cells make the smear difficult to read. Patients should also be advised not to engage in sexual intercourse 24 to 48 hours before the scheduled appointment for the same reason.

Prior to bringing the patient into the examination room for the pelvic exam and Pap, the medical assistant should

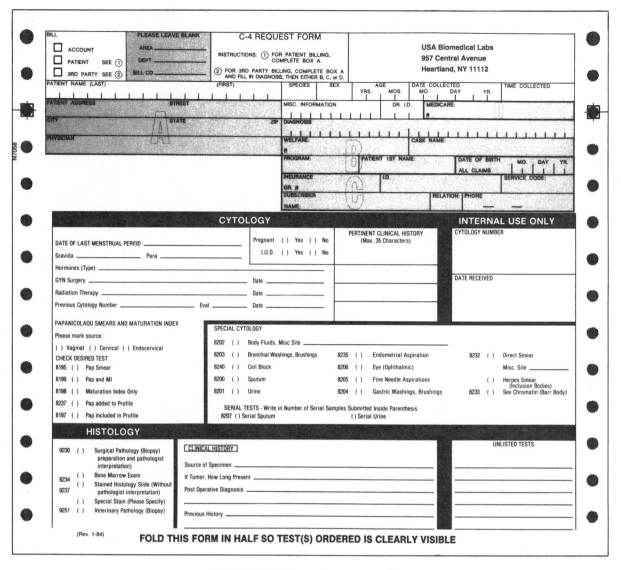

FIGURE 14–43 Cytology request form

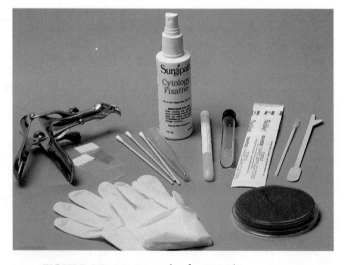

FIGURE 14–44 Example of a GYN/Pap tray setup

make the necessary preparations. You should wash your hands before you begin. The exam table should have a clean protective covering, either table paper or a cloth sheet. Place a gown and drape sheet on the end of the table for the patient (either cloth or disposable paper). On the Mayo tray near the end of the exam table, you should place the instruments and supplies the physician will need to perform the pelvic exam and obtain the Pap smear. In Figure 14–44, the commonly used items for this GYN procedure are displayed. You must learn the names of the instruments and supplies, listed in the GYN procedure, to efficiently assist the physician. To aid in the inspection part of the pelvic exam, a gooseneck lamp should be placed within reach of the examiner's stool at the end of the table.

Escort the patient to the examination room. Before you continue further preparation of the patient, ask if she needs to empty her bladder (using the restroom) and obtain a clean-catch midstream urine specimen if ordered by the physician. Pelvic examinations are uncomfortable for the patients if the bladder is full, besides making the examination difficult for the physician to perform. Examinations that have to be delayed while the patient goes to the restroom disrupt the schedule and are usually unnecessary. Certainly there are exceptions. Some patients may have trouble with bladder control or some other condition that could require frequent trips to the restroom. You should help these patients feel at ease because they will most likely feel embarrassed.

Complete the cytology request form (see Figure 14–43), by making sure that you ask the patient all necessary questions, including complaints she may have and the date of the last menstrual period (LMP, the first day of her last period). Instruct the patient about the procedure, letting her know what to expect, especially if it is her first time having a pelvic exam. *Never* assume that a patient knows about a procedure. Unfortunately, some health care workers can often be remiss in giving important information to patients. Some patients are both afraid and embarrassed to ask questions because they figure they should already know about procedures. Try to make patients feel comfortable and at ease to help them relax for the exam. You should then instruct the patient to undress completely, where to put her belongings, and how to put on the exam gown (opened in front or back). You should politely offer your assistance. Ask her to leave the door unlocked, or slightly opened, when she is gowned. Allow the patient privacy to change for a couple of minutes. When the patient lets you know she is ready, pull out the foot step at the end of the exam table and help her step up to the exam table and sit at the end. Place the drape sheet over the top of her legs. This will give her privacy and warmth. You should remember to push the foot step back in after the patient has been seated to avoid injury to you or the physician.

Alert the physician that the patient is ready to be examined. (If the patient's appointment is for a Pap alone or the physician has ordered a pelvic exam only, you should get everything ready, and then get the patient into the lithotomy position after the doctor arrives in the room, otherwise the patient will become uncomfortable and impatient staying in this position for any longer than necessary.) Most physicians prefer that the medical assistant (or nurse) accompany them into the exam room not only to assist with the procedure, but for legal reasons as well.

Because of the importance of early detection of breast cancer, physicians include the breast exam during the patient's annual appointment for the Pap test and pelvic exam. (Patients should be urged to do a breast self-examination each month following the menstrual period. Giving them a pamphlet of instructions to take with them for this procedure is recommended [Figure 14–45]). Explain to the patient that the exam conducted by the physician with the annual Pap test is certainly

PATIENT EDUCATION

When patients come in for their scheduled appointments, here are a few informative topics you might want to discuss with them.

1. Remind the patient at the time she schedules the appointment for a Pap test that she should not douche or engage in sexual intercourse for 24 to 48 hours before the examination. Because the specimen analysis could be misinterpreted during the menstrual flow, the patient should be advised to schedule the test either before or after her period.

2. Explain to female patients that they should *not* douche routinely because it washes away natural protective vaginal secretions that aid in the resistance of possible invading microorganisms. Douching should be done only with the physician's orders.

3. Those female patients who are sexually active should be instructed to use condoms when engaging in sexual intercourse for protection against both sexually transmitted diseases and unwanted pregnancies.

4. Educate all females to perform breast self-examination at home routinely after her menstrual period. Pamphlets for distribution can be obtained from the American Cancer Society to help patients with the procedure.

5. Remind all female patients over age 35 to schedule a routine mammography for early detection of breast cancer.

6. Explain to female patients that any of the following symptoms could mean that infection or disease are present and that they should call for an appointment: foul vaginal odor, vaginal discharge that is other than clear, unusual bleeding, vaginal itching or soreness, or any other **vaginitis**, pain, or discomfort.

7. Advise female patients to refrain from using perfumed toilet articles such as soaps or bubble baths, vaginal sprays and tampons, toilet tissue, or feminine napkins because they may be irritating to the delicate vaginal tissues. Chronic irritation can lead to infection.

noteworthy but insufficient in detecting abnormal breast tissue between visits to the physician. Most women discover a lump or mass in their breasts themselves and report it to the physician. This leads to early detection and treatment. The physician usually listens to the heart and lungs and does a brief general check of the patient first. Then the patient's gown is lowered to the waist while the patient is still sitting up for the inspection part of the

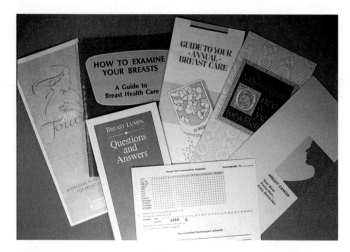

FIGURE 14–45 Breast self-examination (BSE) pamphlets and schedule

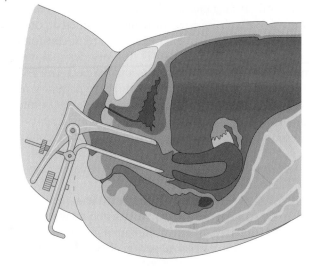

FIGURE 14–46 Lateral view of vaginal speculum in place for inspection and for obtaining specimens

breast exam and palpation for lumps and masses. You should then pull the table extension out to support the lower legs and feet and help the patient lie down in assisting the doctor in further palpation for any abnormalities of the breast tissue (often a towel is placed over the chest to provide a sense of privacy for the patient). The abdominal cavity is examined as the examiner palpates the pelvic area. Remind patients to breathe slowly through the mouth to help relax abdominal muscles during the exam.

Following this portion of the exam, you should help the patient into the lithotomy position. Assist her in getting her feet in the stirrups, adjusting them as necessary, and place the drape sheet over her knees. Ask her to scoot down to the end of the table until the buttocks are just at the edge (place your hand at the edge of the table and ask her to keep moving down until she feels the back of your hand). Be careful in assisting patients into positions because the exam tables are usually rather narrow, and there *is* the possibility of a patient falling *off* of the table. The gooseneck lamp should be adjusted at the end of the table and the stool comfortably into position for the physician. The medical assistant should put latex or vinyl gloves on and hand the physician gloves. The vaginal speculum (after running warm water over it) should be handed to the doctor next for use in inspecting the cervix and in obtaining the smear (Figure 14–46). Hand the physician the spatula to obtain a sample of the vaginal secretions containing the exfoliated cells for analysis. The **endocervical** brush is used to obtain an endocervical tissue specimen. If the physician requests a Pap and **Maturation Index (MI)**, it means that a **hormonal** evaluation is necessary in determining the patient's condition. Hold the slides carefully at the frosted end, and mark each slide accurately (in pencil) as the physician gives them to you: cervical–C, vaginal–V, endocervical–E. Immediately apply the commercial fixative spray to the slide(s) and put in the container, or place in the jar back to back with alcohol-ether solution for transport to the lab. Make sure that you wrap

the completed request form around the container and secure with a rubber band.

The bimanual exam is performed following the collection of specimens (Pap smear, cultures, and so on) so that the lubricant will not interfere in the lab analysis. The examiner inserts one finger (with a small amount of water-soluble lubricant) into the vagina, and palpates the pelvic area with the other hand (Figure 14–47). Normally, the physician does a rectal examination next. You should hand the doctor another latex or vinyl glove and lubricant.

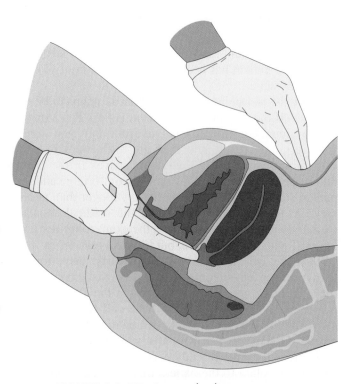

FIGURE 14–47 Bimanual pelvic examination

This is to prevent cross-contamination between the vaginal and rectal tissues. The medical assistant may be asked to write the findings of this examination while the physician conducts the exam. Whichever is your role, you will be a valuable assistant to both physician and patient.

FOLLOW UP PATIENT CARE

When this exam has been completed, offer tissues to the patient to wipe away any residual lubricant. Discard the used tissues in appropriate waste container, remove gloves, and wash hands. Push the stirrups and the extension of the table in, and assist the patient in sitting up. After lying down for the exam, the patient may either feel faint or dizzy; if she attempts to stand up too quickly she may fall. After she has let you know that she has regained her balance, help her down from the table, and ask her to get dressed. Offer assistance to the patient.

Remember to advise her when to expect to receive the results of the Pap test and/or other reports in the mail, or when she should call to find out the report(s) (Figures 14–48 and 14–49). Giving these instructions will decidedly reduce unnecessary phone calls to the office. If the physician requests a return appointment for the patient, politely assist her in scheduling it or direct her to the administrative area. As time permits, you may discuss patient education topics either before or after the exam as appropriate to the age and needs of the patient.

The medical assistant should return to the examination room to clean up the exam area. Wear gloves to protect yourself from disease transmission. Discard all disposables in biohazardous and appropriate containers, remove gloves, and wash hands. Restock the supplies as necessary, making the room ready for another patient to

World Health Organization Class System	Class
Normal	I negative
Atypical—benign squamous or glandular atypia often associated with inflammation, specific infections, radiation, etc.	II doubtful
Dysplasia	
mild	III suspicious
moderate	III
severe	IV highly suspicious
Invasive squamous cell carcinoma	V positive
Adenocarcinoma	V positive
	C insufficient for examination

FIGURE 14–48 This chart shows a sample of current reporting of the cytology of the uterine cervix.

atypical—not typical
CIN—cervical intraepithelial neoplasia
CIS—carcinoma in situ
condyloma—a lesion caused by human papillomavirus
dysplasia—precancerous lesion
epithelial—pertaining to epithelium
epithelium—cellular tissue that covers the surface of a body or that lines a body cavity
glandular—the cell making up the epithelium of a body cavity
HPV—human papillomavirus
lesion—a change in the tissue cells or a wound
malignant—a lesion that spreads out of the epithelium into underlying tissues
reactive changes—changes in cells caused by their reaction to infectious agents or a foreign body
reparative changes—changes in cells as they divide rapidly in an attempt to repair damaged tissue
SIL—squamous intraepithelial lesion (that lies within the squamous epithelium)
squamous—a type of cell that makes up the epithelium, the purpose of which is to protect underlying tissues

FIGURE 14–49 A list of terms and abbreviations used in cytology/Pap smear reports

be seen. Place the specimen(s) in the proper area for pickup by the lab representative.

OBSTETRICS PATIENTS

The same principles apply in assisting with obstetrics patients as apply in assisting with the complete physical examination. You must be complete and efficient in documenting all information regarding patients. This enables the physician to provide quality care to patients.

Of primary concern with obstetrics patients is gaining their compliance with regular checkups. Some of your major responsibilities will be to provide patient education (both verbal and in printed form) and to give emotional support and encouragement. You should refer to Chapter 11, Unit 13, for review of the reproductive system and information regarding **pregnancy**, labor, and childbirth. You should be familiar with the terminology for explanation to the parents and for correct spellings.

Because such convenient home pregnancy tests are available to the public, many women in their childbearing years have already tested their urine at home. Often, even after having performed the home test, they still may not be certain of the results. When patients suspect that they are pregnant, their visit to the doctor is to confirm pregnancy. Usually the patient has missed one or two menstrual periods and suspects pregnancy. The diagnosis is made only after the patient has been given a complete evaluation. This is generally done by (1) interviewing the patient and obtaining a complete **prenatal** health assessment and history; (2) doing a complete physical examination; (3) ordering laboratory tests, such as urinalysis and pregnancy tests, blood tests, and cultures as **warranted**; and (4) performing any other diagnostic test indicated by the patient's condition.

The medical assistant's role in prenatal evaluation and care of patients is to instill the importance of keeping regular appointments, encourage patients to eat a sensible well-balanced diet, alert the doctor with any problems or concerns, and provide patient education materials with explanations. Follow the office policy regarding prenatal and childbirth classes and provide information about times and places of such programs as **Lamaze** classes.

A medical history form (Figure 14–50) and a risk assessment form (Figure 14–51) are used in assessing the health status of pregnant women. Subsequent findings during prenatal visits are recorded on progress notes.

PLEASE USE BALL POINT PEN

NAME_____

ADDRESS_____

PHONE_____ RELIGION_____

AGE_____ GR_____ PARA_____ AB_____

BLOOD TYPE_____ RH_____ SEROLOGY_____

HUSB. BL. TYPE_____ RH_____ GENOTYPE_____

_____

_____

_____

PAP SMEAR_____

SEND TOP (WHITE) COPY TO DEL. ROOM TERM_____

LMP_____ LIFE_____ EDC_____

NURSING_____ PEDIATRICIAN_____

ANESTHESIA_____

REFERRING M.D._____

PRENATAL PREPARATION_____

HUSBAND IN DELIVERY ROOM?_____

_____ RUBELLA TITER_____

MENSTRUAL CYCLE_____

G.C. CULTURE_____

PP AR SE T G.		DATE	WHERE CONFINED	WEEKS GESTATION	LENGTH OF LABOR	INFANT WT.	COMPLICATIONS
	1						
	2						
	3						
	4						

HISTORY AND PHYSICAL

CHILDHOOD_____

FAMILY_____

TRAUMATIC_____

ADULT_____

BLOOD TRANSFUSIONS_____

ALLERGIES_____

SURGERY_____

COMMENTS: _____

_____

MEDICATIONS_____

RH TITERS DATES: _____

HT._____ NORMAL WT._____ NORMAL B.P._____

HEENT_____

HEART & LUNGS_____

BACK & BREASTS_____

ABDOMEN_____

SKIN & EXTREMITIES_____

PELVIC CAPACITY_____

PERIODIC VISITS		DATE	WEIGHT	BP	URINE	FHT	FUNDUS	PELVIC	COMMENTS
	1								
	2								
	3								
	4								
	5								
	6								
	7								
	8								
	9								
	10								
	11								
	12								
	13								
	14								

DELIVERY ROOM - TERM   SIGNATURE: M.D.

FIGURE 14–50 Example of an obstetrics/prenatal history form

PRENATAL RISK ASSESSMENT FORM

Please print or type:

Patient Name	Case Number	ADC Number	E.D.D. month day year
Physician Name	Physician Telephone		

Please check all that apply:

AT RISK OF PRETERM BIRTH

ABSOLUTE FACTORS (one factor puts patient at risk)

OBSTETRICAL HISTORY
- ❑ 1. PRETERM DELIVERY
- ❑ 2. DES EXPOSURE
- ❑ 3. CONE BIOPSY
- ❑ 4. SECOND TRIMESTER ABORTION
- ❑ 5. 1st TRIMESTER SPONTANEOUS ABORTIONS, more than 2

CURRENT PREGNANCY
- ❑ 6. UTERINE ANOMALY OR FIBROIDS
- ❑ 7. MULTIPLE GESTATION
- ❑ 8. ABDOMINAL SURGERY

- ❑ 9. CERVIX DILATED, more than 1.5 cm before 29 weeks
- ❑ 10. CERVIX EFFACED, less than 1 cm before 29 weeks
- ❑ 11. IRRITABLE UTERUS, more than 6 contractions per hr. confirmed
- ❑ 12. POLYHYDRAMNIOS
- ❑ 13. BLEEDING, if significant after 12 weeks
- ❑ 14. PYELONEPHRITIS
- ❑ 15. PRETERM LABOR
- ❑ 16. SMOKING, more than 10 cigarettes per day
- ❑ 17. PROM, confirmed

❑ YES ❑ NO   At least ONE of the above conditions has been checked. Patient is at risk of preterm birth.

AT RISK OF POOR PREGNANCY OUTCOME

ABSOLUTE FACTORS (one factor puts patient at risk)

OBSTETRICAL HISTORY
- ❑ 18. INFANT DEATH, stillborn, neonatal, post neonatal
- ❑ 19. CONGENITAL ANOMALY, major
- ❑ 20. LOW BIRTH WEIGHT, less than 2500g.
- ❑ 21. ECLAMPSIA or severe preeclampsia
- ❑ 22. INCOMPETENT CERVIX

CURRENT PREGNANCY
- ❑ 23. HEART DISEASE, class III or IV
- ❑ 24. DIABETES, insulin dependent
- ❑ 25. SICKLE CELL ANEMIA or other hemoglobinopathy
- ❑ 26. MALIGNANCY or leukemia
- ❑ 27. THYROID DISEASE, confirmed
- ❑ 28. EPILEPSY or on anticonvulsant
- ❑ 29. HEPATITIS or chronic liver disease
- ❑ 30. ASTHMA, on medication
- ❑ 31. TUBERCULOSIS, active
- ❑ 32. PNEUMONIA

- ❑ 33. HYPERTENSION, on medication
- ❑ 34. DEEP VENOUS THROMBOSIS
- ❑ 35. PLACENTA PREVIA, 3rd trimester
- ❑ 36. OLIGOHYDRAMNIOS
- ❑ 37. ECLAMPSIA or preeclampsia
- ❑ 38. ALLOIMMUNIZATION associated with fetal disease
- ❑ 39. RUBELLA EXPOSURE with rising titer
- ❑ 40. POSITIVE SEROLOGY
- ❑ 41. ACTIVE HERPES or positive culture, 3rd trimester
- ❑ 42. PRIMIGRAVIDA, less than 17 years or more than 35 years
- ❑ 43. FAMILIAL GENETIC DISORDER, confirmed
- ❑ 44. PSYCHOSIS
- ❑ 45. MENTAL RETARDATION
- ❑ 46. DRUG OR ALCOHOL ABUSE
- ❑ 47. OTHER_____

❑ YES ❑ NO   At least ONE of the above conditions has been checked. Patient is at risk of poor pregnancy outcome.

RELATIVE FACTORS (two factors put patient at risk)

- ❑ 48. PRIOR C-SECTION
- ❑ 49. PRENATAL CARE NON-COMPLIANCE, most recent pregnancy
- ❑ 50. GRAND MULTIPARA, more than 5 of 20 weeks or more
- ❑ 51. RECENT DELIVERY, less than 1 yr.
- ❑ 52. LATE INITIAL VISIT, after 14 weeks of pregnancy
- ❑ 53. MISSED PRENATAL APPOINTMENTS, 2 consecutive
- ❑ 54. AGE, less than 17 years or more than 35 years
- ❑ 55. Height, less than 5 ft.
- ❑ 56. OBESITY, more than 20% weight for height
- ❑ 57. UNDERWEIGHT, more than 10% weight for height
- ❑ 58. WEIGHT LOSS, continuing after 14 weeks

- ❑ 59. ANEMIA, less than 10 Hgb, or less than 30% Hct.
- ❑ 60. GONORRHEA, positive culture
- ❑ 61. DIABETES, gestational, diet controlled
- ❑ 62. CHRONIC BRONCHITIS
- ❑ 63. TRAUMA, requiring hospitalization
- ❑ 64. ILLITERACY or language barrier
- ❑ 65. DOMESTIC VIOLENCE
- ❑ 66. OTHER_____

❑ YES ❑ NO   At least TWO of the above conditions have been checked. Patient is at risk of poor pregnancy outcome.

Physician's Signature	Date

FIGURE 14–51 Example of a prenatal risk assessment form

Careful attention should be given to sections regarding (1) medications, drugs, alcohol, and smoking (consumption and use); (2) preexisting **risk** factors; and (3) past menstrual and obstetrical health history.

Each time the patient comes in for an appointment you should:

1. Ask her if she has been experiencing any problems and record symptoms.
2. Ask her to empty her bladder and obtain a urine specimen (preferred the first morning specimen).
3. Weigh her and record the findings.
4. Take her vital signs and record.
5. Collect any reports from laboratory findings or other referrals, and place them in the chart for the physician.
6. Assist the patient to the examination table, and position and drape her appropriately.
7. On the Mayo table, place flexible centimeter tape measure, disposable latex or vinyl gloves, lubricant, and **fetal** (pulse) **monitor** (refer to Figure 14–52) (as appropriate for the visit—pregnancy is divided into three sections or **trimesters** of the 9-month [36-week] **gestation** period).
8. Assist with the examination.
9. Assist the patient from the examination table.

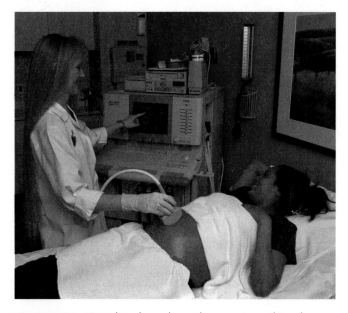

FIGURE 14–52 This photo shows the patient watching the monitor as the physician uses the ultrasound wand to assess the fetus, whose image is shown on the monitor.

After the physician has completed the examination and talked with the patient, you should offer to answer any questions the patient may have. Encourage the patient to make her next appointment before leaving the facility. Give support and assistance by reminding her to call if there are any questions or problems.

To be of further assistance to both physician and patient, you may want to check all Medicare patients' charts to make sure that findings are documented in the SOAP method in a neat and legible manner and signed by the physician. Records may be requested at any time by Medicare to verify the diagnosis and coding. This will lead to more efficient and expedient payment. The medical assistant should return to the exam room to clean up the area. Wear gloves (vinyl or latex) to protect yourself from disease transmission. Note: Especially in an OB-GYN practice, there is the possibility of patients who may hemorrhage or who have an infection that can be transmitted by body fluids and therefore could be a threat to others. Discard all disposables in biohazardous or appropriate waste containers, remove gloves and dispose of them properly, and wash hands. Restock supplies as necessary making the exam room ready for the next patient. Place any specimens in the area for pick up by the lab representative.

PEDIATRIC EXAMINATIONS

When young patients comes in to see the doctor, you must be especially pleasant and show genuine care and understanding. Your attitude may be the deciding factor in their cooperation during the visit. Greeting them with a smile and speaking to them on their developmental level will help to gain their trust and compliance. Often, some

youngsters have had traumatic experiences in emergency care centers because of serious illness or injury, which leaves them fearful of health care providers in general. If you take time, showing consideration and patience, you can establish a rapport with the patients and eliminate this potential problem. Patients of all ages are much more cooperative when they feel welcome.

GENERAL SCHEDULE FOR PRENATAL OR OBSTETRICAL APPOINTMENTS

FIRST TRIMESTER:
Monthly into the second trimester or every four weeks through the 28th week.

THIRD TRIMESTER:
Every two weeks in the 30th–36th weeks. Every week in the 36th+ week up to delivery.

Most medical facilities provide a play area for small children in the reception area or waiting room. This helps the children feel welcome and provides a comfortable environment. A variety of safe, durable, washable, educational toys is suggested. Toys that have many or tiny parts are not recommended because many small objects all over the floor would create an unsafe walkway and could cause others to fall and possibly be hurt. It could also be a potential problem for babies who put everything in their mouths. Keeping the toys clean and contained in one area will be one of your duties. Make it easy on yourself by recommending the purchase of large toys that have minimal accessory parts. Often a child will find an interesting toy while waiting to be called in to the examination room. Obviously the child's cooperation will be greater if the little patient is permitted to bring the toy in with him to keep occupied while awaiting the doctor. It will also help you in performing any necessary procedures for the child in preparation for the doctor's examination. You must make sure that when the child is finished with the toy that it is sanitized properly before returning it to the play area for other children. It should be noted that the play area should ideally be used for well children who are waiting for annual physical examinations or other well visits or for checkups, allergy injections, or immunizations. You should always bring in sick children to an examination room as soon as they arrive so you won't risk the transmission of their disease to others who are present. You must keep an open communication with the administrative medical assistant (receptionist) regarding the scheduling of these ill patients. Because you can never be sure of the health status of anyone, you must be vigilant in the practice of Standard Precautions. Sanitizing and disinfecting items and surfaces in the medical facility as needed is a vital part of your work day. Even when you are frantically busy with an overbooked schedule, remember to follow Standard Precautions. It should become a habit that is second nature to you for your protection and for the protection of patients and other workers. A help in the effort to cut down on disease transmission is a commercial disinfectant spray. You can use this quickly in between patients when you are hurried. The best way to eliminate a potential disease transmission is to remove the item when possible until it can be properly sanitized. Children (and patients of any age) becoming sick and vomiting is a concern you must be aware of in a medical facility. The administrative medical assistant should keep a disposable emesis basin near the window for this potential situation. You should also keep a commercial preparation accessible for use in cleaning up this type of waste material. Latex and vinyl gloves, facial tissues, and biohazardous plastic waste bags should also be easily accessible. A covered waste receptacle lined with a biohazardous plastic bag for disposal of contaminated items should be obtainable. There may be occasions where a parent or caregiver may bring a seriously ill or injured child into the facility unannounced. You must act quickly to provide immediate care to the patient and protect others who may be present from possible disease transmission in an emergency situation.

When you are assisting with the examination of a child, a very important responsibility you will have is relaying information to the doctor from the parent or caregiver, and from the doctor to the patient and parent or caregiver. Your careful observation of the child and the relationship between the parent or caregiver and the child may be critical to the physician in the course of the care and treatment of the patient. You are responsible for reporting any suspected cases of child abuse and neglect to the proper authorities (child protective agency) in your community. Make note of any unusual observations, and advise the physician before the patient is seen.

Many caregivers or parents are unaware of developmental stages and what to expect from their children. Posting a chart regarding these growth and developmental stages of infants and children is most helpful for patient education. Examples of charts are shown in Tables 14–3 and 14–4. While preparing the child for the physician to come into the examination room, it is an ideal time to discuss patient education topics with the caregiver, such as the child's eating habits, sleep and daily activities, immunizations schedules, toilet-training, and taking and recording a temperature. This is a great help to parents and caregivers in caring for their children. Printed booklets and pamphlets on a wide variety of topics should be offered to parents as appropriate to their children's ages.

Cooperation with youngsters is generally obtained by explaining, in a calm, simple manner appropriate to their stage of development, what you and the doctor are going to do and why. If you sense behavior that is not cooperative, then you must ask the parent or caregiver to **intercede**. A child who is unwilling to cooperate with a procedure that is necessary will have to be restrained safely by you and the parent or another health care worker. Doing what has to be done as quickly as possible is the best way to handle a troublesome situation, especially with a child.

Young children are often amused with items that are not ordinary toys during an examination, such as a plastic drinking cup or tongue depressor (with supervision, of course). Giving children nonsharp instruments, such as a percussion hammer, stethoscope, or penlight, to examine may help them to overcome the fear of their use by the doctor during the exam (Figure 14–53). Be sure to clean these items properly when the child has finished with them.

Pediatric patients should be regarded as individuals and given the kindness and respect you give to all patients whom you serve. You may want to make a "poncho" type covering for a little one made by folding a disposable drape sheet in four sections and cutting the point off to make an opening to over the child's head. Young boys and girls are often embarrassed and chilled sitting on the examination table in their underwear, awaiting the doctor. This is an easy way to help them feel more comfortable and keep them warm. They like the special treatment.

Another common practice to help little ones feel special is to provide them with bandages in colorful prints or cartoon characters for their minor cuts and abrasions or for injection sites following immunizations. Most health care providers in medical facilities that treat pediatric patients offer a small token reward, such as stickers, balloons, or trinkets, after their treatment or exam is completed. (Ask the parent or caregiver for approval first). This gives the child positive reenforcement and helps to establish and keep a good rapport between the medical team and the child.

You will also be required to complete many types of forms requesting information derived from health checkups for various facilities, such as schools or day care centers. An example of a comprehensive health care program that requires careful documentation of examination findings is the federally mandated program called **Healthcheck**. This is for eligible Medicaid patients who are between the ages of birth and 21 years. This program requires regular routine health maintenance checkups to detect and treat medical problems. The parent or primary caregiver must accompany the child at each visit. The recommended schedule for examinations is as follows:

AGE	EXAMINATIONS PER YEAR
Birth–12 months	6
1–2 years	2
2–21 years	1

The earlier a medical problem can be detected and treated, the better the prognosis for the child. Health care officials have developed this program for periodic intervals of examinations so that potential problems can be caught before they become serious or beyond treatment stages. The screening procedures are simplified and relatively quick for determining abnormalities or illnesses (the results of these tests determine if further testing is required). This leads to earlier diagnosis and treatment of medical conditions. You should stress the importance of

TABLE 14-3

GROWTH AND DEVELOPMENT DURING INFANCY

Age	Gross Motor	Fine Motor	Language	Sensory
Birth to 1 Month	• Assumes tonic neck posture • When prone, lifts and turns head	• Holds hands in fist • Draws arms and legs to body	• Cries	• Comforts with holding and touch • Looks at faces • Follows objects when in line of vision • Alert to high-pitched voices • Smiles
2 to 4 Months	• Can raise head and shoulders when prone to 45°–90°; supports self on forearms • Rolls from back to side	• Hands mostly open • Looks at and plays with fingers • Grasps and tries to reach objects	• Vocalizes when talked to; coos, babbles • Laughs aloud • Squeals	• Smiles • Follows objects 180° • Turns head when hears voices or sounds
4 to 6 Months	• Turns from stomach to back and then back to stomach • When pulled to sitting almost no head lag • By 6 months can sit on floor with hands forward for support	• Can hold feet and put in mouth • Can hold bottle • Can grasp rattle and other small objects • Puts objects in mouth	• Squeals	• Watches a falling object • Responds to sounds
6 to 8 Months	• Puts full weight on legs when held in standing position • Can sit without support • Bounces when held in a standing position	• Transfers objects from one hand to the other • Can feed self a cookie • Can bang two objects together	• Babbles vowel-like sounds, "ooh" or "aah" • Imitation of speech sounds ("mama," "dada") beginning • Laughs aloud	• Responds by looking and smiling • Recognizes own name
8 to 10 Months	• Crawls on all fours or uses arms to pull body along floor • Can pull self to sitting • Can pull self to standing	• Beginning to use thumb-finger grasp • Dominant hand use • Has good hand-mouth coordination	• Responds to verbal commands • May say one word in addition to "mama" and "dada"	• Recognizes sounds
10 to 12 Months	• Can sit down from standing • Walks around room holding onto objects • Can stand alone	• Picks up and drops objects • Can put small objects into toys or containers through holes • Turns many pages in a book at one time • Picks up small objects	• Understands "no" and other simple commands • Learns one or two other words • Imitates speech sounds • Speaks gibberish	• Follows fast-moving objects • Indicates wants • Likes to play imitative games such as patty cake and peek-a-boo

compliance with this program to the adult who is responsible for the child.

There are 13 areas that constitute the program:

1. Health
2. Developmental history from parent or primary caregiver
3. Complete physical exam (unclothed) (including vital signs ages 3–21 years) and height, weight, and head and chest measurements—plot results on growth charts
4. Nutritional assessment
5. Vision (include color vision acuity)
6. Hearing screening appropriate for the child's age

TABLE 14-4

GROWTH AND DEVELOPMENT DURING TODDLERHOOD				
Age	Gross Motor	Fine Motor	Language	Sensory
12 to 15 Months	• Can walk alone well • Can crawl up stairs	• Can feed self with cup and spoon • Puts raisins into a bottle • May hold crayon or pencil and scribble • Builds a tower of two cubes	• Says four to six words	• Binocular vision developed
18 Months	• Runs, falling often • Can jump in place • Can walk up stairs holding on • Plays with push and pull toys	• Can build a tower of three to four cubes • Can use a spoon	• Says 10 or more words • Points to objects or body parts when asked	• Visual acuity 20/40
24 Months	• Can walk up and down stairs • Can kick a ball • Can ride a tricycle	• Can draw a circle • Tries to dress self	• Talks a lot • Approximately 300-word vocabulary • Understands commands • Knows first name, refers to self • Verbalizes toilet needs	
30 Months	• Throws a ball • Jumps with both feet • Can stand on one foot for a few minutes	• Can build a tower of eight blocks • Can use crayons • Learning to use scissors	• Knows first and last name • Knows the name of one color • Can sing • Expresses needs • Uses pronouns appropriately	

7. Immunization needs using standard schedule
8. Laboratory testing as indicated
9. Anemia or sickel cell tests as indicated
10. Urinalysis
11. Lead poisoning absorption annually for ages one to four years and PRN
12. Tuberculin test annually—Mantoux test on all individuals who have been or are suspected of having been exposed
13. Dental assessment—refer to dentist

Any other laboratory tests, x-rays, and cutlures should be performed as indicated from findings in the health history or during the examination. Your role is to be of assistance in gathering data, documenting information, performing the screening tests as far as your skills and abilities allow, and being of assistance to both patient and physician as needed.

Accuracy in the documentation of each of these components is essential to quality care for these young patients. All screenings must be performed on-site at a

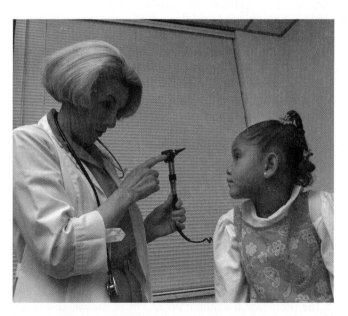

FIGURE 14-53 The medical assistant is explaining to the child how the doctor uses the otoscope to look in her ears

health care facility by qualified medical personnel. Use the time well with parents or caregivers and children by providing patient education as indicated by the child's age and developmental stage at the request of the adult.

ASSISTING WITH THE PEDIATRIC EXAM

The examination of a pediatric patient is basically the same format of the CPE for adults. The physician examines the patient from head to toe. Because little ones may be uncooperative at times, you should assist the doctor by holding the child still until the exam is completed. Often the physician will ask the caregiver to hold the baby while listening to the heart and lungs. The physician will ask the caregiver about the baby's eating and sleeping schedule and how the development is progressing (e.g., at two to three months: is the baby playing with his own hands; at six months: is she crawling). The doctor also observes the mother or caregiver relationship. Part of the examination of babies and children is to observe the child's gait. This is accomplished by placing the little patient across the room and standing behind the child to observe how she walks to the caregiver. Ask the physican about taking the child's vital signs because not all physicians require this to be done at every visit unless there is an indication to request it.

There are some physicians who require that all patients from age two to 100 years have vital signs taken and recorded at every visit regardless of the reason for the appointment. In Chapter 18, you will learn about medications, injections, and immunizations. Refer to this information and the immunization schedule for children. As a part of the pediatric exam, babies and children receive their immunizations. You will be required to have the proper immunizations ready for the physician to administer, or you should be able to administer them. Office policies and physicians differ regarding this procedure. You will be required to record this information on the patient's chart and in the booklet that parents or caregivers keep. Make sure that before the immunizations are given that you give the consent form to the parent or caregiver to sign after you have explained and they have read the possible side effects that are in printed form for them to keep. Instruct them to contact the doctor immediately if a serious reaction should occur from the immunization. If the child has a fever the day of the scheduled appointment, have the physician check the child before giving any immunizations. Be sure to have the physician outline exactly what needs to be done as routine so you will be an efficient medical assistant in having pediatric patients ready for the physician to examine.

PEDIATRIC MEASUREMENTS

The initial part of the pediatric check up and examination is the preparation of the baby or child. As was discussed in Chapter 13, you are responsible for obtaining accurate measurements of patients. Remember to establish a good

rapport with the child and the caregiver by being friendly and relaxed. Ask the caregiver about the child and how everything has been regarding the child's behavior, health, and if there are any problems or questions. Refer back to Tables 14–3 and 14–4 that highlight growth and development during infancy and toddlerhood. At these ages the average child should be able to perform the activities listed. Your medical facility will have this kind of information in a more elaborate and expanded form. You will also have patient education materials for patients to take with them about specific topics, such as sleep disturbances, nutrition for toddlers, and toilet training.

It is essential in the course of the child's examination, diagnosis, and treatment to accurateay record the growth and development of the child on his chart, in the caregiver's record booklet, and on the growth graph. This graph is a valuable visual for the physician because it allows the doctor to easily look at a glance at the child's growth and development pattern. All babies grow at different rates. The growth graph shows the normal growth of infants and children up to 20 years of age. The physician can then compare the child's measurements in relation to the **percentile**, that of other children the same age (this percentile is to the far right of the graph). There is a white curved line section, the one that is closest to the top of the page, where the height, length, and stature are recorded. The white curved line section below that is for plotting the weight of children. If the measurements of a baby or child fall above or below the normal height or weight areas and the family history does not warrant it, there is usually further examination and diagnostic testing scheduled.

The National Center for Health Statistics (NCHS) growth charts become a permanent record of the child's development and are to be filed in the chart. At each subsequent visit, the child's growth should be recorded. These growth graphs aid in the diagnosis of growth abnormalities, nutritional disorders, and diseases of children from birth to 20 years of age. Of course, hereditary factors also influence growth patterns, hence the importance of having a complete family health history in the medical record.

Figures 14–54A, B, C, and D show growth graphs for boys and girls. Two record growth patterns of infant males and females from birth (B) to 36 months, and two record growth patterns of boys and girls from 2 to 20 years of age. This information is printed across the top and bottom of the graph. Each of the squares across the page represents one month. Be sure you use the appropriate chart for the patient, as the normal development and growth patterns are different for males and females. On the front of each of the graphs is a ruled section to record the date, age, length/height/stature, and weight of the child at each appointment. The line for comments is for you to record a brief chief complaint that the caregiver (or the child, if old enough to speak) tells you. By looking at the line provided for the comments, it is vital that you print small and neatly so that it can easily be read. The complaint or problem should also be neatly recorded on the chart.

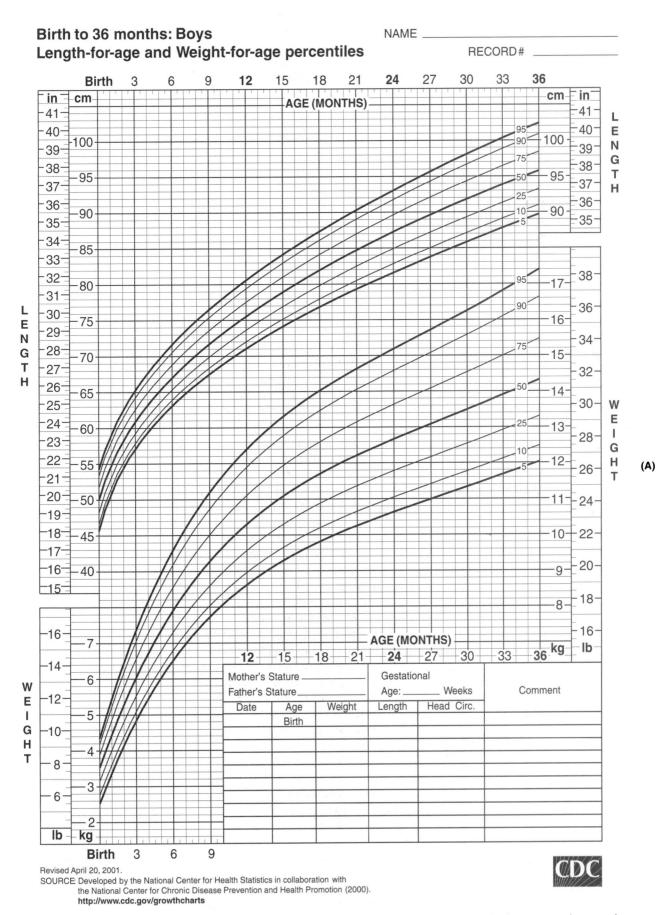

Birth to 36 months: Boys
Length-for-age and Weight-for-age percentiles

NAME _____

RECORD# _____

(A)

Revised April 20, 2001.
SOURCE: Developed by the National Center for Health Statistics in collaboration with
the National Center for Chronic Disease Prevention and Health Promotion (2000).
http://www.cdc.gov/growthcharts

FIGURE 14–54 A and B show growth graphs for boys and girls to record height and weight, ages birth to 36 months. C and D show growth graphs for boys and girls to record height and weight, ages 2 to 20 years.

(Continued)

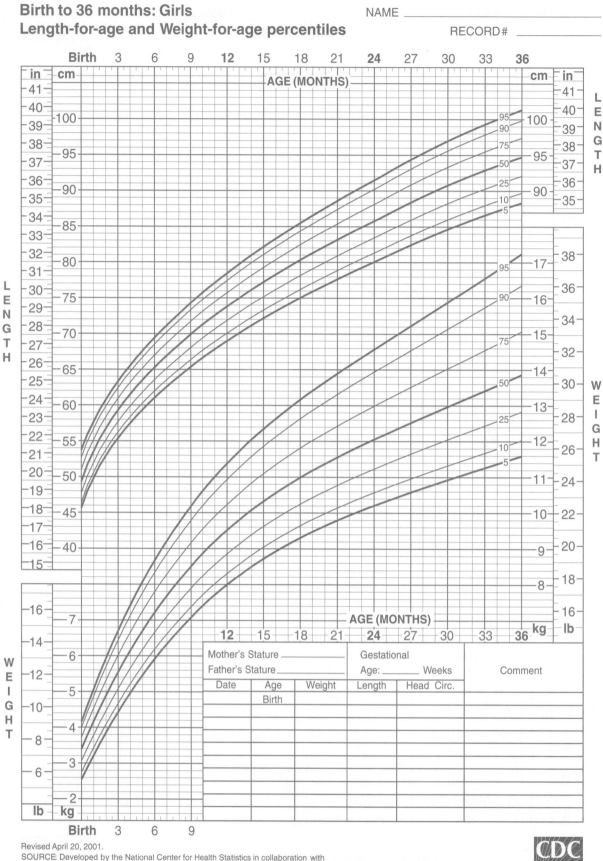

Birth to 36 months: Girls
Length-for-age and Weight-for-age percentiles

NAME _____

RECORD # _____

Revised April 20, 2001.
SOURCE: Developed by the National Center for Health Statistics in collaboration with
the National Center for Chronic Disease Prevention and Health Promotion (2000).
http://www.cdc.gov/growthcharts

FIGURE 14–54 *(continued)*

2 to 20 years: Boys
Stature-for-age and Weight-for-age percentiles

NAME _____

RECORD# _____

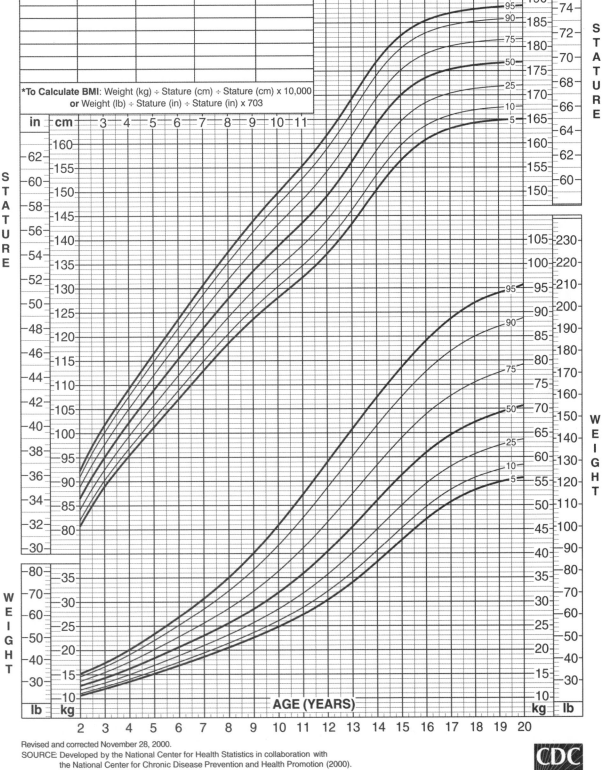

*To Calculate BMI: Weight (kg) ÷ Stature (cm) ÷ Stature (cm) x 10,000
or Weight (lb) ÷ Stature (in) ÷ Stature (in) x 703

Revised and corrected November 28, 2000.
SOURCE: Developed by the National Center for Health Statistics in collaboration with
the National Center for Chronic Disease Prevention and Health Promotion (2000).
http://www.cdc.gov/growthcharts

CDC

FIGURE 14–54 *(continued)*

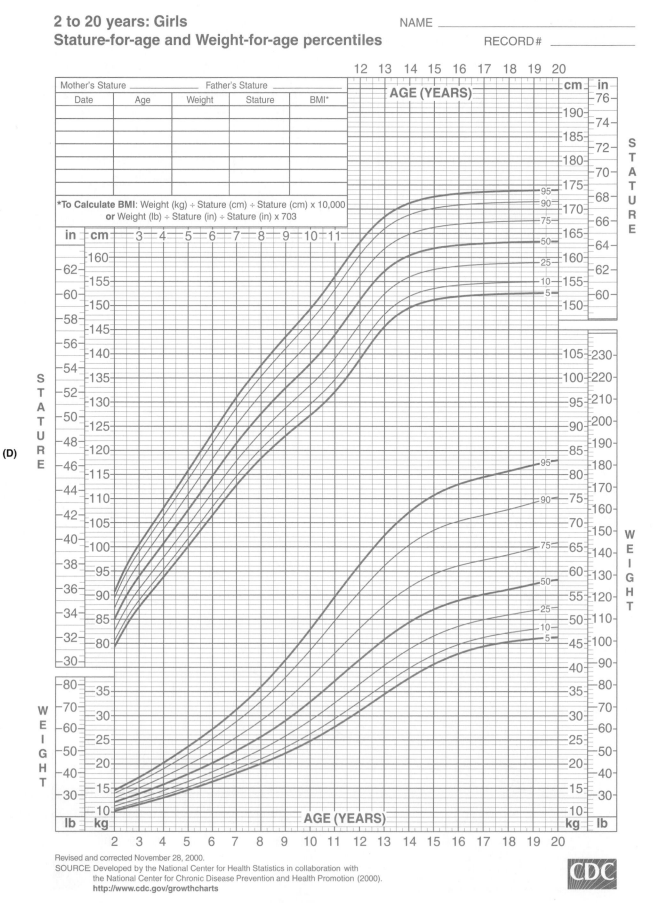

2 to 20 years: Girls
Stature-for-age and Weight-for-age percentiles

NAME _____

RECORD# _____

Revised and corrected November 28, 2000.
SOURCE: Developed by the National Center for Health Statistics in collaboration with
the National Center for Chronic Disease Prevention and Health Promotion (2000).
http://www.cdc.gov/growthcharts

FIGURE 14–54 *(continued)*

MEASURING HEIGHT

Measuring the height of a baby from infancy to 36 months is recomended as the most accurate method of measurement if performed correctly (Refer to Procedure 14–15). The baby should be placed on a pediatric or other examination table with the placement of the baby's head at the headboard. Someone holds the head in position while you stretch the legs out straight (infants tend to stay in fetal position) and measure from the vertex of the head to the heel of the baby. There may be a discrepancy of the length of babies from what was reported as the birth length because babies are sometimes measured from head to toe because the neonate (newborn) curls up into fetal position. Refer to Figure 14–55 to see how to place the baby on the exam table for measuring the length.

After a child reaches the third year or 36 months, you can begin to measure the child's height and weight on the upright scales, or the adult scales as it is sometimes called. The shoes should be removed because you may take both height and weight measurements one after the other. Often the physician will ask for the weight to be taken with the child unclothed except for the underwear. This is a good time for you to make the poncho out of a drape heet, especially for little girls (mentioned earlier).

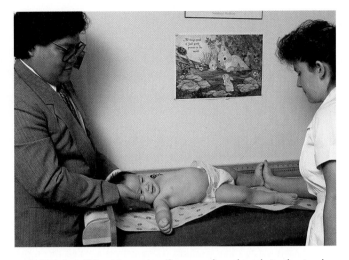

FIGURE 14–55 Measuring the recumbent length is obtained by measuring the vertex of the child's head to the heel.

Remember that children have feelings and may be embarrassed without their clothes, too. It is necessary to have the child hold still to obtain an accurate height measurement. The child must stand in the center of the scales with a measuring bar, or the child may teeter and

---

PROCEDURE

14-15 Measure Recumbent Length of Infant

PURPOSE: To obtain an accurate measurement of recumbent length of an infant to 36 months of age.

EQUIPMENT: Ruled measuring tape, yardstick, or meterstick; patient's chart; parents record booklet; growth graph; pen.

PERFORMANCE OBJECTIVE: Provided with at least three lifelike clinical or toy dolls (or an infant or small child under the close supervision of the parent, guardian, or the instructor) and a pediatric table or examining table along with a ruled measuring device, demonstrate each step required in measuring recumbent length of infants and small children, and obtain a length measurement for each doll. Each length measurement must be within one-eighth inch of each doll's actual length as determined by the instructor beforehand.

1. Wash hands and ask parent to remove infant's shoes and socks or booties.

2. Ask parent to place infant on examination table with the head against the table headboard at the zero mark of ruler. Gently straighten infants' back and legs to line up along ruler. Ask parent to hold infant's head against (end) head-

board of table while you place infant's heels against footboard. If there is no footboard (to place the infant's feet against) use your right hand as one (Figure 14–55). Place your left hand over the child's legs at the knees to secure the child in place and straighten the legs so you can read the recumbent length from the head (vertex) to the heel. **Placing your fingers behind the child's knees with your thumb over the kneecap applying gentle pressure will help to keep the legs straightened out for the procedure.**

3. Read length in inches or centimeters on rule. **NOTE: There may be discrepancies with measurement at birth or from another facility because of difficulty in getting an accurate reading. Infants are so used to fetal position that it is difficult to straighten the legs. The former reading may have been from measuring the infant's length from head to toe, making the measurement of the recumbent length a few centimeters longer or more.**

4. Return infant to parent.

5. Record measurement on growth chart, patient's chart, and parent's booklet of child's growth and development.

PROCEDURE

14-16 Measure Height

PURPOSE: To obtain an accurate measurement of a patient's height.

EQUIPMENT: Upright scale with extension measuring bar, patient's chart, pen (a measuring scale may be fixed to the wall).

PERFORMANCE OBJECTIVE: After the instructor has measured and recorded the height of all students, each student will, in turn, select five other students. Demonstrate on five other students each step in the height measurement procedure to determine the precise height of each of the other five students. The height measurements obtained should not be one-eighth inch more or less than the heights for those five students as measured and recorded by the instructor.

1. Raise measuring bar and extension higher than apparent height of patient. **RATIONALE: Avoids the possibility of striking the patient with the extension when it is raised.**

2. Ask patient to remove shoes. (Patients ready for physical exams will not have on shoes.) Place a paper towel on plat-form of scale. **RATIONALE: Accurate measurement cannot be obtained if shoes are worn. The paper towel provides a clean surface for the shoeless foot.**

3. Help patient onto scale facing you with his back to measuring device. Advise patient to stand erect (Figure 14–56).

4. Slide measuring bar down slowly and carefully to rest on top of patient's head, gently compressing hair. **NOTE: Measurement of height is from the top of the head, not the hair. This can cause a discrepancy in the reading.**

5. Read measurement in inches or centimeters, and tell patient what it is.

6. Help patient down from scale. Tell patient to put shoes back on unless ready for physical exam.

7. Place measuring extension bar back in place, and discard paper towel.

8. Record height measurement on patient's chart.

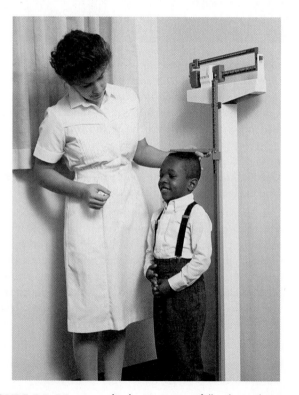

FIGURE 14–56 A medical assistant carefully places the measuring bar at the vertex of the child's head to obtain an accurate measurement of his height.

fall. To reduce the amount of time the child is in place on the platform of the scales, look at the chart and see what the measurement was at the last exam so that you can have an idea where the measurement will be. Follow Procedure 14–16 and refer to Figure 14–56 to see how to place the measuring bar on the top (vertex) of the child's head.

WEIGHING THE PEDIATRIC PATIENT

C Skills Menu:
■ Weighing a Client

It is customary to weigh infants unclothed because the number of inches or centimeters that an infant may gain or lose are as important as the number of pounds gained or lost in older children and adults. If an infant gains or loses weight too quickly it could be a signal of a disease or disorder and should be brought to the physician's attention. It is also important to ask the caregiver about the feeding schedule of the infant or child.

In some offices and clinics, the pediatric scales is kept on a stainless steel cart and simply wheeled to the patient's room. Other facilities may have a pediatric room as in a family or general practice where all infants and children are examined. In the specialty of pediatrics, every patient room may have an infant scales or the scales is

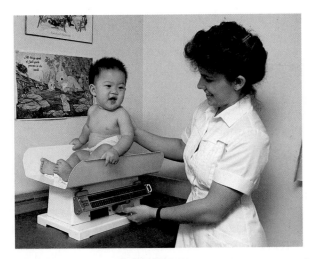

FIGURE 14–57 A baby is weighed in a sitting position on the scales as he holds on to the side while the medical assistant carefully places her hand close to the child for safety.

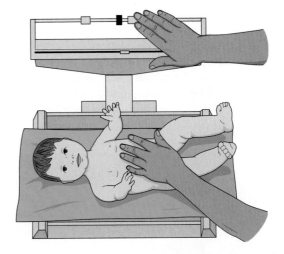

FIGURE 14–58 Infants should be weighed in the recumbent position with the medical assistant giving reassurance in a calm voice to keep the baby as still as possible while obtaining an accurate weight.

kept in a specific location and the little one is carried there. It is best for you to ask the caregiver to transport the baby to the scales and place her on the scales for you. This reduces the possibility of a potential risk of accidental injury to the child on your part. Figures 14–57 and 14–58 show the proper positioning of the baby on the scales. Follow Procedure 14–17 to weigh an infant or baby up to 36 months or 38 pounds.

PROCEDURE

14-17 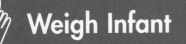 Weigh Infant

PURPOSE: To obtain an accurate weight measurement of an infant.

EQUIPMENT: Infant balance scales, towel, patient's chart, growth graph, parent's record booklet, pen.

PERFORMANCE OBJECTIVE: Provided with at least three lifelike clinical or toy dolls (or an infant or small child under the close supervision of the parent, guardian, or the instructor) and infant scales, demonstrate each step required in weighing infants and very small children by weighing each of the dolls. Each weight must be within one-eighth pound of each weight as determined by the instructor beforehand.

1. Wash hands.
2. Ask parent to remove infant's clothing. **RATIONALE: Alleviates the infant's apprehension and conserves your time.**
3. Place a clean towel on scale cradle to avoid disease transmission and to decrease shock from the cold metal for infant. This will lessen chance that infant will move because of being uncomfortable or afraid. Keep diaper or towel over infant's genital area in case of an elimination.
4. Balance scale at zero with towel in place.

5. Place infant on scale holding one hand over infant (almost touching) to give a sense of security. Talking in a quiet tone will also help keep infant still until reading has been taken. The age of the baby may determine how the child is placed on the scales. Small infants will be easier to weigh lying down; those who can sit up on their own will most likely be more cooperative sitting on the scales (Figures 14–57 and 14–58). In either case, the safety of the baby is primary.
6. Slide weight easily until scale balances, which determines weight of infant. Read scale in pounds and ounces or kilograms.
7. Return infant to parent to dress.
8. Remove towel from scale, place it in proper receptacle, and balance scale at zero mark.
9. Record weight on growth chart, patient's chart, and parent's booklet. **NOTE: If infant is unruly when weight is attempted, a notation should be made on chart that weight is approximate. Other attempts can be made at same visit. If weight is needed to determine nutritional needs or medication dosage, you may have to weigh parent holding infant, then weigh parent, and subtract to get approximate weight of child.**

HEAD CIRCUMFERENCE

On the back of the growth graph for infants is a section to record the head circumference measurement. This is important for alerting the physician of abnormal development. This should be performed and recorded routinely at each office visit until the child is 36 months of age. A

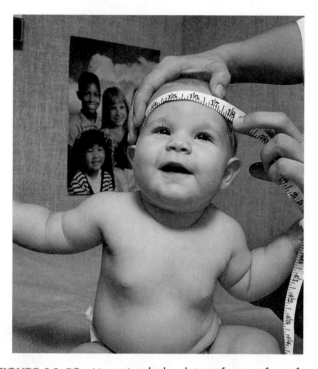

FIGURE 14–59 *Measuring the head circumference of an infant*

flexible measuring tape is required. It is often necessary to ask for assistance in keeping the child from pulling on the tape while you are measuring the head. Place the tape under the head if lying down, about an inch above the ears, and around to the forehead to get an accurate measurement. Refer to Figure 14–59 to see the correct placement of the measuring tape. Procedure 14–18 will help you in performing this measurement.

CHEST CIRCUMFERENCE

The chest circumference is measured by placing the flexible measuring tape around the child's chest just above the nipples (Figure 14–60). Often, it is difficult to keep the baby from moving. As said before, you should ask for assistance from the caregiver or another medical assistant. Place the measuring tape under the child and bring it around the baby's back to the chest to meet the zero mark for easiest measurement. This measurement is not required on the growth graph but should be recorded on the chart. Refer to Procedure 14–19 for measuring infant's chest circumference.

RECORDING MEASUREMENTS

After the measurements of height, weight, and head circumference have been obtained, they are plotted on the graph where the age and the measurement interesect. Refer to Figure 14–61. In this photo, the medical assistant is plotting the weight measurement on the birth to 36 months graph. To record the height measurement, simply follow the age line (vertically) to the child's length measurement

---

PROCEDURE

14-18 Measure Head Circumference

PURPOSE: To obtain an accurate measurement of infants' and small children's head circumference in screening for head growth abnormalities.

EQUIPMENT: Flexible tape measure without elasticity, growth graph, patient's chart, pen.

PERFORMANCE OBJECTIVE: Provided with at least three lifelike clinical or toy dolls and a flexible tape measure, demonstrate each step required in measuring the circumference of heads of infants and small children on each of the three dolls; each circumference measurement must be within one-eighth inch (0.2 cm) of each doll's actual head circumference as determined by the instructor beforehand.

1. Wash hands.

2. Talk to infant to gain cooperation. Infant may be held by parent or may lie on examination table for procedure. Older children of two or three years may stand or sit if they will remain still.

3. Use one thumb or finger to hold tape measure with zero mark against infant's forehead (above eyebrows). With other hand, bring tape around infant's head just above ears to meet in front. **NOTE: Pull tape snugly to compress hair (Figure 14–59).**

4. Read to nearest 0.1 cm or one-half inch.

5. Record on the mesurement on the growth chart, parent's record booklet, and patient record.

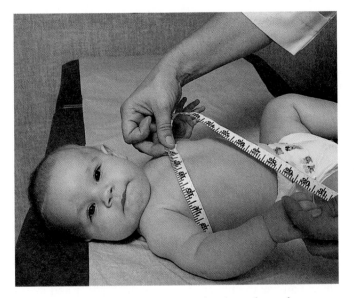

FIGURE 14–60 Measuring the chest of an infant

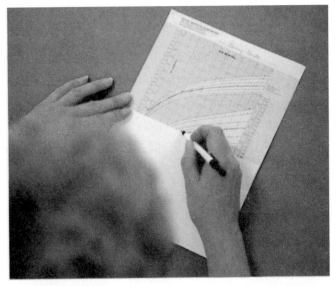

FIGURE 14–61 A medical assistant plotting a weight measurement on a growth graph

(horizontally) on the left, follow the horizontal line to the point at which the two interesect, and place a dot there with your pen. For recording the weight of the infant or child, stay on the vertical (age) line, and look to the right side of the graph. Following the horizontal line from right

to left, place a dot at the intersection of the weight and age lines.

The recumbent length of the child is recorded in inches or centimeters and the weight in either pounds or kilograms. Be consistent when measuring the child to avoid

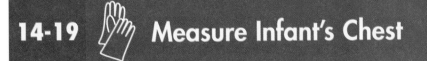

PROCEDURE

14-19 Measure Infant's Chest

PURPOSE: To obtain an accurate measurement of infants' and small children's chests in screening for growth abnormalities.

EQUIPMENT: Flexible tape measure without elasticity, patient's chart, pen

PERFORMANCE OBJECTIVE: Provided with at least three lifelike clinical or toy dolls and a flexible tape measure, demonstrate each step required in obtaining the chest measurement of infants and small children on each of the three dolls. Each chest measurement must be within one-eighth inch (0.3 cm) of each doll's actual chest measurement as determined by the instructor beforehand.

1. Wash hands.
2. Talk to infant or child to gain cooperation. Infant or child may lie down on examination table or be held by parent or guardian for the procedure. Children of 2 or 3 years and older may sit or stand on their own if they will cooperate

and remain still for the procedure. **RATIONALE: Accurate measurement cannot be achieved if the child is crying.**

3. Take the measurement of the chest just above the nipples with the tape fitting around the child's chest under the axillary region. Use one thumb to hold tape measure with zero mark against the infant's chest at the midsternal area. With the other hand, bring the tape around (under) the back to meet the zero mark of the tape in front. If you need assistance in holding the child still, ask the parent or another assistant. The measurement should be taken when the child is breathing normally, not with forced inspiration or expiration (Figure 14–60). **RATIONALE: Measurement would be inaccurate.**

4. Read measurement to the nearest 0.1 cm or one-half inch.

5. Record on parent's chart and in parent's record booklet. **NOTE: This procedure can be used for obtaining the chest measurement of patients of all ages.**

discrepancies. Procedure 14–15 explains how to measure the recumbent length of an infant. Ask for assistance from the caregiver or another medical assistant if necessary.

SIGMOIDOSCOPY

C Skills Menu:
- Proctosigmoidoscopy

Sigmoidoscopy is a **diagnostic** examination of the interior of the sigmoid colon. It is a useful aid in the diagnosis of cancer of the colon, **ulcerations**, polyps, **tumors**, bleeding, and other lower intestinal disorders. The sig-

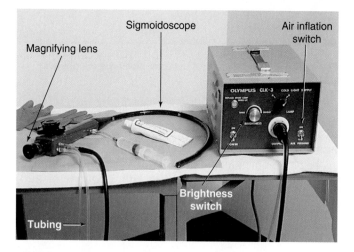

FIGURE 14–62 Parts of the flexible sigmoidoscope are labeled in this photo of a procedure setup. PPE should be worn during this procedure.

moidoscope is a metal or plastic (disposable) instrument with a light source and a magnifying lens, which permits the mucous membranes of the sigmoid colon to be seen.

The metal and plastic types of scopes are still used to examine patients. Recently, another instrument has been gaining in popularity with physicians. It is a **flexible** sigmoidoscope, which is shown assembled with items necessary for the procedure to be performed (Figures 14–62 and 14–63). Because it is flexible, it can be inserted much farther into the colon. This instrument makes it possible to view more of the mucous membranes of the intestines.

An **obturator** is inserted into the sigmoidoscope. The tip of the obturator and scope are lubricated and carefully inserted into the rectum. Then the obturator is removed so that the S shape of the colon can be seen. Patients find this an unpleasant procedure.

As with any examination of the abdominal cavity, you should advise the patient to empty the bladder and **evacuate** the bowel before the procedure begins. This will make the exam easier for both patient and examiner. During the procedure, the patient should be instructed to breathe through the mouth deeply and slowly to relax abdominal muscles. Patients may feel the urge to defecate during any of these colon examinations because of the stretching of the intestinal wall from the instrument passing through and air being introduced with it. If patients use the breathing technique mentioned, this discomfort can be relieved. The procedure should last only a minute or two, especially if patients have followed preparation instructions.

Air is sometimes introduced into the colon (by the examiner's use of the inflation bulb attached to the scope with tubing) to distend the wall of the colon for easier

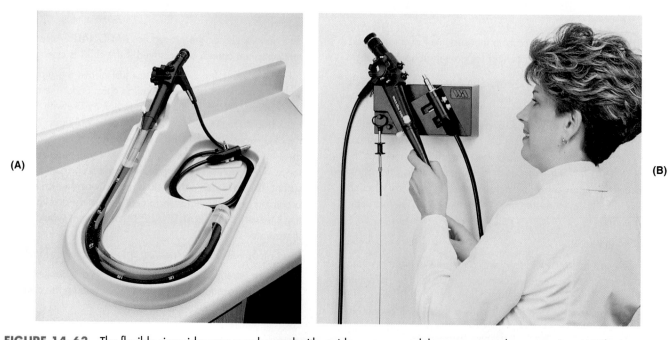

FIGURE 14–63 The flexible sigmoidoscope may be used with a video camera and the exam viewed on a monitor. (A) The instrument is stored and transported in the disinfection tray or (B) stored on the wall hanger after being disinfected. (Courtesy of Welch Allyn, Inc.)

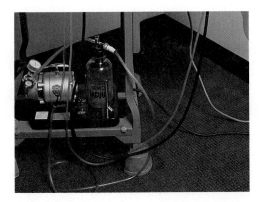

FIGURE 14–64 This suction machine is used with the flexible sigmoidoscope to remove any fecal or enema material for better viewing of the tissues of the colon.

placement of the **lumen** of the **endoscope**. Patients find this to be uncomfortable and sometimes painful. The physician may need to use a **suction** pump to remove mucous, blood, or **fecal** material that is obstructing the view of the colon (Figure 14–64).

Assistance in handing necessary items to the physician and giving support to the patient are your roles during these exams. Refer to Procedure 14–20 for assisting with a sigmoidoscopy.

It is not a common procedure to administer an enema to a patient in the medical office or clinic, but it is sometimes a necessity in the successful completion of a sigmoidoscopy, other rectal examination, or for other reasons. Even though a patient may have received proper instructions and carried them out before the scheduled

PATIENT EDUCATION

It will most often be the medical assistant who tells the patient how to prepare for the **sigmoidoscopy** and explains how the test is performed. For successful examination, proper preparation is essential. In addition to having the patient restrict dairy products, raw fruits and vegetables, and grains and cereals from their diet, she should be encouraged to drink plenty of clear liquids and eat lightly the day before the scheduled appointment for the sigmoid colon exam. A plain Fleet's **enema** should be self-administered at home approximately two hours before the exam. Physicians may vary the instructions according to the patient's condition. It is best to ask the examiner about the patient before proceeding with instructions. If patients are not completely informed about preparations and the exam is attempted with unsatisfactory results, it will have to be repeated, which is both costly and inconvenient. Satisfactory results are obtained by giving patients both oral and written instructions. This practice will also be helpful in reducing phone calls with **trivial** questions.

There are occasions, during an appointment for which the patient was "worked in" to the schedules, when the physician feels that the patient's condition warrants the examination of the sigmoid colon. In this case, the physician will order an enema to be given to the patient in the office. A procedure for both assisting with a sigmoidoscopy and administering an enema will follow in this unit.

Some exams, such as diagnostic sigmoidoscopy and x-rays, require the use of **evacuants** by the patient the day before or the morning of the exam. This may present a problem in the patient's personal or employment schedule if instructions are not made clear before the appointment is scheduled. Most patients are fearful of what the diagnostic examination will **disclose**. Helping them choose a convenient appointment time and explaining the reasons for the preparations they must undergo will usually be appreciated.

When patients come in for rectal or sigmoidoscopy examinations, here are a few informative topics that you may discuss with them.

1. Remind them that laxatives and enemas should only be used by direction of the physician.
2. **Constipation** may be avoided/relieved by including fresh fruits and vegetables and cereals and grains in their diet, drinking plenty of liquids (water), and getting regular exercise.
3. Instruct them that if they have any of the following symptoms persistently, it could mean that a disease or an abnormal condition is present, and consulting the physician is strongly advised: **heartburn** or indigestion, nausea and/or vomiting, constipation or diarrhea, excessive gas or bloating, or **stool** that is **tarry** (black) or other than a normal brown color.
4. Inform patients who are age 40 and over that they should routinely test their stool for **occult** blood every two years for detection of cancer of the colon, or more often if advised by the physician (if family history indicates). All patients over age 50 should test annually.
5. Advise patients to include high-fiber foods in their diets, avoid too much fat (and saturated fats) and cholesterol, and eat red meats sparingly.
6. Urge patients to eat from a variety of foods (from the food pyramid in Chapter 20) and to eat four to six small meals rather than one or two large meals daily to promote better use of nutrients and more energy.
7. Suggest to patients that it is better to select snacks and beverages wisely; for example, choose fruits, vegetables, and juices over coffee, tea, soda pop, and high-calorie sweets or chips.

PROCEDURE

14-20 Assist with Sigmoidoscopy

PURPOSE: To assist in examination of the sigmoid colon to determine its condition.

OSHA GUIDELINES: To comply with Standard Precautions, gloves must be worn if there is any possibility of coming into contact with blood or any body fluids.

EQUIPMENT: Disposable latex or vinyl gloves, water-soluble lubricant, gauze squares, sigmoidoscope, long cotton-tipped swabs, drape sheet (fenestrated-optional), suction machine (container with room temperature water), tissues, (if ordered by physician: biopsy forceps, specimen container for transport to lab, lab request form), pen, patient's chart.

PERFORMANCE OBJECTIVE: With all equipment and supplies provided, demonstrate (insofar as feasible) each of the steps required in assisting with the sigmoidoscopy procedure.

1. Explain procedure to identified patient. **RATIONALE: Speaking to the patient by name and checking the chart ensures that you are performing the procedure on the correct patient.** Ask patient to empty bladder and bowel.

2. Assemble all needed items on Mayo table near end of examination table (Figure 14–65). Plug in cord of light source to make sure it works properly, then unplug. **RATIONALE: If left on it will be uncomfortably warm for patient and may cause a burn. NOTE: If biopsy is scheduled, complete lab request form and label specimen container.**

3. Instruct patient to disrobe from waist down and let you know when ready. Assist patient to sit at end of table and cover with drape sheet.

4. Both medical assistant and physician should wash hands and put on latex or vinyl gloves.

5. Just before physician is ready to begin exam, assist patient into knee-chest or Sims' position, whichever physician prefers. **NOTE: Many physicians have an examining table which permits the patient to kneel on a pad and then be placed in a jackknife position to facilitate the procedure.**

6. Assist physician by applying about two tablespoons of lubricant on gauze square for tip of obturator and tip of gloved fingers. **NOTE: Physician makes digital examination of anus and rectum prior to insertion of endoscope.**

7. As physician finishes digital exam, plug sigmoidoscope into light source. Secure air-inflation tubing and have it ready to hand to physician.

8. As physician inserts sigmoidoscope, be ready to hand items as needed. **NOTE: Have suction machine plugged in and suction tip secured. RATIONALE: Often fecal material or unexpelled enema fluid is present and must be removed before adequate viewing can be accomplished.**

9. If biopsy is indicated, hand biopsy forceps to physician, and have specimen container open so physician can place tissue in it.
   - Place cap on container securely and label properly.
   - Complete lab request form, and attach to specimen container with tape or rubber band.

10. Use tissues to clean lubricant and waste from patient's anal area, and discard into biohazardous waste container. Assist patient to resting prone position.

11. Clean area and place used instruments in basin to soak in detergent solution. Remove gloves and wash hands.

12. Assist patient to a sitting position, allowing time for balance to return before helping down from table. Instruct patient to dress (unless patient has an appointment for additional examinations, such as x-rays in the same office).

13. Disease transmission must be prevented. Wear gloves to clean the exam table and instruments. The metal scope and suction tip should be sanitized and prepared for sterilization (autoclaved). Restock the room, and make ready for the next patient.

14. Record procedure on patient's chart and initial.

CHARTING EXAMPLE:

4/19/XX

Pt tolerated exam well. Return 1 month for recheck. Findings: diverticulitis of the transverse colon.

D. Brown, CMA (CL)

appointment, there is no guarantee that the patient achieved success. In the event that the patient comes in for the appointment and is not sufficiently cleaned out for a sigmoidoscopy, the physician may order a cleansing enema so that the exam can be completed. It is generally best to proceed with the planned procedure, even with the delay of the enema. Usually this works out well for pa-

tient and staff, for rescheduling presents difficulties for everyone.

Often the patient did follow the list of instructions but just did not retain the enema solution long enough for it to work. You will more likely be able to encourage the patient to hold the contents of the enema longer. You may want to explain that the longer the contents are held, the

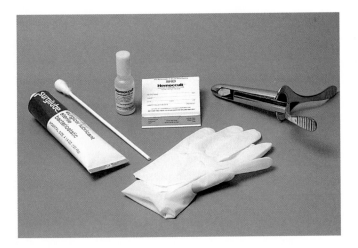

FIGURE 14–65 Basic rectal examination tray setup

more successful the results will be. Otherwise, it may have to be repeated or the exam rescheduled. For the patient's convenience, make sure that you use an examination room that is close to the restroom when you administer an enema. The enema is a simple procedure, one that patients can do at home when advised by the physician. Your patience and understanding are needed here, because most patients are embarrassed to have this done. Procedures 14–20 and 14–21 will provide the information you need to carry out this duty.

Proper positioning of patients during the exam is important for both the physician's viewing of the rectum and sigmoid colon and the patient's comfort. **Proctology** tables are designed especially for this procedure. They provide support of the patient's chest and head with the arm resting against the headboard as the table is tilted to the

---

PROCEDURE

14-21 Administer Disposable Cleansing Enema

PURPOSE: To stimulate elimination of fecal matter from the lower intestinal tract (and in preparation for diagnostic examinations or tests).

OSHA GUIDELINES: To comply with Standard Precautions, gloves must be worn if there is any possibility of coming into contact with blood or any body fluids.

EQUIPMENT: Prepackaged disposable enema (plain Fleet's), water-soluble lubricant, Mayo tray, towel, latex or vinyl gloves, tissues, drape sheet, pen, patient's chart.

PERFORMANCE OBJECTIVE: Provided with an anatomical model of the lower abdominopelvic cavity or a mannequin, and all equipment and supplies required to administer a cleansing enema, first administer the enema to the anatomical model, then the mannequin. In each process, the steps of the procedure must be demonstrated in proper order.

1. Explain procedures to patient. **RATIONALE: Speaking to the patient by name and checking the chart ensures that you are performing the procedure on the correct patient.**

2. Instruct to disrobe from the waist down. Provide drape sheet and assist patient on to exam table.

3. Help patient into Sims' position, asking patient to lie on left side and to bring the right knee up to the waist. Adjust the drape sheet.

4. Wash hands and put on latex or vinyl gloves.

5. Remove the protective covering from the tip of the enema container, and apply a small amount of lubricant if necessary (tip *is* prelubricated) to the tip.

6. With one hand separate the buttocks to expose the anus; with the other hold the enema bottle, and gently insert the tip into the rectum, making sure that the tip points in the direction of the patient's navel. **NOTE: Advise the patient to breathe deeply and slowly through the mouth. RATIONALE: This aids patient to relax and makes instillation easier.**

7. Express the entire contents from the bottle slowly (squeeze from bottom to top of bottle), asking the patient to retain the liquid for as long as possible. **NOTE: Wait five to ten minutes so that the solution will have time to work.**

8. Withdraw the enema tip slowly and provide patient with tissues. **NOTE: Tissues may be used to remove any lubricant or placed against the anus with pressure to aid in maintaining the enema. Discard in a biohazardous waste container if the tissues are left in the room.** Direct patient to restroom as necessary; ask patient to let you check results before flushing. Report to physician.

9. Clean room; discard disposables in appropriate waste containers.

10. Remove gloves and wash hands.

11. Initial chart (signifying that procedure has been completed).

CHARTING EXAMPLE:

10-14-XX

Administered plain Fleet enema to pt, was tolerated well, good results, no remaining abdominal discomfort.

S. Long (HNE)

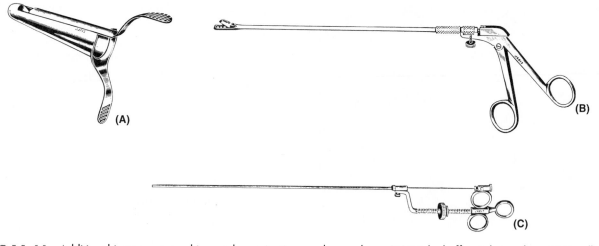

FIGURE 14–66   Additional instruments used in rectal examinations and procedures: (A) Brinkerhoff rectal speculum, (B) Turrell rotating shaft rectal biopsy forceps, (C) Norwood rectal snare (Courtesy of JARIT® Surgical Instruments.)

knee-chest position. Those who cannot tolerate this position are assisted into Sims' position for the exam. Many physicians find this acceptable, and it is certainly more comfortable for the patient. You should ask about the physician's preference in patient position because there are many variations.

The physician may wish to view the intestinal **mucosa** following a normal bowel movement. More often, the patient is instructed to eat a light diet containing plenty of clear liquids and avoiding dairy products for 24 hours before the exam, and to have a plain cleansing enema the morning of, or two hours before, the exam. Still other physicians may wish patients to use laxatives the day before and an enema the night before and also the morning of the exam. Patients have usually eaten little within the past few days because of their abdominal distress.

In the diagnosis of hemorrhoids, fissures, and ulcerations, the physician usually begins investigative procedures by examining the anus and the interior of the rectum with a **proctoscope**. During the sigmoidoscopy, the physician may want to take a biopsy of questionable tissue from the sigmoid colon to aid in confirming the diagnosis. It is a good rule to have all possibly necessary items available. When the patient has been prepared and the examiner is ready to begin the exam, the medical assistant hands the necessary instruments and supplies to the physician as needed. Remember to advise patients to report any problems, such as bleeding, discharge, swelling, or any other unusual discomfort following any procedure. A biopsy lab request form must be completed and accompany the tissue to the lab. Containers for biopsy specimens have a **formaldehyde** solution to preserve the tissue until the analysis is done.

There are many other proctological procedures that may need to be performed by the physician for patients in the office setting. Some of the instruments used in these procedures are shown in Figure 14–66. All instruments and items that come in contact with a body cavity must be sterile. One of the duties that the medical assistant is generally responsible for is to make certain that this is so. Au-

toclaving, which is a method for sterilization of instruments, is discussed in Chapter 12.

ACHIEVE UNIT OBJECTIVES

Complete Chapter 14, Unit 4, in the workbook to help you obtain competency in this subject matter.

A CAAHEP CONNECTION

Preparing patients for specialty examinations is discussed in this unit. Good communication skills in caring for patients and giving empathy and respect is necessary. Giving patients instructions for procedures is helpful to them in relieving their anxiety. It also will help gain better cooperation from them. Your patience and undersanding will be appreciated. Curriculum standards require instruction in **Anatomy and physiology, Medical terminology, Clinical procedures, Communication, Professionalism,** and **Psychology.**

RELATING TO ABHES

Chapter 14 discussed the examination and irrigation of the eyes and ears, visual and hearing tests, preparing and positioning the patient for examination, and assisting with special exams. This content relates to the ABHES accreditation requirements of **Basic clinical skills (e.g., vital signs), Patient examination, Specialties,** and **Universal precautions in the medical office** within the content area of **Medical Office Clinical Procedures.**

Medical-Legal-Ethical Scenario

Suzanne was almost a half hour late this morning. As she approached the time clock and reached for her time card, it was not there but already had been clocked in at her scheduled arrival time. She felt a little uneasy about this and didn't quite know who to talk to about it. It seemed that no one had realized that she was late, except for whoever clocked her card in for her. Knowing that doing this is unethical, besides being dishonest, she began to get really worried about it. Later, as she was bringing a patient in, she passed Jackie who winked at her and whispered, "I won't tell if you don't." It made her feel relieved to know who had done it, but now she was being dishonest with another person. That complicated things even more. Suzanne felt guilty and wondered if this would come up in her annual evaluation with the office manager next week. Jackie acted as though nothing were wrong.

CRITICAL THINKING CHALLENGE

1. What would you do if someone either clocked in for you or asked you to do it for them?
2. What did Suzanne do? Was it anything she shouldn't have done? Why?
3. What do you think Jackie was trying to do?
4. Why do you suppose that Suzanne is worried about this situation?
5. What should Suzanne do about this?
6. Why was Suzanne feeling so guilty and worried?

RESOURCES

A guide for eye inspection and testing visual acuity (1991). National Society for the Prevention of Blindness, Inc.

Corning Metpath Laboratories (1996). Patient education [Pamphlet]. Columbus, OH: Author.

Diagnostic tests, nurse's ready reference (1991). Springhouse, PA: Springhouse Corporation.

WEB LINKS

http://www.cancer.org (American Cancer Society)

Provides information on cancer, breast, and testicular self-exams.

http://www.hearinglossweb.com (Hearing Loss Web)

Provides information for people who are hearing impaired, hard of hearing, late deafened, and oral deaf, including events, issues, support, and technology related to hearing loss.

Specimen Collection and Laboratory Procedures

Foremost regarding the collection of specimens is the safety of all patients and health care providers. As you learned in Chapter 12, prevention of disease is of vital importance in preparation for these clinical tasks. You must be alert and conscientious in the performance of your duties to avoid disease transmission. Remember to practice Standard Precautions with each patient you provide with a service.

In addition to following safety precautions, you should check with your family physician and find out if you need any updating on your own immunizations. Staying current with immunizations is a smart practice. Also, for those who have respiratory conditions, having protection against pneumonia and influenza is generally recommended. Of course, you should have been administered the series of three HBV (hepatitis B virus) injections if in fact you are going to be working directly with patients and there is a potential risk of your coming into contact with blood or other body fluids. The permanent record of this vaccine should be kept in your employee file. If you have not received the HBV, you are hired in to a new position where you supposedly will not be in contact with patients, and your new employer states that it is not necessary for you to have the vaccine, the employer must sign a **waiver** regarding this. This signed document should also be kept in your employee file. There are individuals who are allergic to the contents of the culture media of certain vaccines. If you are allergic, this should be documented also in your employee file. Refer to Figure 15–1 for an example statement to decline the administration of the HBV immunization. When working with patients in the medical field, it makes good sense to be protected from every possible disease because no one knows what will be encountered next with patients.

Further guidelines should be noted regarding safe and efficient practice of procedures in the POL (physician's office laboratory) and in dealing with patients. Pay attention to proper fit when wearing protective barriers. If a gown is too large or too small, the purpose of the gown will be defeated. Latex or vinyl gloves should also fit snugly but not too tight or too loose. These simple problems may seem to be trivial points but could pose a problem situation and a safety risk. Gloves that are too small will most likely tear. Loose clothing or gloves could catch on something and be ripped or snagged, which could present a possible exposure to a dangerous pathogen.

When working with specimens and recording information, you must be careful not to touch items that you would normally touch without gloves, such as light switches, door and drawer handles and pulls, phones, charts, and equipment. Develop the habit of performing (and completing) one task at a time. Complete the procedure that requires gloving and other personal protective equipment (PPE), and then record the results after you have removed the protective barriers. For example, if you are assisting with a sigmoidoscopy wearing all of the PPE, you should complete the assisting, clean up, remove the contaminated barriers, and then perform the charting of the procedure. If you write in the patient's chart with the contaminated gloves still on, you will be contaminating everything you touch and possibly leaving unsightly stains on the patient's permanent record.

Professionalism was discussed in the beginning of the text in Chapter 2. A reminder about jewelry and hair styles must be discussed here for safety reasons. Excessive jewelry is not only inappropriate, but it could also present a dangerous situation; for example, it could get caught on a piece of equipment, or it might harbor pathogens in the crevices of the metal. When you are dealing with babies for their check-ups and often when they are ill, they may be tempted to pull at dangling earrings, necklaces, and bracelets. This is a danger for many reasons: the jewelry could break, which could result in an injury to both you and the child; the pathogens that are on the jewelry could be transmitted to you or the child (little ones like to put things in their mouths); or

you could transmit the microorganisms from one patient to another. Remember that you cannot see germs without a microscope, but they are everywhere. Another safety consideration that is a must is how you wear your hair. Both male and female health care providers who have long hair must keep their hair either worn back and secured or tied back so that it does not fall into the face or into a specimen. Again, there is a chance that a little patient could grab onto your hair. Because babies like to put everything into their mouths, you should make sure that your hair is out of the way (back away from your face if it is long) to avoid this potential problem. Hair jewelry and ribbons should be conservative and, if worn, cleaned periodically to reduce the possibility of disease transmission. These seem to be remote possibilities but could actually happen, and it only takes one exposure to transmit diseases that are opportunistic. Remember: The health statuses of the patients are unknown in most cases. A patient may be susceptible and become infected with a microbe from the medical facility during a routine office call.

The laboratory director in the POL is responsible for the management of the laboratory and for making sure that quality control and quality assurance are provided. The cooperation of the entire staff is necessary for this to be accomplished. Quality control is defined as a process that validates final test results and determines any variations. Every laboratory, including the physician office laboratory, is required by law to have in place a carefully performed, documented, and on-going quality control program. This program ensures both the physician and patient that test results are accurate and is designed to discover and eliminate error.

The quality control program is designed to monitor all aspects of laboratory activity, including specimen collection and processing and the actual testing and reporting of results. It not only monitors the test procedure itself, but

---

Statement of Refusal

I have been given complete information (oral and written) regarding the HBV immunization and the opportunity to receive it at no charge to me. At this time, I have decided not to have it administered. I understand the risk I am taking with possible exposure to hepatitis B, and I realize the seriousness of the disease. I may, at a later date, receive the HBV immunization if I so choose.

_____   _____
        Signature of employee   Date

FIGURE 15-1   This is an example of the form that must be signed by employees who decline the HBV immunization. A copy must be filed in their employee record. The employee must have been given complete information both verbally and in printed form regarding the vaccine and may choose to receive it at a later date.

it also monitors reagents used in testing, equipment, supplies, and personnel.

Thorough and accurate records must be maintained on all equipment used to test patient samples. Temperatures must be checked daily and recorded in a log book on any refrigerators used to store reagents, patient samples, and incubators used for cultures. Automated equipment must be maintained according to the manufacturer's recommendations.

Each test kit used comes with a "control," which is a sample with a known value range to be tested along with the patient specimen. The value range of the control can be a range of numbers or simply a positive or negative result. Controls are tested at specific intervals, usually according to manufacturer's directions. For example, a positive and negative control should be performed with each patient sample when using test kits, such as rapid strep and pregnancy tests. Urine reagent strips should be checked daily and each time a new bottle is opened. Manufacturer's directions should be followed when performing control samples on all automated analyzers.

Carefully maintained records showing consistent and accurate control sample results ensure that test conditions, procedures, and results are accurate.

The credibility of each individual is challenged in compliance of standards and guidelines set by regulatory bodies. In most situations, you are the only one who will know if you did or did not follow Standard Precautions and quality assurance recommendations. You must keep your mind on your work and pay attention to detail to protect yourself and others from possible contamination, and you must focus on accuracy and efficiency of the procedures and charting of information. Expedient and efficient work practices do not mean that you should hurry and make patients feel the brunt of it. Using a methodical and steady pace will help you in accomplishing a great deal of work in a reasonable amount of time. Further guidelines are listed in addition to those in Chapter 12, which all health care providers should follow to ensure that quality and safety in the lab are upheld.

Guidelines for a well-managed and efficient POL:

1. Follow current state and federal regulations, and keep them on file.
2. File correspondences and all other documents regarding the lab.
3. Keep all material safety data sheets (MSDS) regarding all chemicals, reagents, and solutions (such as isopropyl alcohol, disinfectants, and even "whiteout") in a notebook that is readily accessible to all employees.
4. Have a "biohazard communications" manual that includes:
   - a "chemical hygiene plan" (the employer's plan) to prevent employees from being exposed to dangerous chemicals
   - a "biohazard safety" section that includes universal precaution techniques that conform to OSHA and CLIA regulations.

5. File a copy of all biohazard box/bag pick ups.
6. Keep a log of all accidents and what was done for the person (i.e., who used the eye wash station and for what reason).
7. Place all sharps, including intact needles and syringes (do not re-cap), into biohazard sharps container.
8. Keep long hair tied back securely and wear only a minimum amount of jewelry.
9. Keep a 10% bleach solution (made fresh daily) ready for cleanup of infectious wastes.
10. Record all lab work performed in a log with the date, time, name of test, who performed it, the results, and when it was sent to the reference lab and when the results were received.
11. Clearly post Standard Precautions for employees as a safety reminder.
12. Provide adequate lighting in all work areas.
13. Have a fire extinguisher readily available and the directions for use clearly posted with it.
14. Keep hallways and walking paths free of clutter.
15. Have fire/evacuation routes clearly posted.

UNIT 1

The Microscope

OBJECTIVES

Upon completion of the unit, meet the following performance objectives by verifying knowledge of the facts and principles presented through oral and written communication at a level deemed competent. Demonstrate the specific behaviors as identified in the performance objectives of the procedures, observing all aseptic and safety precautions in accordance with health care standards.

1. Spell and define, using the glossary at the back of the text, all the **Words to Know** in this unit.
2. Describe the importance of credibility regarding clinical duties.
3. Explain the reason why a proper fit is necessary regarding PPE.
4. Describe the reasons for wearing conservative jewelry.
5. Explain the reasons for wearing long hair secured back from the face.
6. Identify and discuss the guidelines recommended for the POL. 8 (15 listed)
7. Identify the parts of the microscope and the purpose of each.
8. Adjust and focus the objectives, and state their magnification power.
9. Adjust the light and mirror for proper viewing.
10. Demonstrate how to clean the microscope (lens, stage, and mirror).

11. Explain the general purpose of the microscope in the medical office.

12. Demonstrate the proper way to carry a microscope.

AREAS OF COMPETENCE (AAMA)

This unit addresses content within the specific competency areas of *Fundamental principles, Diagnostic orders, Patient care, Professionalism, Communication skills, Instruction,* and *Operational functions,* as identified in the Medical Assistant Role Delineation Study. Refer to Appendix A for a detailed listing of the areas.

■ WORDS TO KNOW

binocular
compensate
condenser
low-power field (lpf)
high-power field (hpf)
magnify
minute

monocular
objectives
proficient
specimen
technical
waiver

PATIENT EDUCATION

Many patients may be frightened or confused about some of the laboratory procedures requested by the physician to aid in diagnosis. You may perform some of these in the office or clinic setting or send the patient to the lab for tests. If you send patients elsewhere, make sure you give accurate directions on how to get there.

Each test or procedure must be explained clearly and concisely to relieve patients' anxiety. Use language that patients will understand. Most people have little or no knowledge of medical terminology.

Certain lab tests require preparation by patients prior to arrival (e.g., fasting, taking or omitting certain medications). Be sure to instruct patients in these preparations and have clear, concise, written instructions available. Do not presume that patients know all about a procedure even if they have had the test before. Often, new techniques require additional or different instructions for preparation. Medical technology is constantly changing. It is important for health care providers (including medical assistants) to keep abreast of new developments in medicine. Inform patients that some procedures can cause temporary discomfort and how it may be relieved.

Give patients enough time to look over the printed instruction sheet or pamphlet, and make certain you answer all of their questions thoroughly before they leave.

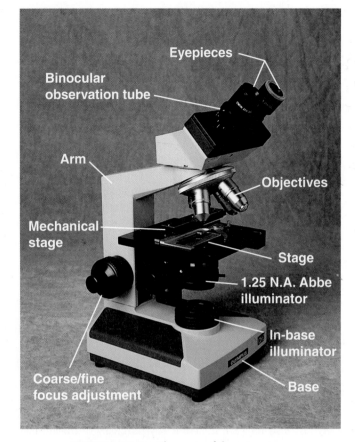

FIGURE 15–2 The parts of the microscope

The microscope is an essential piece of equipment in the laboratory of almost every medical practice. It is used to examine and identify **minute** objects that cannot be seen with the naked eye. Microscopes are fine and expensive **technical** instruments that must be handled with great respect. The operation and care manual should be kept handy for reference because each microscope is slightly different. The amount of routine maintenance required will vary with the amount of use. Each POL must keep a maintenance log of all equipment. Routine inspection and maintenance should be recorded in this maintenance log with information regarding what was done, the date, and the agency that did the required labor to fix it. All maintenance forms or documents should be kept on file.

The part of the microscope that supports the eyepiece is called the arm. Figure 15–2 shows the labeled parts of a **binocular** microscope. The proper way to carry the microscope is to grasp the arm with one hand and place the other hand under the base, holding it at waist level. To secure a microscope while transporting it, the electrical cord for the light source should be loosely wrapped and secured with a twist tie or a rubber band. Wrapping the cord too tightly may cause the enclosed wires to break and lead to a short that could cause an electrical fire. The cord of the microscope should be kept loosely wrapped and out of the work area when not in use. It should always be unplugged by grasping the plug, never by pulling the cord. As when using any electrical appliance, all surrounding surfaces and hands should be dry. Wet hands or floors can lead to electric shock.

PARTS OF THE MICROSCOPE

A binocular microscope has two eyepieces. The **monocular** microscope has only one eyepiece or ocular lens. The eyepiece or ocular lens is in the upper part of the tube of the microscope. The eyepiece contains a lens to **magnify** what is being seen.

The body tube leads to the revolving nosepiece. Attached to the revolving nosepiece are three (sometimes four) small lenses called **objectives**, each of which has a different magnifying power. The shortest has the lowest power. It is called the **low-power field**, or **lpf**. On most microscopes, it will magnify the object to be viewed 10 times, or make it 10X larger than when viewed by the naked eye. The low-power field is the lens used to scan the field of interest and to focus in on the specimen. To position each objective, you simply rotate the nosepiece until you hear a click.

For greater detail in viewing the specimen, turn the nosepiece to the next longer objective, the **high-power field** (**hpf**). It will magnify the object approximately 40 times, or 40X. The longest objective is the oil-immersion objective. This high-power lens, when used with oil, magnifies objects about 100 times, or 100X. Using the fine-focus dial will bring the specimen into good definition.

PROCEDURE

15-1 Use a Microscope

PURPOSE: To gain skill in the use of the microscope.

OSHA GUIDELINES: To comply with Standard Precautions, gloves must be worn if there is any possibility of coming into contact with blood or any body fluids.

EQUIPMENT: Microscope, electrical outlet for light source of microscope, specimen on disposable glass slide with frosted end, cover glass (used usually for wet specimens only), lens cleaning tissues, latex or vinyl gloves.

PERFORMANCE OBJECTIVE: Provided with all necessary equipment and supplies, demonstrate the use of the microscope following the steps in the procedure with the instructor observing each step.

1. Wash hands and put on latex or vinyl gloves.

2. Assemble necessary equipment.

3. Clean ocular lens with lens cleaning tissues. **RATIONALE: Removal of makeup, oil, and eye secretions is necessary to ensure clear viewing and eliminate transmission of disease among office personnel. NOTE: Use only lens tissue paper to prevent damaging the surface of the lens.**

4. Plug microscope light source into electrical outlet, and turn on light switch at front base of microscope.

5. Place specimen slide on stage with frosted end up between clips, and secure over opening of stage. **NOTE: Frosted end is used for labeling the specimen in pencil.**

6. Watch carefully as you raise substage so that it does not come into direct contact with slide.

7. Turn revolving nosepiece to low-power objective (10X) and begin to focus coarse-adjustment dial until a wide shaft can be seen. **NOTE: Regarding microscope lighting—When** you switch from a lower to a higher power objective (or vice-versa), the light will need to be turned up. The light source should be kept at a fairly low level for each objective to improve the clarity of the objects being viewed. Too much light may have a bleaching or glaring effect, and the object may not be seen at all or at least may not be seen well.

8. When outline of specimen is in view, turn fine-adjustment dial until specimen can be seen in detail.

9. Adjust substage diaphragm level or adjust mirror to obtain proper lighting.

10. If sharper detail is needed, carefully turn revolving nosepiece to intermediate-power objective, and adjust fine-focus dial.

11. When using oil-immersion lens objective or hpf (high-power field), oil should be used very sparingly. **NOTE: A disposable cover slide should be used, and the lens must be cleaned after each use. Adjustment must be made for amount of light needed by adjusting diaphragm lever under stage.**

12. When specimen has been identified, turn off light and return all items to proper storage area. **NOTE: Microscope stage should be cleaned and recorded in the maintenance log.**

13. Remove gloves and wash hands. **NOTE: Results of the actual examination should be read and recorded in the laboratory test log by the physician. The medical assistant is responsible for assisting with the preparation of the specimen for microscopic examination unless otherwise instructed by the physician.**

This unit with the introduction discussed the importance of *Asepsis* and *Infection control,* which are components of the Medical Assistant Clinical Procedures curriculum.

The stage of the microscope has two clips which hold the **specimen** slide to be viewed. Just underneath the stage is a substage where a **condenser** is held that regulates the amount of light directed on the magnified specimen. It has a shutter or diaphragm to control the amount of light desired. The substage may be raised or lowered in focusing on the specimen.

A supply of lens tissue paper should be kept nearby to clean the lenses after each use. Makeup, oil, secretions from the eyes, and dust can make it difficult to see through the lens, besides being a possible means of transmitting disease among office personnel. Because there may be several individuals in a medical office who may use the microscope, it is advised to wipe the eyepieces with a disinfectant after each use to avoid the transmission of diseases. Eyeglasses are not necessary when performing microscopic work because the microscope may be focused to **compensate** for all visual defects except astigmatism.

It will take time and patience to learn how to operate the microscope. The supervision of an experienced operator is essential to becoming **proficient** in its use and care. Refer to Procedure 15–1.

ACHIEVE UNIT OBJECTIVES

Complete Chapter 15, Unit 1, in the workbook to help you obtain competency of this subject matter.

UNIT 2

Capillary Blood Tests

OBJECTIVES

Upon completion of the unit, meet the following performance objectives by verifying knowledge of the facts and principles presented through oral and written communication at a level deemed competent. Demonstrate the specific behaviors as identified in the performance objectives of the procedures, observing all aseptic and safety precautions in accordance with health care standards.

1. Spell and define, using the glossary at the back of the text, all the **Words to Know** in this unit.
2. State the purpose of wearing latex or vinyl gloves when performing laboratory procedures.

3. List and describe the regulatory bodies that govern the POL.
4. List and describe the laboratory practices that yield quality assurance in the POL.
5. Define the terms quality assurance and quality control.
6. Explain the reasons for performing capillary blood tests in the medical office.
7. Perform skin puncture procedures to obtain capillary blood specimens.
8. Complete a health department request form for the PKU (phenylketonuria) test, and obtain the blood specimen for it.
9. Obtain hemoglobin and hematocrit levels.
10. Operate a microhematocrit centrifuge.
11. Operate a hemoglobinometer.
12. Perform a blood glucose screening test with glucometer (or color chart on bottle) for reagent strip.
13. Explain the purpose of the glucose tolerance test (GTT).
14. Give instructions and patient education for the preparation of a patient for a GTT.
15. Explain point-of-care testing.
16. Explain quality assurance concerning patient care.
17. Prepare a blood smear for a differential count.
18. List each type of white blood cell, and state the function of each.

AREAS OF COMPETENCE (AAMA)

This unit addresses content within the specific competency areas of *Fundamental principles, Diagnostic orders, Patient care, Professionalism, Communication skills, Instruction,* and *Operational functions,* as identified in the Medical Assistant Role Delineation Study. Refer to Appendix A for a detailed listing of the areas.

WORDS TO KNOW

allosteric	implement
carbohydrates	insulin
centrifuge	laboratory
cholesterol	lancet
differential	low density lipoproteins
diffuse	(LDL)
erythropoiesis	metabolism
gestational	neonate
glucose	pallor
glycohemoglobin	percentage
glycosylation	phagocytosis
Health Care Financing	phenylalanine
Administration	PKU (phenylketonuria)
(HCFA)	polycythemia
hematocrit	Provider Performed
health and human	Microscopy (PPM)
services (HHS)	morphology
high density lipoproteins	puncture
(HDL)	reagent

regulatory   sterile

reticuloendothelial   tolerance

stat   triglycerides

LABORATORY CLASSIFICATION AND REGULATION

The physician's office **laboratory** (POL) falls under many **regulatory** bodies. The complexity of the laboratory tests performed will determine which classification the POL is and under which body it is regulated. The three laboratory classifications under the Clinical Laboratory Improvement Amendments of 1988 (CLIA-88) are Waived, Moderately Complex, and Highly Complex lab tests. **Provider Performed Microscopy** (PPM) means that the physician performs the lab test.

A Certificate of Waiver allows *only* those tests to be performed in a POL that are on the final list of Waived tests. A Waived status (waived by the CLIA-88) is granted according to the difficulty in performing tests. Waived tests that can be performed in a medical office following package insert directions are basically those manufactured for home testing that have been cleared by the FDA. Some of the simplistic testing methods that are used in the medical office are: urinalysis reagent strips or tablets, cholesterol test kits, ESR, occult blood tests, blood glucose testing with glucometer, hemoglobin and hematocrit, H-Pylori, rapid strep, and HCG (pregnancy tests). Application for this certificate is obtained from the Health Care Financing Administration (HCFA) when the facility is registered. Laboratory tests on the certificate of waiver list may be billed to Medicare and Medicaid. This certificate must be renewed every two years for a moderate fee. Tests performed by the medical assistant in the POL must be restricted to this list. All waived and moderately complex tests performed in the POL must follow manufacturer's label instructions and may be performed by non-lab personnel. The HCFA does not stipulate any specific staff requirements, quality control, quality assurance or proficiency tests for waived tests except that the POL must follow good laboratory practices. This refers to quality control and quality assurance.

Moderately Complex laboratory tests must be performed under more strict regulations. PPM tests require even further mandated standards. Included in these requirements are patient test management, stricter staff credentialing, proficiency testing, quality control and quality assurance, keeping logs of all test information, and regulatory agency inspection of the physician's office laboratory. There are extensive laboratory training and educational requirements for personnel for Moderately Complex classification. Any abnormal test results that apply to a previously-undiagnosed condition of a patient must be referred to a Highly Complex lab to be verified.

Regulatory bodies periodically inspect laboratories and medical offices to ensure quality assurance and quality control. Quality assurance in the health care field refers to all evaluative services and the results compared with accepted standards. Quality control implies that operational procedures are used to **implement** the quality assurance program. To determine these standards, many aspects of care are taken into account. First, the cost, place, accessibility, treatment, and benefits of health care are evaluated. The next step is comparing the findings with standard results. Finally, the appropriate recommendations for improving health care are noted.

All laboratories are required to follow quality assurance programs. The purposes of quality assurance programs are to evaluate the quality and effectiveness of health care according to accepted standards and to ensure accuracy and validity in testing procedures. When needed, POLs must also participate in proficiency testing programs for the test procedures that they perform and keep strict records of quality control, temperature readings, and maintenance logs.

Other bodies that provide regulation inspections of a POL are **HCFA** and OSHA. Private agencies also issue accreditations and state licensing for approved operation of the POL. The laboratory may be operated under a provisional certificate, which is issued until the Department of Health and Human Services (HHS) inspects the facility. Certificates must be renewed every two years. Inspections may be made, unannounced, anytime. If OSHA, a separate inspecting body from CLIA, finds a POL in non-compliance of regulations during a visit (scheduled or not), a monetary fine per item, per employee (per visit) applies.

In the POL, no matter what classification, the following practices should be followed to ensure reliable and accurate data and to ensure quality health care to patients. Quality assurance involves *proper:*

1. Patient identification
2. Patient preparation and specimen collection
3. Specimen processing and transportation
4. Instrumental and technical performance
5. Safety
6. In-service training and education of all health care personnel

All state and federal health and safety regulations and laws apply to the POL according to the three lab specifications. It is important to stay abreast of the current regulations that apply to the facility where you are employed.

SKIN PUNCTURE

C **Skills Menu:**
- Skin Puncture

Capillary blood tests are frequently performed in the medical office or clinic because of the small amount of blood required, usually one to a few drops. Because most patients are extremely apprehensive, you must develop skill not only in performing the procedures but in conveying reassurance to the patient. When skin **puncture,** commonly referred to as "finger stick," procedures are done correctly, the patient should feel minimal discomfort. Displaying confidence in carrying out the procedures competently will ensure patient safety and comfort.

Capillaries are minute blood vessels which convey blood from the arterioles to the venules. At this level, blood and oxygen diffuse to the tissues, and products of metabolic activity enter the bloodstream. For this reason, capillary blood is an ideal sample for the screening of **hematocrit**, hemoglobin, blood glucose, PKU levels, and other screening tests that require a very small amount of blood. Refer to Procedure 15–2.

Capillary blood is just under the surface of the skin. The most practical sites to use are the ring and great fin-

---

PROCEDURE

15-2 Puncture Skin with Sterile Lancet

PURPOSE: To obtain a few drops of capillary blood for screening tests.

OSHA GUIDELINES: To comply with Standard Precautions, gloves must be worn if there is any possibility of coming into contact with blood or any body fluids.

EQUIPMENT: Latex or vinyl gloves, sterile lancet, Figure 15–4, alcohol, cotton balls, sharps container, Mayo table.

PERFORMANCE OBJECTIVE: Provided with all necessary equipment and supplies, and using other students as patients, demonstrate the skin puncture procedure following all steps to obtain capillary blood for test(s) specified by the physician or instructor. The instructor will observe each step.

1. Identify the patient. **RATIONALE: Speaking to the patient by name and checking chart ensures that you are performing the procedure on the correct patient.**

2. Explain the procedure to the patient.

3. Inspect patient's fingers (or other puncture sites) and select most desirable site. **NOTE:**
   - Main sites are ring or great finger, earlobe, infant's lateral areas of heel.
   - Some patients have a preference for a particular site.
   - Earlobe is less sensitive to pain than fingers.
   - Do not use areas that are bruised, calloused, or injured.

4. Wash hands, put on latex or vinyl gloves, and assemble needed items on Mayo table.

5. Wipe desired site with an alcohol-saturated cotton ball and let dry. Do not blow the skin to expedite drying: **RATIONALE: You may contaminate the skin with microorganisms in the exhaled air.**

6. Take sterile lancet out of package without contaminating point. **NOTE: Another must be used if point is touched.**

7. Hold patient's finger (or other site) securely between your thumb and great finger. In your other hand hold lancet, pointed downward, with thumb and index or great finger. Puncture site quickly with a firm, steady, down-and-up motion to approximately a two-mm depth. **NOTE: Control entry and exit of lancet in same path to avoid ripping skin. To obtain a better blood sample, puncture across fingerprints not parallel to them.**

8. Discard first drop of blood by blotting away with dry gauze square. **RATIONALE: First drop may contain traces of alcohol or tissue fluid that would dilute sample and make test inaccurate.**

9. Keep applying gentle pressure on either side of puncture site until necessary amount of blood has been obtained. **NOTE: Too much pressure will cause tissue fluid to mix with blood resulting in diluted sample and incorrect test results.**

10. Wipe site with cotton ball and ask patient to gently hold it for a minute or two. **NOTE: Check site to be sure bleeding has stopped. Determine if patient is allergic to adhesive before applying bandage to puncture site (use gauze square and hypoallergenic tape if allergic).**

11. Remove gloves, wash hands, and discard used items in proper receptacle.

12. Record procedure on patient's chart.

NOTE: A solution of approximately one-fourth cup bleach per gallon of tap water (a 1:100 dilution of common household bleach) should be made fresh daily and kept readily available for clean up of accidental spills of blood or body fluids.

CHARTING EXAMPLE:
8-5-XX
Rt. ring finger punctured, filled two microhematocrit tubes with capillary blood; Hct 37%; Hgb 12.4.

J. Watkins, CMA (CL)

PATIENT EDUCATION

Most patients, especially youngsters, are apprehensive about having blood taken. The medical assistant must calmly explain to each patient that screening tests, such as a hemoglobin or a blood glucose, are performed with a small amount of blood taken from the finger, earlobe, or infant's heel. Let the patient know ahead of time what you are going to do to gain cooperation. You should tell the patient that there will be a little pain or discomfort during the initial skin puncture, but it will not last long. Reassure the patient that this procedure is short-lived and necessary for the physician to aid in making a diagnosis or evaluating the condition. Remember to advise the patient to keep the puncture site clean and dry for 24 hours with a fresh bandage as necessary.

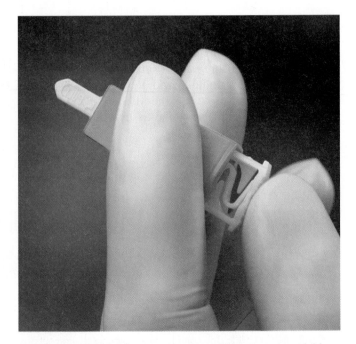

FIGURE 15–4 BD Microtainer™ Brand lancets are available in different types for various purposes. To use, position lancet firmly against puncture site. Hold lancet between fingers and place thumb on white activation button. Press the white button to activate lancet. Do not pull lancet away from puncture site until after activation. Dispose of used lancet in appropriate sharps container. (Courtesy BD Vacutainer Systems.)

ger, the earlobe, and in infants the heel (Figure 15–3A and B).

The sterile lancet is widely used by diabetic (and other) patients in their homes for simple blood tests that require capillary blood. You may be given the duty of instructing patients in use of one of the skin puncturing devices shown in Figure 15–4. Patients who use this technique daily should simply wash the puncture site thoroughly with soap and water. Alcohol tends to toughen the skin if used for extended periods. Patients should be provided with a sharps container to keep at home to dispose of the lancets after use. Encourage them to return the three-fourths full container to your facility where you can properly autoclave it and dispose of it safely.

With strict regulations regarding quality control and quality assurance, you are required to keep a log book to record all specimens and the results of the tests performed. The log should include:

1. Date
2. Patient's name
3. Test performed
4. Results of the test
5. Your initials
6. Any kit, reagent strip, or **reagent** lot numbers and expiration dates

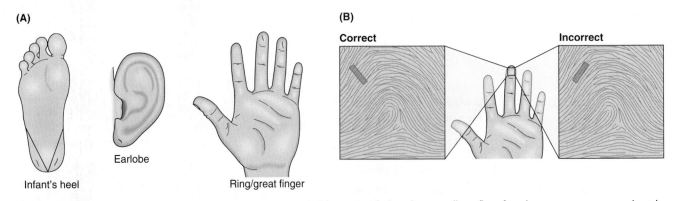

(A)

Infant's heel

Earlobe

Ring/great finger

(B)

Correct

Incorrect

FIGURE 15–3 (A) These skin puncture sites are recommended because of abundant capillary flow for obtaining a specimen, besides being a convenient site for patients. (B) Skin punctures should be made across fingerprints, not parallel to them.

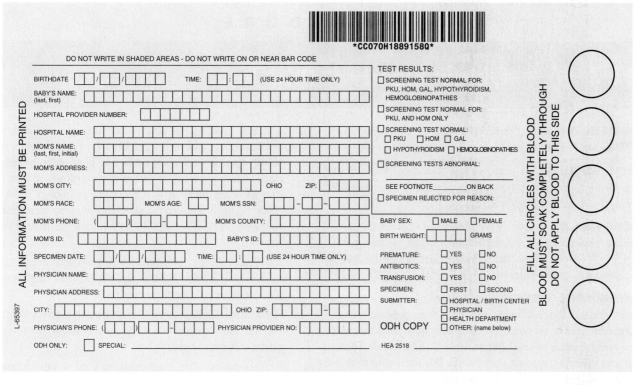

(A)

PKU Test

A screening test done with capillary blood from an infant's heel is the **PKU** (**phenylketonuria**). Phenylketonuria is a congenital disease caused by a defect in the **metabolism** of the amino acid, **phenylalanine**. This unmetabolized protein, phenylalanine, accumulates in the bloodstream and can prevent the brain from developing normally. If this condition goes undetected and untreated, the result is mental retardation. This screening is required by law in most states and all Canadian provinces, either by blood test or urinalysis. The blood test requires that a few drops of the infant's blood be soaked through the outlined circles (from the back) of the treated paper attached to the health department form (Figure 15–5). This duplicated form must be completed accurately. Parents usually bring the form with them on the infant's first office visit if the procedure was not performed at the hospital. After completion of the instructions, the form (intact with all copies) should be mailed to the health department. Obtaining and returning the PKU testing cards varies throughout the country, so it is wise to check with the standard procedure in your state. With the Ohio Department of Health, for instance, the ODH PKU log is sent in to have the test cards replaced at no charge if the physician purchases and supplies the tests. A report of the results of the screening test is mailed back to the physician to be filed in the infant's chart. This test is limited to newborns (**neonates**) and their biological parents. Refer to Procedure 15–3 for obtaining infant's blood for PKU screening.

INSTRUCTIONS FOR NEWBORN SCREENING SPECIMENS

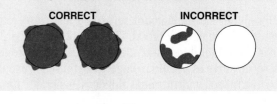

1. Cleanse infant's heel with alcohol swab.
2. Puncture heel in fleshy lateral or medial posterior portion with sterile disposable lancet. Wipe puncture site with dry sterile swab.
3. Allow large blood droplet to form. Touch blood droplet to center of circle on **ONE SIDE** of filter paper card **ONLY**. Observe reverse side of card and insure that blood has soaked completely through before removing card from infant's heel.
4. Repeat step 3 to fill **ALL FIVE CIRCLES**. **DO NOT** squeeze heel excessively to obtain blood.
5. Allow card to **AIR DRY** 2 hours at room temperature on a non-absorbent surface. **DO NOT** stack cards together while drying.
6. After blood spots are completely dry, place card in ODH self-addressed laboratory mailing envelope. **MAIL** within **48 HOURS**.

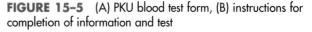

CORRECT   **INCORRECT**

(B)

FIGURE 15–5   (A) PKU blood test form, (B) instructions for completion of information and test

PROCEDURE

15-3 Obtain Blood for PKU Test

PURPOSE: To obtain a blood specimen for determination of PKU (phenylketonuria) level in blood.

OSHA GUIDELINES: To comply with Standard Precautions, gloves must be worn if there is any possibility of coming into contact with blood or any body fluids.

EQUIPMENT: PKU health department form, Autolet or sterile lancet, latex or vinyl gloves, cotton balls, alcohol, gauze squares, round adhesive bandage, patient's chart, pen, stamped envelope addressed to health department.

PERFORMANCE OBJECTIVE: Provided with all necessary equipment and supplies, and using other students as patients, demonstrate the steps of the procedure for obtaining a blood specimen for determination of phenylketonuria level in the blood. The instructor will observe each step. **NOTE: This procedure may be simulated by using a clinical lifelike doll and milk colored with red food coloring for practice.**

1. Wash hands, put on latex or vinyl gloves, and assemble needed items on Mayo table.

2. Identify the patient. Ask parent to name patient and check chart to avoid error.

3. Explain procedure to parent and ask for necessary information to complete form. Be sure to write the exact birth weight of the infant on the form and the date and time the test was performed. **RATIONALE: Accurate results depend on the ratio of findings to birthweight.** Ask for their assistance in holding infant still during procedure.

4. Wipe desired site with alcohol prep or cotton ball and let dry.

5. Take sterile lancet out of the package without contaminating point.

6. Secure infant's lateral heel with your great finger and thumb, and gently apply pressure to produce a large drop of blood. Carefully blot onto one of outlined circles on end of form soaking the test paper from the back of the form. **NOTE: Repeat until each circle has been entirely saturated.** Newborn blood is thick and flows slowly so it may stop bleeding (clot). It is not uncommon that a second "stick" is required because all circles must be completely saturated (soaked) through from the back to the front of the test card.

7. Wipe puncture site with cotton ball and apply dry gauze square. Ask parent to hold against puncture site. Then place small round bandage over area.

8. Place completed test form into protective envelope and then into an envelope addressed to health department with physician's return address.

9. Remove gloves, wash hands, discard used items in proper receptacle, and return items to proper storage area.

10. Record procedure on patient's chart. Refer to charting example below.

11. Record on the required log sheet and/or other collection log. **NOTE: Check with the regulations of the health department in your state regarding documentation.**

12. File report in patient's chart when received in return mail after physician has checked the results.

LOG BOOK EXAMPLE:

DATE	PATIENT'S NAME	TEST	RESULTS OBTAINED BY
3-18-XX	Brittani C. Jones	PKU	J. Watkins, CMA

CHARTING EXAMPLE:
5-30-XX
PKU test completed with all 5 circles saturated with blood from infant's L heel; mailed to health dept.

J. Watkins, CMA (CL)

HEMOGLOBIN AND HEMATOCRIT

Hemoglobin and hematocrit screening tests also require a few drops of capillary blood. Usually the ring or great finger is used in children and adults because these fingers are not so sensitive as the index finger. The thumb is usually too tough-skinned, and the little finger is generally too small and would not yield an adequate amount. The patient's age or preference will help you decide which site to choose.

Hematocrit is a screening test to determine anemia. Anemia is a condition in which there is a lack of circulating red blood cells. Erythrocytes transport oxygen to the entire body. When there are not enough of them to supply all of the cells, symptoms of paleness, fatigue, drowsiness, among others, begin to be apparent in patients. **Polycythemia** may be indicated by an abnormally high reading. Polycythemia is a condition of having an excessive number of erythrocytes. Some of the symptoms are similar to anemia—weakness and fatigue. Redness of the skin (opposite of anemia) and pain of the extremities, often with black and blue spots, is observed in some patients with polycythemia. You should become familiar with all of the symptoms of the diseases for which you perform screening

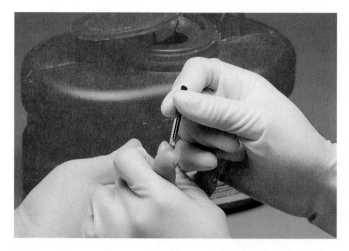

FIGURE 15–6 Skin puncture (finger stick) is made with sterile lancet with capillary puncture device across fingerprints.

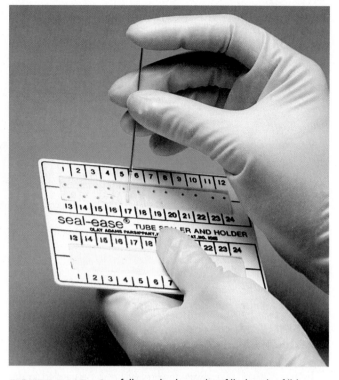

FIGURE 15–8 Carefully push glass tube (filled to the fill line with capillary blood) into clay to seal one end before placing in the microhematocrit centrifuge.

tests so that you may alert the physician to any changes that patients may tell you. Often patients disclose important information to you and then do not say anything to the doctor because they think you have already reported it.

To perform a microhematocrit screening test, you begin by cleansing the skin site with alcohol using a gauze square or cotton ball. A sterile lancet is used to puncture the skin (Figure 15–6). Very small glass tubes, called microhematocrit tubes, are used to collect the blood sample (Figure 15–7). Many of them are marked with a fill line at about the three-quarter point. The tube fills very quickly by capillary action if the puncture site is deep enough, usually about two mm. A small amount of clay sealant is carefully placed in one end of the microhematocrit tube to seal the opening so that blood will not leak out as shown in Figure 15–8. Make sure that there is no trace of red visible around the end of the tube with clay (even a minute hairline path of red will cause *all* of the blood in the tube to spin out during centrifugation).

The tube is then placed in a microhematocrit **centrifuge**, as in Figure 15–9, where spinning for approximately three minutes will separate the blood components by centrifugal force. The tube after centrifugation has

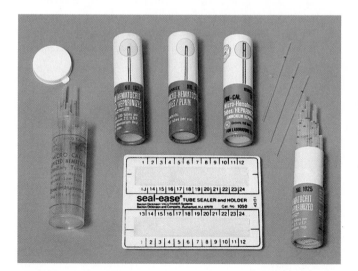

FIGURE 15–7 Microhematocrit (capillary blood) tubes with clay sealant.

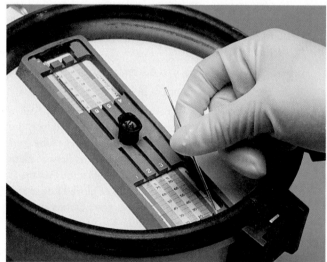

FIGURE 15–9 There are grooved slots for up to six microhematocrit tubes to be centrifuged at once. Be sure to note the space number for each patient's hematocrit tube, and write it down to avoid confusion. The clay sealant tray also has numbers along the side to help you keep track of several specimens. Note: You may want to use the same number on the tray as in the centrifuge for each patient when there are two or more. Carefully place sealed end of tube (toward you) against the padding of the centrifuge wall.

three layers: plasma, a thin yellowish layer called the buffy coat, and packed red blood cells (Figure 15–10). Contained in the buffy coat are the white blood cells and the platelets. Refer to Procedure 15–4.

The hematocrit is expressed as the **percentage** of the total blood volume made up of red blood cells (erythrocytes) or as the volume in cubic centimeters (cc) of erythrocytes packed by centrifugation in 100 cc of blood. The

---

PROCEDURE

15-4 ✋ Determine Hematocrit (Hct) Using Microhematocrit Centrifuge

PURPOSE: To determine the volume of packed erythrocytes in whole blood.

OSHA GUIDELINES: To comply with Standard Precautions, gloves must be worn if there is any possibility of coming into contact with blood or any body fluids.

EQUIPMENT: Autolet or sterile lancet, microhematocrit tube(s), sealing clay, microhematocrit centrifuge, latex or vinyl gloves, cotton balls, alcohol, patient's chart, pen (if hemoglobin is done by this procedure, conversion chart will also be needed to determine Hb), Table 15–1.

PERFORMANCE OBJECTIVE: Provided with all necessary equipment and supplies, and using other students as patients, demonstrate the steps in the procedure for determining hematocrit (Hct) readings using the microhematocrit centrifuge. The instructor will observe each step.

1. Assemble needed items on Mayo table. Check to see that centrifuge is plugged into the electrical outlet.

2. Identify patient and explain procedure. **RATIONALE: Speaking to the patient by name and checking chart ensures that you are performing the procedure on the correct patient.**

3. Wash and dry hands, and put on latex or vinyl gloves.

4. Follow desired skin puncture procedure.

5. Hold microhematocrit tube as you would hold a pencil or pen, horizontally with opening next to drop of blood that appears at puncture site. **RATIONALE: Holding tube horizontally slightly tilted downward assists the flow of blood to enter the tube by capillary action until it reaches the fill line or three-quarter point. Hold tip of gloved finger over Hct tube to keep blood from flowing out. Obtain as many tubes as ordered, usually one or two. Avoid bubbles in the capillary tube.**

6. Wipe outside end of glass tube with gauze square while still holding it horizontally. Carefully seal *only one end* of the tube by placing it into the clay and turning it until the entire end is solid clay. **NOTE: Do not apply too much pressure or the glass tube will break (Figure 15–8).** Only a very small amount of clay is needed. You may leave the

tube standing up in the tray until you are finished tending to the needs of the patient.

7. Have patient hold dry gauze square on puncture site. **NOTE: Check to make sure bleeding has stopped.** Offer patient a bandage.

8. Secure sealed end of tube against rubber padding in centrifuge (clay end of tube is always toward you). Balance centrifuge with another tube opposite it. **NOTE: If two or more patients' tubes are placed in centrifuge at same time, make sure that you note numbers of spaces to avoid a mix-up (Figure 15–9). RATIONALE: Accurate identification is essential to assigning results to proper patient.**

9. Close inside cover carefully over tubes, and lock into place by turning dial clockwise. Then close and lock outside cover. Listen for it to click into place.

10. Turn timer switch to three to five minutes. (Most timing switches indicate that you turn past desired time and then back to time you want set.) It will automatically turn off.

11. Wait until centrifuge has completely stopped spinning and unlock covers. (Opening a centrifuge before it stops spinning is most dangerous—centrifugal force pulls objects, such as hair, jewelry, or loose sleeves of lab coats, into it.)

12. Read results by placing bottom line of packed RBCs (red blood cells) (up to buffy coat but not including it) against calibrated chart in centrifuge where tube is resting (Figure 15–11). (There is usually a magnifying glass attached to centrifuge to assist in reading Hct accurately.) Keep cover of centrifuge closed when not in use.

13. Discard used items in proper waste receptacles, remove gloves, and wash hands.

14. Record reading in patient's chart and on log sheet as a percentage.

CHARTING EXAMPLE:
4-21-XX
Finger stick of L ring finger for capillary blood for Hct—reading is 47%

S. Davis, RMA (DV)

15. Return items to proper storage areas.

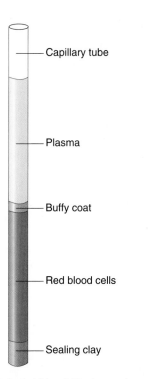

FIGURE 15–10 Capillary tube — Plasma — Buffy coat — Red blood cells — Sealing clay

FIGURE 15–10 A labeled blood-filled microhematocrit tube after centrifugation

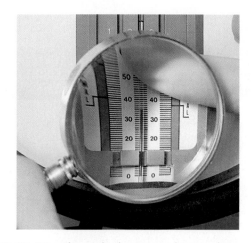

FIGURE 15–11 The medical assistant obtains a hematocrit reading by looking down onto the tube against the values chart within the centrifuge. After centrifugation, the hematocrit reading is obtained by placing the sealed end of the tube against the padding, making sure that the line between the packed red blood cells and the clay is at "0" (zero). Read the hematocrit at the bottom of the meniscus (the curved line where the red blood cells and the buffy coat meet). The reading in this photo is 35%.

normal hematocrit range for adult males is 40 to 54% and for adult females 37 to 47%.

Finger puncture or venous blood samples can be analyzed to provide the following values:

- hematocrit
- platelet count
- total white blood cell count
- total granulocyte count
- percentage granulocytes
- total lymph/mono count
- percentage lymphs/mono

Hematocrits are read by looking down onto the tube against the values chart within the centrifuge. Refer to Figure 15–11 for a close look into the centrifuge. After the blood tube has been centrifuged, the reading is done by placing the sealed end of the tube against the padding, making sure that the line between the packed red cells and the clay is at "0" (zero). Read the hematocrit at the bottom of the meniscus (the curved line where the red cells and the buffy coat meet). Using a magnifying lens to read the hematocrit is advised for accuracy. There is also a method of reading hematocrits by using a "crit" reader. Often, this is used for tubes that are not adequately filled to the fill line. The physician can get an approximate reading in this case to decide if further blood studies are indicated.

Figure 15–12 shows the QBC STAR, which is a centrifugal hematology system that provides cost-effective, quantitative CBC results quickly while the patient waits.

This method of testing is important in point-of-care testing for better patient compliance. Combining the physician's examination and on-site test results and discussing the test report and treatment plan with the patient all in one visit, when possible, is an ideal way to care for patients.

In determining the hemoglobin (Hb) level of the blood, a conversion chart may be used when the hematocrit percentage (Hct %) is known; it may also be used to check

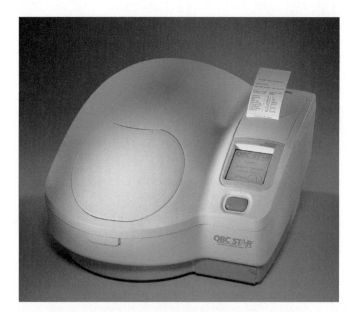

FIGURE 15–12 The QBC STAR offers efficient and accurate point-of-care tests in hematology. (Courtesy Becton, Dickinson and Company.)

TABLE 15–1

APPROXIMATE RELATIONSHIP BETWEEEN HEMATOCRIT, RED BLOOD CELL COUNT, AND HEMOGLOBIN IN ADULTS

For Red Blood Cells of Normal Size— To Be Used for Checking Purposes Only*

Hematocrit (%)	Red Blood Cell Count (×1 million per cubic millimeter of blood)	Hemoglobin (in grams per 100 cc)
30	3.4	9.8
31	3.6	10.4
32	3.7	10.7
33	3.8	11.0
34	3.9	11.3
35	4.0	11.6
36	4.1	11.9
37	4.3	12.4
38	4.4	12.8
39	4.5	13.1
40	4.6	13.3
41	4.7	13.6
42	4.8	13.9
43	4.9	14.2
44	5.1	14.8
45	5.2	15.1
46	5.3	15.4
47	5.4	15.7
48	5.5	16.0
49	5.6	16.2
50	5.7	16.5
51	5.9	17.1
52	6.0	17.4
53	6.1	17.7
54	6.2	18.0
55	6.3	18.3
56	6.4	18.6
57	6.6	19.1
58	6.7	19.4
59	6.8	19.7
60	6.9	20.1
61	7.0	20.3

NORMAL HEMATOCRITS	NORMAL RED BLOOD CELL COUNTS	NORMAL HEMOGLOBINS
Men: Range 40–54% Aver. 47%	Men: Range 4,600,000–6,200,000 Aver. 5,400,000	Men: Range 14.0–18.0 grams Aver. 15.8 grams
Women: Range 37–47% Aver. 42%	Women: Range 4,200,000–5,400,000 Aver. 4,800,000	Women: Range 11.5–16.0 grams Aver. 13.9 grams

*The relationship shown between hematocrit and red blood cell count is based on normal cells (which have an average mean corpuscular volume of 0.87). The relationship between hemoglobin and red blood cell count is based on normal cells (with a mean corpuscular hemoglobin of 29). These relationships do not hold true in cases of microcytic or macrocytic anemias, which probably will not be more than 5% to 10% of blood examined by clinical laboratories and blood banks.

the red blood cell count when hemoglobin and hematocrit (H & H) are known (Table 15–1). Hemoglobin is an **allosteric** protein found in erythrocytes, which transports molecular oxygen in the blood. Red blood cells carry oxygen to the tissues of the body and carry carbon dioxide back to the lungs where it is exhaled from the body. A most reliable and simple way to determine hemoglobin level is with the hemoglobinometer (Figures 15–13 and 15–14). The normal range of hemoglobin for males is 14 to 18 grams per 100 ml of blood, and for females, 12 to 16. Physicians may order an H & H to get a more definite idea of the patient's red blood cell volume. The hemoglobinometer shown in Figure 15–13 is considered to be a Moderately Complex test. Still on the list of Waived tests for hemoglobin readings is an electronic readout device. Check with the physician when reading the results of these tests. Refer to Procedure 15–5 for Hb determination using the hemoglobinometer.

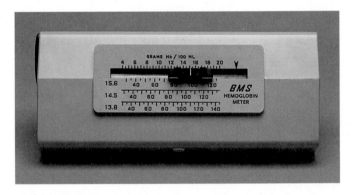

FIGURE 15–13 The hand-held hemoglobinometer is used in POCT.

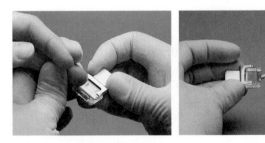

(A)

(B)

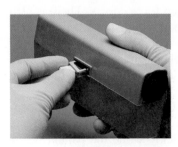

(C)

FIGURE 15–14 (A) Place capillary blood on glass chamber. (B) Mix (hemolyze) blood with hemolysis applicator (wooden stick). (C) Push chamber into the clip, and place into the slot in the side of the hemoglobinometer.

P R O C E D U R E

15-5 Hemoglobin (Hb) Determination Using the Hemoglobinometer

PURPOSE: Estimating the amount of Hb (iron-carrying protein) in the blood.

OSHA GUIDELINES: To comply with standard precautions, gloves must be worn if there is any possibility of coming into contact with blood or any body fluids.

EQUIPMENT: Hemoglobinometer, glass chamber slide, hemolysis applicator (plastic or wooden), Autolet or sterile lancet, cotton balls, alcohol, latex or vinyl gloves, gauze squares, Mayo table, batteries and light bulbs (as needed), patient's chart, pen.

PERFORMANCE OBJECTIVE: With all necessary equipment and supplies provided, and using other students as patients, demonstrate the steps required to perform a hemoglobin determination using the hemoglobinometer. The instructor will observe each step.

1. Assemble all needed items on Mayo table, check batteries and light bulb in hemoglobinometer, and change if needed.

2. Explain procedure to identified patient. **RATIONALE: Speaking to the patient by name and checking chart ensures that you are performing the procedure on the correct patient.**

3. Wash hands and put on latex or vinyl gloves. Follow the desired skin puncture technique (procedure in this unit).

4. Pull the glass chamber out of the side of the hemoglobinometer and fix the lower part of the slide so that it is slightly offset.

5. Place a large drop of blood directly onto the offset glass chamber surface from the patient's finger (or other puncture site) (Figure 15–14A). Wipe the patient's finger with a cotton ball, and give patient a dry gauze square to hold over the puncture site. **NOTE: Check to be sure bleeding has stopped.**

6. Mix the blood on the slide with the hemolysis applicator to break down the cell membranes to release the hemoglobin. **NOTE: This is seen when the appearance of the blood becomes clear from cloudy and will take up to 45 seconds (Figure 15–14B).**

7. Push the chamber into the clip and place into the slot on the left side of the hemoglobinometer (Figure 15–14C).

8. Hold the hemoglobinometer in your left hand at eye level while using your left thumb to turn on the light by depressing the button on the bottom of the instrument. Look into the instrument to see a split green field.

9. Slide the button on the right side of the meter with your right thumb and index finger while still looking into the meter until a matching solid green field occurs. Leave the sliding scale on the calibrated line where the solid green field appeared.

10. Read the hemoglobin level at the top calibration scale for which it is most frequently used (there are four on the scale). It is read in grams of hemoglobin per 100 mL of blood.

11. Wash chamber (and hemolysis applicator if reusable) with a detergent solution, rinse, dry, and return to the hemoglobinometer for the next use. Discard disposable items in proper receptacle, return items to proper storage area.

12. Remove gloves and wash hands. Place gloves in the proper receptacle.

13. Record the reading in the patient's chart, (e.g., 14.5 g/100mL, initial). Refer to charting example.

14. Record the results in the log book.

CHARTING EXAMPLE:

4-21-XX
Finger stick of Rt. ring finger for capillary blood for Hgb—reading is 14.7

S. Davis, RMA (DV)

LOG BOOK EXAMPLE:

DATE	PATIENT'S NAME	TEST	RESULTS	OBTAINED BY
5-21-XX	Melody C. Jones	Hgb	14.7	J. Watkins, CMA (DV)

BLOOD GLUCOSE SCREENING

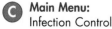

Main Menu:
Infection Control

Skills Menu:
■ Measuring Blood Glucose

Another capillary blood test performed in most medical practices today is the blood **glucose** screening. It is done with a drop of blood obtained from a skin puncture. A drop of blood is applied directly to a chemically-treated reagent strip. After timing (as directed by the manufacturer), the strip is blotted and read by comparing the color of the reagent strip with the color chart on the bottle. A more accurate reading may be obtained by reading the reacted reagent strip in a glucometer (Procedure 15–6). There are several types that can be used for reliable test-

PROCEDURE

15-6 Screen Blood Sugar (Glucose) Level

PURPOSE: To determine the sugar (glucose) level of the blood.

OSHA GUIDELINES: To comply with Standard Precautions, gloves must be worn if there is any possibility of coming into contact with blood or any body fluids.

EQUIPMENT: Sterile lancet, reagent strips, bottle (for color chart) glucometer, latex or vinyl gloves, cotton balls, alcohol, gauze squares, watch or clock, facial tissue.

PERFORMANCE OBJECTIVE: Provided with all necessary equipment and supplies, and using other students as patients, demonstrate the steps required in the procedure for determining blood glucose levels. The instructor will observe each step.

1. Assemble all needed items on Mayo table. **NOTE: If glucometer is to be used, make sure it has been turned on required time and has been calibrated for accuracy (follow manual of instruction).**

2. Identify patient and explain procedure. **RATIONALE: Speaking to the patient by name and checking chart ensures that you are performing the procedure on the correct patient. NOTE: If test is to be for a fasting blood sugar level, be certain patient has not had anything by mouth for the past 8 to 12 hours.**

3. Wash hands and put on latex or vinyl gloves. **NOTE: As you converse with the patient during his scheduled appointment, be sure to inquire about the medications (both prescription and OTC), any home remedy that has been taken, and his diet, and record all information on the patient's chart. Most diabetics are encouraged to keep a record (or diary) of one's daily routine of medicines, blood glucose readings, nutritional intake, and exercise, especially if one's condition has been unruly. Reporting this information to the physician is valuable in assessing the patient's condition and plan of treatment because there are substances that can affect the accuracy of the readings of some blood glucose monitors.**

4. Follow desired skin puncture procedure.

5. Open reagent strip bottle and take one of plastic strips out without touching chemically treated pads. **RATIONALE:**

Heat and moisture from skin may alter results. Reclose bottle.

6. Apply large drop of blood from patient's finger so that pad is completely covered.

7. Begin timing *immediately* (**stat**) for *exactly* the amount of time specified by the manufacturer. Give patient dry gauze square to hold over puncture site after wiping it with alcohol-saturated cotton ball.

8. After the specified time, immediately blot pad firmly and quickly. **NOTE: Follow manufacturer's instruction precisely for timing and blotting.**

9. Immediately place the reagent strip into glucometer and close the door. **NOTE: Color begins to fade after a few seconds. Delay may cause inaccurate reading of results.** The number displayed is the blood glucose level (Figure 15–15).

10. Discard all used items in proper receptacle, remove gloves, and wash hands. You should perform a capillary puncture for a glucose reagent strip from an FBS (fasting blood sugar) sample. (You may use whole blood from a red or lavender top tube but not from a gray top tube.)

11. Record in patient's chart (e.g., 98 mg/100 mL of blood, initial). Refer to charting example.

12. Record in the log book the lot number and the expiration date of the reagent test strips.

CHARTING EXAMPLE:
6-12-XX
Finger stick of L great finger for capillary blood for FBS—reading is 98 mg/100ml of blood.

S. Davis, RMA (DV)

LOG BOOK EXAMPLE:

DATE	PATIENT'S NAME	TEST	RESULTS	OBTAINED BY
6-12-XX	Mark J. Stanford	FBS	98 mg/100ml	S. Davis, RMA (DV)

glucose reagent strips Lot #875913-42 Exp 9/30/XX

ing. Unless the machine has an automatic calibration mechanism incorporated within it, you should calibrate the glucose meter and follow directions for use according to the manufacturer's specifications. A known quality control specimen should be run daily and recorded in the laboratory test log. The operation manual and directions should be kept near the instrument for reference. For management of glucose monitoring there is a system called Precision Link (Figure 15–16). This convenient hand-held monitor is easily used by the patient at home.

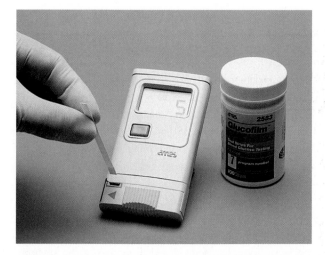

FIGURE 15-15   Insert reagent strip into glucometer with the color pad toward the screen, and read glucose level after hearing the beep at 22 seconds (here five seconds are left before the glucose reading appears on the screen).

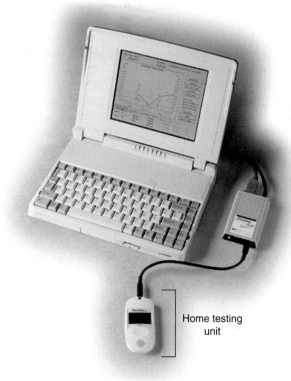

Home testing unit

FIGURE 15-16   The Precision Link Blood Glucose Data Management System provides the patient with a simple glucose meter that stores up to 125 readings. At the patient's next office visit, it is attached to the computer for a graph of those results to be displayed on the monitor. (Courtesy Abbott Diagnostics.)

The monitor is brought in by the patient for the health care provider to link it to the computer for a display of the last 125 glucose readings for a comprehensive look at the effectiveness of treatment.

There are various convenient home testing devices on the market. One type of glucose monitoring device uses a minute blood sample obtained from the top of the forearm to check blood glucose levels. This is especially convenient, particularly with children, for those who must test several times a day to manage their diabetes. The slight minimal discomfort using this product rather than a finger stick is a far better experience for both adults and children.

The normal fasting blood glucose range is from 70 to 126 mg/100 dl blood. The term *fasting* means that the patient has had nothing to eat or drink for a specific period of time, usually for 8 to 12 hours prior to the test. Fasting means that the patient should not even chew gum, eat mints, smoke, or drink water (a sip is ok). Any stimulation of the digestive system may alter the results of the scheduled laboratory test.

A recent finding in older adult patients with diabetes is that a high percentage of them did not have adequate cholesterol screening, regular eye examinations, or testing for glycohemoglobin. **Glycohemoglobin** is a modified form of hemoglobin that is elevated when blood glucose is high. A simple finger stick blood test helps determine how well the diabetes patient's glucose level has been during the last two or three months or so (this is often the amount of time since the last office visit). Even though diabetic patients generally check their blood sugar levels at home daily (type I generally twice a day and type II as their physician recommends) and bring in their readings, this additional diagnostic test can be of help in monitoring the patient's condition. Hemoglobin A1c is the

stable molecule that is formed when sugar and hemoglobin bond together. This process is called **glycosylation**. Hemoglobin is the oxygen-carrying protein found in red blood cells. Glycohemoglobin, or GHBA1c, testing should be performed on type II diabetics every six months, and for those with type I diabetes, at least every three months.

During triage and assessment portions of the patient's office visit, the physician may order a fasting blood sugar (FBS) after determining an abnormal GHB level. Physicians may use this diagnostic aid during routine office visits to assess the control of the diabetic patient. It is also of value in checking the accuracy of the existing diagnostic testing methods.

The medical assistant can be a great influence in the care of the patient with diabetes by reminding them periodically of the need for regular eye examinations and encouraging them to pay special attention to their nutritional needs. Remind them also of the importance of keeping their **cholesterol** level within normal ranges as much as possible. Usually, the physician will order a lipid profile that includes **triglycerides**, the "good" cholesterol (**high density lipoproteins [HDL]**) and the "bad" cholesterol (**low density lipoproteins [LDL]**) to periodically monitor this. Patients who have high levels of triglycerides and cholesterol should be encouraged to stay on the diet that the doctor has recommended for them and exercise regularly according to their capability. There are patients who have elevated levels of cholesterol even when they follow doctor's orders. Those patients may have a hereditary tendency toward high cholesterol levels. These are the patients who are prescribed medication to bring the cholesterol levels down to a safe range. Those patients who require medication for treatment of hyperlipoproteinemia must have more frequent testing to monitor their condition.

GTT—GLUCOSE TOLERANCE TEST

The standard glucose **tolerance** test (GTT) determines a patient's ability to metabolize **carbohydrates**. This test is used primarily to aid in the diagnosis of diabetes mellitus and hypoglycemia. Usually, the patient is advised to eat a high-carbohydrate diet for three days before the scheduled GTT. The night before the procedure, the patient is required to have nothing to eat or drink from midnight on, or to fast for 8 to 12 hours before the test begins. A small amount of water is generally permitted; however, you should check with the physician before instructing the patient to ingest anything.

Fasting samples of blood and urine are obtained from the patient to begin this procedure. (Note: If the patient's FBS is 150 mg/dl or higher, inform the physician and DO NOT administer glucola to the patient. Higher than 150 mg/dl of glucose is diagnostic of diabetes mellitus [DM], and giving glucola could be harmful to the patient.) Then, the patient is given glucose (commercial preparation) orally. The ordered amount will vary with the age of the patient. A half hour after the patient has consumed the glucose drink, samples of blood and urine are taken. Every hour thereafter, both blood and urine samples are taken for up to six hours, or for whatever period the physician has ordered. Because accuracy is critically important in this test, timing and precise readings of the tests are vital in assessing glucose metabolism.

A GTT is performed routinely most often at six months into pregnancy to check for **gestational** diabetes. This test may be ordered at any time during pregnancy if there are symptoms that are associated with diabetes, such as extreme thirst, visual difficulties, fatigue, weight loss, dehydration, and, of course, an abnormally high glucose reading. Women who have miscarried or have delivered large babies at birth seem to be most at risk for having gestational diabetes. If the patient is a known diabetic, regular home glucose tests should be done. Frequent office exams and glucose testing to monitor the patient's condition are required to prevent complications that can occur during pregnancy.

With today's highly skilled laboratory technicians, you will probably do few blood tests in the medical office.

Some offices have their own labs in which laboratory technicians are employed to carry out tests that the medical assistant is not trained to do or is not licensed to do by law. The blood screening tests already mentioned are simple and require a minimal amount of instruction to perform. Proficiency in performing these minor tests will come with practice.

BLOOD CELL COUNT

Be sure to determine if it is lawful and within laboratory governing regulations before performing *any* diagnostic laboratory tests. Many of these tests must be performed only by licensed clinical laboratory technicians. These regulations have been made for quality assurance purposes. When the physician wants to know a patient's red or white blood cell count immediately to aid in diagnosis, blood cell counts can be performed in the office for convenience to the physician and the patient. Medical offices or clinics may have mechanical/automated devices specifically designed to perform blood cell counts, such as the hematology analyzer shown in Figure 15–19. In-service training should be provided by your employer.

Red Blood Cells A red blood cell (erythrocyte) count is ordered when symptoms indicate possible anemia. Automated cell counting equipment in the POL make it simple to quickly produce results, which leads to faster diagnosis and treatment of the patient. Performing diagnostic

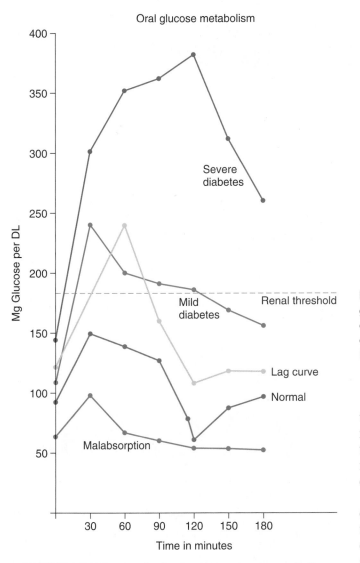

FIGURE 15–17   Graph of a three-hour glucose metabolism

DATE	PATIENT		ADDRESS	
GLUCOSE TOLERANCE TEST			HOURS	
TIME	BLOOD SUGAR	URINE SUGAR	ACETONE	PATIENT'S CONDITION (SYMPTOMS)
FASTING	mg/100ml			
1/2 HR	mg/100ml			
1 HR	mg/100ml			
2 HR	mg/100ml			
3 HR	mg/100ml			
4 HR	mg/100ml			
5 HR	mg/100ml			
6 HR	mg/100ml			
PHYSICIAN		PHONE	TECHNOLOGIST	

FIGURE 15–18   Laboratory report form for GTT (glucose tolerance test)

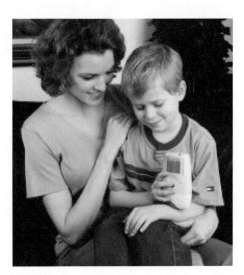

FIGURE 15–19   The child in this picture is using the Sof-Tact glucometer to obtain a blood glucose sample from his arm. This device does both a skin puncture and a read-out of the blood glucose results from a non-traditional test site. (Courtesy of Abbott Laboratories.)

tests simply and quickly for physicians to treat patients is referred to as point-of-care testing (POCT). A decrease in the number of RBCs constitutes a form of anemia. The normal RBC count range for males is 4 to 6 million per cubic millimeter of blood, and for females, 4 to 5 million.

The function of the RBC is to transport oxygen to and carry carbon dioxide from the cells. It also contributes to the acid–base balance of the blood. If there is an insufficient number of RBCs in the bloodstream, the patient's symptoms will be lack of energy, fatigue, and, in severe cases, shortness of breath (SOB), pounding of the heart, rapid pulse, and **pallor**.

The iron-carrying protein, hemoglobin, gives the RBC its color. Erythrocytes have a biconcave disk shape and no nucleus when mature. They are formed in the red bone marrow of adults (**erythropoiesis**) and in the liver, spleen, and bone marrow of the fetus. The average life span of the RBC is about 120 days. The **reticuloendothelial** system, mostly the liver, bone marrow, and spleen, removes the worn-out red blood cells from the circulatory system.

White Blood Cells

A white blood cell (leukocyte) count is done when symptoms indicate possible infection in the body. An increase in WBCs (white blood cells) signifies that the process of **phagocytosis** (WBCs combating infection by engulfing microorganisms or other foreign particles or cells and forming pus) is taking place. The normal leukocyte count for males and females is from 5 to 10 thousand per cubic millimeter of blood. Leukocytes are formed in the bone marrow, lymph

TABLE 15-2

CATEGORIES OF WHITE BLOOD CELLS AND THEIR FUNCTIONS

White Cell Type	Percent in Normal WBC	Function
Granulocytes:		
Neutrophils		Phagocytosis and killing of bacteria; release of pyrogen that produces fever
Segmented	56 ± 10	
Band	3 ± 2	
Eosinophils	2.7 ± 2	Phagocytosis of antigen-antibody complexes; killing of parasites
Basophils	0.3 ± 1	Release of chemical mediators of immediate hypersensitivity
Lymphocytes:	34 ± 10	
B lymphocytes		Humoral immunity; production of specific antibodies against viruses, bacteria, and other proteins
T lymphocytes		Cell-mediated immunity including delayed hypersensitivity and graft rejection; regulation of immune response
Monocytes	4 ± 3	Phagocytosis of microorganisms and cell debris; cooperation in immune response

nodes, spleen, and the lining of various visceral organs. The chief function of the WBCs is to aid in the body's defense against disease. Because all manual blood counts are no longer performed in medical facilities, several automated cell counting devices have become both practical and necessary in POCT management of patients. Point-of-care testing is simply those lab tests that can be performed for the patient at the medical facility. A blood cell analyzer provides quick and easy complete blood cell counts with a minimal amount of whole blood. Even if it is difficult to draw blood from patients (especially pediatric patients), an automated method makes testing easier and efficient.

Differential Count

One of the most vital tests generally performed with the complete blood count (CBC) is the **differential** count. This count determines the number and percentage of each of the five different types of white blood cells (leukocytes). Each has a specific function as outlined in Table 15–2. Preferably, the differential count is made from a fresh whole blood specimen. This blood smear is usually sent to a clinical or hospital laboratory where it is stained by a skilled certified laboratory technician who also determines the estimated platelet count. The **morphology** (which refers to the study of the size and shape of cells, especially during their development) of the erythrocytes is also noted during this microscopic examination. Figure 15–20 is a drawing of normal blood cells.

Most laboratories provide an apparatus for slide preparation of blood smears (which can be demonstrated at your request). A blood smear can be obtained from capillary or venous blood by placing a small drop of blood on

A CAAHEP CONNECTION

In this unit, instruction in basic laboratory procedures and specimen collection is discussed. The areas included in the Medical Assistant curriculum are **Medical terminology, Communication, Clinical procedures**, and **Medical law and ethics.**

a glass slide (frosted side up) and labeling it with pencil. A second glass slide is used to distribute the blood cells evenly over three-fourths of the slide, ending in a feathered tip. Practice is necessary in developing skill and proficiency in making good blood smears.

The procedure for making a blood smear for the purpose of a differential count includes directions regarding methods of obtaining blood specimens. See Procedure 15–7.

All medical staff who are involved with POCT must be aware of safety and standard precautions with laboratory procedures. Keeping good records of tests and quality assurance and quality control procedures are essential in having an efficient and competent physician office laboratory.

ACHIEVE UNIT OBJECTIVES

Complete Chapter 15, Unit 2, in the workbook to help you obtain competency of this subject matter.

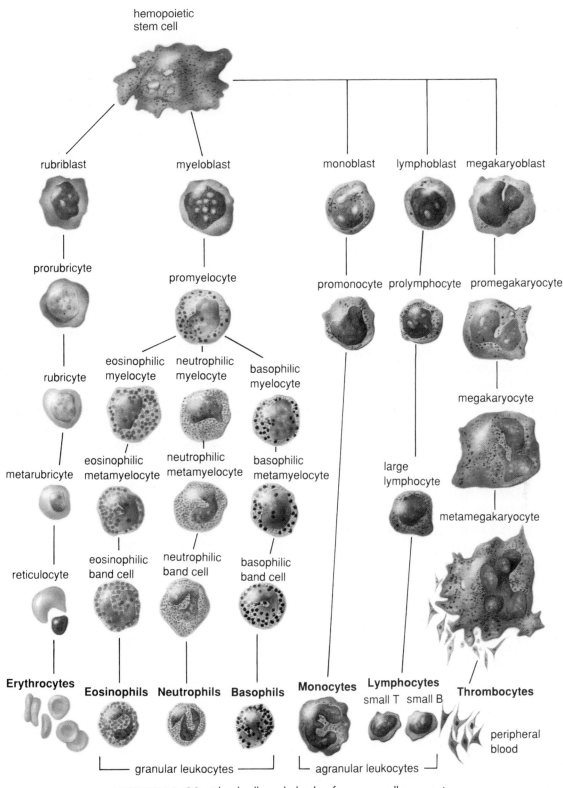

FIGURE 15–20   Blood cells and platelets from stem cell to maturity

PROCEDURE

15-7 Making a Blood Smear

PURPOSE: To make an adequate blood smear for a *differential* white blood cell count.

OSHA GUIDELINES: To comply with Standard Precautions, gloves must be worn if there is any possibility of coming into contact with blood or any body fluids.

EQUIPMENT: Latex or vinyl gloves, sterile lancet (or skin puncture device with sterile lancet) or CBC (lavender top) blood collection tube with needle adapter attached, or needle and syringe (for venipuncture procedure), alcohol, cotton balls or gauze squares, fresh clean glass slides with frosted ends, pencil, pen, laboratory request form, patient's chart, sharps container.

PERFORMANCE OBJECTIVE: Provided with all necessary equipment and supplies, demonstrate the steps required to make an adequate blood smear for a differential white blood cell count. The instructor will observe and check each step.

1. Explain procedure to identified patient. Complete laboratory request form. Print patient's name and date on the frosted end of the glass slide with the pencil. This appropriately identifies slide in case multiple slides are in the laboratory area.

2. Assemble all needed items on Mayo table near patient.

3. Wash hands and put on latex or vinyl gloves.

4. Perform desired method for obtaining blood specimen (either capillary or venous blood may be used).

5. Place a small drop of blood approximately one-fourth inch from the frosted end of the glass slide (the drop of blood should be approximately one-eighth inch in diameter) (Figure 15–21).
   NOTE:
   - If blood is obtained from the patient's finger, touch the drop of blood carefully to the slide (do not press the blood onto the slide or smudging will occur).
   - If the blood is obtained by needle and syringe, depress plunger to allow a drop of blood to fall onto the end of the glass slide.
   - If the blood is obtained from the needle and adapter, press in on the CBC blood tube attached (within the adapter) to allow a drop of blood to fall onto the glass slide.

6. a. Hold the corners of the frosted end of the glass slide down on a flat surface with the thumb and index finger of one hand, and with the other hand hold the second glass slide with the thumb and index (or great) finger at a 45° angle. **NOTE: If smear is too thick, the angle of spreading should be decreased; if too thin, increased.**

   b. Rest the spreader slide against the first one, and move it back carefully into the drop of blood. The blood will follow the edge of the slide evenly across the glass.

   c. Move the angled slide toward the frosted end quickly and gently (pressure will hemolyze blood cells). (The second glass slide is used to evenly spread the blood over the first slide, thereby distributing the blood cells for the differential white blood cell count. Or a blood smear can be made in the same way, only the spreader slide can be turned lengthwise and placed at the edge of the frosted area of the slide and backed into the blood to spread to the end of the slide making a feathered tip. It usually takes a considerable amount of practice to make a good blood smear for a differential count. Use the method that works best for you.) **NOTE: The smear should have a feather-edge.** This is the area of the blood smear where the technician examines the cells. If the slide has been prepared properly, the red blood cells will be in an even monolayer, and the white blood cells will be evenly distributed. It should not be too thick or cells are overly crowded, making counting difficult; if too thin, it results in an inadequate number of cells to count.

7. Allow the blood smear to air dry, or *carefully* fan it in the air to expedite drying. **RATIONALE: Quickly drying helps cells maintain their shape and size. Note: Avoid blowing on the smear to dry. It may disturb the cells.**

8. Place blood smear into appropriate container (attach completed lab request form) for transport to laboratory. Generally, the slide will accompany a CBC request with a lavender top blood-filled tube.

9. Remove latex or vinyl gloves and wash hands. Discard all waste in appropriate containers.

10. Initial procedure on patient's chart.

CHARTING EXAMPLE:

4-11-XX

Two blood smears made for differential count and packaged for lab pick-up.

S. Davis, RMA (DV)

NOTE: Because there are insurance companies that require health care team members to sign after each order is performed as "S. Davis," the physician checks off the chart by writing his initials in parentheses to indicate that orders were completed as directed: (DV).

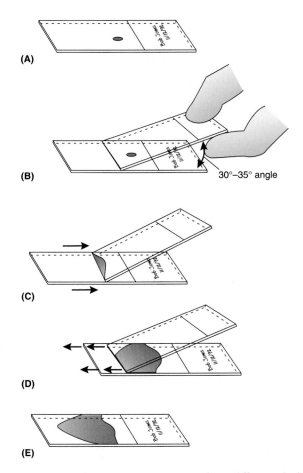

(A)

(B) 30°–35° angle

(C)

(D)

(E)

FIGURE 15–21 Making a blood smear for a differential white blood cell count

UNIT 3

Venous Blood Tests

OBJECTIVES

Upon completion of the unit, meet the following performance objectives by verifying knowledge of the facts and principles presented through oral and written communication at a level deemed competent. Demonstrate the specific behaviors as identified in the performance objectives of the procedures, observing all aseptic and safety precautions in accordance with health care standards.

1. Spell and define, using the glossary at the back of the text, all the Words to Know in this unit.
2. Prepare blood specimens to be sent to a reference laboratory.
3. Perform a venipuncture by the sterile needle and syringe method and the vacuum method.
4. Explain how to obtain serum from whole blood.
5. Determine an erythrocyte sedimentation rate (ESR).
6. List the different colors used to code blood specimen tubes and what they stand for.

WORDS TO KNOW

elasticity
gauge
hematoma
hemolysis
heparin
meniscus
oxygenate

prothrombin
sedimentation
tourniquet
venipuncture
venous

AREAS OF COMPETENCE (AAMA)

This unit addresses content within the specific competency areas of *Fundamental principles, Diagnostic orders, Patient care, Professionalism, Communication skills, Instruction,* and *Operational functions,* as identified in the Medical Assistant Role Delineation Study. Refer to Appendix A for a detailed listing of the areas.

Venous means pertaining to the veins. As veins return blood to the heart and lungs to be **oxygenated** and recirculated, they carry the waste products of the body. Venous blood tests permit measurement of the kind and amount of those waste products.

VENIPUNCTURE

When more than a few drops of blood are required to perform tests, a venipuncture is performed. **Venipuncture** is the surgical puncture of a vein.

Usually, the patient is seated in a chair with the arm supported for the venipuncture procedure. In the event that a patient faints from this position, first remove the **tourniquet**, withdraw the needle, and hold a bandage over the puncture site. Then the patient must be helped carefully to the floor. Spirits of ammonia may be used to help revive the patient. The physician should check the

PATIENT EDUCATION

Explaining the procedure and making the patient comfortable is of great importance. If the patient shows any signs of apprehension, ask the patient to lie down and try to relax. This eliminates the possibility of a patient falling as the result of fainting during the procedure. Some patients experience a queasy (nauseated) feeling, so it is a good idea to keep an emesis basin nearby. Displaying competency and efficiency in carrying out the procedure will gain the patient's confidence and cooperation.

patient before you proceed further. Patients who say they feel faint should put their head down between their knees. Usually this will help within a few minutes, and the procedure can be accomplished with no further interruptions. Often, following a complete physical examination, the patient may still be lying on the examination table. This makes an ideal work area for the medical assistant, and the position for the patient is most comfortable. In case the patient feels faint, there is no worry of accidental falling when the patient is lying down. The law regarding who performs venipuncture varies from state to state. Usually the physician is aware of it and will not ask you to perform the procedure unless it is lawful.

The area of choice for venipuncture is most often the inner arm at the bend of the elbow (Figure 15–22). The veins in this area are the median basilic and the median cephalic (commonly referred to as antecubital veins). A means of promoting better palpation and sometimes visual position of the veins is a tourniquet. Tourniquets are available in many materials. Soft, flat vinyl/rubber tubing is probably most popular and economical. Some medical facilities use a tourniquet only once and then discard it with the gloves they remove after drawing blood samples. It comes in widths of one to two inches and can be cut into any length desired, usually from 12 to 16 inches. Thinner vinyl or rubber tubing is also popular, but it tends to pinch the skin. If the hair on the patient's arm is especially thick, it may be wise to apply the tourniquet over the patient's sleeve, or you can place a thin towel around the arm and apply the tourniquet over the cloth. This will keep the tourniquet from pinching and pulling the hair, and the patient will most likely be more cooperative with your thoughtfulness. Tubing is easily washed with a detergent solution and quickly cleaned with alcohol and a cotton ball. Velcro tourniquets are cloth strips, approximately one and one half to two inches wide. They are not so easily cleaned and are not elasticized, so they cannot be used on patients with larger than average arms. Wiping them off

with alcohol will help prevent most of the staining problems. In very difficult to draw patients, you may try using a blood pressure cuff as a tourniquet. Be careful not to inflate it too tightly on the patient's arm or you may cut off the circulation completely and cause unnecessary discomfort to the patient. Be sure that the cuff size is appropriate for the size of the arm. Care also must be taken to avoid getting blood on the cuff. It must be discarded (or sanitized and sterilized before reuse) if it does become contaminated. Tourniquets that are very worn or permanently visibly soiled (even after washing) should be discarded.

The tourniquet is placed on the patient's upper arm, about three to four inches above the elbow. Before applying the tourniquet, it is a good idea to check both arms of the patient or simply ask which arm is better for this procedure. Many patients have had the procedure performed and know that one arm is better. Some patients will have a preferred arm because of their work or planned activities. Some patients are extremely difficult to obtain blood from. It may be necessary in these cases to draw the sample from a vein on the back of the hand using a smaller gauge needle. These veins are small and the procedure is painful. The tourniquet should be applied just above the wrist in this case. A method that may be used in this type of situation is called the "butterfly" needle method (Figure 15–23). A skilled phlebotomist can perform this procedure successfully alone; however, this procedure is commonly performed with two persons as a team effort. One performs the actual venipuncture while the other pulls back on the plunger and changes tubes as necessary. Refer to Procedure 15–8. Venipuncture must always be done carefully to

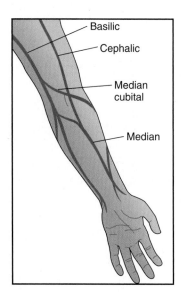

Basilic

Cephalic

Median cubital

Median

FIGURE 15–22 The veins of the arm. The median cephalic vein is the most often used for venipuncture.

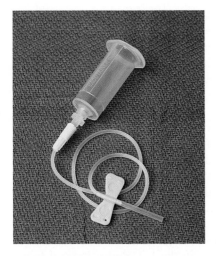

FIGURE 15–23 Butterfly needle assembly

avoid causing a **hematoma** (collection of blood just under the skin). When the needle is inserted into the vein it punctures the wall of the vein and blood can then leak out into surrounding tissues. This bleeding causes discoloration and sometimes swelling. If the vein has been punctured from the needle going completely through the vein (in one side and out the other) then the chances of a hematoma are even greater. Consult with the physician about applying ice, which can be helpful in reducing discomfort and swelling. Gentle pressure applied immediately on withdrawing the needle will help avoid this problem.

Use a cotton ball saturated with alcohol to swab the entire area. The alcohol will help make the skin more sensitive to your touch. Slowly move your fingertip across the patient's arm at the bend of the elbow. Veins

---

PROCEDURE

15-8 Obtain Venous Blood with Butterfly Needle Method

PURPOSE: To obtain venous blood specimen(s) of infants, children, or of patients with veins that are difficult to draw (veins are not easily seen or felt). Suggested sites to obtain blood are antecubital or lower arm, and the back of the hand.

OSHA GUIDELINES: To comply with Standard Precautions, gloves must be worn if there is any possibility of coming into contact with blood or any body fluids.

EQUIPMENT: Sterile butterfly needle (22G), syringe (or vacuum tubes and needle adaptor), appropriate specimen tube(s), pen, patient's chart, lab request form, spirits of ammonia, emesis basin, tourniquet, latex or vinyl gloves, alcohol prep, cotton balls or gauze squares, bandage, Mayo tray table, biohazard sharp's container.

PERFORMANCE OBJECTIVE: Provided with all necessary equipment, and using a training model, demonstrate the steps necessary for obtaining blood specimen(s) using the butterfly method. The student must achieve a satisfactory score on the evaluation checklist. (Often, this procedure is performed by two persons: one can insert the needle, and the other can pull back on the plunger of the syringe or change vacuum tubes using the adaptor as the other person secures the needle.)

1. Wash hands.
2. Identify the patient, and complete the appropriate lab request form.
3. Assemble all necessary equipment on Mayo tray table next to the patient.
4. Securely attach the butterfly needle to the syringe.
5. Put gloves on.
6. Palpate vein and clean venipuncture site of arm/hand with alcohol prep, and dry with cotton/gauze.
7. Apply tourniquet approximately three inches above the needle insertion site.
8. Ask patient to make a fist and hold it until you say to release it.
9. Remove needle guard and quickly insert the butterfly needle into the vein.
10. Push any air out of syringe before using to draw blood specimen.
11. Pull back on the plunger of the syringe slowly until adequate amount of blood is obtained, and then ask patient to release fist. (Fill appropriate vacuum tube[s] without forcing it to prevent hemolysis stat and to avoid clotting, keeping in mind the correct order of draw.)
12. Release tourniquet and withdraw needle quickly.
13. Apply gentle pressure over site with cotton or gauze, and ask patient to hold arm slightly up for a few minutes to help prevent a hematoma.
14. Attend to patient and apply bandage to site. **NOTE: Ask if patient has an allergy to adhesive.**
15. Place the used needle and all other contaminated supplies in biohazard sharps container or bag.
16. Place specimens in appropriate lab transport container.
17. Remove gloves and discard in biohazard container or bag.
18. Wash hands.
19. Record procedure on patient's chart and initial.

have **elasticity** and will give somewhat when depressed. Feeling the subtle spring-back movement will help you find a suitable vein for the procedure. You should ask the patient to clench the fist only if the vein does not stand out. This pressure of the clenched fist may interfere with some chemistry tests. A few gentle slaps to the antecubital area with two of your fingers will also help the vein stand out for better view and access. Another method to encourage blood flow in difficult draw patients is to place a warm compress on the antecubital area for a few minutes before you begin the procedure. This will help make the veins stand out to the touch if not to the sight.

There are two methods of performing this procedure: (1) the syringe/sterile needle method (refer to Procedure 15–9), and (2) the vacuum tube/sterile needle method (refer to Procedure 15–10). Sterile technique must be used because a foreign object is introduced directly into the vein.

A 19-23 **gauge** needle is generally used. The gauge must be large enough to allow blood to flow through the needle without causing **hemolysis** (breakdown of blood cells).

The needle and syringe method is always used when very small veins are involved because it is less damaging to the tissues than the vacuum method (Figure 15–24). The size of the syringe will vary according to the amount of blood needed. Usually a 10- to 20-cc syringe is used when drawing several tubes, each 5 to 15 mL.

The vacuum method is probably the most popular because it is so convenient. Blood specimens enter directly into the tubes for the desired tests rather than having to be transferred. It is vital that the correct tubes be used, however.

Specimen test tubes are color coded for the various hematology departments in the lab. Red-stopped tubes come in sizes ranging from 3 to 15 mL. They are used to

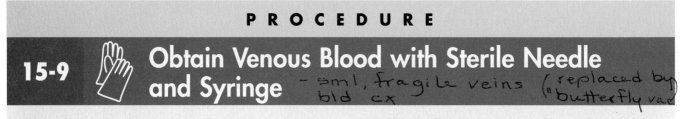

PROCEDURE

15-9   Obtain Venous Blood with Sterile Needle and Syringe

[handwritten annotation: – sml, fragile veins (replaced by "butterfly vac bld cx]

PURPOSE: To obtain venous blood specimens when the amount needed is more than a few drops.

OSHA GUIDELINES: To comply with Standard Precautions, gloves must be worn if there is any possibility of coming into contact with blood or any body fluids.

EQUIPMENT: Sterile needle (19–23 G, one to one and one-half inch in length) 10–20 cc syringe for specimen tubes, laboratory specimen packaging materials, pen, patient's chart, alcohol, latex or vinyl gloves, cotton balls, tourniquet, lab request form (labeled appropriately with the vacuum blood specimen tubes that were ordered), gauze squares, adhesive bandage, spirits of ammonia, emesis basin, biohazardous waste container (should be within reach), and sharps container.

    NOTE: A utility bucket is a convenient way to carry all necessary items for venipuncture procedures. It should be stocked with lab request forms, specimen tubes, cotton balls, alcohol dispenser, syringes, sterile needles, sharps container, latex or vinyl gloves, tourniquet, frosted-end slides, adapter for vacuum tube method, pen and pencil, gauze squares, spirits of ammonia, and bandages. This handy carrier may be set next to the patient. It should be restocked daily during routine checking of supplies.

PERFORMANCE OBJECTIVE: Provided with all necessary equipment and supplies and using a training arm model, demonstrate the steps necessary for obtaining venous blood using the sterile needle and syringe method. The instructor will observe each step. **NOTE: The instructor will determine the student's skill in the per-**

formance of this procedure on other students as patients. Use the picture guide in Figure 15–24 to help you with this procedure.

1. Identify the patient. **RATIONALE: Speaking to the patient by name and checking chart ensures that you are performing the procedure on the correct patient.**

2. Wash hands and put on latex or vinyl gloves. Assemble all needed items on Mayo table next to patient. **NOTE: Label all required specimen tubes and complete lab request form.**

3. Explain procedure to patient, and ask if there is a preferred venipuncture site. If patient has no preference, visually check both arms and select a vein which can be palpated (felt) easily with your fingertip after application of alcohol. Ask a patient who is eating or chewing gum to remove the contents from his mouth before you begin to eliminate any possibility of the patient's choking in the event that he faints or becomes ill during the procedure. **NOTE: Ask patient to lie down if there is any sign of apprehension. Most often, patient will be sitting down with arm extended and supported on arm rest of chair or on a table. Providing a comfortable position will relax the patient and elicit better cooperation.**

4. Secure needle onto syringe by holding needle guard in one hand and turning syringe barrel clockwise. Push in plunger of syringe all the way to release any air from barrel. It is a good practice to pull back one-half to one-third of the way and then forward to push out all of the air. This makes it easier to start pulling back once you are in the vein. It is also less traumatic to the patient.

(Continues)

PROCEDURE

15-9 Obtain Venous Blood with Sterile Needle and Syringe (continued)

5. Apply tourniquet to patient's upper arm, about three inches above bend in elbow. **RATIONALE: The tourniquet slows down blood flow, increasing volume within the vein and thereby aiding palpation and visualization of the blood vessel.**
   a. Bring ends of tourniquet up evenly and cross them.
   b. Switch, so that you are holding an end in each hand comfortably.
   c. Stretch end in your right hand to apply gentle pressure over area of arm while you hold other end against patient's arm.
   d. Tuck any excess of stretched end under section that is held against arm so that there is nothing in way of puncture site. **NOTE: Proceed quickly, as tourniquet should not be left on longer than one minute. If tourniquet is applied too tightly, it will prevent blood flow and patient will be most uncomfortable.**

6. Clean site lightly with alcohol-saturated cotton ball, and let it air dry. **RATIONALE: Blowing on site to dry it will contaminate tissue.** You should ask the patient to clench the fist only if the vein does not stand out. This pressure of the clenched fist may interfere with some chemistry tests. A few gentle slaps to the antecubital area with two of your fingers will also help the vein stand out for better view and access. Another method to encourage blood flow in difficult draw patients is to place a warm compress on the antecubital area for a few minutes before you begin the procedure. **RATIONALE: This will assist further in making vein stand up.** Take off needle guard and, with the bevel of needle up, insert needle tip into vein with a quick and steady motion, following path of vein at approximately 15° angle. **NOTE: Holding skin at site to stretch it slightly will help keep vein from moving as puncture takes place. Needle should be inserted no more than one-fourth to one-half inch, or it may pass through the vein. RATIONALE: This helps maintain position of vein.**

7. Hold barrel of syringe in one hand and with other hand pull plunger back slowly and steadily until barrel is filled with amount of blood needed to fill specimen tubes. As you observe blood flow into the syringe, ask the patient to slowly open the fist, and then release the tourniquet. Release tourniquet by quickly pulling up on end of portion which is tucked in.

8. Pull needle out in same path as it was inserted and place gauze square over site as needle is withdrawn. **NOTE: Have patient apply gentle pressure and slightly elevate arm.**

9. Blood tubes that are to be filled from the syringe should be placed in a secure holder. Quickly fill required specimen tubes by inserting needle into rubber-stoppered end. Gently push plunger of syringe to fill. Angle the needle toward the top of the tube so that blood runs down the side to prevent hemolysis. **RATIONALE: Forcing blood into tubes will cause hemolysis. Vacuum tubes fill easily because vacuum draws in blood. NOTE: Specimen tubes must be filled quickly, for clotting will begin within minutes in the syringe and needle.** Fill tubes with blood from syringe into blood culture tubes in the following order: red, blue, green, lavender, and gray. **RATIONALE: Blood in syringe contains no anticoagulant.** Blood smears should be made at this time if needed. **NOTE: Before filling the tubes containing powdered additives, you should tap the tube(s) gently to allow any of the contents that may have collected around the top to fall to the bottom of the tube. Check with the laboratory manual regarding the required amount of blood for test(s) ordered by the physician that contain additives. Test results may be false or inaccurate if there is a ratio imbalance of blood and additive.**

10. Stand red-stoppered tubes vertically to clot so that serum can be drawn after centrifugation. **NOTE: Do not shake blood or hemolysis will occur.** In tubes that contain an anticoagulant, use a figure eight motion to gently mix the blood.

11. Deposit needle and syringe intact in sharps biohazardous waste container. DO NOT RECAP the needle. Wrap labeled specimen tubes together with lab request form and secure with rubber band. **NOTE: Keep near centrifuge so that serum-only transfer tube(s) may be added when completed.** The completed lab request form is usually placed in one side of the lab-provided biobag and the specimens in the other protected (sealed and leak-proof) side to be sent to a reference lab for analysis.

12. Attend to patient's needs; apply bandage over puncture site.

13. Discard disposables in proper receptacle. Remove gloves, wash hands, and return items to proper storage area.

14. Record procedure in log book and on patient's chart and initial. Refer to charting example.

LOG BOOK EXAMPLE:

DATE	PATIENT'S NAME	NUMBER	TEST	SENT	RESULTS	FILED BY
4-18-XX	Bernie L. Mitchell BD 7-18-61	7843	CBC	4-18-XX		

CHARTING EXAMPLE:

5-30-XX
One CBC tube drawn from Mr. Mitchell's L arm: packaged for reference lab pick-up.

J. Watkins, CMA (CL)

PROCEDURE

15-10 Obtain Venous Blood with Vacuum Tube

PURPOSE: To obtain venous blood specimens when the amount needed is more than a few drops.

OSHA GUIDELINES: To comply with Standard Precautions, gloves must be worn if there is any possibility of coming into contact with blood or any body fluids.

EQUIPMENT: Multiple sample sterile needles (19–23 G, one to one and one-half inch length), plastic adapter (a shielded blood needle adapter is recommended for safety), labeled specimen tubes (vacuum), alcohol, latex or vinyl gloves, sharps container, cotton balls, gauze squares, tourniquet, lab request forms, pen, patient's chart, bandages, biohazardous waste container, and laboratory specimen packaging material.

PERFORMANCE OBJECTIVE: Provided with all necessary equipment and supplies and using a training arm model, demonstrate the steps necessary for obtaining venous blood using the vacuum tube method. The instructor will observe each step. **NOTE: The instructor will determine the student's skill in the performance of this procedure on other students as patients.**

1. Identify the patient.
2. Wash hands and assemble all needed items on Mayo table next to the patient. **Note: Label all required specimen tubes and complete lab request form before gloving. Put on latex or vinyl gloves.**
3. Secure needle onto adapter by screwing grooved end of needle into grooved tip of adapter, holding needle guard and turning adapter in clockwise motion. Set aside.
4. Explain procedure to patient, and ask if there is a preferred venipuncture site. Ask patient if he has any questions before you proceed. If there is no site preference, visually check both arms, and select a vein which can be palpated (felt) easily with your fingertip after applying alcohol. **NOTE: Ask patient to lie down if there is any sign of apprehension. Generally the patient will be sitting down with the arm extended and supported on arm rest of chair or on a table. Providing a comfortable position will help to relax the patient and elicit better cooperation.** If the patient is eating or chewing gum, ask him to remove the contents from his mouth before you begin to eliminate any possibility of the patient's choking in the event that he faints or becomes ill during the procedure.
5. Clean site with lightly alcohol-saturated cotton ball, and let air dry. (Blowing on site to dry it will contaminate skin.)
   a. Push rubber-stoppered end of vacuum tube into adapter until needle is inserted just into rubber to hold tube in place.
   b. Apply tourniquet to patient's upper arm, about three inches above the bend in the elbow. **RATIONALE: The tourniquet slows down blood flow, increasing volume within the vein and thereby aiding palpation and visualization of the blood vessel.**
   c. You should ask the patient to clench the fist only if the vein does not stand out. This pressure of the clenched fist may interfere with some chemistry tests. A few gentle slaps to the antecubital area with two of your fingers will also help the vein stand out for better view and access. Another method to encourage blood flow in difficult draw patients is to place a warm compress on the antecubital area for a few minutes before you begin the procedure. This will assist further in making vein stand up.
   d. Take off needle guard and, with bevel of needle up, insert tip of needle into vein with a quick and steady motion, following path of vein at approximately a 15° angle.

NOTE: Holding skin at site to stretch it slightly will help keep vein from moving as puncture takes place. Needle should be inserted no more than one-fourth to one-half inch, or it may pass through vein.

6. Hold adapter with one hand and with other hand place your index and great fingers on either side of protruding edges of adapter. Push vacuum tube completely into adapter with your thumb, allowing needle to puncture stopper. Blood will flow into tube by vacuum force if other end of needle is in vein properly. As you observe blood flow into the syringe, ask the patient to slowly open the fist, and then release the tourniquet. When tube is filled, pull it out of adapter by holding it between your thumb and great finger and pushing against adapter with your index finger. **NOTE: Fill required number of tubes for tests ordered by physician.** Begin with blood culture tubes first, then red, red/black, green, lavender, gray, and blue, in that order. **NOTE: Before filling the tubes containing powdered additives, you should tap the tube(s) gently to allow any of the contents that may have collected around the rubber stopper to fall to the bottom of the tube. Check with the laboratory manual regarding the required amount of blood for test(s) ordered by the physician that contain additives. Test results may be false or inaccurate if there is a ratio imbalance of blood and additive. RATIONALE: This order will prevent any possible traces of additive from entering the "serum-only" specimen tube.** Remember to mix blood with additive gently using a figure eight motion.
7. Remove tourniquet by pulling on the end that was tucked under then, pull needle out of vein in path of insertion, and

(Continues)

PROCEDURE

15-10 Obtain Venous Blood with Vacuum Tube (continued)

place gauze square over site as needle is withdrawn. Ask patient to elevate arm slightly to help stop bleeding, and apply gentle pressure. **NOTE: If a blood smear is needed for a differential, turn CBC (lavender) tube (if still attached to adapter) upside down and gently press tube down to release drop ential, turn CBC (lavender) tube (if still attached to adapter) upside down, and gently press tube down to release drop of blood onto glass slide.** Make blood smear or as many as have been ordered, label frosted end with pencil, air dry quickly, and send with other specimens. If using a blood analyzer system such as the Coulter A^cT diff 2 shown in Figure 15–25, you should place the lavender stopper tube in the closed vial to run the test.

8. Set red tubes vertically to clot so that serum can be obtained by centrifugation for serum-only tests.

9. Same as steps 10–14 for needle and syringe procedure except for disposing of needle from plastic adapter carefully into biohazardous waste or sharps container. If Saf-T Clik® is used, dispose of the entire locked unit in the biohazardous waste or sharps container. Table 15–3 lists laboratory normal value ranges of commonly performed venous blood test results.

10. Stand red stoppered tubes vertically to clot so that serum can be drawn after centrifugation. **NOTE: Do not shake blood or hemolysis will occur.** In tubes that contain an additive, use a figure eight motion to gently mix the blood.

11. Deposit needle and syringe intact in sharps biohazardous waste container. Place labeled specimen tubes with lab request form securely in the appropriate specimen container for safe transport to the lab. **NOTE: Keep near centrifuge so that serum-only transfer tube(s) may be added when completed.** The completed lab request form is usually placed in one side of the lab-provided biobag and the specimens in the other protected (sealed and leak-proof) side to be sent to a reference lab for analysis.

12. Attend to patient's needs; apply bandage over puncture site.

13. Discard disposables in proper receptacle. Remove gloves and wash hands. Return items to proper storage area.

14. Record procedure in log book and on patient's chart. Refer to charting example.

LOG BOOK EXAMPLE:

DATE	PATIENT'S NAME NUMBER	TEST SENT	RESULTS	FILED BY
5-28-XX	Bernie L. Mitchell BD 7-18-61	7843	CBC 5-28-XX	

CHARTING EXAMPLE:

5-30-XX

One CBC tube drawn from Mr. Mitchell's L arm: packaged for reference lab pick-up.

J. Watkins, CMA (CL)

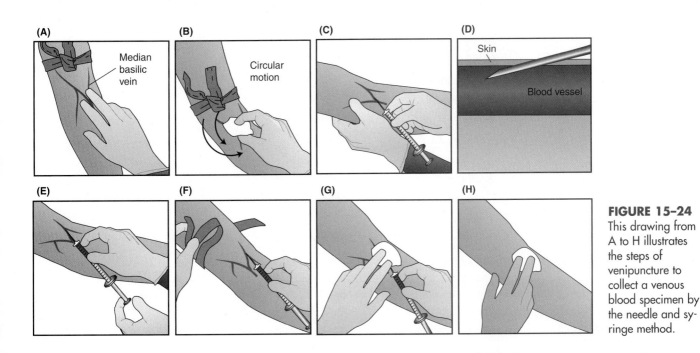

(A) Median basilic vein

(B) Circular motion

(C)

(D) Skin / Blood vessel

(E)

(F)

(G)

(H)

FIGURE 15–24
This drawing from A to H illustrates the steps of venipuncture to collect a venous blood specimen by the needle and syringe method.

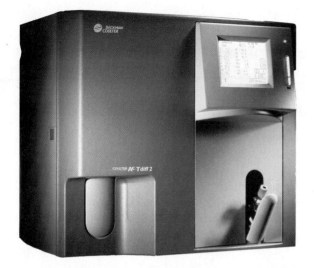

FIGURE 15–25 The COULTER A^CT diff 2 uses a closed vial system with results of tests in less than a minute. A printed document is generated with a list of tests and results. (Courtesy Beckman Coulter.)

collect whole blood that is allowed to clot so that the serum can be drawn off by centrifugation. The serum can be drawn out by a disposable pipette and deposited into a transfer tube, which is labeled for the particular test to be done. There are other methods to easily transfer serum from the centrifuged tube. The most efficient way is to use the red/black stoppered tube, which has a gel in the bottom. During centrifugation, the gel liquifies and travels to the center of the tube separating the red cells from the serum. You can then carefully pour the serum into a transfer tube and label for analysis. Another method is to place a slender rubber-tipped tube down carefully into the centrifuged tube (pushing the tube down forcefully will result in hemolysis) just to the **meniscus** of the packed red blood cells. The screened filtered opening at the rubber end of the inner tube allows the serum to fill the tube, leaving the red blood cells at the bottom. Then, pour off the serum into a transfer tube and label for analysis. Lavender-stoppered tubes contain ethylenediamienetetraacetic acid additive (EDTA) and are generally called CBC tubes. They are usually 5 or 10 mL in size and are also used to collect whole blood specimens. Gray-stoppered tubes are used in blood glucose tests and are usually five mL. They contain oxalate. Blue-stoppered tubes must be completely full because of the large amount of citrate. These tubes are most often the 5-mL size and are used for testing **prothrombin** times and *p*H levels. For accurate test results, the test should be performed within two hours from the time it is drawn. The green-stoppered tubes generally are the 5-mL-sized tubes that contain **heparin** and are used to determine the level of blood gases. The blood specimen vacuum tubes that are used for pediatric patients are the same as the tubes used for adults, except for the sizes which are between two cc and three cc. Tests drawn in the blue tubes should be performed within two hours for accurate results or centrifuge. Freeze the plasma until testing may be performed.

When several blood specimens are ordered, they should be drawn into the color-coded stoppered tubes in the following order: yellow (for blood cultures), red or

TABLE 15–3

NORMAL VALUES OF COMMONLY PERFORMED LABORATORY TESTS

Chemistry		Hematology	
Total cholesterol	130–200 mg/dl	White blood cell count	5,000–10,000/mm3
HDL cholesterol	45–65 mg/dl	Red blood cell count	3.5–5.5 × 10/mm3
LDL cholesterol	90–130 mg/dl	Hemoglobin	12–16 g/dl
Glucose	70–120 mg/dl	Hematocrit	35.5–49%
Triglyceride	40–150 mg/dl	Sedimentation rate	0–10 mm/hr
Creatinine	0.7–1.4 mg/dl	Platelet count	150,000–350,000/mm3
Uric acid	3.5–7.5 mg/dl	Coagulation Prothrombin time	
BUN	8–20 mg/dl		
Sodium	132–142 mEq/L	Adult	10–15 seconds
Potassium	4–5 mEq/L	Newborn	<17 seconds
Chloride	98–106 mEq/L	Child	11–14 seconds
CO_2	25–32 mEq/L		

Note: All reference laboratories have established normal values or controls that are based on the system or method and the reagents used in the performance of tests. A test may be considered within the normal range if there is an outcome that is within two seconds of the control determined by the laboratory.

red/black (red-gray), blue, green, lavender, and gray. The red or red/black tubes do not contain additives and should be drawn first in multiple sample draws to prevent possible contamination from the additives in the other tubes. In cases that require only one blue stoppered tube, there should be a five-mL red stoppered tube drawn first and discarded. This will prevent thromboplastin from the site of the draw from interfering with the results of coagulation testing.

Blood in specimen tubes that contain an anticoagulant must be mixed immediately in a figure eight motion 8 to 10 times. Gentle mixing will prevent hemolysis. The tubes with the red stoppers must be allowed to stand vertically and undisturbed for at least 20 to 30 minutes to allow clotting to occur. The tube(s) must then be properly balanced in a centrifuge and spun for 20 to 30 minutes. The serum, which is a clear, light yellow liquid, is then carefully drawn off with a pipette (usually disposable ones provided by the laboratory) or by using one of the methods discussed earlier.

Blood collection tubes and supplies must be checked for the expiration date, and if out of date, not used. This is in compliance with quality control and quality assurance regulations. A log book must be kept of all specimens collected and sent for analysis. The log book must contain the following information:

1. Date collected
2. Patient's full name, DOB, social security number, or records number
3. ~~Date sent to lab~~
4. Test requested
5. Date results received
6. Test results—may not be kept in specimen log book unless the test is being performed "in house." Generally, a copy is filed in the patient's chart and a copy in the lab file in order of the date collected.

A lab request form, such as the one in Figure 15–26, must be completed and sent with the specimen(s) and listed in the log book.

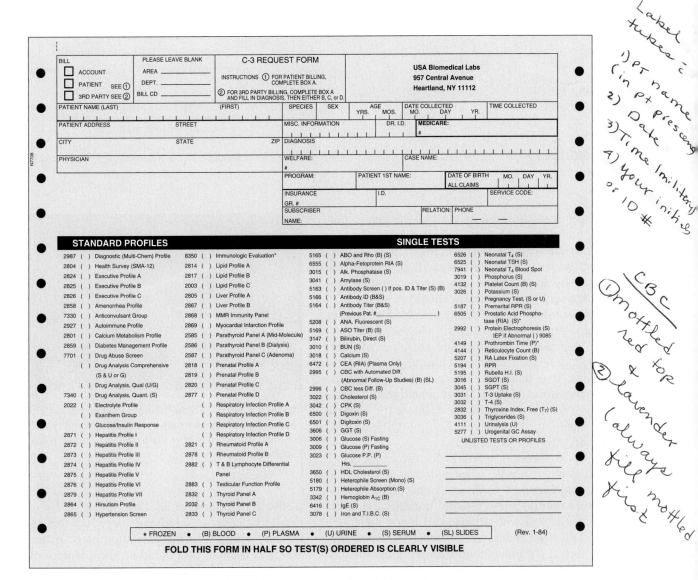

FIGURE 15–26 Laboratory request form for hematology tests

Saf-T Clik Shielded Blood Needle Adapter

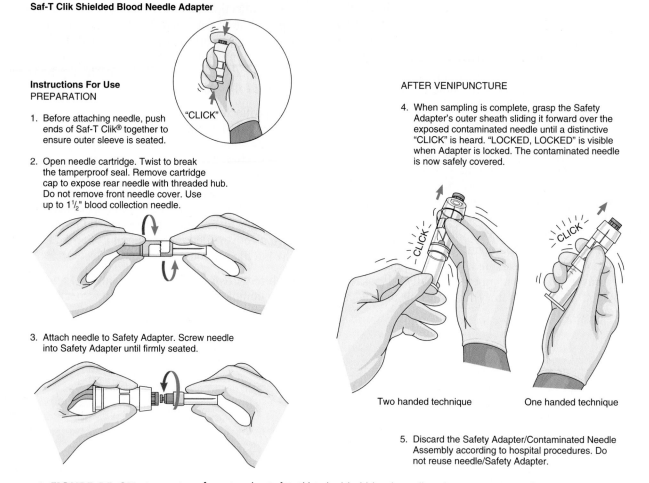

Instructions For Use
PREPARATION

1. Before attaching needle, push ends of Saf-T Clik® together to ensure outer sleeve is seated.

2. Open needle cartridge. Twist to break the tamperproof seal. Remove cartridge cap to expose rear needle with threaded hub. Do not remove front needle cover. Use up to 1½" blood collection needle.

3. Attach needle to Safety Adapter. Screw needle into Safety Adapter until firmly seated.

AFTER VENIPUNCTURE

4. When sampling is complete, grasp the Safety Adapter's outer sheath sliding it forward over the exposed contaminated needle until a distinctive "CLICK" is heard. "LOCKED, LOCKED" is visible when Adapter is locked. The contaminated needle is now safely covered.

Two handed technique   One handed technique

5. Discard the Safety Adapter/Contaminated Needle Assembly according to hospital procedures. Do not reuse needle/Safety Adapter.

FIGURE 15–27 Instructions for using the Saf-T Clik® shielded blood needle adapter (Courtesy of MPS Acacia.)

Often, specimens are sent by mail or shipped to out-of-town or out-of-state laboratories for analysis. The federal government requires that specimens are shipped/transported in securely-closed, watertight containers. Blood tubes should be enclosed in a second durable watertight container. Then specimens should be wrapped in layers of paper towels to absorb any possible breakage or leakage during transportation. The doubly-secured specimens are then placed in a shipping container of fiberboard, wood, or heavy cardboard with a label stating it is biohazardous. It is then ready for safe transport to the reference laboratory. A second label should read: In case of breakage, send to this address: Centers for Disease Control, Attention: Biohazards Control Office, 1600 Clifton Road, Atlanta, GA 30333.

Figure 15–27 shows instructions for use of the Saf-T Clik shielded blood needle adapter. It was designed to protect the phlebotomist from accidental needle injury, thereby reducing possible disease transmission. This adapter may be used with all standard blood collection needles and does not change the procedure for venipuncture. After its use, the phlebotomist simply slides the pro-

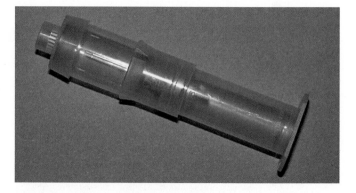

FIGURE 15–28 Eclipse™ Safety Shielding Blood Collection needle helps protect the user from accidental injury. The shield is activated immediately after the needle is withdrawn from the vein. (Courtesy of MPS Acacia.)

tective sheath forward until the "click" is heard, and the needle is safely covered and locked so that there is no danger of injury to the phlebotomist or patient. Figure 15–28 is a photo of a blood needle adapter covered and locked after use. Both types of needle adapters are completely disposable and must be discarded in the biohazardous sharps waste receptacle.

ERYTHROCYTE SEDIMENTATION RATE

The erythrocyte **sedimentation** rate is also known as the ESR, the sed rate, and the SR. It is the rate at which red blood cells settle in a particular calibrated tube within a given time, usually one hour. The purpose of the test is to determine the degree of inflammation in the body. When inflammation is present, red blood cells become heavier than normal. The ESR may be performed in the medical office or clinic. Whole blood is required, and the usual procedure is to draw blood into a lavender stoppered tube that contains an anticoagulant. The test should be performed within two hours of being drawn for accurate results. The erythrocyte sedimentation rate is useful in the diagnosis and evaluation of diseases of the respiratory tract and in cancer, arthritic, and Collagen's patients. It may also be used in determining the extent of dehydration in burn victims. Sed rates are performed with several different types of calibrated cylindrical tubes. The most common methods and their normal ranges are:

ESR Method	Males	Females
SEDIPLAST WESTERGREN	0–15 mm/hr (under 50) 0–20 mm/hr (over 50)	0–20 mm/hr (under 50) 0–30 mm/hr (over 50)
SEDIPLAST WINTROBE	0–9 mm/hr (all ages)	0–20 mm/hr (all ages)
COULTER	0–8 mm/hr (all ages)	0–10 mm/hr (all ages)

Since the dawn of managed care by OSHA and CLIA regulations, there has been a steady rise in technically advanced laboratory testing for the medical office. Safety for the patient and medical personnel is of vital importance. Diagnostic tests that are safe and convenient with accurate results are in demand. The National Committee for Clinical Laboratory Standards has recommended the Westergren ESR (Erythrocyte Sedimentation Rate) system as the standard as it is more sensitive. With POCT, the convenience for both patient and physician is another positive consideration for use in medical offices. Figure 15–29 shows the Sediplast ESR System, and Figure 15–30 shows its simplistic instructions. This system has many advantages over former methods. There is an automatic self-zeroing cap and reservoir that protects the user from blood leakage, overfilling, and spraying from the pipette. It is a completely closed system and eliminates manual techniques.

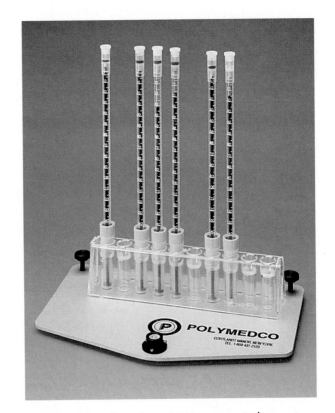

FIGURE 15–29 The SEDIPLAST Westergren Sedimentation method is a completely closed system that provides safety for the user and reliable results. (Courtesy Polymedco, Inc.)

The normal rate at which red blood cells fall is one mm every five minutes. Because the readings vary according to which method is used, it is essential that the method be recorded with the results on the patient's chart. Females tend to have higher readings than males, especially during menstruation and in pregnancy.

ACHIEVE UNIT OBJECTIVES

Complete Chapter 15, Unit 3, in the workbook to help you obtain competency of this subject matter.

A CAAHEP CONNECTION

This unit discussed instruction in venous blood specimen collection. The areas included in the Medical Assistant curriculum are *Anatomy and physiology, Medical terminology, Psychology, Communication, Clinical procedures,* and *Medical law and ethics.*

SEDIPLAST® ESR SYSTEM is easy to use:

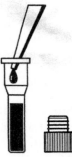

1 - Remove the stopper on the pre-filled vial, and fill to the indicated line with blood. Replace stopper and invert several times to mix.

2 - Insert the pipette through the pierceable stopper, and push down until the pipette touches the bottom of the vial. The pipette will autozero the blood, and any excess will flow into the closed reservoir compartment.

3 - Let the pipette stand for one hour, and then read the numerical results of the ESR.

Normal values		Specifications	
Male (under 50)	0–15 mm/hr	Overall length	200 mm
Male (over 50)	0–20 mm/hr	Graduations	0–150 mm
Female (under 50)	0–20 mm/hr	Bore Size (I.D.)	2.55 mm
Female (over 50)	0–30 mm/hr	Uniformity of Bore	± 0.05 mm

FIGURE 15–30 SEDIPLAST ESR system instructions (Courtesy Polymedco, Inc.)

UNIT 4

Body Fluid Specimens

■ OBJECTIVES

Upon completion of the unit, meet the following performance objectives by verifying knowledge of the facts and principles presented through oral and written communication at a level deemed competent. Demonstrate the specific behaviors as identified in the performance objectives of the procedures, observing all aseptic and safety precautions in accordance with health care standards.

1. Spell and define, using the glossary at the back of the text, all the **Words to Know** in this unit.

2. Explain the methods of urine collection: clean-catch midstream, catheterization, infant collection, and random.

3. Perform routine urinalysis: physical, chemical, and microscopic examination.

4. Instruct patients in collection of urine, sputum, and stool for analysis.

5. Assist with a catheterization urine specimen from a female patient.

6. Describe the reagent strips used in chemical urinalysis.

7. Describe the proper storage of urine specimens until analysis can be performed and the reasons for it.

8. Complete a lab request form.

9. Record the results of a urinalysis on the patient's chart.

10. Describe patient education regarding respiratory, digestive, and urinary systems. 2 only on urin. syst only

11. Explain the collection process of specimens sent for drug and/or alcohol analysis. "chain of custody"

12. Explain the reason for a Hemoccult® Sensa® test and the procedure to be followed.

13. Perform and interpret a Hemoccult® Sensa® slide test.

WORDS TO KNOW

amber
cancer
caustic
chemical
clarity
crenated
dextrose
feces
guaiac reagent
in vivo
last menstrual period
(LMP)

laxative
occult
physical
random
renal threshold
stability
supernatant   *Urinary (meatus)*
turbidity
urinalysis
urinary tract infection
(UTI)
urination

micturition   void

In addition to obtaining blood specimens and preparing them for laboratory tests, the medical assistant will probably be responsible for collecting specimens of other body fluids from patients or instructing the patients to do so. The specimens that you must obtain and prepare for analysis most often are urine, sputum, and stool. The same standard information (the patient's name, age, sex, etc.) should accompany each specimen on the appropriate laboratory request form. In addition, specimens must be obtained and sent to the lab in the proper containers to avoid misunderstanding by lab personnel.

Most specimens should be refrigerated if there is a delay in transporting them to the laboratory. Many specimen containers already have a preservative added to prevent deterioration so that refrigeration is not necessary. A laboratory procedure manual should be kept at hand for reference on how to prepare specimens.

URINE SPECIMENS

(C) Main Menu:
Infection Control

Skills Menu:
- Clean-Catch Urine Sample
- Testing Urine

Urinalysis is probably the most frequently performed test in the medical office. Examination of urine consists of three major areas of testing: **physical, chemical,** and microscopic (Figure 15–31).

Specimens for urinalysis are usually collected in plastic disposable containers (Figure 15–32). The time that

PHYSICAL EXAMINATION:

Appearance   *CLEAR, STRAW-COLORED*
pH   *4.5 To 7.5*   Specific Gravity   *1.010 To 1.025*

CHEMICAL ANALYSIS:

Albumin (protein) *NONE To TRACE*   Urobilinogen *NEG.*
Sugar (glucose, dextrose) *NONE*   Porphyrins *NEG.*
Ketones (acetone) *NONE*   PKU *NEG.*
Bilirubin   *NONE*   Occult Blood *NEG.*

MICROSCOPIC EXAMINATION:

Cells: Epithelial *FEW*
          WBC's   *0 To 4*
          RBC's *FEW TO OCCASIONAL*

Casts: Hyaline *NEG.*
          Epithelial *NEG.*
          Blood *NEG.*

Crystals: *FEW*
Other: *NEG.*

FIGURE 15–31   This lab report form shows normal values for a routine urinalysis.

the urine specimen was obtained should be noted on the container with the patient's name, the date, and the test to be performed on the specimen. Ideally, urinalysis should be performed within ~~two hours~~ *30'* of collection to avoid bacterial growth and the decomposition of cells. If there is a delay, the specimen should be refrigerated.

The first morning **urination** is the most concentrated and therefore most often the choice for accurate test results. In addition, patients usually have little difficulty in obtaining **random** urine specimens upon request in the medical office. Random refers to nonscheduled and/or no preparation required. Most physicians prefer that the specimen be a midstream sample. Partial voiding before catching the specimen will clear the urethra of any sloughed off cells, bacteria, mucus, or other debris that could interfere with accurate test results. Patients should be instructed to wash the genital area with soap and water, rinse well, wipe the genitals with several antiseptic-soaked cotton balls from front to back (usually zephrin chloride is used), begin to void into the toilet, and after a few seconds, catch about three ounces in the urine container.

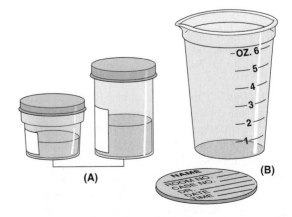

FIGURE 15–32   Plastic disposable urine specimen containers with identification label/lids

In the management of insulin-dependent diabetic patients, many physicians are requesting a double-voiding urine sample when they come in for their regular checkups to test for glucose and acetone content. To do this, the patient is asked to void a clean catch specimen and then repeat in one hour. This practice provides the physician with more information in assessment of the patient's condition.

The 24-Hour Urine Specimen

On occasion, a 24-hour urine specimen will be called for. Usually, a written laboratory order will be given to the patient, and instruction will be given by the laboratory technician, but you may be given this responsibility. Printed instruction sheets are most helpful in this procedure. The patient is given a large container with a preservative already added. Check the lab test manual if necessary for proper instructions for any tests you are not sure of to be accurate. This container will hold all of the urine the patient voids in a 24-hour period and must be refrigerated throughout this time. The patient must keep a record of the date and exact time that the collection begins, which should be at the second urination of the day. Then every time the patient voids, day and night, for the next 24 hours, the patient should urinate into a clean smaller container and add the urine to the larger container. The last specimen included in the test period is the first urination of the next morning. When completed, the specimen should be taken to the laboratory as soon as possible and kept cool during transporting with ice in a portable cooler. Again, it is necessary to check the lab manual for directions in preparing specimens because some 24-hour urine samples should not have the preservative added.

Pediatric urine collection bags fit over the genital area of either gender and are secured with adhesive (Figure 15–33). The infant's skin should be washed and dried thoroughly before application if the bag is to stay in place. You have to instruct the parent in the procedure so that it can be done at home. It may be necessary to transfer the urine into a regular specimen container for transporting. You should advise the parent to label the specimen with the baby's name and the date and time of the urine collection.

The lab report will be given to the physician within a few days depending on the type of tests performed. As with any lab test, the patient will be anxious to know the results and should be notified as soon as possible.

Catheterization   You may be asked to either perform or assist with the procedure of urinary bladder catheterization, the introduction of a catheter (tube) through the urethra into the bladder for withdrawal of urine. If the physician wants female catheterizations performed by the medical assistant, then the physician will teach the proper method of performing this procedure. The learner's skills will be observed by the physician to determine if the medical assistant may perform catheterization of female patients without further supervision (documentation of this teaching and evaluation is advised).

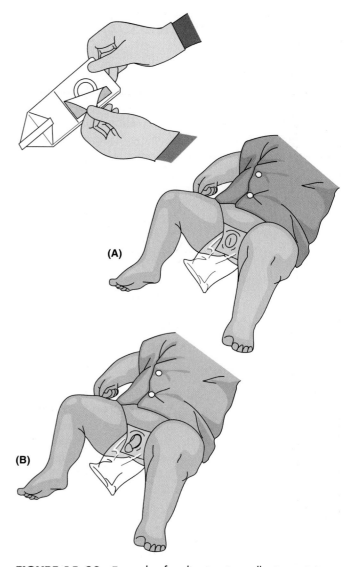

FIGURE 15–33 Example of pediatric urine collection unit in proper position

There are basically three reasons for catheterizing patients:

1. to obtain a sterile urine specimen for analysis
2. for relief of urinary retention
3. to instill medication into the bladder after the bladder is emptied

This procedure is not performed routinely. In most cases, it is done by a urologist, a physician who specializes in diseases of the urinary system. However, some physicians in obstetrics-gynecology and general and family practice may delegate this duty to the medical assistant to aid in the diagnosis of the patient. Generally, the physician will order a culture and sensitivity analysis of the urine obtained from catheterization. This is done to determine what microorganism is present and what medication will be effective in treatment. You must be authorized by the physician to perform the procedure. The physician generally will have you observe several catheterizations to become familiar with the procedure. After you have demonstrated the skill under the direct supervision of the physician, you will be authorized to perform catheterizations alone. See Procedure 15–11. If any doubt or problem occurs during the catheterization procedure, the physician should be notified immediately.

Generally, physicians will catheterize male patients because it is a more difficult procedure and sometimes painful. Assistance in assembling the necessary items and helping the physician during the procedure may be the medical assistant's role.

Sterile technique must be maintained throughout the procedure. Contamination of any of the items during the procedure is possible, and these should be discarded and another sterile item used to continue the procedure. Carelessness may result in severe bladder infection or injury

---

PROCEDURE

15-11 Catheterize Urinary Bladder

PURPOSE: To obtain a sterile urine specimen from the urinary bladder for laboratory analysis.

OSHA GUIDELINES: Remember to wear gloves later when handling any items that have come into contact with blood or any body fluids.

EQUIPMENT: Sterile tray covered with sterile towel, sterile gloves, sterile towels, sterile specimen container with lid, sterile basin to catch excess urine, sterile catheter (French type, sizes 12–16), sterile cotton balls, sterile medicine cup, sterile 4 x 4-inch gauze squares, sterile forceps, sterile plastic sheet, antiseptic solution, sterile lubricant, sterile gloves, gooseneck lamp, Mayo table, biohazard bag.

PERFORMANCE OBJECTIVE: With all equipment and supplies provided, and using a female training model or mannequin in lieu of a patient, demonstrate the steps required to perform a urinary bladder catheterization. The instructor will observe each step. **NOTE: To prevent injury, disease transmission, or embarrassment, this procedure should not be practiced before other students. Simulation should be made by the instructor if models are not available.**

1. Place catheter kit on Mayo table next to examination table, and explain procedure to identified female patient. Adjust position of lamp and turn on.

2. **NOTE: Normally, patient to be catheterized has already been examined and gowned or is covered below the waist with a drape sheet.** Assist her into dorsal recumbent position with her feet in stirrups. Drape patient with sheet and expose external genitalia.

3. Pull out the footrest. Place sterile kit on footrest and open outer wrapping. Touching only corners, place sterile plastic sheet under patient's buttocks. Ask patient to keep her knees apart.

4. Wash and dry hands and put on sterile gloves, being careful not to contaminate your gloved hands. Pour antiseptic solution over cotton balls in medicine cup. Open urine specimen container and keep on sterile field. Apply sterile lubricant to one of gauze squares.

5. With left hand, spread labia and wipe genitalia once with each of three antiseptic-soaked cotton balls (front-to-back motion). Using right hand, discard onto Mayo table. Keep left hand in place, and do not touch sterile items with it because it is now contaminated. Place tip of catheter in lubricant and other end of catheter tube into basin.

6. Holding catheter tube about four inches from lubricated tip with your right thumb and index finger, insert tip gently into urinary meatus (located below clitoris and above the vaginal opening) about two to three inches (Figure 15–34). Patient should be instructed to breathe slowly and deeply to relax abdominal muscles and tissues so that procedure is not painful. Tell patient that uncomfortable feeling will last only a few minutes until tube is withdrawn. Procedure should not be painful to the patient. Any unusual complaints should be brought to physician's attention immediately.

7. After inserting tip of catheter, urine should begin to flow immediately into basin. Flow may be stopped by closing metal clamp attached to tubing. Position other end of tube into specimen container, and release clamp to collect urine specimen. Allow remainder of urine from bladder to flow into basin.

8. Withdraw catheter tip gently once specimen is obtained, and dry area with sterile gauze squares or cotton balls. Secure lid onto urine specimen container and set aside. Turn lamp off and return it to usual position. Remove all items from footrest.

9. Assist patient to sitting position then from table to dress.

10. Place any reusable items in basin of cold water to soak until you have time to wash and sterilize them. Clean off examining table. Discard gloves and disposable items in biohazardous waste bag.

11. Wash hands. Label specimen for analysis, and complete request form if sending it to outside lab.

12. Record procedure on patient's chart and initial. Include information about physical properties of urine, rate of flow, and any abnormal or significant observations.

During the patient's office visit, you may have an opportunity to discuss a few of the following areas which may help the patient better understand proper health habits in regard to urinary problems.

1. Remind patients to avoid using perfumed toilet articles (i.e., tissue, tampons, or soaps) that are irritating to delicate vaginal tissues.
2. Advise patients to void when they feel the urge because delay can cause bladder stress and irritation.
3. Instruct female patients to practice Kegel exercises to increase the sphincter control of the bladder to improve urine retention. This exercise is done by pushing down with the lower pelvic muscles (as in forcing urination), counting to 10, and then squeezing back, counting down to 1. Repeating this routine several times a day helps to strengthen muscle control.
4. Remind patients that they should drink plenty of fluids, avoiding caffeine drinks.
5. Remind patients (especially females) that taking a shower instead of a tub bath reduces the possibility of infection. (Bubble baths should be taken rarely because they irritate delicate vaginal tissues.)
6. Advise female patients that wearing pants that are too tight and nylon underwear may be irritating to delicate vaginal tissues. Cotton is recommended because it breathes, allowing heat and moisture to escape.

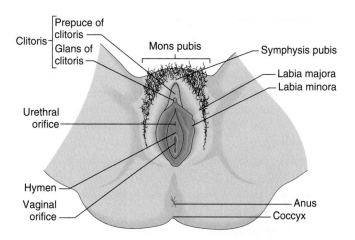

FIGURE 15-34 External female genitalia

zation kits are available that contain all necessary items to perform the procedure. Some have only the catheter tube, which attaches to the sterile specimen container directly. This is convenient for obtaining a sterile urine specimen. Other items must be assembled to properly carry out the procedure.

Physical Urinalysis

Physical properties of urine include the appearance (color), specific gravity, **turbidity** (**clarity**), and color. Standard color descriptors are light straw, straw (yellow), dark straw, light **amber**, amber, and dark amber. Clarity is described as clear, slightly cloudy, cloudy, and very cloudy. Specific gravity indicates the concentration of urine. It can be measured with a refractometer or with some reagent strips. The weight of substances contained in the urine is assessed by comparing the specific gravity of urine with that of distilled water, which is 1.000. The specific gravity of urine is normally from 1.003 to 1.035. Lighter colored urine usually has a lower specific gravity, and darker urine a higher one.

The color of urine can be affected by disease, some medications, and food. Urine with a strong ammonia-like odor may be alkaline from a high concentration of bacteria. Urine with a high glucose level (glycosuria) may have a fruit-sweet odor. Glycosuria is caused by a high glucose level in the blood, which spills into the urine when the **renal threshold** is reached.

Blood in the urine *(hematuria)* may give the specimen a red or rusty color. However, foods with strong color, such as beets, also produce redness in the urine and stool. Patients should be advised that this is only temporary and told not to worry. If medication is known to cause urinary discoloration, the patient should be told in advance to avoid undue stress.

Chemical Urinalysis

Any urine specimen that has been refrigerated should be returned to room temperature before testing.

Reagent strips are convenient and relatively inexpensive diagnostic tests that reveal the presence of abnormal substances in the urine. The reagent strips provide both qualitative and quantitative assessment. Qualitatively, they reveal the presence of an abnormal substance; quantitatively, they determine how much of the substance is present. The substances include sugar (glucose), protein (albumin), ketone (acetone), bilirubin, urobilinogen, blood, nitrate, *p*H, leukocytes, and specific gravity. The treated paper end of the reagent strip reacts chemically with the urine, and if a sufficient amount of a substance is present in the urine, the strip changes color. The strip is then compared with the color chart on the bottle.

Fresh urine specimens should be used, and exact timing of the tests is vital. Adequate lighting is also important to view the colors of the reagent strips and the changes that may occur. If there is no reaction (no change in color), the results are recorded as negative.

to the patient. You should follow the procedure for putting on sterile gloves given later in the text.

French catheters are used in performing simple catheterizations. The Foley catheter is used when the catheter will remain in the urinary bladder. Sterile, disposable catheteri-

Care must be taken to protect the reagent strips from exposure to light, heat, and moisture. Reagent strip bottles must be capped immediately after use and stored in a dry, cool area (but not refrigerated). The strips are bottled in light-resistant plastic with a moisture-absorbent agent included. They must not be used after the expiration date on the bottle. The date when the bottle is opened should be noted on the side of the bottle. You should not exceed open vial **stability** to ensure accuracy

of the testing. Always check the package insert for current information.

Many companies manufacture urine tests. One test that is commonly used because of its wide range is the Multistix 10 SG reagent strip test (Bayer Diagnostics). Each reagent strip bottle has a package insert with instructions, which should be precisely followed. Refer to Procedure 15–12.

The Multistix® 10 SG is also used in the Clinitek 50 urine chemistry analyzer (Figure 15–35). This instrument

---

PROCEDURE

15-12 Test Urine with Multistix® 10 SG

PURPOSE: To detect pH, protein, glucose, ketones, blood, bilirubin, urobilinogen, leukocytes, and specific gravity in urine.

OSHA GUIDELINES: To comply with Standard Precautions, gloves must be worn if there is any possibility of coming into contact with blood or any body fluids.

EQUIPMENT: Multistix® 10 SG reagent strips, fresh urine specimen, disposable gloves, watch or other timepiece, tongue depressor, patient's chart, pen, adequate lighting to read color chart on reagent bottle (for accurate test results, use before expiration date on the bottle).

PERFORMANCE OBJECTIVE: Provided with all necessary equipment and supplies, demonstrate the steps required to perform the procedure for using Multistix® 10 SG. The instructor will observe each step.

1. Wash hands, put on gloves, and assemble all needed items on cleared counter.

2. Stir urine with tongue depressor to evenly distribute solutes throughout the specimen.

3. Remove cap from bottle, and take out one reagent strip without touching test paper end. Place cap securely back on bottle. **NOTE: Study times are given on bottle for reading each test section.**

4. Dip test paper end of reagent strip into urine specimen. With reagent side of strip down, pull across inside of specimen container opening to remove excess urine. **RATIONALE: If strip is too saturated, treated test paper chemicals will run together and make results inaccurate.**

5. a. Place reagent strip next to color chart on bottle by holding bottom of bottle in left hand and strip by right thumb and index finger.
   b. Read results by comparing color of reacted reagent strips with color chart on bottle.
   c. Place bottle on its side, and hold it at bottom with left hand.
   d. Hold reagent strip in right hand with thumb and index finger, and line up with color chart on bottle.

   e. Read test results from bottom to top in order of shorter to longer timings. Proper timing is essential for accurate results.

6. Begin timing tests immediately. **NOTE: The scale below is in the same order as reagents on strip and on color chart on bottle when properly aligned and observed from left to right.**

   2 minutes—leukocytes
   60 seconds—nitrite
   60 seconds—urobilinogen
   60 seconds—protein (albumin)
   60 seconds—pH
   60 seconds—blood
   45 seconds—specific gravity
   40 seconds—ketone
   30 seconds—bilirubin
   30 seconds—glucose (quantitative)
   ~~10 seconds—glucose (qualitative)~~

7. Discard used reagent strip, gloves, and other disposables into proper receptacle. Wash hands. Return Multistix® 10 SG to proper storage area.

8. Record results as indicated for each section on patient's chart and in log book. Refer to charting example.

LOG BOOK EXAMPLE:

DATE	PATIENT'S NAME	NUMBER	TEST	SENT	RESULTS	FILED BY
7-17-XX	Marcene Mitchell BD 8-8-63	7539	UA Clinitek 50	7-17-XX	large amount of leukocytes	J. Watkins, CMA (CL)

CHARTING EXAMPLE:

5-30-XX
Clean-catch urine specimen from Marcene Mitchell tested with Clinitek 50 shows clear yellow urine positive for leukocytes, all other tests negative.

J. Watkins, CMA (CL)

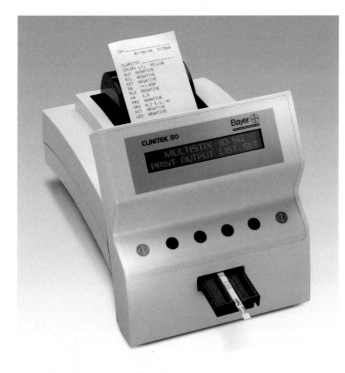

FIGURE 15–35 The Clinitek 50 urine chemistry analyzer (Courtesy of Bayer Diagnostics.)

provides standardized readings of reflectance photometry on a screen (with abnormal results highlighted) and a printed record for the patient's file.

The pH range for normal urine is from 5.0 to 7.0 (Figure 15–36). Above 7.0 is considered alkaline, and below 5.0 is acid. If a urine specimen has a pH over 7, it probably contains a great number of bacteria, which make the urine alkaline. This will destroy the urinary casts that are formed in the kidney. Urinary casts are important in the diagnosis of a patient's condition.

Diseases of the kidney and **urinary tract infections (UTI)** produce protein (albumin) in the urine that is not normally present. A patient with a trace or reading of 1+ or more of protein on a random specimen will probably

be asked to have a first morning sample checked to see if the protein is in the concentrated urine.

Ketone (acetone) bodies are not normally present in the urine. They are the result of fat metabolized in the digestive tract. Their presence could indicate severe diabetes mellitus, starvation, a high-fat diet, or body wasting. A highly concentrated amount of ketones is called ketonuria. Some patients who have been fasting before coming in to the medical office for blood and urine tests may show a high ketone urine level, which is usually insignificant.

Bilirubin (bile) is an orange or yellowish pigment that is a product of degenerated RBCs that release hemoglobin in the liver. This waste product is normally excreted through the intestines. In patients who have liver damage or disease, bilirubin will appear in the urine, often before they develop symptoms and appear jaundiced.

Urobilinogen is bilirubin that has been converted in the intestines by coli bacteria. This chemical reaction gives feces its brown color. Urobilinogen is excreted through the intestines normally. Large amounts are produced when the heart, spleen, and liver are diseased or dysfunctioning.

Blood in the urine is termed hematuria. Presence of blood in the urine indicates damage of the kidney from injury or from disorders and diseases of the urinary tract. Blood is found normally in the urine specimens of menstruating females. If the specimen is necessary immediately for a diagnosis, a catheterized specimen may be required.

Nitrite is present in urine that contains microorganisms. The action of the invading bacteria converts nitrates in the normally sterile urine to nitrite **in vivo.** Bacteria increase in number and the contents of urine that has been left unrefrigerated for more than two hours may begin to deteriorate. This is why urinalysis should be done as soon as possible after collection.

Phenistix is a reagent strip that detects the presence of phenylketonuria (PKU) in infants. This test may be done like the others by dipping the reagent strip into a fresh urine specimen and timing the reaction.

Glucose (sugar, **dextrose**) is not normally present in the urine, but it may spill out from the kidney when the bloodstream is saturated. Female patients may have a high glucose level during pregnancy and postpartum. Further tests should then be performed to determine the cause. Glucose in the urine may indicate presence of the disease diabetes mellitus. Some patients have a low renal threshold, which may explain the presence of glucose in the urine. Patients with a high glucose level are usually asked for several specimens from different times of the day, with blood tests. The results are evaluated by the physician with other findings from the patient's history before a final diagnosis is made.

Another reliable way to determine the amount of glucose in the urine is with the Clinitest tablet. Instructions for use are enclosed with each kit and may be used by di-

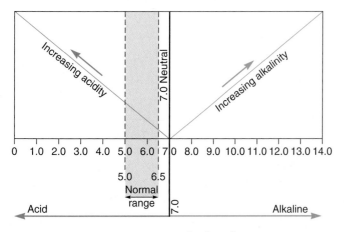

FIGURE 15–36 Scale of pH for urine

abetic patients in daily monitoring of their glucose level at home. Bottles which contain Clinitest tablets are light-resistant and should be kept in a dry, cool storage area to ensure accurate test results. As with all medications and chemical preparations, Clinitest should be kept out of the hands of children. These tablets should not come in contact with skin, or a **caustic** reaction with the skin's moisture will result in a burn. Patients who use Clinitest or other home test kits keep a record of the results and either phone the medical office or bring the report in to be filed in their chart. See Procedure 15–13.

Pregnancy tests are often performed with urine specimens. Female patients usually bring a urine specimen into the medical office in their own containers. They should be instructed to wash, rinse, and dry these carefully before using.

The ideal urine specimen for pregnancy testing is obtained from the first morning urination, which contains the greatest concentration of chorionic gonadotropin, the hormone on which most pregnancy tests are based. The patient should be instructed to discontinue medications, or the test results may be inaccurate. If the patient is pregnant, only those medications ordered by the physician should be taken because the developing embryo would be at risk from possible side effects. You should caution patients tactfully with this information so that you do not frighten them.

If pregnancy tests are performed in the medical office, the package insert instructions should be followed exactly. Most are simple and easy to complete. Pregnancy tests performed in the medical office take only a few minutes, and patients may want to wait for the results. If the

PROCEDURE

15-13 Determine Glucose Content of Urine with Clinitest Tablet

PURPOSE: To determine the glucose content of urine.

OSHA GUIDELINES: To comply with Standard Precautions, gloves must be worn if there is any possibility of coming into contact with blood or any body fluids.

EQUIPMENT: Clinitest tablets with color chart for test result (must be used before expiration date to ensure accurate results), disposable glass test tubes, eyedropper, fresh urine specimen, disposable latex or vinyl gloves, small container of water, test tube rack, tongue depressor, watch or timepiece, proper lighting, biohazard bag.

PERFORMANCE OBJECTIVE: Provided with all necessary equipment and supplies, demonstrate the steps in the procedure for using Clinitest tablets. The instructor will observe each step.

1. Wash hands, put on gloves, and assemble needed items on adequate counter space.
2. Stir urine with tongue depressor, and fill dropper halfway with urine. **RATIONALE: Stirring mixes liquid and solutes in urine for more accurate testing.**
3. Hold test tube near top between thumb and index finger, and with other hand, release five drops of urine into test tube.
4. Rinse dropper and fill halfway with water. Release 10 drops of water into test tube. Shake gently to mix.
5. Set test tube in rack and open Clinitest bottle. Without touching tablets, shake one tablet directly into Clinitest bottle cap. **RATIONALE: Moisture on hands may cause a**

chemical reaction with the tablet, causing a burn. Recap the bottle.

6. Watch reaction (Figure 15–37). As soon as boiling stops, allow exactly 15 seconds before carefully grasping test tube at top, gently tilting it back and forth and swirling contents, and then comparing color of mixture in bottom of test tube with closest color on chart (Figure 15–38). Results are determined in percentage of milligrams per deciliter.
7. Return items to proper storage. Discard disposable items. Remove disposable gloves and discard in proper receptacle. Wash hands.
8. Record reading on patient's chart and in log book.

LOG BOOK EXAMPLE:

DATE	PATIENT'S NAME	NUMBER	TEST	SENT	RESULTS	FILED BY
7-17-XX	Marcene Mitchell	7539	UA	7-17-XX	large	J. Watkins,
					amount of	CMA (CL)
	BD 8-8-63		Clinitek 50		leukocytes	
			Clinitest Tablet		2+	

CHARTING EXAMPLE:

7-17-XX

Clean-catch urine specimen from Marcene Mitchell tested with Clinitek 50 shows clear yellow urine positive for leukocytes, all other tests negative, except for Clinitest tablet glucose 2+.

J. Watkins, CMA (CL)

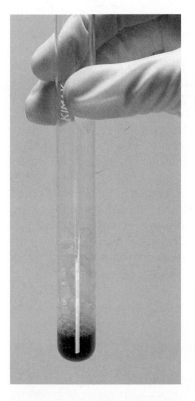

FIGURE 15–37 Carefully hold the test tube at the top to avoid being burned from boiling caused by chemical reaction of Clinitest tablet with urine and water solution.

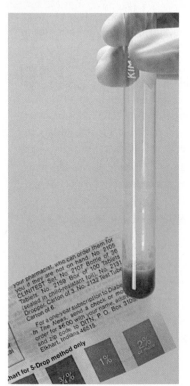

FIGURE 15–38 Compare reaction color with chart 15 seconds after boiling stops and after gently swirling the tube to mix the contents.

test is positive (meaning that pregnancy is evident), the patient may have several questions and may wish to consult further with the physician. Routine scheduling of an appointment is advised.

Patients are usually advised to bring a urine specimen for a pregnancy test no earlier than 10 days after the first missed menstrual period. Refrigeration is necessary if the specimen cannot be taken directly to the laboratory. The laboratory request form and patient's chart should contain the age of the patient and the date of the first day of the **last menstrual period (LMP)** along with the standard information requested.

Microscopic Examination of Urine

Although the medical assistant may not read and interpret the microscopic examination of urine, she may need to prepare urine for this type of examination. Refer to Procedure 15–14 and Figure 15–39.

Collection of Specimens for Substance Analysis

You may be given the responsibility of collecting specimens for drug (chemical) and alcohol analysis. You must be sure to explain the procedure thoroughly before you have the patient complete and sign the consent/release form for the blood or urine test (or both). The form, called *chain of custody,* will state that the purpose of the test is to screen for the presence of drugs, alcohol, and chemical substances. The signature of the patient on this form gives authorization for you to collect the specimen(s) for this purpose, prepare it for transport to the laboratory for analysis, and release the results to the agency (employer) where it was requested. The chain of custody form shown in Figure 15–40 is necessary for all pre-employment and Department of Transportation (DOT) testing. Generally, this information is an employment requirement. It can also be required for legal reasons. These specimens should be collected very carefully. The consent form and the test request form must accompany the specimens to the laboratory. Information regarding the samples includes:

1. Purpose of the test
2. Number of specimens
3. Comments about: (urine) color, temperature, *p*H, and specific gravity
4. Collector's name
5. Site of collection/date/time

The signature of the collector then verifies that the sealed specimen sent is the same one that was received from the patient (at the site) whose name is on the request and consent forms. This multiple (five) copy form is color-coded for routing purposes. Copies are given to:

1. Medical review officer
2. Laboratory
3. Patient
4. Collector
5. Employer

Patients should be informed that all medications, drugs, and alcohol that have been consumed within the last 30 days prior to the test will be revealed by the test-

P R O C E D U R E

15-14 Obtain Urine Sediment for Microscopic Examination

PURPOSE: To obtain urine sediment to determine microscopic contents of urine.

OSHA GUIDELINES: To comply with Standard Precautions, gloves must be worn if there is any possibility of coming into contact with blood or any body fluids.

EQUIPMENT: Fresh urine specimen, disposable latex or vinyl gloves, two glass test tubes, centrifuge, frosted-end glass slides with cover glass, tapered pipette, patient's chart, pen, pencil, tongue depressor, microscope with light source, urine sediment chart, timer or timepiece, sharps container.

PERFORMANCE OBJECTIVE: Provided with all necessary equipment and supplies, demonstrate all steps required in the procedure for obtaining urine sediment. The instructor will observe each step.

1. Wash hands, put on gloves, and assemble all needed items on cleared counter surface near centrifuge.

2. Stir urine specimen with tongue depressor, and pour equal amounts (approximately 10 cc) into each of two test tubes, or use plain water in one of test tubes. **NOTE: Remember that equal weight is required for proper operation of centrifuge.**

3. To balance centrifuge, place test tubes on opposite sides. Urine should be spun at 1500 revolutions per minute for three to five minutes. **NOTE: Set timer or write down time.**

4. When centrifuge has completely stopped, lift out tube containing urine specimen and carefully pour off urine (**supernatant**).

5. There will still be a few drops of urine in the bottom of test tube with sediment. Gently tap bottom of tube on counter or against your palm to mix urine and sediment together. **NOTE: Make sure that all sediment is thoroughly mixed.**

6. Obtain a drop or two of urine sediment with a tapered pipette and place it on a clean frosted-end glass slide.

7. Place a cover slip over specimen, allow it to settle, and place on microscope stage.

   Unless you are highly experienced in this area, the physician will conduct the examination from this point on. Consult with your employer about the office policy in this matter before proceeding with the examination.

8. View slide under low-power objective first. Scan for casts and epithelial cells (Figure 15–39). **NOTE: Use dim light. RATIONALE: Dim light enhances visualization; bright light causes glare, interfering with vision.**

9. Change to high-powered objective to view structures, such as red and white blood cells, bacteria, and crystal cells. At least 10 different fields should be viewed. Turn light off when finished. **RATIONALE: Heat from light will dry out slide and destroy specimen.**

10. Record microscopic observations on patient's chart and on the log sheet. Casts and epithelial cells are counted as few, moderate, or many; for example:

    blood casts—few/lpf
    epithelial cells—many/lpf

    Red and white blood cells and bacteria are counted by number seen under microscope using high-power objective or by terms *occasional* or *loaded* (to describe too many to count); for example:

    WBCs—loaded/hpf
    bacteria—occ/hpf

    Red blood cells that are shrunken, or crenated, will appear smaller than average and will have a jagged surface.

11. Rinse glass items, wash in detergent solution if not disposable, rinse well, and dry on paper towels. Test tubes may be placed bottom-up to drain on paper towels. Return items to proper storage area. Remove disposable gloves and discard in the proper receptacle. Wash hands.

---

ing process. OTC (over the counter) medications are included. Explain that concealing information is certainly not advised because it would only make a possible problem situation worse for them. A section of the form allows the patient to list all substances consumed in the last month. Patients should be advised to be specific and state what was taken and how much. Ask patients to think about this before completing the form so that they can remember exactly to complete the form accurately.

Discarding specimens may present a problem, with odor caused by the bacterial growth. Pouring urine specimens down the sink is a common practice, but it should be done carefully and only down a "special discard" sink used solely for the purpose of disposing contaminated items. Running cold water for a few seconds will flush the trap under the sink. Routine daily use of a few tablespoons of baking soda will keep the drain clean and help eliminate odors.

CRYSTALS FOUND IN ACID URINE

| URIC ACID (BRIGHTFIELD) | URIC ACID (POLARIZED) | TYROSINE (BRIGHTFIELD) | LEUCINE (BRIGHTFIELD) | CYSTINE (BRIGHTFIELD) | CYSTINE (POLARIZED) |

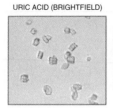 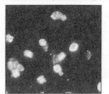 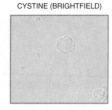

CRYSTALS FOUND IN ALKALINE URINE

| TRIPLE PHOSPHATE (BRIGHTFIELD) | AMMONIUM URATES (BRIGHTFIELD) |

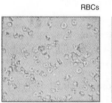 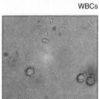

CRYSTALS FOUND IN ACID, NEUTRAL, AND ALKALINE URINE

| HIPPURIC ACID (BRIGHTFIELD) | CALCIUM OXALATE (BRIGHTFIELD) |

 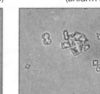

CELLS FOUND IN URINE

| RBCs | WBCs | RENAL TUBULAR & WBC (SEDI-STAIN) | RENAL TUBULAR | TRANSITIONAL | SQUAMOUS |

CASTS AND ARTIFACTS FOUND IN URINE

| GRANULAR | HYALINE | WBC CASTS | RBC CASTS |

BACTERIA, FUNGI, PARASITES FOUND IN URINE

| BACTERIA | YEAST | TRICHOMONAS VAGINALIS |

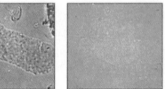 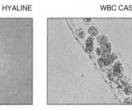 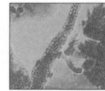
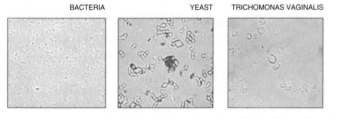

FIGURE 15–39 Crystals, cells, and casts found in urine sediment (Courtesy of Bayer Diagnostics.)

SPUTUM SPECIMENS

C Skills Menu:
- Collecting Specimens

Sputum specimens are sent to the laboratory for analysis of the secretions from the patient's lower respiratory tract. The patient is instructed to obtain the specimen from deeply coughing up the secretions from the bronchial tubes, the trachea, and the lungs into a sterile specimen container. Saliva and mucus from the mouth and nasal passages are not the desired secretions for the sputum analysis and interfere with the test results. The physician may wish to induce coughing in some patients to obtain the specimen in the medical office. Otherwise the patient should be instructed to collect the secretions at home. The patient must understand that the most productive cough will probably occur in the morning soon after waking. This specimen will be the most concentrated. Explain why it is important to follow directions in obtaining a sputum specimen and that the physician needs accurate information to make a diagnosis. Instruct the patient that this procedure will help identify certain

USA LABS
ID#

Referred by

Health Care Provider
Address
Phone

**DO NOT WRITE
IN THIS AREA**

C
H
A
I
N

O
F

C
U
S
T
O
D
Y

STEP 1 — TO BE COMPLETED BY EMPLOYER/COLLECTOR.
DONOR IDENTIFICATION—PLEASE PRINT

LAST NAME

FIRST NAME   M.I.

SOC. SEC. NO. _____ — _____ — _____

EMPLOYEE NO.

DONOR I.D. VERIFIED   ☐ PHOTO I.D.

☐ EMPLOYER REPRESENTATIVE

SIGNATURE OF EMPLOYER REP.

REASON FOR TEST (CHECK ONE)

☐ (1) PRE-EMPLOYMENT ☐ (2) POST ACCIDENT ☐ (3) RANDOM

☐ (4) PERIODIC ☐ (5) REASONABLE SUSPICION/CAUSE

☐ (6) RETURN TO DUTY

☐ (99) OTHER (SPECIFY)

TESTS REQUESTED: TOTAL TESTS ORDERED

SPECIMEN   ☐ Urine   ☐ Blood   (SUBMIT ONLY ONE SPECIMEN WITH EACH REQUISITION)

STEP 2—COLLECTOR, FOR URINE SPECIMENS, READ TEMPERATURE WITHIN FOUR MINUTES OF COLLECTION.
CHECK THE BOX IF TEMPERATURE IS WITHIN THE SPECIFIED RANGE ☐90°–100°F / 32°–38°C

OR RECORD ACTUAL TEMPERATURE HERE: _____

STEP 3—TO BE COMPLETED BY COLLECTOR.   COLLECTION SITE

COLLECTION DATE _____ TIME _____ ☐ AM PM _____
                                                        ADDRESS

REMARKS _____
                                                        CITY   STATE   ZIP
_____
                                                        ( )
                                                        PHONE

I certify that the specimen identified on this form is the specimen presented to me by the employee identified in Step 1 above, and was collected, labeled and sealed in the donor's presence.

COLLECTOR'S NAME PRINT (FIRST, M.I., LAST)   SIGNATUE OF COLLECTOR

STEP 4—TO BE INITIATED BY THE DONOR AND COMPLETED AS NECESSARY THEREAFTER.

PURPOSE OF CHANGE	RELEASED BY SIGNATURE	RECEIVED BY SIGNATURE	DATE
A. PROVIDE SPECIMEN FOR TESTING			
B. SHIPMENT TO LABORATORY			
C.			

COMMENTS:

Self-stick   identification
Labels for sealing specimen:

(123) (123) (123) (123)

SPECIMEN PACKAGE INTEGRITY WAS ☐ACCEPTABLE ☐UNACCEPTABLE WHEN RECEIVED IN LAB.

RECEIVER'S INITIALS

FOR OFFICE USE

FIGURE 15–40 Sample of a Chain of Custody form

PROCEDURE

15-15 Instruct Patient to Collect Sputum Specimen

PURPOSE: To instruct patients in collection of an adequate sputum specimen for laboratory analysis.

EQUIPMENT: Sputum specimen container and lid, label, pen, patient's chart, lab request form, note pad, rubber band, printed instruction sheet (optional).

PERFORMANCE OBJECTIVE: Provided with all necessary equipment and supplies and using other students as patients, demonstrate the steps of the procedure for instructing a patient in the collection of a sputum specimen for analysis. The instructor will observe each step.

1. Assemble items next to patient.

2. Write patient's name on specimen cup label, and complete lab request form.

3. Explain physician's orders to identified patient. Give printed instructions, or write out if you feel patient has a difficult time understanding you.

4. Instruct patient to remove lid from sterile specimen container and to expel secretions from a first morning coughing episode into the center of cup, being careful not to touch inside of cup. Container should not be more than half full.

5. Instruct patient not to allow saliva, tears, sweat, mucous from nose or mouth, or any other substance to enter cup. **NOTE: Secretions must be coughed up (expectorated) from lower respiratory tract (lungs, bronchial tubes, and trachea), or test will not be acceptable.**

6. When secretions have been obtained and cup sealed with its cover, patient should write time and date that it was obtained on label and lab request form and bring it to lab or medical office as soon as possible. **NOTE: If patient cannot bring specimen in within two hours after collection, it should be refrigerated.**

7. Secure completed lab request form to specimen container with a rubber band or tape. Send to lab. **NOTE: If patient prepares specimen at home, show patient how to do this.**

8. Record that instruction was given to patient in sputum collecting.

CHARTING EXAMPLE:

5-30-XX
Verbal and printed instructions for collection of sputum specimen given to Jaren.

J. Watkins, CMA (CL)

---

organisms that might not be diagnosed otherwise. Be sure to answer all questions about the process of obtaining the specimen.

The sterile specimen cup (usually a disposable cardboard or plastic container) should be prelabeled with the patient's name and other standard information. The patient should be instructed to fill in the time and date of the specimen and transport it to the medical office as soon as possible. The container should be no more than half full and securely sealed. If it will be more than an hour until the specimen is received by the lab, it should be refrigerated. Refer to Procedure 15–15.

PATIENT EDUCATION

When you are giving instructions to patients concerning the collection of sputum specimens, you may also want to advise them about health habits regarding the respiratory tract. Some of the areas you may want to remind them of are listed.

1. Advise patients not to smoke; give advice about stop-smoking programs.

2. Instruct patients to drink plenty of fluids, especially if they have a respiratory ailment.

3. Remind patients to help diminish transmission of viruses and other germs by using disposable paper products at home when a family member is sick.

4. Advise patients to wash hands often, especially when they are infected or when another family member is sick.

5. Urge them to take all the prescribed medication, as directed, for infections to avoid a recurrence of the illness.

6. Advise patients to get proper rest and diet to help them regain strength and resistance to disease.

BILL
☐ ACCOUNT
☐ PATIENT SEE ①
☐ 3RD PARTY SEE ②

PLEASE LEAVE BLANK
AREA ______
DEPT. ______
BILL CD ______

C-5 REQUEST FORM
INSTRUCTIONS ① FOR PATIENT BILLING, COMPLETE BOX A.
② FOR 3RD PARTY BILLING, COMPLETE BOX A AND FILL IN DIAGNOSIS, THEN EITHER B, C, or D.

USA Biomedical Labs
957 Central Avenue
Heartland, NY 11112

PATIENT NAME (LAST) (FIRST) | SPECIES | SEX | AGE YRS. MOS. | DATE COLLECTED MO. DAY YR. | TIME COLLECTED
PATIENT ADDRESS STREET | MISC. INFORMATION | DR. I.D. | **MEDICARE:** #
CITY STATE ZIP | DIAGNOSIS
PHYSICIAN | WELFARE: # | CASE NAME:
PROGRAM: | PATIENT 1ST NAME: | DATE OF BIRTH ALL CLAIMS MO. DAY YR.
INSURANCE GR. # | I.D. | SERVICE CODE:
SUBSCRIBER NAME: | RELATION: | PHONE

N5961

VIROLOGY

VIRUS ISOLATION

9325 ( ) GENERAL VIRUS
9326 ( ) INFLUENZA VIRUS
9327 ( ) HERPES SIMPLEX VIRUS
9328 ( ) CYTOMEGALOVIRUS

9329 ( ) CHLAMYDIA CULTURE
9330 ( ) ROTAVIRUS ANTIGEN SCREEN
9332 ( ) C DIFFICILE TOXIN SCREEN

CLINICAL INFORMATION

VIRUS SUSPECTED
SOURCE OF SPECIMEN ______
DATE COLLECTED ______
IS PATIENT PREGNANT YES ___ NO ___
PATIENT SYMPTOMS ______
EPIDEMIOLOGIC FACTORS ______
SIMILAR ILLNESS IN FAMILY ______
LOCAL EPIDEMICS ______
RECENT TRAVEL ______
ANIMAL CONTACT ______
IMMUNIZATION (SPECIFY TYPE AND DATE OF LAST DOSE)
POLIO ______ INFLUENZA ______ OTHER ______
MISCELLANEOUS INFORMATION

MICROBIOLOGY

SOURCE OF SPECIMEN ______

9219 ( ) ACID FAST CULTURE & SMEAR
9220 ( ) ACID FAST SMEAR ONLY
9245 ( ) ANAEROBIC CULTURE
9209 ( ) BETA STREP (A), FA
9214 ( ) BLOOD CULTURE
9226 ( ) FECES, FAT & MUSCLE FIBER
9225 ( ) FECES, OCCULT BLOOD
9309 ( ) FECES, OVA & PARASITES
9221 ( ) FUNGUS CULTURE
9204 ( ) FUNGUS, ID. COMPLETE
9222 ( ) FUNGUS, KOH PREP
9232 ( ) GENERAL CULTURE
9215 ( ) GONOCOCCUS CULTURE
9218 ( ) GRAM STAIN ONLY
9207 ( ) LEGIONELLA CULTURE
9228 ( ) PINWORM EXAM
9241 ( ) POST VASECTORY EXAM

9233 ( ) SALMONELLA & SHIGELLA SCREEN
9203 ( ) SPUTUM CULTURE
9227 ( ) STOOL, COMPREHENSIVE
9208 ( ) STREP SCREEN, THROAT
9202 ( ) UPPER RESPIRATORY TRACT CULTURE
9212 ( ) URINE, COMPREHENSIVE CULTURE
9213 ( ) URINE, SCREEN CULTURE
9234 ( ) UROGENITAL CULTURE

UNLISTED TESTS

ADDITIONAL CLINICAL INFORMATION

SENSITIVITIES ARE PERFORMED AS PART OF THE ROUTINE CULTURE AT NO ADDITIONAL CHARGE WHERE ORGANISMS ARE CONSIDERED PATHOGENIC. SENSITIVITIES ARE NOT PERFORMED ON NORMAL FLORA, ALPHA STREPTOCOCCUS, PNEUMOCOCCUS OR BETA STREPTOCOCCUS ROUTINELY.

(Rev. 1-84)

FOLD THIS FORM IN HALF SO TEST(S) ORDERED IS CLEARLY VISIBLE

FIGURE 15–41 Example of a laboratory request form for study in determining different types of microorganisms

Some sputum specimens require collection of secretions of the patient's productive coughing episodes over a period of 24 hours or up to 72 hours. In this case, the secretions will be placed in a larger container and must be refrigerated and appropriately labeled. The appropriate laboratory request form (Figure 15–41) must be completed with important information regarding the specimen and the patient and accompany the specimen to the lab for proper analysis.

The sputum specimen is analyzed for fungal infections, tuberculosis, and pneumonia. **Cancer** is detected from sputum by the Papanicolaou stain. This test requires a special request form identifying the source of the specimen (Figure 15–42). This specimen usually should be sent in the appropriate container with a 70% isopropyl alcohol solution. Always check with the laboratory manual or test directory for proper instructions or when you are not sure for accuracy of testing.

Stool Specimens

Stool specimens (**feces**) are probably the most difficult to instruct patients to obtain. There is a certain amount of embarrassment for both the patient and the medical assistant in regard to this procedure. Nevertheless, it is an extremely important specimen. Microbial organisms, ova, and **occult** (otherwise invisible and/or hidden) blood may be determined from careful examination of the fecal material.

Patients are instructed to obtain the stool specimen at home, usually within a few days of the request. For the pa-

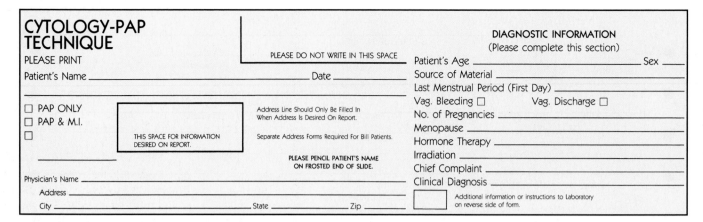

FIGURE 15–42 Example of cytology request form.

tient who has a daily bowel movement, this will be no problem. For patients who have difficulty with daily elimination, it may take a few days. Patients should use **laxatives** only by order of the physician. Straining during a bowel movement may cause hemorrhoids and is never recommended. You may suggest that the patient drink plenty of fluids to help avoid constipation. Refer to Procedure 15–16.

A very small amount of stool is required for laboratory tests. The patient is usually advised to use a tongue depressor or similar stick that can be disposed of to get a sample of stool (the size of a half dollar) from the toilet after a bowel movement. Female patients should be careful not to contaminate the specimen with urine or blood. The stool should be placed in a container that has been labeled

---

PROCEDURE

15-16 Instruct Patient to Collect Stool Specimen

PURPOSE: To instruct patients to obtain an adequate stool specimen for laboratory analysis.

EQUIPMENT: Specimen container with lid, lab request form, pen, patient's chart, label, rubber band, printed instructions (optional), tongue depressors, note pad.

PERFORMANCE OBJECTIVE: With all necessary equipment and supplies and using other students as patients, demonstrate the steps of the procedure for instructing a patient in collecting an adequate stool specimen for laboratory analysis. The instructor will observe each step.

1. Assemble items next to patient.

2. Write identifying information on request form and label (usually cover), and affix to specimen cup.

3. Identify patient and explain physician's orders. **RATIO-NALE: Speaking to the patient by name and checking chart ensures that you are performing the procedure on the correct patient.** Give printed instructions or write out if necessary.

4. Instruct patient to obtain a small amount of stool (about three or four tablespoons) from next bowel movement,

within next few days. Explain that nothing else should be placed in cup besides stool (no tissue paper, urine, and so on). Patients may defecate onto a paper plate and obtain a small specimen from plate, which is then discarded. Or, they may use a tongue depressor to obtain specimen from toilet bowl.

5. Instruct patient to place specimen in cup, secure cover tightly and write date and time specimen was obtained on cover of cup; then bring specimen to lab or medical office with request form as soon as possible. **NOTE: To prevent bacterial growth, specimen should be refrigerated if it cannot be received by lab within two hours.**

6. Record that the patient was given instructions.

CHARTING EXAMPLE:
5-30-XX
verbal and printed instructions to collect stool specimen given to Sarah

J. Watkins, CMA (CL)

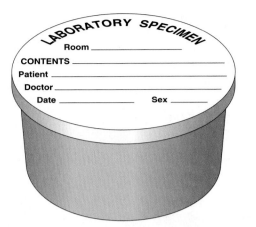

FIGURE 15–43 Laboratory stool specimen container with identification lid

with the date and time of collection (Figure 15–43). If the specimen cannot be taken directly to the lab or brought to the medical office, it may need to be refrigerated to prevent bacterial growth. Check with lab for instructions.

HEMOCCULT SENSA TESTS

Hemoccult sensa is the trademark for a **guaiac reagent** strip test used to detect the presence of occult blood (Figure 15–44). The test may detect bleeding in the digestive tract that is otherwise not detectable. It is a diagnostic aid in the detection of cancer of the colon. Hemoccult Sensa tests are usually given routinely to patients aged 40 and over, following a complete physical exam or if the patient's symptoms indicate their use. Hemoccult Sensa slides are recommended for both men and women who

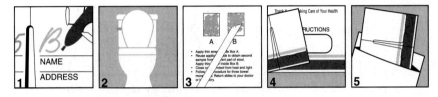

1. Remove slide from paper dispensing envelope. Using a ball-point pen, write your name, age, and address on the front of the slide. **Do not tear the sections apart.**
2. Fill in sample collection date on section 1 before a bowel movement. Flush toilet and allow to refill. You may use any clean, dry container to collect your sample. Collect sample before it contacts the toilet bowl water. Let stool fall into collection container.
3. Open front of section 1. Use one stick to collect a small sample. Apply a thin smear covering Box A. Collect second sample from different part of stool with same stick. Apply a thin smear covering Box B. Discard stick in a waste container. **DO NOT FLUSH STICK.**
4. Close and secure front flap of section 1 by inserting it under tab. Store slide in any paper envelope until the next day. **Important: This allows the sample to "air dry."**
5. Repeat steps 2-4 for the next two days, using sections 2 and 3. After completing the last section, store the slide overnight in any paper envelope to air dry.
   The next day, remove slide from the paper envelope and place in the Mailing Pouch, if provided. Seal pouch carefully and **immediately return to your doctor or laboratory.**
   Note: Current U.S. Postal Regulations prohibit mailing completed slides in any standard paper envelope.

IMPORTANT NOTE: Follow the procedure exactly as outlined above. Always develop the test, read the results, interpret them and make a decision as to whether the fecal specimen is positive or negative for occult blood BEFORE you develop the Performance Monitors®. Do not apply Developer to Performance Monitors® before interpreting test results. Any blue originating from the Performance Monitors® should be ignored in the reading of the specimen test results.

READING AND INTERPRETATION OF THE HEMOCCULT® TEST
the world's leading test for fecal occult blood

Negative Smears*

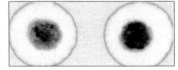

Sample report: negative
No detectable blue on or at the edge of the smears indicates the test is negative for occult blood.
(See **LIMITATIONS OF PROCEDURE.**)

Negative and Positive Smears*   **Positive Smears***

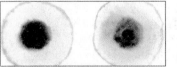   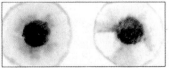

Sample report: positive
Any trace of blue on or at the edge of one or more of the smears indicates the test is positive for occult blood.

FIGURE 15–44 Hemoccult Sensa test (Courtesy of Beckman Coulter, Inc.)

have a personal or family history of colorectal cancer, polyps, or ulcerative colitis. It is also advised as a screening for people who have a personal history of inflammatory bowel disease. Bleeding may be caused by peptic ulcers, hemorrhoids, polyps, and other conditions of the bowel tract. It can also be an early symptom of cancer of the colon. This test was designed to help detect hidden blood in the stool early enough for corrective measures to be taken. Because cancer of the colon is one of the leading cancer killers in the United States, it makes sense to follow the simple, easy-to-use screening test that could help save one's life. Instruct patients how to collect specimens at home and to return them in the double-layered, leak-proof mailing envelope as soon as possible; otherwise people have a tendency to forget.

The Hemoccult Sensa test is easy to complete. It requires proper lighting to compare the color change of the reagent paper to the control. Two drops of developer are applied to each stool smear, A and B, and one drop to the control area. If the test area turns blue as compared to the positive control, then the Hemoccult Sensa is reported as positive. Further studies will then be ordered by the physician to determine where in the colon the bleeding is occurring. See Procedure 15–17.

Intestinal bleeding may be intermittent (not all the time). Giving the patient three slides with smears of two sections of stool for each increases the detection of the presence of blood in the bowel tract. Ask patients to carefully follow instructions printed on the envelope.

ACHIEVE UNIT OBJECTIVES

Complete Chapter 15, Unit 4, in the workbook to help you obtain competency of this subject matter.

A CAAHEP CONNECTION

This unit discussed instruction in various body fluid specimen collection. The areas included in the Medical Assistant curriculum are *Anatomy and physiology, Medical terminology, Psychology, Communication, Clinical procedures,* and *Medical law and ethics.*

PROCEDURE

15-17 Perform a Hemoccult Sensa Test

PURPOSE: To determine the presence of occult blood in the stool.

OSHA GUIDELINES: To comply with Standard Precautions, gloves must be worn if there is any possibility of coming into contact with blood or any body fluids.

EQUIPMENT: Hemoccult Sensa slide(s) prepared by patient, developer, timer or timepiece, patient's chart, pen, biohazard bag, latex or vinyl gloves.

PERFORMANCE OBJECTIVE: Provided with all necessary equipment and supplies and using samples obtained from own stool, demonstrate each step in the Hemoccult Sensa testing procedure.

1. a. Wash hands and assemble items needed for testing on counter.
   b. Put on gloves.
2. Open test side of Hemoccult Sensa paper slide.
3. Remove cap from bottle of developer.
4. Place two drops of developer on each of the sections of reagent paper slide: A, B.

5. Immediately begin timing for one minute. At 30 seconds, watch closely for any change of color which may be developing. Read at 60 seconds.
6. Compare test with control color and read results.
7. Place one drop of developer between positive and negative control. Read within 10 seconds.
8. a. Discard test in biohazardous bag.
   b. Remove gloves and wash hands.
9. Record test results on patient's chart and log sheet as either positive or negative, and sign. **NOTE: Positive reading means that there is occult blood in the stool. Negative means that no occult blood is present. If first slide is negative and second and third are positive, record as:**

CHARTING EXAMPLE:
7-24-XX
Hemoccult Sensa slides: 1. neg
2. pos
3. pos

J. Watkins, CMA (CL)

Instructing patients in the collection of stool specimens is a good opportunity to give helpful advice in regard to bowel problems. The following is a list of suggestions for discussion with patients.

1. Advise patients to drink plenty of fluids to help reduce the incidence of constipation.
2. Urge patients to refrain from using laxatives, enemas, or suppositories unless specifically ordered by the physician.
3. Instruct patients regarding straining during a bowel movement, which could cause hemorrhoids (and other problems). Sitting or standing for prolonged periods can also be a factor in the development of hemorrhoids.
4. Remind patients that a change in bowel habits should be reported to the physician.
5. Advise patients that a proper well-balanced diet (from the food guide pyramid), consistent meal times, and exercise are the best way toward regularity regarding bowel habits.
6. Remind patients to wash hands with soap and water before *and* after the bathroom each time to avoid spreading germs.

UNIT 5

Bacterial Smears and Cultures

OBJECTIVES

Upon completion of the unit, meet the following performance objectives by verifying knowledge of the facts and principles presented through oral and written communication at a level deemed competent. Demonstrate the specific behaviors as identified in the performance objectives of the procedures, observing all aseptic and safety precautions in accordance with health care standards.

1. Spell and define, using the glossary at the back of the text, all the **Words to Know** in this unit.
2. Obtain a smear for bacteriological examination.
3. Heat-fix a smear for staining.
4. Explain the reason for heat-fixing specimens.
5. Complete a Gram's stain.
6. List common diseases caused by gram-positive and gram-negative bacteria.
7. Obtain a throat culture and streak on agar plate.

8. Describe growth media for cultures.
9. Label specimens for analysis.
10. Record information concerning specimens on the patient's chart.

AREAS OF COMPETENCE (AAMA)

This unit addresses content within the specific competency areas of *Fundamental principles, Diagnostic orders, Patient care, Professionalism, Communication skills, Legal concepts,* and *Operational functions,* as identified in the Medical Assistant Role Delineation Study. Refer to Appendix A for a detailed listing of the areas.

WORDS TO KNOW

agar	gram-positive
exudate	microscopic
gram-negative	

The possibility of disease transmission is extremely high in handling any type of specimen, especially those of patients suspected of having infections. Proper handwashing and sterile technique must be used at all times to break the cycle of the infection. Eating, drinking, chewing gum, smoking, and any other hand-to-mouth gesture should be avoided to prevent possible self-contamination. Any items used must be carefully washed or properly disposed of to prevent others from becoming infected. Disposable items are almost exclusively used in medical practice today for this reason.

BACTERIOLOGICAL SMEAR

C Main Menu:
Infection Control
Skills Menu:
■ Hand Washing
■ Collecting Specimens
■ Wound Specimens

Identification of microorganisms that cause disease is accomplished by obtaining a smear or a culture from the area of the body that appears to be infected. To make a smear, a sample of the **exudate** (drainage) is taken from the throat, mouth, ear, eye, nose, vagina, anus, the surface of the skin, or from within a wound by introducing a sterile cotton swab into the area (Figure 15–45). The swab is then rolled over two-thirds of a frosted-end slide (Figure 15–46). The smear is air dried at room temperature and then *heat-fixed* (Figure 15–47). This seals the specimen to the glass so that it will not wash off during the staining process.

After preparation of a bacteriologic smear, determination of the microorganism causing the infection must be

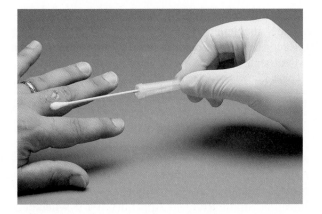

FIGURE 15–45 Use a sterile swab to obtain a specimen from a wound.

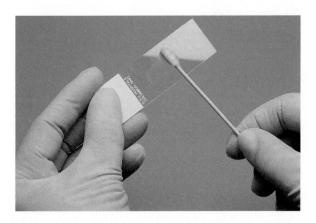

FIGURE 15–46 Apply the specimen onto the glass slide by rolling the swab from left to right, covering two-thirds of the area.

made by the physician. Your role is that of obtaining and preparing the smear (see Procedure 15–18).

CULTURING

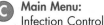

Main Menu:
Infection Control

Skills Menu:
- Hand Washing
- Sterile Gloves and Gowns
- Removing Contaminated Items

Culturing is a means of isolating a disease-causing microorganism for identification. It takes far longer than a bacteriologic smear but is still a relatively simple procedure. A specimen is obtained and placed in a culture medium, which contains nutrients comparable to human tissue to encourage growth of microorganisms. The medium is **agar**, a gelatinlike substance, mixed with sheep's blood or other nutrients.

Explain to the patient that a throat culture is necessary to identify certain organisms. Be sure to tell the patient that there might be some momentary discomfort in obtaining the specimen, and answer all questions about the process of obtaining the specimen. Refer to Procedure 15–19. The specimen is taken directly from the affected area of the patient with a sterile swab and distributed over the agar in a Petri dish of clear plastic, using the pattern shown in Figure 15–48. Many cultures are streaked with a fine-wire loop (pictured in the foreground of Figure 15–47), which is sterilized by flame to prevent cross-contamination when distributing the specimen. The culture plate is then placed

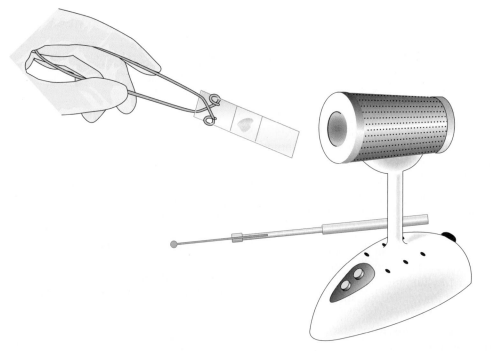

FIGURE 15–47 Heat-fix the specimen onto the glass slide (in the forefront of this photo is the wire loop used to streak agar plates).

PROCEDURE

15-18 Prepare Bacteriological Smear

PURPOSE: To adhere a specimen to a glass slide for examination under the microscope.

OSHA GUIDELINES: To comply with Standard Precautions, gloves must be worn if there is any possibility of coming into contact with blood or any body fluids.

EQUIPMENT: Specimen (on labeled cotton swab), disposable gloves, clean frosted-end glass slide, forceps, Bunsen burner, matches, slide staining rack, pencil, pen, patient's chart, (if sent to outside lab: slide holder, lab request form, rubber band or tape).

PERFORMANCE OBJECTIVE: With all necessary equipment and supplies provided, demonstrate the steps of the procedure for preparing a bacteriological smear for microscopic analysis. The instructor will observe each step.

1. Wash hands and put on latex or vinyl gloves. Assemble all needed items on counter space. Pencil patient's name on frosted end of glass slide. Complete lab request form, including source of specimen.

2. Prepare as many smears of specimen as ordered by physician by rolling cotton swab evenly over two-thirds of glass slide, holding slide with thumb and great finger.

3. Light Bunsen burner or other source for flame and adjust to a blue flame. **RATIONALE: Blue flame is hottest.**

4. Hold frosted part of slide with your thumb and index finger or with forceps and pass specimen portion of slide through blue part of flame, smear slide up, slowly (taking about two seconds) two or three times. Avoid burning yourself. **RATIONALE: The yellow portion must be avoided as it leaves carbon deposits on slide, obscuring visualization. NOTE: Excessive heating will destroy specimen.** Turn Bunsen burner or other source off.

5. Place heat-fixed smear on staining rack to cool for staining procedure or place on microscope stage for observation by physician.

6. Discard used disposables and return other items to proper storage area. Remove disposable gloves and discard in the proper receptacle. Wash hands.

PATIENT EDUCATION

As you obtain throat cultures from patients, you may want to give them some helpful advice concerning their condition. Generally, when a person has a sore throat, it is associated with other respiratory symptoms as well. The following suggestions may provide some relief from discomfort and help them toward better health.

1. Advise patients to drink plenty of liquids (fruit juices) and to eat sensibly from the basic food groups.
2. Urge patients to get extra rest and dress comfortably (according to the weather/temperature outside).
3. Suggest use of gargles or throat lozenges (or both) to relieve painful sore throat.
4. Remind them to avoid tobacco/smoking.
5. Instruct them to cough/sneeze into tissue and discard into proper waste container wherever they are to prevent the spread of germs.
6. Remind them not to eat or drink after others and to use disposables at home when there is illness.

in an incubator for 24 to 48 hours to provide the proper temperature for bacterial growth. (Note: Make sure you check the incubator for proper temperature setting.) Many physicians in pediatrics, general, and family practice obtain, incubate, and read their own cultures, not only for the patient's convenience, but for their own.

The Petri dish must be properly labeled for identification purposes. This includes the patient's name, the date and time the specimen was taken, and the source of the specimen. This information should be written on the bottom of the Petri dish with a wax crayon or label.

Petri plates and other types of transport media for culturing specimens should be prepared according to the outside laboratory's directions. The culture media are disposable and should be discarded in securely tied biohazardous plastic bags in the proper receptacle.

GRAM'S STAINING

Main Menu:
Infection Control

Skills Menu:
- Hand Washing
- Sterile Gloves and Gowns
- Removing Contaminated Items

PROCEDURE

15-19 Obtain a Throat Culture

PURPOSE: To isolate a disease-causing organism to determine effective treatment of the patient.

OSHA GUIDELINES: To comply with Standard Precautions, gloves must be worn if there is any possibility of coming into contact with blood or any body fluids.

EQUIPMENT: Culture plate (Petri dish), sterile cotton swabs, sterile tongue depressor, disposable gloves, pen, patient's chart, penlight (optional), wax crayon or label for culture plate (if sent to outside lab, request form and label for culture plate, clear tape, tissues).

PERFORMANCE OBJECTIVE: Provided with all necessary equipment and supplies, and using a lifelike clinical doll infant or small child under close supervision or other students as patients, demonstrate the steps required to perform the procedure for obtaining a throat culture. The instructor will observe each step.

1. Assemble needed items near identified patient. Label culture plate and complete request form if required. Wash hands and put on gloves.

2. Identify patient. **RATIONALE: Speaking to the patient by name and checking chart ensures that you are performing the procedure on the correct patient.**

3. Explain procedure to patient, and assist patient to comfortable position. Sitting is usual position for adults. It may be easier to work with children if they are lying down. Assistance may be necessary.

   NOTE: If you must obtain a throat culture from a small child or infant without assistance, it may prove easier if you sit with child on your lap. Place child's right arm under your left arm. Hold child's left wrist with your left hand and cradle head between your left wrist and left shoulder. This will free your right hand to obtain specimen. Encourage mouth to open. With your right hand, hold swab securely, quickly insert it, and swab back of throat with a rolling motion. (Insert swab at corner of mouth behind teeth to prevent child from biting it.) Use flexible swabs (wooden stick swabs may break if bitten, and splintering is a danger when working with small children or infants). Touch only back of throat.**

4. Open sterile swab, and ask patient to open mouth as wide as possible. Quickly examine with light source.

5. Depress tongue with sterile tongue depressor held in one hand. Hold sterile swab in other. Ask patient to say "ah" to assist depression of tongue (this also prevents patient from feeling gag reflex by diverting attention). Quickly insert swab into back of throat and roll over at least two areas, touching areas with obvious exudate.

6. Remove swab and depressor from patient's mouth. **NOTE: Some physicians order a nasopharyngeal culture (NPC) in which a specimen is obtained from the nasal passages and throat. This is accomplished by inserting a sterile swab into nasal cavities (one for each nostril) and applying each to culture plate, or into a transport media if sent to a lab** (Figure 15–49). Attend to patient, offer tissues. Tearing may result from procedure.

7. Immediately apply specimen to agar in Petri dish, smearing it as shown in Figure 15–50 or place swab into container for transportation to lab. Tape request form securely.

8. Place identification label on bottom of Petri dish, or write patient's name, date, time, and source on bottom with wax crayon. Secure cover with clear tape.

9. Discard all disposable items in proper receptacle. Place culture in incubator agar side up. **RATIONALE: The growth of microorganisms releases moisture that collects on cover and will drip onto agar, drowning microorganisms if agar is on bottom** (Figure 15–51).

10. Remove gloves and wash hands.

11. Record procedure on patient's chart and initial.

The purpose of Gram's staining is to make heat-fixed bacteria visible for **microscopic** identification (Figure 15–52). The two most common divisions of bacteria are **gram-positive** and **gram-negative**. The infectious diseases most commonly caused by these bacteria are:

- *Gram-positive bacteria:* botulism, diphtheria, lobar pneumonia, rheumatic fever, staph infection, streptococcal sore throat, tetanus

- *Gram-negative bacteria:* bacillary dysentery, cholera, gonorrhea, meningitis, pertussis, plague, typhoid fever, most UTIs

Bacteria have certain characteristic formations and are identified by their size and shape. Cocci appear in clusters. Staphylococci form grapelike clusters. Bacteria that form pairs are called diplococci. Those that form chains are streptococci. Bacteria with capsule-like coverings are called spore-forming.

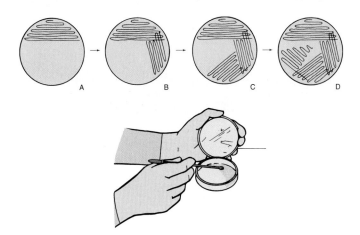

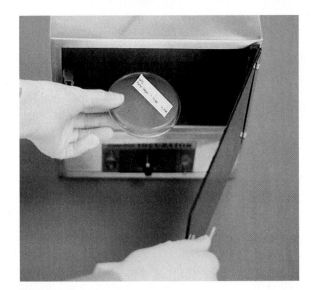

FIGURE 15–48 Pattern for smearing an agar plate with a specimen using a wire loop. Notice the rotation of the plate in a counter-clockwise pattern.

FIGURE 15–51 Place the culture plate in the incubator, agar side up. To identify the culture plate, the label should be placed on the agar side.

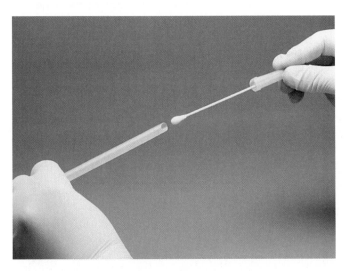

FIGURE 15–49 Place swab with specimen into transport container with culture media for laboratory analysis.

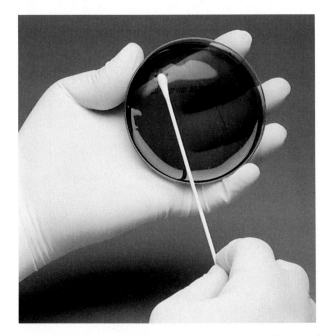

FIGURE 15–50 Smear culture plate with specimen from swab. Refer also to Figure 15–49.

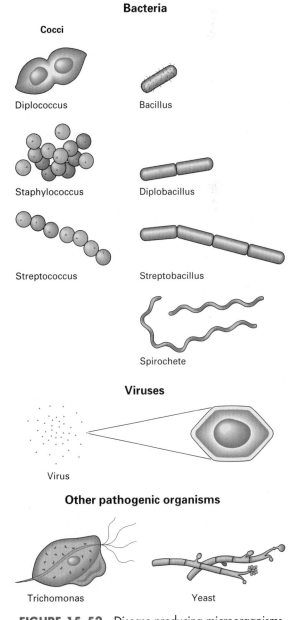

Bacteria

Cocci

Diplococcus

Bacillus

Staphylococcus

Diplobacillus

Streptococcus

Streptobacillus

Spirochete

Viruses

Virus

Other pathogenic organisms

Trichomonas

Yeast

FIGURE 15–52 Disease producing microorganisms

15-20 Prepare Gram's Stain

PURPOSE: To stain a heat-fixed bacteriological smear for microscopic identification.

OSHA GUIDELINES: To comply with Standard Precautions, gloves must be worn if there is any possibility of coming into contact with blood or any body fluids.

EQUIPMENT: Heat-fixed slide (frosted end labeled), slide rack and tray, crystal (or gentian) violet dye, water wash bottle, forceps, Gram's iodine, alcohol (or acetone), safranine solution (or dilute fuchsin), timer or timepiece, immersion oil, microscope with light source, pen, patient's chart, pencil, cover glass slides, eyedroppers, paper towels; disposable latex or vinyl gloves and plastic apron (optional).

PERFORMANCE OBJECTIVE: Provided with all necessary equipment and supplies, demonstrate the steps in the procedure for preparing a Gram's stain. The instructor will observe each step.

1. Assemble all needed items on counter and wash hands. **NOTE: Apron and disposable gloves are to be used; put them on now.**

2. Place heat-fixed slide on staining rack, specimen side up, over tray. **NOTE: Recap all solutions immediately after each use to avoid accidents.**

3. Open crystal violet (gentian) dye and fill dropper. Apply over entire specimen area of the slide, and time for 60 seconds (Figure 15–53).

4. Hold frosted end of slide with forceps or thumb and index finger, and tip slide to allow stain to run off into tray. Wash slide with water, letting flow begin at top and run down.

5. Place slide flat on rack. Fill dropper with Gram's iodine and apply over entire specimen. Leave on for 60 seconds. Tilt slide to allow iodine to run off into tray.

6. Wash slide with water, tilting to direct runoff into tray, and replace flat on rack.

7. Apply alcohol (or acetone) with dropper for a few seconds until purple color in excess runoff is gone.

8. Tilt slide and wash with water immediately. Return flat to rack.

9. Apply safranine solution with dropper to counterstain specimen, and wash off with water immediately.

10. Hold slide by frosted end, and wipe excess solutions from back. Tap side of slide onto paper towel to help remove excess liquid. Allow slide to air dry. **NOTE: Slide may be blotted between paper towels, but be careful not to rub slide or specimen may be destroyed.**

11. Apply small drop of immersion oil to specimen, and place on microscope stage to view under oil-immersion objective. Ask physician to observe and read the Gram's-stained slide. (Turn light on to view and turn off when finished.) A slide cover may be used to help preserve specimen for future viewing.

12. Discard disposables, wash used items, and return items to proper storage. Wash hands.

13. Record procedure and results on patient's chart and on log sheet and sign.

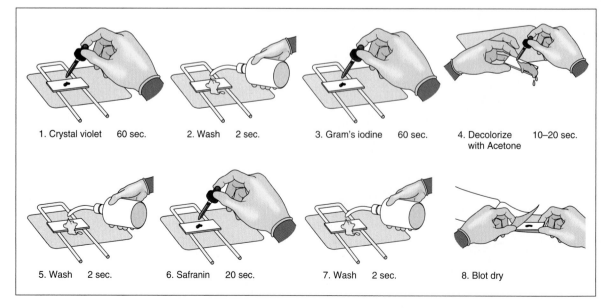

1. Crystal violet   60 sec.   2. Wash   2 sec.   3. Gram's iodine   60 sec.   4. Decolorize   10–20 sec. with Acetone

5. Wash   2 sec.   6. Safranin   20 sec.   7. Wash   2 sec.   8. Blot dry

FIGURE 15–53   Gram's staining procedure

TABLE 15–4

SOME IMPORTANT PATHOGENIC BACTERIA AND THEIR REACTION TO THE GRAM'S STAIN

Gram-Positive Reaction (+) (Reaction of Purple Stain)		Gram-Negative Reaction (−) (Loss of Purple Stain)		Gram-Variable Reaction (+/−)	
Bacterium	Disease It Causes	Bacterium	Disease It Causes	Bacterium	Disease It Causes
Bacillus anthracis	Anthrax	Bordetella pertussis	Whooping cough	Mycobacterium leprae	Leprosy
Clostridium botulinum	Botulism (food poisoning)	Brucella abortus (bovine strain)	Infectious abortion in cattle and undulant fever in man	Mycobacterium tuberculosis	Tuberculosis
Clostridum perfringens	Gas gangrene, wound infection	Brucella melitensis (goat strain)			
Clostridium tetani	Tetanus (lockjaw)	Brudella suis (porcine strain)			
Corynebacterium diphtheriae	Diphtheria	Escherichia coli	Urinary infections		
Staphylococcus aureus	Carbuncles, furunculosis (boils), pneumonia, septicemia	Haemophilus influenzae	Meningitis, pneumonia		
Streptococcus pyogenes	Erysipelas, rheumatic fever, scarlet fever, septicemia, strep throat, tonsillitis	Neisseria gonorrhoeae	Gonorrhea		
		Neisseria meningitidis	Nasopharyngitis, meningitis		
Streptococcus pneumoniae	Pneumonia	Pseudomonas aeruginosa	Respiratory and uro-genital infections		
		Rickettsia rickettsii	Rocky mountain spotted fever		
		Salmonella paratyphi	Food poisoning, paratyphoid fever		
		Salmonella typhi	Typhoid fever		
		Shigella dysenteriae	Dysentery		
		Treponema pallidum	Syphilis		
		Vibrio cholerae	Cholera		
		Yersinia pestis	Plague		

Gram-positive bacteria take a violet (purple) color from the Gram's stain procedure. Gram-negative bacteria take a red or pink color from the counterstain. Without the staining process, the bacteria are colorless. In preparing the slide, you should avoid getting the crystal (or gentian) violet dye on the hands, clothing, or counter because it is difficult (sometimes impossible) to remove. Alcohol and acetone are helpful in removing the dye in some cases. Refer to Procedure 15–20 for steps to prepare a Gram's stain.

Refer to Table 15–4 for examples of how different bacteria stain the particular color of purple (positive) or pink (negative).

ACHIEVE UNIT OBJECTIVES

Complete Chapter 15, Unit 5, in the workbook to help you obtain competency of this subject matter.

Medical-Legal-Ethical Scenario

Dr. Long asked Judy to draw a Lipid Profile on Mr. Peterson. She went to the room to get everything ready for the draw and realized that there were no gloves in her size in the storage cupboard. Because Judy was running behind already, and she thought Mr. Peterson seemed to be a good person, she went ahead and drew the blood tubes without wearing gloves. Mr. Peterson chatted while she was drawing the blood tubes and mentioned that he had just broken up with his wife a month ago but that he already had a new girlfriend.

CRITICAL THINKING CHALLENGE

1. What was Judy's thinking when she realized there were no gloves in the room?
2. What should she have done?
3. Why was she in such a hurry?

4. How do you think she felt when she realized that she could have been at risk?
5. Should the doctor be notified?
6. What would you have done in this situation?

RELATING TO ABHES

Chapter 15 discusses the parts and use of the microscope; obtaining and testing of blood, urine, sputum, and stool specimens; and the obtaining and preparation of material for smears and cultures. This content is related to the ABHES accreditation requirements of *Orientation, Urinalysis, Hematology, Basic blood chemistries, HIV/AIDS and blood borne pathogens,* and *OSHA compliance rules and regulations* within the content area of **Medical Laboratory Procedures.**

A CAAHEP CONNECTION

This unit discussed instruction in various culture specimen collection. The areas included in the Medical Assistant curriculum are *Anatomy and physiology, Medical terminology, Psychology, Communication, Clinical procedures,* and *Medical law and ethics.*

RESOURCES

Heller M. and Krebs C. (1997). Clinical handbook for health care professionals. Clifton Park, NY: Delmar Learning.

Kovanda, B.M. (1998). Multiskilling: Point of care testing: capillary puncture for the health care professional. Clifton Park, NY: Delmar Learning.

WEB LINKS

http://www.fda.gov/cdrh/clia **(Clinical Laboratory Improvements Amendments)**

Provides information on quality standards for all laboratory testing.

Diagnostic Tests, X-Rays, and Procedures

Diagnostic tests, x-rays, and procedures will be discussed in this chapter. The medical assistant has a multiple role in these diagnostic aids. You will be responsible for instructing and preparing patients for procedures, tests, and x-rays. In some cases, you will either carry out the test(s) or procedure(s) or assist the primary care physician. After completion, you will alert the physician of the results, and from the order of the doctor, notify the patient. Then, you will file the report of the results in the patient's chart.

Often, as a part of the CPE, the physician may order certain tests or other procedures (e.g., chest x-ray, mammography, intravenous pyelogram). If these diagnostic tests are performed on site, the results may often be determined while the patient is still present. If referrals must be made for diagnostic tests and so on, patients may be asked to return within a week to 10 days for a final report of the findings. This gives the medical assistant and the physician time to gather reports in the patient's chart for review and evaluation. You may want to advise the patient to bring a list of his concerns so he will not forget to ask necessary questions. This practice may reduce the number of phone consultations required.

UNIT 1

Diagnostic Tests

▮ OBJECTIVES

Upon completion of the unit, meet the following performance objectives by verifying knowledge of the facts and principles presented through oral and written communication at a level deemed competent. Demonstrate the specific behaviors as identified in the performance objectives of the procedures, observing all aseptic and safety precautions in accordance with health care standards.

1. Spell and define, using the glossary at the back of the text, all the **Words to Know** in this unit.
2. Describe scratch, patch, and intradermal skin tests; state their purpose; and perform each test under supervision.
3. Describe the schedule and instructions for administering allergy injections.
4. Describe patient education concerning allergies and treatment.

AREAS OF COMPETENCE (AAMA)

This unit addresses content within the specific competency areas of *Fundamental principles, Diagnostic orders, Patient care, Professionalism, Communication skills, Legal concepts,* and *Instruction,* as identified in the Medical Assistant Role Delineation Study. Refer to Appendix A for a detailed listing of the areas.

▮ WORDS TO KNOW

adrenalin	histamine
adverse	hypersensitive
anaphylactic	immune
antibody	interpret
antigen	mock
contact dermatitis	obsolete
desensitizing	systemic
eosinophil	venom
epinephrine	wheal
extract	

SKIN TESTS

Three procedures are commonly used to determine allergic reactions in patients. They are the scratch, intradermal, and patch tests. The physician determines the diagnosis by evaluating the results of the tests along with the patient's medical history, physical exam, and other laboratory tests. The medical assistant may assist the physi-

cian in performing these tests or may perform them by order of the physician. Tests should always be performed under the direct supervision of the physician.

The tests involve introducing an **antigen** directly into the patient's skin to induce a reaction. If the reaction is negative (normal), there will be no change in the appearance of the skin following testing. A normal **immune** reaction occurs in the body when an antigen and **antibody** unite and the foreign substance is excreted by the body.

A positive allergic reaction to a test is shown by a raised area on the skin, much like a mosquito bite, called a **wheal** (hive). This is caused by interaction of the antigen and antibody, which releases **histamine** and is termed a **hypersensitive** reaction. Histamine is naturally produced by the body to attach itself to certain cells to cause dilation of blood vessels and contraction of smooth muscles. Most cells release histamine during allergic reactions. As a part of the normal inflammatory response of the body, histamine protects tissue against injury (the scratch test), and it is the reason that redness and a wheal are produced. The inflammatory response of the body is specific in that it is the whole body's defense against infection, chemicals, or other physical factors.

Besides histamine, researchers are still finding that other chemicals are released during the allergic response. Millions of people have allergies to a variety of substances, including certain foods, pollens, dust, drugs (medications), chemicals, **venom** of stinging insects, animal dander, molds, pollutants, and other allergens. In addition to the allergy causing substances mentioned, there are some that are not so well known. It is very important to realize that cockroaches and their egg casing and fecal matter are major sources of allergens in large cities. The extermination of these roaches is of concern because the chemicals that can eliminate them can cause serious problems for those who have allergies and respiratory diseases. Asthma patients are most sensitive to these sprays and other methods of getting rid of the roaches. The allergen is still there even after the roaches are killed. Thorough cleaning is necessary to rid the home of the allergen as much as possible after extermination has been completed. Advising patients of the risks is extremely important. Often there is a family member or friend who will allow the patient to stay at their home while the treatment is being done to rid the home of insects.

Certain irritants can make allergies worse. These irritants can be caused by smoke (from campfires and tobacco products), paint fumes, perfumes, insect sprays, gasoline, cleaning materials, and personal grooming products (hair sprays, soaps, lotions, etc.). Sensitivity to these irritants is most likely to cause a problem for those who have allergies. The best advice for such patients is to avoid being around these substances. Reaction to these substances ranges from slight to severe. Severe reactions can be life-threatening. A life-threatening reaction must be counteracted with an injection of **adrenalin** immediately to prevent **anaphylactic** shock. Symptoms of anaphylactic shock initially include intense anxiety, weakness, sweating, and shortness of breath. Symptoms may continue to include hypotension, shock, arrhythmia, respiratory congestion, laryngeal edema, nausea, and diarrhea.

For example, those who have known allergies to the venom of stinging insects or to certain foods that produce intense life-threatening allergic reactions are instructed to carry an anaphylactic shock kit with them at all times. The kit contains a self-injecting dose of adrenalin for emergency use. Instruct patients with food allergies to read the contents (ingredients) on all labels of foods and over the counter medications to avoid adverse reactions. Herbal remedies, when combined with prescribed medications and foods, can produce health risks. Check with the pharmacist before taking such combinations of off-the-shelf medicines and prescriptions from your physician. It is also a good practice to advise patients to ask the server or the dinner host about the contents of some foods on the menu, such as soups, breads, and deserts. Some of these foods may contain ingredients that may result in an allergic reaction to those who are sensitive to these substances. You may also want to inform these patients, if they do not already wear them, to get a medic alert bracelet or necklace. These are very helpful in the event that a medical emergency occurs; the medic alert tag informs others of their condition if they are not able to speak or if they are found unconscious.

Treatment for many allergy patients consists of an allergy immunotherapy program. Over a considerable period, which can be indefinite, this therapy gradually provides immunization against the substance that the person is allergic to. Increasing amounts of the allergen are injected as long as the patient can tolerate each dose. Treatment generally takes a few years. It is usually effective in reducing symptoms of most allergies. Often patients bring their serum from the allergy specialist to the family doctor's office or clinic for administration. All allergy serum should be refrigerated unless otherwise specified. These **desensitizing** injections of allergy serum (which patients refer to as "allergy shots") should always be administered under the direct supervision of a physician because anaphylactic shock can occur within seconds even in unsuspecting individuals. Following any injection, the patient must be observed for 20 minutes for possible reaction. Any reaction or unusual symptom must be reported to the physician and noted on the patient's chart and on the schedule sheet accompanying the allergy serum. An example of this schedule is shown in Figure 16–1.

Company's Name
(maker of serum)

Physician's Name/Allergist
Address and Phone Number

Patient's Name   Lot Number of Serum
Account Number   Expiration Date

INSTRUCTIONS FOR ADMINISTRATION

—Preparations should always be made for physician to treat anaphylaxis should it occur.
—Patients who are being treated with beta-blocker medications should not be given allergy serum.
—Use 27G one-half inch needle.
—Administer three-eighths to one-half inch into subcutaneous tissue between deltoid and biceps muscle (but not into the muscle).
—Aspirate plunger of syringe to ensure needle is not in a blood vessel.
—Reschedule patient for injection if he or she is feverish or is wheezing.
—Observe patient for possible reaction for 20 minutes following injection.
—Administer cold packs on site if local redness, itching, or wheal develops—alert physician for administration of antihistamine PRN.
—If a systemic or general reaction occurs, such as hives, sneezing or wheezing, alert physician for dosage and administration of epinephrine (subcutaneous).
—**Contact allergist for rescheduling instructions if systemic reaction occurs.**

SCHEDULE

Administer allergy serum injections every _____ days. If no adverse reaction occurs, resume scheduled dose. If adverse local reaction occurs, resume schedule with the last well-tolerated dose. Proceed with the following schedule until maximum dose is reached and well-tolerated. Then repeat maximum dose tolerated until vial is empty.

Dose	Date Administered	Adverse Reaction
0.10 cc	month/day/year	type of reaction
0.15 cc	initials of one who	if any (note the
0.20 cc	administered the	severity and
0.30 cc	injection	symptoms of
0.40 cc	and which arm	the patient)
0.50 cc	was injected	
*0.50 cc	Rt or L	

*Reorder before last dose is administered. Allow two weeks for delivery.

FIGURE 16–1 Example of schedule and instructions for allergy serum injections

Because patients generally continue this therapy once a week (or even more frequently) over a few years, it is wise to change the injection sites frequently. A practical method of keeping a record of where the allergy serum is injected each time is by alternating arms and numbering the injection sites. This pattern allows up to 18 injection sites, and then it can be repeated. This may help in preventing tissue damage from recurring frequent injections of the same area. Keep track of the pattern on the schedule that comes with the allergy serum, or in the patient's chart by recording which arm, the number of the injection site, and of course, the date and your initials.

Figure 16–2 shows an illustration of (A) a suggested clockwise pattern and (B) charting method. Refer to Chapter 18 for the procedure for administering injections.

The size of the wheal is **interpreted** by the physician after a timed 20- to 30-minute period. Wheals are measured in centimeters by using a tape measure or by comparison (Figure 16–3). A trained skin tester may observe the reaction and make an interpretation by inspection alone.

Extracts of substances that are commonly the cause of allergy in patients are manufactured in applicator bottles. These should be refrigerated and the expiration date noted for accurate test results. Many of the skin testing extracts vary in strength from one company to another. Because specific allergens may also differ geographically, skin tests are sometimes unreliable. Standardization would be helpful. New methods are being researched, and skin testing may one day become an **obsolete** procedure.

Scratch Test

Desirable sites for the scratch test are the arms and the back, depending on the number of tests to be performed and, in some cases, the preference of the patient. Small children are easier to restrain if they are lying face down while the test

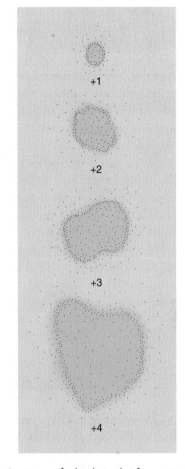

FIGURE 16–3 Sizes of wheals (welts) from +1 to +4 in reaction to scratch testing of allergens.

is being administered. The area to be tested should be comfortably accessible to both patient and physician or assistant. The patient must stay in the same position for at least 20 minutes, so comfort is essential for compliance.

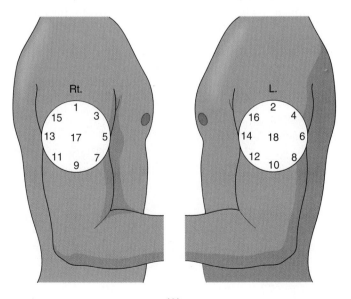

(A)

(B)

FIGURE 16–2 (A) The alternating pattern shown here allows 18 sites to help prevent tissue damage. (B) Example of charting allergy serum injection on a patient's chart.

The tests should be numbered in a pattern with washable ink on the surface of the skin. Explain to the patient that there will be some discomfort when administering either the scratch test or the intradermal test, but it will not last long. Instruct the patient to inform you of any itching, redness, or swelling at the site of injection. Advise the patient to avoid scratching the area for accurate interpretation following the prescribed timing of the test(s). Several extracts may be applied to the patient's skin in rows from evenly spaced applicators that have been dipped into various bottles of allergen substances. The applicator provides a small drop of the substance on the skin in preparation for the scratch test. Figure 16–4 shows a medical assistant applying seven different extracts on the patient's skin. Usually, the

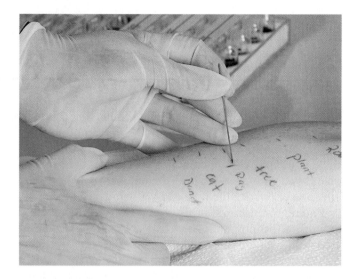

FIGURE 16–5 Each extract is labeled with ink for identification. The medical assistant uses a sterile fine-pointed needle or lancet to scratch the surface of the skin to allow the extract to enter the epidermis.

skin is prepared with alcohol and allowed to air-dry. Alcohol may also be used to remove the ink after the test is completed. A sterile needle or lancet is used to tear the surface of the skin in a scratch of about one-eighth inch or less to allow a drop of the antigen to enter the epidermis (Figure 16–5). Some test materials are packaged in sealed glass capillary tubes, the contents of which are shaken onto the skin after the tube is snapped. Only a small drop should be used. Otherwise, antigens may run together, and test results will be inaccurate. The scratches should be from one and one-half to two inches apart, allowing possible reactions to spread without interfering with each other. A control is used for comparison in interpreting the results. This is a nonallergy-producing plain base fluid. See Procedure 16–1.

Reactions usually occur within the first 20 minutes. (Itching at the test site may be relieved by application of cold or ice packs after the test site has been evaluated by the physician. Look at the examples in Figure 16–6 of

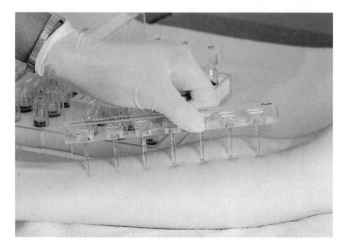

FIGURE 16–4 A medical assistant is placing allergy extracts on the skin with the multiple applicator.

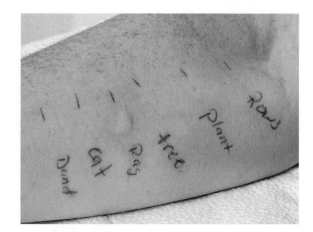

FIGURE 16–6 After timing the skin tests for 20 minutes, observe the reaction and record it on the patient's chart. Pictured here is a +3 reaction to ragweed.

PROCEDURE

16-1 Perform a Scratch Test

PURPOSE: To determine an allergy-causing substance.

OSHA GUIDELINES: To comply with Standard Precautions, gloves must be worn if there is any possibility of coming into contact with blood or any body fluids.

EQUIPMENT: Sterile needle(s) or lancet(s), allergen (extract), cotton balls, alcohol, pen, patient's chart, timer or timepiece, control, biohazard sharps container and bag, and disposable latex or vinyl gloves.

PERFORMANCE OBJECTIVE: Provided with all necessary instruments and supplies and a suitable simulated skin surface (such as an orange), demonstrate each of the steps required in the scratch test procedure. Each step will be observed by the instructor.

1. Assemble all needed items on Mayo table near patient, wash hands, and put on gloves.

2. Explain procedure to the identified patient as you prepare test site with alcohol-saturated cotton ball. Sites most commonly used are upper arm and back. Help patient into comfortable position.

3. Apply small drop of extracts onto site, and continue until all extracts are applied.

4. Mark site(s) with initial abbreviation or number of extract in pen if more than one test is to be administered. Leave about one and one-half to two inches between test sites. **RATIONALE: Adequate area for possible reaction must be allowed.**

Accurate assessment requires measurement of individual reaction areas, which might come together if placed too close.

5. Remove sterile needle or lancet from package without contaminating it. Make one-eighth inch scratch in surface of skin.

6. Begin timing 20-minute period.

7. Discard disposables and gloves in proper receptacle, return items to proper storage area, and wash hands.

8. As soon as the 20-minute time period is up, re-glove and check each site after cleansing with alcohol-saturated cotton ball. **NOTE: Be careful not to wipe off the identification of the extract until after interpretation of reaction has been made by tester or physician.**

9. Compare reaction of site with package insert drawings or measure in centimeters. **NOTE: This step cannot be realistically carried out when a simulated surface is used. However, until the new medical assistant gains experience on the job, the physician will probably make this comparison personally. Cold packs or ice bag may be applied to site to relieve itching.** Repeat step #7 and then proceed to step #10.

10. Record test results on patient's chart.

CHARTING EXAMPLE:

5-12-XX

Patricia Marie Stevens tested +3 reaction 10 minutes after application of ragweed extract, L forearm.

S. Davis, RMA (DV)

---

graduated sizes of reactions to allergy testing.) Many physicians wish to recheck the test sites in 24 hours for delayed reactions. If the physician's interpretation of the skin tests is consistent with the patient's history and phys-ical examination findings, more advanced studies will not be necessary. It is not advisable to perform intradermal tests on patients who have had positive scratch tests.

Occasionally, there will be patients who will need to be cleaned with soap and water to prepare the skin testing site. Patients should be made to feel like this is the procedure for all patients. This way the patient does not feel embarrassed about not being clean. Remind the patient after the procedure to pay special attention to the tested area during daily bathing. This may encourage more routine personal hygiene with patients. In some cultures and ethnic groups, daily bathing has never been a part of their day. You should approach this issue with kindness and understanding in caring for all patients.

A CAAHEP CONNECTION

To ease a patient's anxiety about having the diagnostic scratch testing, try to talk with the patient about some current event, movie, or TV program, and allow the patient to calm down. Preparing the set up regarding the procedure should include giving the patient printed patient education materials. Often there are pictures of how the procedure is done. Explaining what will happen will return a more cooperative patient and make your job easier.

Intradermal Test

The intradermal test, thought to be more accurate, is often performed if the scratch test is negative or unclear. Although the solutions used for intradermal tests are about

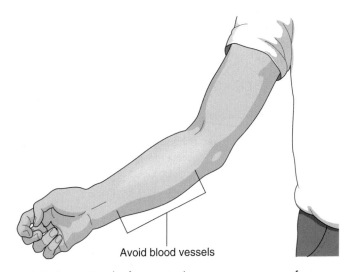

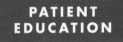
Avoid blood vessels

FIGURE 16–7 The forearm is the most common area for up to 14 sites for intradermal skin tests.

100 times more dilute than those used for scratch tests, they are still potentially dangerous. Severe reactions may occur, however, with either method. Generally, the diluted solutions used prevent **systemic** reactions. Intradermal test sites are performed at spaced intervals on the forearm

PATIENT EDUCATION

During the allergy patient's visit, especially if recently diagnosed as such, giving the patient advice concerning the condition and the prevention of further problems will be well received. The following are a few suggestions for discussion with patients who have allergies.

1. Urge patients to follow the allergy serum desensitizing schedule closely to help build up immunity to the substance to which they are allergic.

2. Advise them to avoid what they are allergic to if at all possible.

3. Instruct patients to read all labels carefully (household products, clothing, consumable products, and so on) to identify possible allergens.

4. Urge them to develop and practice good health habits, such as following a sensible, well-balanced diet, proper rest, and exercise. The should also be encouraged to wash their hands frequently with soap and warm water for 20 seconds (approximately the length of time it takes to sing the "Happy Birthday" song at a traditional pace) and teach their families to do so.

5. Advise them to take only prescribed medication and to avoid OTC medications unless advised by the physician.

6. If patients have a known severe reaction to a particular substance, remind them to carry their kit with them at all times.

(Figure 16–7) or scapular area. In the event of a severe **adverse** reaction, a tourniquet can be applied proximal to the site when the arm is used. The intradermal test can also be referred to as the *subcutaneous test*. Serum or vaccine is sometimes used in intradermal testing. If the initial test is negative, it is often repeated with a stronger solution. Usually, the reaction time is 15 to 30 minutes. **Epinephrine** should be administered about an inch above the site by order of the physician if severe reaction occurs.

In performing an intradermal test, a fine-gauge needle (usually 26 G and three-eighths to five-eighths inches long) is used. The antigen is introduced into the dermal layer of the skin in minute dosages of 0.01 to 0.02 cc by sterile technique. The area will appear as a small blister from the fluid raising the skin. The reaction period is up to 30 minutes, and the interpretation of the results is the same as in the scratch tests. Some antigens such as fungi and bacteria produce delayed reactions from 24 to 48 hours after administration. Be sure to impress upon the patients the importance of comparing the reaction to something well known, (e.g., size of welt [size of a dime], redness, itching), and record all symptoms of the reaction with the date and time, especially if it is at a time when the office is closed. Provide an emergency phone number or instructions to call EMS (911 where applicable) in case a severe or life-threatening reaction should occur.

Intradermal tests are sometimes used by physicians to determine medication sensitivity or immunization needs. Follow the procedure for intradermal injections in Chapter 18.

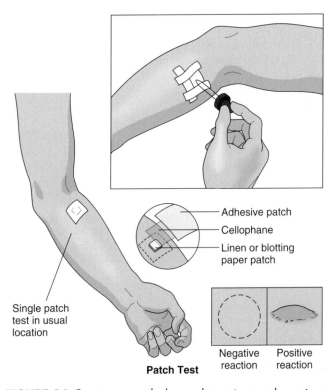

Adhesive patch
Cellophane
Linen or blotting paper patch

Single patch test in usual location

Negative reaction　Positive reaction

Patch Test

FIGURE 16–8 As you apply the patch test, instruct the patient to keep the patch clean and dry and to keep it intact until the results are read by the physician. The control patch is placed next to the test patch.

PROCEDURE

16-2 Apply a Patch Test

PURPOSE: To determine the causative substance of suspected contact dermatitis.

OSHA GUIDELINES: To comply with Standard Precautions, gloves must be worn if there is any possibility of coming into contact with blood or any body fluids.

EQUIPMENT: Commercially prepared paper with suspected substance or gauze saturated with substance and **mock** control substance, latex or vinyl gloves, alcohol, cotton balls, gauze squares, biohazardous waste bag, nonallergenic tape, pen, patient's chart.

PERFORMANCE OBJECTIVE: After practicing with water in lieu of the suspected substance, students will be provided with all necessary supplies, including the suspected substance. Using another student as a patient, demonstrate each of the steps required in carrying out the skin patch test, including the 48-hour recheck. The instructor will observe each step.

1. Assemble items on Mayo table next to patient, wash hands, and put on gloves.

2. Explain procedure while assisting identified patient to comfortable sitting position.

3. Clean test site with alcohol-saturated cotton ball, and let air dry.

4. Apply suspected substance to test site and mock control substance next to it, and secure with nonallergenic tape. **NOTE: Usually it is placed near unaffected area in patients with contact dermatitis.** Remove gloves and wash hands.

5. Record date, time, substance, and area tested on patient's chart.

6. Schedule patient to return in 48 hours.

7. Instruct patient to keep area clean and dry until return appointment.

8. Remove patch with gloved hands; read the results and record. **NOTE: Discard gloves and the patch in biohazardous waste bag.**

CHARTING EXAMPLE:

7-21-XX

Verita Joan Stevens—patch test for adhesive applied on L forearm; Verita was instructed to return for evaluation in 24 hours.

S. Davis, RMA (DV)

Patch Test

The patch test is done to determine the cause of **contact dermatitis**. A patch consisting of a gauze square saturated with the suspected allergy-causing substance is placed on the surface of the skin and secured with nonallergenic tape (Figure 16–8). The arm is the usual site of choice for convenience. The results are read after a 24-hour period and then repeated at a 48-hour period. A control is thought necessary and should be placed on the arm near the patch if the substance of the patch test is not a known skin irritant. Redness or swelling of the area indicates a reaction, and its interpretation is based on grading as for scratch and intradermal tests. Refer to Procedure 16–2.

Nasal Smear

A helpful aid for years in the diagnosis of allergies has been a smear done with nasal secretions to observe the **eosinophil** count. If there are many and they are clumped together, there is a strong indication of allergy. This is a simple means of screening for an allergy and is usually the first step in the testing program.

ACHIEVE UNIT OBJECTIVES

Complete Chapter 16, Unit 1, in the workbook to help you obtain competency of this subject matter.

UNIT 2
Cardiology Procedures

OBJECTIVES

Upon completion of the unit, meet the following performance objectives by verifying knowledge of the facts and principles presented through oral and written communication at a level deemed competent. Demonstrate the specific behaviors as identified in the performance objectives of the procedures, observing all aseptic and safety precautions in accordance with health care standards.

1. Spell and define, using the glossary at the back of the text, all the **Words to Know** in this unit.

2. Explain the reasons for performing an ECG.
3. Describe the electrical conduction system of the heart.
4. Apply limb and chest electrodes properly.
5. Describe methods of and perform a routine 12-lead ECG.
6. Define *artifacts* and list their causes on an ECG.
7. Describe the reason for mounting an ECG tracing.
8. State the purpose of a Holter monitor, and explain the procedure to a patient.
9. Demonstrate the procedure for proper hook-up of a Holter monitor.
10. State the purpose of defibrillation.
11. Describe cardiac stress testing, and discuss the proper placement of the electrodes.
12. State the purpose of cardiac stress testing.
13. Describe patient education regarding the heart.

AREAS OF COMPETENCE (AAMA)

This unit addresses content within the specific competency areas of *Fundamental principles, Diagnostic orders, Patient care, Professionalism, Communication skills, Legal concepts, Instruction,* and *Operational functions,* as identified in the Medical Assistant Role Delineation Study. Refer to Appendix A for a detailed listing of the areas.

■ WORDS TO KNOW

amplifier	interpretive
arrhythmia	interval
artifacts	limbs
atrial depolarization	mechanical
augmented	multichannel
cardiology	precordial
computerized	Purkinje
countershock	reliable
current	repolarization
defibrillator	sedentary
electrocardiogram	segment
electrocardiograph	simultaneous
electrode	somatic
electrolyte	standardization
galvanometer	stylus
Holter monitor	trace
impulse	treadmill
interference	voltage
intermittent	

In family and general practice, internal medicine, and **cardiology**, a procedure frequently used in the diagnosis of heart disease and dysfunction is the **electrocardiogram**. This procedure is painless and safe, and patients should be told so to eliminate apprehension.

A CAAHEP CONNECTION

To a patient who has never had an ECG, it could be quite intimidating with all the wires and electrodes that are attached. A patient may fear the electrical hook up and be afraid of being electrocuted. Even if the patient does not verbally express these feelings, the medical assistant should be aware that this is a normal reaction and that the look on the patient's face may give the fear away. Try to reassure the patient that the procedure of an ECG is perfectly safe and that the machine is grounded so that nothing harmful will happen. Think of the way you felt when you first saw the machine and your reaction. Most people do wonder what it might do to them.

You will obtain the electrocardiogram (recording) (EKG/ECG) by operating the **electrocardiograph** (machine). Figures 16–9 and 16–10 show three widely used models of ECGs.

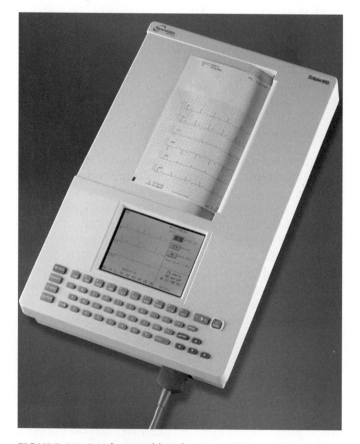

FIGURE 16–9 The portable Eclipse 850 electrocardiograph. (Courtesy of Spacelabs Medical, Inc.)

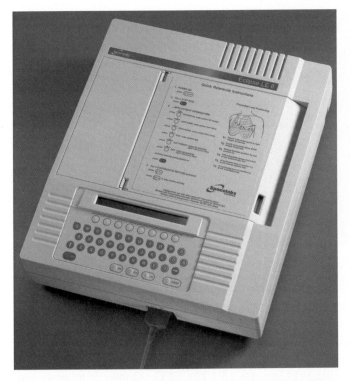

FIGURE 16-10 The multi-channel Eclipse LE II electrocardiograph. (Courtesy of Spacelabs Medical, Inc.)

Through a process of electrical transmission, this machine **traces impulses** of the heart on paper to create a permanent record of its activity.

All muscle movement produces electrical impulses. The ECG is a recording of the electrical impulses of the heart muscle. To accomplish this **electrodes** are placed on the patient's **limbs** and chest, which pick up the electrical **current** produced by the contractions of the heart. Some electrodes and **electrolytes** (for use with metal electrodes) are pictured in Figures 16–11 and 16–12. These minute impulses are transmitted by the electrocardiograph by metal tips (or clips) of the patient cable (wires) attached to the electrodes. Figure 16–13 displays AstroTraceClips, sometimes referred to as the "universal clip" because they can be used with most types of electrodes. The current enters the electrocardiograph through the wires to reach the **amplifier**, which enlarges the impulses. They are transformed into **mechanical** motion by the **galvanometer**. The **stylus** produces a printed representation on ECG paper. ECG paper is made for the different types of machines, standard, single, and **multichannel** (Figure 16–14). As the heated stylus moves against the tracing paper, the impulses given off by the heart are recorded. The tracing paper should be handled carefully to protect it from being accidentally marked. Dot matrix paper makes tracings easy to read and copy because they are clear and legible.

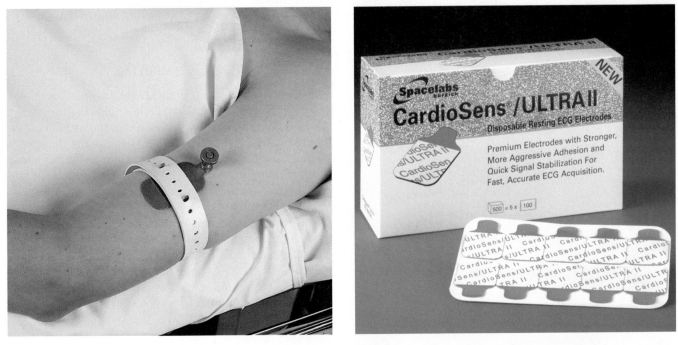

(A)

(B)

FIGURE 16-11 (A) Metal limb leads and rubber straps that have been used successfully for many years with electrolyte pads shown in Figure 16–12A are being replaced with disposable ECG electrodes (Figure 16–11B). (Courtesy of Spacelabs Medical, Inc.) (B) Cardio-Sens Ultra II disposable sensors and others that are similar have widespread use in obtaining electrocardiograms. (Courtesy of Spacelabs Medical, Inc.)

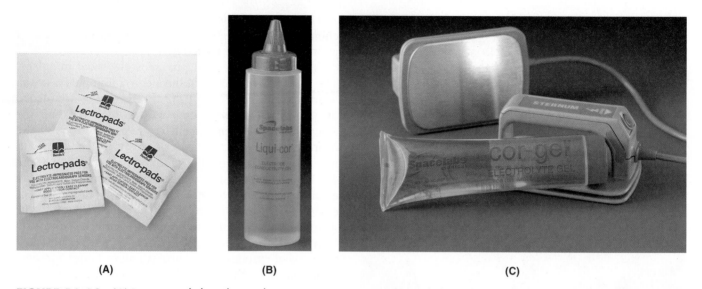

(A)   (B)   (C)

FIGURE 16-12 (A) Presaturated electrolyte pads are convenient to use with metal electrodes. (B) Electrolyte lotion or gel can be used with metal electrodes. (C) Electrolyte gel is applied to the paddles of the defibrillator that is shown in Figure 16–31. (Courtesy of Spacelabs Medical, Inc.)

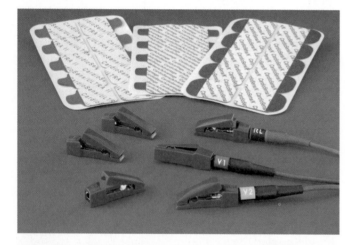

FIGURE 16-13 AstroTrace clips (Courtesy of Spacelabs Medical, Inc.)

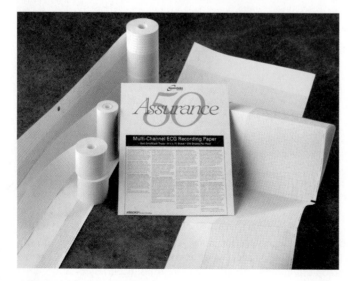

FIGURE 16-14 ECG blush coat paper (Courtesy of Spacelabs Medical, Inc.)

Some ECGs are mounted onto permanent folders for filing (Figure 16–15). The ECG trimmer is a handy tool for cutting the ECG tracings in preparation for mounting.

The ECG is interpreted by the physician, usually the one who ordered the procedure. Some physicians prefer to have a cardiologist interpret the ECG and send the results in the form of a written report with a copy of the tracing. The physician will read the ECG and compare the measurement, rate, rhythm, duration of the electrical waves, **intervals**, and **segments** with known normal ECG readings.

PATH OF ELECTRICAL IMPULSES

The heart is a four-chambered pump that produces minute electrical current by muscular contraction (Figure 16–16). An electrical impulse originates in the modified myocardial tissue of the sinoatrial (SA) node, causing the atria to contract (Figure 16–17). This contraction is the beginning of **atrial depolarization**, which is the first part of the cardiac cycle. The first impulse as recorded on the graph paper is termed the P wave. The impulse continues through the heart tissue to the atrioventricular (AV) node, to the bundle of His, and spreads to the **Purkinje** fibers. These fibers cause the muscles of the ventricles to contract and produce the QRS complex of waves on the ECG paper. The T wave on the graph paper follows, representing the **repolarization** of the ventricles, or the time of recovery before another contraction.

ROUTINE ELECTROCARDIOGRAPH LEADS

C Skills Menu:
  ■ Administering an EKG

The routine ECG consists of 12 leads, or recordings of the electrical activity of the heart from different angles. The

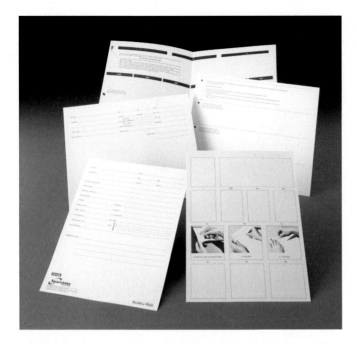

FIGURE 16–15   Various types of mounts for ECG tracing paper for patient's permanent record (Courtesy of Spacelabs Medical, Inc.)

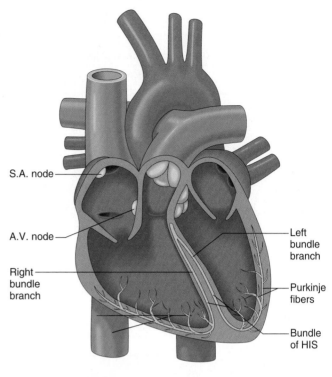

FIGURE 16–16   Anatomy of the heart

first three leads are called standard or bipolar leads and are labeled with Roman numerals I, II, and III. These leads are obtained by placing limb electrodes on the fleshy part of the upper outer arms (refer back to Figure 16-12) and the inner lower calves (Figure 16–18). Lead I records the electrical voltage difference between the right arm and left

arm. Lead II records the difference between the right arm and the left leg. Lead III records the **voltage** difference between the left arm and left leg (Figure 16–19).

The **augmented** leads are the next three in the standard 12-lead ECG. They are aVR, aVL, and aVF. aVR is the recording of the heart's voltage difference between the

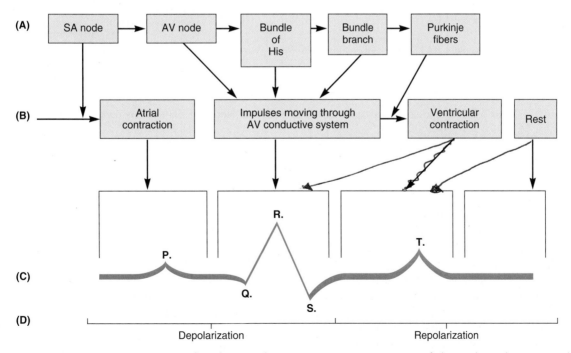

FIGURE 16–17   Diagramatic representation of cardiac impulses on ECG tracing: (A) Course of electrical impulses, (B) Cardiac muscle reaction to impulses, (C) ECG tracing of impulse waves, (D) Phases of cardiac cycle (Courtesy of Spacelabs Medical, Inc.)

LEAD ARRANGEMENT AND CODING

STANDARD LIMB LEADS

LEAD MARKING CODE	LEAD	ELECTRODES CONNECTED	COLOR CODE			
					BODY	INSERT
●	LEAD 1	LA and RA	RL		GREEN	GREEN
	LEAD 2	LL and RA	LL		RED	RED
			RA		WHITE	GRAY
	LEAD 3	LL and LA	LA		BLACK	GRAY

AUGMENTED LIMB LEADS

LEAD MARKING CODE	LEAD	ELECTRODES CONNECTED	COLOR CODE			
					BODY	INSERT
● ●	aVR	RA and (LA-LL)	RL		GREEN	GREEN
	aVL	LA and (RA-LL)	LL		RED	RED
			RA		WHITE	GRAY
	aVF	LL and (RA-LA)	LA		BLACK	GRAY

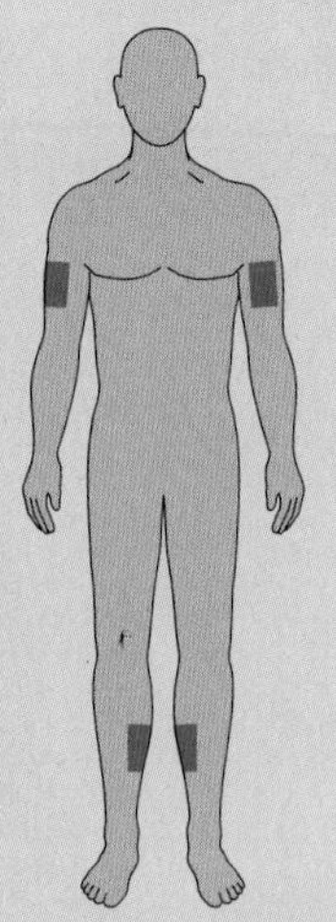

CHEST LEADS

LEAD MARKING CODE	LEAD	ELECTRODES CONNECTED	COLOR CODE			
					BODY	INSERT
● ● ●	V_1	V_1 and (LA-RA-LL)	V_1		BROWN	RED
	V_2	V_2 and (LA-RA-LL)	V_2		BROWN	YELLOW
	V_3	V_3 and (LA-RA-LL)	V_3		BROWN	GREEN
● ● ● ●	V_4	V_4 and (LA-RA-LL)	V_4		BROWN	BLUE
	V_5	V_5 and (LA-RA-LL)	V_5		BROWN	ORANGE
	V_6	V_6 and (LA-RA-LL)	V_6		BROWN	VIOLET

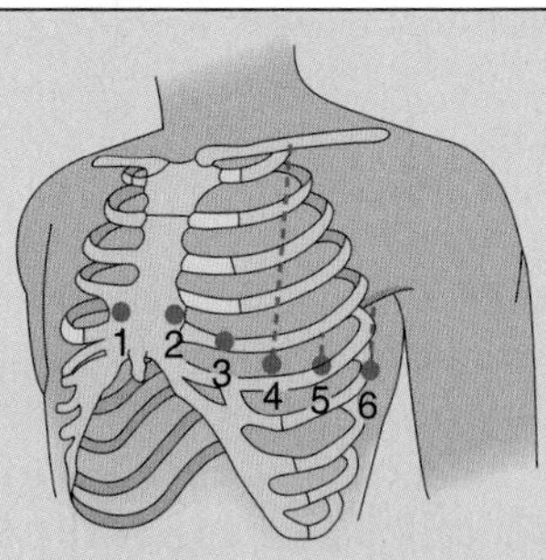

V_1 Fourth intercostal space at right margin of sternum

V_2 Fourth intercostal space at left margin of sternum

V_3 Midway between position 2 and position 4

V_4 Fifth intercostal space at junction of left midclavicular line

V_5 At horizontal level of position 4 at left anterior axillary line

V_6 At horizontal level of position 4 at left midaxillary line

FIGURE 16–18   Proper placement of electrodes for the standard routine 12-lead ECG and lead markings (Courtesy of Spacelabs Medical, Inc.)

right arm electrode and a central point between the left arm and the left leg (augmented voltage right arm). aVL is the recording of the heart's voltage difference between the left arm electrode and a central point between the right arm and the left leg (augmented voltage left arm). aVF is the recording of the heart's voltage difference between the left leg electrode and a central point between the right arm and left arm (augmented voltage left leg or foot). The term augmented means to become larger. Because these three leads are produced by such small impulses, the amplifier of the ECG machine augments their size sufficiently for recording them on the graph paper.

The six standard chest or **precordial** leads are obtained by moving the electrode to the anatomical positions shown in Figure 16–20.

The lead selector switch must be set for each different chest lead to obtain the correct code. Some electrocardiographs have an automatic lead marker to identify each of the 12 standard leads as the selector switch is turned. Others require the operator to mark each lead of the ECG. A standard marking code is recommended for use either with the manual or automatic method. Some physicians prefer other codes. It is best to follow the policy where you are employed. Refer to Procedure 16–3.

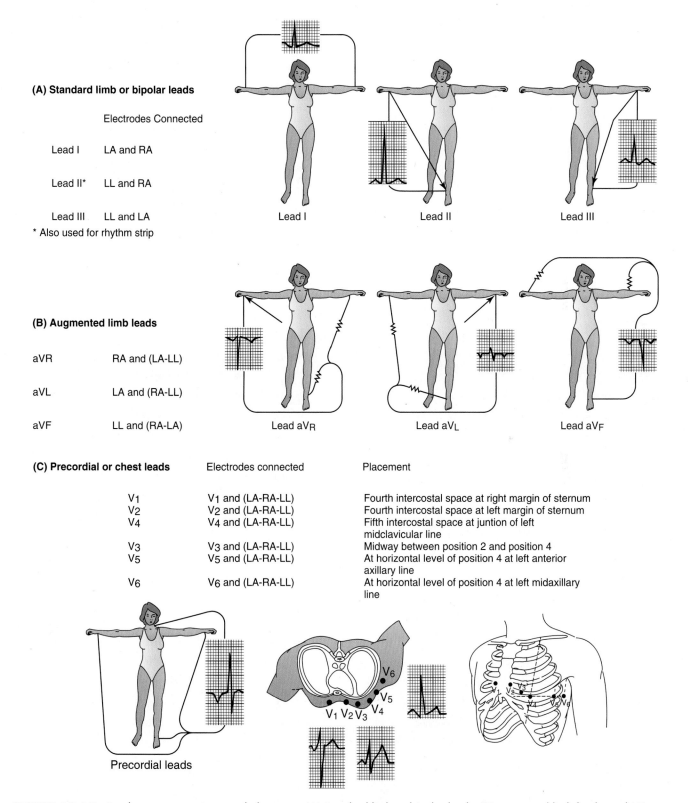

(A) Standard limb or bipolar leads

Electrodes Connected

Lead I	LA and RA
Lead II*	LL and RA
Lead III	LL and LA

* Also used for rhythm strip

Lead I   Lead II   Lead III

(B) Augmented limb leads

aVR	RA and (LA-LL)
aVL	LA and (RA-LL)
aVF	LL and (RA-LA)

Lead aV$_R$ Lead aV$_L$ Lead aV$_F$

(C) Precordial or chest leads

	Electrodes connected	Placement
V$_1$	V$_1$ and (LA-RA-LL)	Fourth intercostal space at right margin of sternum
V$_2$	V$_2$ and (LA-RA-LL)	Fourth intercostal space at left margin of sternum
V$_4$	V$_4$ and (LA-RA-LL)	Fifth intercostal space at juntion of left midclavicular line
V$_3$	V$_3$ and (LA-RA-LL)	Midway between position 2 and position 4
V$_5$	V$_5$ and (LA-RA-LL)	At horizontal level of position 4 at left anterior axillary line
V$_6$	V$_6$ and (LA-RA-LL)	At horizontal level of position 4 at left midaxillary line

Precordial leads

V$_6$ V$_5$ V$_4$ V$_1$ V$_2$ V$_3$

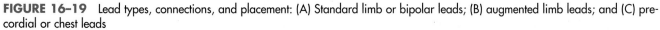

FIGURE 16–19   Lead types, connections, and placement: (A) Standard limb or bipolar leads; (B) augmented limb leads; and (C) precordial or chest leads

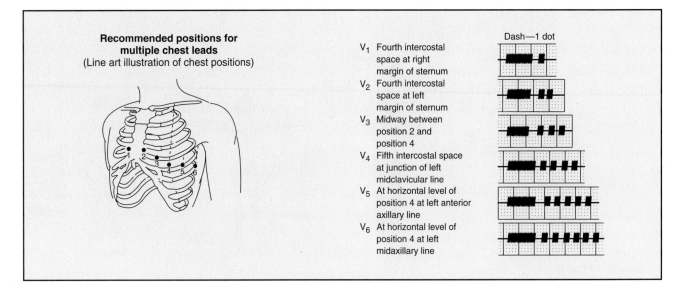

Recommended positions for multiple chest leads
(Line art illustration of chest positions)

V₁ Fourth intercostal space at right margin of sternum
V₂ Fourth intercostal space at left margin of sternum
V₃ Midway between position 2 and position 4
V₄ Fifth intercostal space at junction of left midclavicular line
V₅ At horizontal level of position 4 at left anterior axillary line
V₆ At horizontal level of position 4 at left midaxillary line

Dash—1 dot

FIGURE 16–20 Example of common coding system for ECG leads that must be manually coded on older electrocardiographs by pressing the lead marker button appropriately (Courtesy of Spacelabs Medical, Inc.)

PROCEDURE

16-3 Obtain a Standard 12-Lead Electrocardiogram

PURPOSE: To obtain a graphic representation of the electrical activity of the patient's heart.

EQUIPMENT: Electrocardiograph, ECG paper, four metal limb electrodes and straps, or disposable pregelled adhesive electrodes as appropriate for use with patient cable of ECG machine—lead wires with snaps, clips, or tips (use chest strap if necessary) to attach to electrodes, patient cable, electrolyte (pads, cream, or gel), chest strap, treatment table, pillow, drape sheet, tissues, paper towels, ECG mount, footstool, tongue depressor, patient's chart, pen, disposable razor.

PERFORMANCE OBJECTIVE: Provided with an electrocardiograph and all essential equipment and supplies and using other students as patients, demonstrate each of the steps required in obtaining a standard 12-lead ECG reading. The instructor will observe each step. **NOTE: The specified disrobing may be simulated.**

1. Plug in ECG machine to outlet away from known electrical interference. Plug in patient cable wire to machine. Assemble electrodes and attach to straps. Apply electrolyte pads and set aside. Turn machine on. Wash hands.

2. Ask identified patient to disrobe from waist up and remove clothing from lower legs. Provide privacy and show patient where to put belongings. Explain procedure.

3. Assist patient onto treatment table and cover with drape sheet. Ask patient to lie down. Pull out leg rest. Adjust pillow under patient's head for comfort.

4. Apply chest strap by placing hard plastic end under patient's left side and weighted end against right side of patient's chest. Re-cover chest with drape sheet.

5. Place arm electrodes (with electrolyte) on fleshy outer area of upper arm with connectors pointing toward shoulders. Straps should be moved one space tighter than relaxed. Leg electrodes (applied with electrolyte) should be placed on fleshy inner area of lower leg near calf, connectors pointing toward upper body. **RATIONALE: Placement of electrodes eliminates friction from examining table and body movement.** If gel or cream is used, use a small amount, the size of a dime, and spread with tongue depressor. **NOTE: Especially when disposable electrodes are used, it is very important to use a tongue depressor or gauze square to rub sites vigorously to increase circulation and promote better contact of the electrodes.**

6. Connect lead wire tips to appropriate electrodes by screwing tightly into place with all pointing down, or by snapping or clipping electrodes securely in place. **NOTE: Power cord and patient cable must not be allowed to touch.** Figure 16–26 shows a patient with electrodes properly placed for a 12-lead ECG.

(continues)

PROCEDURE

16-3 Obtain a Standard 12-Lead Electrocardiogram—continued

7. Place chest electrode (electrolyte side up) under chest strap and secure until needed, or attach all six pregelled disposable adhesive chest electrodes V_1 through V_6 (shaving dense chest hair as necessary for placement of electrodes) (Figure 16–27).

8. Turn lead selector switch to STD, and adjust stylus to center of graph paper.

9. Move record switch to 25-mm/second position, and run for a few seconds to adjust centering of stylus. Make standardization mark 2 mm wide and 10 mm high. Then turn machine off, or with computerized electrocardiograph (single and multichannel), press "auto" and run the 12-lead ECG. Proceed to appropriate instructions for steps 13 through 17.

10. Turn lead selector switch to lead I and run 8 to 12 inches of tracing. Proceed in same manner for leads II and III. Run four to six inches each of leads aVR, aVL, and aVF. **NOTE: Lead selector switch should be allowed a second or two to pause between leads to allow for adjustment. RATIONALE: This permits steadier centering of tracing.** Standardization should appear at beginning of each lead if requested by physician; otherwise at beginning of tracing and whenever sensitivity switch is changed to either reduce or enlarge size of cardiac cycles. **NOTE: Each lead should be marked accordingly, either manually or automatically by the machine.**

11. Turn lead selector switch either to V or V_1 depending on machine you are using. Place chest electrode in proper position and standardize. Run four to six inches of recording. Turn switch to AMP OFF when changing electrode posi-

tions. **RATIONALE: This allows stylus to remain steady.** Move chest electrode to V_2 for second chest lead and run four to six inches of recording, then to V_3, and so on. **NOTE: Turn the run switch to AMP off after each of the chest or precordial leads. RATIONALE: Allows the stylus to adjust to next lead by pausing a few seconds so that centering is certain and standardized as instructed. NOTE: Mark each lead.**

12. Turn lead selector switch back to STD slowly, one lead at a time, to avoid stripping of dial gears. Run recording out until baseline only appears and turn machine off.

13. Tear off tracing from machine. **NOTE: Immediately mark it with patient's name, age, day's date, and your initials.** Roll or loosely overlap tracing back and forth, carefully secure with paper clip, and set aside. **NOTE: This is not required with computerized ECG printout.**

14. Remove tips of lead wires from limb electrodes by unscrewing ends. Remove chest electrode and strap, limb straps, and electrodes from patient. Clean sites with a warm, wet paper towel and dry. Discard used towels in proper receptacle.

15. Assist patient to sitting position and then down from table when ready. Assist patient in dressing if necessary.

16. Change table paper and pillow cover, and discard used disposables. Wash hands.

17. **NOTE: Alert physician of any complaints or unusual findings at once.** Place tracing and initial ECG order in patient's chart for physician to interpret. Record appropriate entry on patient's chart (e.g., pt experienced SOB while lying flat).

INTERFERENCE

As with any procedure, a full explanation must be given to the patient to gain cooperation. Providing privacy and adequate draping of the patient during the procedure will ease patient apprehension and avoid chills. The patient must be relaxed for a good tracing to be obtained, as any movement of the patient may cause **interference** on the tracing. Shivering from nervousness or cold can produce muscle voltage artifacts for example. This additional activity is called **somatic** tremor. Arm electrodes should be placed close to the shoulders of the upper outer arms to

decrease the possibility of muscle voltage **artifacts** and arrhythmias (Figure 16–21).

Other artifacts which may appear on the ECG, called AC interference, are caused by electrical activity. The latest models of electrocardiographs have sensitive filtering devices that eliminate most of the interference, but it is still recommended that a room with a minimum of electrical wiring be used for the ECG procedure. All power cords should be kept away from the patient, and the patient table should be away from the wall to eliminate the possibility of interference from electrical wiring within the wall. The patient must be properly connected with the

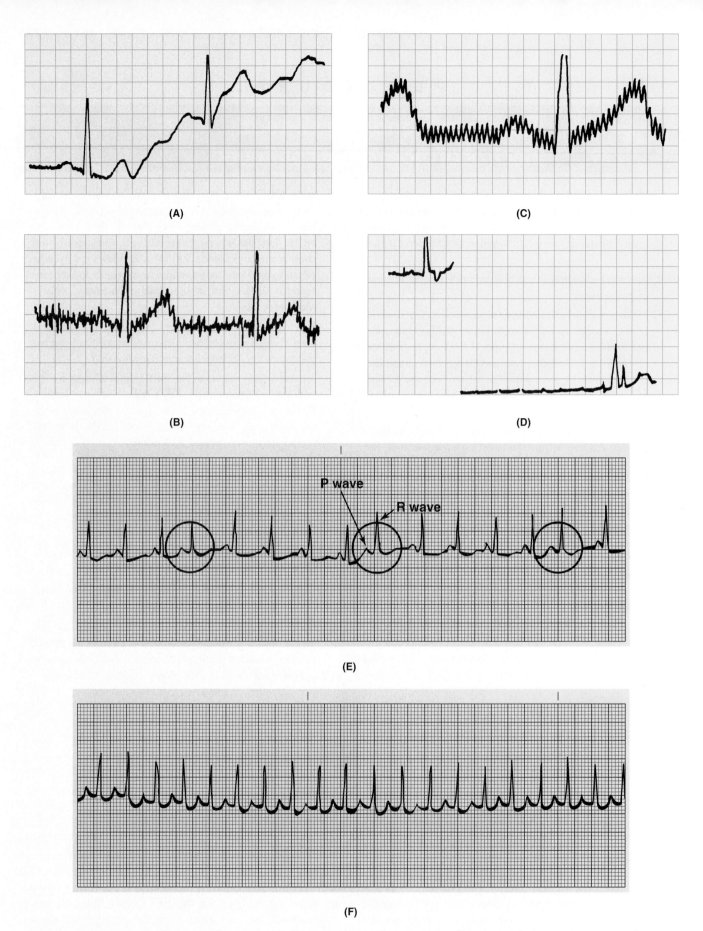

FIGURE 16-21 ECG interference artifacts and arrhythmias: (A) Somatic tremor or involuntary muscle movement, (B) AC (alternating current), (C) wandering baseline, (D) interrupted baseline, (E) premature atrial contractions (PAC), (F) paroxysmal atrial tachycardia (PAT), (G) atrial fibrillation, (H) premature ventricular contractions, (I) ventricular tachycardia, (J) ventricular fibrillation

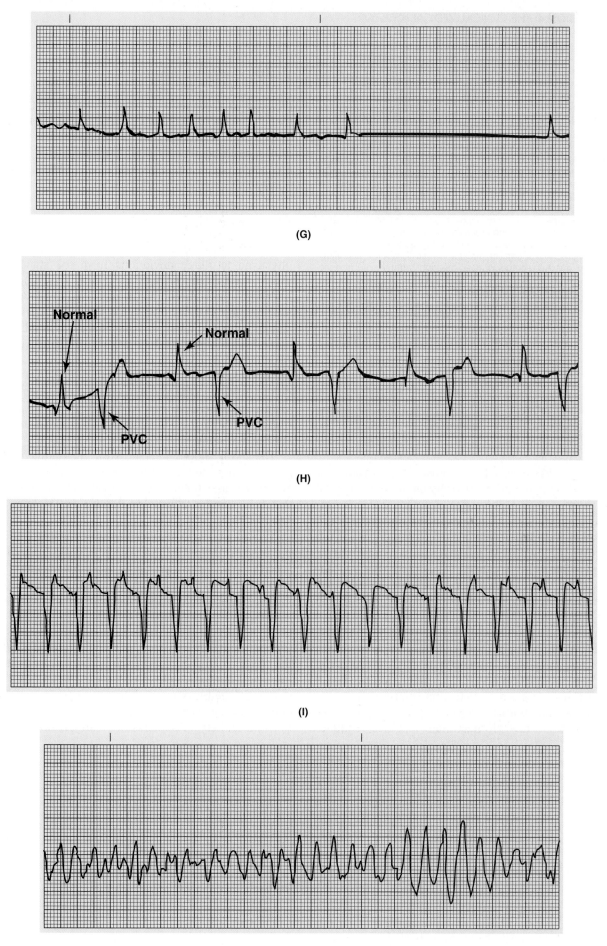

(G)

(H)

(I)

(J)

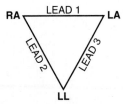

LOCATION OF SOURCE OF ARTIFACTS
Leads 1, 2, and 3 can be helpful in locating the source of interference. Refer to the triangle. Notice that each limb electrode is involved in recording two of the three leads. This means that if an artifact is observed in two leads but not in the third, the artifact is probably caused by a condition at or near the electrode that is common to the two leads. Examples: tremor on leads 1 and 3 and not on lead 2 indicates that the left arm is the probable source since it is common to leads 1 and 3. Similarly, a large amount of AC interference appearing in leads 1 and 2 and a smaller amount in lead 3, would most likely indicate that the AC source is near the right arm. If interference problems cannot be readily solved, contact your Burdick dealer or The Burdick Corporation for the name of your nearest Burdick field representative. They have equipment to help you find the interference source and can offer suggestions to eliminate or reduce the problem.

FIGURE 16–22 Sources of artifacts from leads. (Courtesy of Spacelabs Medical, Inc.)

electrodes and properly grounded (Figure 16–27). Using good technique will also reduce AC interference. The sources of artifacts from different leads is shown in Figure 16–22.

Wandering baseline can be caused by corroded or improperly applied electrodes or by an unequal amount of electrolyte on the electrodes. Another cause is improperly cleaned skin. Oils, creams, and lotions should be removed from the patient's skin with alcohol, or the conduction of electrical impulses will be impaired. Interrupted baseline is caused by an electrode becoming separated from the wire or by a broken lead wire. Follow manufacturer's instructions for repairing the electrocardiograph.

To further ensure a good ECG, the operator must use clean electrodes. Metal electrodes should be cleaned with a mild detergent solution after each use and with scouring powder and a cloth as needed. The rubber straps should also be washed with a mild detergent solution after each use. A proper amount of electrolyte must be used with each electrode to provide maximum electrical conduc-

tion. Individual packets of pretreated disposable pads are available for convenience.

Many offices and clinics still use a standard electrocardiograph with the metal electrodes and limb straps. All of the **computerized** channel ECG machines require the disposable electrodes and electrolyte pads. These are widely used because of their convenience. Because they are obviously more expensive, you should use them wisely and avoid unnecessary waste.

STANDARDIZATION

The **standardization** of the ECG is necessary to enable a physician to judge deviations from the standard. The usual standardization mark is 2 mm wide and 10 mm high. This mark should begin each lead to provide a **reliable** reading. If the tracing is too large, the sensitivity dial should be turned down to ½ to produce a standardization mark 5 mm high and 2 mm wide. If the tracing is too small, the sensitivity dial can be turned up to 2, making the impulse 20 mm high and 2 mm wide. You must pay close attention to the tracing as it is being run to make adjustments as needed. Figure 16–23 shows the standardization marking from an electrocardiograph with the sensitivity dial set at ½, 1, and 2.

The stylus should be centered in the middle of the paper. The baseline will allow you to observe the centering and make adjustments as necessary. The temperature of the stylus can be adjusted to control the thickness of the line.

The tracing paper is normally run at a speed of 25 mm per second. If the ECG cycles are too close together, the speed can be changed to 50 mm per second (Figure 16–24). This adjustment should be noted in pen on the tracing.

The physician may order a standard 12-lead ECG with a rhythm strip. This simply means that you should record a long strip, usually 12 inches, or for a period of seconds (generally 30, or however long the physician orders for the rhythm strip) of lead II in addition to the standard tracing. This gives the physician a better look at the rhythm of the heartbeat and how often an irregularity occurs. Be sure to explain to the patient what you are doing to avoid anxiety. A patient may worry unnecessarily if a

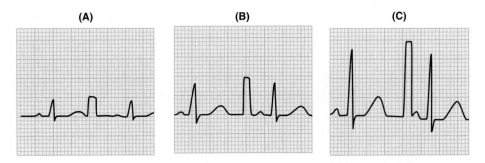

FIGURE 16–23 Standardization markings with sensitivity dial set on: (A) ½, (B) 1, and (C) 2 (Courtesy of Spacelabs Medical, Inc.)

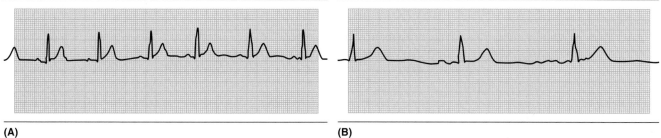

(A)   (B)

Illustrated below are a normal ECG and a normal artery.

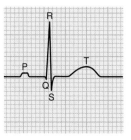

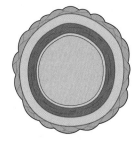

The artery narrows as the atheroma, fatty deposits, (atherosclerosis) becomes larger and hardens, causing a decrease in circulation (arteriosclerosis) in the heart. This condition causes heart pain (angina pectoris).

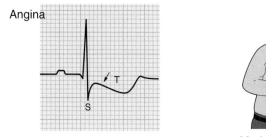

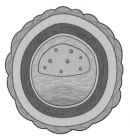

Moderate
myocardial ischemia
↓
Angina pectoris

Moderate atherosclerotic
narrowing of lumen

The ECG shows what happens during an MI (myocardial infarction) or heart attack caused by a coronary occlusion (blockage) from deposits of calcium in the arteries.

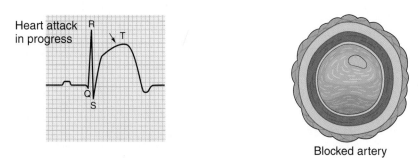

(C)

Blocked artery

FIGURE 16–24 ECG paper: (A) Lead II run at 25 mm/second, (B) lead II run at 50 mm/second (lead II is also known as a rhythm strip). (C) ECG examples and progression of coronary artery disease

procedure is somewhat different from what was remembered from the last visit.

Any obvious abnormality should be brought to the physician's attention immediately if the patient is experiencing pain or discomfort at the time it is observed.

The ECG is an extremely important procedure. Every detail must be performed accurately.

It is extremely important that the patient be relaxed and comfortable during the ECG procedure. Reassure the patient by answering any questions. Explain that the machine does not "put electricity" into the body. Your calm, efficient manner will help the patient relax.

The computerized electrocardiographs have many timesaving features. They have **simultaneous** 12-lead **interpretive** analysis. Data are not only printed out but also stored in its memory. The entire ECG tracing is generated in about one minute. There is no time involved in mounting. A manual mode provides additional leads, such as the rhythm strip of lead II. These machines are relatively light weight and can be easily moved if necessary.

The ECG can detect damage from previous heart attacks, enlargement of the heart muscle, disturbances in the rhythm, and other abnormal conditions. Three examples of the heart's electrical activity are shown in the illustration in Figure 16–24. This may give you a better understanding of what happens during normal beating of the heart and when it is in crisis. As you can see, the changes in the normal pattern can aid the physician in detecting many heart conditions. Before the physician can confirm a diagnosis, an examination that considers the patient's symptoms, medical history, and other diagnostic tests are necessary. It is usually recommended for patients between the ages of 35 and 40 to establish a base reading. Physicians may then refer to this ECG in the event of later problems. Most often an ECG is performed along with the routine annual physical examination every 5 to 10 years after a baseline normal reading has been established. Some physicians prefer to have a tracing more often, even annually, for patients who have a history of hypertension, are smokers, are obese, or have a high serum cholesterol level. Another factor in heart problems is a **sedentary** lifestyle, which is usually accompanied by obesity.

Zymed Medical Instrumentation provides a computerized ECG with only five leads. The electrodes are placed only on the patient's chest. This ultra efficient electrocardiogram provides the same information as the standard 12-lead. Figure 16–25 shows the electrocardiograph and the placement of the electrodes. This technology offers a multichannel tracing that can be viewed on a monitor to assess the heart's activity. This method also keeps a memory of ECGs for review of the patient's condition and the progress of treatment.

STRESS TESTS

ECG stress tests are done by some physicians on a routine basis for patients with a high risk of developing heart disease. They are more often done in a limited manner for patients interested in starting a strenuous exercise program or those who continue to have heart pain even after

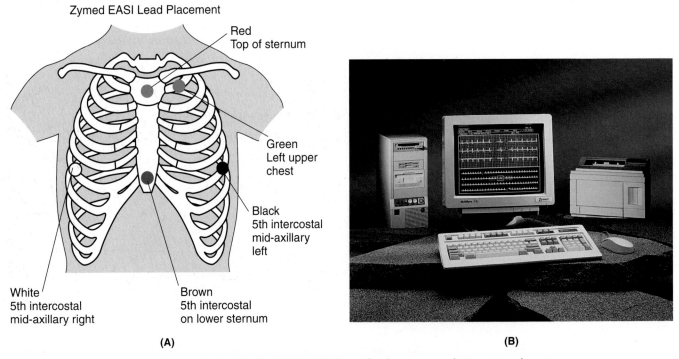

FIGURE 16–25 Zymed 5 lead ECG: (A) Electrode placement, and (B) computed tracing

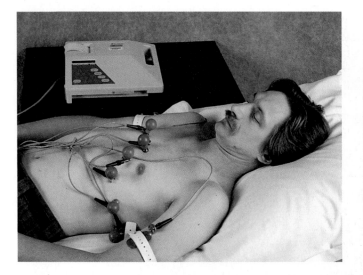

FIGURE 16–26 Patient with electrodes placed properly for standard 12-lead ECG

a routine ECG has been read as normal. Figure 16–28 illustrates the BaseLine prep kit and instructions for cardiac stress testing. The stress test ECG is done while a patient is exercising either on a bicycle or **treadmill** under careful supervision. Figure 16–29 shows a physician reading the computerized printout of a stress test in progress. The medical assistant monitors the patient's blood pressure while he exercises on the treadmill. The purpose of this test is to detect the unknown cause of the patient's heart trouble. (Refer to Chapter 11, Unit 8, for discussion regarding additional cardiovascular testing.) Even with ECGs and other diagnostic tests, the physician cannot predict future heart attacks.

HOLTER MONITORING

Patients who have normal routine ECGs but still have **intermittent** or irregular chest pain or discomfort, are often tested over a period of 24 hours or more by a device known as a **Holter monitor**. This method of recording the electrical activities of a patient's heart for a time is

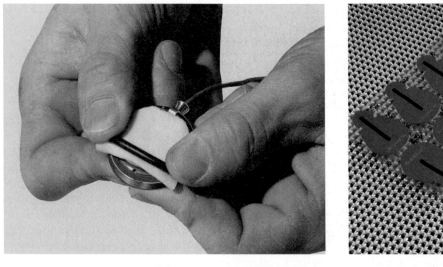

(A)

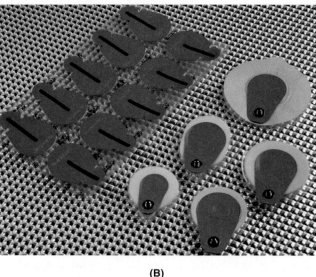

(B)

FIGURE 16–27 (A) Chest electrode that is held in place with chest strap (Courtesy of Spacelabs Medical, Inc.), (B) adhesive pregelled disposable electrodes (Courtesy of Spacelabs Medical, Inc.)

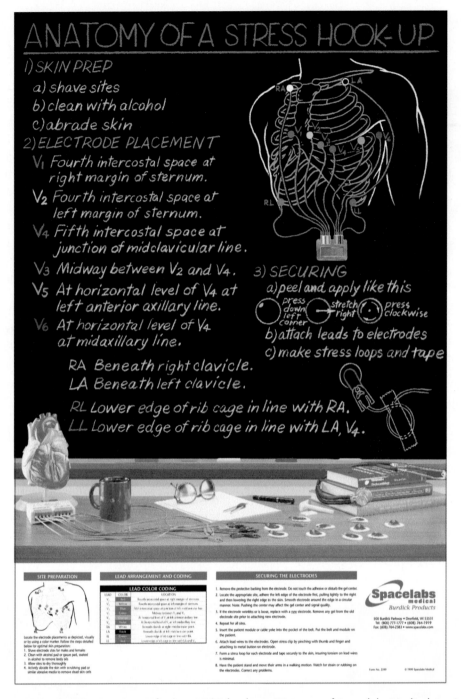

FIGURE 16–28 Instructions for stress ECG hook up. (Courtesy of Spacelabs Medical, Inc.)

also referred to as an ambulatory (walking) or "24-hour ECG." The ECG electrodes are attached to the patient's chest wall. A portable cassette recorder (monitor) is attached to a belt worn around the patient's waist. During the prescribed time, usually 24 hours, the patient's heart action is recorded. The patient is asked to keep a diary of all activities and note any pain or discomfort experienced during this monitoring. Figure 16–30 shows the medical assistant giving instructions to the patient about recording any problems. The patient is instructed to press the "event button" when any cardiac symptoms are experienced. At the end of the test period, the patient returns to have the

electrodes and monitor removed. The cassette is then placed in a computerized analyzer for a permanent printout of the results (or sent to a laboratory for interpretation). Evaluation of the 24 hour tracing reveals any cardiac **arrhythmias**, chest pain, and effectiveness of cardiac medications and correlates any symptoms with the patient's activity at the time it occurred. You should instruct patients to carry on with all routine daily activities during this test. Advise patients to take a "sponge bath" and not to get into a tub or shower while conducting this monitoring heart test. Ask patients to avoid using electric blankets or being around metal detectors, mag-

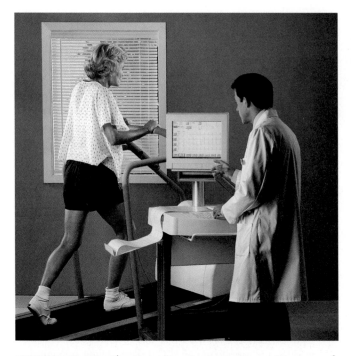

FIGURE 16–29 The Quest Exercise Stress System (Courtesy of Spacelabs Medical, Inc.)

nets, and high-voltage areas because these might interfere with the recording. This method of monitoring is also used in evaluating the status of recovering cardiac patients. See Procedure 16–4.

Another version of this test permits the patient to activate the recording device only when experiencing symptoms. This patient-activated monitor can be worn for several days.

OTHER CARDIOVASCULAR EQUIPMENT

Many medical offices, clinics, and emergency centers are equipped with a **defibrillator** (Figure 16–31). These units are designed to provide **countershock** by a trained individual to convert cardiac arrhythmias into regular sinus rhythm. Part of your routine duties may be to check this, and other equipment and supplies, to ensure that they are in proper working order and that everything is ready in case of a cardiac emergency. Employers offer in-service training periodically to all employees in assisting with emergency procedures. All employees should have current cardiopulmonary resuscitation (CPR) certification. Echocardiography is a noninvasive diagnostic tool that is the recording of the sound waves that are reflected through the heart. A transducer (similar to a microphone) sends and receives these sound waves and records them. Measurements are calculated to determine abnormalities within the heart. See Figure 16–32 for an example of this diagnostic technology.

ACHIEVE UNIT OBJECTIVES

Complete Chapter 16, Unit 2, in the workbook to help you obtain competency of this subject matter.

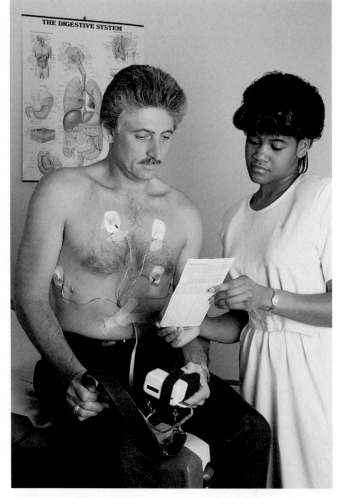

FIGURE 16–30 The medical assistant shows the patient the diary and gives instructions regarding the Holter monitor before securing it around his waist.

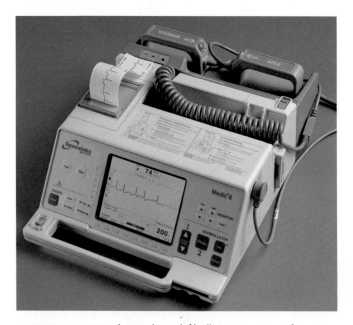

FIGURE 16–31 The Medic 6 defibrillator (Courtesy of Spacelabs Medical, Inc.)

PROCEDURE

16-4 Holter Monitoring

PURPOSE: To detect chest pain and cardiac arrhythmias, to evaluate chest pain and cardiac status following pacemaker implantation or after an acute myocardial infarction, and to determine correlation of symptoms and activity.

EQUIPMENT: Disposable razor and shaving cream, alcohol and swabs, pregelled adhesive electrodes, lead wires, appropriate batteries and tape recorder, standard ECG, diary for patient, belt for recorder, nonallergenic adhesive tape to secure electrodes PRN, drape sheet, patient's chart, pen.

PERFORMANCE OBJECTIVE: With all equipment and supplies provided, demonstrate the steps of the procedure for hooking up a patient for the Holter monitor. The instructor will observe each step.

1. Explain procedure to the identified patient. Ask patient to remove clothing from the waist up (provide a drape sheet). Assist patient to sit at the end of the examination table.

2. Wash hands and assemble equipment and supplies on Mayo table near patient.

3. Test Holter monitor for proper working order, and replace with new batteries if indicated. **RATIONALE: Batteries must function for entire test period.**

4. Use shaving cream and razor to remove chest hair if necessary. **RATIONALE: Smooth area provides optimal skin contact.** Rinse and dry electrode sites, and clean with alcohol swabs.

5. Rub each site vigorously with gauze square or skin rasp, and apply electrodes and lead wires carefully, making sure there is good skin contact. Use extra tape to secure electrodes and wires. Refer to Figure 16-31.

6. Place the belt around the patient's waist, and advise patient about care of recorder and precautions (refer to text). Assist patient in dressing to help avoid disturbing wires and electrodes. Remind patient not to take a tub bath or shower during 24-hour period.

7. Instruct patient to go about routine daily activities but to be sure to note in diary any symptoms or problems experienced (include the time it occurred and how long it lasted). **RATIONALE: Accurate reporting and recording is essential to correct interpretation of ECG findings when compared with activity taking place when symptoms occurred.**

8. Record date and time that monitor began on patient's chart and in the patient's diary, and initial.

9. Give patient diary to take with her, and arrange a return appointment time.

10. When patient comes in for appointment the next day, assist in disrobing. Remove electrodes and wires, clean electrode sites, and place cassette from recorder in computerized ECG for printout of tracing. Place diary and recording of ECG in patient's chart for evaluation by physician and initial.

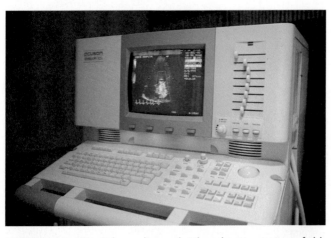

FIGURE 16–32 Echocardiograph (Photo by Marcia Butterfield, courtesy of W.A. Foote Memorial Hospital, Jackson, MI.)

UNIT 3

Diagnostic Procedures

■ OBJECTIVES

Upon completion of the unit, meet the following performance objectives by verifying knowledge of the facts and principles presented through oral and written communication at a level deemed competent. Demonstrate the specific behaviors as identified in the performance objectives of the procedures, observing all aseptic and safety precautions in accordance with health care standards.

1. Spell and define, using the glossary at the back of this text, all the **Words to Know** in this unit.

2. Describe a spirometry test, and state the purpose of it.
3. Instruct a patient about the spirometer, and demonstrate how to use it.
4. Explain what magnetic resonance imaging (MRI) is.
5. List reasons for contraindication of the MRI.
6. Describe ultrasound and state the purpose of it.
7. Explain the patient preparation for ultrasound procedures.
8. Describe patient education concerning the procedures in this unit.

AREAS OF COMPETENCE (AAMA)

This unit addresses content within the specific competency areas of *Fundamental principles, Diagnostic orders, Patient care, Professionalism, Communication skills, Legal concepts, Instruction,* and *Operational functions,* as identified in the Medical Assistant Role Delineation Study. Refer to Appendix A for a detailed listing of the areas.

■ WORDS TO KNOW

claustrophobia	noninvasive
diagnostic	oscilloscope
echocardiography	resonance imaging
echoes	sonogram
electromagnetic	sophisticated
implants	spirometer
magnetic	transducer
maturity	ultrasonic scanning

VITAL CAPACITY TESTS

Vital capacity is defined as the greatest volume of air that can be expelled during a complete, slow, unforced expiration following a maximum inspiration. Vital capacity should equal inspiratory capacity plus expiratory reserve. Vital capacity is usually reported in both absolute values and statistically derived values based on the age, sex, and height of the patient. The statistical value is reported as a percentage.

Several devices are used to measure the capacity of the lungs. Many physicians prefer to use the hand-held **spirometer,** which comes with vital capacity charts.

Vital capacity testing is performed to evaluate patients who are suspected to have pulmonary insufficiency. The spirometer is an instrument used to test the capacity of the lungs. Vital capacity testing aids in the diagnosis of and degree of functional or obstructive abnormalities. It also helps the physician find the cause of dyspnea and evaluate the effectiveness of medication and therapy.

When scheduling patients for these tests of vital capacity, it is important to advise them to eat lightly and not to smoke for at least six hours before the appointment. Patients should refrain from routine treatment, and medication should not be taken until after the test is completed.

In preparing to perform this diagnostic procedure, instruct the patient regarding the necessary steps and demonstrate the use of the spirometer. Routine procedures, such as height, weight, and vital signs, should be taken and recorded on the patient's chart. Showing the patient how to hold the instrument and what is expected will yield a more accurate test result. Disposable mouthpieces are used to prevent disease transmission. Most spirometers are computerized and have a printout of the results within minutes of administering the test. You should type in the patient's name, age, height, race, gender, account number, and any other information if applicable, before you start the test.

Figure 16–33 pictures the medical assistant coaching a patient through the procedure. A clip is placed on the patient's nose to force the expired air out of the lungs directly into the mouthpiece (make sure patient's mouth is sealed around the mouthpiece) and into the spirometer.

A CAAHEP CONNECTION

In performing the procedures in this unit, the medical assistant must be aware of explaining what is expected of the patient in cooperating with the steps of the procedures. Unless the patient knows exactly what to do and how to do it, the test outcome will be inaccurate and useless to the physician in diagnosis of the patient's medical problem(s). Good communication skills are vital to the success of diagnostic procedures. Observing the patient for non-verbal and verbal responses is necessary in completing procedures in an efficient and expedient manner. Taking this important skill into your career will help patients feel confident in your abilities and appreciate your concern for their well being.

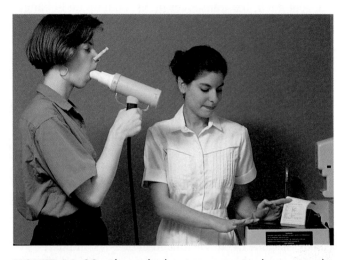

FIGURE 16–33 The medical assistant operates the computed spirometer while the patient blows exhaled air from the lungs into the disposable mouthpiece.

Instruct the patient to stand up straight and to take in a slow deep breath. Coach the patient to expel all the air from the lungs quickly until he cannot exhale any more, within approximately 15 seconds. Give the patient a couple of practice runs before beginning the official test because it is an awkward procedure for most people. Follow each of the expirations with a few seconds of resting for the patient. Watch for signs of stress, dizziness, coughing, or other problems the patient may have during the test. Generally three to five expirations are tested. The results are analyzed by the computerized instrument and the diagnostic data are printed for evaluation by the physician. Test results below 80% are usually considered abnormal. This spirometry reading is placed in the patient's chart, along with a notation of any symptoms or problems the patient may have had during the test and your initials. Spirometry tests should not be performed when the patient has been diagnosed with angina, acute coronary insufficiency, or recent myocardial infarction. Allow the patient to sit and relax to wait for consultation with physician. Instruct the patient to resume medication and therapy routine as directed by the physician.

You may be instructed to schedule patients for further pulmonary function studies to be performed by a pulmonary and thoracic specialist. More **sophisticated** equipment may be necessary to evaluate a patient's condition.

SONOGRAPHIC STUDIES

Sonograms are records obtained by **ultrasonic scanning**. Ultrasonography is a technique in which internal structures are made visible by recording the reflections, or **echoes**, of ultrasonic sound waves directed into the tissues. These high-frequency sound waves are conducted through the use of a **transducer** (a hand-held instrument resembling a microphone). While the transducer is held against the body area to be tested, it sends sound waves through the skin to various organs. As the echoes are sent back, the transducer picks them up and changes them into electrical energy. This energy is transmitted into an image on a monitor, or printed out on paper in wavy lines. The picture formed on the screen represents a cross-section of the organ. Photos of these images are taken for permanent records. The physician interprets these images to aid in the diagnosis and treatment of the patient. **Echocardiography** is a technique used to examine the heart: echoes are converted into electrical impulses, which create a picture of the tissues being examined on an **oscilloscope**.

Ultrasonography is useful in examination of the abdominopelvic cavity to locate aneurysms of the aorta and other blood vessel abnormalities. The size and shape of internal organs can also be determined with ultrasound. It can be of value in the identification of cysts and tumors of the eye and in the detection of pelvic masses and obstructions of the urinary tract. In obstetrics and gynecology, where the radiation of x-ray examination is avoided, ultrasound is useful in the diagnosis of multiple pregnancies

and in determining the size, **maturity**, and position of the fetus. Patient preparation may vary, but usually the patient is instructed to drink a large amount of water, up to a quart. This will distend the bladder, help to push the uterus into place, and increase the conduction of the sound waves. Sonograms are not useful in viewing the lungs, for echoes are not created by structures containing air.

When scheduling patients for this type of study, you should give them a few important instructions. They should avoid eating foods that produce gas and drink plenty of fluids (specific amounts are required for certain tests) as mentioned earlier (Figure 16–34). Check with the radiology facility regarding what the patient may drink. Some facilities allow other liquids besides water. However, no alcoholic beverages are permitted. Further instruct the patient *not* to void following drinking the water (or other liquids). Explain to the patient that she will be asked to lie down on an examination table and that the procedure lasts approximately 45 minutes to an hour. It is an accurate and painless diagnostic tool. A gel or lotion is used to produce better sound wave conduction and to allow the transducer to glide more easily across the skin.

Besides being a diagnostic procedure, ultrasound is used in the treatment of diseased or injured muscle tissue. Sound waves vibrate into the tissues producing heat, which helps to relieve inflammation and pain. It also increases circulation, which speeds up healing of injured muscle tissues. Another common use of ultrasound is in dentistry. Sound vibrations make it possible for tartar to be painlessly removed from the teeth.

Specific in-service training is necessary before using this instrument because the patient can be burned if precautions are not followed precisely.

must keep wand moving! (avoid per burn)

MAGNETIC RESONANCE IMAGING — MRI

A technique to view the structures inside the human body is called **magnetic resonance imaging** or MRI. This method allows physicians to examine a particular area of the body without exposing the patient to x-rays or surgery. This **noninvasive** procedure, which may range from 30 to 60 minutes, requires that the patient lie on a padded table that is moved into a tunnel-like structure (Figure 16–35).

There is no advance patient preparation required for this examination. The MRI procedure becomes an *invasive* procedure only when an intravenous contrast media is administered to the patient under certain conditions.

---

(1) ABDOMINAL ULTRASOUND: Take nothing by mouth after midnight. No breakfast on the morning of the examination.

(2) PELVIC ULTRASOUND: Drink 24–30 ounces of fluid one hour before the examination. Do not urinate after drinking the fluid.

(3) FETAL ULTRASOUND: Drink 24–30 ounces of fluid one hour before the examination. Do not urinate after drinking the fluid.

FIGURE 16–34 Preparation for ultrasound procedures

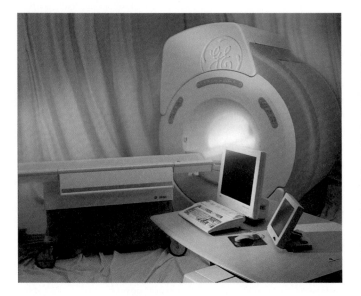

FIGURE 16–35   Magnetic resonance imaging (MRI) system shows computer screen. (Courtesy of GE Medical Systems.)

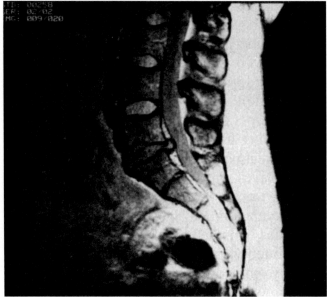

FIGURE 16–36   MRI shows a herniated disc in the lumbar spine. (Courtesy of GE Medical Systems)

This *contrast enhanced* technique is done during the last series of images of the examination to detect certain pathologies. The patient may resume normal activity following the procedure. There are no known harmful effects to the patient from this imaging technique.

The magnetic resonance machine scans all planes of a body structure to produce an image processed by a computer, without moving the patient. Radio signals are sent from the scanner that are influenced by strong magnetic fields to which the body responds. Figure 16–36 shows an image of the lumbar spine in the sagittal plane. Note the herniated disc and the clarity of the image. The MRI has reduced a great number of diagnostic exploratory surgeries. It is most useful in helping to diagnose brain and nervous system disorders, cardiovascular disease, cancer, and diseases of the visceral organs. Magnetic resonance imaging can be performed for particular areas of the body, such as the hip, shoulder, or neck. This specific imaging of small areas takes less time, approximately a half hour. Whatever the time requirement for the patient's appointment, explain this to the patient as a courtesy. The patient may better plan their transportation if the time of the appointment and the length of time the test takes is known. MRI is also used to help monitor the effectiveness of treatment. Since the MRI uses a strong **electromagnetic** field, it is extremely important that any metal objects be removed before the procedure is performed. The technician will request that the patient remove all metallic objects including jewelry, hairpins, and nonpermanent dentures before being placed in the tunnel for the MRI. Patients should be interviewed thoroughly regarding their health history. Inform the patient that at the facility where the MRI will be performed, they will generally be asked to sign a consent form prior to the procedure. Female patients should refrain from even wearing mascara since tiny metallic flakes may be present in it. During the procedure, these minute pieces of metal may become hot and burn the patient.

PATIENT EDUCATION

Assure the patient that the studies are done in a controlled environment. Always provide clear and concise oral *and* written instructions for examinations that require advance preparation. Be sure that the patient understands the necessary preparations. Answer all questions. Emphasize the importance of being on time for the radiological appointment to avoid unnecessary delays because some examinations are very long.

If the patient is not familiar with the facility where the x-ray studies are scheduled, give specific instructions (and a map) of how to get there and where to park. Patients appreciate this courtesy. Often, this information is printed on the appointment/information sheet the facility provides to medical offices and clinics for referral appointments.

If x-rays are considered as a part of the assessment of their condition, it is of vital importance that you advise all female patients who are of childbearing age to inform you if they are pregnant, or could possibly be. X-rays are contraindicated in pregnant females, especially in the first trimester because radiation is damaging to the fetus. During triage you should always ask females for the date of the first day of menstrual flow of their last menstrual period (LMP) for documentation in their chart. This will help in preventing any misunderstanding concerning a possible pregnancy. Other **diagnostic** exams can be performed that are safe for the fetus during this time as necessary.

During the process the many repetitive noises sound like clanging and banging, humming, and whirring. This is just the sound of the electromagnetic field. There are no sensations of pain and no known side effects. The patient must be still and relax for the test to be properly completed. The technician observes the patient during the entire time. Patients may speak to the technician by the use of a microphone inside the tunnel.

The MRI procedure is contraindicated in patients who have pacemakers, have metallic **implants**, are in the first trimester of pregnancy, are severely claustrophobic, or are obese. The **claustrophobia** can be handled by counseling and/or the use of a sedative administered by a physician before the procedure is begun.

ACHIEVE UNIT OBJECTIVES

Complete Chapter 16, Unit 3, in the workbook to help you obtain competency of this subject matter.

UNIT 4

Diagnostic Radiological Examinations

OBJECTIVES

Upon completion of the unit, meet the following performance objectives by verifying knowledge of the facts and principles presented through oral and written communication at a level deemed competent. Demonstrate the specific behaviors as identified in the performance objectives of the procedures, observing all aseptic and safety precautions in accordance with health care standards.

1. Spell and define, using the glossary at the back of the text, all the **Words to Know** in this unit.
2. Instruct patients in preparation for radiological studies.
3. Explain the importance of diet in preparation of x-rays.
4. Explain why pregnant women should not have x-rays.
5. Describe x-rays that require no preparation.
6. Explain the importance of patient education in scheduling a mammography.

AREAS OF COMPETENCE (AAMA)

This unit addresses content within the specific competency areas of *Fundamental principles, Diagnostic orders, Patient care, Professionalism, Communication skills, Legal concepts, Instruction,* and *Operational functions,* as identified in the Medical Assistant Role Delineation Study. Refer to Appendix A for a detailed listing of the areas.

WORDS TO KNOW

absorb	fluoroscope
artifact	intravenous pyelogram
compression	(IVP)
computed transaxial	iodine
tomography (CTAT)	KUB (kidneys, ureters,
conjunction	bladder)
contract	lesion
contrast	mammography
cystoscope	planes
distends	radioactive
electromagnetic	radiograph
radiation	radiologist
electron	radiopaque
enema	residual barium
evacuate	retrograde
flatus	roentgen
flexible	therapeutic

RADIOLOGICAL STUDIES

Radiology is a mysterious realm to most patients. The perceptive medical assistant can sense that patients exhibit a fear of what is going to happen to them during the radiology procedure(s) and even more frightening is what the radiologist may find. Generally, patients know if there is something seriously wrong with them. These patients and all others need to feel a comforting touch. The medical assistant should show genuine caring and compassion to patients who are in pain and discomfort. When they are in your care and you can see that they are confused and unsure of what will happen next, you can offer them support and reassurance. Often, just talking to them for a few minutes can ease their fears and uncertainties. Many times, the patient has never been to a radiological facility and is somewhat frightened and uneasy about being there. Checking the patient's medical history and simply talking

A CAAHEP CONNECTION

As patients come in for office visits and disclose their symptoms, they do not always know the severity of their medical problems. Again, it should be stressed that effective communication is of utmost importance. Often the patient senses that there is something very seriously wrong and they may already be somewhat depressed. Your responsibility to both patient and physician is to communicate information and to record findings appropriately on the patient's chart. You must show compassion and understanding to patients regardless of their problems. Each patient should be treated as an individual with respect and dignity.

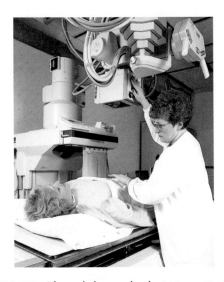

FIGURE 16–37 The radiology technologist is positioning the patient and adjusting the x-ray tube over the patient. (Photo by Marcia Butterfield, courtesy of W.A. Foote Memorial Hospital, Jackson, MI.)

to the patient will give you this information. Asking the patient if she has ever had an x-ray before is certainly the first question you should pose. If you can give the patient an idea of what to expect and describe what it is like, you can lessen the stress and anxiety of the patient. Figure 16–37 shows a technologist getting a patient positioned and adjusting the angle of the beam of the x-ray tube. When the physician orders x-rays to aid in the diagnosis of their condition, it could be the patient's first encounter with this process. Children especially can be apprehensive about what is going to happen to them. You can explain to a child that having x-rays taken is just like having pictures taken with a camera; the x-ray machine is really a great big metal camera taking a picture of the inside of their body. Explain that you have to be very still when having an x-ray taken just like when you have a photograph taken so that the picture does not get blurred and out of focus. The child will be more cooperative when given an explanation of what to expect. Explain that a big lead apron will be put over him to protect the reproductive organs from the x-rays. Visual aides are helpful to show patients what radiological equipment looks like. Generally, the radiology technologist will be very understanding with children and will show the child the x-ray film when it is processed. The x-ray the physician has ordered will determine the extent of what patient education is indicated. Some radiological studies require preparation before they can be performed. You must make sure that the patient understands all instructions clearly to avoid misunderstandings and time delays. Often the explanation will be quite simple because the patient already knows there is an obvious problem, such as an injury. For example, Figure 16–38 shows a severe fracture of the femur.

All radiology departments have signs prominently displayed in several areas of their facility that tell female patients to inform the radiology technologist or radiologist

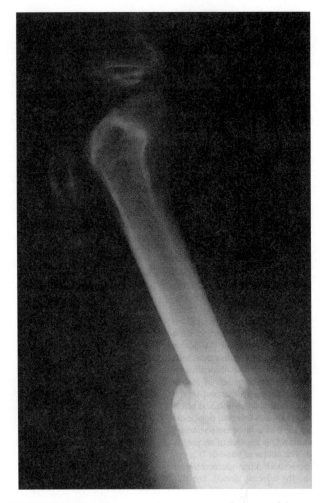

FIGURE 16–38 This x-ray shows a severe fracture of the femur.

physician if they are pregnant or if they possibly could be pregnant. X-rays can be damaging to an unborn child, especially in the first three months of pregnancy (first trimester), sometimes before the patient is even aware she is pregnant. Before scheduling any female patient whose age indicates that she is within the childbearing years, you must always ask if she could be pregnant.

Radiological studies are made by the use of x-rays (**roentgen** rays), which are high-energy **electromagnetic radiation** produced by the collision of a beam of **electrons** with a metal target in an x-ray tube. An x-ray photograph is taken of the requested part of the patient's body, and a permanent film picture is made. Patients must follow preparation instructions for certain radiological studies. Bone studies do not require preparation and are performed to aid in the diagnosis of tumors, fractures, and other disorders and diseases. Chest x-rays do not normally need advanced preparation. When the physician orders an x-ray of the chest (Figure 16–39), the patient is asked to hold still in the positions shown in Figure 16–40 so that a permanent film (upon inspiration of breath) can be taken and evaluated by the radiologist. A report of the radiological studies is sent to the primary physician. The

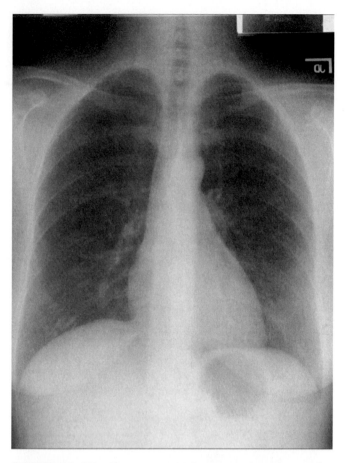

FIGURE 16–39 Chest x-ray—AP (anterior posterior) view of the chest.

physician may request to view the films. **Therapeutic** x-rays are used in the treatment of cancer. Following are the most commonly ordered radiological studies for which

you may be responsible in scheduling and preparing patients. It is very important to review the preparation instructions for various radiological and sonographic studies when you schedule the patient's appointment because techniques and preps can vary from one facility to another and are also subject to change with technology.

Gallbladder—Imaging

The gallbladder stores bile that is produced in the liver to break down fat in the digestive process. When the gallbladder malfunctions, the patient experiences abdominal discomfort (nausea) and pain. The cholecystogram enables the physician to diagnose the cause of the patient's distress. Even though this procedure is rarely performed, there may be occasions when the physician may still order a patient to have a cholecystogram. Providing the necessary information for the patient to follow will help the radiology technologist produce a quality film for the radiologist to evaluate. The oral cholecystogram is also referred to as a gallbladder series and a double dose gallbladder. Refer to Figure 16–41, which shows gallstones present on the permanent film of the cholecystogram.

An imaging technique that has replaced the cholecystogram is the abdominal ultrasound. Ultrasound, or sonography, is a process of using sound waves with a frequency of over 20,000 vibrations per second to produce images of the internal structures of the body. An image is produced when continuous sound waves are projected toward the desired area to measure and record the reflected image. This procedure requires a 12-hour fast for a morning appointment. This generally means that the patient should have nothing to eat or drink past midnight the

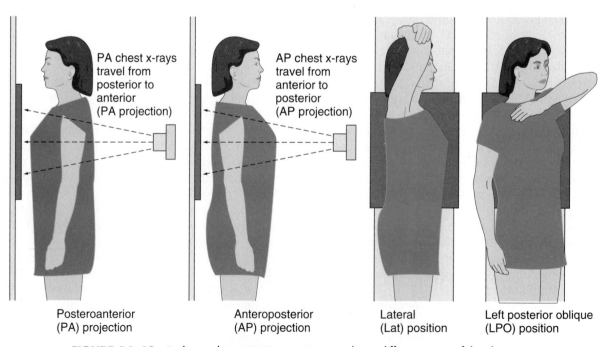

Posteroanterior
(PA) projection

Anteroposterior
(AP) projection

Lateral
(Lat) position

Left posterior oblique
(LPO) position

FIGURE 16–40 Radiographic projection positions to obtain different views of the chest

night before the scheduled ultrasound and no breakfast the morning of the appointment. Some radiology facilities offer afternoon appointments for abdominal ultrasounds. To prepare for this, the patient is instructed to have a fat-free liquid breakfast before 9:00 AM the day of the appointment with nothing to eat or drink until after the ultrasound. The abdominal ultrasound includes gallbladder, pancreas, liver, and other visceral organs. Sonograms are very useful in aiding in the diagnosis of gallstones, tumors, heart defects, and fetal abnormalities.

In addition to abdominal ultrasound examinations, you may be required to give patients necessary information about pelvic and fetal ultrasound procedures. In the procedure for a pelvic ultrasound, a vaginal probe is used to aid in visualizing internal structures. It is helpful for patients to be aware of this before it is done so that they will be prepared. Refer to Unit 3 of this chapter for review.

In preparation for this study of the gallbladder, the patient must follow a prescribed diet and take prescribed medications (a **contrast** medium) to make the gallbladder visible on the x-ray film (Figure 16–41 and 16–42). Generally, the patient is advised to avoid drinking alcoholic and carbonated beverages the day before the exam be-

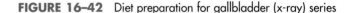

1. Two days prior to exam, starting at 6 P.M., take one tablet of Oragrafin every five minutes until six tablets have been taken.
2. On day prior to exam, repeat step 1.
3. Day prior to exam, take 4 oz. of Neoloid or three Dulcolax 5 mg tablets from 2–4 P.M.
4. Evening before exam, eat a fatfree meal—dry toast, tea, fruit, jello.
5. Nothing by mouth after midnight.
6. No breakfast.

FIGURE 16–42 Diet preparation for gallbladder (x-ray) series

cause these drinks may produce **flatus** (gas). Unless otherwise specified by the physician, you should remind patients to take their regularly prescribed medication(s).

The preparation for the gallbladder ultrasound is minimal in comparison to the cholecystogram. The preparation for the sonogram is much easier for the patient because it only requires preparation on the same day as the appointment. You should still advise patients regarding

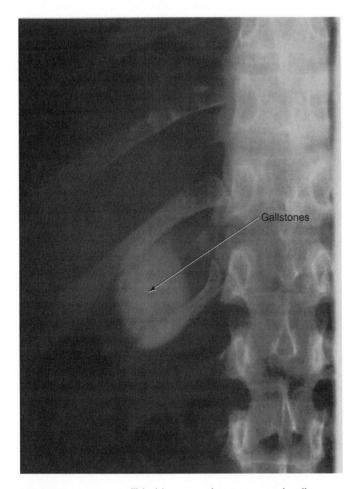

FIGURE 16–41 Gallbladder x-ray showing several gallstones (cholelith)

PATIENT EDUCATION

Most patients with gallbladder trouble already know they should avoid fatty foods. The usual preparation for a cholecystogram is a nonfatty evening meal the night before the scheduled appointment. Foods which are permitted are fresh fruits and vegetables, lean meat (broiled), toast, bread, jelly, and coffee or tea. Fatty foods will cause the gallbladder to **contract** and empty the contrast medium, which the patient usually takes following the evening meal.

The medication is usually in pill form, with directions to swallow one tablet every five minutes with a minimum amount of water until all are consumed. Repeating this a second night is necessary to define the gallbladder sufficiently. This takes approximately half an hour. Spreading the consumption of the contrast medium out over this time allows the gallbladder to **absorb** the substance. The patient is instructed to eat or drink nothing after midnight the night before the cholecystogram is performed. In addition to these preparations, many physicians request an **enema**, laxative, or both to help remove fecal material and gas, which could cause shadows, blockages, or other **artifacts**.

Often, when the series of **radiographs** is completed, patients are given a drink called "fatty meal" or are instructed to return after a meal containing fats to observe radiographs that show how the gallbladder functions during digestion of fats.

PATIENT EDUCATION

UGI preparation requires that the patient eat a light evening meal of only clear liquids (see Figure 16–42). The patient should have nothing to eat or drink from midnight until after the x-ray series the next day. Prescribed medications must not be consumed until after the films have been taken, or the view of the structures could be impaired. Dairy products, carbonated beverages, and alcohol are not permitted. The digestive tract should be clear of all foods to avoid blockage of or shadows on the anatomical structures to be observed.

Constipation may result from the barium, and patients should be advised to drink plenty of clear liquids to help relieve it. You should also mention that their stool may appear lighter than usual from the white barium, and that this should not be a cause for concern. Laxatives are ordered only by the physician. Patients should phone the medical office if any problem arises.

ESOPHAGUS, UPPER GI SERIES

1. Nothing by mouth after midnight.
2. No breakfast.

IF SMALL BOWEL

1. Day prior to exam—Take 4 oz. of Neoloid or three Dulcolax 5 mg tablets from 2–4 P.M.
2. Nothing by mouth after midnight.
3. No breakfast

FIGURE 16–43 Preparation for UGI (upper gastrointestinal) series.

their diet and what to expect during the visit to the radiology facility.

Upper GI Series—Barium Swallow

For this study, the patient must drink the contrast medium during the examination while the **radiologist** observes the flow of the substance directly by means of a **fluoroscope**. The contrast medium is a mixture of barium and water, usually flavored to increase palatability. In radiology, it is now a custom to use "Fizzy's" that are crystals similar to Alka-Seltzer combined with a small amount of water to add air to the stomach. This is called a "double contrast." Next, a thickened barium mixture is ingested by mouth. Then, to examine further the esophagus and duodenal bulb, a thin barium mixture is given to the patient. Radiologic films are taken for a permanent record of the upper digestive tract. During the study, the patient is positioned so that different angles of the digestive organs can be seen.

The physician observes the functioning of the esophagus, stomach, duodenum, and small intestine as the barium passes. Such disorders or diseases as hiatal hernias, peptic or duodenal ulcers, and tumors may be diagnosed as a result of the upper GI series. Adherence to a restricted diet the day before and on the day of the exam is also necessary (Figure 16–43).

Lower GI Series—Barium Enema

Patients who are scheduled for this radiological study should follow the preparation listed in Figure 16–44 very

strictly. Stress the avoidance of milk and all dairy products for better visualization of the colon. Be sure to explain the importance of adequate preparation for these studies. Improper preparation could result in the need to repeat the tests.

In this examination, barium sulfate is the contrast medium. It is introduced into the colon by an enema tube, and the radiologist observes the flow into the lower bowel. Many physicians order a barium enema with air-contrast. This procedure **distends** the barium-filled colon with air to make the structures more visible by fluoroscopy. Permanent radiographs are taken periodically

BARIUM ENEMA OR COLON EXAMINATION.

a. Beginning the morning of the day before the examination, change to an all liquid diet*, as outlined below. Do not take any more solid food until after the examinations.

b. At 12:30 P.M., or half an hour after lunch on the day before the examination, drink entire contents of a bottle of Citrate of Magnesia (10 oz.).

c. At 1:00 P.M., drink one glass of fluid.

d. At 3:00 P.M., take two Dulcolax tablets with a large glass of water.

e. At 4:00 P.M., drink one large glass of fluid.

f. At 5:00 P.M., or as close as possible, liquid dinner.

g. At 6:00 P.M., drink one large glass of fluid.

h. Bedtime—drink one large glass of fluid.

i. You may have one cup of coffee, tea, or water on the morning of the examination.

*ALL LIQUID DIET

You may have any of the following: coffee, tea, carbonated beverages, clear gelatin desserts, strained fruit juice, bouillon, clear broths, tomato juice. Do not drink milk of any kind.

Please call office if you have any questions regarding above instructions.

FIGURE 16–44 Preparation for barium enema

during the procedure. This study is helpful in diagnosing diseases of the colon, tumors, and **lesions**.

The barium enema procedure generally takes several minutes and produces discomfort and some pain. Patients should be told to breathe through the mouth slowly and deeply to help relax the abdominal muscles. A strong urge to defecate is normal, and patients often cannot resist the urge. After several films have been taken and the study of the lower bowel is completed, the patient is allowed to use the toilet.

Patients should be encouraged to drink plenty of liquids for the next few days to help evacuate the **residual barium** sulfate in the lower colon.

Intravenous Pyelogram

In studies of the genitourinary system, the **intravenous pyelogram (IVP)** (Figure 16–45) requires that the patient prepare with laxatives, enemas, and fasting (Figure 16–46). The IVP consists of an intravenous injection of **iodine**, the contrast medium, to define the structures of the urinary system. **CAUTION:** Patients who have a known iodine allergy should alert the radiology department personnel so that non-iodine preparation may be used in their x-ray studies. Patients who are suspected of having an allergy to iodine should be tested by order of the physician. This information should be obtained during the medical

PATIENT EDUCATION
Patients must prepare for this study by precisely following instructions, usually beginning the day before the appointment. The instructions generally include laxatives and enemas to clear the bowel of fecal matter and gas. The patient should eat lightly, avoid dairy products, and drink plenty of clear liquids to encourage more comfortable **evacuation**. Patients should have nothing to eat or drink past midnight the night before the x-ray (see Figure 16–43). On the day of the appointment, the patient should have an enema two hours before the scheduled appointment.

history interview and documented accurately. Allergies should be recorded or circled in red ink so that attention is brought to this vital information. A **retrograde** pyelogram is a study of the urinary tract done by inserting a sterile catheter into the urinary meatus, through the bladder, and up into the ureters. The **radiopaque** contrast medium then flows upward into the kidneys. This diagnostic test is usually done in **conjunction** with **cystoscopy**. Patients should have iodine-sensitive tests prior to the examination to determine the possibility of an allergic reaction. A voiding cystogram may be ordered in conjunction with an IVP. In this case, the contrast medium is injected into the bladder by catheter, and no special patient preparation is needed.

KUB

The **KUB (kidneys, ureters, bladder)** is an x-ray of the patient's abdomen, sometimes termed "flat plate of abdomen." This requires no patient preparation and is used in the diagnosis of urinary system diseases and disorders. It may also be useful in determining the position of an intrauterine device (IUD) or in locating foreign bodies in the digestive tract. In some cases, surgery is indicated to remove an object that may block the normal digestive flow, but many small objects are easily passed with solid

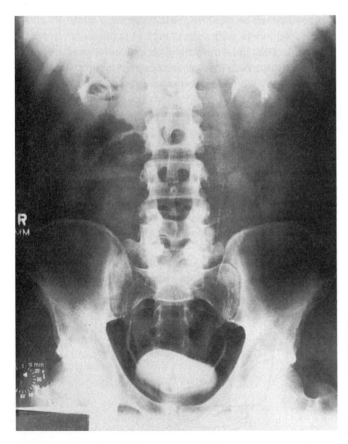

FIGURE 16–45 Radiologic x-ray of kidneys, ureters, and bladder (IVP)

ALL LIQUID DIET
You may have any of the following: coffee, tea, carbonated beverages, clear gelatin desserts, strained fruit juice, bouillon, clear broths, tomato juice. Do not drink milk of any kind.
1. Day prior to exam—three Dulcolax 5 mg tablets from 2–4 P.M.
2. You may drink only one glass of liquid on the morning of the exam.

FIGURE 16–46 Preparation for intravenous pyelogram (IVP)

PATIENT EDUCATION

The medical assistant should schedule the mammography during the first week following the patient's menstrual cycle because the breasts must be compressed firmly during the procedure to obtain a satisfactory image for diagnostic purposes (Figure 16–47). During this time, the patient would experience less discomfort. Because this procedure is often very uncomfortable and even sometimes painful in many women, there are other suggestions that may be helpful in reducing the discomfort. For instance, it is advisable to tell patients to omit caffeine from their diets for 7 to 10 days prior to this examination to reduce the possible effects of swelling and soreness that caffeine often produces. **Compression** of the breasts during this procedure requires less radiation to be used. It also allows a much clearer picture to be taken of the breast tissue. Following this exam, some areas of the breast(s) may sometimes become temporarily discolored. However, it does not damage the breast tissue and should not be alarming. At the advice of the physician, a mild analgesic may be taken to relieve any discomfort or aching that may be experienced by the patient.

Explaining these details to the patient and requesting their cooperation with the radiology technician during this procedure will be most helpful in obtaining a quality mammogram for diagnostic study by the physician. It is also important to let the patient know when the results will be available so that they will not have to contend with unnecessary worry. Remind patients again of the importance of breast self-examinations on a continuing basis. The mammography is not a substitute for this important means of detection.

foods, especially in young children whose internal structures are more **flexible**. The physician ultimately makes this decision in patient care.

Mammography

Mammography aids in the diagnosis of breast masses, some of which may be as small as one cm in size or less. Women who practice self-examinations regularly each month and find lumps in breast tissue early have a much better cure rate if a malignancy is found. Breast self-examination (see Chapter 14, Unit 3) and regular examinations by the physician should be strongly reinforced to female patients in addition to their scheduled mammography. The American Cancer Society recommends a baseline mammography at the age of 35 for all women. After age 40, women are urged to have a mammography every year. Some insurance companies will not pay for this exam before a woman is 40 without a written order from the patient's physician. However, most insurance providers will pay for a mammography at any age if it is diagnostic.

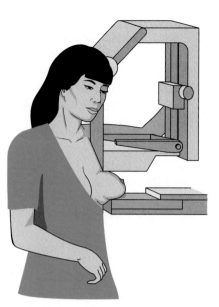

FIGURE 16–47 Breasts are compressed by plates during mammography to produce a clearer image of structures.

At any time a lump is found, patients should be advised to see the physician at once for examination. This procedure requires the patient to move into various positions so that different angles of the breast tissue may be x-rayed (Figure 16–47). The x-ray pictures are called mammograms. Patients are usually advised to wear slacks or a skirt for ease in preparation for the procedure Figure 16–48) because it is necessary to undress to the waist for the examination. The only preparation required is that the patient wash the chest and underarms and rinse and dry thoroughly. No deodorants, perfumes, or powders are to be used on the day of the mammography because the film on the skin from these substances could interfere with the radiograph. As a courtesy to patients, most diagnostic facilities provide soap, towels, and spray deodorant for patients to use after their mammography is completed. You may remind patients to bring their own preferred toiletry items.

To ensure the best results for your mammogram, please follow these procedures prior to your appointment:

a. BE SURE TO NOTIFY OUR PERSONNEL IF YOU ARE PREGNANT.

b. Please shower or bathe as close to your appointment time as possible.

c. Do not use deodorants, powders, perfumes, and etc. on the breast or underarm areas.

d. You will only have to undress to the waist, so wear an easily removable top such as a blouse.

FIGURE 16–48 Instructions for mammography preparation

Body Scans

Rapid scanning of single-tissue **planes** is performed by a process that generates images of the tissue in "slices" about one cm thick. Figure 16–49 illustrates how different parts of the body are sectioned for the image. This

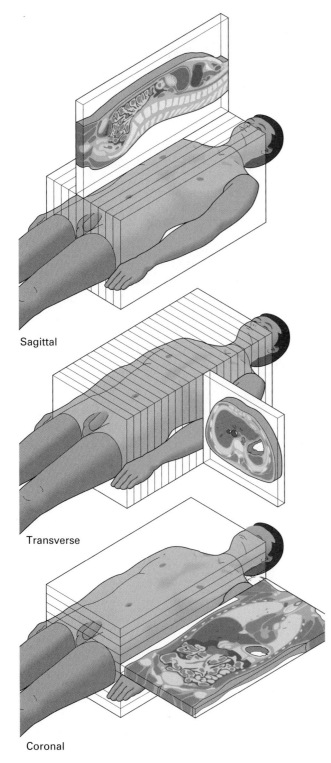

Sagittal

Transverse

Coronal

Computed Tomography (CT)

FIGURE 16–49 Computed tomography provides a three-dimensional view of the internal structures of the body.

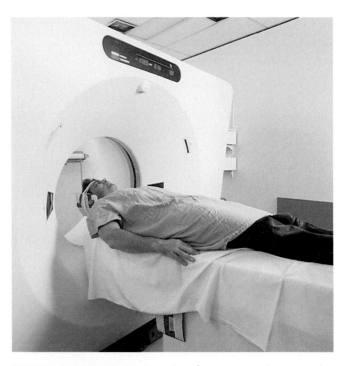

A CAAHEP CONNECTION

It is very important for the medical assistant and other health care providers to realize that in some cultures and religions, women are to keep themselves covered at all times when they are in public and in the presence of men. A breast examination and mammography would be especially problematic for the patient unless a female physician or technologist conducted the exam or the mammography. Be sure that you explain to the patient or ask an interpreter to explain the preparation, examination, and the imaging to prepare the patient for this experience. Relieving anxiety about this matter will help the patient understand and not be afraid of what to expect.

method of radiology is called the CAT or CT (computed axial tomography) scan or **CTAT (computed transaxial tomography)**. These procedures can be performed in seconds and aid in diagnosis of diseases and disorders of the breast or other internal organs (Figure 16–50).

The branch of medicine that uses radionuclides in the diagnosis and treatment of disease is nuclear medicine. Almost any organ of the body may be viewed and recorded by having the patient ingest, or be injected with, radioactive material.

Uptake studies refer to procedures in which patients ingest a **radioactive** substance under careful supervision and return within 24 hours to have the amount of

FIGURE 16–50 Patient in position for a computed tomography

radioactive substance in a particular organ measured. For example, the radioactive thyroid uptake determines the function of the thyroid gland. Tumors of the thyroid may also be determined by this method. In female patients, pregnancy should be determined prior to the radioactive thyroid uptake, for it is seriously damaging to the fetus, especially within the first trimester of pregnancy.

ACHIEVE UNIT OBJECTIVES

Complete Chapter 16, Unit 4, in the workbook to help you obtain competency of this subject matter.

RELATING TO ABHES

Chapter 16 discusses the various diagnostic skin tests, procedures to evaluate cardiac performance, assessment of lung function, and routine radiologic studies. This content is related to the ABHES accreditation requirements of *Patient examination, Medical equipment,* and *Specialties* within the content area of **Medical Office Clinical Procedures.**

RESOURCES

Columbus Radiology, Grant Livingston Location, 3341 East Livingston Avenue, Columbus, Ohio 43227.

Diagnostic tests, nurse's ready reference (1990). Springhouse, PA: Springhouse Corporation.

Mosby's medical, nursing, and allied health dictionary (4th ed.). (1994). St. Louis: Mosby.

Radiology Inc., 1375 S. Hamilton Rd., Columbus, Ohio 43232.

Siemens Burdick, Inc., Schaumburg, Illinois 60173.

Wendt-Bristol Diagnostic Center, 1550 Kenny Road, Columbus, OH.

WEB LINKS

http://www.sinuses.com (Sinusitis)

This web site is maintained by Wellington S. Tichenor, M.D. It explores the symptoms and treatment of sinusitis, and other sinus diseases and the interrelated problems of allergy and asthma.

Medical-Legal-Ethical Scenario

Johnetta was working with patients one afternoon when her clinical supervisor asked her to schedule a patient, Leslie Drake, for a barium enema. Because Johnetta was in the middle of getting an infant ready for a six-month examination at the time, she told her supervisor she would do it as soon as she finished with the baby. When she came out of the room, Dr. Lane asked Johnetta to do an ECG. After completing it, she was asked to explain the prep for an IVP to an elderly patient. Johnetta's day kept going with one thing after another. Forgetting to schedule the barium enema, she mistakenly put Ms. Drake's chart with the others to be filed. To help finish up so the all staff could go home, Johnetta helped file charts. She was exhausted by the time they closed the office.

The next day there was a call from Leslie Drake asking about her appointment for the barium enema.

Johnetta was embarrassed because she forgot to schedule it and had filed her chart yesterday at the end of the day. When Johnetta phoned the radiology department to schedule the appointment, the soonest she could make it was in two weeks. She was also upset when she read the physician's note on the chart that said "schedule BaE stat." Johnetta was told that if she had called yesterday (Wednesday) the appointment could have been on Thursday because there was a cancellation. She asked if they could please squeeze in this patient the next day, but this was not possible. When Johnetta called and informed Ms. Drake when the appointment was, she was upset that it would be so long to wait but agreed to take the appointment. Johnetta did not tell the doctor.

CRITICAL THINKING CHALLENGE

1. What was Johnetta's first mistake?
2. When should she have made the appointment?
3. Did she even look at the chart before filing it?
4. Why didn't she tell the physician?
5. How serious is this situation?
6. What should Johnetta do?
7. Is the clinical supervisor at fault for anything?
8. What would you have done in this situation?

Minor Surgical Procedures

As a clinical medical assistant, you may assist with a variety of sterile procedures. Maintaining medical asepsis is vital to prevent the transmission of diseases *before, during,* and *following* any of the invasive surgical procedures performed in the medical office or clinic. In compliance with Standard Precautions, proper barriers, such as latex or vinyl gloves, gown, and face mask or shield, must be worn to protect the health care staff from possible **contamination** while performing these procedures. All disposable waste must be placed in a plastic biohazardous bag or in a sharps container and discarded properly to prevent disease transmission.

Setup for various procedures may vary slightly according to the physician's preference. However, sterile technique will always remain the same for any invasive procedure. The basic information for assisting both the physician and patient is covered in this chapter.

OBJECTIVES

Upon completion of this chapter, meet the following performance objectives by verifying knowledge of the facts and principles presented through oral and written communication at a level deemed competent. Demonstrate the specific behaviors as identified in the performance objectives of the procedures, observing all aseptic and safety precautions in accordance with health care standards.

1. Spell and define, using the glossary at the back of the text, all the **Words to Know** in this chapter.
2. Explain scheduling and preop and postop instructions of patients for minor office surgery.
3. Explain the importance of obtaining the consent form for the surgical procedure.
4. Demonstrate skin preparation procedure for surgical site.
5. Prepare treatment room and minor surgical tray setup.
6. Describe various procedures that require sterile technique.
7. Demonstrate procedure for assisting with minor surgery.
8. Demonstrate how to assist with suturing a laceration.
9. Demonstrate how to put on and remove sterile gloves properly.
10. Describe proper care of surgical instruments.
11. Demonstrate proper way to remove sutures.
12. Describe important information that should be recorded on patient's chart.

AREAS OF COMPETENCE (AAMA)

This unit addresses content within the specific competency areas of *Fundamental principles, Diagnostic orders, Patient care, Professionalism, Communication skills, Legal concepts,* and *Instruction,* as identified in the Medical Assistant Role Delineation Study. Refer to Appendix A for a detailed listing of the areas.

WORDS TO KNOW

adverse	dominant
anesthesia	electrocautery
anesthesiologist	electrocoagulation
anesthetic	eschar
antiseptic	expiration
appropriate	fenestrated
authorize	hemophilia
biopsy	histology
coagulation	hypoallergenic
contaminate	incision and drainage
cryosurgery	(I & D)
debridement	invasive

microbial	stress
polyp	suture
postoperative (postop)	taut
preoperative (preop)	wart
schedule	

Laceration Repair

The medical assistant is usually responsible for **scheduling** minor office surgery. Surgery may include removal of a sebaceous cyst, **wart**, or foreign object; circumcision; vasectomy; skin biopsy; **incision and drainage (I & D)**; out-patient dilation and curretage (D & C); insertion of an IUD; and many other out-patient surgeries.

You may be asked to schedule an appointment for a patient to have a surgical procedure as an out-patient at a large medical center or hospital. Be sure to check with the person who makes the appointment regarding the preparation for the patient because it may be different from what your instructions are. When you write the appointment date and time for the patient, make certain the patient has directions to the facility if he is not familiar with the area. The assistant in the hospital or surgeon's office generally phones the patient the day before the surgery to confirm the appointment. You should also get a pre-certification from the patient's medical insurance company, unless you know definitely that the patient is responsible for this or the surgeon's office assistant is.

PATIENT EDUCATION

Preop

In scheduling, advise patient of:

1. Approximate length of time for procedure
2. Appropriate clothing to wear at appointment
3. Amount of time to fast as instructed by physician
4. Arranging for someone to accompany him
5. Anticipated time to take off work or arranging for home care
6. The surgical procedure by providing printed education materials

When patient arrives for appointment:

1. Provide written instructions regarding the surgical procedure and follow-up care
2. Explain surgical consent form, and obtain patient's signature
3. Answer any questions concerning procedure
4. Ascertain if the patient has any allergies to any medications, including topical preparations, latex products, and adhesive tapes.

Be mindful of the amount of time required for each type of surgical procedure you schedule. Advise patients as you make their appointments how long they should plan to be at the office on the day of their minor surgery. Depending on the type of procedure being performed, patients may need to make arrangements for someone to bring them for the appointment and take them home. Occasionally patients do not feel well enough following a surgical procedure to drive or travel alone and should have some assistance for at least a few hours. Because it is unpredictable how an individual patient may react to even a minor surgical procedure, it is best to advise *all* patients to arrange for assistance to ensure their safety and well-being. You should also advise them about possibly taking appropriate time off from work or arranging for home care, depending on the procedure scheduled.

You should first be sure that the patient understands the procedure and the instructions regarding **preoperative** (**preop**) and **postoperative** (**postop**) care. Most medical facilities have printed instructions for patients. Be mindful that some patients you see are either non-English speaking or cannot read. You need to explain as well as you can verbally and observe the patient's reactions to your instructions. Printed instructions in other languages and the services of an intrepreter should be made available to the patient. Information regarding this can be obtained through the local medical association in your area. This eliminates any misunderstandings, and patients feel more at ease knowing they can refer to it. Patients should be advised of the **appropriate** clothing to be worn on the day of the surgery. Loose-fitting clothing, clothing easy to put on and take off, and clothing that is not their "Sunday best" should be suggested as appropriate for the anatomical area of surgery. It is a good practice to phone the patient the day prior to the appointment, not only to reassure the patient and answer any questions but to confirm the physician's schedule.

The day before the scheduled surgery, you should get all the necessary surgical instruments and supplies ready. A routine inventory of all supplies and sterile items is vital so that a sterile tray set-up can be made for any emergency surgical procedure. Having whatever is needed in an emergency situation lessens stress and allows for more efficient and expedient care in an emergency.

All surgical instruments must be properly labeled and autoclaved. Most of the instruments will already have been sterilized as they should be after each use. The basic setup for most minor surgical procedures includes the following sterile items: scalpel handle and blades, hemostats (straight or curved), needles holder, needles and **suture** material (catgut or silk), suture scissors, thumb forceps, probe, gauze squares, sponges, vial of anesthetic medication, syringes, needles, towels, and bandages. Some of these supplies may be wrapped and sterilized together. All sterile packages must be labeled with the contents, date package was sterilized, and the signature of the person who prepared and sterilized it. Items that need to be added

are dropped onto the sterile field after the wrap has been carefully unfolded on the Mayo table by sterile technique. Autoclaved items remain sterile if they have been properly processed and have been protected from moisture for 30 days. Packages should be checked before use for any tears or other signs of tampering to ensure sterility.

Most items used today are disposable and come already sterile in the manufacturer's packaging. You must make sure that the package has not been torn or punctured to ensure sterility. The sterilization of the product is guaranteed only to a certain date marked on the package, and this date must be checked.

A variety of minor **invasive** surgical procedures are performed in the medical office, and each requires several instruments. Figure 17–1 shows an example of a surgical instrument tray setup and supplies commonly used in minor office procedures. You must become familiar with the physician's preference for particular items and the way they are to be arranged for use. Until you are certain about the details of a particular procedure, you may want to keep a notebook handy for reference.

When the patient arrives for the surgery, the consent form must first be explained to the patient and completed. An example is shown in Figure 17–2. You should allow the patient time to ask any questions about the procedure and answer them adequately. The patient's signature must be on the consent form, which is filed in the chart. If the patient is a minor, or incompetent, the person **authorized** to give consent must sign for the patient following an explanation of the procedure and answering any questions. The patient's vital signs should be taken, and any complaints or problems should be recorded on the patient's chart. The patient should then empty the bladder before being positioned and draped for the procedure.

Place items on tray in order of use.

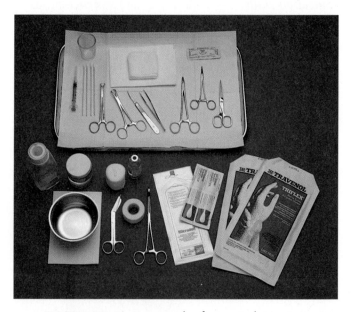

FIGURE 17–1 An example of a surgical setup tray

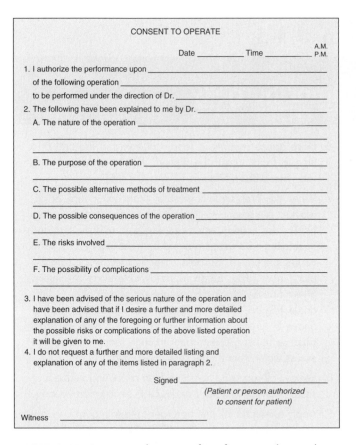

```
                    CONSENT TO OPERATE

                                                      A.M.
            Date _____ Time _____          P.M.

1. I authorize the performance upon _____
   of the following operation _____
   to be performed under the direction of Dr. _____
2. The following have been explained to me by Dr. _____
   A. The nature of the operation _____
   _____
   _____
   B. The purpose of the operation _____
   C. The possible alternative methods of treatment _____
   D. The possible consequences of the operation _____
   E. The risks involved _____
   F. The possibility of complications _____
   _____
3. I have been advised of the serious nature of the operation and
   have been advised that if I desire a further and more detailed
   explanation of any of the foregoing or further information about
   the possible risks or complications of the above listed operation
   it will be given to me.
4. I do not request a further and more detailed listing and
   explanation of any of the items listed in paragraph 2.

                    Signed _____
                           (Patient or person authorized
                               to consent for patient)
Witness _____
```

FIGURE 17–2 A sample consent form for surgical procedure

Most procedures are performed under local **anesthesia**. A physician always administers the **anesthetic**. Large group practices may have a qualified **anesthesiologist** on staff. A careful medical history must be taken from the patient to determine possible allergic or **adverse** reactions. This helps avoid complications during and after the procedure.

If the patient discloses a family history of **hemophilia**, (a serious blood clotting disease in which there is the absence of one of the necessary blood clotting factors for blood to coagulate) or is himself a hemophiliac, you should bring it to the physician's attention immediately. This information should be marked in red ink on the patient's chart. Hemophilia is a sex-linked hereditary trait that occurs mostly in males. Patients who have this diagnosis must have surgery of any type *only* at a completely equipped, well-staffed medical-surgical hospital for their safety and well-being.

In procedures requiring that a **biopsy** be taken for analysis, careful labeling and handling of the specimen is vital. The laboratory provides a formalin solution container for preservation of the tissue specimen. This container is sterile, and the specimen must be placed directly in the solution with sterile transfer forceps. A completed lab request form must accompany the specimen for analysis.

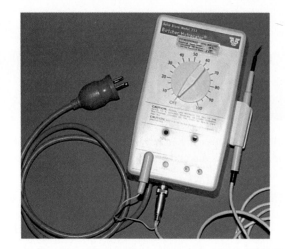

FIGURE 17–3 The Hyfrecator, an electrocautery unit that is used to seal blood vessels to stop bleeding, following surgical removal of a mole or skin tag

In certain surgical procedures, such as in removing warts or **polyps**, an **electrocautery** device may be used. Often this is used to control bleeding of the surgical site by **electrocoagulation**. Controlled high-frequency current is applied by the physician to the surgical area to **coagulate** the blood to close the incision. If the reusable tips are preferred by the physician for surgical procedures, they must be autoclaved to prevent possible cross-contamination. Disposable tips are available. Figure 17–3 illustrates a Hyfrecator.

Another method used in removing skin tags, warts, and other skin disorders and growths is by **cryosurgery**. Often, certain gynecological treatments and surgical procedures are performed with this instrument. This process uses subfreezing temperature to destroy or remove tissue. Generally, the substances used are solid carbon dioxide or

A CAAHEP CONNECTION

Patients who are having any type of surgery, from removal of a mole or a gallbladder, are likely to be apprehensive about it. Your professionalism and confidence in meeting the needs of the patient will help to make the patient feel more at ease. Offering printed information about the surgical procedure and discussing what to expect with the patient and family members gains cooperation. Assisting patients with their insurance coverage and pre-certification is a necessity that is most appreciated. If you remain calm and courteous during this stressful time for patients, plans will go smoothly in most cases.

PROCEDURE

17-1   Prepare Skin for Minor Surgery

PURPOSE: To remove hair from surgery site to prevent infection and to clean the skin and apply antiseptic solution to reduce microbial growth.

OSHA GUIDELINES: To comply with Standard Precautions, gloves and other protective barriers must be worn if there is any possibility of coming into contact with blood, or any body fluids.

EQUIPMENT: Small basin for soap solution, 4 × 4-inch gauze squares (sponges), safety razor and blades, scissors, antiseptic soap solution, emesis basin for disposables, gooseneck lamp, sterile drape sheet or towels (or fenestrated drape sheet), sterile latex or vinyl gloves, Mayo table, sterile forceps and container, sterile water for irrigation, Figure 17–4.

PERFORMANCE OBJECTIVE: Provided with all necessary equipment and supplies and other students to act as patients, demonstrate each of the steps required in the skin prep procedure. **NOTE: In the instructional setting, preparing the forearm may be sufficient; moreover, the shaving process may be demonstrated by using a razor with no blade.**

1. Wash and glove hands, and assemble all needed items.

2. Identify the patient. **RATIONALE: Speaking to the patient by name and checking chart ensures that you are performing the procedure on the correct patient.**

3. Explain procedure to patient. Ask patient to remove necessary clothing. Explain where patient should put belongings. Assist patient if necessary.

4. Assist patient into proper position on treatment table and drape with sheet or light bath blanket as directed by physician.

5. Position Mayo table over patient near surgical site. Adjust gooseneck lamp to light area to be shaved.

6. Place gauze squares in soapy solution and use one at a time to soap area to be shaved. After use, discard each into emesis basin (Figures 17–5 and 17–6).

7. When skin prep site is covered by scalp hair, beard, or pubic hair, use scissors to clip hair in preparation for shaving. **NOTE: Use caution when clipping hair with scissors and in shaving with razor to avoid both self-injury and harm to the patient.** If reusable razor is used, very carefully place new razor blade in razor to prevent self-injury. Shave hair by placing razor against skin at about a 30° angle (Figure 17–7). Hold skin taut for easier shaving. Shave in direction hair grows. Wipe soap and hair from razor with tissue. Swish razor through soapy water, shake excess water from it, and shave next area.

8. Remove all soap and hair from area by wetting steril gauze square with sterile water. Dry area with sterile gauze squares.

9. Apply antiseptic solution to surgery site with gauze square held by transfer forceps. **NOTE: Begin application in center of site and move outward in a circular motion** (see Figure 17–6). **RATIONALE: This pattern of continuous movement ensures total coverage without contamination from untreated areas.**

10. Cover the prepared area with sterile drape sheet or towel until physician is ready to begin. **NOTE: Instruct patient not to touch sterile field (either the sterile field of surgical site or instrument tray setup).**

11. Discard disposable items and return other items to proper storage area. Remove gloves and wash hands.

12. Attend to patient's comfort. Patients are usually apprehensive about even most minor surgical procedures. Reassurance at this time is most important.

---

liquid nitrogen. It is sometimes referred to as cold cautery. Refer to Procedure 17–1 for preparing patient's skin for minor surgery.

SKIN PREPARATION

Preparation of the area of skin that will be affected by the surgical procedure is called skin prep. Because body hair encourages **microbial** accumulation, it is usually shaved.

The skin cannot be completely sterilized, or the cells would be destroyed, but an **antiseptic** is used to reduce microbial growth.

Many physicians still prefer the use of a stainless steel razor with disposable blades, but there are also disposable skin-prep kits that contain all the necessary items for this procedure. If a reusable razor is preferred for hair removal in preparation for the surgery site, it must be autoclaved to prevent possible disease transmission. A new

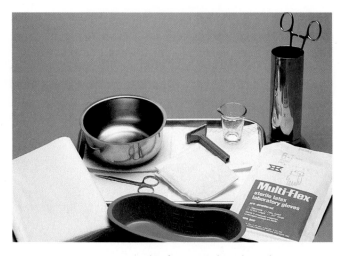

FIGURE 17-4 An example of a surgical scrub or skin prep tray

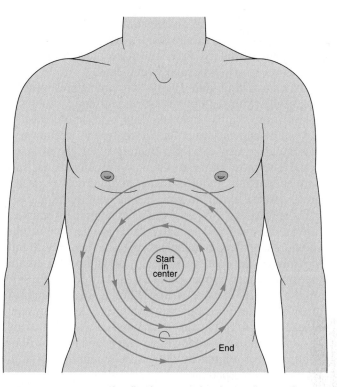

FIGURE 17-6 Apply all solutions to the skin in this circular pattern. Prepping the skin with an antiseptic solution should begin at the center of the incision site and proceed outward in one continuous circular motion as shown.

blade must be used for each patient. To protect yourself and the patient from possible disease transmission, you should wear latex or vinyl gloves during the skin prep procedure.

You must be extremely careful to avoid nicking the patient's skin. Microorganisms can enter the body through a

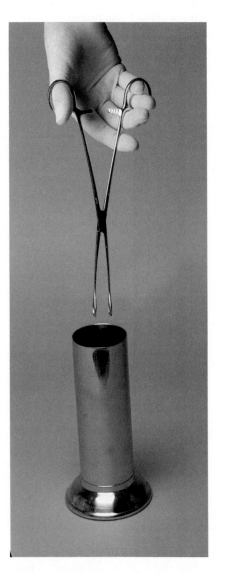

FIGURE 17-5 Remove transfer forceps from the container without touching the sides.

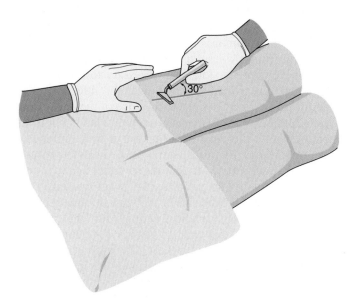

FIGURE 17-7 Angle for shaving a surgery site (or for suture insertion)

break in the skin, and an infection could develop from carelessness. If this should happen, the physician must be notified immediately. Practice in the procedure for this skill is necessary to become proficient.

When assisting with acupuncture procedures, preparation of the skin is simply to use an antiseptic, such as alcohol (if the skin is obviously dirty, you should wash the area with soap and water and dry before proceeding).

Acupuncture is used for treating a variety of conditions. The most common use is pain control. Assisting with acupuncture requires that sterile needles are used to prevent disease transmission just as with traditional surgical procedures. Some of the needles used in acupuncture are as small as a human hair. These delicate needles should not go deep into the patient's skin but only slightly to stimulate the energy force (chi) of the body. A competent practitioner of acupuncture uses these needles to restore a healthy balance of the contradicting forces of yin and yang. This type of therapy can be used to compliment other therapies in patient treatments. The success of one or more therapies used together with acupuncture will depend on the communication between practitioners in the total care of the patient.

Some other surgical procedures that you may assist with are: incision and drainage (I&D), removal of a cyst, moles/skin tag, laceration care and suture, and injection of a painful joint. The physician or clinical supervisor will teach you the procedures with which you do not know how to assist. Ask questions as necessary so that you will know what is required in assisting efficiently with all procedures.

DEBRIDEMENT

In assisting the physician with the many duties of sterile technique in surgeries and other important procedures, you may be asked to assist with or perform **debridement**. Debridement simply means that you use a sterile scissors and a splinter forceps, using sterile technique, to trim dead skin from a wound or a burn. Because microorganisms thrive on dead skin, it is necessary to remove it in stages as the wound heals to prevent infection. The necrotic tissue is cut off just to the edge of the intact skin. The scab of a wound is termed **eschar**. This is not to be confused with the dead skin that needs to be removed. The eschar is an important stage of the healing process. This will slowly come off, and it may result in a scar. It is generally thought that an antibiotic cream applied to the eschar will diminish the size of the scar. Be sure to check with the physician for instructions for the patient. Reschedule the patient every other day for a re-check of the wound. Your assessment should be evaluated also by the physician at intervals to determine the frequency of follow up visits and treatment. Patients who have severe burns or serious wounds are prone to infection. Be sure to advise the patient in proper care of the wound at home. Often, the physician will give the patient bandaging ma-

terials and topical medication to change the dressings at home. Make her appointment at times when the reception area is not too populated, so she does not have to wait for assessment and re-dressing. Remind the patient to keep the bandage clean and dry when taking care of the wound at home. When the physician approves the patient's release, show the patient how to continue care for the wound at home.

STERILE GLOVES

Ⓒ **Main Menu:**
Infection Control

Skills Menu:
- Handwashing
- Sterile Gloves and Gown
- Gloves and Gown

If the physician wishes you to assist directly with the surgical procedure, sterile gloves must be worn (Figure 17–8). Dressing changes should also be performed wearing sterile gloves to protect both yourself and the patient. In addition, you may assist with needle biopsies, IUD insertions, and lacerations resulting from injuries. All of these procedures require sterile techniques.

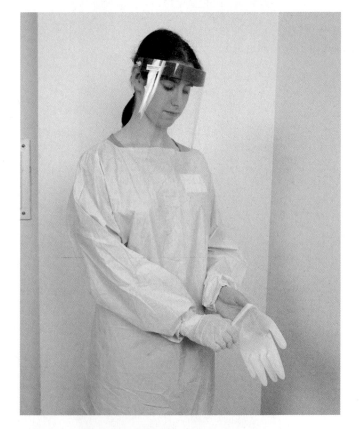

FIGURE 17–8 The medical assistant shown in this picture is wearing PPE (face shield, gown, and gloves) in preparation for assisting with a procedure that may involve contact with blood or body fluids.

Before you put sterile gloves on, you must perform a complete and careful hand washing to remove as many microorganisms as possible. Refer to the procedure and figures for proper hand washing in Chapter 12. Routine hand washing should take 20 seconds. There are a few ways to make sure you have spent the whole 20 seconds actually washing your hands. You can sing the popular "happy birthday" song or one of your choosing at a normal pace. Watch the sweep hand and sing at the pace it will fill for 20 seconds. Timers are nice, but if your hands are soiled you should not touch them to set the time for 20 seconds. Do not just rinse your hands: you should always remember to use soap. Your initial hand washing before you begin to work each day, and in between handling obviously contaminated materials, should last for approximately one minute. Keeping a timer and setting it for the amount of time for the appropriate hand washing procedure will be of great help to you because it is easy to misjudge how long you take in performing this procedure. A

thorough surgical scrub should be performed for six minutes. If it has been within 48 hours since the last surgical scrub was performed, three minutes is sufficient. Just before you begin to assist with surgery, after you have properly washed your hands and before putting on sterile gloves, you should put on the appropriate personal protective equipment. This may include face shield or face mask, eye protectors (goggles), and gown (Figure 17–8). Additional pairs of sterile latex or vinyl gloves should be kept nearby during the surgical procedure in case of an accidental tear or puncture. Refer to Procedure 17–2 for instructions for properly putting on sterile gloves.

ASSISTING WITH PROCEDURES

Assisting with surgical procedures requires basic knowledge in several areas. The medical assistant should learn anatomy and physiology, medical terminology, the names and uses of the instruments used in minor office proce-

PROCEDURE

17-2 Put On Sterile Gloves

PURPOSE: To protect both patient and medical assistant from contamination.

OSHA GUIDELINES: To comply with Standard Precautions, gloves and other protective barriers must be worn if there is any possibility of coming into contact with blood, or any body fluids.

EQUIPMENT: Package of sterile latex or vinyl gloves of proper size and biohazardous waste bag.

PERFORMANCE OBJECTIVE: After practicing with clean gloves, each student will be provided with a package of sterile gloves. Standing in front of a clean, clear counter surface, demonstrate the correct method of putting on sterile gloves. The instructor will observe each step.

1. Remove wristwatch, rings, and other jewelry from hands and wrists, and perform surgical scrub using nail brush. Thoroughly dry hands with sterile towels. **NOTE: Hands are now clean but unsterile.**

2. Tear seal and open package of sterile gloves as you would open a book (Figure 17–9A). Place on clean counter surface with cuff end toward your body. **NOTE: Do not touch inside of package. RATIONALE: Hands would contaminate inside of sterile package.**

3. Grasp glove for your dominant hand by fold of cuff with finger and thumb of your nondominant hand (Figure 17–9B). Insert dominant hand, carefully pulling glove on

with other hand, keeping cuff turned back. **NOTE: Dominant hand is now gloved and sterile (Figure 17–9C).**

4. Place gloved fingers under cuff of other glove and insert nondominant hand (Figure 17–9D). Put glove on by pulling on inside fold of cuff (Figure 17–9E). Avoid touching thumb of dominant hand to outside cuff of other glove where it has been contaminated.

5. Now both hands are gloved and sterile. Place fingers under cuffs to smooth gloves over wrists (Figure 17–9F) and smooth out fingers for better fit. **NOTE: Check for tears and holes (Figures 17-9G [1] & [2]). RATIONALE: Any break in the integrity of the glove would not maintain sterility.**

6. Keep hands above waist level. Do not touch anything other than items in sterile field. **NOTE: Contact with any nonsterile object or surface will contaminate gloved hand(s) requiring removal and regloving.**

7. Remove gloves by pulling glove off dominant hand with thumb and fingers (Figure 17–9H). Hold outside cuff and pull glove off inside-out. Slip ungloved hand into palm of gloved hand, and slip glove off inside-out (Figure 17–9I). **NOTE: Be careful not to touch contaminated side of gloves when removing.**

8. Deposit gloves in biohazardous waste bag.

9. Wash hands.

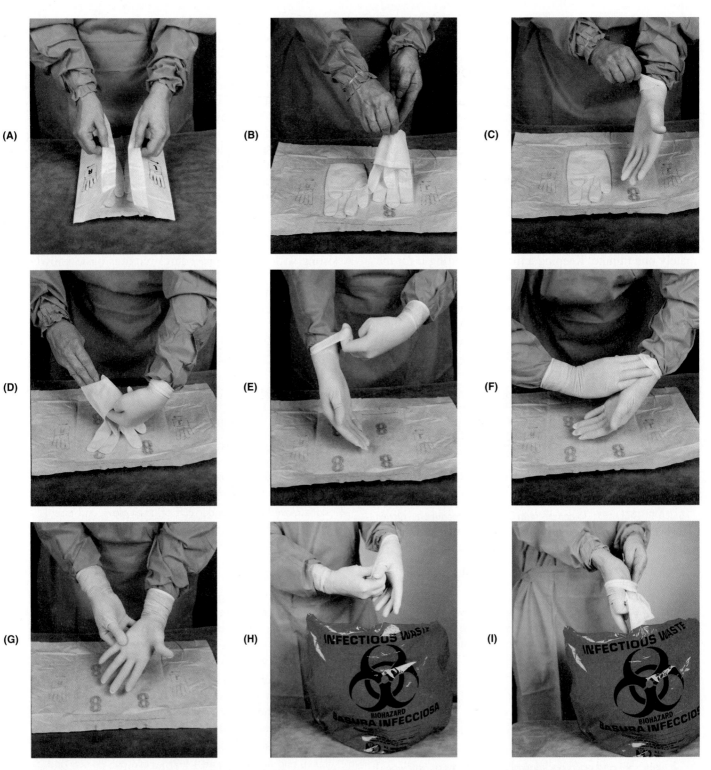

FIGURE 17–9 (A) Open the package by pulling on the center paper folds. (B) Grasp the fold of the inside cuff of the gloves with the thumb and fingers of your dominant hand. (C) Insert your nondominant hand into the glove, and pull the glove on with your dominant hand by the turned-down cuff. (D) Insert the fingers of your gloved nondominant hand under the folded-down cuff of the glove, and insert your dominant hand. (E) Place the gloved fingers of your nondominant hand under the folded-down cuff of the glove to pull the glove on your dominant hand up over the cuff of the gown. (F) Place the gloved fingers of your dominant hand (palm down) under the cuff of your gloved nondominant hand to push over the cuff of the gown. (G) Check the gloves for tears, holes, and imperfections. Inspect both palm-sides-up and down for proper fit. **To remove the gloves:** (H) Pull the glove off from your nondominant hand by grasping the outside of the glove, and hold with your gloved dominant hand. (I) Slip the fingers of your ungloved hand under your gloved hand (at the base of the palm), fold over the glove held in your hand, and slip it off the hands into the biohazard bag. Wash hands with antibacterial soap, and dry thoroughly.

dures, and sterile or aseptic technique. Procedures and additional surgical instruments are presented in Table 17–1. You should also develop skills in human relations. With experience, you will become more sensitive and aware of the patient's needs. The more knowledge you acquire about procedures and the items necessary to perform them, the more perceptive you will be in assisting the physician.

TABLE 17–1

INSTRUMENTS USED IN MINOR OFFICE SURGICAL PROCEDURES

Figure Number	Category: Description	Use
	Operating Scissors:	
A	*Deaver 5½″ (14 cm) straight, sharp-sharp*	Cut tissue and suture
B	*Sistrunk 5½″ (14 cm) slightly curved, blunt-blunt*	Same
C	*Deaver 5½″ (14 cm) straight, sharp-blunt, and curved, sharp-blunt*	Same
	Bandage Scissors:	
D	*Lester 5½″ (14 cm) sidecurved*	Cut dressings, tape
E	*Knowles finger 5½″ (14 cm)*	Same
F	*Spencer suture 3½″ (8.75 cm)*	Cut suture
G	*Littauer stitch 5½″ (14 cm)*	Same
	Petit-Point Hemostats:	
H	*Mosquito 4¾″ straight-curved*	Grasp tissue to hold, clamp, or pull out of the way
I	*Mosquito 3½″ straight curved*	Same
	Towel Forceps:	
J	*Backhaus (clip) 3½″ (8.75 cm)*	Grasp towels, dressing; hold drape towels in place (use caution—will puncture skin)
K	*Jones (clip) 3″*	Same
L	*Knife Handle #3 5″ (12.5 cm) holds blades 10, 11, 12, 15*	Accept blades
M	*Blades*	Cut tissue
	Sponge-Holding Forceps:	
N	*Forrester 7″ (18 cm) straight-smooth jaws or serrated*	Pick up and hold dressings
	Needle Holders:	
O	*Brown 5¼″ (13.5 cm)*	Grasp suture needle
P	*Collier 5″ (13 cm)*	Same
	Dressing and Tissue Forceps:	
Q	*Thumb 4″ (10 cm) serrated*	Pick up dressings, delicate tissue
R	*Tissue 4½″ (11 cm) 1 × 2 teeth*	Grasp tissue securely for control during dissection or suturing
S	*Adson serrated, extra delicate, 0.8 mm-wide tip*	Pick up delicate tissue
T	*Semken dressing 4¾″ (12 cm) serrated*	Pick up dressings
U	*Cushing 7¼″ (18.5 cm) serrated handle, scraper end, bayonet, 1 × 2 teeth*	Close skin
V	*Plain splinter 3½″ (8.75 cm)*	Remove splinters
W	*Judd-Allis tissue 6″ (15 cm)*	Grasp tissue

(Continued)

TABLE 17–1

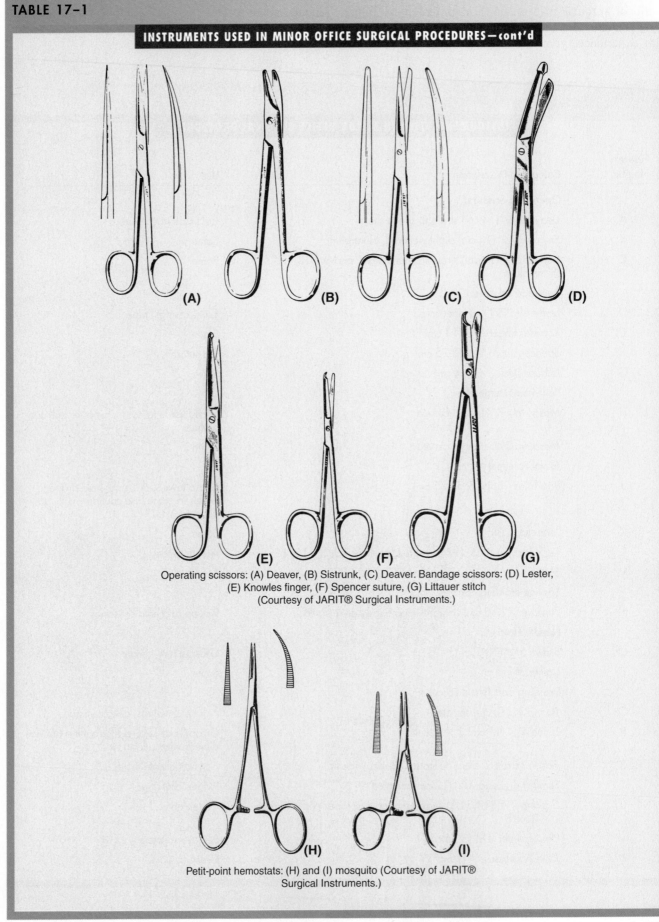

INSTRUMENTS USED IN MINOR OFFICE SURGICAL PROCEDURES—cont'd

(A) (B) (C) (D)

(E) (F) (G)

Operating scissors: (A) Deaver, (B) Sistrunk, (C) Deaver. Bandage scissors: (D) Lester,
(E) Knowles finger, (F) Spencer suture, (G) Littauer stitch
(Courtesy of JARIT® Surgical Instruments.)

(H) (I)

Petit-point hemostats: (H) and (I) mosquito (Courtesy of JARIT®
Surgical Instruments.)

(continues)

TABLE 17–1

INSTRUMENTS USED IN MINOR OFFICE SURGICAL PROCEDURES—cont'd

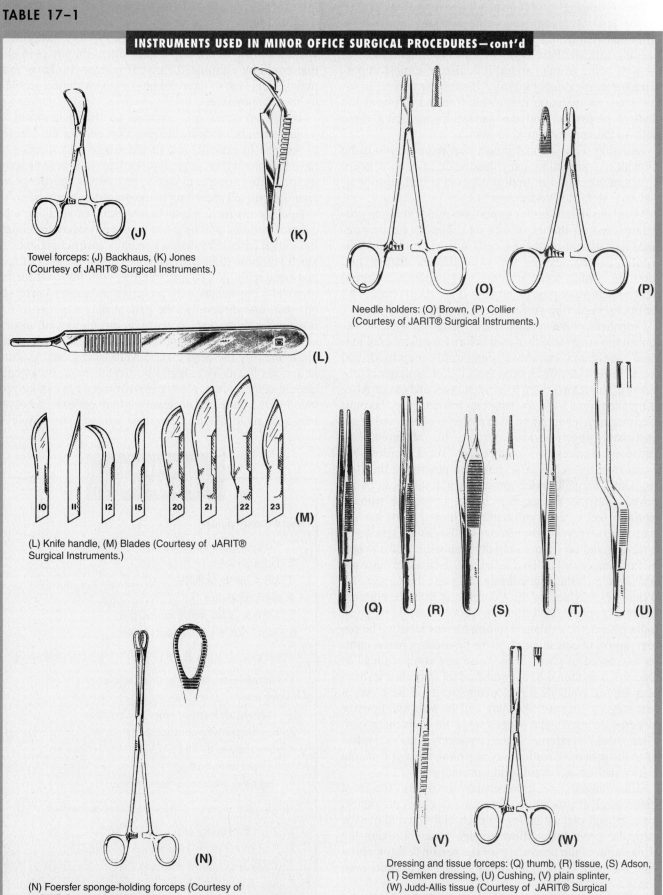

Towel forceps: (J) Backhaus, (K) Jones
(Courtesy of JARIT® Surgical Instruments.)

Needle holders: (O) Brown, (P) Collier
(Courtesy of JARIT® Surgical Instruments.)

(L) Knife handle, (M) Blades (Courtesy of JARIT®
Surgical Instruments.)

(N) Foersfer sponge-holding forceps (Courtesy of
JARIT® Surgical Instruments.)

Dressing and tissue forceps: (Q) thumb, (R) tissue, (S) Adson,
(T) Semken dressing, (U) Cushing, (V) plain splinter,
(W) Judd-Allis tissue (Courtesy of JARIT® Surgical
Instruments.)

The following procedures in assisting with minor surgery and suture and skin staple removals are valuable skills that require self-discipline and personal integrity. Keeping a sterile field is of monumental importance for the well-being of the patient. It is also of utmost importance for medical-legal reasons. If sterile technique is not practiced, an infection can result. You must respect the medical profession and the patient in practicing these skills to the very best of your ability.

Assisting with surgical procedures requires you to be efficient in completing many details. Of primary concern is patient education in both preoperative and postoperative care. Refer to Procedure 17–3.

Many physicians prefer to perform minor surgical procedures first on the day's schedule. The doctor may require that patients fast for a certain time before the procedure. Fasting lessens the possibility of nausea and vomiting, which some patients may experience during and following any type of surgery. It is best to check with the doctor regarding preference in preop instructions.

Outpatient, or ambulatory, surgery in recent years has become more acceptable than ever before for a number of reasons. Anesthesia has been significantly improved and causes fewer side effects in patients following surgical procedures. This allows them to awaken faster and easier. Also, the required time for many surgeries has decreased because of advances in instruments, such as the "scopes" used in sophisticated surgeries. For example, the abdominal laparoscopy requires two to three very small incisions for insertion of the scope, a suction, and possibly a third instrument. The gallbladder, growths, and tumors can be removed with this advanced technology. Because patients naturally feel more comfortable at home, following the "same day surgery," most patients of all ages are sent home to recover and do so more rapidly than when in the hospital. Post-surgery infection rate has also declined in those patients who go home immediately following the surgery. All of this is highlighted by the reduced cost from the elimination of a hospital stay. Printed instructions should be given to the patient and explained to him and his family. The patient should, of course, be given the physician's phone number and urged to phone if there are any complications or concerns. You should have a standard set of printed instructions readily available for telephone triage of those outpatient surgery patients who may call in with questions or concerns. Any calls that suggest a serious problem or condition should be referred to the physician immediately. Refer to the patient education box regarding what you should caution patients about following any surgery.

Often patients are apprehensive about even the most minor surgical procedure. You must display confidence, concern, and understanding to each individual about the particular procedure. Allow enough time following the explanation of the procedure for the person to think about what was said. Offer to answer questions of patients even if they do not ask.

Make sure that return appointment visits are confirmed and reminder cards are given to patients before they leave the office. Phoning patients the next day is an excellent way to follow-up and reassures them that you and the physician are genuinely concerned about their progress. It will also bring to the physician's attention any problems that could be eliminated early. If patients do have complaints, it is best to have the physician check the problem as soon as possible.

Follow-up visits are essential so that assessment of progress can be made by the physician and for the removal of sutures. In general, you should advise all patients who have had any minor surgical procedure to limit their activity for at least a couple of weeks, or however long the physician has ordered according to the procedure performed.

Specific instructions, such as soaking or applying topical medications, will be given by the physician for certain individual cases. Physicians generally instruct patients (or teach you how to instruct patients) about packing or special bandaging procedures, such as with ingrown toenail removals. Physicians may prescribe an analgesic for minor pain and discomfort the patient may experience following the procedure. Where you are employed, always check the policy regarding the types of emergencies that are treated by the physician. Severe lacerations resulting in serious blood loss should be treated in an emergency trauma center where more extensive services can be provided to the patient if necessary. Many patients, however, may seek medical care from their primary care physician

---

PATIENT EDUCATION

Usual care of patient:

1. Keep site clean and dry
2. Place no stress on the area
3. Drink plenty of fluids
4. Get proper rest
5. Eat a sensible well-balanced diet
6. Return for follow-up appointment

Patients should report to the physician any of the following:

1. Unusual pain, burning, or other uncomfortable sensation
2. Swelling, redness, or other discoloration
3. Bleeding or other discharge
4. Fever above 100°F (37.7°C)
5. Nausea and vomiting
6. Any other problem or symptom

Following suture removal patients should be advised to:

1. Keep the site dry for at least 24 hours
2. Cover the area to keep it clean
3. Apply supportive bandaging PRN
4. Report any sign of infection immediately to physician

17-3 Assisting with Minor Surgery

PURPOSE: To assist physician in the performance of a surgical procedure and to provide support for the patient.

OSHA GUIDELINES: To comply with Standard Precautions, gloves and other protective barriers must be worn if there is any possibility of coming into contact with blood or any body fluids.

EQUIPMENT: Basic sterile setup: needle and syringe, needle holder, appropriate suture, scalpel handle and blade, thumb forceps, surgical scissors, hemostats, retractor, three or four pairs of latex or vinyl gloves, gauze squares, cotton-tipped applicators, alcohol pad, fenestrated sheet or towels, towel clamps, bandages, bandage scissors, tape, ordered anesthetic, antiseptic (small glass container for antiseptic solution), plastic biohazardous sharps container and waste bag (and waste receptacle), patient's chart, pen, histology request form for laboratory analysis if a biopsy is indicated, Mayo tray table, and proper lighting (extra back-up sterile setup).
NOTE: Table 17–1A, B, and C show surgical scissors. These are termed sharp-sharp, blunt-blunt, and sharp-blunt referring to the tip of the scissor blades. The physician will usually request scissors by these terms and, of course, the length for various procedures.

PERFORMANCE OBJECTIVE: Provided with all necessary equipment and supplies, with the instructor role-playing as physician and the students role-playing as patients, demonstrate (insofar as possible) each of the steps required in assisting with minor surgery. The instructor will observe each step. **NOTE: Some steps will need to be simulated in the instructional setting.**

1. Wash hands.

2. Assemble appropriate equipment and supplies on counter or table near Mayo tray. Position the Mayo tray table next to treatment table, and check condition and expiration dates of sterile items. **RATIONALE: If an item is expired or package shows signs of improper conditions, items may no longer be sterile.**

3. Bring scheduled patient into treatment room. Advise patient to empty bladder. **RATIONALE: This ensures patient's comfort during procedure. Anxiety often results in the urge to void.** When patient returns, take vital signs and record. **RATIONALE: Vital signs must be within acceptable limits to proceed with procedure.** Explain procedure to patient and obtain signature on consent form. **RATIONALE: A signature on consent form is absolutely essential before any invasive procedure is performed.** If biopsy is to be taken, complete lab request form for histology analysis.

4. Instruct patient to disrobe as necessary for procedure, and advise where to place belongings. Assist patient if needed. Allow privacy and ask patient to let you know when ready for positioning.

5. Assist patient to treatment table and into desired position for surgery. Perform skin prep procedure. Give patient support and understanding, and answer any questions at this time. Drape patient appropriately.

6. Place sterile towel on Mayo tray by holding the underneath sides of it (the top side must be untouched). Open all sterile items (as ordered by physician for scheduled surgery) carefully by holding them at the tabs; drop them onto the sterile field without touching them.

7. Put on sterile vinyl or latex gloves. Arrange instruments and other sterile items in the order that they will be used in the procedure. **NOTE: Do not reach, cough, sneeze, wave, talk, or cross over the sterile field or it will become contaminated. Carefully cover field with a sterile towel until physician is ready to begin.** Remove gloves and wash hands.

8. When physician is ready to begin the surgical procedure, remove the sterile towel from the prepared sterile setup. Assist physician by handing sterile gloves, use alcohol prep to wipe the top of the anesthetic vial, and hold it for physician to draw out the amount needed (Figure 17–10).

9. If you are to assist with surgical procedure, wash hands and put on sterile latex or vinyl gloves. Hand instruments and other sterile items to physician as needed, mop excessive blood with gauze sponges as needed PRN. **NOTE: If a biopsy is to be performed, special care must be taken to preserve the specimen. According to the physician's preference, the tissue may be placed on a gauze square to be handled later or deposited directly into an open specimen container. Label and attach completed laboratory requisition when procedure is completed.** You may assist the physician in suturing the incision by clipping each individual suture after the knot is tied by the physician (Figure 17–11). You should perform any other assistance as directed by physician during the procedure PRN. If additional sterile items are needed during the procedure, open the package and hand to physician for removal, or drop onto the center of the sterile field. Table 17–1 describes various surgical instruments used in minor office procedures.

10. When surgery is completed, assist in (or perform) cleaning and bandaging the surgery site, remove gloves, and wash hands. Tend to the patient by helping into sitting position to regain balance, and when stable, from the table. Assist in dressing if necessary. Give patient education regarding any return visit, care of surgery site, and any other orders from physician. Ask patient if allergic to adhesive; if so, use hypoallergenic tape to secure bandage.

11. Put on gloves to clean up treatment table, discard disposable items in biohazardous bag, place instruments in detergent solution to soak after rinsing with cold water, remove gloves and wash hands, restock room.

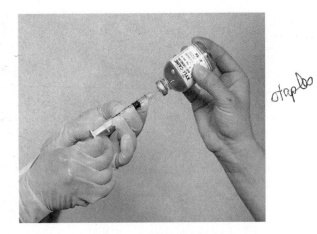

FIGURE 17-10 Hold the anesthetic solution in a convenient position so that the physician can fill the syringe without contamination.

for minor lacerations sustained in an accident or injury. The patient should be seen as soon as possible for treatment to lessen the possibility of infection at the site of injury. Because this situation can occur at any time, you should always have a suture pack and all necessary supplies and materials on hand to accommodate patients.

The term *suture* means a type of thread that is used to join skin of a wound, either an accidental laceration or a surgical incision, together. A type of suture, called catgut, is eventually absorbed by the body and does not need to be removed (generally used in major surgeries). It is made from the intestines of sheep. Suture is also made of a material such as silk, nylon, or other man-made substances that must be removed in a matter of days depending on the area of the body where they are inserted. For convenience, most physicians prefer to use suture that has a needle already attached. Figure 17–12 shows examples of different types of suture materials and needles used in closing wounds.

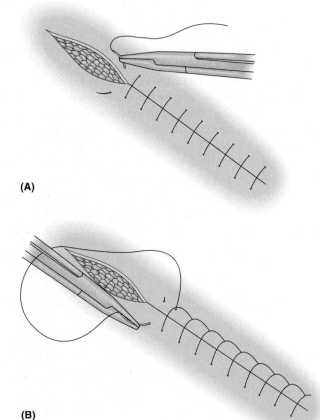

FIGURE 17-11 Two examples of suturing techniques: (A) interrupted (individual) sutures and (B) continuous sutures

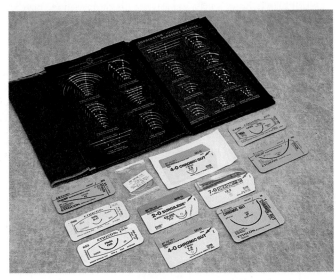

(A)

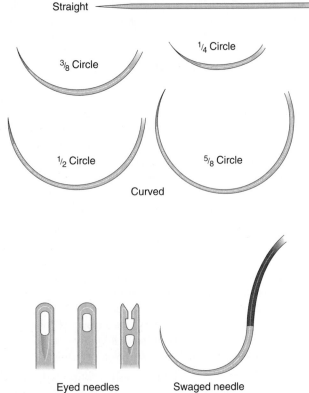

(B)

Straight

³/₈ Circle   ¹/₄ Circle

¹/₂ Circle   ⁵/₈ Circle

Curved

Eyed needles   Swaged needle

FIGURE 17-12 (A) A variety of suture packs and curved and straight surgical needles, (B) various needle shapes used in the insertion of sutures to close wounds

Working cases into an already full schedule can present delays for other patients waiting for scheduled appointments. Having a good rapport with the administrative medical assistant is very important. Communication regarding how the schedule is going is a must, especially when emergencies arise. Knowing this information will help you in altering patient flow to avoid further problems with the schedule and smooth patient flow. Try to have several patients prepared for the physician prior to the time when the physician begins suturing the laceration so that as soon as the procedure is finished, and while you tend to the patient and clean up, the physician can continue to see scheduled patients without additional interruption of the schedule. Your efficiency and expedient preparation of setting up the treatment room will be appreciated by both the physician and the patient in this situation. Follow the steps in Procedure 17–4 for assisting with suturing a laceration. Always make sure that you record the number of sutures (stitches) that the physician inserts and the anatomical location. Go over patient education and any additional instructions from the physician with the patient before she leaves the office. If the patient is given instructions by the physician to redress and bandage the wound at home, show the patient how to do this. Alert patients to call with any questions or concerns.

PROCEDURE

17-4 Assisting with Suturing a Laceration

PURPOSE: To close a wound (laceration or incision) with a sterile material until it is healed.

OSHA GUIDELINES: To comply with Standard Precautions, gloves and other personal protective barriers must be worn if there is any possibility of coming into contact with blood, or any body fluids.

EQUIPMENT: Items needed for skin prep (refer to Procedure 17–1) alcohol, cotton balls, PPE, biohazard bag, gauze squares, bandages and tape, bandage scissors, antiseptic, ordered anesthetic, tetanus toxoid PRN, patient's chart, pen; sterile items: swabs, needle and syringe, latex or vinyl gloves, fenestrated drape, ordered suture material, gauze squares, hemostats, needle holder, scissors. **NOTE: Suture packs containing all necessary items except suture material are generally already made and kept readily available for emergency use. NOTE: Check expiration date of items. (Restraints may be necessary for a child. A cloth sheet may be used to wrap around the child's arms and legs to immobilize him during the procedure; a papoose (restraining) board can also be used for small children.)**

PERFORMANCE OBJECTIVE: Provided with all necessary equipment and supplies and other students to act as patients, demonstrate each of the steps required in the procedure to assist with suturing a laceration. **NOTE: In the instructional setting, the instructor will pose as physician and simulate the procedure with a mannequin to check the steps of the procedure.**

1. Wash hands and assemble all needed items.

2. Identify the patient. **RATIONALE: Speaking to the patient by name and checking the chart ensures that you are performing the procedure on the correct patient.**

3. Explain procedure to patient. Advise patient to empty bladder.

4. When patient returns, take and record vital signs. **RATIONALE: The patient may have lost a considerable amount of blood which could alter vital signs. The patient may experience weakness and may not feel well enough to be left alone.**

5. Ask patient to remove necessary clothing. Explain where patient should place belongings.

6. Assist patient into appropriate position for skin prep of wound. Proceed with steps for preparing skin for minor surgery because the area for suture insertion must be prepared the same way. Drape patient appropriately.

7. Assemble unsterile items on Mayo tray table. Answer patient's questions as you prepare for the procedure.

8. Open sterile pack or place a sterile towel on Mayo tray by holding the underneath sides of it or at the tabs. Drop additional sterile items carefully onto the sterile field as necessary (i.e., suture material).

9. Put on PPE and sterile latex or vinyl gloves. Arrange instruments and other sterile items in the order that the physician will use them. **NOTE: Do not reach, cough, sneeze, wave, talk, or cross over the sterile field, or it can become contaminated. Carefully cover the sterile field with a sterile towel until physician is ready to begin.** Remove gloves and wash hands.

10. When physician is ready to begin the suturing procedure, remove the sterile towel from the prepared setup. Hand sterile gloves to physician and use alcohol prep to wipe the top of the anesthetic vial. Hold the vial for the physician to draw out desired amount. Refer to Figure 17–10. If you assist with the suturing procedure, wash hands and put on sterile gloves. Hand instruments and other sterile items to

(continues)

PROCEDURE

17-4 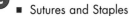 Assisting with Suturing a Laceration—continued

physician as needed, mop excessive blood from wound with sterile gauze PRN. Assist physician by clipping each individual suture as directed by physician.

11. When the wound has been closed with sutures, assist with or perform cleaning and bandaging the site as physician orders (you may need to reglove to keep from getting the dressing and bandage soiled), remove gloves, dispose in biohazard waste bag, and wash hands. **NOTE: Some individuals are allergic to adhesive. Be sure to ask patient before applying tape. Hypoallergenic tape may be preferred.**

12. Administer tetanous toxoid if ordered. Tend to the patient. Assist with sitting up, getting dressed, helping from treat-

ment table, and so on. **NOTE: Allow patient sufficient time to regain balance before standing alone because dizziness may occur.**

13. Instruct patient in care of sutures and provide return appointment for their removal. Refer to the patient education box: Patients can develop infections following a wound sustained in an accident.

14. Put on latex or vinyl gloves to clean up treatment table, discard disposables in biohazard bag/sharps container, place instruments in detergent solution after rinsing with cool water, remove gloves and PPE, and dispose of in biohazard bag. Wash hands and re-stock treatment room.

15. Record procedure on patient's chart and initial.

SUTURE REMOVAL

C Skills Menu:
- Sutures and Staples

Patients usually see the family/general practitioner for suture removal following laceration repair from an injury. You may have this duty to perform. It is vital that you check the emergency center's report regarding the number of sutures put in, so you can be sure to remove all of them.

Be sure to remove the same number of sutures as were inserted by the primary care physician. Suture that is not removed will become infected, so care in removing all of the material is vital. Patients sometimes report that one or two stitches have already come out during a bandage change at home. This should also be noted on the patient's chart. Follow the steps in the procedure for suture removal. Removal of staples is performed with a staple extractor as described in Procedure 17–5 for suture removal. Check the report also for a tetanus booster and record on the patient's chart to bring the immunization record up to date. Before you remove the sutures, check the number of days that the physician who put them in recommended as the time to wait before removal. Ask the physician to inspect the healing wound. Physicians generally order additional closure materials to cover healing incisions/lacerations following suture removal (Figure 17–16). A support skin closure may be necessary to keep the skin together until the wound is completely healed. The type of supportive closure should be noted on the pa-

tient's chart. New advances in skin closures offer a sutureless substance applied to small lacerations. This type of closure is an adhesive material and is used frequently with children who may already be frightened and thus uncooperative. A sutureless procedure is much quicker and less traumatic for the child and staff as well. Skin closures give support to the wound and offer the patient more flexibility. The type of bandage that the physician orders will vary and should be appropriate for the wound and the patient. For patients who are very active or who are employed in activities that could further injure or cause the wound to become dirty or wet, the wound should be wrapped in a very thick dressing to cushion and protect it and to allow it to heal. Make sure you advise the patient to keep the dressing clean and dry. Remind the patient to place a plastic bag over the extremity to keep it dry during shower or bath. If the wound is on the trunk of the body, taking a shower or bath should not be done unless the physician has approved it. Usually a sponge bath is preferred until the bandage comes off. This is important in minimizing the possibility of infection. If an infection should occur, you may be asked to obtain a specimen for laboratory analysis and culture. Simply use a sterile cotton swab and insert the tip into the center of the infected area of the wound. Then transfer the swab with the specimen into the culture medium. Provide patient education regarding care of the site and when to return for a follow-up appointment. Additionally, physicians advise using an elastic bandage to offer more protection and support of surgical areas of the extremities, especially for pediatric

PROCEDURE

17-5 Removing Sutures

PURPOSE: To remove suture(s) from healing laceration or incision.

OSHA GUIDELINES: To comply with Standard Precautions, gloves and other protective barriers must be worn if there is any possibility of coming into contact with blood, or any body fluids.

EQUIPMENT: Sterile: thumb forceps, suture-removal scissors (or staple extractor), gauze squares, latex or vinyl gloves, cotton-tipped applicators, butterfly or steristrip closures; antiseptic solution, hydrogen peroxide, basin with warm soapy water, bandages, tape, towels, biohazardous waste bag, bandage scissors, patient's chart, pen.

PERFORMANCE OBJECTIVE: Provided with all necessary equipment and supplies, and using a mannequin or model as the patient, demonstrate the steps required to remove sutures. The instructor will observe each step. Simulation should be made by the instructor.

1. Wash hands and move Mayo table next to treatment table, or to where patient will be during the procedure.

2. Assemble all necessary items on Mayo table tray (Figure 17–13). Ask if patient is allergic to adhesive. If so, use hypoallergenic tape to secure bandage (ask also about allergies to topical preparations, such as povidone-iodine mixture, or any medications).

3. Bring scheduled patient to treatment room. Ask patient about healing condition of incision or laceration, take vital signs, and record on patient's chart. (If sutures resulted from a laceration injury, ask appropriate questions regarding where and when injury occurred and when a tetanus booster was administered [file ER report in chart].) Record.

4. Ask patient to remove appropriate clothing for inspection of healing incision (offer to help PRN).

5. Assist patient to treatment table and into required position and drape appropriately. Explain procedure and answer any questions.

6. Put on gloves and remove bandage. Clean incision with antiseptic solution using cotton-tipped applicators. **NOTE: If bandage has stuck to the incision (record condition of site on chart [i.e., excessive blood, or drainage]), apply gauze squares that have been soaked with soapy warm water soloution, or hydrogen peroxide, to the area for a few minutes to loosen the bandage from the sutures and scab.** This will make removal of the bandage easier. (Pulling off a stuck bandage may reopen the wound or pull out sutures.) Either result would be very painful. Advise physician that the incision site is ready to be checked.

7. After physician orders suture removal, open sterile package containing the necessary instruments on the Mayo tray and proceed. Grasp the knot of the suture material with thumb forceps, and gently but firmly pull up making just enough space to place the suture removal scissors to clip the suture as close to the skin as possible (Figure 17–14). Pull the suture with the forceps (back) toward the healing incision so that no **stress** is put on it. **RATIONALE: Pulling the suture away from the site could possibly pull the incision open. CAUTION:** Do not pull a suture that has been on the surface of the skin (exposed to the outside) through the path of the suture being removed, or infection may develop. Continue in this manner until all sutures are removed.

8. Apply antiseptic solution to site, and allow to air dry. Apply steristrips or butterfly closure if necessary for support during healing process, and bandage.

9. Remove gloves and wash hands.

10. Instruct patient to keep the bandage clean and dry for 24 to 48 hours, or as directed by physician. **RATIONALE: A dirty or wet dressing allows microorganisms to enter the tiny openings where sutures were removed until they are healed.** Advise patient to avoid undue stress for appropriate amount of time for the anatomical area. Give patient education regarding home care and follow-up appointment if ordered by physician.

11. Record on progress notes in patient's chart: (1) anatomical area of incision or laceration; (2) condition of site; (3) number of sutures removed; (4) type of antiseptic applied; (5) support closures applied; (6) type of bandage applied, and your signature. Be sure to include the ER report if sent from facility where injury was treated, and record date of tetanus booster if applicable.

    NOTE: If skin staples (or clips) are to be removed, the physician may perform the procedure. However, you may be instructed to do so. Basically, skin staples are removed in the following manner: Follow steps 1 through 6 above.

    Place the sterile staple extractor under staple (one at a time), and squeeze handles of extractor completely closed (Figure 17–15). (Explain to patient that a tugging sensation may be felt.) Lift staple away from skin and place in biohazardous waste container. Continue process until all are removed. Resume procedure above with step 8.

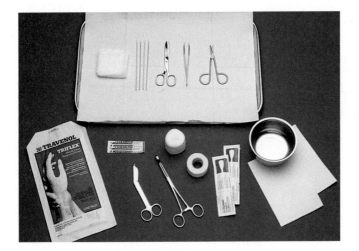

FIGURE 17-13 An example of a suture-removal tray setup

A CAAHEP CONNECTION

Chapter 17 discusses preparation, gloving, sterile technique, instrument identification, and assisting with minor surgical procedures in the office. This content is related to the ABHES accreditation requirements of **Medical asepsis/sterilization and minor office surgery** and **Universal precautions in the medical office** within the content area of **Medical Office Clinical Procedures.**

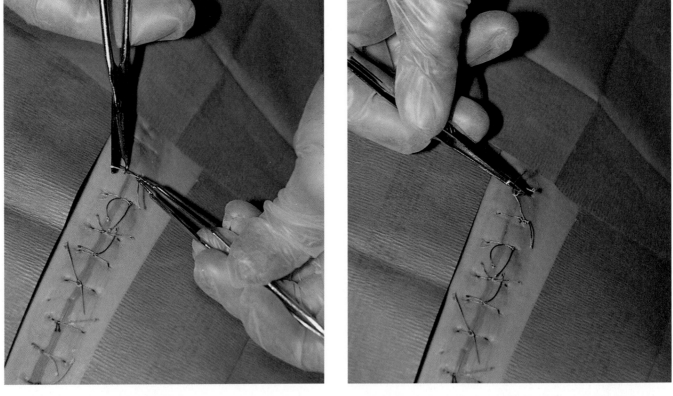

(A)   (B)

FIGURE 17-14 Suture removal. (A) Grasp the suture knot with thumb forceps, and place the curved tip of the suture-removal scissors just next to the skin under the suture and clip; (B) gently pull the suture knot up and toward the incision with the thumb forceps to remove (pulling the suture away from the incision may pull the incision open).

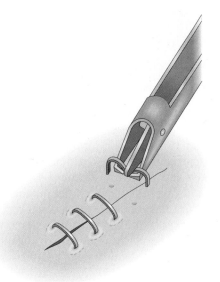

FIGURE 17–15   Removal of a staple. The staple extractor reforms the staple (clip). Then, the staple is lifted from the incision.

and physically active patients. Application of an Ace wrap increases circulation of the area, which hastens the healing process.

Until you are confident in assisting with various office surgeries, it is suggested that you keep a notebook or file cards to help you learn the instruments and steps required for each procedure.

ACHIEVE UNIT OBJECTIVES

Complete Chapter 17 in the workbook to help you obtain competency of this subject matter.

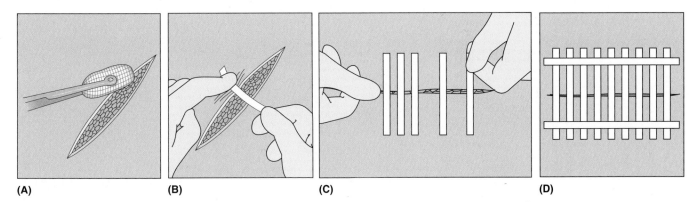

(A)   (B)   (C)   (D)

FIGURE 17–16   Care of an incision/wound with a closure applications: (A) Use transfer forceps with sterile gauze to apply antiseptic, (B) apply steristrip closure to center of incision, and (C) apply closures to each side for evenness, then fill in and cover full wound area. If ordered, apply topical medication and a sterile bandage. (D) For additional support, closures may also be applied parallel to the incision/wound.

Medical-Legal-Ethical Scenario

Barry was the medical assistant assigned to assist with a cyst removal scheduled immediately following the lunch break. Before Barry went to lunch, he asked Renita to set up the surgical room because he might be late getting back from running errands, and she was not leaving for lunch anyway. Renita reluctantly agreed and began setting up the room for the surgical procedure. As she removed the sterile packet from the drawer, she noticed that it was the last one. She placed all the instruments (still wrapped) on the Mayo stand next to the exam table. Barry returned late, just before the physician came out of her office. Barry quickly washed his hands, finished setting up the tray of instruments and supplies, and brought the patient in for the procedure. He asked Mr. Case to remove his shirt and lie on the exam table. Barry performed the skin prep and placed the fenestrated drape sheet over the patient just before the doctor came in to begin the procedure. During the surgery, the physician asked Barry to get another sterile pack from the drawer. Barry returned and reported that there were none in the drawer. The physician was upset about this and had to make do with what she had. After the patient was taken care of and left the room, the doctor spoke sternly to Barry about not being prepared for the procedure. Barry wanted to say that it was Renita's fault, but decided not to because she really did a favor for him.

CRITICAL THINKING CHALLENGE

1. Who was at fault here?
2. What was Barry's first mistake?
3. Was Renita responsible for any problems?
4. What should Barry have done?
5. Do you think Barry handled the reprimand from the doctor well?
6. Because Barry didn't know that there were no sterile packs in the drawer, should the doctor blame him?
7. Did Renita really do Barry a favor?

RESOURCES

JARIT® Surgical Instruments, 9 Skyline Drive, Hawthorne, New York 10532.

Outpatient surgery: a sign of progress, regarding women and healthcare (Spring 1994). Columbus, OH: Mount Carmel Health.

WEB LINKS

http://www.jarit.com (JARIT® Surgical Instruments)

This site provides information about surgical instruments.

http://www.ethiconinc.com/wound_management/index.htm (Ethicon, Inc. Wound Management)

This site provides information on wound closure and suturing techniques.

Assisting with Medications

Administering medications is one of the most sensitive and important duties that the medical assistant will perform.

You must first become familiar with the medications that are most frequently given to patients. Knowing the properties of the medications will help in answering patients' questions and recognizing common side effects that patients may exhibit. The *Physicians' Desk Reference,* or PDR, and the *Physicians' Desk Reference for Nonprescription Drugs* will become valuable resources. Because these resources are frequently referred to, they should be kept in a central accessible place for use by all members of the health care team. You should also become familiar with the many terms and abbreviations used in administering medications. Some of the most common ones are included in this chapter and in the Appendix.

The laws may vary from state to state in regard to your administering medications. You should check with your employer about this matter. Some physicians prefer always to administer medications to patients themselves, thereby lessening a possible medical-legal concern.

A review of the basic math skills will be helpful in preparing medications. The areas in which to practice are addition, subtraction, multiplication, division, fractions, decimals, percentages, and ratio–proportion. Refer to Table 18–6 for examples of these math problems. Accuracy and care must always be taken in assisting with and administering medications to patients.

UNIT 1

Prescription and Nonprescription Medications

◼ OBJECTIVES

Upon completion of the unit, meet the following performance objectives by verifying knowledge of the facts and principles presented through oral and written communication at a level deemed competent. Demonstrate the specific behaviors as identified in the performance objectives of the procedures, observing all aseptic and safety precautions in accordance with health care standards.

1. Spell and define, using the glossary at the back of the text, all the **Words to Know** in this unit.
2. Demonstrate how to use PDRs for both prescription and nonprescription medications.
3. Explain how to properly phone in prescriptions to a pharmacist.
4. Demonstrate how to write a prescription as ordered by the physician.
5. Describe the drugs that are under federal regulation according to category, or Schedules I through V.
6. Define abbreviations commonly used in regard to medications.
7. Demonstrate how to record medications properly on the patient's chart.
8. Explain how to categorize medications used in the medical office.
9. Describe medical/legal/ethical concerns regarding medications.
10. List and discuss the necessary information required when recording medications.

AREAS OF COMPETENCE (AAMA)

This unit addresses content within the specific competency areas of *Fundamental principles, Patient care, Professionalism, Communication skills, Legal concepts,* and *Instruction,* as identified in the Medical Assistant Role Delineation Study. Refer to Appendix A for a detailed listing of the areas.

◼ WORDS TO KNOW

accuracy
administer
auxiliary
Drug Enforcement
  Administration (DEA)
dispense
expertise
facility
license
narcotic

over-the-counter (OTC)
Physician's Desk
  Reference (PDR)
pharmaceutical
prescribe
prescription
reference
resource
vial

COMMONLY PRESCRIBED MEDICATIONS

Because of the nature of each type of medical practice, certain medications will be more commonly prescribed than others. It is a good idea to keep a list of these medications handy with the most often questioned information. This list should include the usual dosage and possible side effects. The entire staff should become knowledgeable about these medications.

The list in Table 18–1 is meant as an introduction. The common names of some of the drugs are listed. Consulting a **PDR (Physician's Desk Reference)** or other resource for complete information is suggested.

PHARMACEUTICAL REFERENCES

The PDR is a valuable **resource** that the medical assistant should keep handy in the medical office. The purpose of the PDR is to provide accurate, reliable, and current information about most prescribed medications and related products. You may need to consult the PDR for the proper spelling, strength, or other information concerning medications that are not given frequently to assist the physician in accurately prescribing medications.

One of your responsibilities may be to order the current edition of the PDR so that the practice may keep abreast of the newest **pharmaceuticals** approved by the Food and Drug Administration (FDA). This reference book is published annually. A supplement with the latest information is sent to subscribers quarterly. There are six sections:

1. Manufacturer's index (white)
2. Brand and generic index (pink)

PATIENT EDUCATION

Many patients are very anxious about receiving medication, whether by mouth, injection, or any of the other means of administration. Careful and complete explanation of the procedure and the need for medications is essential for reassuring the patient. The patient must understand when and how to take prescribed medications to receive the full benefits of these medications. Some medications are to be taken before meals or after meals, with certain fluids or excluding certain fluids, and in the presence or absence of certain foods or other medications. Carefully explained verbal and written instructions are essential for the patient's compliance. The patient must understand that the medication dosage cannot be changed without first consulting the physician. Emphasize also that the medication should be continued or finished as directed, even if the patient begins to feel better.

TABLE 18–1

SELECTED DRUG CLASSIFICATIONS

Classification	Action	Examples
Analgesic	An agent that relieves pain without causing loss of consciousness	acetaminophen (Tylenol), aspirin, morphine, ibuprofen (Advil, Motrin)
Anesthetic	An agent that produces a lack of feeling. May be local or general depending on the type and how administered	lidocaine HCL (Xylocaine), procaine HCL (Novocaine)
Antacid	An agent that neutralizes acid	Amphojel, Gelusil, Mylanta, Aludrox, Milk of Magnesia
Antianxiety	An agent that relieves anxiety and muscle tension	benzodiazepines: diazepam (Valium) and chlordiazepoxide HCL (Librium)
Antiarrhythmic	An agent that controls cardiac arrhythmias	lidocaine HCL (Xylocaine), propranolol HCL (Inderal)
Antibiotic	An agent that is destructive to or inhibits growth of microorganisms	penicillins (Pentids, Duracillin, Polycillin, Pipracil, Augmentin), cephalosporins (Keflin, Mandol, Rocephin)
Anticholinergic	An agent that blocks parasympathetic nerve impulses	atropine, scopolamine, trihexyphenidyl HCL (Artane)
Anticoagulant	An agent that prevents or delays blood clotting	heparin sodium, Dicumarol, warfarin, sodium (Coumadin)
Anticonvulsant	An agent that prevents or relieves convulsions	carbamazepine (Tegretol), phenytoin (Dilantin), ethosuximide (Zarotin)
Antidepressant	An agent that prevents or relieves the symptoms of depression	monoamine oxidase (MAO) inhibitors: isocarboxazid (Marplan), phenelzine sulfate (Nardil), amitriptyline HCL (Elavil), imipramine HCL (Tofranil)
Antidiarrheal	An agent that prevents or relieves diarrhea	Lomotil, Pepto-Bismol, Kaopectate
Antidote	An agent that counteracts poisons and their effect	naloxone (Narcan)
Antiemetic	An agent that prevents or relieves nausea and vomiting	Tigan, Dramamine, Phenergan, Reglan, Marinol
Antihistamine	An agent that acts to counteract histamine	Dimetane, Benadryl, Seldane
Antihypertensive	An agent that prevents or controls high blood pressure	methyldopa (Aldomet), clonidine HCL (Catapres), metoprolol tartrate (Lopressor)
Anti-inflammatory	An agent that counteracts inflammation	naproxen (Naprosyn), aspirin, ibuprofen (Advil, Motrin)
Antimanic	An agent used for the treatment of the manic episode of manic-depressive disorder	lithium
Antineoplastic	An agent that kills or destroys malignant cells	busulfan (Myleran), cyclophosphamide (Cytoxan)
Antipyretic	An agent that reduces fever	aspirin, acetaminophen (Tylenol)
Antitussive	An agent that prevents or relieves cough	codeine, dextromethorphan
Bronchodilator	An agent that dilates the bronchi	isoproterenol HCL (Isuprel), albuterol (Proventil)
Contraceptive	Any device, method, or agent that prevents conception	Enovid-E 21, Ortho-Novum 10/11-21; 10/11-28 Triphasil-21
Decongestant	An agent that reduces nasal congestion and/or swelling	oxymetazoline (Afrin), epinephrine HCL (Adrenalin), phenylephrine HCL (Neo-Synephrine), pseudoephedrine HCL (Sudafed)
Diuretic	An agent that increases the excretion of urine	chlorothiazide (Diuril), furosemide (Lasix), Mannitol (Osmitrol)

(continues)

TABLE 18-1 *(continued)*

SELECTED DRUG CLASSIFICATIONS—continued

Classification	Action	Examples
Expectorant	An agent that facilitates removal of secretion from bronchopulmonary mucous membrane	guaifenesin (Robitussin)
Hemostatic	An agent that controls or stops bleeding	Humafac, Amicar, vitamin K
Hypnotic	An agent that produces sleep or hypnosis	secobarbital (Seconal); chloral hydrate ethchlorvynol (Placidyl), flurazepam (Dalmane)
Hypoglycemic	An agent that lowers blood glucose level	insulin; chlorpropamide (Diabinese), glyburide (Micronase)
Laxative	An agent that loosens and promotes normal bowel eliminations	Metamucil powder, Dulcolax
Muscle relaxant	An agent that aids in relaxation of skeletal muscle	Robaxin, Norflex, Paraflex, Skelaxin, Valium
Sedative	An agent that produces a calming effect without causing sleep	amobarbital (Amytal), butabarbital sodium (Buticaps), phenobarbital
Tranquilizer	An agent that reduces mental tension and anxiety	Thorazine, Mellaril, Haldol
Vasodilator	An agent that produces relaxation of blood vessels; lowers blood pressure	isorbide dinitrate (Isordil), nitroglycerin
Vasopressor	An agent that produces contraction of muscles of capillaries and arteries; elevates blood pressure	metaraminol (Aramine), norepinephrine (Levophed)

(Adapted from Rice, *Principles of Pharmacology for Medical Assistants,* 2nd ed., copyright 1994, Clifton Park, NY: Delmar Learning.)

3. Product category index (blue)
4. Product identification guide (gray)
5. Product information section (white)
6. Diagnostic product information (white)
7. Miscellaneous:
   a. Key to Controlled Substances Categories
   b. Key to FDA Use-in-Pregnancy Ratings
   c. U.S. Food and Drug Administration Telephone Directory
   d. Common Laboratory Test Values
   e. Poison Control Centers
   f. Adverse Event Report Form (MedWatch)

Guidelines for Using the PDR:

1. The pink section alphabetically lists brand and generic names of medicines and products. The manufacturer of the product provides either one or two page numbers. The first page number refers you to the picture section for identification of the product, and the next page number is for product information in the white section.
2. The blue section contains products in alphabetical order according to their classification.

3. The last white section contains current information about diagnostic products also listed in alphabetical order.

Note: The medical assistant should become familiar with the PDR's contents page with each new edition to become proficient in assisting the physician with needed information. The *Physicians' Desk Reference for Nonprescription Drugs* is also another valuable resource that can be of great assistance in identifying over-the-counter (**OTC**) medicines that patients use for self-medication. The format of this reference book is similar to the PDR for prescription products. Sections on patient education material, support groups, and diagnostic home use products are also included.

Getting familiar with the arrangement of both PDRs will prove its worth very quickly when a difficult situation is encountered in the medical practice.

Many other sources of information about pharmaceutical products are used by physicians. Most offices have more than one **reference** for this purpose. *The National Formulary,* the *Pharmacopoeia of the United States of America* (USP), and the *Pharmacopoeia Internationalis* are three reference books that contain facts and comparisons of a vast variety of pharmaceutical products.

Do not give cost. info

WRITING PRESCRIPTIONS

Finance:
Prescriptions

A **prescription** is a written order for a particular medication or treatment for a particular patient by a **licensed** physician. It is a legal document. Most prescriptions are hand written by the physician, especially those for **narcotics**. However, some physicians delegate the task of writing the information on the prescription blank to the medical assistant. The physician will then check the prescription and sign it. In many states, for instance, prescriptions for controlled substances can only have one drug, the controlled substance, written on it. It is now required that the quantity be in both numerical and written form. Any medication that is **prescribed** must be recorded on the patient's chart. Figure 18–1 shows examples of prescription blanks. When the physician prescribes only one medication for a patient, the single medication prescription pad is used. With the advancement in health information software, prescriptions may now be printed by selecting a particular drug, its strength and dosage, and the amount ordered. Special prescription paper with tamper-proof watermark is used to print the document. Computer generated prescriptions reduce the possibility of forgery and also help to eliminate errors from illegible handwriting. Physicians use the multiple medication prescription pads for those patients whose condition requires several medications to be prescribed at a time. This eliminates having to write in the patient's name, date, and other information on each single prescription order. It also saves the doctor from having to sign each individual sheet.

The prescription should contain the:

- Date
- Patient's full legal name and complete address
- Rx symbol (means recipe, or "take thou")
- Drug name and amount in numerical and written form
- Pharmacist's instructions
- Patient's instructions
- Signature of physician
- Physician's full name, address, and phone number
- Physician's DEA number
- Number of refills
- DAW (dispense as written) option

This standard information helps the pharmacist fill the prescription. It is much easier for pharmacists today to fill prescriptions because of prepared and prepackaged medications. Although it is rare, some medications must still be prepared by the licensed pharmacist from the directions on the prescription. When phoning in prescriptions, you must give the pharmacist all the information that the prescription contains. To ensure **accuracy**, you should ask the pharmacist to repeat the information. This practice will help avoid dangerous misunderstandings.

When patients have their prescriptions filled by a pharmacist, the container often has an **auxiliary** label(s) on it. Pharmacists frequently use one or more of these labels to alert the patient of special instructions or warnings regarding a particular medication ordered by the doctor. Warning labels are made in a variety of bright colors to attract attention to their messages (Figure 18–2). Encourage patients to read and comply with the warning labels. Patients who take many medications every day can often become so used to seeing the warning labels that they may be ineffective. Your gentle reminders can be helpful in possibly preventing a serious problem. The instruction "DAW" written on a prescription means that the physician does not want the medication prescribed to be substituted—it should be exactly what was written for the patient.

All physicians who prescribe, **dispense**, or **administer** medications in the United States must register with the United States Department of Justice, **Drug Enforcement Administration (DEA)**, under the Controlled Substances Act of 1970. A form must be filled out with the physician's state license number and signature and accompanied by a standard fee (Figure 18–3). If the physician moves the medical practice, this change of address must be reported in writing to the nearest DEA field office. Registration must be renewed every three years. The certificate must be filed at the registered location and be available for inspection by officials on request. If the physician practices med-

```
DEA NUMBER (MAY BE PRINTED)          TELEPHONE NUMBER
                  PHYSICIAN'S NAME
                   ADDRESS ZIP
PATIENT'S NAME _____ DATE _____
ADDRESS _____
Rx
Sig:
Refill _____ Times
Please label (   )
                              _____
                                    PHYSICIAN'S SIGNATURE
```

DEA NUMBER (MAY BE PRINTED)			TELEPHONE NUMBER
PHYSICIAN'S NAME, ADDRESS, ZIP			
PATIENT'S NAME _____ DATE _____			
ADDRESS _____			
Sig: **LABEL MEDICATION**	**mg/cc**	**Quantity**	**Refills**
Rx 1.			
Rx 2.			
Rx 3.			
Rx 4.			
Rx 5.			
PHYSICIAN'S SIGNATURE			

FIGURE 18–1 Sample prescription blanks for single medication and multiple medications

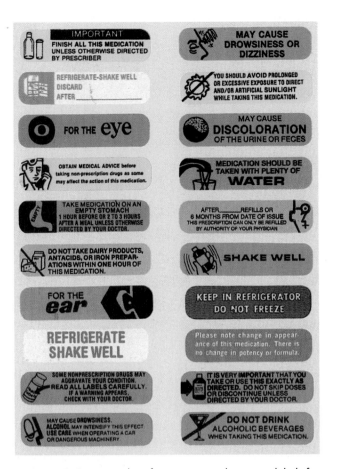

FIGURE 18-2 Examples of instruction and warning labels for prescription medications

icine in one or more locations, as long as it is within the same state, individual registration must be filed for each address only if controlled substances are administered or dispensed at each place. If prescriptions only are written at other locations, registration needs to be filed with the DEA just for the primary location. Physicians must be in compliance with these requirements of the 1984 Diversion Control Amendments to administer, dispense, or prescribe any controlled substance. A current printed schedule of controlled substances is enclosed with the application, and this should also be kept on file. Table 18–2 lists the drugs that are under federal control according to their actual or potential level for abuse or addiction in five categories or schedules.

Because there is no medical use for any of the drugs in Schedule I, prescriptions are prohibited. Drugs in Schedule II must have a written or typed prescription order with the physician's personal signature and DEA registry number. These medications may not be refilled. If a genuine emergency situation arises, the doctor may phone in a limited amount of medication to the pharmacist for the patient. A written, signed prescription order must be presented to the pharmacist within 72 hours for the controlled substance in compliance with DEA regulations. In Schedules III and IV of controlled substances, medica-

tions may be ordered by phone or written prescription to the pharmacist. Five refills may be ordered within a six-month period. Schedule V medications are subject to state and local regulations. A written prescription for these medicines is not necessarily required.

RECORDING MEDICATIONS

You will be expected to read and record many types of medications. Accurately recording the medication(s) administered to patients is absolutely necessary. When following the physician's orders in giving medications to patients, you should always prepare, administer, and record each one yourself. In situations where the physician is present and giving the order while you are preparing an injectable, each of you should check the specific medicine, the dose, the expiration date, and any other necessary details. The one who administers the injection should record and sign the patient's chart. It is never recommended that you document a medication for anyone else or have anyone else do this for you. The person who records the medication on the chart is the one responsible for the action (of administering the medication) and any possible reaction the patient may experience.

Never admin a med. you did not personally prepare

Many factors need to be included in recording medication information on the patient's chart. The following is a list of the details that should be included in recording medications. Ask yourself the traditional approach of who, what, how (much), where, when, and why, to make it easier for you to remember all the information every time.

Who—Answers the question of whoever ordered the medication and who should take it. Include the physician's name accurately and correctly spelled out.

What—Answers what medication is given. The name of it should be recorded accurately and legibly; *how* much, meaning the strength and dose of the substance, should also be recorded.

When—The date the medication is administered should be recorded, and the time as it may be applicable. This can also help you to check the expiration date of the medication before administering it.

Where—Refers to the route of the administration of the medication: oral, sublingual, topical, or parenteral. If administered by injection, the site must be noted.

Why—Answer this question for the patient verbally and with printed patient education material as necessary.

Memorizing the commonly used abbreviations and symbols given in Table 18–3 will prepare you to carry out this responsibility. Because medications can be prescribed in either metric, apothecary, or household measurements, it is important to know equivalents among all three to calculate the dose of prescribed medication. Note that some apothecaries' measurements are also household

Form **DEA** (Jun 1990) **— 224** OMB No. 1117-0014

APPLICATION FOR REGISTRATION
UNDER
CONTROLLED SUBSTANCES ACT OF 1970

Please PRINT or TYPE all entries.

No registration may be issued unless a completed application form has been received (21 CFR 1301.21).

NAME

PROPOSED BUSINESS ADDRESS

CITY STATE ZIP CODE

RETAIN Copy 3. Mail Orig. and 1 copy with FEE to:

UNITED STATES DEPARTMENT OF JUSTICE
DRUG ENFORCEMENT ADMINISTRATION
CENTRAL STATION
P. O. Box 28083
WASHINGTON, D.C. 20038-8083
For INFORMATION, Call: (202) 307 7255

See "Privacy Act" Information on reverse

THIS BLOCK
FOR DEA
USE ONLY

REGISTRATION CLASSIFICATION: Submit Check or Money Order Payable to the **DRUG ENFORCEMENT ADMINISTRATION** in the amount of $ 60.00 (3 year registration period)

1. BUSINESS ACTIVITY: *(Check ☑ ONE only)* *(Specify Medical Degree, e.g., DDS, DO, DVM, MD, etc.)*

● FEE MUST ACCOMPANY APPLICATION

A ☐ RETAIL PHARMACY   B ☐ HOSPITAL/CLINIC   C ☐ PRACTITIONER   D ☐ TEACHING INSTITUTION *(Instructional purposes only)*

2. SCHEDULES: *(Check ☑ all applicable schedules in which you intend to handle controlled substances. See Schedules on Reverse of Instruction Sheet.)*

SCHEDULE II	SCHEDULE II	SCHEDULE III	SCHEDULE III	SCHEDULE IV	SCHEDULE V
☐ NARCOTIC	☐ NONNARCOTIC	☐ NARCOTIC	☐ NONNARCOTIC	☐	☐

3. ☐ CHECK HERE IF YOU REQUIRE ORDER FORMS.

4. ALL APPLICANTS MUST ANSWER THE FOLLOWING:

(a) Are you currently authorized to prescribe, distribute, dispense, conduct research, or otherwise handle the controlled substances in the schedules for which you are applying, under the laws of the **State** or jurisdiction in which you are operating or propose to operate?

☐ YES - **State** License No. _____
  ☐ Not Applicable   ☐ Pending

☐ YES - **State** Controlled Substance No. _____
  ☐ Not Applicable   ☐ Pending

(b) Has the applicant ever been convicted of a crime in connection with controlled substances under State or Federal law, or ever surrendered or had a Federal controlled substance registration revoked, suspended, restricted or denied, or ever had a State professional license or controlled substance registration revoked, suspended, denied, restricted or placed on probation?   ☐ YES   ☐ NO

(b) If the applicant is a corporation (other than a corporation whose stock is owned and traded by the public), association, partnership, or pharmacy, has any officer, partner, stockholder or proprietor been convicted of a crime in connection with controlled substances under State or Federal law, or ever surrendered or had a Federal controlled substance registration revoked, suspended, restricted or denied, or ever had a State professional license or controlled substance registration revoked, suspended, denied, restricted or placed on probation?   ☐ YES   ☐ NO   ☐ NOT APPLICABLE

IF THE ANSWER TO QUESTIONS 4(b) or (c) is YES, include a statement using the space provided on the REVERSE of this part.

● ATTACH CHECK HERE

Print or Type Name Here - Sign Below   Applicant's Business Phone No.

SIGN HERE ▶
_____   _____
Signature of applicant or authorized individual   Date

Title (If the applicant is a corporation, institution, or other entity, enter the TITLE of the person signing on behalf of the applicant (e.g., President, Dean, Procurement Officer, etc....))

5. CERTIFICATION FOR FEE EXEMPTION
☐ CHECK THIS BLOCK IF INDIVIDUAL NAMED HEREON IS A FEDERAL, STATE, OR LOCAL OFFICIAL.

The Undersigned hereby certifies that the applicant herein is an officer or employee of a Federal, State or local agency who, in the course of such employment, is authorized to obtain, dispense, or prescribe controlled substances or is authorized to conduct research, instructional activity or chemical analysis with controlled substances, and is exempt from the payment of this application fee.

Signature of Certifying Official   Date

Print or Type Name

Print or Type Title

Name of Institution or Agency

WARNING: **SECTION 843(a)(4) OF TITLE 21, UNITED STATES CODE, STATES THAT ANY PERSON WHO KNOWINGLY OR INTENTIONALLY FURNISHES FALSE OR FRAUDULENT INFORMATION IN THIS APPLICATION IS SUBJECT TO IMPRISONMENT FOR NOT MORE THAN FOUR YEARS, A FINE OF NOT MORE THAN $30,000.00 OR BOTH.**

Mail the Original and 1 copy with FEE to the above address. Retain 3rd copy for your records.

FIGURE 18–3 A DEA physician registration form

TABLE 18-2

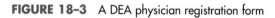

SCHEDULES OF CONTROLLED SUBSTANCES

Drug Category	Potential for Abuse (Addiction)	Medical Use	Potential for Dependence	Example
Schedule I	High	—Unaccepted —Limited to research	High	Heroin, LSD, marijuana, peyote
Schedule II	High	—Accepted —Tightly restricted	Severe psychic or physical	Amphetamines, morphine,
Schedule III	Less than I or II Low to moderate	Acceptable	High psychological	Certain opioids, barbiturates, and some depressants
Schedule IV	Low	Acceptable	Limited physical and psychological	Phenobarbital propoxyphene
Schedule V	Low	Acceptable	Limited physical and psychological	Small amounts of codeine in cough preparations and analgesics

(continues)

TABLE 18-3 *(continued)*

ABBREVIATIONS AND SYMBOLS COMMONLY USED IN ADMINISTERING MEDICATIONS

Abbreviation	Meaning	Abbreviation	Meaning
@	at	K	potassium
aa	of each	kg	kilogram
ac	before meals	L	liter, left
ad	up to	lb, LB(S)	pound(s)
AD	right ear	m, min	minim
adde	add, let it be added	M	mix
ad lib	as much as needed, as desired	μg, MCG	microgram
agit	shake, stir	mg, MG	milligram
AgNO₃	silver nitrate	mL, ML	milliliter
alt dieb	alternate days	noct	night
alt hor	alternate hour	non rep	do not repeat
alt noc	alternate nights	NPO	nothing by mouth
am	morning	q h	every hour
a, ante	before	q m	every morning
aq	water	OS	left eye
AS	left ear	OD	right eye
AU	in each ear, both ears	OU	in each eye, both eyes
Ba	barium	oz, ℥	ounce
bid, BID	twice a day	pc	after meals
BSA	body surface area	pil	pill
/c, c	with	po	by mouth
CAP(S)	capsule(s)	prn, PRN	as necessary, whenever necessary
cc	cubic centimeter	pt	patient
comp	compound	pulv	powder
contra	against	qd	every day
coq	boil	qh	every hour
DC, Disc	discontinue	q (2,3,4) h	every (2, 3, 4) hours
dil	dilute	qid, QID	four times a day
div	to be divided	qns	quantity not sufficient
dos	doses	qod, QOD	every other day
dr, ʒ	dram	qs	quantity sufficient
EENT	eye, ear, nose and throat	rep	let it be repeated
elix	elixir	R	right
emul	emulsion	Rx, ℞	take, recipe
et	and	s̄	without
ext	extract	sat	saturated
Fe	iron	sc, sub cu, SC, Subc	subcutaneous (under the skin)
fl	fluid	Sig, Sig, S	write on label, give directions
G	gauge	sol	solution
garg	gargle	ss	one-half
GI	gastrointestinal	stat, STAT	immediately
g, G, Gm, gm	gram	suppos	suppository
GR	grain	syr	syrup
gt	drop	T, tbsp	tablespoon
gtt	drops	TAB	tablet
GU	genitourinary	tid, TID	three times a day
guttat	drop by drop	tr, tinct	tincture
h	hour	t, tsp	teaspoon
H₂O₂	hydrogen peroxide	u	unit
hs	bedtime, hour of sleep	ung	ointment
IM	intramuscular	i, ii, iii, etc.	1, 2, 3 capsules, tablets, pills, and so on
inj	injection		
IV	intravenous		

measures. However, in the apothecary's system, 12 ounces is equal to 1 pound; in the household system, 16 ounces is equal to 1 pound. See Tables 18–4 and 18–5.

As with any medication given either at the medical facility or elsewhere, any reaction or side effect observed by a health care professional or reported by the patient must be documented on the patient's chart.

TABLE 18–4

Metric	Apothecary	Household
	Dry	
60 mg	1 gr	
1 Gm	15 gr	1/4 tsp
15 Gm	4 dr	1 tbsp (3 tsp)
30 Gm	1 oz	1 oz (2 tbsp)
	12 oz	1 lb (16 oz)
1 kg		2.2 lb
	Liquid	
	1 m	1 gt
1 mL	15 m	15 gtt
(1 cubic centimeter)		
5 mL	1 fldr	1 tsp
15 mL	4 fldr	1 tbsp (3 tsp)
30 mL	1 oz (8 fldr)	1 fl oz (2 tbsp)
500 mL	(1 pt)	(1 pt or 2 cups)
1000 mL	(1 qt or 2 pts)	4 cups (1 qt)
	Length	
2.5 cm		1 in
1 m		39.37 in

TABLE 18–5

Apothecaries' Unit of Weight		
60 grains (gr)	is equal to	1 dram (dr)
8 drams (dr)	is equal to	1 ounce (oz)
12 ounces (oz)	is equal to	1 pound (lb)
Apothecaries' Units of Liquid Volume		
60 minims (m)	is equal to	1 fluidram (fldr)
8 fluidrams (fldr)	is equal to	1 fluid ounce (fl oz)
16 fluid ounces (fl oz)	is equal to	1 pint
2 pints (pt)	is equal to	1 quart
4 quarts (qt)	is equal to	1 gallon (gal)

Immunizations require even further documentation. In addition to the aforementioned, the name of the medication and the name of the pharmaceutical company who manufactured it must be clearly written out. Companies that produce massive quantities of a particular immunization must assign a lot number to each batch of the product. The lot numbers can be used to keep track of and report to the manufacturer any unusual side effects or other problems experienced by a patient who received the medication. The manufacturer can then conduct an evaluation to find the cause of the patient's problem. The lot number provides the means of the trace. The expiration date is also very important. The manufacturer states that the medication or drug is guaranteed for its intended effect only until the expiration date printed on the container. Finally, the physician's name and complete address must be written on the chart and the form the patient provides for legal documentation. So that you do not have to use so much time and effort in repeating this task, a name/address stamp is most practical. Figure 18–4 gives an example of a medication properly recorded on a patient's chart.

Basic math skills should be among your many areas of **expertise.** These skills may mean monetary savings to your employer because there are competitive prices for everything, including medical supplies and medications. When ordering injectables, for instance, you may find that a multiple-dose **vial** is more economical for the needs of the practice than a single-dose vial. Determining what is cost effective for the practice and shopping for the best values will make you an asset to the practice. Table 18–6 provides examples of the common math problems you may encounter in determining costs, dosages, and other mathematical calculations in the medical setting.

Pharmaceutical representatives will undoubtedly visit the medical **facility** from time to time, bringing detailed information concerning prices and the newest products. These representatives are always willing to answer questions. Many of these companies offer support in the area of education for members of the American Association of Medical Assistants and the American Registry of Medical Assistants.

Steven C. James (patient)

9-23-XX:

Energix-B 0.5 ml IM L deltoid
per Dr. Elizabeth R. Evans, 100 E. Main St
Suite 205, Yourtown, US 98765-4321
SKB Lot #345 exp 1 yr. S. Markey (EE)

FIGURE 18–4 A sample recording of an immunization on a patient's chart

TABLE 18-6

REVIEW EXAMPLES OF MATH PROBLEMS

Addition

$$\begin{array}{r} 876 \\ 493 \\ + 521 \\ \hline 1890 \end{array}$$

Subtraction

$$\begin{array}{r} 691 \\ - 98 \\ \hline 593 \end{array} \qquad \begin{array}{r} 581 \\ - 98 \\ \hline 483 \end{array}$$

Fractions $\frac{\text{numerator}}{\text{denominator}}$

Addition
$$\frac{2}{5} + \frac{4}{5} = \frac{6}{5} = 1\frac{1}{5}$$
$$\begin{array}{l} \frac{1}{5} = \frac{3}{15} \\ + \frac{1}{3} = \frac{5}{15} \\ \hline \frac{8}{15} \end{array} \qquad \begin{array}{l} 1\frac{7}{8} = 1\frac{35}{40} \\ + 7\frac{7}{10} = 9\frac{28}{40} \\ \hline 10\frac{63}{40} = 11\frac{23}{40} \end{array}$$

Multiplication

$$\begin{array}{r} 437 \\ \times 25 \\ \hline 2185 \\ 874 \\ \hline 10925 \end{array}$$

To Prove
Divide your
answer by
437

$$\begin{array}{r} 25 \\ 437\overline{)10925} \\ 874 \\ 2185 \\ 2185 \end{array}$$

Division

$$\begin{array}{r} 56.80 \\ 70\overline{)3976.00} \\ 350 \\ \hline 476 \\ 420 \\ \hline 560 \\ 560 \end{array}$$

To Prove
Multiply
your answer
by 70

$$\begin{array}{r} 56.80 \\ \times 70 \\ \hline 3976.00 \end{array}$$

Subtraction
$$\frac{3}{5} - \frac{1}{3} = \frac{9}{15} - \frac{5}{15} = \frac{4}{15}$$
$$3\frac{7}{16} - 2\frac{1}{8} = 3\frac{14}{32} - 2\frac{4}{32} = 1\frac{10}{32} = 1\frac{5}{16}$$

Multiplication
$$\frac{1}{5} \times \frac{7}{\cancel{16}} = \frac{1}{5} \times \frac{7}{8} = \frac{7}{40}$$
$$\frac{1}{5} \times \frac{7}{10} = \frac{1}{5} \times \frac{7}{10} = \frac{7}{50}$$

Division
$$\frac{1}{12} \div \frac{2}{3} = \frac{1}{12} \times \frac{3}{2} = \frac{1}{8}$$
$$1\frac{1}{4} \div 3 = \frac{5}{4} \times \frac{1}{3} = \frac{5}{12}$$

Decimals

Addition	Subtraction	Multiplication	Division

Addition
$$\begin{array}{r} 87.43 \\ + 39.57 \\ \hline 127.00 \end{array}$$

Subtraction
$$\begin{array}{r} 796.37 \\ - 55.62 \\ \hline 740.75 \end{array}$$

Multiplication
$$\begin{array}{r} 394.75 \\ \times 68.29 \\ \hline 3552.75 \\ 7895 \\ 315800 \\ 236850 \\ \hline 26957.4775 \end{array}$$

Division
$$\begin{array}{r} 272.52\frac{1}{5} \\ 35\overline{)9538.27} \\ 70 \\ \hline 2538.27 \\ 2450.00 \\ \hline 088.27 \\ 70 \\ \hline 18.27 \\ 17.5 \\ \hline .77 \\ 7 \end{array}$$

Percentages   To find out what percent (%) one number is to another, use the number following the word "of" as a denominator and make a fraction. Divide the numerator by the denominator, for example:

25 is what percent of 35?

$$\frac{25}{35} = \frac{5}{7} = \begin{array}{r} .70 = 70\% \\ 7\overline{)5.00} \\ 49 \\ \hline 10 \end{array}$$

Ratio   Ratios show how one quantity relates to another and are separated by a colon (:), for example:

$20 : 100 = \frac{20}{100} = .20$ parts or 20%

Proportion A set of two equal ratios is a proportion. In the equation, a double colon (::) separates each of the equal ratios, for example:

To mix a cleaning solution knowing the correct portions for a small amount, you can find out how much baking soda to use to make a larger amount, using *x* for the unknown amount.

$\frac{1}{2}$ cup baking soda : 16 oz. water :: *x* amount of baking soda : 32 oz. water

$$\frac{1}{2} : 16 :: x : 32$$
$$.5 : 16 :: x : 32$$
$$16x = 32 \times .5$$
$$16x = 16$$
$$x = 1 \text{ cup baking soda}$$

Example of figuring dosage calculation for children using the nomogram shown in Figure 18–9 (A):

Child's ht—42″, wt—40#—use to find the child's BSA on nomogram

(Adult strength medication 220 mg)

child's dose = m (child's BSA) × (drug dose) mg
child's dose = .7 × 220 mg
child's dose = .49 × 220 mg
child's dose = 107.8 mg

STORING MEDICATIONS

"A place for everything and everything in its place" is the rule for storing medications. Many necessary forms, prescription blanks, and records must be kept. Commonly used medications must be rotated according to their expiration dates. The most practical way to store medications is to categorize them by their classification as in Table 18–1. Medications may also be stored alphabetically. Labeling shelves increases efficiency, as do pull-out shelves. The medication storage cabinet, closet, or room must be locked and accessed only by a qualified member of the health care team.

Sample medicines are a very helpful way for the physician to introduce a new medication to a patient to determine if the person can tolerate the substance, or as a consideration to give the patient a few complimentary doses. When samples are given to patients, they must be recorded on the patient's chart just as if it were a prescription. All information must be charted each time a sample medication is given for any reason. Keeping samples in order is an ongoing task. Storing them according to category, ailment, or alphabetically are some of the common ways to organize them. You should pay careful attention also to the product's expiration date and properly discard outdated substances. Check with local regulatory agencies on how to discard. A common practice is to flush old meds down the toilet or to place them in biohazard containers for waste removal.

Special attention needs to be given to the many medicines that require refrigeration, such as antibiotics and immunizations. Sometimes refrigeration is necessary only after the bottle or vial has been opened or after it has been reconstituted. There are also medications that must be stored in the freezer, such as the polio vaccine. Remember to check freezer and refrigerator temperatures daily to comply with MSDS (Material Safety Data Sheet) regulations. It is most important to check labels, directions, and package inserts to determine the proper method of storage for all products, as storage requirements may change.

■ ACHIEVE UNIT OBJECTIVES

Complete Chapter 18, Unit 1, in the workbook to help you obtain competency of this subject matter.

UNIT 2
Methods of Administering Medications

■ OBJECTIVES

Upon completion of the unit, meet the following performance objectives by verifying knowledge of the facts and principles presented through oral and written communication at a level deemed competent. Demonstrate the specific behaviors as identified in the performance objectives of the procedures, observing all aseptic and safety precautions in accordance with health care standards.

1. Spell out and define, using the glossary at the back of the text, all the **Words to Know** in this unit.
2. List and describe the various methods of medications.
3. Demonstrate how to instruct patients in the method of medication ordered by the physician.
4. Explain how to apply a transdermal patch medication properly.
5. Describe precautions in applying a transdermal patch medication.
6. Explain the importance of checking medications prior to administration.
7. Explain patient education to females regarding vaginal medications.
8. List considerations regarding drug action in the body.

A CAAHEP CONNECTION

Among your duties as a medical assistant, you will be responsible for medication inventory, proper storage and security, ordering, documentation, and administration. Included in the security and storage is the prescription pad. These must be accounted for every minute of the day because theft and forgery are real concerns. It is also advised to keep current reference materials regarding medications and their side effects and adverse reactions and other important information. Communication with patients in explaining their medication schedules and answering their questions is a very important part of medical assisting. Offering your support to patients will be encouraging to them and will result in better compliance of the physician's orders.

AREAS OF COMPETENCE (AAMA)

This unit addresses content within the specific competency areas of *Fundamental principles, Patient care, Professionalism, Communication skills, Legal concepts,* and *Instruction,* as identified in the Medical Assistant Role Delineation Study. Refer to Appendix A for a detailed listing of the areas.

WORDS TO KNOW

body surface area (BSA)   sacrilege
buccal   salve
douche   sublingual
infusion   suppository
interaction   tolerance
nomogram   topical
ointment   transdermal
parenteral   unwittingly

ADMINISTERING MEDICATION

C Skills Menu:
  - ~~Rectal Medications~~

There are many methods of medicating patients, and even though you may not administer every type, you should know something about each one. You will also assist in the preparation of different types of medications for patients and in the instruction of patients in specific directions for taking medications. The methods of administering medications are: oral, ~~including~~ sublingual and buccal; inhaled; topical; sprays, including transdermal; vaginal; rectal and urethral; and injected. (parenteral)

When administering any medication to a patient, you should follow a standard format checklist to make certain that you are accurate and efficient. Develop the habit of using the checklist that follows to help you to achieve this standard quality patient care.

Before you administer the medication, always be sure that you have the correct:

1. Patient
2. Medication
3. Dose/amount
4. Route/method /Technique
5. ~~Technique~~ Documentation
6. Time/schedule

It may seem unlikely that one would make a mistake and administer a medication to a patient in error. However, care must be taken in identifying the patient for whom the medication is intended before it is administered, or this could be possible. Many offices and clinics care for so many patients in the course of the daily schedule, with multiple family members being seen in the same treatment room; therefore, if particular attention is not given, an error could result.

Reading the label of the ordered medication and the amount or dose when you obtain it from storage, as you prepare it, just before you administer it, and again after you have administered it will safeguard you from committing an error. If an error is made, necessary steps must be taken immediately to report it to the doctor for emergency care to be given if necessary.

The route or method of administering medication is equally important. Carefully reading the order provides instruction in how the physician wants the medication to be administered (e.g., topical—applying a cream or other preparation to the skin; by injection—intramuscular, subcutaneous, intradermal; transdermal—skin patch; or

---

It is common practice and sound advice to follow these precautions when giving any medications:

- Compare the medication order to the container when taking the container from storage (Figure 18–5A)
- Compare the medication order to the container when preparing the medication
- Compare the medication order to the container before administering the medication
- ~~Compare the medication order to the container just after administering the medication to the patient~~

This practice ensures accuracy in giving any medication.

If there is ever a chance that a medication was given in error, the necessary action must be taken immediately. Admitting such a mistake is not a pleasant experience, but it is necessary for the well-being of the patient. Reporting the error to the physician at once is essential.

Properly instructing the patient about how a medication should be taken is extremely important. If the pa-

tient does not understand the directions or the need for carrying out the physician's orders, then the medication will be virtually useless and may be dangerous because the patient may not take it or may take it incorrectly. Patients who are given medication that may induce drowsiness should be made aware of the dangers of driving or operating machinery while taking the medication. Even though the physician may give these instructions to patients, you should make sure the information is clearly understood before the patient leaves the office. You should be mindful of recording all medications given to patients, including sample packages. On the patient's chart, record the name of the medication, the strength, directions for use, and how many dispensed. Writing the directions for use for the patient will eliminate possible confusion for the patient. Package inserts enclosed with all medication contain the necessary information. This same information is found in the PDR. If there is any further question, the PDR should be consulted.

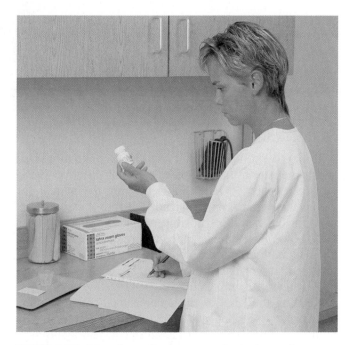

FIGURE 18–5A The medical assistant checks the medication label as she takes it from the shelf.

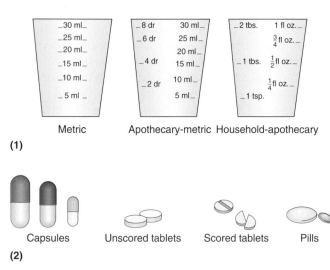

FIGURE 18–5B Means of administering oral medication: (1) medicine cups for liquids/syrups, and (2) capsules, caplets/ tablets (scored and unscored), and pills.

orally—buccal or sublingual). All of these are certainly very different.

Technique refers to how the method is administered (e.g., skill in giving the different types of injections, the manner in which you apply a topical preparation, or the way in which you administer an inhalation treatment to a patient).

Attention must be given to time and schedule in administering medicines. For example, immunizations must be given within a certain time frame for maximum effectiveness in the immunity process of the patient. The time

---

A CAAHEP CONNECTION

Patients from all over the world may present themselves for medical care in your facility. It is of paramount importance that communication is conveyed precisely. Often, when someone does not understand what is being said, the person smiles and nods his head up and down, making the communication confusing. When there is a language barrier between you and the patient, an interpreter is a must! Remember to be polite and compassionate with patients and their families. Generally, there is one family member who is the interpreter. Allow enough time for the family to discuss the information you are giving about the medication before proceeding. There should be no question or confusion concerning the patient when you are administering any medication.

---

a medication is administered is also important to the well-being of the patient. For instance, some medicines should not be taken when the stomach is full, and some should not be taken when the stomach is empty. Determining the time the patient has eaten last is important. Time also should remind you to check the expiration date of the medication to be sure of its quality strength.

Most oral medications are intended for absorption in the small intestine. The remaining methods are **parenteral**, or intended for absorption outside the digestive system.

Oral Administration

 Skills Menu:
- Oral Medications

One of the most common methods of administering medications is the oral method. These medicines are in the form of pills, tablets, capsules, caplets, lozenges, syrups, sprays, and other liquids, which are swallowed, Figure 18–5B. These medications are usually given to patients as prescriptions, although they may be administered in the office (see Procedure 18–1). For example, an analgesic may be given to a patient while in the office for relief of pain. The OPV (oral live polio vaccine) is given orally to infants and children in the medical office by the physicians or the medical assistant. This vaccine immunizes children against polio myelitis which is discussed in Unit 3 of this chapter.

Patient education is not only vitally important, it can be very helpful and practical as well. In the case of new parents who are uneasy about giving medicine to their in-

PROCEDURE

18-1 Obtain and Administer Oral Medication

PURPOSE: To obtain the ordered oral medication and administer it to the patient.

EQUIPMENT: Ordered oral medication (for practice, any tiny candies), medicine cup (disposable), disposable paper cup filled with water, medicine tray.

PERFORMANCE OBJECTIVE: Provided with all necessary equipment and supplies and using other students as patients, demonstrate the steps required to obtain the ordered oral medication, and administer it to the patient. The instructor will observe each step.

1. Obtain medication from storage area, and read label carefully, comparing it with order. **NOTE: Work in a well-lighted area, and avoid distractions.**

2. Calculate dosage if necessary, and wash hands.

3. Take bottle cap off, and place inside up on counter. **RATIONALE: The counter top is considered contaminated and must not come into contact with inside of cap. Likewise, touching inside of bottle or cap will result in contamination.** Read label of medication container.

4. If in pill or capsule form, pour desired amount into cap. Then pour medication into medicine cup. If liquid medicine, pour directly into measuring device to calibrated line of ordered amount. **NOTE: Hold measuring device at eye level with thumbnail placed at desired amount (Figure 18–6).** Syrup or liquid medications may also be given in disposable plastic measuring spoons. Liquids should be poured from the opposite side of the bottle's label to prevent the contents from dripping and discoloring the label.

5. Place medication container on tray and ordered dose in medicine cup. Place cup of water on tray for patient to take with medicine. Read label of container again.

6. Take medication tray to patient and confirm patient's identification. Explain procedure.

7. Give patient medication and offer cup of water. Observe patient taking medicine and report any reaction or problem to physician.

8. Discard any disposables and return medication container and tray to proper storage area. **NOTE: Read label of medication container again.**

9. Record information on patient's chart.

CHARTING EXAMPLE:

3-19-XX
Two tsp Robitussin® administered orally at 2:35 PM for nasal congestion and cough; instructed to take medicine two oz bottle home and take two tsp q4hr

S. Davis, RMA (DV)

---

fant, it is crucial that you give proper instruction for the child's well-being. As the child gets to be of an age where the medication could be spilled or knocked over, instruct the parents to approach the child with the dosage only and not the whole bottle. This can save you and the parents with expending unnecessary time, effort, and expense. If you give or dispense medication to the parents (patients) to give to their child to take at home, it is the same as a prescription because the physician prescribed it. Medication given in this manner is dispensed.

Oral medications have many advantages. An obvious one is their convenience. If a patient exhibits an intolerance or an adverse reaction to an oral medication, the remedy may be to just discontinue the medicine. The reaction to a single oral dose would certainly be much less dangerous than if the medication were given by injection. They are also easily stored and are economical for the medical practice and the patient.

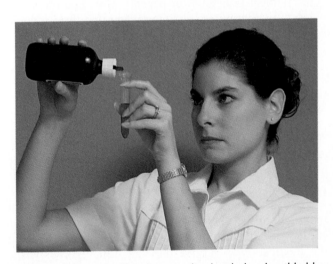

FIGURE 18–6 Pour liquids at eye level with thumbnail held at the point of the amount needed as this medical assistant is showing.

Sublingual and Buccal

The sublingual method of administering medication involves placing the medication, usually tiny tablets or spray, under the tongue. This introduces the medication immediately into the bloodstream. An example is nitroglycerine, which is usually prescribed for patients who suffer from angina. Tiny tablets or spray is also administered by the buccal method, that is, placed or sprayed in the mouth between the gum and the cheek. The medication is then absorbed through the mucous membranes. Patients should avoid eating, drinking, or chewing while the medication is in place. Instruct patients how to use these medications properly because sublingual and buccal medications should not be swallowed whole, or their intended action would be delayed and ineffective.

Inhalation Administration

Ⓒ **Skills Menu:**
- Nebulized Medications

Medications given to patients by the inhalation method are in the form of gases, sprays, fluids, or powders to be mixed with liquid and used with equipment that will produce a mist or vapor. These are breathed into the respiratory tract. The patient usually self-administers the medication at home. After being instructed properly, the patient should feel comfortable in doing so. Manufacturers prepare instruction material on the proper use and care of their equipment. You should keep a file of these for the most commonly prescribed medications.

A form of inhalation medication that should be kept in every medical practice is oxygen. Although it is not given often in most practices, it should be available for emergency use. Many companies offer instruction in the use and care of such equipment. They also offer various home oxygen treatment programs for patients who need this treatment daily. Setting aside a time when this service could benefit the entire medical staff would be advantageous.

Topical Administration

Ⓒ **Skills Menu:**
- Skin/Topical Medications

Topical medications are used in treating diseases or disorders of the skin by application to the skin in some form. They come in sprays, lotions, creams, **ointments**, paints, **salves**, wet dressings, and transdermal patches.

Topical medications must be applied as instructed for maximum effect. For example, a patient should apply a medication to reduce itching with gentle single strokes. If the medication is rubbed into the skin vigorously, the itching will increase from the heat produced from the friction, which increases the circulation.

The patch type of medication, commonly called the *transdermal patch,* is a convenient method of choice for medicating patients for many medical conditions. It is painless and ensures patient compliance. The patch is placed on the skin according to the directions of the pharmaceutical company. It then releases minute dosages of the desired medicine into the patient's tissues, which carry it into the circulatory system. The patient receives timed-release treatment without worrying about when to take medication. Patients return as scheduled or as indicated to have the effectiveness of the medication evaluated. Patients should be properly instructed to apply the transdermal patch themselves. When applying the transdermal patch, one must be extremely careful when handling it to avoid getting the medication on the fingers. A priming dose of medication is the adhesive edge of the patch. The medication intended for the patient can also be absorbed by the person who applies it. If one is not careful to wash the hands with soap and water immediately after application of the transdermal medicating patch, the effects could be undesirable or even dangerous to the one who applied it. Traces could also be transferred to another person, which could also present problems. Wearing disposable gloves when applying transdermal patches is a suggested practice, especially when a potential adverse reaction is possible for the person who applies the patch.

Several commonly prescribed medications are available as transdermal systems. Figure 18–7 shows the once-a-day Nitro-Dur® patch to help control the pain of angina. The instructions for use of another transdermal nitroglycerin infusing system are shown in Figure 18–8.

Transdermal patches containing time-released amounts of nicotine have become popular as a means of quitting cigarette smoking. These are intended to curb the craving for nicotine. Patients may obtain the patches OTC; they supply decreasing doses of nicotine over a three-month period. The patch is changed every 24 hours. Before recommending the transdermal patches, a thorough interview with the patient regarding the extent of nicotine addiction is vital. Many patients have tried to stop smoking and have already reduced their intake of nicotine. Often, the initial dose of the transdermal patches contains more nicotine than the patient is used to and will cause potentially serious side effects. Many patients also do not realize the serious effects of smoking while wearing the patches. A high dose of nicotine could produce dangerous consequences, such as elevated blood pressure and heart dysfunction. Some of the side effects experienced by patients include insomnia, racing and pounding heart, hyperactivity, and irritability. In discussing the dosage that is specific to each patient, be sure that you stress to the patient that adjusting the dosage in individual patient cases can control unnecessary problems. You can be instrumental in communicating these concerns to both patient and physician. As you prepare patients for examinations and re-checks and they disclose that they are smokers, you can make patients aware that there are OTC nicotine patches available as an option to help them stop smoking. They are relatively expensive, but the initial expense is a sound investment in the long run for good health.

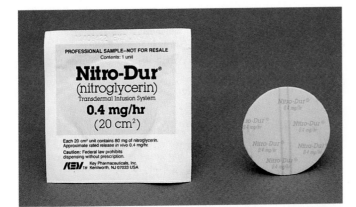

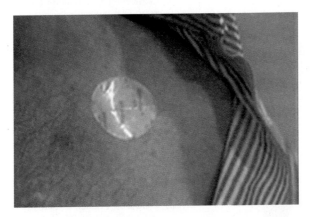

FIGURE 18–7 (A) The Nitro-Dur® skin patch is applied once a day. It helps prevent the pain of angina by delivering a steady level of nitroglycerin to the body. The patch provides medication without interfering with a patient's daily activities. (Courtesy Novartis Pharmaceuticals Corporation.)

(B) When applied to the skin, Nitro-Dur® delivers nitroglycerin at a constant and predetermined rate through the skin directly to the bloodstream. One patch gives 24-hour protection against the pain of angina pectoris caused by coronary artery disease. (Courtesy Novartis Pharmaceuticals Corporation.)

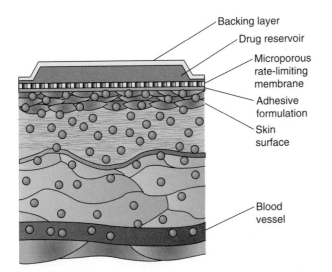

Backing layer
Drug reservoir
Microporous rate-limiting membrane
Adhesive formulation
Skin surface
Blood vessel

C) The Nitro-Dur® is a multi-layered unit. It consists of a blocking layer, a reservoir of nitroglycerin, a rate-controlling membrane, and an adhesive layer that has a priming dose of nitroglycerin. (Courtesy Novartis Pharmaceuticals Corporation.)

Vaginal Administration

Vaginal medications are applied as creams, **suppositories**, tablets, **douches**, foams, ointments, tampons, sprays, and salves.

PATIENT EDUCATION

You must make sure the patient understands the proper method of self-administration of vaginal medications because many women are embarrassed about asking. For example, many women may not know that vaginal medications should be used during the menstrual flow because this is an ideal time for growth of microorganisms.

Vaginal medications may seem undesirable because they tend to be messy. Most vaginal medications are ordered for use at bedtime, so better patient compliance is gained. You may also advise patients to use disposable panty liners or, with the advice of the physician, to insert a tampon to hold the medication in the vaginal canal.

Stress to female patients the importance of completing the prescribed treatment plan that the doctor has ordered. Remind patients who have STDs (sexually transmitted diseases) to have their partners seek medical attention and follow treatment if necessary. Some infections can be harbored in the partner with no symptoms and the patient may **unwittingly** be re-infected if the partner is not treated. Often, patients stop using a medication after a few doses or a few days because the symptoms seem to clear up. Unless all of the prescribed medication is used, the condition or problem could return. Many self-medications are available for women with gynecological symptoms. You should urge patients to seek advice from the physician if their complaints do not improve with the use of these OTC products because they may have a serious condition.

You may also want to instruct female patients in good personal hygiene. Advertising has made women believe that they should be clean "inside and out." But frequent douching or bathing with perfumed soaps or other toilet articles may leave the body open to infection by washing the natural body secretions away or irritating the delicate vaginal tissues. Patients should be aware that vaginal sprays and douches are really not necessary. Daily showering or bathing should be sufficient. Excessive odor and vaginal discharge are symptoms of infection and should be brought to the attention of the physician. Guard against giving your own personal recommendations to patients regarding treatments and medications. For instance, never suggest to a patient that you used a particular medication once and it did nothing for you. Maintain professionalism at all times, and follow office policy and your job description, in the extent of patient education.

CAUTIONS

If your physician has prescribed "under-the-tongue" nitroglycerin tablets in addition to Nitro-Dur, you should sit down before taking the "under-the-tongue" tablet. If dizziness should occur, notify your physician. This may be an indication that the "under-the-tongue" tablet dosage needs to be reduced.

POSSIBLE SIDE EFFECTS

The most common side effect experienced by people taking nitroglycerin is a headache. Your physician may tell you to take a mild analgesic to relieve the headache.

Some people may experience dizziness. This is due to a slight decrease in blood pressure, which is usually experienced when a person changes position, from lying flat to sitting upright or from sitting to standing. If this occurs, sit down until the dizziness stops, then notify your physician. He may wish to reduce your Nitro-Dur dosage.

In some people, nitroglycerin preparations may cause the skin to feel flushed or the heart to beat faster. If this should occur, notify your physician; again, he may wish to change your Nitro-Dur dosage.

Nitro-Dur II is a unique drug that depends on direct contact with the skin to work. For this reason, the skin should be reasonably hair-free, clean and dry.

INSTRUCTIONS FOR USE
PLACEMENT AREA

☐ Select a reasonably hair-free application site. **Avoid** extremities below the knee or elbow, skin folds, scar tissue, burned or irritated areas.

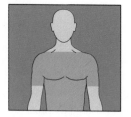

APPLICATION

☐ Wash hands before applying.

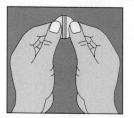

☐ Hold the unit with brown lines facing you, in an up and down position.

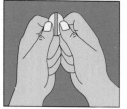

☐ Bend the sides of unit away from you.

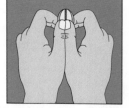

☐ Then bend the sides toward you, until the clear plastic backing "snaps" down the middle.

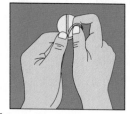

☐ Peel off both halves of the clear plastic.

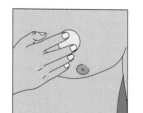

☐ Apply the sticky side of the unit to the selected body site.

☐ Wash hands to remove any drug.

☐ It is important to use a different application site every day.

REMOVAL

☐ Gently lift unit and slowly peel away from skin.

☐ Wash skin area with soap and water. Towel dry. Wash hands.

SKIN CARE

1. After you remove Nitro-Dur, your skin may feel warm and appear red. This is normal. The redness will disappear in a short time. If the area feels dry, you may apply a soothing lotion.

2. Any redness or rash that does not disappear should be called to your physician's attention.

OTHER INFORMATION

1. Allow Nitro-Dur to stay in place for 24 hours unless otherwise instructed by your physician.

2. Showering is permitted with Nitro-Dur in place.

3. Apply your Nitro-Dur the same time every day, preferably before going to bed. This allows it to adhere firmly to your skin while you are sleeping, when body movement is minimal.

4. Nitro-Dur should be kept out of reach of children and pets.

5. Store at controlled room temperature—15–30° C (59–86° F). Do not refrigerate.

6. Nitro-Dur is boxed so that you have a 30-day supply. Be sure to check your supply periodically. Before it runs low, you should visit your pharmacist for a refill or ask your physician to renew your Nitro-Dur prescription.

7. It is important that you do not miss a day of your Nitro-Dur therapy. If your schedule needs to be changed, your physician will give you specific instructions.

8. Nitro-Dur has been prescribed for you. Do not give your medication to anyone else.

9. Nitro-Dur is for prevention of angina; not for treatment of an acute anginal attack.

10. Notify physician if angina attacks change for the worse.

If you have any questions about Nitro-Dur, ask your physician or pharmacist.

FIGURE 18–8 Transdermal infusion system for the administration of nitroglycerin. (Reproduced with permission of Key Pharmaceuticals, Inc. All rights reserved.)

Disease conditons

CONSIDERATIONS OF DRUG ACTION

Several considerations may affect how the body responds to a drug. These are age, weight, **body surface area (BSA)**, method of administration, **tolerance**, allergies, time, and **interaction**. Pediatric and geriatric patients and some individuals usually require a smaller dose than an average adult. Special medications, such as chemotherapy drugs, are determined by the BSA, which is derived by plotting the patient's height and weight on a **nomogram**. Refer to Figure 18–9. To achieve a specific blood level of a medication, the dosage must be calculated according to the patient's weight. An example of figuring dosage calculation for children using the nomogram in Figure 18–9:

> Child's ht—42 inches, wt—40 pounds—use to find the child's BSA on nomogram
> (Adult strength medication 220 mg)
> child's dose = m (child's BSA) × (drug dose) mg
> child's dose = .7 × 220 mg
> child's dose = .49 × 220 mg
> child's dose = 107.8 mg

The different methods of administering medications and the rate at which the body uses them varies. Medications given by injection are circulated in the bloodstream rapidly; transdermal patch **infusion** systems deliver small amounts of medication in a sustained time-release manner; oral medicines take considerable time before they are

FIGURE 18–9 The information derived from the Nomogram is useful in calculating dosage. Refer to Table 18–5 for an example.

absorbed by the small intestines. If a patient has to take a particular medication for a long time, a tolerance may develop. An increase in the amount or a change in medicine may be necessary for the desired effect to take place. An

---

Medical-Legal-Ethical Scenario

It is a practice of some religious beliefs to fast for a period during the year. This situation may present itself to you in your career. Within the time of fasting, the patient tells you that he cannot take prescribed medication because taking anything during that time would be a **sacrilege**. Taking the medicine orally would bring a terrible anxiety for the patient about being disrespectful toward the holy day. No matter what you try, the patient says he cannot take the medicine. You realize that there is a language barrier besides the religious observance. You know how crucial it is that he take the antibiotic for his pneumonia and drink plenty of fluids. The observance of the holy days begins in 24 hours.

CRITICAL THINKING CHALLENGE

1. What should be done in this situation?
2. Is it that critical that a patient take a prescribed medication?
3. Do you need an interpreter to help make the patient understand?
4. Can you go to the physician and ask him to take this problem?
5. What might an option to his treatment be?
6. Should you have printed instructions? In what language?
7. What would you do in order of importance?

allergy to a medication may occur at any time in an individual. Careful attention must be given to the medical history and to the patient's responses during the interview. Further, the medical assistant must be alert to notice any notations in red ink signifying allergies. If a patient phones you to let you know that a medication that was taken (prescribed the day before) gave her a reaction, it must be determined exactly what the reaction is (was) and the extent of it and then carefully recorded on the patient's chart. Occasionally a patient may have an intolerance of a medication and not a reaction. A medication intolerance (e.g., vomiting it) should also be charted. Many patients take several medications daily. Helping the patient determine what to take medicine with and when to take it will encourage the desired result.

ACHIEVE UNIT OBJECTIVES

Complete Chapter 18, Unit 2, in the workbook to help you obtain competency of this subject matter.

UNIT 3

Injections and Immunizations

OBJECTIVES

Upon completion of the unit, meet the following performance objectives by verifying knowledge of the facts and principles presented through oral and written communication at a level deemed competent. Demonstrate the specific behaviors as identified in the performance objectives of the procedures, observing all aseptic and safety precautions in accordance with health care standards.

1. Spell and define, using the glossary at the back of the text, all the **Words to Know** in this unit.
2. Correctly identify the parts of a syringe and needle.
3. Name the tissue layers and sites of injection for intradermal, intramuscular, and subcutaneous injections.
4. Demonstrate how to administer intradermal, intramuscular, and subcutaneous injections properly.
5. Demonstrate how to reassure an apprehensive patient in preparation for an injection.
6. Demonstrate how to recap a needle properly after filling a syringe from a vial or an ampule.
7. Demonstrate the proper way to discard a used needle and syringe.
8. List and explain the immunization schedule for normal infants, children, and adults.
9. Explain the importance of informing patients or the responsible party for a minor, verbally and in writing, of both the benefits and the risks of immunizations before they are administered.
10. Discuss the importance of patient education regarding medications.

11. Demonstrate how to instruct patients in self-administration of insulin injections.
12. Identify the various sites for administering insulin injections.

AREAS OF COMPETENCE (AAMA)

This unit addresses content within the specific competency areas of *Fundamental principles, Patient care, Professionalism, Communication skills, Legal concepts,* and *Instruction,* as identified in the Medical Assistant Role Delineation Study. Refer to Appendix A for a detailed listing of the areas.

WORDS TO KNOW

ampule	intravenous
anaphylactic	lethal
antitoxin	measles
attenuated	meningitis
booster	mumps
catarrhal stage	paroxysmal stage
cholera	pertussis
debridement	photophobia
decline stage	polio
diphtheria	retardation
epiglottitis	rubella
epinephrine	rubeola
flu	series
haemophilus	sensitivity
hepatitis B	subcutaneous
haemophilus influenza	tetanus
type B (HIB/Hib)	toxin
immunization	toxoid
incubation	trimester
influenza	typhoid
insulin	vaccine
intradermal	vial
intramuscular (IM)	Z-tract IM

INJECTIONS

 Main Menu:

Skills Menu:
- Withdrawing from an Ampule
- Medication from a Vial
- Mixing Medication from Vials

You will be helping to prepare and possibly to administer medications in the form of injections. Because this method of medication introduces the substance directly into the tissues, where it quickly enters the patient's bloodstream, extreme caution must be practiced. The proper technique must be learned under supervision. Latex or vinyl gloves should be worn to administer an injection. Medication should only be given to patients when a physician is avail-

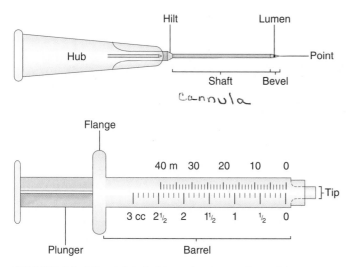

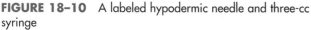

FIGURE 18–10 A labeled hypodermic needle and three-cc syringe

able nearby should the patient exhibit any adverse reaction. There is always a possibility of **anaphylactic** shock. Refer to Chapter 16, Unit 1, for symptoms of anaphylactic shock. In the event that this situation occurs, the physician should be notified to administer the immediate treatment of injecting **epinephrine** just above the initial injection site. Following the injection into the muscle or subcutaneous tissue, the area should be massaged. This is to aid in speeding the distribution of the epinephrine into the circulatory system as fast as possible. You should keep taking the patient's vital signs until the patient is stable. Provisions should always be made for emergency situations. Even though the patient's past history reveals no **sensitivity** to a particular drug, there is no guarantee of what the next dose may do. This information regarding an allergic episode must be recorded on the patient's chart. There should also be a flag (sticker) of the medication allergy to place on the outside and inside of the patient's chart. Advise the patient to wear an identification bracelet containing this information about the medication allergy.

The term *hypodermic* simply means under the skin. You must become familiar with the parts of the syringe and needle and proficient in handling them. Figure 18–10 pictures a needle and syringe with labeled parts. Practice with different types of syringes and needles; filling the syringe with varying amounts of sterile water from a **vial** and **ampule** will give you confidence (see Procedures 18–2 and 18-3).

PROCEDURE

18-2   Withdraw Medication from Ampule

PURPOSE: To withdraw an ordered amount of medication into a syringe from an ampule.

EQUIPMENT: Ampule of medication (sterile water for injection), medication tray, sterile gauze square, sterile needle and syringe, filter needle, disposable gloves, and needle resheather.

PERFORMANCE OBJECTIVE: Provided with all necessary equipment and supplies, demonstrate each of the steps required to withdraw medication (sterile water for instructional purposes) from an ampule; the procedure will be repeated three times, each time withdrawing a specific quantity of fluid as predetermined by the instructor. **NOTE: Injectables obtained from an ampule should be withdrawn with a filter needle to prevent minute particles of glass from entering the syringe and mixing with the injectable substance. The filter needle is then taken off (using a needle resheather) and the needle to be used during the injection attached. Avoid using the last few drops of the substance to further eliminate particles. Using a new needle also ensures a sharp point for swifter insertion, causing less pain for the patient.**

1. Place sterile gauze square over middle of ampule and hold ampule between thumb and index finger of one hand (Figure 18–11). **RATIONALE: Sterile gauze will keep any fragments of glass from flying.**

2. Flick pointed end of ampule with index finger to release medication into bottom of ampule before opening.

3. Grasp tip of ampule and snap it off. Discard tip.

4. Make sure that syringe and filter needle are secured by turning barrel to right while holding needle guard. Remove guard by placing in needle resheather, as shown in Figure 18–13.

5. Expel air from syringe by pushing down on plunger. Insert tip of needle into solution while holding ampule in upright position. **NOTE: Do not touch the rim of ampule to maintain sterile technique.**

6. Draw back plunger quickly and steadily to fill syringe with medication (Figure 18–12). Keep needle point below meniscus level of liquid to avoid air bubbles entering syringe. (**NOTE: If air bubbles do enter, turn syringe pointing up and gently tap the barrel to free the bubbles to the top. Gently push plunger up to release the air bubbles.**)

7. Place the filter needle of the syringe into the needle resheather and twist it off of the syringe. Place the original capped needle onto the syringe securely, and remove the cap just before administering the injection. Maintain sterility and safety. Place filled syringe on medication tray.

8. Discard ampule and gauze in proper receptacles.

Use Quick-✓ Hand-out **PROCEDURE**

18-3 Withdraw Medication from Vial

PURPOSE: To withdraw an ordered amount of medication into a syringe from a vial.

EQUIPMENT: Multiple- and single-dose vials (sterile water for injection), alcohol-saturated cotton balls, sterile needle and syringe, medication tray.

PERFORMANCE OBJECTIVE: Provided with all necessary equipment and supplies, demonstrate each of the steps required in withdrawing medication (sterile water for instructional purposes) from multiple- and single-dose vials. The procedure will be repeated three times, each time withdrawing a specific quantity of fluid as predetermined by the instructor.

1. Calculate dosage if required and wash hands.

2. Use alcohol-saturated cotton ball to clean rubber-topped vial.

3. Secure needle onto syringe by holding needle guard and turning barrel of syringe to right.

4. Remove needle guard, and pull back on plunger to fill syringe with same amount of air as medication that has been ordered. **RATIONALE: This prevents vacuum from forming in vial and thus makes it easier to withdraw solution.** There are some injectible medications that should not have air injected into the vial. You should refer to the package insert for direction in this step of the procedure.

5. Hold syringe by barrel between thumb and fingers and with other hand hold vial upside-down (Figure 18–13). Insert needle into rubber top and push plunger in, expelling air into vial.

6. Pull back on plunger so desired amount of medication will flow into syringe, keeping needle below level of solution to avoid air bubbles. **NOTE: Air takes up space where medication should be, and the dosage would not be correct if air remained.** To release air bubbles if they appear, flick barrel of syringe with finger in quick, hard motion. They will be released into hub of syringe. Push plunger carefully to make sure they are out of needle. Withdraw needle from vial.

7. Let go of plunger. Hold barrel of syringe and pull needle out of vial, keeping syringe in vertical position. Check for air bubbles. Replace needle guard by carefully scooping it onto the needle, as shown in Figure 18–15, or by placing in needle resheather, as shown in Figure 18–13, to keep needle sterile and for safety.

8. Keep medication with loaded syringe on medication tray to ensure proper identification. Place alcohol-saturated cotton ball with syringe to administer medication.

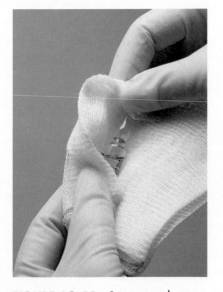

FIGURE 18–11 Snap open the ampule using sterile gauze for protection from possible flying glass fragments.

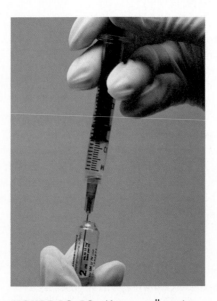

FIGURE 18–12 Keep needle point below meniscus of the liquid with ampule upright.

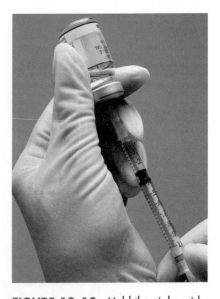

FIGURE 18–13 Hold the vial upside down at eye level, and insert needle into the rubber-topped vial.

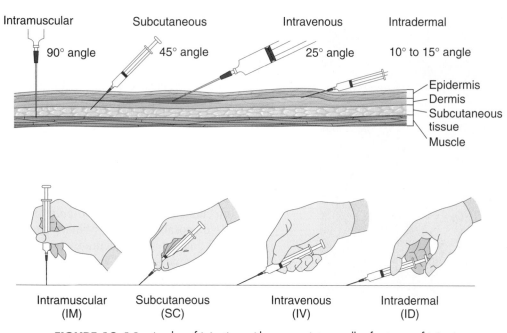

FIGURE 18-14 Angles of injection with appropriate needles for types of injection

Use an orange to practice inserting different needle lengths at different angles of injection (Figure 18–14). This should be done under supervision for instruction, practice, evaluation, and correction in developing proper technique. While becoming proficient in handling the syringe and needle confidently and thereafter, one must use caution to avoid dangerous needle sticks. It is recommended that to prevent injuries, needles should *never* be recapped. Used needles and syringes should be discarded intact in the biohazardous sharps waste container. Even though you are strongly urged to never recap needles, in reality it may be necessary in certain circumstances to do so. For your safety, you should recap a needle by placing your nondominant hand behind your back, and holding the syringe and needle intact, "scoop" the cap onto the needle (Figure 18–15). Keeping your other hand behind you will lessen the chance of being tempted to use it to recap the needle, the point at which most needle sticks occur. The only time it may even be necessary to recap a needle is *before* the injection is given. If a needle stick would occur before the injection were to be given, the needle and syringe should be discarded and the procedure repeated or the patient could become infected from the contaminated needle. In addition to the scoop method of recapping a needle and syringe, there are now many ways to prevent such accidental needle sticks from happening. Figure 18–16 is an example of a needle re-

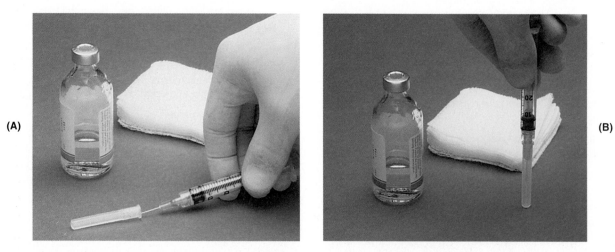

(A)   **(B)**

FIGURE 18-15 (A) Keeping one hand behind your back, "scoop" the needle into the needle cover carefully so it does not become contaminated, and to prevent a needle stick. (B) Secure the cap/cover onto the hub of the needle by pressing the tip against a hard surface (keep your other hand behind your back to help you resist using it to secure the cover). It may be helpful to press the tip of the cover against a weighted object.

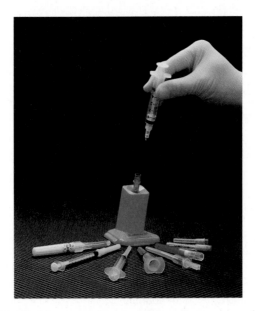

FIGURE 18–16   A needle resheather used to uncap and recap needles to help prevent accidental needle stick injuries (Courtesy Ingenious Technologies Corp., Osprey, FL 34229-8863, 800-470-4482.)

sheather, which is a stationary device that holds the sheath of the needle while you fill the syringe. Recapping the needle can be safely done with one hand so that the chance of a needle stick during the process is avoided. Some needle and syringe units have a shield that locks into place over the used needle to prevent injury to the user. There are also safety devices that activate by the touch of a finger to click a shield over the used needle or retract the needle into a sleeve on the syringe. Another safety device to protect health care team members from contaminated needle sticks is a sheath cover that clicks into place to completely cover the used needle.

Injectable medications also come in single-dose, prefilled, disposable sterile syringes and cartridges. This method guarantees an accurate dosage and is also convenient and time-saving. The single-dose units are assembled by inserting the cartridge into a reusable injector.

The administration techniques for injecting medications are extremely important. Improper injection techniques can result in infection and cause damage to nerves, blood vessels, and tissues. These can lead to legal action. When proper technique is used, however, giving medica-

---

PATIENT EDUCATION

General Guidelines for Teaching Patients about Medications

The following are general considerations patients need to know about taking prescribed medication:

1. Take only the medicine that has been prescribed by the physician for you.
2. Never share your medicine with anyone else, not even family members.
3. Take your prescribed medication when and only as directed, not more or less, to maintain proper blood level for its desired effect in your treatment.
4. Keep *all* medicines (or any chemicals) out of the reach of children.
5. Phone the physician's office immediately if you experience any reaction (regardless of how minor) to any medication or immunization.
6. Report any OTC or home remedy medication that you are taking to the physician.
7. Eat a well-balanced diet and include plenty of fluids while taking your medication. (Avoid foods/beverages that you have been instructed to stay away from because they may interfere with the action of the medicine.)
8. Refrain from alcoholic beverages or any other drugs (both OTC and home remedy–type) that are not prescribed by the physician while you are taking prescribed medication to avoid dangerous side effects.

9. Women should report to the physician if they are pregnant, plan to become pregnant, or are nursing mothers before taking any medication.
10. Remind female patients who are receiving contraceptive injections that it is vitally important for them to be on time, once every three months, for the injection to be effective. Being early for it is acceptable, but if late, remind the patient to use an additional birth control method.
11. Never save some of your prescription for a later date (i.e., antibiotics, take only as directed).
12. Throw old medicines away—flush down the toilet—after they are six months old.
13. Direct questions that patients have regarding diet, activity, dosage, or any concern about their medications to the physician's attention immediately.
14. To avoid confusion and gain compliance, explain to patients that many generic products and brand name products will produce the same effects.
15. Caution patients about taking medications that could cause them to become sleepy, interfere with their concentration, or affect their ability to operate machinery or drive.

tions by injection can be a minimally painful experience for the patient.

You can relieve the patient's anxiety by explaining the procedure. Being honest with patients is most important. In the case of children's immunizations, for example, it is far better to explain that the injection will hurt for a minute than to say it will not. You may give the child a simplified explanation of the disease for which the immunization is meant. This may help the child understand how it is really better in the long run to hurt for a minute rather than suffer the dreaded disease. If the child shows extreme apprehension, it is advisable to have assistance in restraining the child before proceeding with the injection. Instructing parents in how they can explain injections to their children can be helpful. Some pharmaceutical companies provide badges of courage or other awards to pediatric patients who display bravery in receiving their immunization injections. This gives the child a sense of pride in good behavior and makes future visits much easier for all concerned.

Authorization forms should be in order before immunizations are administered to minors. You should allow sufficient time for parents (or those responsible for the child) to read the information regarding the vaccine and have all questions answered before obtaining the authorization signature. This form must be filed in the patient's chart.

The site to be injected should be free from restricting clothing. Patients should be asked to remove these items of clothing while the medication is being prepared.

Follow correct gloving procedure before you begin to administer the injection. Proper preparation of the skin at the site of injection is necessary before and after injecting the medication because microorganisms can enter the body through a break in the skin. Alcohol is the antiseptic usually used, because it is least irritating to the skin and is economical.

Proper disposal of used needles and syringes is also of vital importance in preventing possible accidents to the medical and custodial staff of the facility and avoiding transmission of disease. Nondisposable needles and syringes must be properly sanitized and autoclaved before using again. Disposable syringes and needles should be used only once and discarded properly. Keep the needle guard on the needle until just before you are ready to administer the injection. (Again, this is a situation where recapping a needle may be necessary. Remember to scoop the cap onto the needle; do not use your other hand or you risk a needle stick, besides risking contamination of the needle before it is to be used for injecting the patient.) Afterward dispose of the entire syringe and needle intact in the biohazardous sharps container according to Standard Precautions recommendations. *Do not recap.* Remove latex or vinyl gloves before handwashing.

Before you can become proficient in injecting medications, you must first learn to withdraw medications into the syringe accurately. Medications for injection are available in single-dose and multiple-dose ampules or vials.

Intradermal Injections

C Skills Menu:
  ■ Intradermal Medications

Intradermal (ID) injections are used in allergy and tuberculin testing. The intradermal injection is administered just under the surface of the skin with a fine-gauge needle (26G or 27G). The bevel of the needle should be facing upward so that the substance will be expelled into the dermis. The needle is generally three-eighths to five-eighths inches in length, and the angle of the insertion into the skin is 10° to 15° (Figure 18–17). The sites for this type of injection are usually the anterior forearm and the mid-back area. Proper positioning of patients is vital for the accuracy of results and for the patient's comfort. Make sure the patient's forearm is supported on the treatment table and that the patient is sitting comfortably, or have the patient lie down on the treatment table.

A small wheal should develop at the site of the injection to give evidence that the medication is in the dermal layer of the skin. Very small amounts of medication, from

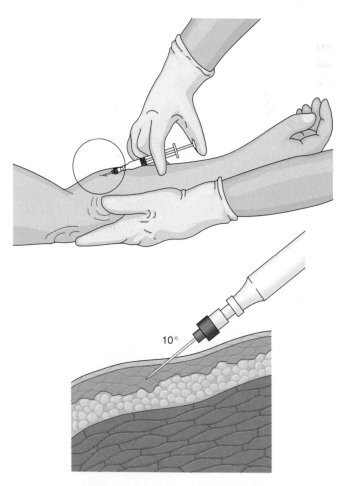

FIGURE 18–17   Intradermal injection

0.01 to 0.05 cc, are administered by this method of injection. The speed of the reaction and the size of the wheal should be recorded. The patient should be watched carefully and any reaction reported to the physician at once; however, most allergy testing is performed under the direct supervision of the physician. The patient must be observed for 20 minutes or more after the injection is administered. In the event of a hypersensitive reaction, a preparation of epinephrine may be injected by order of the physician. Refer to Procedure 18–4 for administering intradermal injections.

Subcutaneous Injections

C Skills Menu:
- Subcutaneous Medications

Subcutaneous (sub q) injections are used to administer small doses of medication, usually not more than 2.0 cc. The injection is most often given in the upper outer part of the arm (deltoid area), abdominal area, or upper thigh (midvastus lateralis area) (Figure 18–19). The length of the needle ranges from one-half to five-eighths inches and the gauge from 25G to 27G. Subcutaneous injections are

---

PROCEDURE

18-4  Administer Intradermal Injection

PURPOSE: To inject liquid solutions of 0.01 cc and 0.05 cc into the dermal layer of tissue for allergy and immunity testing of patients.

EQUIPMENT: Medication (sterile water for injection in vial/ampule), cotton balls, adhesive bandage (or hypoallergenic tape), sterile needle and syringe (needle is usually three-eighths to five-eighths inches length and 25G to 27G), medication tray, alcohol prep, patient's chart, pen, latex or vinyl gloves.

PERFORMANCE OBJECTIVE: Provided with all necessary equipment and supplies, demonstrate each of the steps required in administering an intradermal injection; three injections will be administered to a latex training arm with the instructor observing each step. The dosage amount will be determined by the instructor each time.

1. Wash and glove hands. **CAUTION:** Be extremely careful when using the "scoop" method for recapping the needle by always placing the hand you are not using behind your back, so you will not be tempted to help with the procedure. Prepare syringe with ordered amount of medication. Replace needle guard by carefully scooping it onto the needle. **NOTE: Read label of medication, and compare with order.**

2. Place medication tray near patient. Compare medication order with patient's chart, identify patient, and explain procedure.

3. Use alcohol prep to clean injection site. Allow alcohol to air dry. Do not blow on the area to dry. **RATIONALE: The area may be contaminated by microorganisms in the exhaled air.**

4. Remove needle guard. Hold patient's skin taut between thumb and fingers to steady area to be injected. With other

hand insert needle at a 10° to 15° angle of insertion and slowly expel medication from syringe by depressing plunger. **NOTE: Bevel of needle should be up; this allows the material to produce a wheal by infiltrating the dermal layer of the skin.**

5. Remove needle quickly by the same angle of insertion and wipe site with cotton ball. **NOTE: Do not massage injection site. RATIONALE: Massaging distributes the material throughout the tissues.**

6. Observe patient and time reaction. Give patient instructions as ordered, and answer any questions. Determine if patient is allergic to adhesive before applying a bandage. Hypoallergenic tape is recommended.

7. Wash and prepare any reusable items for sterilization. Discard any disposable items and gloves into biohazardous waste bag. (Place entire syringe and needle intact into the biohazardous sharps container according to Standard Precautions recommendations. If using a click-in-place shield/cover over used needle, secure the cover and drop entire needle and syringe intact into the biohazard sharps container (Figure 18–18). Wash hands. Return medication and tray to proper storage area.

8. Record information.

CHARTING EXAMPLE:
7-21-XX
0.1 mL ID (intradermal) L forearm MSTA (Mumps Skin Test Antigen) Pt advised to have site evaluated within 48–72 hours

S. Davis, RMA (DV)

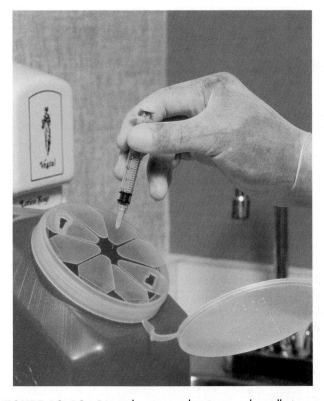

FIGURE 18-18 Discard entire used syringe and needle intact into biohazardous sharps container to prevent dangerous needle sticks.

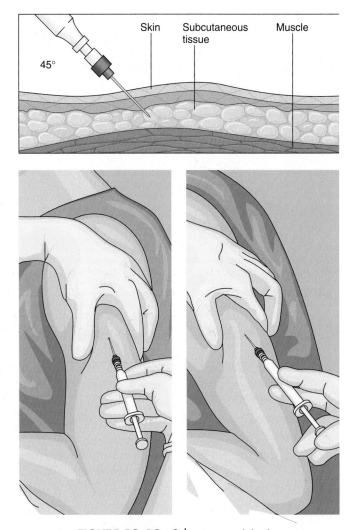

FIGURE 18-19 Subcutaneous injection

administered at a 45° angle of insertion. See Procedure 18–5. Many medications, including allergy injections, insulin, and immunizations are administered by the subcutaneous method. Refer to Chapter 16, Unit 1, for specific details in giving allergy injections. The patient should be asked to sit or lie on the treatment table for safety.

Intramuscular Injections

C Main Menu:

Skills Menu:
- Intramuscular Medications
- Z-track Injection

As the name suggests, **intramuscular (IM)** injections are made into muscle tissue. The most common sites for this method of injection are the deltoid (upper outer arm), gluteus medius (upper outer portion of the hip), ventrogluteal (lateral outside portion of the hip), and vastus lateralis (midportion of the thigh) (Figures 18–20 and 18–21). Proper positioning of patients is important. For injections in the deltoid area, the patient should be sitting. If the site is the gluteus muscle, ask the patient to lie in prone position on the treatment table with the toes pointed inward or to lean over the treatment table and stand on the non-injection-site leg. This will allow the muscle to relax and make the procedure much easier. For

injection of the vastus lateralis site, the patient may be sitting or lying in the horizontal recumbent position.

The site of injection must be recorded so that injection sites can be rotated. This practice is necessary when patients receive injections routinely, to reduce the possibility of muscle tissue damage. See Procedure 18–6.

In the administration of IM injections, the needle is from one to three inches in length or longer, for it must penetrate many layers of tissue. The angle of injection is 90°. IM injections are indicated when large doses of medication or oil-based, non-water based, or thicker medications must be given. Dosage may vary from 0.5 to 3.0 mL. Medications given by IM method are absorbed quickly by the rich blood supply of the muscle tissue.

The gauge of the needle ranges between 18G and 23G to accommodate the density of the substance. In giving injections intramuscularly to pediatric patients, the gauge and length of the needle may be smaller.

For injecting substances that may cause discoloration of the subcutaneous tissues, the **Z-tract IM** method is used. Tissue is displaced by holding it to the side of the

18-5 Administer Subcutaneous Injection

PURPOSE: To inject aqueous solutions of 0.5 to 2.0 cc into the subcutaneous tissue.

EQUIPMENT: Medication (sterile water for injection in vial or ampule), alcohol preps, adhesive bandage (hypoallergenic tape), sterile needle and syringe (needle is usually one-half to five-eighths inches, 25G), latex or vinyl gloves.

PERFORMANCE OBJECTIVE: Provided with all necessary equipment and supplies, demonstrate each of the steps required in administering a subcutaneous injection. Three injections will be administered to a latex training arm with the instructor observing each step. The dosage amount will be determined by the instructor each time.

1. Compare orders with medication, and wash and glove hands. **CAUTION**: Prepare syringe and place it on medication tray.

2. Compare medication order with patient's chart, identify patient, explain procedure, and ask patient to remove clothing if necessary.

3. Use alcohol prep to clean injection site. Remove needle guard.

4. Hold patient's skin taut between thumb and fingers of one hand and with other hand hold syringe securely.

5. Insert needle (bevel down) at a 45° angle with a steady penetration. Let go of patient's skin.

6. With one hand, hold barrel of syringe while pulling back on plunger slightly with other hand to make sure a blood vessel has not been penetrated. If no blood appears in syringe, proceed by slowly pushing down on plunger to expel medication into issues. **NOTE: If blood appears in syringe, pull needle out carefully at angle of entry. Discard medication, syringe, and needle. Replace with new syringe and medication. RATIONALE: Blood in the needle indicates the possibility of the needle placement being within a blood vessel. Medication injected directly into the bloodstream causes rapid absorption and may cause undesirable as well as dangerous results.**

7. Pull needle out at angle of insertion, wipe injection site with cotton ball, and gently massage area. **RATIONALE: Massaging the site helps distribute medication throughout the tissue.**

8. Observe patient for possible reaction and report to physician if a reaction occurs. Be sure that the patient is comfortable and can easily be observed by a member of the health care team in case of a reaction. Extra caution must be taken when giving desensitizing allergy injections. Reactions may take 15 to 20 minutes to develop. Instruct patient to wait for a full 20 minutes in case of a possible reaction. Answer any questions. Determine if patient is allergic to adhesive before applying a bandage. Hypoallergenic tape is recommended.

9. Discard all used disposable items. (Place entire syringe and needle in sharps container. If using a click-in-place shield/cover over used needle, secure the cover and drop entire needle and syringe intact into the biohazard sharps container.) Wash and sterilize all reusable items, remove gloves, and wash hands. Return medication and tray to proper storage area.

10. Record information.

CHARTING EXAMPLE:
7-28-XX
0.6 cc SC (sub q) Rt arm Allergy serum advised to wait for 20 min to be evaluated before leaving

S. Davis, RMA (DV)

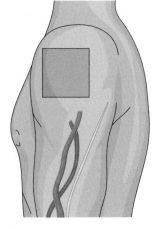
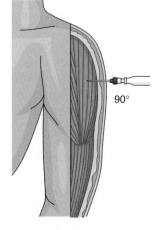
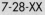
90°
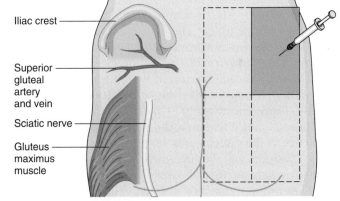

Iliac crest

Superior gluteal artery and vein

Sciatic nerve

Gluteus maximus muscle

FIGURE 18–20 IM sites, deltoid and gluteus medius

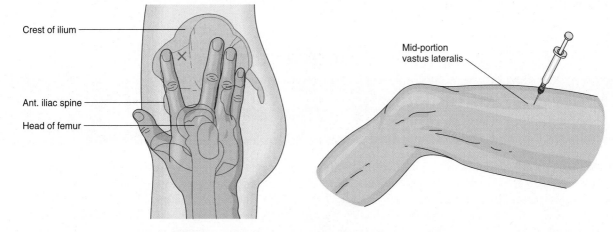

FIGURE 18–21 IM sites, ventrogluteal and vastus lateralis

Crest of ilium

Ant. iliac spine

Head of femur

Mid-portion
vastus lateralis

PROCEDURE

18-6 Administer Intramuscular Injection

PURPOSE: To inject large amounts of medication, 0.5 cc to 3.0 cc, and oil-based substances or irritating solutions which are more easily tolerated in the muscle tissue.

EQUIPMENT: Medication (sterile water for injection in vial or ampule), cotton balls, alcohol preps, adhesive bandage (or hypoallergenic tape), sterile needle and syringe (needle usually is one to three inches length, 18G to 23G), medication tray, patient's chart, pen, latex or vinyl gloves.

PERFORMANCE OBJECTIVE: Provided with all necessary equipment and supplies, demonstrate each of the steps required in administering an intramuscular injection. Three injections will be administered to a latex training arm with the instructor observing each step. The dosage amount will be determined by the instructor each time.

1. Wash and glove hands. **Caution:** Prepare syringe with ordered amount of medication. Replace needle guard by the scoop method as shown in Figure 18–12. Place medication on tray. **NOTE: Read label of medication and compare with order.**

2. Compare medication order with patient's chart. Identify patient and explain procedure. Ask patient to remove any clothing if necessary.

3. Use alcohol prep to clean injection site. **NOTE: Allow alcohol to dry. Remove needle guard.**

4. Secure a large area of skin (to accommodate large amount of medication) between thumb and fingers of one hand. With other hand, grasp syringe midway as you would a dart and hold over site at 90° angle. Insert needle quickly with firm and steady action. **NOTE: Avoid force when injecting to keep bruising to a minimum.** Pull back plunger to make sure a blood vessel has not been penetrated. If no blood is seen in barrel of syringe, proceed by pushing down on plunger and expelling medication into muscle. **NOTE: If blood appears in syringe barrel, pull out needle at angle of insertion. Discard syringe, needle, and medication and begin again with new syringe and medication. RATIONALE: Blood in the needle indicates the possibility of the needle placement being within a blood vessel. Medication injected directly into the bloodstream causes rapid absorption and may cause undesirable and dangerous results.**

5. Pull need out at angle of insertion carefully and quickly. Wipe injection site with cotton ball, and gently massage area. **RATIONALE: Massaging the site helps distribute medication throughout the tissue.**

6. Observe patient for any reaction, and report to physician if needed. Determine if patient is allergic to adhesive before applying a bandage. Hypoallergenic tape is recommended.

7. Discard disposable items. (Place entire syringe and needle in sharps container. If using a click-in-place shield/cover over used needle, secure the cover and drop entire needle and syringe intact into the biohazard sharps container.) Wash and sterilize reusable items, remove gloves, and wash hands. Return medication and tray to proper storage area.

8. Record information.

CHARTING EXAMPLE:
12-4-XX
1,000 units/kg Sterile Bacitracin IM (intramuscular) Rt hip
Parent advised to wait with child for 20 min to be evaluated before leaving

J. Watkins, CMA (CL)

PROCEDURE

18-7 Administer Intramuscular Injection by Z-Tract Method

PURPOSE: To inject substances (which may be irritating or discoloring to the tissues) deep into the muscle layer of tissue. Some substances would cause tissue discoloration and irritation if given in the subcutaneous tissues from leakage in following the path of the needle when administered. The site of injection is in the gluteal muscle of the buttocks (upper outer quadrant; for some medications the deltoid muscle may be used). Dose is from 0.5 cc to 3.0 cc.

EQUIPMENT: Medication (sterile water for injection in vial/ampule), cotton balls, alcohol preps, adhesive bandage (or hypoallergenic tape), sterile needle and syringe (needle usually is two to three inches, 19G to 21G), sterile gauze square, medication tray, patient's chart, pen, latex or vinyl gloves.

PERFORMANCE OBJECTIVE: Provided with all necessary equipment and supplies, demonstrate each of the steps required in administering a Z-tract intramuscular injection using a clinical mannequin. Three injections will be administered with the instructor observing each step. the dosage will be determined by the instructor.

1–3. Same as for intramuscular injection (Figure 18–22).

4. Use gauze square to securely hold patient's skin at injection site to one side to displace skin and tissues until injection is completed. Insert needle into gluteal muscle of buttocks or deltoid at a 90° angle, holding syringe as you would a dart. First and second fingers may be used to aspirate while thumb and ring finger hold syringe near needle end. If no blood is seen in barrel of syringe, proceed by expelling medication into muscle. Wait a few seconds before removing needle. **NOTE: If blood is seen in barrel of syringe, pull needle out quickly at angle of insertion.** Discard syringe, needle, and medication, and begin again with new syringe and medication. **RATIONALE: Blood in the needle indicates the possibility of the needle placement being within a blood vessel. Medication injected directly into the bloodstream causes rapid absorption and may cause undesirable and dangerous results. NOTE: Read package insert of medication carefully. There may be additional instructions for certain medications.** Some Z-tract injection instructions suggest that 0.5 cc of air be in syringe to follow medication to prevent leakage from needle track.

5. Pull needle out at angle of insertion and let go of skin quickly so that displaced tissue will cover needle track and prevent it from leaking into surrounding subcutaneous tissues. Cover injection site with cotton ball, and hold it in place for a few seconds. **NOTE: Do not massage area. RATIONALE: Massage causes distribution of the medication, which is undesirable with Z-tract injections because of the tissue irritating properties of the medication.**

6–8. Same as for intramuscular injection.

injection site. Following injection of the medication, the tissue is moved back over the site blocking any residual substance. Using this technique prevents the medication from following the path of the needle and leaking out into the tissues. Refer to Procedure 18–7. After Z-tract IM administration, the injection site should *not* be massaged because this action would encourage the irritating substance to circulate into the subcutaneous tissues.

Injections that are given to infants and small children need special attention. The size of the child's arm or leg will help you decide the size of the underlying muscle, which determines the needle length appropriate for the muscle thickness. The gauge of the needle is determined by the viscosity of the medication. The vastus lateralis is the preferred injection site for infants and young children. You must be sure to aspirate between 5 and 10 seconds (tiny blood vessels take time to flow) before injecting the medication to prevent entering a blood vessel which would be critical in a child. If you do enter a blood vessel while aspirating, you must withdraw the needle and start over. For injecting the left vastus lateralis, place your palm on the head of the femur (see Figure 18–21) so that your index finger points to the crest of the ilium; then, spread your fingers so that your index finger and your great finger form a "V." Lightly prepare the tissue with an alcohol prep, and proceed with assistance in holding the child during the procedure. Administer the injection carefully in the center of the "V" by holding the tissue between your thumb and finger to secure the site to be injected.

You must tell the child what you are going to do and include that it may hurt for a few seconds. Explain to a child who can understand that holding still will help you do it quicker and more easily and will keep it from hurting as much. Always ask the parent or caregiver to help hold the child to prevent an undue injury during the injection procedure. Try to distract the baby or child with a story, a toy, or other amusement to keep them from feel-that the child will be afraid of health care professionals and that it makes your job more difficult when children come in for immunizations and other procedures. Ask them to please refrain from this means of discipline.

Intravenous Injections

The **intravenous**, or IV, method of injection is used by the physician usually in an emergency situation. You are not qualified to administer medications by this method but may prepare medications to be given intravenously. IV medications have an immediate effect on the patient for they are introduced directly into the bloodstream. Needles are one to one and one-half inches in length and are usually 20G to 21G. Intravenous preparations vary in amount from a few mL to much larger doses, which are given by IV drip. The items needed are needle and syringe, medication, tourniquet, alcohol preps, adhesive bandage, and IV stand if necessary.

Usually you will draw up medication in the syringe for an intravenous injection. After filling the syringe, be sure to carefully recap the needle by the scoop method to avoid contaminating the needle. You then place the vial or ampule on the medication tray so that the physician can check to be certain it is correct. You may be asked to stay

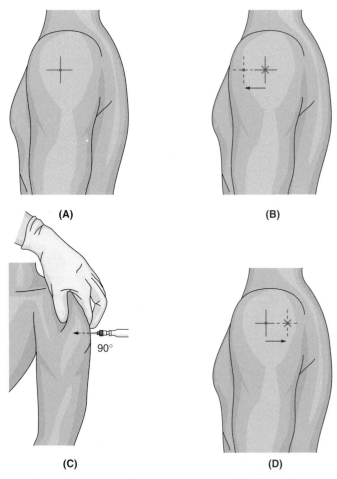

FIGURE 18–22 (A) The upper outer arm (deltoid muscle) shows the site for the Z-tract injection at the (B) Skin (tissue) is moved over to the left and held (C) during the administration of a 90° IM injection into the muscle. (D) A few seconds after the injection is given, the skin is released to cover the path of the needle, preventing leakage of medication into the subcutaneous tissues. The X shows where the actual puncture site occurred; beneath the + is actually where the medication was injected into the muscle.

ing the discomfort. You can ask the parent or caregiver who is holding the child to reposition the child immediately after you are finished with the injection to further distract her from what just happened. You can quickly talk to the child in a pleasant tone and with a smiling face. When this tactic is orchestrated, tears are often very short-lived. Keeping the mind off the discomfort is the key. Offer the child a token of appreciation for the cooperation you received. For instance, tell the child "thank you" for helping give the medicine to keep him from getting sick. Many offices give stickers and other small rewards. For a child who is very apprehensive and unruly, you must ask for help in securing the child's position in this case, or possible injury could result to the child and others as well. Restraint is in the best interest of all to prevent a dangerous situation from happening.

Discourage parents and other caregivers from threatening children who are misbehaving with "getting a shot from the doctor." Explain to those who speak this threat

PATIENT EDUCATION

It is vitally important that all patients are instructed properly in safety regarding storage, use, and disposal of used syringes and needles. The medical assistant must stress that all of these materials must be kept safely out of reach of children. The potential danger of used and discarded needles must be stressed to avoid possible accidents. Remind patients not to remove the needle from the barrel of the syringe after use. Provide patients with sharps containers. Advise patients to keep these containers in a safe place at home and to return them to their medical facility when they return so the medical assistant can dispose of them properly. Having patients follow this safety procedure will help avoid unnecessary punctures to the skin. This is an especially important precaution for diabetics, who are prone to develop infections from such punctures.

It is also of vital importance to remind the diabetic patient to record daily blood glucose levels, ketone test results, and the dosage amount of insulin. Impress on the patient how important it is to bring this record to the next appointment for the physician to review. This daily information, along with an interview, examination, and laboratory findings, help the physician to make adjustments as necessary in the treatment plan for each patient.

Preparing and Injecting the Dose of Insulin

Preparing the Dose of Insulin

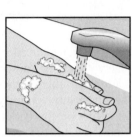

1

Wash your hands.

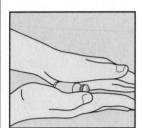

2

Gently mix the insulin. You can mix it by rolling the bottle between the palms of your hands, by turning the bottle over from end to end a few times, or by shaking the bottle gently.

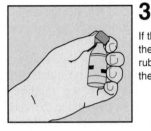

3

If this is a new bottle of insulin, remove the flat, colored cap. Do not remove the rubber stopper or the metal band under the cap.

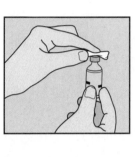

4

Clean the rubber stopper with an alcohol swab.

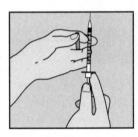

5

Remove the cover from the needle. Pull the plunger back until the tip of the plunger is at the line for correct dosage (units). This will pull air into the syringe.

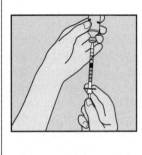

6

Push the needle through the rubber stopper. Press in the plunger to push the air into the bottle of insulin.

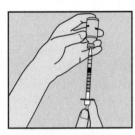

7

Turn the bottle and syringe upside down. Hold the bottle with one hand. The tip of the needle should be in the insulin. Use the other hand to pull back on the plunger until its tip is at the line for correct dosage (units). This will pull insulin into the syringe.

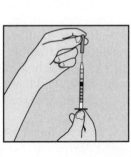

8

Look at the insulin in the syringe. Are there any air bubbles? If so, use the plunger to push the insulin back into the bottle. Then slowly pull insulin into the syringe again. Pull the plunger back to the line for your dose of insulin. Repeat this until there are no large air bubbles in the syringe.

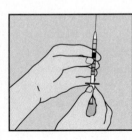

9

Make **sure** the tip of the plunger is at the line for correct dosage (units). Double-check your dose. Magnifiers that connect to your syringe are available if needed. They can help you see the lines on the syringe more clearly.

10

Pull the needle out of the rubber stopper. (If you need to lay the syringe down before taking your shot, put the cover back on the needle to protect it.)

FIGURE 18–23 Instructions for self-administration of insulin (Courtesy of Eli Lilly and Company.)

Injecting the Dose of Insulin

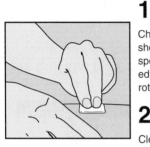

1

Choose a site for your shot. Each shot should be given in a different spot. Ask your doctor or diabetes educator to discuss injection site rotation with you.

2

Clean the skin at that place with an alcohol swab.

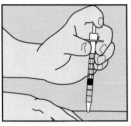

3

"Pinch" up a large area of skin. Push the needle into the skin, going straight in (at a 90 degree angle). Be sure the needle is all the way in.

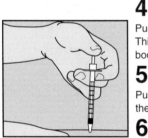

4

Push the plunger all the way down. This will push the insulin into your body. Release pinched skin.

5

Pull the needle straight out. Don't rub the place where you gave your shot.

6

Safely dispose of used needles and syringes. Your doctor, pharmacist, or diabetes educator can show you how.

FIGURE 18–23 (continued)

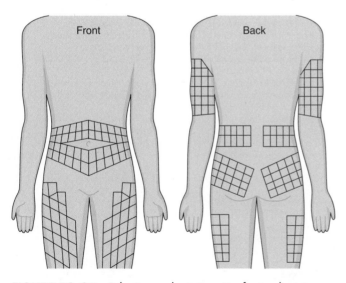

FIGURE 18–24 Selection and rotation sites for insulin injections (Courtesy of Eli Lilly and Company.)

with the patient while waiting for the emergency squad or ambulance to transport the patient to the hospital. Observing the patient for signs of distress and reactions to the administered medication is an important responsibility. The physician must be notified immediately of any complications. All information should be recorded on the patient's chart.

The medical assistant is often the one who will give instruction to the diabetic patient in the technique of self-administration of daily **insulin** injections. You may be of great help in demonstrating the proper method of filling a syringe, preparing the injection site, and acquiring skill in injecting the insulin. Figure 18–23 shows a step-by-step self-injection outline for the patient who needs daily insulin injection. Generally, the physician teaches the patient initially about diet, dosage, and the different types of insulin. You may be delegated to do follow-up patient education in this area. Because the insulin-dependent diabetic patient must administer this injection at home to herself at least once each day, you should instruct the patient to follow a pattern of rotation of injection sites, an example of which is shown in Figure 18–24. Explain to the patient to number each area of the body that is injected each time in the boxes in an alternating rotation pattern. This method offers the patient the means to develop her own personal schedule. Printed patient education material for patients is available from most pharmaceutical companies to help patients gain an understanding of their diabetes. You may also want to refer patients to educational programs held at local hospitals or through the American Diabetes Association.

IMMUNIZATIONS Not on test ↓

Our immune system responds immediately to the invasion of disease-causing microorganisms. If the exposure to the disease is slight and our susceptibility is low, our immune response may defend us from coming down with the disease itself. However, if we are susceptible to the disease, meaning our resistance is low, we develop the disease, experience the symptoms, and are sick. Antibodies are produced to protect us, making us resistant from further attacks of the specific pathogen that has made us sick. For instance, if one gets mumps, the body produces antibodies to destroy the mumps-causing organisms. After recovery from the illness, antibodies against mumps will protect one from coming down with it again. This is a process which is called *natural immunity.*

Artificial immunity is produced by administering **immunizations** or **vaccines** made from the dead or harmless infectious agents that trigger the immune response in the body to manufacture antibodies against the particular disease-causing agent. Occasionally, one has a slight reaction during this process by experiencing mild symptoms of the disease or having a slight fever. In this process, one becomes immune (resistant) to the disease. The immunization schedule (Table 18–7) is the recommendation of

TABLE 18-7

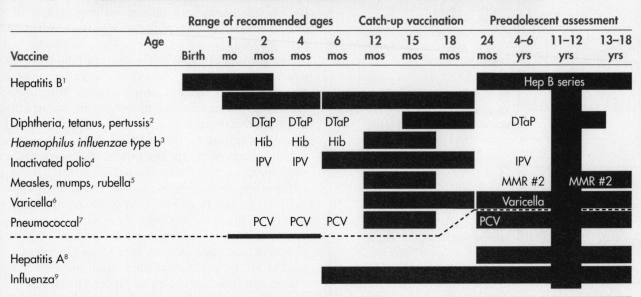

RECOMMENDED CHILDHOOD IMMUNIZATION SCHEDULE UNITED STATES, 2002

Vaccine \ Age	Birth	1 mo	2 mos	4 mos	6 mos	12 mos	15 mos	18 mos	24 mos	4–6 yrs	11–12 yrs	13–18 yrs
			Range of recommended ages			Catch-up vaccination			Preadolescent assessment			
Hepatitis B[1]											Hep B series	
Diphtheria, tetanus, pertussis[2]			DTaP	DTaP	DTaP					DTaP		
Haemophilus influenzae type b[3]			Hib	Hib	Hib							
Inactivated polio[4]			IPV	IPV						IPV		
Measles, mumps, rubella[5]										MMR #2		MMR #2
Varicella[6]										Varicella		
Pneumococcal[7]			PCV	PCV	PCV					PCV		
Hepatitis A[8]												
Influenza[9]												

This schedule indicates the recommended ages for routine administration of currently licensed childhood vaccines, as of December 1, 2001, for children through age 18 years. Any dose not given at the recommended age should be given at any subsequent visit when indicated and feasible. ▬ Indicates age groups that warrant special effort to administer those vaccines not previously given. Additional vaccines may be licensed and recommended during the year. Licensed combination vaccines may be used whenever any components of the combination are indicated and the vaccine's other components are not contraindicated. Providers should consult the manufacturers' package inserts for detailed recommendations.

1. **Hepatitis B vaccine (Hep B).** All infants should receive the first dose of hepatitis B vaccine soon after birth and before hospital discharge; the first dose may also be given by age two months if the infant's mother is HBsAg-negative. Only monovalent hepatitis B vaccine can be used for the birth dose. Monovalent or combination vaccine containing Hep B may be used to complete the series; four doses of vaccine may be administered if combination vaccine is used. The second dose should be given at least four weeks after the first dose, except for Hib-containing vaccine which cannot be administered before age six weeks. The third dose should be given at least 16 weeks after the first dose and at least eight weeks after the second dose. The last dose in the vaccination series (third or fourth dose) should not be administered before age six months.

   Infants born to HBsAg-positive mothers should receive hepatitis B vaccine and 0.5 mL hepatitis B immune globulin (HBIG) within 12 hours of birth at separate sites. The second dose is recommended at age one to two months and the vaccination series should be completed (third or fourth dose) at age six months.

   Infants born to mothers whose HBsAg status is unknown should receive the first dose of the hepatitis B vaccine series within 12 hours of birth. Maternal blood should be drawn at the time of delivery to determine the mother's HBsAg status; if the HBsAg test is positive, the infant should receive HBIG as soon as possible (no later than age one week).

2. **Diphtheria and tetanus toxoids and acellular pertussis vaccine (DTaP).** The fourth dose of DTaP may be administered as early as age 12 months, provided 6 months have elapsed since the third dose and the child is unlikely to return at age 15–18 months. **Tetanus and diphtheria toxoids (Td)** is recommended at age 11–12 years if at least five years have elapsed since the last dose of tetanus and diphtheria toxoid-containing vaccine. Subsequent routine Td boosters are recommended every 10 years.

3. *Haemophilus influenzae* **type b (Hib) conjugate vaccine.** Three Hib conjugate vaccines are licensed for infant use. If PRP-OMP (Pedvax HIB® or ComVax® [Merck]) is administered at ages two and four months, a dose at age six months is not required. DTaP/Hib combination products should not be used for primary immunization in infants at ages two, four, or six months, but can be used as boosters following any Hib vaccine.

4. **Inactivated polio vaccine (IPV).** An all-IPV schedule is recommended for routine childhood polio vaccination in the United States. All children should receive four doses of IPV at ages two months, four months, six to eighteen months, and four to six years.

5. **Measles, mumps, and rubella vaccine (MMR).** The second dose of MMR is recommended routinely at age four to six years but may be administered during any visit, provided at least four weeks have elapsed since the first dose and that both doses are administered beginning at or after age 12 months. Those who have not previously received the second dose should complete the schedule by the 11–12 year old visit.

6. **Varicella vaccine.** Varicella vaccine is recommended at any visit at or after age 12 months for susceptible children, i.e. those who lack a reliable history of chickenpox. Susceptible persons aged greater than 13 years should receive two doses, given at least four weeks apart.

7. **Pneumococcal vaccine.** The heptavalent **pneumococcal conjugate vaccine (PCV)** is recommended for all children age 2–23 months. It is also recommended for certain children age 24–59 months. **Pneumococcal polysaccharide vaccine (PPV)** is recommended in addition to PCV for certain high-risk groups. See *MMWR* 2000;49(RR-9):1–35.

8. **Hepatitis A vaccine.** Hepatitis A vaccine is recommended for use in selected states and regions, and for certain high-risk groups; consult your local public health authority. See *MMWR* 1999;48(RR-12):1–37.

9. **Influenza vaccine.** Influenza vaccine is recommended annually for children age greater than six months with certain risk factors (including but not limited to asthma, cardiac disease, sickle cell disease, HIV, diabetes; see *MMWR* 2001;50(RR-4):1–44), and can be administered to all others wishing to obtain immunity. Children aged less than or equal to 12 years should receive vaccine in a dosage appropriate for their age (0.25 mL if age 6–35 months or 0.5 mL if age greater than or equal to three years). Children aged less than or equal to eight years who are receiving influenza vaccine for the first time should receive two doses separated by at least four weeks.

For additional information about vaccines, vaccine supply, and contraindications for immunization, please visit the National Immunization Program Web site at www.cdc.gov/nip or call the National Immunization Hotline at 800-232-2522 (English) or 800-232-0233 (Spanish).

Approved by the Advisory Committee on Immunization Practices (www.cdc.gov/nip/acip), the American Academy of Pediatrics (www.aap.org), and the American Academy of Family Physicians (www.aafp.org).

public health officials in the United States against the usual childhood diseases (UCHD) and suggested vaccines for adults (especially high-risk patients). Immunization schedules may vary in other countries for infants, children, and adults. You should make sure before administering any immunization that the patient does not have an active illness or fever. If this is the case, the vaccine should be rescheduled when the patient is well. Also, check the patient's health/medical history to be sure the patient has no past history of convulsions or allergies of any kind. If an allergy is known, bring it to the attention of the physician *before* the vaccine is administered. You may want to look the immunization up in a medications reference book for contraindications, precautions, and warnings. It is strongly advised that the parent/patient be made aware of the benefits and risks of all vaccines. Sufficient time should be given to the responsible person to read printed material after a verbal explanation is given regarding the vaccine(s). An opportunity must be provided for any questions of the parent/patient to be answered by the doctor before administration of immunization(s). When more than one dose of a vaccine is necessary to reach adequate immunization against a particular disease, such as the DPT injections, it is referred to as a primary "**series**." Each of these should be given with at least six to eight weeks between each dose within a reasonable period. The primary series requires a **booster** for the immunization to be most effective and complete. In years past, these diseases were dreadful illnesses that affected children and adults and often caused death. In the following text is a brief description of each of the diseases, the symptoms, the method of transmission, **incubation** period, and its treatment. This is to help you in answering questions about the diseases in the immunization schedule when patients ask "why" they need to have the vaccine. Certainly a few seconds/minutes (or even hours) of discomfort are well worth the minor suffering to gain protection from a potentially fatal disease.

The anatomy and physiology section of this text (Chapter 11) provides information regarding pneumonia and influenza, which are diseases affecting the respiratory system. A brief description follows.

Influenza   Commonly referred to as "the **flu**," **influenza** is a disease caused by a myxovirus that affects the respiratory tract. It is spread by direct contact, by droplet infection from the vapor of coughing and sneezing from an infected person, and by indirect contact from handling soiled items (such as used tissues) of the patient. The incubation period is between one and four days. Symptoms include sudden onset of fever, chills, sore throat, cough, muscle aches and pains, general malaise, and weakness. Treatment for the flu consists of bed rest, increased intake of fluids, antipyretics, and mild analgesics. Immunization against some strains of influenza is recommended for high-risk patients, such as the elderly, those with chronic illness, respiratory distress, or other conditions that warrant protection from infectious disease.

Pneumonia   This is an acute inflammation of the lungs. Eighty-five percent of pneumonia cases are caused by the *pneumococcus* bacterium. Pneumonia may also be caused by other bacteria, a virus, rickettsiae, and fungi. The *pneumococcus* bacterium disease (pneumonitis) is spread by droplet infection and direct contact with an infected person. The incubation period is only a few hours after exposure to the bacteria. The symptoms are abrupt in onset and include severe chills, high fever, headache, chest pain, dyspnea, rapid pulse, cyanosis, and cough with blood-stained sputum. Bed rest, increased fluid intake, analgesics, antipyretics, and in many cases, oxygen are necessary for successful treatment of the patient. Pneumovax is a vaccine to protect high-risk patients from contracting the disease generally. Only one immunization is required for life protection, although boosters may be considered after 10 years. Those age 65 and over are encouraged to get this vaccine.

Haemophilus influenza type B   Hemophilus or **haemophilus**, also known as **Hib** and **HIB**, is a disease caused by a small gram-negative, nonmotile parasitic bacterium that leads to severe destructive inflammation of the larynx, trachea, and bronchi. The disease is transmitted by droplet airborne infection. Incubation is from one to three days. The symptoms are sudden onset of fever, sore throat, cough, muscle aches, weakness, and general malaise. General care is bed rest, increased fluid intake, antipyretics, antibiotics, and analgesics as necessary. Because this particular disease affects infants and small children, immunization is recommended to this population. Each year, this illness attacks one in every 200 infants in the United States; the most at-risk group is between the ages of six months and five years. With the rise in popularity of day care centers, immunization against the Hib bacterium is a most sensible way to prevent this often resistant-to-antibiotic disease from spreading through the very young population in the United States. Complications of this childhood disease include **meningitis**, which could result in damage to the nervous system or in mental **retardation**; **epiglottitis**, which could cause a child to choke to death if immediate treatment is not given; joint infections; and forms of crippling arthritis. The Hib vaccine is administered in a series of three subcutaneous or intramuscular injections at two, four, and six months (see Table 18–7). A booster is given at 18 months.

Measles, mumps, and rubella   The MMR vaccine protects children from all three childhood diseases. **Measles** is medically termed **rubeola**. It is also referred to as "old-fashioned" and 10-day measles. It is spread by direct contact, droplet infection, and by indirect contact from infected items of a patient. It has a 10- to 21-day incubation period. In the prodromal stage (earliest), the patient exhibits fever, malaise, runny nose, cough, sometimes conjunctivitis, and progresses with loss of appetite, **photophobia**, sore throat, and eventually Koplik's spots (the red skin rash). The cause is the rubeola virus, which is an acute and highly contagious viral disease involving the respiratory tract. Complications of measles can result in deafness, brain damage, and pneumonia. Treatment for measles is bed rest, increased fluid intake, antipyretics, antibiotics, cough medicine, and calamine lotion. The patient should be kept in isolation to prevent transmission to others. Quiet activity is suggested for the patient during recovery time, usually a few days.

Mumps is an acute contagious febrile disease that causes inflammation of the parotid and salivary glands. Parotitis is transmitted by droplet infection or direct contact with an infected person. The usual incubation period is from 14 to 28 days. Symptoms include chills and fever, headache, and pain below and in front of the ear(s) for five to seven days' duration. Another symptom is pain between the ear and the angle of the jaw with drinking or eating acidic substances. Bed rest and a soft diet, including increased fluid intake, is recommended. Application of cold packs to control swelling of the glands of the neck, and in males, of the testicles in orchitis, is advised.

Rubella, also called German measles or three-day measles, is an acute contagious viral disease characterized by an upper respiratory infection. If a female acquires rubella during the first **trimester** of pregnancy, fetal abnormalities may result. You should remind female patients in childbearing years of this concern and to be tested for a rubella antibody titer, and/or to be vaccinated before becoming pregnant. *Females should not be vaccinated during pregnancy.* Be sure to determine this before administering the vaccine. Rubella is transmitted by droplet infection and by direct contact. The incubation period is from 12 to 23 days. Symptoms include slight fever, sore throat, drowsiness, malaise, swollen glands and lymph nodes, arthralgia, and a diffuse fine red rash (Figure 18–25). Treatment is bed rest, liquids, antipyretics, and sponge baths. Complications of rubella can result in blindness, deafness, brain damage, heart defects, enlarged liver, and bone malformation.

Diphtheria This acute infectious disease is caused by *Corynebacterium diphtheriae,* which is a gram-positive, nonmotile, nonspore-forming, club-shaped bacillus. **Diphtheria** diagnosis is confirmed by throat culture. Transmission is by direct and indirect contact. The incubation period is between two and five days. Symptoms include headache, malaise, fever, and sore throat with a yellowish white or gray membrane. Treatment consists of adequate liquids and a soft diet, antibiotics, bed rest, and in some cases, a tracheostomy. The Schick test is an interdermal injection of a minute amount of the diphtheria toxin used to determine the degree of immunity to the disease. Little or no reaction indicates immunity (the presence of antibodies).

Pertussis Whooping cough, or **pertussis**, is an acute infectious disease characterized by respiratory drainage, then a peculiar paroxysmal cough, which ends in a whooping inspiration (sounds like a shrill trumpeting cry;

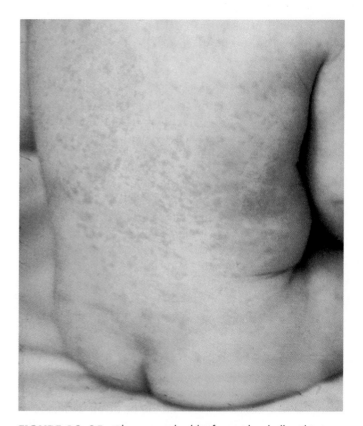

FIGURE 18–25 Eleven-month-old infant with rubella. This infant has typical discreet macupapular erythematous rash indistinguishable from that seen in other viral illnesses.

the name comes from the whooping crane that makes this sound). This disease is most common in children under four years, although it can affect children of all ages if they have not been immunized against it. Pertussis is caused by the small, nonmotile, gram-negative bacillus *Bordetella pertussis.* It is transmitted by direct and indirect contact. The incubation period is from 7 to 14 days. Symptoms of whooping cough include: in the **catarrhal stage**—an increase in leukocyte count marked by lymphocytosis, respiratory drainage, sneezing, slight fever, dry cough, irritability, loss of appetite; in the **paroxysmal stage**—violent cough with whooping inspiration sounds, forceful vomiting that can evoke hemorrhaging from various portions of the body from the straining; and in the **decline stage**—decline in coughing and return of appetite. A trace cough may last for several months to two years.

Rabies This viral disease is transmitted in the saliva of infected animals (nonvaccinated animals, such as dogs, cats, bats, foxes, raccoons, and skunks in the wild) and through airborne transmission, which is possible in heavily-infested bat caves. Human symptoms of the disease may include fever, pain, aggressive behavior, hallucinations, extreme weakness, and thirst. For the unfortunate victim who has been bitten by a rabid animal, a vaccine that consists of a series of five injections is very effective in combating the disease. There do not seem to be any side effects of this vaccine. If one is not treated with the vaccine until after the symptoms appear, it is always a fatal disease. The rabies vaccine for animals is still the best means of prevention. You may help in educating patients about this potential problem by reminding them about getting their pets protection against this disease with the rabies vaccine and keeping them from roaming unsupervised. Further alert them that wild animals, even the cute little ones, have the potential risk of carrying rabies and are to be considered dangerous. Explain that people, especially unsuspecting children, should not approach wild animals even if they appear mild-mannered. Another point for those who are planning to travel to rural areas of foreign countries is that they should check about getting pre-immunization shots against rabies in addition to the established list of required immunizations. Health officials are hopeful that this will help prevent serious illness and death around the world as people heed the warnings.

Tetanus This acute, potentially fatal, infectious disease affects the central nervous system. **Tetanus** was commonly referred to as "lockjaw." It is caused by the bacillus *Clostridium tetani,* the **toxin** of which is one of the most **lethal** poisons known. The bacillus is found in superficial layers of the soil. It is a normal inhabitant of the intestinal tracts of horses and cows. Tetanus affects only wounds that contain dead tissue, transmitted commonly in puncture wounds, abrasions, lacerations, and burns. Immediate cleaning of the wound and **débridement** are necessary initially in treatment. There is a short incubation period of 3 to 21 days, and a longer one of four to five weeks. The symptoms of tetanus are stiffness of the jaw, esophageal muscles, and sometimes neck muscles. Progressing rigidity follows soon with fixed jaw (thus lockjaw), altered voice, fever, painful spasms of all body muscles, irritability, and headache. Motor nerves transmit impulses from the infected central nervous system to muscle. Maintaining an airway and administering **antitoxin** are vital. Additionally, treatment consists of sedation, controlling muscle spasms, maintaining fluid balance, penicillin G, tracheostomy, and oxygen as necessary. The patient must be in a quiet room to prevent the triggering of muscle spasms.

Rotavirus The rotavirus is a disease that affects infants and small children, causing diarrhea and vomiting in many cases. This virus strikes over 500,000 children under the age of three years in the United States each year. It also is cause to hospitalize approximately 50,000 each year because of dehydration from the effects of the disease. Every year, approximately 20 children die from rotavirus. The child or infant who has the rotavirus should be given medical attention immediately because dehydration can be a serious threat to the child's life. Maintaining

the child's fluid levels is vital. The means of transmission is from an infected child. Often, children have no symptoms for a couple of days before they begin the diarrhea, and for a couple of days after the diarrhea stops, the child seems to be better. Even during these times when the child or infant does not seem to be sick, the virus can be passed on to other children. Child day care center workers should strive to prevent this virus by frequent hand washing of the children and of themselves.

There is a rotavirus vaccine that can be given to infants along with other immunizations at ages two, four, and six months of age. If an infant has not had the vaccine by the age of seven months, it is thought to be unnecessary. This rotavirus vaccine has not yet been added to the recommended childhood immunization schedule, but is available to physicians who recommend it for their patients.

Varicella zoster Better known as "chickenpox," this virus is highly contagious and is spread by direct contact and droplets from the respiratory tract in the prodromal stages or in the early stages of the rash. It is a member of the herpes virus family and is often called herpes zoster. It primarily affects young children. The rash develops into vesicular fluid eruptions that are infectious until they become dry scabs. Incubation is between two to three weeks. Symptoms include highly pruritic rash, fever, headache, loss of appetite, and general malaise, which last from a few days to two weeks. The treatment is baking soda paste for the itching eruptions, bed rest, liquids, antipyretics, and oral antihistamines if necessary for control of the itching. There is a relatively new vaccine for the prevention of this disease. The VZV vaccine is given to children between 12 and 18 months by injection, with an additional dose given between 11 and 12 years. The most common complication of chickenpox is secondary infections. Many children are also affected with respiratory ailments and ear infections.

Hepatitis A Hepatitis A is also referred to as infectious hepatitis. The symptoms of hepatitis are much the same as hepatitis B. A vaccine consisting of two injections six months apart is available, but it is generally recommended only for those who travel to countries that are in distant continents. You can find further information about hepatitis A in Chapter 11, Unit 10.

Hepatitis B This is a highly contagious, potentially fatal, form of viral hepatitis. It is caused by the **hepatitis B** virus (HBV). It has been known as "serum hepatitis." Hepatitis B is transmitted by contaminated serum in blood transfusions or by using contaminated needles or instruments. It has an incubation period of 14 to 50 days. The symptoms are slow at onset with fever, malaise, loss of appetite, nausea, and vomiting, progressing to include jaundice, weakness, dark urine, and whitish stool. Bed rest and a forced-fluid diet are recommended. Alcohol and fats should be eliminated from the patient's diet. The hepatitis B vaccine is urged for all who may be at risk, especially *all health care workers*. It is thought to be in widespread proportions everywhere and immunization is strongly urged to protect the country's population and to prevent a massive epidemic. The hepatitis B virus vaccine, Hep B, is given to neonates whose mothers have not had the disease before leaving the hospital. The second dose is given between one and four months of age, and the third dose between six and eighteen months. A booster dose is recommended for children between 11 and 12 years. Protecting the very young from this often fatal disease is a sensible means of control of possible epidemics.

Meningitis (Bacterial)

In the 1990s, there was an increase in the number of cases of bacterial meningitis among young adults between the ages of 15 and 24 years. Bacterial meningitis is a highly contagious disease that can cause serious and long-lasting effects on the nervous system. Death within 24 to 48 hours after contracting the disease is a very real possibility. Fortunately, this type of meningitis can be prevented with a vaccine. Persons who have an altered immune system, a serious health condition, or women during pregnancy should not have this vaccine. For most people, the vaccine is safe and results in minor reactions, such as slight soreness at the injection site and mild fever. These reactions are true of most vaccines. Viral meningitis is not as serious an illness and has no vaccine at this time.

Inactivated Polio Vaccine

In addition to the oral polio vaccine you will read about next, there is a higher-potency killed polio vaccine, IPV (inactivated polio vaccine), that is given by injection. Parents are to be given the information about each type of vaccine that their child may receive before it is administered. In this way, the parents can make a decision about what they want for their children based on facts presented them. Infants are given two injections in their first year with eight weeks between them. Children should have another injection at 18 months, when they begin school, and every five years until the child is 18 years old. IPV is recommended for those who have a low resistance to serious infections, for those in close daily contact with them, or for adults who have never been vaccinated against polio when their children are given the oral vaccine.

As with any parenteral administration of medications, it is important to instruct the patient to relax as much as possible during the procedure. Tense or tight muscles around the site of injection will make not only the procedure itself an unpleasant experience, but will have an after-effect of unnecessary soreness of the area. Becoming proficient in technique, besides developing a good rapport and educating the patients you serve, is fundamental.

Other vaccines

All of the immunizations mentioned thus far are vaccines administered by injection.

A vaccine administered orally is the **polio** immunization. It is kept frozen until just before it is to be administered. It should never be refrozen. As you can see in the immunization schedule, this vaccine is administered to infants and young children. It is made from the pathogenic microorganisms and is **attenuated**, which makes it less virulent. The disease it protects against is known as infantile paralysis, or poliomyelitis, which is the acute infection and inflammation of the gray matter of the spinal cord caused by the polio virus. Children are more susceptible than adults. It is transmitted by the oral-fecal route. Incubation is usually from 7 to 12 days (and can be from 5 to 35).

The symptoms begin with fever, malaise, headache, nausea and vomiting, slight abdominal discomfort, and general paralysis (if respiratory muscles are involved, it is likely to be fatal). Treatment consists of relieving symptoms, bed rest, mild analgesics, sedatives as necessary, fluid and salt balance, laxatives or enemas as necessary to relieve constipation, oxygen, respirator, and tracheostomy if necessary. Physical and occupational therapy are needed as the patient recovers. In the United States, there have been cases of polio reported in children whose immunization records have not been completed or have not included the polio vaccine. Generally, schools require that children are immunized against the communicable diseases (listed in the schedule in Table 18–7) before they are admitted to school. Local health services offer free immunizations to the public to those who cannot afford the cost. Direct patients to their municipal officials for a schedule and further information regarding this service. Remind parents of the importance of keeping their immunization appointments as recommended by the CDC to protect their children from unnecessary childhood diseases and to prevent the return of epidemics.

Remind patients to protect themselves and their families against all of these diseases to prevent the return of epidemics. There are other diseases, such as **cholera** and **typhoid**, for which there are vaccines to prevent dangerous epidemics that have the potential to wipe out entire populations. Many underdeveloped countries have such situations even today. Immunizations other than what appears in the schedule in Table 18–7 are not recommended on a routine basis in most Western countries. It has been said that an ounce of prevention is worth a pound of cure. The prevention of disease often means saving lives and, in many cases, also improving the quality of life. Health officials advise immunizations as determined necessary. Check with your family physician to keep abreast with new recommendations of the CDC regarding vaccines. Refer to Table 18–8 for vaccines listed that are recommended for adults. Travel to some countries requires immunizations against particular diseases before entry is permitted. To provide up-to-date immunization information

TABLE 18-8

SUMMARY OF ADOLESCENT/ADULT IMMUNIZATION RECOMMENDATIONS

Agent	Indications	Primary Schedule	Contraindications	Comments
Tetanus and diphtheria toxoids combined (Td)	All adults All adolescents should be assessed at 11–12 or 14–16 years of age and immunized if no dose was received during the previous five years.	Two doses 4–8 weeks apart, third dose 6–12 months after the second. No need to repeat doses if the schedule is interrupted. Dose: 0.5 mL intramuscular (IM) Booster: At 10-year intervals throughout life.	Neurologic or severe hypersensitivity reaction to prior dose.	WOUND MANAGEMENT: Patients with three or more previous tetanus toxoid doses: (a) give Td for clean, minor wounds only if more than 10 years since last dose; (b) for other wounds, give Td if over five years since last dose. Patients with less than three or unknown number of prior tetanus toxoid doses; given Td for clean, minor wounds and Td and TIG (Tetanus Immune Globulin) for other wounds.
Influenza vaccine	a. Adults 50 years of age and older. b. Residents of nursing homes or other facilities for patients with chronic medical conditions. c. Persons greater than or equal to six months of age with chronic cardiovascular or pulmonary disorders, including asthma. d. Persons greater than or equal to six months of age with chronic metabolic diseases (including diabetes), renal dysfunction, hemoglobinopathies, immunosuppressive or immunodeficiency disorders. e. Women in their second or third trimester of pregnancy during influenza season. f. Persons six mo.–18 years of age receiving long-term aspirin therapy. g. Groups, including household members and care givers, who can infect high risk persons.	Dose: 0.5 mL intramuscular (IM) Given annually each fall and winter.	Anaphylactic allergy to eggs. Acute febrile illness.	Depending on season and destination, persons traveling to foreign countries should consider vaccination. Any person greater than or equal to six months of age who wishes to reduce the likelihood of becoming ill with influenza should be vaccinated. Avoiding subsequent vaccination of persons known to have developed GBS within six weeks of a previous vaccination seems prudent; however, for most persons with a GBS history who are at high risk for severe complications, many experts believe the established benefits of vaccination justify yearly vaccination.

(continues)

Adapted from the recommendations of the Advisory Committee on Immunization Practices (ACIP). Foreign travel and less commonly used vaccines such as typhoid, rabies, and meningococcal are not included.

TABLE 18-8 *(continued)*

SUMMARY OF ADOLESCENT/ADULT IMMUNIZATION RECOMMENDATIONS—continued

Agent	Indications	Primary Schedule	Contraindications	Comments
Pneumococcal polysaccharide vaccine (PPV)	a. Adults 65 years of age and older. b. Persons greater than or equal to two years with chronic cardiovascular or pulmonary disorders including congestive heart failure, diabetes mellitus, chronic liver disease, alcoholism, CSF leaks, cardiomyopathy, COPD or emphysema. c. Persons greater than or equal to two years with splenic dysfunction or asplenia, hematologic malignancy, multiple myeloma, renal failure, organ transplantation or immunosuppressive conditions, including HIV infection. d. Alaskan Natives and certain American Indian populations.	One dose for most people* Dose: 0.5 mL intramuscular (IM) or subcutaneous (SC) *Persons vaccinated prior to age 65 should be vaccinated at age 65 if five or more years have passed since the first dose. For all persons with functional or anatomic asplenia, transplant patients, patients with chronic kidney disease, immunosuppressed or immunodeficient persons, and others at highest risk of fatal infection, a second dose should be given—at least five years after first dose.	The safety of PPV during the first trimester of pregnancy has not been evaluated. The manufacturer's package insert should be reviewed for additional information.	If elective splenectomy or immunosuppressive therapy is planned, give vaccine two weeks ahead, if possible. When indicated, vaccine should be administered to patients with unknown vaccination status. All residents of nursing homes and other long-term care facilities should have their vaccination status assessed and documented.
Measles and mumps vaccines**	a. Adults born after 1956 without written documentation of immunization on or after the first birthday. b. Health care personnel born after 1956 who are at risk of exposure to patients with measles should have documentation of two doses of vaccine on or after the first birthday or of measles seropositivity. c. HIV-infected persons without severe immunosuppression. d. Travelers to foreign countries. e. Persons entering postsecondary educational institutions (e.g., college).	At least one dose. (Two doses of measles-containing vaccine if in college, in health care profession or traveling to a foreign country with second dose at least one month after the first). Dose: 0.5 mL subcutaneous (SC)	a. Immunosuppressive therapy or immunodeficiency including HIV-infected persons with severe immunosuppression. b. Anaphylactic allergy to neomycin. c. Pregnancy. d. Immune globulin preparation or blood/blood product received in preceding 3–11 months. e. Untreated, active TB.	Women should be asked if they are pregnant before receiving vaccine, and advised to avoid pregnancy for 30 days after immunization.
Rubella vaccine**	a. Persons (especially women) without written documentation of immunization on or after the first birthday or of seropositivity. b. Health care personnel who are at risk of exposure to patients with rubella and who may have contact with pregnant patients should have at least one dose.	One dose. Dose: 0.5 mL subcutaneous (SC)	Same as for measles and mumps vaccines.	Women should be asked if they are pregnant before receiving vaccine, and advised to avoid pregnancy for three months after immunization.

**These vaccines can be given in the combined form measles-mumps-rubella (MMR). Persons already immune to one or more components can still receive MMR.

(continues)

TABLE 18-8 *(continued)*

SUMMARY OF ADOLESCENT/ADULT IMMUNIZATION RECOMMENDATIONS—continued

Agent	Indications	Primary Schedule	Contraindications	Comments
Hepatitis B vaccine	a. Persons with occupational risk of exposure to blood or blood-contaminated body fluids. b. Clients and staff of institutions for the developmentally disabled. c. Hemodialysis patients. d. Recipients of clotting-factor concentrates. e. Household contacts and sex partners of those chronically infected with HBV. f. Family members of adoptees from countries where HBV infection is endemic, if adoptees are HBsAg+. g. Certain international travelers. h. Injecting drug users. i. Men who have sex with men. j. Heterosexual men and women with multiple sex partners or recent episode of a sexually transmitted disease. k. Inmates of long-term correctional facilities. l. All unvaccinated adolescents.	Three doses: second dose one to two months after the first, third dose four to six months after the first. No need to start series over if schedule interrupted. Can start series with one manufacturer's vaccine and finish with another. Dose (<u>Adult</u>): intramuscular (IM) Recombivax HB®: 10 μg/1.0 mL (green cap) Engerix-B®: 20 μg/1.0mL (orange cap) Dose (<u>Adolescents 11–19 years</u>): intramuscular (IM) Recombivax HB®: 5 μg/0.5 mL (yellow cap) Engerix-B®:10 μg/0.5mL (light blue cap) Booster: None presently recommended.	Anaphylactic allergy to yeast.	a. Persons with serologic markers of prior or continuing hepatitis B virus infection do not need immunization. b. For hemodialysis patients and other immunodeficient or immunosuppressed patients, vaccine dosage is doubled or special preparation is used. c. *Pregnant women should be sero-screened for HBsAg and, if positive, their infants should be given post-exposure prophylaxis beginning at birth.* d. Post-exposure prophylaxis: consult ACIP recommendations, or state or local immunization program.
Poliovirus vaccine: IPV—inactivated vaccine; OPV—oral (live) vaccine	Routine vaccination of those greater than or equal to 18 years of age residing in the U.S. is not necessary. Vaccination is recommended for the following high-risk adults: a. Travelers to areas or countries where poliomyelitis is epidemic or endemic. b. Members of communities or specific population groups with disease caused by wild polioviruses. c. Laboratory workers who handle specimens that may contain polioviruses. d. Health care workers who have close contact with patients who may be excreting wild polioviruses. e. Unvaccinated adults whose children will be receiving OPV.	Unimmunized adolescents/adults: IPV is recommended—two doses at 4–8 week intervals, third dose 6–12 months after second (can be as soon as 2 months). Dose: 0.5 mL subcutaneous (SC) or intramuscular (IM). Partially immunized adolescents/adults: Complete primary series with IPV (IPV schedule shown above). OPV is no longer recommended for use in the United States.	<u>IPV</u>: Anaphylactic reaction following previous dose or to streptomycin, polymyxin B, or neomycin.	In instances of potential exposure to wild poliovirus, adults who have had a primary series of OPV or IPV may be given one more dose of IPV. Although no adverse effects have been documented, vaccination of pregnant women should be avoided. However, if immediate protection is required, pregnant women may be given IPV in accordance with the recommended schedule for adults.

(continues)

TABLE 18-8 *(continued)*

SUMMARY OF ADOLESCENT/ADULT IMMUNIZATION RECOMMENDATIONS—continued				
Agent	Indications	Primary Schedule	Contraindications	Comments
Varicella vaccine	a. Persons of any age without a reliable history of varicella disease or vaccination, or who are seronegative for varicella. b. Susceptible adolescents and adults living in households with children. c. All susceptible health care workers. d. Susceptible family contacts of immunocompromised persons. e. Susceptible persons in the following groups who are at high risk for exposure: - persons who live or work in environments in which transmission of varicella is likely (e.g., teachers of young children, day care employees, residents and staff in institutional settings) or can occur (e.g., college students, inmates and staff of correctional institutions, military personnel) - nonpregnant women of childbearing age - international travelers	For persons less than 13 years of age, one dose. For persons 13 years of age and older, two doses separated by four to eight weeks. If greater than eight weeks elapse following the first dose, the second dose can be administered without restarting the schedule. Dose: 0.5 mL subcutaneous (SC)	a. Anaphylactic allergy to gelatin or neomycin. b. Untreated, active TB. c. Immunosuppressive therapy or immunodeficiency (including HIV infection). d. Family history of congenital or hereditary immunodeficiency in first-degree relatives, unless the immune competence of the recipient has been clinically substantiated or verified by a laboratory. e. Immune globulin preparation or blood/blood product received in preceding five months. f. Pregnancy.	Women should be asked if they are pregnant before receiving varicella vaccine, and advised to avoid pregnancy for one month following each dose of vaccine.
Hepatitis A vaccine	a. Persons traveling to or working in countries with high or intermediate endemicity of infection. b. Men who have sex with men. c. Injecting and non-injecting illegal drug users. d. Persons who work with HAV-infected primates or with HAV in a research laboratory setting. e. Persons with chronic liver disease. f. Persons with clotting factor disorders. g. Consider food handlers, where determined to be cost-effective by health authorities or employers.	HAVRIX®: Two doses, separated by 6–12 months. Adults (18 years of age and older)—Dose: 1.0 mL intramuscular (IM); Persons 2–17 years of age: Dose: 0.5 mL (IM). VAQTA®: Adults (18 years of age and older): Two doses, separated by 6 months. Dose: 1.0 mL intramuscular (IM); Persons 2–17 years of age: Two doses, separated by 6–18 months; Dose: 0.5 mL (IM)	A history of hypersensitivity to alum or the preservative 2-phenoxyethanol	The safety of hepatitis A vaccine during pregnancy has not been determined, though the theoretical risk to the developing fetus is expected to be low. The risk of vaccination should be weighed against the risk of hepatitis A in women who may be at high risk of exposure to HAV.

by country, computer databases have been established. One such program containing health information for travelers in over 200 countries is available from Immunization Alert, Storrs, Connecticut. Current information may also be obtained at local and state health departments. You should provide the patient with a card or booklet to accurately record each immunization and the month, day, and year for each (Figure 18–26). Record each vaccine on the patient's chart, as was discussed earlier in this chapter. Any reaction to the vaccine, no matter how slight, must also be recorded on the patient's chart. Remind patients to make appointments and carry the immunization record (or a copy) with them at all times.

Because of the continuing research and advances in the production of vaccinations against many infectious diseases, these illnesses are rarely experienced in developed countries, except in severely poverty-stricken areas. Unfortunately, however, third world nations are still constantly fighting a losing battle against communicable diseases. Deaths from them are staggering in number. This is mainly caused by inadequate education, poor living conditions, and lack of funding for vaccines.

ACHIEVE UNIT OBJECTIVES

Complete Chapter 18, Unit 3, in the workbook to help you obtain competency of this subject matter.

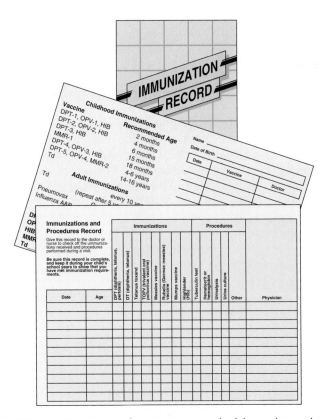

FIGURE 18–26 Sample immunization schedules and record booklets

RELATING TO ABHES

Chapter 18 discussed commonly prescribed medications, pharmaceutical references, drug classifications, and the prescribing, recording, storing, and administering of various forms of medications. It also discussed the vaccines used for and the scheduling of immunizations. This content relates to the ABHES accreditation requirements of *Occupational math and metric conversions (drug calculations)*, *Use of PDR's and medication books, Common abbreviations used in prescription writing, Legal aspects of writing prescriptions, FDC and state laws,* and *Medications prescribed for the treatment of illness and disease based on a systems method* within the content area of **Pharmacology**; and *Basic clinical skills (e.g., vital signs)*, and *Injections (dosage calculations)* within the content area of **Medical Office Clinical Procedures.**

A CAAHEP CONNECTION

Informing patients about medications, injections, immunizations, and the risks will help to settle their anxiety. Explaining the informed consent forms for vaccines and securing the caregiver's signature is necessary for the immunization to be given to a minor. Because patients may ask questions regarding medications and injections, the medical assistant should be able to answer intelligently regarding immunizations, the diseases they prevent, and the methods and schedules for their administration. Patients appreciate empathy and understanding because the injection method of medication administration is a real fear and concern to them. Developing good communication skills and learning about basic psychology will prepare the medical assistant to better serve patients and their needs.

Medical-Legal-Ethical Scenario

Darlene was the medical assistant assigned patients in the clinical area for the day. She was having a busy morning with many infants and children having exams and getting their immunizations. When Mrs. Jackson brought her baby, Kenya, for her four-month check up, she told Darlene that the baby had been coughing a lot. Darlene, wanting to go to lunch as soon as Kenya was ready for the doctor, said that the cough was probably from the dust in the house. Darlene weighed and measured Kenya and plotted the measurements on the growth graph. Darlene checked the immunization schedule and got out the DTP, Hib, and the OPV. Darlene gave the immunizations to the baby and told Mrs. Jackson that Dr. Lane would be in soon. Then she left for lunch. As Dr. Lane examined the baby, she noticed that Kenya felt warm. When she took an axillary temperature and it read 103.2°F, she explained to Mrs. Jackson that the baby was sick. She would have to bring Kenya back for her immunizations after she finished the antibiotic she was prescribing for bronchitis. Mrs. Jackson told the doctor that Darlene had already given them to Kenya just before she left the office to go to lunch. Darlene had not even recorded that she gave the immunizations. Dr. Lane looked quite concerned.

CRITICAL THINKING CHALLENGE

1. What happened here?
2. What do you suppose will happen when Darlene returns from lunch?
3. What is Darlene guilty of?
4. Will Darlene be fired for doing what she did?
5. What do you think Mrs. Jackson will do?
6. Is Mrs. Jackson at fault for this situation? Why or why not?
7. Who is responsible if the baby has a serious reaction?
8. Do you think Darlene noticed the baby's fever?
9. What would you do about this situation?

RESOURCES

Heller M. and Krebs C. (1997). Clinical handbook for health care professionals. Clifton Park, NY: Delmar Learning.

Miller, B.F., and Keane, C.B. (1997). Encyclopedia and dictionary of medicine, nursing, and allied health (6th ed.). Philadelphia, W.B. Saunders.

Physician's desk reference (56th ed.). (2002). Montrale, NJ: Medical Economics.

Physician's desk reference for nonprescription drugs and dietary supplements (22nd ed.) (2001). Oradell, NJ: Medical Economics.

Protecting yourself against prescription errors (1996, January). *Health After 50.*

Venes, T. (2001). Taber's cyclopedic medical dictionary (19th ed.) (2001). Philadelphia, PA: F.A. Davis.

WEB LINKS

http://www.cdc/gov/ **(The Centers for Disease Control and Prevention National Immunization Program website)**

Provides information on the importance of vaccines.

Emergencies, Acute Illness, Accidents, and Recovery

Individuals working in health care can expect to be confronted with emergency or accident situations. Patients may be brought into the physician's office, you may be witness to an incident in your community or neighborhood, and almost certainly you will be responding to phone calls concerning injuries or sudden illness. When anything happens within your family or immediate neighborhood, your relatives and neighbors will probably expect you to be the "resident authority" just because you are a medical assistant. It is important for you to acquire first aid skills and have a working knowledge of appropriate actions to take in common accident or illness situations. It is your responsibility to maintain current certification to provide the Basic Life Support Measures involving **obstructed** airway, resuscitation, or CPR.

If you should happen upon a situation where an unknown person has become ill or lost **consciousness**, check for a universal emergency medical identification symbol (Figure 19–1). This symbol was designed by the American Medical Association as a means for individuals with certain medical conditions to alert health care workers of their conditions when they are unable to. The tag is worn around the neck, wrist, or ankle. Some may identify the particular problem the person has, others may not. If a tag is found, the person should have an information card on his person, usually inside a wallet, which identifies his condition and provides some directions to follow (Figure 19–2). All patients who have conditions that could have emergency episodes, such as heart conditions, diabetes, epilepsy, allergies, or a laryngectomy, should be encouraged to wear a **universal emergency medical identification** tag.

This chapter deals with emergency care in cases of acute illness, accident, or injury. It also discusses care within the physician's office and first aid outside the health care setting. The last unit covers the use of exercise, supporting devices, and equipment to assist an individual to recover and obtain mobility following illness or injury. This information will be of value not only in your professional life but also in your personal life.

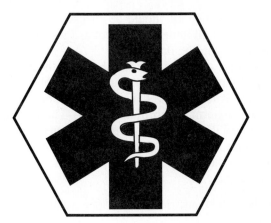

FIGURE 19–1 Universal emergency medical identification symbol

---

EMERGENCY

I am a laryngectomee (no vocal cords).

I breathe through an opening in the neck, not through the nose or mouth.

If artificial respiration is necessary:

1. Keep neck opening clear of all matter.
2. Don't twist head sidewise.
3. Apply oxygen only to neck opening.
4. Don't throw water on head.
5. Mouth-to-opening breathing is effective.

FIGURE 19–2 Emergency medical information card

UNIT 1

Managing Emergencies in the Medical Office

OBJECTIVES

Upon completion of the unit, meet the following performance objectives by verifying knowledge of the facts and principles presented through oral and written communication at a level deemed competent.

1. Spell and define, using the glossary at the back of the text, all the **Words to Know** in this unit.
2. Define a medical emergency.
3. Explain the purpose of the universal emergency medical identification symbol.
4. List 11 items that might be found in an emergency kit.
5. Identify nine items of information usually obtained on an incident report.
6. Explain the purpose of an AED and its three capabilities.

AREAS OF COMPETENCE (AAMA)

This unit addresses content within the specific competency areas of *Fundamental principles, Patient care, Professionalism,* and *Legal concepts,* as identified in the Medical Assistant Role Delineation Study. Refer to Appendix A for a detailed listing of the areas.

WORDS TO KNOW

bandage	ipecac
certification	obstructed
consciousness	post mortem
coroner	resuscitation
emergency	trauma
emetic	universal emergency
incident report	medical identification

EMERGENCY PROVISIONS IN THE MEDICAL OFFICE

A physician's office must always be ready to react to an **emergency** situation. A medical emergency is any situation in which an individual suddenly becomes ill or has an injury or circumstances calling for decided action. This can involve a patient already in the office or one that is brought in already experiencing problems. A patient receiving a medication or injection may have a severe reaction and quickly present an emergency. Someone may be injured just outside the office and brought in for treatment. Patients may bring in very ill or injured family members. Knowing how to respond and how to assist the physician in treating the individual is very important. Swift and appropriate action can affect the outcome of the situation. Remember, you will not be expected to perform at the level of **trauma** or trained medical emergency personnel, only to a standard of care equal to that of any person with like training and experience.

Emergency Kits

As part of your preparation for emergency care, you and your employer should make a list of the supplies and equipment that are necessary to handle any emergency that might come under your care. These items should be collected and set aside in a special place where they will always be ready for use. This could be in the form of a small suitcase or a cart. All office employees should know this location and how to use the materials. Perhaps the

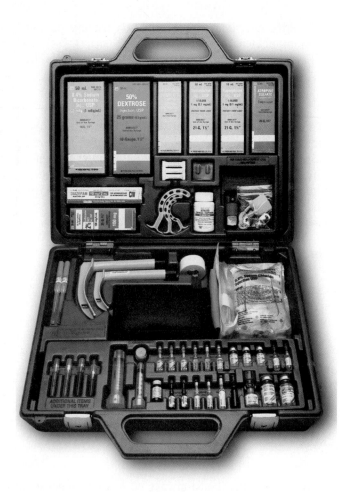

FIGURE 19–3 Prepared emergency kit (Courtesy of Banyan International Corporation.)

easiest way to assemble a kit would be to purchase a prepared one that is available from most medical supply dealers (Figure 19–3).

Equipment and supplies in an emergency kit would include at least the following:

- alcohol wipes
- stethoscope
- penlight
- easily activated hot and cold packs
- disposable syringes with adrenaline, narcotics, and antihistamines
- **ipecac**, (an effective **emetic** to achieve vomiting)
- oxygen tank with a mask
- aromatic spirits of ammonia
- sterile dressings
- paper and pen
- airways of differing sizes
- blood pressure cuff
- **bandage** material
- adhesive tape
- bandage scissors
- glucose to treat hypoglycemia

The emergency kit should be checked occasionally to be certain that all items are present and no dated material is past its expiration date.

In addition to the kit or a "crash cart," offices should be equipped with a defibrillation unit to be able to respond to cardiac emergencies. One type of defibrillator is the automated external defibrillator (AED). These are used in addition to CPR if the heart is in fibrillation or arrest. This type of unit is easily operated and can be used in the office even in the absence of the physician. The unit is computerized and can:

- analyze the heart rhythm of a person in fibrillation or arrest
- recognize a shockable rhythm
- advise the operator through lights and voice prompts if shock is indicated
- with built-in diagnostic capability, permit life saving intervention without the operator needing to evaluate the situation or interpret an ECG. (Fibrillation was discussed in Chapter 11, Unit 8, the circulatory system.)

DOCUMENTING EMERGENCY PROCEDURES

Every office must identify who is responsible for recording the detailed information regarding an emergency situation and its handling. This report is called either an accident or an **incident report**. Remember, this becomes part of a patient's record, and all patient records can be used in court, so the form must be complete and accurate.

The usual information necessary on an incident report is:

- full name of injured or ill party
- date and time of accident or emergency
- address and phone number of injured party
- notation as to whether the individual is a patient, visitor, or office staff member
- location of where incident occurred
- name, address, and signature of any witness(es) to the accident
- detailed description of the incident and conditions surrounding it
- description of action taken, medications given, physician who examined the injured person, and the disposition of the patient
- signature of person preparing report, with date and time of day

A printed form should be available with the above information. It should be approved by both the physician and the liability insurance company. After the incident report is completed, it should be handled as determined in the office policy manual. The office legal council should advise about whether to place the form in the patient's chart or place it in a special incident file. Emergencies, sudden illness, and accidents can also occur among personnel while they are working in the medical office. It is

---

A CAAHEP CONNECTION

This content on preparing for and responding to emergencies addresses the curriculum standard requirement to deal with clinical procedures as they relate to *Medical emergencies.* It also involves dealing with incident documentation, *Risk management* and the dynamics of the workplace in responding to emergencies of patients, the public, or office personnel.

---

equally important to document the circumstances surrounding the incident. Persons experiencing at-work injuries may be eligible for benefits under Worker's Compensation if the injury occurred while performing job responsibilities. Employee forms may be placed in the employee's personal file and in the office personnel file.

Office Policy Manual

The office policy manual should have guidelines to follow when dealing with emergencies. An emergency plan with assigned responsibilities should be developed and made known to each employee (such as who should call 911). All staff members should be capable of administering first aid and cardiopulmonary **resuscitation** (CPR) and hold current **certification** in CPR. The goal for emergency care in an office is to get the patient stable to release them to her family or send her to a hospital for further treatment.

EMERGENCY SERVICES

When severe injury or sudden critical illness occurs, a patient should have the advantages of trauma and critical care facilities as soon as possible. Often, the first hour is so important that it directly correlates with prognosis and the possibility of recovery. Major urban areas have emergency medical services (EMS) available, usually provided by the police and/or fire departments. These services can be activated by telephoning 911. Outside metropolitan areas, these systems may not be available, and the 911 service may not be in place. Smaller cities or towns often contract with private ambulance services who employ trained personnel to provide emergency coverage. In rural areas, the only assistance may come from volunteer firefighters, local law enforcement officers, or the state police. Of course, their response time is much longer because they have to cover large areas.

You should know how to summon assistance in your area. If not, contact providers to identify the appropriate service and determine what help is available and the quickest way to obtain emergency assistance. A list of all emergency numbers should be posted by every phone in the physician's office. All office staff should be aware of this information. (This is helpful at home as well.) When an actual emergency occurs, an individual tends to become "absorbed" in the situation and often experiences difficulty finding numbers in a phone directory. Posted information also saves critical time. Some offices may place a card containing this information with the emergency kit. In a situation where the physician and the medical assistant are both involved in administering first aid and there are no other office personnel present, the card can be handed to a family member to summon help.

If life-saving procedures are not effective and the patient dies in the office, arrange for the body to be removed through a back door and not the reception room entrance. If the physician has not been in attendance, it may be necessary to notify the local law enforcement agency who will in turn notify the **coroner** to pick up the body for **post mortem** examination. Regulations differ and will be determined by local statutes. Normally, if the patient has not been examined by a physician within a fairly recent time frame, an autopsy is required to establish the cause of death to be recorded on the death certificate. If the individual was a patient, be certain the specifics regarding the death are recorded on the chart and notations made upon other records so that no inappropriate correspondence is sent to the residence.

ACHIEVE UNIT OBJECTIVES

Complete Chapter 19, Unit 1, in the workbook to help you obtain competency of this subject matter.

UNIT 2

Acute Illness

OBJECTIVES

Upon completion of the unit, meet the following performance objectives by verifying knowledge of the facts and principles presented through oral and written communication at a level deemed competent.

1. Spell and define, using the glossary at the back of the text, all the **Words to Know** in this unit.
2. Identify seven descriptive terms that describe the severity or onset of a disease or disorder.
3. List, in order of occurrence, the "chain of events" that might happen with a seizure.
4. Compare 10 symptoms of diabetic coma to insulin reaction.
5. Identify nine symptoms of a heart attack.
6. Differentiate the symptoms of heat stroke and heat exhaustion.

7. Name six symptoms of frostbite.
8. Identify the distinguishing characteristics of capillary, vein, and arterial bleeding.
9. List eight symptoms of internal bleeding.
10. Discuss seven instances when respiratory emergencies may develop.
11. List six symptoms of shock.
12. Identify eight signs of possible stroke.
13. Demonstrate mouth-to-mouth resuscitation.
14. Demonstrate cardiopulmonary resuscitation for adults and infants.

AREAS OF COMPETENCE (AAMA)

This unit addresses content with the specific competency areas of *Fundamental principles, Patient care, Professionalism, Communication skills,* and *Legal concepts,* as identified in the Medical Assistant Role Delineation Study. Refer to Appendix A for a detailed listing of the areas.

■ WORDS TO KNOW

acute	ingested
ammonia	insidious
aspiration	insulin shock
cessation	intubation
chronic	poison
diabetic coma	prophylactic
diaphoresis	resuscitation
exhaustion	seizure
flushed	syncope
hyperglycemia	urgent
hypoglycemia	

DISTINGUISHING SEVERITY OF ILLNESS

Several terms are used to describe the severity and length of time for onset of disease or illness. Some of the more common terms and explanations are:

- **Chronic**—long, drawn out, not acute. Some diseases have a slow chronic phase but can quickly change into acute episode.
- **Insidious**—hidden, not apparent, treacherous. Often disease conditions have a slow, hidden beginning, then quickly develop symptoms.
- **Urgent**—a situation requiring intervention as soon as can be arranged. This term may be applied to the need for care when experiencing a blocked ureter by a kidney stone.
- **Sudden**—occurring quickly and without warning. Onset of headaches or allergies may be sudden.
- **Acute**—having a rapid onset, severe symptoms, and short course. Heart attacks are an example of acute illnesses.

- **Severe**—extensive, advanced. When injuries are severe, it usually implies multiple sites and requires considerable medical attention. The term is also applied to an illness that requires aggressive action and is potentially irreversible.
- **Life threatening**—may cause death. Extensive trauma and massive circulatory or respiratory involvement that may be beyond medical intervention are deemed life threatening.

Almost any injury or illness could be manifest in most of the above classifications. Consider a cut that is bleeding: it could be oozing, a slow flow, a pulsating flow, or a hemorrhage that is life threatening. In this unit, the following conditions are examples of disorders, diseases, or situations that may present emergency events if in an acute phase.

Convulsions (Seizures)

Seizures may occur when the patient has high body temperature, head injuries, brain disease, or a brain disorder, such as epilepsy. A **seizure** is a severe involuntary contraction of muscles that first causes the patient to become rigid and then to have uncontrollable movements. The patient becomes unconscious and may be injured during the seizure. The face and lips may become cyanotic, and the patient may stop breathing. He may also lose bladder and bowel control and bite the tongue. When the seizure has stopped, the patient may be confused and complain of headache and **exhaustion**.

During the convulsive phase, do not restrain movement. Move objects out of the way that might cause injury. Do not force any object between the patient's teeth or it could cause vomiting, **aspiration**, or spasm of the larynx. Following the convulsion, turn the head to the side to prevent choking from profuse salivation. Allow the patient to rest or sleep after the seizure is over. Artificial respiration should be given if necessary. Provide emotional support as the patient regains composure because this situation can cause the person to feel embarrassed.

Diabetic Coma (Hyperglycemia) and Insulin Shock (Hypoglycemia)

Diabetic patients may present emergency situations by going into **diabetic coma** or **insulin shock** (Table 19–1). A diabetic coma (**hyperglycemia**) is caused by an increased amount of sugar in the blood. This may be caused by consuming excess carbohydrates, an infection, fever, emotional stress, or failing to take adequate insulin. The patient may complain of confusion, dizziness, weakness, or nausea. Vomiting may occur. Respiration may be rapid and deep. The skin may be dry and **flushed**. The patient's breath has a sweet or fruity odor, which may be evident some distance away. The patient can lapse into unconsciousness and may die if not treated quickly. The patient

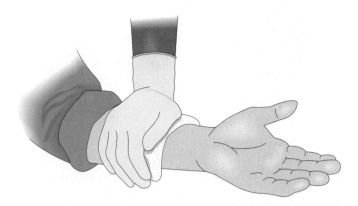

FIGURE 19–4 Direct pressure

times, especially with arterial bleeding, this is not sufficient, and pressure must be exerted at the pressure point proximal (Figure 19–5), to the wound to stop the flow of blood to the area. Any bleeding from capillary damage will produce a steady ooze from the wound area. This type of bleeding will often clot without first aid measures being taken.

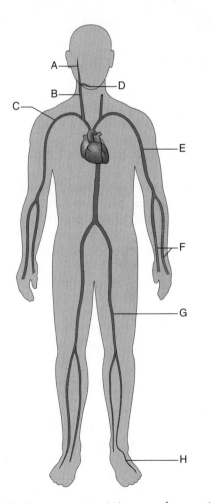

FIGURE 19–5 Pressure points: (A) temporal artery, (B) carotid artery, (C) subclavian artery, (D) facial artery, (E) brachial artery, (F) radial artery, (G) femoral artery, (H) dorsalis pedis

Internal bleeding causes symptoms similar to those of shock. The patient may have a rapid weak pulse, shallow breathing, cold clammy skin, dilated pupils, dizziness, faintness, thirst, restlessness, and a feeling of anxiety. Internal hemorrhage will need to be controlled by surgery. The patient must be kept in a recumbent position with strictly limited movement until the surgery can be performed.

Internal bleeding may be difficult to detect unless it produces symptoms or external signs. The patient who coughs up bright red blood may have a lung hemorrhage. Vomiting bright red blood could mean an ulcer has started bleeding. If the patient is vomiting what looks like coffee grounds, it could indicate chronic slow bleeding of the stomach. If the patient notices coal-black stools, there is probably a loss of blood in the intestines. If the patient has bright red rectal bleeding, it is likely to be from a lesion in the rectum or lower colon. A patient with severe abdominal pain from trauma may have internal bleeding from a ruptured organ, such as a kidney, liver, or spleen. Internal bleeding that causes symptoms of shock and produces pain will probably require surgical intervention to correct. Slow bleeding, once the cause has been determined, may be treated with medication and if intestinal, by altering the diet to allow the area to heal. The hemorrhage that occurs with the rupture of various types of aneurysms was discussed in Chapter 11, Unit 8, The Circulatory System.

Epistaxis (nosebleed) may be the result of excessively dry air over a prolonged period, hypertension, injury, or simply blowing the nose too hard (see Chapter 11, Unit 3). First aid for epistaxis is to elevate the head and pinch the nostrils closed for at least six minutes. Keep the patient in a sitting position with the head tilted forward so that the blood will not trickle down the throat unseen. The use of a cold compress over the nasal area or on the back of the neck may be helpful. A piece of gauze may be placed between the lips and gums with pressure against this area for several minutes. Specially treated gauze is best to use for nasal packing because it is less difficult to remove. A physician should be consulted if bleeding is not easily controlled. Sometimes the addition of humidity to the air will relieve the patient who has recurrent epistaxis.

If a pregnant patient experiences vaginal bleeding, it is necessary to determine the kind of flow. If there is heavy bleeding, the patient should lie down immediately with feet elevated, and emergency medical services should be called. If there has been a discharge of clots or tissue substance, this should be taken to the hospital for analysis. Your employer will let you know how these emergencies should be handled.

Poisoning

Skills Menu:
- Accidental Poisoning

Poison can be **ingested**, absorbed, inhaled, injected, and acquired from bites and stings.

If someone calls regarding a possible ingestion of **poison**, you should always ask what was taken, how much was taken, and the time it was taken. You should learn the location and the telephone number of the local Poison Control Center so that you can direct callers to the best source of help. If an antidote is on the label of the poison, the patient should be given the antidote only after approval or order of the Poison Control Center or the physician. It is usually safe to dilute the poison with water or milk. If the substance is one that should be removed after diluting, you may use Ipecac, large amounts of warm water, or activated charcoal to induce vomiting. The area at the back of the tongue known as the gag reflex may be touched to cause vomiting. If table salt is available, you may add a small amount to warm water to induce vomiting. The patient should not be encouraged to vomit if a strong alkali, acid, or petroleum product has been ingested.

For poisoning from plants such as mushrooms or from bacterial-contaminated shellfish, the emergency treatment is to induce vomiting and then keep the patient as quiet as possible.

Poisoning by inhalation may be caused by the use of cleaning fluids and sprays in a poorly ventilated area. Carbon monoxide poisoning may be caused by a faulty exhaust system in an automobile or home heating system. First aid for inhalation poisoning is pulmonary resuscitation, 100% oxygen, and immediate care in a hospital.

Poisoning by injection is usually the result of drug abuse. The patient may exhibit symptoms from confusion to excitement to hallucinations to convulsions. These patients need hospitalization for proper treatment.

RESPIRATORY EMERGENCIES

Obstructive Airway

C Skills Menu:
  ■ Heimlich Maneuver

One of the most common medical emergencies is an obstructed airway. The most usual cause in adults is food that is aspirated while eating. This occurs when partially chewed food is sucked into the trachea when talking, laughing, or coughing while eating. Children, on the other hand, can get toys, toy parts, buttons, or candy and a variety of other objects caught in their throats and obstruct their airway. Pieces of food are also a problem for children. Most everyone is familiar with the dangers of filmy plastic sacks and bags because of all the warning labels, but one of the most common airway obstructers is the latex balloon. Safety authorities believe no young child should have a balloon unless it is made of mylar. Children ages four to eight require supervision if playing with or trying to inflate latex balloons.

The obstruction, if complete, must be cleared away immediately because brain damage may result in about four minutes from lack of oxygen. A person who is choking usually places her hand at her throat (the universal dis-

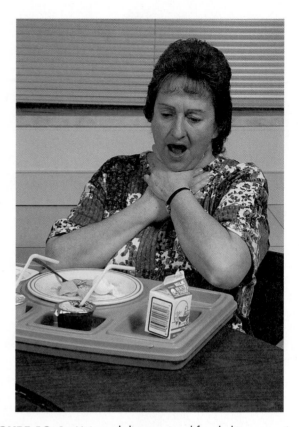

FIGURE 19-6 Universal distress signal for choking: grasping neck between thumb and index finger

tress signal) (Figure 19–6). The individual may not be able to cough or speak but simply falls from the chair if nothing is done.

The method used to relieve an obstructed airway is a manual thrust, or subdiaphragmatic abdominal thrust also known as the Heimlich maneuver. While standing behind the victim, reach around the waist. Clench one hand to make a fist, and grasp your fist with the other hand. Place the thumb side of the fist against the midline of the victim's abdomen between the waist and the rib cage (Figure 19–7). Thrust fist inward and upward in quick, firm movements to move air out of the lungs with enough force to dislodge the obstruction. The abdominal thrust may be performed on an unconscious supine victim by sitting astride the victim's thighs. With fingers pointed towards the head, place the heel of one hand flat on the victim's abdomen, slightly above the navel. Place your other hand in a like position over the first. With the elbows straight, press inward and upward with quick thrusts to dislodge the obstruction. A choking victim who is alone may use the abdominal thrust with the fist or may thrust against a chair back or any hard object of appropriate height.

If a patient is in the advanced stage of pregnancy or is very obese, abdominal thrusting will not be possible. A chest thrust may be used to dislodge the material. If standing, from the back, place arms around the victim di-

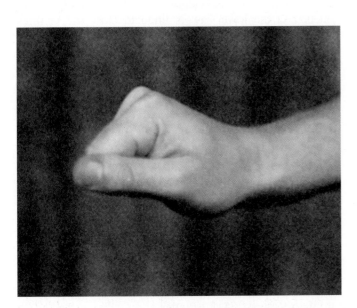 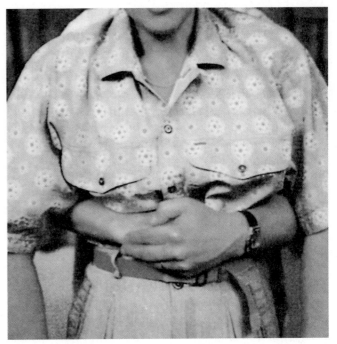

FIGURE 19–7 Hand placement for abdominal thrust

rectly under their axillae. Using the abdominal clenched fist technique, place the thumb over the sternum, place your other hand over the fist, and give firm thrusts, pulling straight back toward yourself. Chest thrusts to the supine victim are given like external chest compressions for CPR.

If the thrusts have dislodged the obstruction but not expelled it from the victim's mouth, then a finger sweep is performed. Open the victim's mouth by tilting the head back with one hand and moving the jaw forward to lift the tongue away from the back of the throat. Insert an index finger along the inside of the cheek and sweep deeply into the mouth in a hooking action. Be careful not to push an obstruction deeper into the throat. If it is possible to dislodge an obstruction, be sure to remove it from the mouth. If dentures are worn, it is helpful to remove them. If the patient has vomited, it is extremely important to turn the patient on the side to keep an open airway and prevent aspiration of material into the lungs.

Accidental, Allergic, and Drug-Induced Distress

Respiratory problems can also arise from other conditions, as follows:

1. A patient suffering from severe edema of the vocal cords as a result of an allergic reaction to food or stings of bees or wasps must be hospitalized as quickly as possible.
2. The victim of a drowning must receive artificial respiration immediately. This can be given before the

patient is taken from the water if there is help to support the patient while mouth-to-mouth resuscitation is given. A person surviving drowning needs to be hospitalized for follow-up observation.
3. Poisoning by toxic gases, such as carbon monoxide, or suffocation may also require immediate artificial respiration.
4. A person having an asthma attack may have great breathing difficulty. The physician must determine the treatment needed, but you can be helpful in attempting to calm the patient. Emotional upset often starts an asthma attack.
5. Some medications will cause a slowing or **cessation** of breathing.
6. Electric shock may cause respiratory paralysis. The victim must be moved away from the source of the electricity by indirect means (never touch the victim) and then be given artificial respiration and CPR if necessary.

CARDIOPULMONARY RESUSCITATION (CPR)

Ⓒ Skills Menu:
■ Administering CPR

All medical assistants should take CPR and a standard first aid course.

CPR is best learned in a course taught by a certified instructor. Procedures are constantly being refined, and the procedure you learn should be the one you practice. There is currently a recommendation that a one-way valve face piece be used in a health care environment as a guard against communicable diseases. If that is not available, the mouth-to-nose method is recommended.

CPR AND DISEASE TRANSMISSION

Much concern has been voiced regarding the safety of the layperson rescuer. Statistics show that the most likely place of providing CPR is in the home where 70 to 80% of respiratory and cardiac arrest occurs. The greatest concern over the risk of disease transmission should be directed to persons who perform CPR frequently, such as health care providers, prehospital emergency personnel, lifeguards, and others whose job-defined duties require them to perform first-response medical care. The layperson who responds to an emergency of an unknown victim should be guided by the moral and ethical values of preserving life and assisting those in distress balanced against the risk that may exist. It is realistic to believe that any emergency situation involves exposure to certain body fluids and has the potential for disease transmission. These can be minimized by using a face shield or face mask barrier device. They may provide a degree of protection. Masks without one-way valves, including the S-shaped devices, offer little if any protection and should not be considered for routine use. Obviously, **intubation** and bag compression by trained medical emergency personnel is more effective and highly desirable because it does not require personal contact.

The probability that a rescuer will become infected with HBV or HIV as a result of performing CPR is minimal. Although some incidents have been documented from blood exchange or penetration of the skin, infection during mouth-to-mouth has not been documented. HBV positive saliva has not been shown to be infectious even to oral mucous membranes. Saliva has not been implicated in the transmission of HIV even after bites, percutaneous inoculation, or contamination of cuts and open wounds with HIV-infected saliva. The theoretical risk of infection is greater for salivary transmission of herpes simplex and airborne diseases, such as tuberculosis and other respiratory infections. Rare instances of herpes simplex transmission during CPR have been reported. Rescuers with impaired immune systems may be particularly at risk of acquiring tuberculosis and should be tested initially and about 12 weeks after a known exposure. Performance of mouth-to-mouth when blood is apt to be exchanged, such as in trauma cases, does pose a theoretical risk of HBV or HIV transmission. Because of this concern, public safety and health care personnel should follow the guidelines established by the CDC and OSHA. These involve the use of latex or vinyl gloves and mechanical ventilation equipment. Rescuers who themselves are ill should not perform the procedures if other methods of ventilation are available.

An alternative method of mouth-to-nose **resuscitation** is effective and is especially recommended when it is impossible to ventilate through the mouth because of serious injury or if a tight mouth-to-mouth seal cannot be achieved, such as with absence of teeth. To do this, the rescuer's mouth is sealed over the victim's nose, the head tilt is maintained, and the lower jaw is lifted to close the victim's mouth. After the breaths are given, the rescuer must remove the mouth from the victim to allow expiration. (The author found no reference to indicate this method was safer for the rescuer.)

The perceived risk of disease transmission during CPR has reduced the willingness of laypersons to provide mouth-to-mouth in unknown cardiac arrest victims. If a lone rescuer refuses to initiate mouth-to-mouth ventilation, he should at least access the EMS system, open the airway, and perform chest compressions until a rescuer arrives who is willing to provide ventilation or until EMT or paramedics can use the necessary barrier devices.

Activating Medical Services

It is also imperative to activate the emergency medical services immediately when an adult has respiratory or circulatory arrest. A bystander should be instructed to make a call while the rescuer begins BLS procedures. If the rescuer is the only person available, the call must be done *prior* to starting BLS. Research has shown that a single rescuer often performs CPR longer than anticipated, delaying the call to an EMS system and the necessary advanced lifesaving care. Witnesses often spend time calling neighbors, relatives, or family physicians before activating the EMS system, which delays critical defibrillation. The majority of adults (80 to 90%) are in ventricular fibrillation when the initial ECG is obtained. The time from collapse to defibrillation is critical. The window of opportunity for survival of sudden cardiac arrest is very narrow. The chain of survival involves the following sequence of event occurring as quickly as possible:

1. recognition of early warning signs
2. activation of the EMS system
3. basic CPR
4. early defibrillation
5. intubation
6. intravenous administration of medications

With infants and children, the prime concern is usually respiratory. A lone rescuer in this situation is currently advised to first give appropriate BLS for approximately one minute and then break to summon the EMS system.

CPR Procedure

The American Heart Association has issued the following statement in the *Guidelines 2000 for CPR and Emergency Cardiovascular Care:* "All professional rescuers (BLS ambulance providers, health care providers, and appropriate laypersons, who have a duty or obligation to respond, such as lifeguards and police) should learn both the one- and two-rescuer techniques. When possible, air-

PROCEDURE

19-1 Give Mouth-to-Mouth Resuscitation

PURPOSE: To provide a victim who is not breathing with sufficient oxygen to maintain life until self-breathing returns or mechanical ventilation is functioning.

EQUIPMENT: (For simulation) Training mannequin, gauze squares, sanitizing material.

PERFORMANCE OBJECTIVE: In a course taught by a certified instructor, using a training mannequin, demonstrate mouth-to-mouth resuscitation. Perform the steps as instructed following recommended Standard Precautions.

1. Determine whether unresponsive victim is breathing.

2. Position victim on back on firm surface.

3. Rescuer is positioned at victim's side near head and shoulders.

4. Open airway. **NOTE: Use head tilt, listen for air exchange at mouth and nose, and sense for exhaled air on rescuer's cheek. RATIONALE: Often, in the absence of muscle tone, the tongue may obstruct the airway; tilting the head is all that is required to permit breathing.** If not effective, continue with procedure.

5. Check for mouth obstruction. **NOTE: Foreign matter and vomitus that is visible in the mouth should be removed, but excessive time must not be taken to do this. Liquids should be wiped out with covered middle and index fingers; solid material is swept out with a hooked index finger. RATIONALE: This procedure is necessary to clear mouth area before ventilation.**

6. Use head tilt-chin lift maneuver thereby moving tongue from back of throat. **RATIONALE: This opens victim's airway and determines whether victim is breathing independently.** Continue with procedure if there is no evidence of breathing.

7. Pinch victim's nostrils together with fingers of one hand while placing heel of hand on forehead to keep the head tilted. **RATIONALE: This prevents escape of air through nose and maintains open airway.**

8. Take a deep breath, then seal your mouth over victim's, and breathe two slow breaths into the victim's mouth. Take a breath after each ventilation. **NOTE: Breathe at rate of one to one and one-half seconds for each breath. NOTE:**
   - If mouth is injured, hold it shut and breathe into nose.
   - With small child, place your mouth over mouth and nose and breathe into both, adjusting the force of your breaths for the size of the child.

9. Turn head to one side and listen for return of air. Watch chest for movement. **NOTE: If inflation has not occurred, adjust the victim's head tilt and chin lift, and try again. If still not successful, recheck for obstruction, ensure that your mouth seal is adequate, and reventilate.**

10. Repeat the cycle of breathing and listening with approximately 12 breaths per minute for adults and 20 for children until breathing is fully restored or other medical help takes over.

CHARTING EXAMPLE
6-24-XX
Rosie suffered an allergic reaction from an injection of Cefanoal at 2:48 PM and stopped breathing. Called for assistance. Mouth-to-mouth resuscitation was administered for one minute before she responded. Dr. Long examined and treated. She was observed for 45 minutes before being released to husband to take home. Given instructions to follow if reoccurred.

S. Santino, RMA (RL)

---

way adjunct methods, such as mouth-to-mouth devices, should be used."

The CPR procedure has some variations when used for a child or infant. Infants are generally considered to be under one year of age and children ages one to eight. Adult procedure would be used for anyone over eight.

Basic lifesaving (BLS) procedures of mouth-to-mouth resuscitation (Procedure 19–1) and cardiopulmonary resuscitation (CPR) (Procedures 19–2 for adults and 19–3 for infants and children) are included for your information; however, appropriate instruction and performance evaluation requires a certified instructor.

The CPR procedure assumes the lone rescuer is a person without the benefit of devices to observe Standard Precautions. If you were in a situation where this procedure would be anticipated, such as in a physician's office, additional equipment should be available. For example, gloves should be put on prior to step 5, which involves placing a finger or fingers within the victim's mouth. A ventilation barrier device of some form should also be accessible to prevent acquiring organisms from the victim. This device would be inserted or applied prior to step 6. If a second rescuer should arrive, then the responsibility can be shared with one person continuously giving the

PROCEDURE

19-2 Give Cardiopulmonary Resuscitation (CPR) to Adults

PURPOSE: To provide the victim with adequate oxygen and circulation of blood when respiratory collapse and cardiac arrest have occurred, until breathing and heart action can be restored.

EQUIPMENT: (For simulation) Training mannequin, gauze squares, sanitizing material.

PERFORMANCE OBJECTIVE: In the course taught by a certified instructor, using a training mannequin (Figure 19–8), demonstrate the procedure. Perform each step as instructed, following recommended precautions.

1. Gently shake victim and ask "Are you OK?" Call for help. **NOTE: Call to another person, or phone 911 or local emergency service before beginning resuscitation. RATIONALE: This summons assistance while you are attempting to revive the victim.**

2. Position mannequin on its back on floor.
   NOTE:
   ■ Victim must always be in recumbent position on firm surface (floor or ground).
   ■ Never practice this procedure on a person.

3. Rescuer is positioned at victim's side near head and shoulders.

4. Open airway. **NOTE: Use head tilt, listen for air exchange at mouth and nose, and sense for exhaled air on rescuer's cheek (Figure 19–9). RATIONALE: Often, in the absence of muscle tone, the tongue may obstruct the airway; tilting the head is all that is required to permit breathing.** If not effective, continue with procedure.

5. Check for mouth obstruction. **NOTE: Visible foreign matter and vomitus should be removed quickly. Liquids should be wiped out with covered middle and index fingers; solid material is swept out with a hooked index finger.**

6. Position victim to open airway; pinch nostrils together with fingers while placing heel of hand on forehead to maintain head tilt.

7. Take a deep breath, seal your mouth over victim's, and breathe two slow breaths into victim's mouth. Take a breath after each ventilation.

8. Turn your head to one side, listen, and feel for return of air. Watch chest for movement. **NOTE: If inflation has not occurred, adjust the victim's head tilt and chin lift, and try again. If still not successful, recheck for obstruction, and ensure that your mouth seal is adequate, and reventilate.**

9. Check for carotid pulse by placing index and middle fingers into natural groove at side of victim's neck. Check carefully because pulse will probably be weak (Figure 19–10). The pulse check should be done in conjunction with assessment for signs of circulation, which includes evaluation of victim for breathing, coughing, or movement. This assessment should take no more than 10 seconds.

10. If victim has a pulse, continue mouth-to-mouth respirations at rate of one breath every five seconds (12 times per minute). **NOTE: Correct timing can be obtained by counting one, one thousand; two, one thousand; three, one thousand; four, one thousand; then breathe.** Go to step 19.

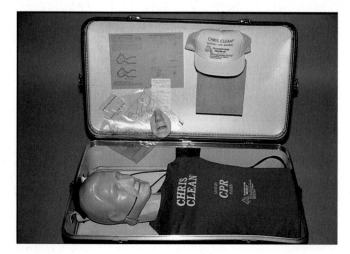

FIGURE 19–8 Chris Clean CPR training mannequin with disposable parts

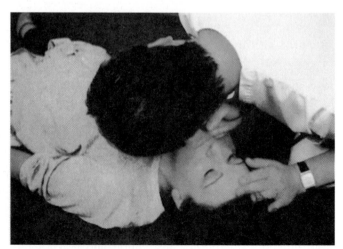

FIGURE 19–9 After opening the airway, look, listen, and feel for breathing; if victim is not breathing, give two slow, full breaths.

PROCEDURE

19-2 Give Cardiopulmonary Resuscitation (CPR) to Adults—continued

11. If victim does not have a pulse, chest compression must be started. Locate lower margin of victim's rib cage and follow it to notch where ribs meet sternum in center of chest.

12. Place index finger on lower end of sternum.

13. Heel of hand closest to head is then placed on lower sternum next to index finger of first hand.

14. Place heel of hand that located notch over hand on sternum and lock fingers. Hold fingers high, away from body.

15. Rise on your knees so your shoulders are directly over hands on victim's sternum. Lock your elbows and keep arms straight (Figure 19–11).

16. Use a smooth, even motion to push straight down on chest and compress about one and one-half to two inches for a count of 15 compressions. A count of one and, two and, three and, etc. will help you obtain correct time. (The rate of compressions is approximately 100 times per minute.)

17. After administering 15 compressions, give victim two mouth-to-mouth resuscitations or ventilations. **Key Point: Do this without moving from your position beside body.**

18. Repeat four cycles of compressions and respirations before pausing to check for breathing, signs of circulation, and presence of carotid pulse.
    Key Points:
    ■ If no pulse is felt, resume compressions and respirations.
    ■ Check every few minutes.

19. You must not discontinue CPR unless victum recovers, someone takes over for you, or a physician pronounces the victim dead.

20. Use alcohol or Zephiran to clean mannequin. **NOTE: It is recommended that mannequins with disposable mouthpieces and air bags are used in training for CPR, as shown in** Figure 19–9, **to prevent disease transmission.** For those mannequins that have no disposable parts, they must be carefully and faithfully cleaned after each use with a clean gauze pad soaked in a liquid chlorine bleach and water solution, or with rubbing alcohol. The soaked gauze pad should remain in contact with the area for at least 30 seconds and then wiped clean. It should be dried with a clean gauze pad.

CHARTING EXAMPLE:

9-23-XX

Mohammed was reported collapsed on the sidewalk outside the office at 2:15 PM. Dr. Long was not in the office. Patient found without respiration or heartbeat. EMS summoned by Maria. CPR administered for six minutes. EMS arrived and took over resuscitation efforts. Stabilized and transported to First Hospital at 2:48 PM.

S. Seiple, CMA

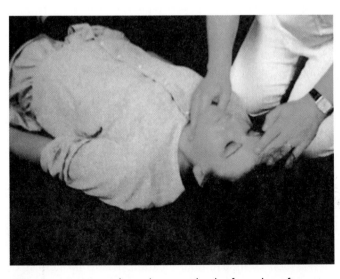

FIGURE 19–10 Palpate the carotid pulse for at least five seconds to determine whether the heart is beating.

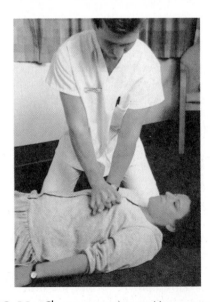

FIGURE 19–11 Chest compression position; use smooth, even motions to compress the chest straight down, about one and one-half to two inches in an adult.

PROCEDURE

19-3 Give Cardiopulmonary Resuscitation (CPR) to Infants and Children

PURPOSE: To provide an infant or child who is not breathing with sufficient oxygen to maintain life until self-breathing or mechanical ventilation is functioning.

EQUIPMENT: (For simulation) Training mannequin, gauze squares, sanitizing material.

PERFORMANCE OBJECTIVE: In a course taught by a certified instructor, using a training mannequin, demonstrate the procedure by performing each step with 100% accuracy following Standard Precautions.

1. Gently shake and call to a child, or flick bottom of foot of an infant to check for consciousness.

2. Call to another person to phone 911 or local emergency service, and begin resuscitation. **RATIONALE: Summons assistance while you are attempting to revive the victim. If alone, provide CPR for approximately one minute, then summon EMS.**

3. Place infant or child on back on firm surface.

4. Tip victim's head back and lift chin to open airway (Figure 19–12). **NOTE: Be careful not to tip head too far back because this can cause obstruction of airway in infant.**

5. Listen and watch for breathing. Place ear by mouth to listen. Also, sense if breath is felt on your cheek, and watch chest for breathing.

6. If no breathing is observed, give two slow breaths, one to two seconds each.
   - For infants, cover nose and mouth with your mouth, and breathe gently.
   - For a child, cover mouth, pinch nostrils, and carefully give breaths.

7. For a child, check carotid pulse as for an adult. Check pulse in conjunction with assessment for signs of circulation, which includes evaluating victim for breathing, coughing, or movement. This assessment should take no more than 10 seconds. For an infant, check pulse over brachial artery by putting your middle fingertips on inside of upper arm halfway between elbow and shoulder. At the same time, keep airway open.

8. If pulse is present, continue one breath every three seconds for an infant and one breath every four seconds for a child.

9. If no pulse is present, start cardiac compression. For an infant, use two fingers to compress middle of sternum to one inch at rate of 100 per minute. For a child, use adult hand position, but use only the heel of one hand. Compress a depth of one-half to one inch at rate of not less than 100 times per minute. Give one breath for every five compressions.
   - Be sure infant or child is on a firm surface or is being supported in back while administering compressions.
   - Correct rate for infants could be counted as one, two, three, four, five, breathe.
   - Correct rate for child would be one and two and three and four and five and breathe.

10. Do 10 cycles of compressions and breaths, and then check for signs of circulation and pulse. **NOTE: Do not take more than five seconds for this check.**

11. If there are no signs of circulation or pulse, give one breath, and continue cycle until help arrives.

12. Sanitize the mannequins used in training for CPR. **NOTE: Use a solution of one-fourth cup bleach to a gallon of water, or according to manufacturer's instructions.**

CHARTING EXAMPLE

4-23-XX

Maria was carried into the office from the apartment next door because she was found not breathing in her crib. Mouth-to-mouth resuscitation was started at 3:15 PM. Dr. Long was involved in a joint aspiration. The baby responded and started crying at 3:18 PM. After initial examination by Dr. Long and observation for 30 minutes, she was determined stable and taken by her parents to nearby Children's Hospital for further evaluation.

S. Mitchell, CMA (RL)

chest compressions while the second gives a breath immediately following each fifth compression. Perform any variables to the procedure as may be indicated by a certified instructor of CPR.

Also, remember if the procedure is provided by the physician or an employee within the office, it must be recorded on a chart. If the victim is not a patient, a new chart should be established and the incident recorded. As soon as care is provided, a doctor–patient relationship is established, and there are legal responsibilities.

The guidelines previously have indicated that CPR should continue until the rescuer is exhausted and can no longer continue. This has been modified for those situations, such as in a remote location, where no help is or

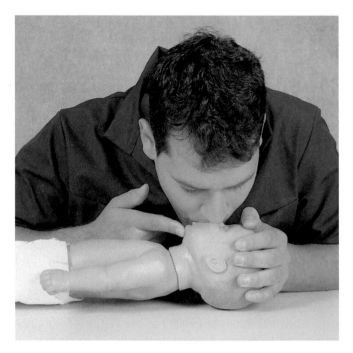

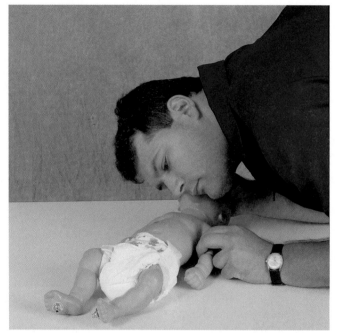

FIGURE 19-12   Basic CPR for infants

will be available. If no signs of life occur after 15 minutes, the chance that CPR alone can restore heartbeat is very slim, the victim has for all purposes died, and there is no possibility of meaningful survival. The key to this evaluation is "no signs of life," which means no pulse, no gasping respirations, no maintenance of body temperature with progressive mottling (bluish spotting) of the skin, increased dependent livido (bluish-gray coloring), and persistently fixed and dilated pupils. As hard as it may be to accept, continuation of CPR will not change the outcome.

Defibrillation

In addition to initial lifesaving methods of resuscitation and CPR, for the past several years, health care facilities and EMS providers have been using defibrillation machines to respond to cardiac emergencies. This technology has now become practical for use by general health care workers and laypersons.

The automated external defibrillator (AED) consists of two large electrodes (pads that are placed on the patient's chest) and cables that connect to the machine. A battery package serves as the source of power so that the equip-

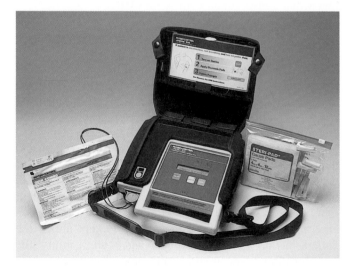

FIGURE 19-13A   The automated external defibrillator (AED)

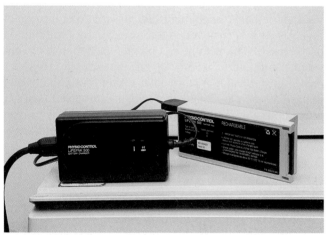

FIGURE 19-13B   The rechargeable battery is the power source for the AED.

ment can operate in any location (Figure 19-13A and B). (Some units have a self-contained battery.) The AED is indicated only when the victim is unresponsive, is not breathing, and has no pulse. There are four universal steps to follow. This description is not intended to be operating instructions because some differences exist between different machines, and those must be followed. The AED is used in connection with CPR when cardiac function is not responding.

AED Universal Steps
- Turn on the power.
- Attach the electrode pads of the AED to the victim's chest (must be against dry bare skin and may require cutting or shaving of hair. Usually, a disposable razor is with the equipment).
- Analyze the rhythm. Some machines respond automatically, others require a button to be pushed. Stop CPR. It is critical that no one touches the victim while the rhythm is being analyzed.
- Charge the AED if so advised by the AED message; some charge automatically.
- Advise everyone to stay clear, and then push the shock button if the AED so indicates.
- If victim responds, leave electrodes in place in case of re-arrest. If no response, repeat the analyze and shock sequence.
- Continue efforts until emergency medical services arrive.

Because of ease of operation, defibrillators are being placed in many public buildings, health clubs, recreational facilities, and airplanes. In a physician's office, designated personnel should be trained to operate the equipment to be prepared to respond to life threatening emergencies. Accurate recording of time, actions, and the use of the defibrillator is very important to document emergency response and provide for risk management. Equally important is the scheduled equipment check to assure the battery is charged, the cables are intact, and the dated electrode package remains sealed and has not expired. Successful lawsuits have been awarded for unsuccessful resuscitation as the result of inoperable equipment. Each minute of ventricular fibrillation results in an approximate 10% decrease in survival. CPR provided within four minutes and defibrillation in less than eight minutes still gives a patient only about a 43% chance of survival. Survival of cardiac arrest depends upon immediate response. With cardiac arrest, every minute is critical.

Caution is needed with the use of AED equipment in certain situations:

- Not for children under 8 years of age because the electric energy setting is too high
- Victim must not be in water; drag from area before using
- If has implanted pacemaker or defibrillator, place electrode at least 1 inch to the side.

- Remove and wipe dry any area with a transdermal patch that interferes with electrode placement

Cervical Spine Injury

With injuries from falls, vehicles, gymnastic equipment, diving, and athletics, there is always the chance of cervical spine injury. A person who requires emergency ventilation or CPR following an injury needs to be in a supine position on a firm, flat surface to receive proper care. If the victim is lying face down or on his side, the rescuer must roll the victim in such a way that the head, shoulders, and torso move together as a unit, *without twisting*. This maneuver is also know as "logrolling." This is especially critical to help prevent any additional spinal injury. If two persons are available, one should move the head and neck as the other turns the rest of the body. The head should not be tilted to open the airway; instead, a procedure called "jaw thrust" is indicated. This can be accomplished by grasping the angles of the victim's lower jaw and lifting with both hands, one on each side, displacing the jaw forward without tilting the head. When efforts to provide resuscitation fail to ventilate the victim, try adjusting the hand positioning and jaw displacement airway opening maneuver, and recheck for a missed obstruction. Remember, if there is an inadequate seal over the victim's mouth, efforts to ventilate will not provide an adequate amount of air. This can occur when the victim has ill-fitting or dislodged dentures or complete absence of teeth. Readjust or remove dentures and try again. If efforts are still inadequate, use the mouth-to-nose technique.

When there is a spinal injury and ventilation or CPR is not required, and when the person is not in any danger from their surroundings, it may be best to provide emotional support and not move them. As with any injury, always watch for signs of shock. When EMS personnel arrive, they will be able to attach a collar to support the neck and position the person on a board to prevent any additional back or neck injury when transporting to emergency care.

Shock

Shock may be associated with many different kinds of injuries and is a serious depressor of vital body functions. Symptoms include a rapid, thready, weak pulse; shallow, rapid respirations; dilated pupils; ashen color; and cool, clammy skin. All of these result from decreased blood volume because there is diminished cardiac output and the blood pressure drops. It is possible for shock to cause death even when the injury causing the shock is not life threatening. First aid measures include placing the patient in recumbent position with feet elevated unless there is a head injury, in which case the patient is kept flat. If the patient has difficulty breathing or has a chest injury, the head and shoulders should be elevated. It is best to place a blanket under and over the patient to maintain body warmth but not to overheat.

Shock can be caused by various circumstances. It can be associated with a heart attack or respiratory collapse. It frequently follows trauma or physical injury. Extensive burns, electrical shock, hemorrhage, near drownings, and severe infection can all result in shock. Another type, an anaphylactic shock, is an acute allergic reaction to a foreign substance, which may include certain foods, bee stings, or injections of therapeutic or **prophylactic** substances. The patient may have dyspnea, cyanosis, and seizures. Epinephrine and oxygen should be immediately available for use by the physician or by the medical assistant under the direction of the physician. No patient should be given an allergy injection and then be allowed to leave the office immediately because anaphylactic shock may result from these injections. Patients may also have severe reactions to penicillin, aspirin, serums, vaccines, local anesthetics, salicylates, and x-ray contrast medias.

Stroke

The common terms for a cerebrovascular accident (CVA) are stroke or apoplexy. A CVA is the result of a ruptured blood vessel in the brain. A CVA can also be caused by an occlusion of a blood vessel. The patient may have a light stroke with very little damage or a more extensive one with immediate paralysis in the form of sagging muscles on one side of the face or the inability to use an arm or leg. One entire side of the body may be paralyzed. The patient may complain of numbness. The pupils of the eyes may be unequal in size. There may be mental confusion, slurred speech, nausea, vomiting, or difficulty in breathing and swallowing. Control of urine and bowels may also be lost. Avoid any unnecessary movement of the patient. Keep in mind that the patient who appears to be unconscious or is unable to speak may be able to hear what is being said. If a patient is experiencing a CVA, loosen the clothing and be sure the patient is positioned so as not to choke on excess saliva. Strokes are now considered to be emergency situations. (See Chapter 11, Unit 8.) The patient who exhibits

any of the warning signs of stroke needs immediate emergency assistance to ensure optimal recovery. Remember, approximately one-third of patients with a complete stroke die as a result of the condition. Quick, appropriate intervention in many cases reverses damage caused by blood vessel occlusion and restores patients to prior state of health. The American Heart Association has adapted a series of actions to take for EMS and emergency personnel to evaluate and react to stroke similar to that of cardiac response. It involves initial field evaluation criteria, rapid transportation, medical evaluation, CT scan interpretation, and injection with fibrinolytics if ischemic stroke and actions for acute hemorrhage if not.

■ ACHIEVE UNIT OBJECTIVES

Complete Chapter 19, Unit 2, in the workbook to help you obtain competency of this subject matter.

UNIT 3
First Aid in Accidents and Injuries

■ OBJECTIVES

Upon completion of the unit, meet the following performance objectives by verifying knowledge of the facts and principles presented through oral and written communication at a level deemed competent. Demonstrate the specific behaviors as identified in the performance objectives of the procedures, observing all aseptic and safety precautions in accordance with health care standards.

1. Spell and define, using the glossary at the back of the text, all the **Words to Know** in this unit.
2. Describe the symptoms of an allergy to stings.
3. Explain the classifications of burns.
4. Describe how to remove a foreign body from the eye.
5. Describe how to remove a foreign body from the ear.
6. List three first aid measures to take when dealing with an open fracture.
7. Explain the effects of cold applications.
8. Explain the effects of heat applications.
9. Describe four types of wounds.
10. Demonstrate the proper method of cleaning a wound.
11. Demonstrate application of dressing and recurrent turn bandages.
12. Demonstrate application of dressing and open spiral bandage.
13. Demonstrate application of dressing and closed spiral bandage.
14. Demonstrate application of dressing and figure-eight bandage to the hand.
15. Demonstrate application of cravat bandage to the head.
16. Demonstrate application of triangular bandage to the head.

A CAAHEP CONNECTION

The curriculum standards indicate that information on **Medical emergencies** as listed under the category of **Medical assisting clinical procedures** musst be included in a medical assisting program. This unit covers many acute illness conditions, such as diabetic coma or shock, heart attack, hemorrhage, stroke, and situations requiring rescue breathing and CPR. This content and the instructions for performing lifesaving procedures are addressed in this unit. It has further stressed the need for professional growth by obtaining and retaining CPR credentials from a certified instructor.

■ WORDS TO KNOW

abrasion	laceration
anaphylactic	molten
chemical	puncture
electrical	recurrent
foreign body	shock
friction	splinter
immobilize	superficial
incision	thermal

SUDDEN ILLNESSES AND INJURIES

Knowing what to do when an accident or injury occurs is very helpful not only in your professional life but also in your personal life. When you have a basic understanding of first aid, you can quickly and efficiently respond to the sudden incidents that may occur without becoming overly anxious or upset. As you come into contact with injury incidents, you will begin to learn when they can be handled with simple first aid and when they require the assistance of a physician or advanced emergency medical services. As stated in Unit 1, many illnesses and injuries can occur in varying degrees of severity. As an example, consider a burn. A burn confined just to the skin surface can probably be managed without medical assistance unless it covers extensive body surface, whereas a relatively small area of burn can require medical attention if it extends into underlying tissue. If you are ever called on to make a judgment, it is always better to "err" on the conservative side and seek medical or advanced emergency services than to underestimate the severity of an injury.

Bee, Wasp, and Hornet Stings

Bees, wasps, and hornets cause deaths every year. If the victim is not sensitive to the sting, the result may only be a painful swelling with redness and itching. When several stings are received at one time, the victim may become quite ill. The patient may develop severe hives or generalized edema.

When a patient is severely allergic to stings, they can cause acute illness. The patient may become restless, complain of headache, have shortness of breath, or have mottled blueness of the skin. In the cases where shortness of breath is not apparent, the victim may appear to be in shock and have severe nausea, vomiting, and bloody diarrhea. The severely allergic patient should always have a special emergency kit close at hand when there is a possibility of a sting. (Refer to Chapter 16, Unit 1, for a discussion about **anaphylactic** shock and stings.) If there is evidence of anaphylactic shock, epinephrine should be given as a lifesaving measure.

A honeybee leaves the stinger in the skin, and it should be immediately removed by scraping it out carefully with a sharp object. Never grasp the stinger with your fingers or a tweezers, as that would inject more of the venom. Wasps, hornets, and yellow jackets retain their stingers and can sting repeatedly.

Bites

An animal bite may tear skin and cause a bruise. The bite is dangerous because of the possibility of infection or rabies. The wound should be thoroughly cleansed with an antiseptic soap and rinsed well. The area should be bandaged and immobilized, and the victim should be examined by a physician as soon as possible. The animal should be held for observation for at least 15 days to see if it is rabid. The bite must be reported to the police or local health authorities, who will examine the animal for rabies. The decision must be made regarding the use of antirabies serum. If the skin is broken and the animal cannot be tested, antirabies serum should be used. When the animal can be observed and is found to be free of rabies, no serum is necessary.

There is also concern regarding human bites because of HIV and hepatitis B. The only way HIV could be transmitted in this manner is if the bite breaks the skin and the person doing the biting has bleeding gums. It is still necessary to cleanse the wound thoroughly, cover with a sterile bandage, and have a physician examine the area. Patients who have sustained such a bite from another person should be advised to have injections to be immunized against hepatitis B.

BURNS

Burns are terrible injuries. Extensive burns require painful treatment and a long period of rehabilitation. They often result in permanent disfigurement and physical and emotional problems. About two million people per year suffer burns. About 300,000 people are burned seriously; approximately 6,000 burn victims die.

Types of Burns

Burns are basically of three types: **thermal, chemical,** and **electrical,** with thermal being the most common.

Thermal—Caused by residential fires, automobile accidents, playing with matches, accidents with gasoline, space heaters, electrical sources (such as faulty wiring, firecrackers, scalding water from the stove or tub), and children coming into contact with curling irons, stoves, or clothing irons. Some childhood burns, such as with cigarettes, can be traced to deliberate abuse. Sunburn results from overexposure to sunlight.

Chemical—From contact with, ingestion, inhalation, or injection of acids or alkalines.

Electrical—Occur after contact with faulty electrical wiring, a child chewing on an electrical cord, or from high-voltage power lines. Though rare, an electrical burn can also come from a lightening strike.

Classification of Burns

Burns are classified by three methods. One is by the percentage of body surface area (BSA) involved in the burn. The Rule of Nines illustrated in Figure 19–14A and the Lund and Browder chart in Figure 19–14B are methods used to estimate the size of the burn. These methods establish a standard by which all injuries can be estimated. Note that the Lund and Browder chart is more specific and has a way to estimate areas for different age groups because body proportions are quite different for infants and small children as compared to adults.

A familiar classification reflects the extent of burn as a relationship to the layer of skin involved and is estimated from one to four degrees (Figure 19–15). A first-degree burn is a **superficial** injury primarily to the epidermis, resulting in reddening of the skin and moderately severe pain. A sunburn or contact with boiling water or steam may cause this type of burn (Figure 19–15B). A second-degree burn involves the epidermis and part of the dermis. The leakage of plasma and electrolytes from the capillaries damaged by the burn into the surrounding tissues raises up the epidermis to form blisters and results in mild to moderate edema and pain (Figure 19–15C). A third-degree burn involves the epidermis, dermis, and subcutaneous skin layers. No blisters appear, but white, leathery tissue and thrombosed vessels are visible. A fourth-degree burn indicates that the damage extends through the subcutaneous tissue into muscle and bone. The tissue appears deeply charred (Figure 19–15D).

Another classification of burns measures the severity of a burn by a combination of two methods. It correlates

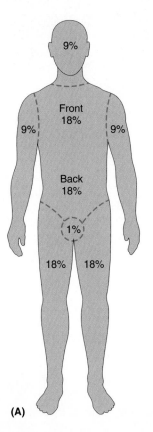

(A)

(B)

Relative percentages of areas affected by growth

	At birth	1 yr	5 yr	10 yr	15 yr	Adult
A: Half of head	9½%	8½%	6½%	5½%	4½%	3½%
B: Half of thigh	2¾%	3¼%	4%	4¼%	4½%	4¾%
C: Half of leg	2½%	2½%	2¾%	3%	3¾%	3½%

FIGURE 19–14 (A) Diagram for use in calculating the extent of burns or other injuries for an adult. (B) Lund and Browder chart for estimating the extent of burns. Because this chart takes proportional age-size differences into account, it can be used for infants and children and for adults. (Redrawn from CP Artz and JA Moncrief. The Treatment of Burns, ed. 2, Philadelphia, WB Saunders Company, 1969, used with permission.)

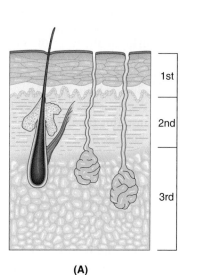

(A)

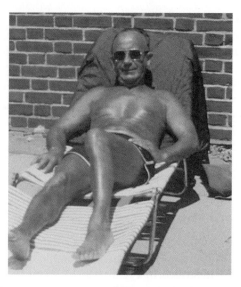

(B)

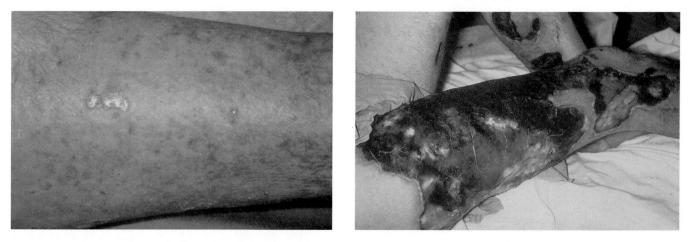

(C)   **(D)**

FIGURE 19–15   (A) Layers of skin in relation to degree of burn (B) First-degree burns involve the top layer of skin. (Courtesy of the Phoenix Society of Burn Survivors, Inc.) (C) Second-degree or partial thickness burns affect the top layers of skin. The healing process is slower, and scarring may occur. (Courtesy of the Phoenix Society of Burns Survivors, Inc.) (D) Fourth-degree or deep, full-thickness burns are the most serious, affecting or destroying all layers of skin plus the fat, muscle, bones, and nerves. (Courtesy of the Phoenix Society of Burns Survivors, Inc.)

the burn's depth with its size (BSA) to determine its severity, which is then classified as a minor, moderate, or major burn.

■ A *minor* burn has less than 2% of BSA at the third-degree level and burns on less than 15% for adults and 10% for children at the second-degree level.
■ A *moderate* burn is one where third-degree burns cover 2% to 10% of BSA; second-degree burns cover from 15% to 25% on adults or over 10% on children.
■ A *major* burn is one where a third-degree burn covers more than 10% of BSA or second-degree burns cover more than 25% in adults or 20% in children; burns of the hands, feet, or genitalia are also major burns; burns

that are complicated by fractures, affect poor risk patients, or are electrical are also major burns.

The Phoenix Society of Burn Survivors, Inc., states that some professionals are no longer using the term "degree" to designate extent of burns. Instead, they refer to burns as:

Partial thickness burns = second-degree
Full thickness burns = third-degree
Deep full thickness burns = fourth-degree

The classification of burns used will probably be at the discretion of the physician or the treatment facility involved.

Treatment of Burns

The first priority in the treatment of burns is to "stop the burning process." If burns are minor, they will heal without special treatment. Applying cold water to the area should stop the pain and may even keep the burn from progressing into deeper tissue layers. The application of butter or ointments is contraindicated for two reasons: it will hold in the burn and cause more pain, and it will be difficult to remove when the burn is being evaluated and treated. In addition, butter contains salt, which would be painful if the skin surface was broken. The use of ice is also considered to be contraindicated because of the chance of frostbite to the damaged tissue. Treatment of first-degree burns may involve the use of an antiseptic preparation that can be easily removed and a dressing to protect the area. A victim of severe sunburn would be encouraged to soak in a tub of cool water and drink large amounts of fluids. Patients who are on photosensitive drugs need to be warned about their increased danger from exposure to the sun and the need to wear protective sunscreen and clothing. Pharmacists generally place a warning label on the prescription bottles containing these drugs.

In second-degree burns, first aid may involve treatment for **shock**, removal of any jewelry because edema may be severe, providing ample amounts of liquid to drink, and covering the burned area with a sterile dressing. Healing may be facilitated if the blisters are opened by the physician under aseptic conditions and the area covered with a sterile dressing. Patients should be cautioned to refrain from breaking blisters and peeling the skin because this leaves the area open to infection.

Third-degree burns should receive immediate medical treatment. If over 10% of the BSA is involved, it is considered a major burn and will require surgical intervention, IV fluids for fluid replacement, medication for pain, and probably tetanus antitoxin or a toxoid booster shot. The only first aid that is appropriate is to cover the burned area with sterile dressings and treat the patient for shock. Remember to avoid applying a dressing to second- and third-degree burns with any material that could adhere to the area because it will cause pain and tissue damage when it has to be removed. No attempt should be made to remove clothing that is in contact with the burn. The patient will need surgical care to remove the burned fabric, clean the area, and dress the wound.

Some physicians use the term "fourth-degree burn" for burns involving all layers of the skin, muscle, and bone. This can result from an industrial injury, such as contact with **molten** metal. The intense heat of a burning building or a chemical fire could also cause this type of injury. Of course, this is extremely severe and requires immediate treatment similar to third-degree burns.

Treating Electrical and Chemical Burns

When burns are caused by electricity or chemicals, other factors need to be considered before first aid can be given. An electrical burn results from contact with electrical wiring, power lines, or lightning. The first concern is to remove the victim from the source of electricity but only AFTER the electrical source has been turned off. This situation requires evaluation. If the electrical source is from the wiring within a home, the main electrical supply coming into the house can be shut off at the electrical box, thereby making rescue safe. If the electrical source is power lines, the electric company must be summoned. If the person and the electrical source are in a wet area, keep in mind that electricity conducts well through water. If you come into contact with the water, you could receive a severe shock or be electrocuted. EMS personnel have been electrocuted trying to rescue people from situations involving downed wires and water. Because of this potential for a lethal accident, policy states that they summon the electric company or the fire department to deal with the electrical source prior to any rescue attempt.

If the voltage is of a sufficient amount, it is possible for the victim to suffer circulatory and respiratory arrest, which will necessitate administering CPR and obtaining advanced medical care. The everyday electrical burn is treated like any other burn; however, the extent of the damage may not be readily observable. Electrical burns can cause extensive internal damage along the conduction pathway, which may take a few days to manifest itself. Persons struck by lightning will need CPR and immediate emergency treatment. They may have hallmark "ferning" markings on their body, which are characteristic of lightning burns.

Chemical burns are treated by removing any clothing from the area and then immediately flooding the burn area with water for at least 15 minutes. A dry chemical should first be brushed off carefully before flushing the patient's skin because some chemicals, such as lime, are activated by water. Following the flooding of water, chemical burns, like all other burns, should be covered with a sterile dressing. A chemical burn of the eye should be flooded with water continuously for at least 20 minutes (refer to Figure 12–10). A physician should always examine eye burns immediately.

A CAAHEP CONNECTION

Curriculum for approved medical assistant programs must contain instruction in *Asepsis, Patient care,* and *Medical emergencies.* This unit discusses first aid, initial care, and evaluation of illness and injuries to determine the presence of an emergency situation.

FIRST AID FOR COMMON INJURIES
Dislocations

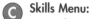
Skills Menu:
- Applying a Splint

At least half of all dislocations involve the shoulder, but dislocations are possible of any freely moving joint. When a bone end slips out of the socket or when the capsule surrounding a joint is stretched or torn, a dislocation is likely to occur. There is usually severe pain and obvious deformity of the joint area. There may be loss of function of the affected limb. There is also noticeable swelling. Dislocations are best treated by a physician. The only first aid measure is to **immobilize** the dislocation during the trip to the medical office or hospital. Treat all sprains, strains, and dislocations as if a fracture. The injured extremity should be carefully supported in the position in which it was found to avoid additional injury. This involves splinting from the joint above and to the joint below the injury. With a shoulder involvement, this will probably involve immobilizing the affected arm by wrapping it to the body for support.

Foreign Bodies

Foreign bodies are substances or objects that become lodged in any part of the human body where they do not belong. It is fairly common for a speck of dirt, soot from a fire, or an eyelash to lodge in the eye, for example. Always wash your hands before touching the eyes. A foreign body under the lower lid can usually be seen easily and can be removed with a bit of cotton or a fold of tissue moistened with water. If a foreign body is under the upper lid, it may be possible to remove it by pulling the upper lid down over the lower lid. If this procedure is not successful, it may be necessary to grasp the eyelashes and carefully turn back the upper lid over a cotton swab (Figure 19–16). When the object is located under the upper lid it may be removed with a folded piece of moistened sterile gauze. If the material cannot be easily removed or is on the cornea, try flushing with large amounts of water to dislodge (see eye irrigation in Chapter 14). Any object imbedded on the cornea will require removal by a physician. A sterile compress should be placed over both eyes to help keep the injured eye from moving, which will cause discomfort and additional irritation, until the object can be removed. The patient must be warned not to rub the affected eye, which would only imbed the object deeper into the cornea. When chemicals, either liquid or powder, get in the eyes, use a sterile eye irrigation solution to dilute and neutralize the chemical. This solution should be continuously dripped into the eye for 20 minutes. Prepacked solutions should be kept in the physician's office for emergency use. When in a situation where a sterile solution is not available, use any clean tap

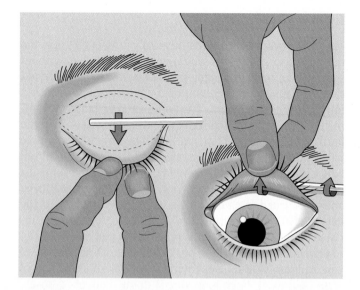

FIGURE 19–16 Remove a foreign object from the upper eyelid by turning the eyelid back over a cotton-tipped swab or the stem of a wooden kitchen match.

or bottled water to flush the eye. Eye injuries should be evaluated by a physician as soon as possible.

First aid for an object lodged in the ear consists of placing several drops of warm olive oil, mineral oil, or baby oil into the ear and pulling back on the earlobe to straighten the external canal while the head is tilted toward the unaffected side (Figure 19–17). Then let the oil run out and see

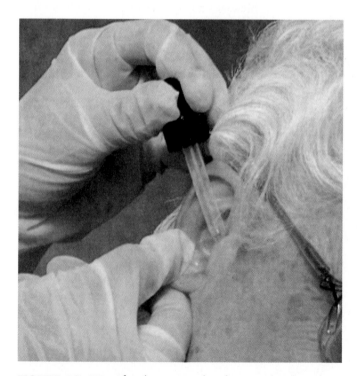

FIGURE 19–17 After the patient's head is tipped to the side, pull back on the earlobe to straighten the external canal and instill eardrops.

if the object will come out with it. Never try to dig an object out of the ear; damage can be done to the external canal or tympanic membrane. If first aid measures are not successful, a physician should examine the patient.

Children are notorious for putting things, such as beans, pebbles, buttons, or marbles, in their ears or up their noses. Instilling oil in the ear when there are large, smooth objects to be removed may make them more difficult to grasp and retrieve. Often, these can be removed from the nose with forceps or irrigated out of an ear by directing water against the wall of the external canal. However, water should never be used with any object, such as beans or peas, which would swell, thereby causing pain and making removal much more difficult.

You may get a call from a parent who is frightened because a child has swallowed a small object. It is best for the physician to perform a fluoroscopic examination to see if the object is actually in the stomach. If the object is

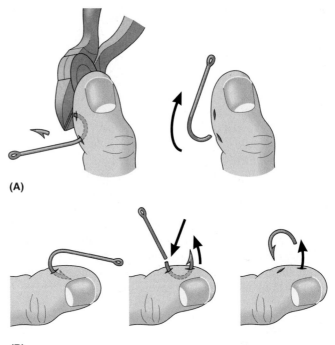

(A)

(B)

FIGURE 19–19 (A) Removing a fish hook by cutting the barb or (B) cutting the shank

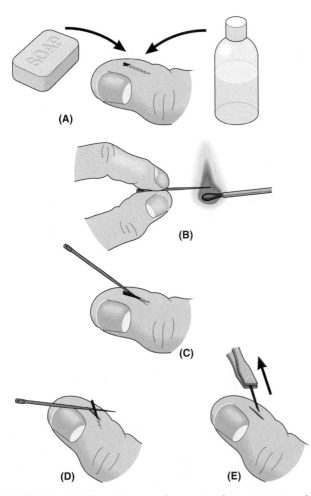

(A)

(B)

(C)

(D)

(E)

FIGURE 19–18 Removing a splinter: (A) Clean area around splinter, (B) heat needle in flame and let cool, (C) open the skin over the splinter, (D) lift the end of the splinter from the skin, and (E) remove the splinter with tweezers.

not sharp, it will probably pass on through the intestinal tract and be eliminated in the stool.

Splinters can generally be removed with a needle at home or with a splinter thumb forceps in the office (Figure 19–18). The skin should be washed with soap and water. The needle should be held over a flame until it is thoroughly heated and then cooled before making a slit over the splinter. Lift the end of the exposed splinter with the needle, and remove by grasping with a pair of tweezers. If a splinter or thorn is under a fingernail, it is best to have a physician remove it. After the splinter or thorn is removed, the area should again be washed with soap and water and covered with an adhesive bandage.

One of the hazards of fishing, or of being around individuals who are casting for fish, is that hooks may become embedded in fingers, backs, scalps, or any part of the anatomy that is exposed. It is best for a physician to use a local anesthetic for such removal. If you do not have a physician near, you should push the barb on through the flesh and then cut if off with a pair of nipper pliers (Figure 19–19). After this is done, you can back out the remainder of the hook. The other possibility is to cut off the shank of the hook and pull out the barbed end. After the hook is removed, the area should be carefully cleaned and a dry dressing applied. If the removal is done away from the office, the patient should be seen by a physician. A tetanus toxoid booster or tetanus antiserum may be needed. The physician may also prescribe an antibiotic.

Fractures

Ⓒ **Skills Menu:**
■ Assisting with Casting
■ Cast Care and Comfort

Fractures are breaks in bone caused by trauma or bone disease. In a *closed* or *simple fracture,* there is no open wound. In an *open* or *compound fracture,* there is an open wound. First aid for an open fracture is to control bleeding and to splint without moving the bone ends. The patient may also need to be treated for shock. You should check the pulse and motor and sensory reflexes (PMS). Capillary refill of the distal area to all fracture sites on an injured limb will be impaired. To ensure good perfusion and nonimpaired neurologic function, treatment must be administered as soon as possible. A fracture can be accurately diagnosed only by an x-ray unless bone ends can be seen in an open wound or a severe deformity is present. A physician is the only person who should attempt to straighten, or reduce, a fracture.

Strains and Sprains

Strains are the result of overuse of a muscle or group of muscles. They may be caused by improper lifting or by slipping while moving a heavy object. Muscle strain is common after engaging in any strenuous activity that you are not accustomed to doing. First aid is to rest the injured muscles in a comfortable position. Application of ice and then heat will help to relieve muscle strain. The physician may prescribe an analgesic or muscle relaxant.

Sprains are injuries to ligaments surrounding a joint. They are usually the result of twisting the joint and are sometimes so severe that a fracture may also occur. A common site is the ankle. Treatment as soon as possible after the injury is to elevate the sprained area and apply ice for the first 24 hours. An elastic bandage is helpful for support but should not be put on too tightly. Temporary support may be given to an ankle by use of a cravat bandage, which may be applied over the shoe (Figure 19–20). (Note: A cravat is a folded, triangular bandage.)

Applying Heat and Cold Treatments

Ⓒ **Skills Menu:**
■ Applying Dry Heat
■ Applying a Cold Treatment

In the treatment of injuries, often physicians order the application of a heat or cold pack. The physician will give specific instructions concerning the length of time and where to apply the treatment.

Many offices and clinics today use disposable heat and cold packs because of their convenience (Figure 19–21). These plastic packs contain chemicals that are activated by either squeezing the bag or mixing the contents to produce cold or by bending a metal disc to initiate heat.

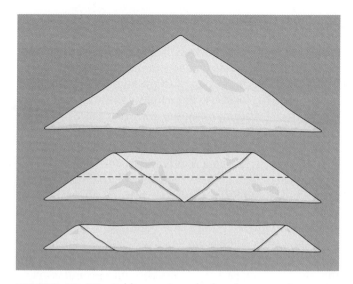

FIGURE 19–20 Folding a triangular bandage to make a cravat bandage

Many of these disposable packs are reusable by boiling or freezing them, which is of further convenience to the patient. When using these packs, it is recommended that they be placed in a cloth covering or a disposable towel to protect the skin. If the physician requests moist heat or cold treatment, you should use a clean, moist cloth towel between the plastic pack and the skin. Moisture facilitates conduction to tissues. Moist heat is less likely to cause burns of the skin, and it also provides deeper penetration to tissues. Unless otherwise ordered by the physician, the pack should be left in place for 20 minutes at a time. Generally, the standard instruction is on for 20 minutes and off 10. This may be repeated to increase circulation, but constant hot or cold is never advised.

Application of cold decreases local circulation temporarily, bacterial growth, and body temperature. It also is a temporary anesthetic, relieves inflammation, helps con-

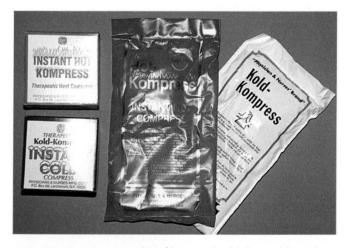

FIGURE 19–21 Examples of heat and cold disposable packs before activating the chemicals

trol bleeding, and reduces swelling. The average temperature is between 50° and 80°F (10° to 26.7°C). Cold applications are used in burns, sprains, strains, and bruises and in the initial treatment of injuries to the eye.

Heat applications are used to increase tissue temperature, circulation, and rate of healing. When heat is applied to an injured area, pain decreases. The average temperature is between 105° and 120°F (40.6° to 49°C). Heat treatments are used to relieve congestion in deep muscle layers and visceral organs and muscle spasms. The heat dilates blood vessels, which helps to increase circulation and reduce localized swelling after the initial 24 to 48 hours following the injury.

WOUNDS

 Skills Menu:
- Skin Puncture

It is important to know the characteristics and be able to identify and treat many types of wounds. **Abrasions** involve a scrape of the epidermis with dots of blood and possibly the presence of foreign material, such as dirt or gravel. First aid is to carefully clean the area with soap and water, apply an antiseptic solution or ointment, and cover with a dressing. If the abrasion resulted from contact with rusty metal or an unusually dirty object, an injection of tetanus toxoid or antitoxin may be required.

A wound caused by a sharp object that leaves a clean cut is called an **incision** and may need sutures to close. Some people prefer to use tape steristrips for closure rather than sutures if the wound is not too long or in an area that bends. The area must be carefully cleaned with soap and water, and an antiseptic may be applied before covering with a sterile dressing. A **laceration** is a tearing of body tissue and is more difficult to clean and suture properly. Special care must be taken to avoid infection. In the first aid care of an incision or laceration, the first concern must be control of bleeding. This is accomplished with direct pressure to the wound area and elevation of the extremity. If direct pressure is not effective, indirect pressure on the appropriate pressure point should be used.

A **puncture** wound is one made with a pointed object, such as an icepick, knife, or nail. First aid is to clean the wound area and if necessary enlarge the hole with a probe to allow for irrigation with antiseptic solutions. A puncture wound may also be the result of an animal or human bite. It is usually possible to identify the type of bite by looking at the shape of the wound. A human bite is identified by the shape of the denture and needs to be carefully cleaned. An animal bite may result in a laceration. A snake bite will show a two-fang wound. Treatment has changed from past practices. Recommended first aid is:

Do not apply cold packs or ice.
Do not apply a tourniquet.
Do not cut into the wound or attempt to suck out venom.
Do not apply any form of electric shock.

These past practices do little good and may cause additional harm. Instead, cleanse the area to remove any surface venom, and immobilize the victim. If the bite is located on an extremity, try to maintain the extremity *below* the level of the heart.

Initially, all bites should be thoroughly cleansed with soap and water and covered with a dressing. Any human or animal bite where the skin is broken should be seen by a physician.

A gunshot wound entrance will be a small deep puncture site with evidence in some cases of powder burns. The exit area may be considerably larger and have irregular borders. This type of wound needs to be treated by a physician. First aid would be to keep the patient in shock position and carefully monitor vital signs while taking measures to control hemorrhage. Gunshot and stab wounds must be reported to the police. The location of either of these wounds would dictate the first aid measures to be taken. If a lung puncture is suspected, do not remove the piercing object; call EMS or send the patient immediately to an emergency facility.

Cleaning and Bandaging Wounds

 Skills Menu:
- Bandaging
- Dry Dressing
- Elastic Bandages

Human skin cannot be sterilized, but the microorganisms that may be harmful can be washed off the skin's surface with soap, water, and **friction**. Applying a disinfectant following the washing will make the skin essentially germ free. The procedure of cleaning a wound is usually the responsibility of the medical assistant and is presented in Procedure 19–4.

When the wound does not bleed excessively and does not involve tissues below the skin, the area can be thoroughly cleaned. If a wound is superficial and will heal well with simple cleaning and protection from contamination, there is no need for sutures. Some clean cuts may be closed with adhesive steristrips or butterfly closures.

When bleeding has been severe, no attempt should be made to clean the area because it may restart the bleeding. Because the patient will need additional medical care, it can be cleaned then. A pressure bandage should be applied securely and the patient taken for emergency medical care immediately. (A pressure bandage usually consists of multiples layers of gauze squares or pads tightly fastened to the skin with tape or bound with roller bandage, ace bandage, or a cravat.) If such a patient comes to your office, wait for instructions from the physician before removing the pressure dressing. You will be responsible for having a suture set up for use when the physician is ready. You may question the patient or a relative to find out what caused the wound and how large and deep it is. You should also inquire about the most recent tetanus immunization booster

PROCEDURE

19-4 Clean Wound Areas

PURPOSE: To remove blood, debris, and surface microorganisms from the area of injury.

OSHA GUIDELINES: Standard Precautions require gloves to be worn if there is any possibility of coming into contact with blood, body fluids, or wound drainage. All contaminated materials are to be placed in biohazardous waste container.

EQUIPMENT: Basin, mild detergent, warm water, sterile gauze sponges, sterile sponge forceps, latex or vinyl gloves, sterile water, irrigation syringe, biohazardous waste bag, and bandage.

PERFORMANCE OBJECTIVE: Provided with all necessary equipment and supplies, demonstrate cleansing wounds, following procedure steps and Standard Precautions.

1. Assemble equipment and materials.
2. Wash hands and put on latex or vinyl gloves.
3. Grasp several gauze sponges with sponge forceps.
4. Dip into warm detergent water. **NOTE: Make certain water is at a comfortable temperature.**
5. Wash wound and wound area to remove microorganisms and any foreign matter. **NOTE: Be careful not to injure patient further with instrument. Clean wound area with sponges only working from inner to two to three inches around wound as you would for surgical prep. RATIONALE: This prevents bringing microorganisms from surrounding skin into open wound.**

6. Discard sponges into biohazardous waste bag or other disposable container.
7. Irrigate wound thoroughly with sterile water.
8. Blot wound dry with sterile gauze, and dispose in container with cleansing sponges.
9. Cover with dry sterile dressing, and bandage in place.
10. Advise patient to call physician immediately if evidence of infection develops. **NOTE: Patient should be told to watch for redness, swelling, and sensation of pain or fever. Typed instructions should be given to patient for follow-up care.**
11. Clean up work area. Place all used materials and gloves in the biohazardous waste bag and into proper receptacle for safe disposal.
12. Wash hands.
13. Record and initial procedure on patient's chart.

CHARTING EXAMPLE:

5-3-XX
Extensive wound over knee and lateral surface of right leg from fall off bicycle onto gravel area by road. Also jagged 10 cm laceration from broken glass fragment. Wound cleansed thoroughly in preparation for glass removal and suture.

S. Davis RMA (JDS)

---

and record the information on the patient's chart. The physician will write the orders for the necessary immunization(s). You should not proceed with any medication or injection until the order has been written by the physician.

After the physician has treated the wound, it may become your responsibility to apply the dressing. The following illustrations and procedures will provide you with guidelines to satisfactorily care for the patient.

- An injury to fingers or toes or an amputation can be effectively covered with the use of a non-stick dressing over the wound area, which is held in place with **recurrent** turns bandaging (as shown in Figure 19–22 and Procedure 19–5).
- An injury on the arms or legs will require the dressing to be held in place with an open or closed spiral bandage (as shown in Figure 19–23 and Procedure 19–6).

- A wound on the palm or back of the hand may be protected with a dressing and a figure-eight bandage (as shown in Figure 19–25 and Procedure 19–7).
- When applying a dressing to the forehead, ears, or eyes, a cravat may be used to hold the dressing in place (Figure 19–26 and Procedure 19–8). A cravat can be made from a triangular bandage (see Figure 19–20 and Procedure 19–9).
- A bandage that is particularly useful in keeping a dressing in place over a large head wound or a burn is the triangular bandage (Figure 19–27).
- The easiest and probably quickest way to bandage arms, legs, fingers, and toes is with tubular gauze bandage (Figure 19–28). This is accomplished with the use of an appropriately-sized cylindrical cage applicator. The amount of tube gauze you expect to use is stretched over the applicator and placed over the extremity. By

PROCEDURE

19-5 Apply Bandage in Recurrent Turn to Finger

PURPOSE: To hold dressing in place.

OSHA GUIDELINES: To comply with Standard Precautions, gloves must be worn if there is any possibility of coming into contact with blood or any body fluids.

EQUIPMENT: Scissors, dressing, bandage, latex or vinyl gloves, and biohazardous waste bag.

PERFORMANCE OBJECTIVE: Provided with all necessary equipment and supplies, apply recurrent turn bandage, following procedure steps and Standard Precautions. **NOTE: This procedure explains how to apply a dressing to a wound and then cover with bandage.***

1. Wash hands.
2. Assemble supplies.
3. Put on gloves
4. Carefully open dresisng without contaminating, and place over injury area.
5. Secure dressing with bandage of gauze. **NOTE: Start at the proximal end of the finger on the palm side and then directly over the finger to the proximal end on the back of the hand, and repeat several times.**

(*Omit step 4 to eliminate dressing application.)

6. Hold recurrent turns in place with spiral turns.
7. Secure by tying off gauze at wrist. **NOTE: Tie off using a figure-eight turn.**
   a. From the finger, take the end of the bandage diagonally across the back of the hand to the wrist.
   b. Circle the wrist once or twice.
   c. From the opposite side of the wrist, continue back to finger and loop.
   d. Repeat the figure eight several times and tie off at wrist, or tape in place. **NOTE: It is difficult to tear and handle tape while wearing gloves.**
8. Discard contaminated materials and gloves in biohazardous waste bag.
9. Wash hands.
10. Record and initial procedure on patient's chart.

CHARTING EXAMPLE:
1-12-XX
Recurrent turn bandage applied over dressing on right thumb.

J. Finelli, RMA (BAS)

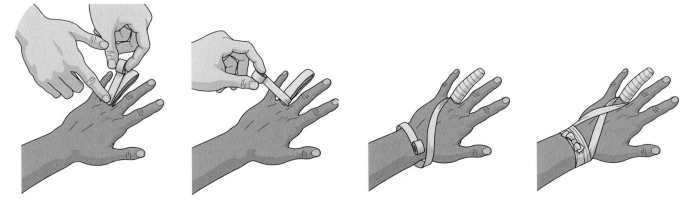

FIGURE 19–22 Recurrent turn bandage on finger

manipulating the cylinder around the extremity, grasping the tube gauze, withdrawing the cylinder, twisting the gauze, and repeating the sequence, a snug gauze bandage can be placed over the dressing.

ACHIEVE UNIT OBJECTIVES

Complete Chapter 19, Unit 3, in the workbook to help you obtain competency of this subject matter.

PROCEDURE

19-6 Apply Bandage in Open or Closed Spiral

PURPOSE: To support and cover a dressing. **NOTE: This procedure describes how to apply a dressing to a wound and then cover with bandage.***

OSHA GUIDELINES: To comply with Standard Precautions, gloves must be worn if there is any possibility of coming into contact with blood or any body fluids.

EQUIPMENT: Bandage, adhesive tape, scissors, sterile dressing, bandage, scissors, and biohazardous waste bag.

PERFORMANCE OBJECTIVE: Provided with all necessary equipment and supplies, apply open- and closed-spiral bandage, so that the dressing is secure, following procedure steps and standard precautions guidelines.

1. Wash hands.
2. Assemble needed supplies.
3. Put on gloves.
4. Carefully open dressing, without contaminating, and place over wound area.
5. Anchor bandage by placing end of bandage on bias at starting point (Figure 19–23A).
6. Encircle part, allowing corner of bandage end to protrude (Figure 19–23B). **CAUTION: Take care not to wrap extremities straight around because it impedes circulation to the distal part of the extremity.**
7. Turn down protruding tip of bandage (Figure 19–23C).
8. Encircle part again (Figure 19–23D).

(*Omit step 4 to eliminate dressing application.)

9. Continue to encircle area to be covered with spiral turns spaced so that they do not overlap. *OR* form closed spiral by continuing to encircle with overlapping spiral turns until all open spaces are covered (Figure 19–23E & F).
10. Complete bandage by tying off or taping in place (Figure 19–23G).
    NOTE:
    ■ Tape should be long enough to hold bandage snugly in place and applied to run in opposite direction from body movement.
    ■ Tearing adhesive tape is difficult while wearing gloves. You may find it necessary to first remove gloves and discard them into proper container (Figure 19–24).
11. If gloves are removed, reglove to clean area.
12. Discard contaminated materials and gloves in biohazardous waste bag.
13. Wash hands.
14. Record and initial procedure on patient's chart.

CHARTING EXAMPLE:
4-18-XX
Open spiral bandage applied over dressing on left lower leg.

C. Spatz CMA (JAS)

NOTE: Because there are insurance companies that require health care team members to sign after each order is performed as "C. Spatz," the physician checks off the chart by writing his initials in parentheses to indicate that orders were completed as directed: (JAS).

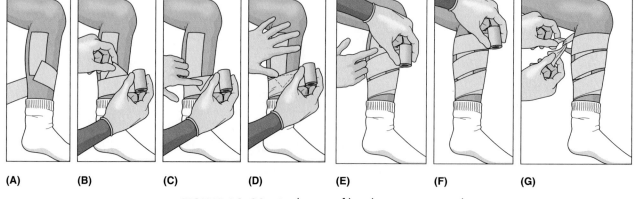

(A) (B) (C) (D) (E) (F) (G)

FIGURE 19–23 Application of bandage in open spiral

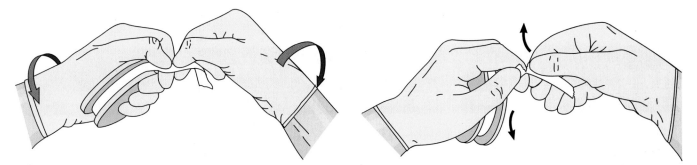

FIGURE 19–24 Tearing adhesive tape is much simpler when grasping the edge of the strip between the thumbnails and forefingers and using a quick rotary motion of the hands in the opposite directions.

PROCEDURE

19-7 Apply Figure-Eight Bandage to Hand and Wrist

PURPOSE: To hold dressing securely on hand. **NOTE: This procedure describes how to apply a dressing to a wound and then cover with bandage.***

OSHA GUIDELINES: To comply with Standard Precautions, gloves must be worn if there is any possibility of coming into contact with blood or any body fluids.

EQUIPMENT: Sterile dressing, bandage, latex or vinyl gloves, bandage, scissors, and biohazardous waste bag.

PERFORMANCE OBJECTIVE: Provided with all necessary equipment and supplies, apply a figure-eight bandage to hand and wrist neatly to secure dressing following procedure steps and Standard Precautions.

1. Wash hands.
2. Assemble needed supplies.
3. Put on gloves.

(*Omit step 4 to eliminate dressing application.)

4. Apply dressing. Do not contaminate any part that will touch wound area.
5. Anchor bandage with one or two turns around palm of hand.
6. Roll gauze diagonally across front of wrist and in figure-eight pattern around the hand (Figure 19–25).
7. Tie off at the wrist. **Caution: Do not impair circulation.**
8. Discard contaminated materials and gloves in biohazardous waste bag.
9. Wash hands.
10. Record and initial procedure on patient's chart.

CHARTING EXAMPLE:
6-14-XX
Figure-eight bandage applied to right hand.
                                    M. Gomes, CMA (PEP)

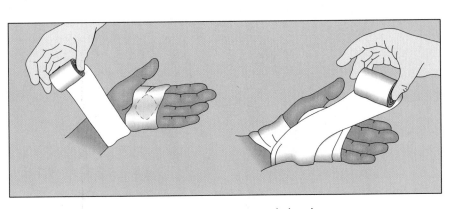

FIGURE 19–25 Figure-eight bandage

PROCEDURE

19-8 Apply Cravat Bandage to Forehead, Ear, or Eyes

PURPOSE: To hold a dressing neatly and securely in place. **NOTE: This procedure explains how to apply a dressing to a wound and then cover with a cravat bandage.***

OSHA GUIDELINES: To comply with Standard Precautions, gloves must be worn if there is any possibility of coming into contact with blood or any body fluids.

EQUIPMENT: Sterile dressing, cravat bandage, latex or vinyl gloves, and biohazardous waste bag.

PERFORMANCE OBJECTIVE: Provided with all necessary equipment and supplies, apply a cravat bandage to the head following procedure steps and standard precautions.

1. Wash hands.
2. Assemble needed supplies.
3. Put on gloves.

(*Omit step 4 to eliminate dressing application.)

4. Carefully place dressing over wound taking care not to contaminate area which will be over wound.
5. Place center of cravat over dressing.
6. Take ends around to opposite side of head and cross them. Do not tie (Figure 19–26).
7. Bring ends back to starting point and tie them.
8. Discard contaminated materials and gloves in biohazardous waste bag.
9. Wash hands.
10. Record and initial procedure on patient's chart.

CHARTING EXAMPLE:
8-28-XX
Cravat bandage applied over dressing on head.

S. Cimenella, CMA (RAK)

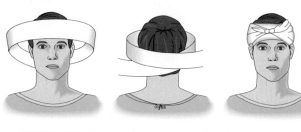

FIGURE 19–26 Applying a cravat bandage to the head

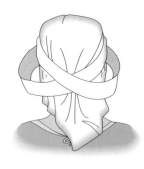

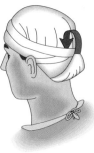

(D)

(E)

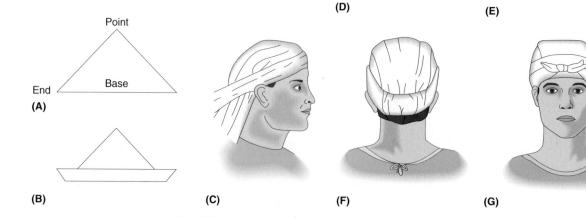

(A) Point / End / Base

(B)

(C)

(F)

(G)

FIGURE 19–27 Applying a triangular bandage to the head

PROCEDURE

19-9 Apply Triangular Bandage to Head

PURPOSE: To cover and support a dressing on the head. **NOTE: This procedure explains how to apply a dressing to a wound and then cover with a triangular bandage.***

OSHA GUIDELINES: To comply with Standard Precautions, gloves must be worn if there is any possibility of coming into contact with blood or any body fluids.

EQUIPMENT: Triangle bandage, sterile dressing, latex or vinyl gloves, and biohazardous waste bag.

PERFORMANCE OBJECTIVE: Provided with the necessary equipment, apply a triangular bandage to the head, following procedure steps and Standard Precautions so that the dressing is neat and secure.

1. Wash hands.

2. Assemble needed supplies.

3. Put on gloves.

4. Carefully place dressing over wound area without contaminating.

5. Fold a hem about two inches wide along base of bandage (Figure 19–27B).

(*Omit step 4 to eliminate dressing application.)

6. With hem on outside, place bandage on head so that middle of base is on forehead close to eyebrows and point hangs down back (Figure 19–27C & D).

7. Bring two ends around head above ears, and cross them just below bump at back of head.

8. Draw ends snugly around head, and tie them in center of forehead.

9. Steady head with one hand, and with other hand, draw point down firmly behind to hold dressing securely against head. Grasp point, and tuck it into area where bandage ends cross (Figure 19–27E).

10. Discard contaminated materials and gloves in biohazardous waste bag.

11. Wash hands.

12. Record and initial procedure on patient's chart.

CHARTING EXAMPLE:
9-14-XX
Triangular bandage applied over dressing on head wound.

M. Jackson, RMA (CST)

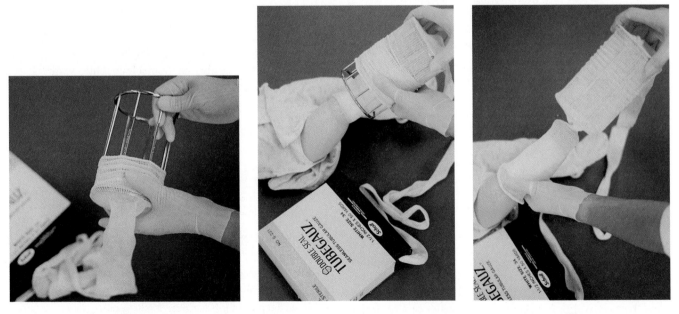

(A) **(B)** **(C)**

FIGURE 19–28 (A) Push Tubegauz onto cylinder and allow for excessive amount; (B) carefully place cylinder with Tubegauz over injured extremity; (C) hold end of Tubegauz gently above injury, and pull cylinder away from extremity, twisting the gauze. Repeat applications as desired for protection of wound.

UNIT 4
Recovering Function and Mobility

■ OBJECTIVES

Upon completion of the unit, meet the following performance objectives by verifying knowledge of the facts and principles presented through oral and written communication at a level deemed competent. Demonstrate the specific behaviors as identified in the terminal performance objectives of the procedures, observing all aseptic and safety precautions in accordance with health care standards.

1. Spell and define, using the glossary at the back of the text, all the **Words to Know** in this unit.
2. Explain why it is important to role-play being a patient.
3. Identify situations when the use of mobility equipment is indicated.
4. Role play instruction of range of motion exercises.
5. Demonstrate application of a sling.
6. Demonstrate fitting and instruction in use of a cane.
7. Demonstrate fitting and instruction in use of crutches.
8. Demonstrate instruction in use of a walker.
9. Demonstrate movement of patient from wheelchair to and from examination table.

AREAS OF COMPETENCE (AAMA)

This unit addresses content with the specific competency areas of *Patient care, Communication skills, Legal concepts,* and *Instruction,* as identified in the Medical Assistant Role Delineation Study. Refer to Appendix A for a detailed listing of the areas.

■ WORDS TO KNOW

ambulate	quad-base
angle	range-of-motion (ROM)
axilla	sling
balance	stabilize
crutches	support
flexibility	triangular bandages
gait	wheelchair
mobility	

This unit discusses the various devices that may be indicated in the process of recovering and gaining mobility and provides procedures covering the most common ones. Not only should you learn to instruct others in the proper use or application of the various pieces of equipment, but you should also participate in the patient's experience. Practice being the medical assistant and the patient so that you can appreciate the patient's dependence and understand the constraints involved. Few people realize the amount of strength and energy required to walk a long hallway or climb a stair using crutches. Spending a few hours in a wheelchair can also prove to be a very enlightening experience.

INDICATIONS FOR MOBILITY DEVICES

Ⓒ Skills Menu:
■ Safe Falling

Many times, following a serious illness or an accident, some form of supporting device or equipment is needed to allow a person to have as much **mobility** as possible. This may take the form of only a splint or a **sling** to support extremities or it may be nearly complete reliance in the form of a **wheelchair.** Examples of situations when the use of some type of device may be needed are as follows:

■ After an accident or injury—Sprains, fractures, and dislocations require temporary **support** and absence from use to permit healing.
■ Following a stroke—If there has been a loss of use of the extremities or if the person has become somewhat unsteady on his feet, something may be needed to help him maintain **balance**.
■ After surgery—When joints are replaced, supportive devices are necessary until muscles are strengthened around the new implant and the person is allowed to bear her own weight when she **ambulates**.
■ With a severe medical condition—Patients with congestive heart failure, emphysema, or similar debilitating illnesses frequently use supportive devices to aid their mobility.
■ Arthritis sufferers—The use of a cane or **crutches** to support a portion of the body weight reduces the discomfort in the knees, hips, and lower back.
■ The aged—The elderly often become unsteady on their feet and, because of the fear of falling, use a cane or walker to help **stabilize** themselves while walking.
■ Physically challenged—Persons with physical disabilities often require supportive devices to assist them with mobility.

A CAAHEP CONNECTION

The importance of precise *Verbal and non-verbal communication* is critical when instructing patients to perform exercises to restore function or using supporting devices to achieve mobility. It is also necessary to consider the stage of life the patient is in because it relates to his ability to comply with those instructions. This content addresses those requirements for medical assistant program curriculum.

Range-of-Motion Exercises

 Skills Menu:

- ROM Exercises

In addition to the use of mobility devices, patients can benefit greatly by improving their strength and **flexibility**. This can be accomplished with participation in a regular program of exercise. Regular exercise improves circulation and muscle tone and relieves tension. People who have followed an exercise routine regularly report that they experience a better outlook on life, have more energy, and feel healthier. The degree of exertion in any exercise routine will vary with individuals, and the physician's advice should be taken.

For patients who cannot engage in strenuous exercise, walking and **range-of-motion** exercises (**ROM**) are suggested to improve circulation, flexibility, and promote muscle tone (Figure 19–29).

ROM is defined as any body action involving muscles, joints, and natural directional movements, such as abduction, adduction, extension, flexion, pronation, and rotation. Such exercises are usually applied actively or passively in the treatment of orthopedic deformities, assessment of injuries and deformities, and athletic conditioning. These movements help to move each joint through its full range. Patients who have arthritis, bursitis, and other disabilities can be helped by these exercises.

Study the illustrations in Figure 19–29, and perform the motions yourself. Patients are frequently sent to a physical therapist for treatment and instruction, but the medical assistant is often responsible for showing the patient how to perform the exercises.

Flexibility Exercises

Flexibility exercises are designed to increase muscle strength and make the body more flexible. These exercises work specific flexor/extensor groups to improve their function. Flexibility exercises increase muscle tone and flexibility and also relieve tension (refer to Figure 20–6). You should be familiar with these exercises so that you can teach them to patients if they do not go to a physical therapist, engage in a structured exercise program, or use a personal trainer. This type of muscle stretching can be used prior to engaging in exercise routines to "warm up" muscles and thus prevent injury. Stretching muscles is also beneficial following exercise to engage in a "cooling down" period, which helps muscles return to a normal state of contraction.

Arm Sling

 Skills Menu:

- Applying an Arm Sling
- Elastic Bandages

A sling is often used to support an arm after a fracture or injury to the shoulder or arm. This aids the patient by supporting and protecting the injured extremity so that most activities can be continued until it is healed. It is important to learn the correct way to apply a sling with the pa-

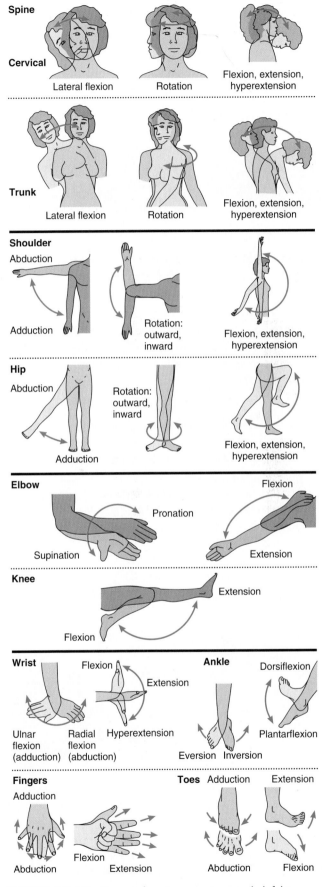

FIGURE 19–29 Range-of-motion exercises are helpful to patients who have limited physical activity. They improve circulation, increase flexibility, and promote improved muscle tone.

tient standing, sitting, or lying down. Care must be taken to elevate the head properly to assist the return of circulation and avoid swelling. You must also be sure that the sling is tied to one side and never over the spine where a knot becomes extremely uncomfortable.

Triangular bandages may be made from muslin or purchased in individual packages. Some physicians like to use a print material for children. The standard adult sling is about 55 inches across the base and 36 to 40 inches along the sides. See Procedure 19–10.

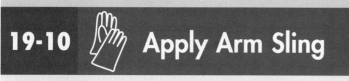

PROCEDURE

19-10 Apply Arm Sling

PURPOSE: To provide support for injured arm or shoulder.

OSHA GUIDELINES: To comply with Standard Precautions, gloves must be worn if there is any possibility of coming into contact with blood or any body fluids.

EQUIPMENT: Triangle and/or buckle type sling.

PERFORMANCE OBJECTIVE: Provided with the necessary equipment, demonstrate the steps in the procedure for applying an arm sling so that the arm is supported properly and the sling is correctly tied.

1. Wash hands.
2. Place one end of bandage over shoulder on uninjured side and let other end hang down over chest (Figure 19–30).
3. Pull point behind elbow of injured arm.
4. Pull end of bandage that is hanging down up around injured arm and over shoulder. Elevate hand four to five inches above elbow. **RATIONALE: Elevation aids in return**

circulation, which reduces swelling and discomfort. Tie ends together at side of neck (never over spine).

5. Bring point of bandage at elbow over front of sling, and pin to sling with safety pin.

NOTE:
- If pin is not available, twist point until it is snug against the elbow, and tie a single knot.
- Be sure ends of finger extend slightly beyond edge of sling. **RATIONALE: It is necessary to be able to observe fingers for signs of impaired circulation, such as swelling or discoloration.**

CHARTING EXAMPLE:
6-23-XX
Triangular sling applied to left arm for support following fall. Fingers elevated and extended from sling. No swelling observed, color normal.

P. Blair RMA, (JKR)

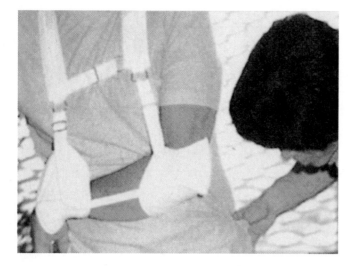

(A)

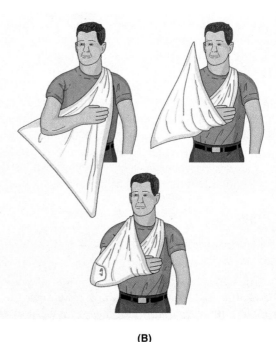

(B)

FIGURE 19–30 (A) Buckle type of arm sling for support, (B) applying an arm sling

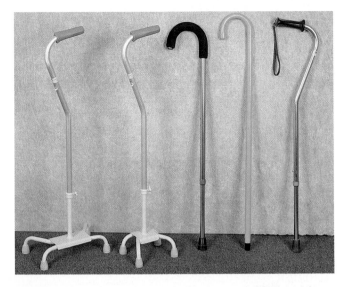

FIGURE 19–31 Types of standard canes: quad canes and single-tip canes

A Cane

C Skills Menu:
- Assisting with a Cane

The patient who needs only a cane for support should have one that is the proper length to fit comfortably in the hand with the arm hanging naturally at the side and the elbow flexed at about a 25° to 30° **angle**. The handle should be just below hip level. Many canes are adjustable; if not, they must be fitted to the correct length. Canes come in a variety of materials and types (Figure 19–31). An elderly patient usually has less trouble with a **quad-base** cane because its four "feet" provide a stable base that gives better support. The patient should carry the cane on the strong or uninjured side. The cane should swing forward with the injured extremity. Part of the weight is carried by the cane being firmly placed on the floor simultaneously with the injured extremity. Refer to Procedure 19–11.

P R O C E D U R E

19-11 Use a Cane

PURPOSE: To measure cane height and teach patient proper and safe use of cane.

EQUIPMENT: Cane.

PERFORMANCE OBJECTIVE: Provided with a cane, demonstrate adjusting the length of a cane, and provide patient with instruction to properly and safely use a cane. The cane will be the appropriate length, and the patient will demonstrate correct usage.

1. Identify patient, and confirm physician's orders. **RATIONALE: Speaking to the patient by name and checking chart ensures that you are performing the procedure for the correct patient.**

2. Assemble equipment. Check cane for intact rubber tip. **NOTE: Patient must be wearing nonskid shoes or foot coverings. RATIONALE: This helps prevent slipping or falling.**

3. Adjust height of cane so that patient's elbow is flexed comfortably at approximately a 25° to 30° angle, and check that the handle of the cane is positioned just below hip level of the uninjured or strong side.

4. Demonstrate for the patient the **gait** ordered for safe ambulation.
   a. Move the cane and injured extremity forward simultaneously.
   b. Then, move the strong or uninjured extremity forward.

5. Allow patient to practice the procedure. **NOTE: Observe patient, and be alert to assist patient and rescue in case of fall.**

6. Demonstrate going up stairs, and have patient practice. Move the uninjured extremity up first. Then move injured extremity up. Remind patient to use cane for support.

7. Demonstrate going down stairs, and have patient practice. Move uninjured extremity down first. Then, move injured extremity down. Remind patient to use cane for support.

8. Instruct patient to take small, slow steps. **RATIONALE: This aids in maintaining balance. NOTE: Answer questions patient may have and give emotional support.**

9. Ensure that cane height is correct and that patient is using cane correctly.

10. Record and initial on patient's chart.

CHARTING EXAMPLE:
7-23-XX
Cane adjusted for proper height. Rubber tip securely in place. Proper use of cane demonstrated to Julio, and he correctly returned the demonstration. Practiced on level floor and short flight of stairs. Advised him regarding selection of appropriate shoes to prevent slipping or falling.

B. Cox, CMA (REW)

Crutches

C Skills Menu:
- Assisting with Crutches

It is often necessary for a patient to walk with crutches to give a foot, ankle, knee, or leg injury or surgery an opportunity to heal. It is important for the crutches to be adjusted to the correct height (Figure 19–32A). This is accomplished by holding the crutches up to the side of the patient and adjusting them so that the underarm pad is two to three inches below the axilla. The handhold should be adjusted so that the hands fit comfortably with the arms extended. The axillary piece and the handhold should be foam padded for comfort. The patient should be instructed to stand on the uninjured foot while swinging the injured leg forward as the crutches are moved forward (Figure 19–32B). The weight of the body should be on the hands and never on the axillary area because over time, prolonged pressure on the axillary nerves can cause nerve damage.

Crutches can be used in three different gait or step patterns (refer to Procedure 19–12). The four-point gait shows the right crutch being positioned first, followed by moving the left foot. Then, the left crutch is moved forward, followed by the right foot. This makes for good stability but requires practice to coordinate the movements. The three-point gait positions both crutches and the left foot forward, then brings up the right foot. (The foot moved with the crutches depends upon which extremity is injured.) The two-point gait matches the crutch to the opposite foot moving them together. Practice all three gaits following the procedure until you are certain you could instruct a patient in the safe use of crutches.

Other varieties of crutches are designed for special situations. Lofstrand or forearm crutch (Figure 19–32C) eliminates axillary pressure and with the forearm cuff is more stable. This type would be used for long term rehabilitation. The platform crutch, (Figure 19–32D) is used when a patient's hand or forearm is not able to bear her body's weight.

Walker

C Skills Menu:
- Assisting with a Walker

A walker is useful for patients who, because of age or physical condition, cannot safely use crutches. The walker may be adjusted to proper height for the patient. The patient must be cautioned not to step too far into the walker because it makes it difficult to maintain balance. The patient should move the walker forward and then step into the walker while leaning slightly foward (Figure 19–34 and Procedure 19–13).

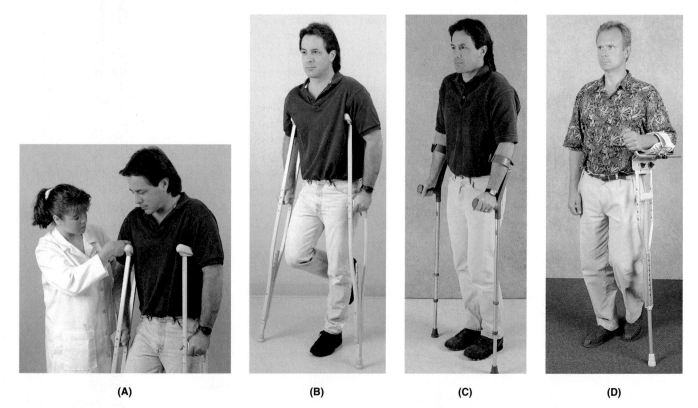

(A)   (B)   (C)   (D)

FIGURE 19–32 Types of crutches. (A) Measuring for axillary crutches. Note the height is about two to three fingers below the patient's armpit. (B) Axillary crutches. (C) Lofstrand or forearm crutches. (D) Platform crutch. This is an ideal substitute for a cane if the patient cannot bear weight on the forearm or hand.

PROCEDURE

19-12 Use Crutches

PURPOSE: To adjust crutches' length and teach patient to correctly and safely use crutches.

EQUIPMENT: Crutches, hand pads, rubber tips.

PERFORMANCE OBJECTIVE: Provided with all necessary equipment and supplies, adjust the length of the crutches, and demonstrate the steps of this procedure to instruct a patient in the correct use of crutches. The crutches will be the correct length, and the patient will be able to demonstrate the proper and safe use of crutches.

1. Identify patient, and confirm physician's orders. **RATIONALE: Speaking to the patient by name and checking chart ensures that you are performing the procedure for the correct patient.**

2. Assemble equipment. Make sure crutches are intact (hand pads and rubber tips) and stable.

3. Stabilize patient upright near wall or chair for support. **NOTE: Patient must be wearing non-skid shoes or foot coverings. RATIONALE: This helps prevent slipping or falling.**

4. Adjust length of crutches for patient so that the handles are comfortable with a 30° angle bend of the elbows with two inches between the area under the arm and the top of the crutches.

NOTE:
- Explain to the patient to support her weight at the handle and not under the arm. Rationale: Pressure in the axilla from upper body weight may damage nerves.
- Tell patient to take small steps slowly to avoid getting off balance and possibly falling.
- Instruct patient to stand on his uninjured foot while swinging the injured leg forward with crutches.

Crutches should be placed approximately four to five inches in front and four to five inches to the side of the patient's heels. Use Figure 19–33 to show the ordered gait for walking safely with crutches.

5. Demonstrate proper use of crutches.

6. Allow patient to practice the procedure to ensure correct use.

7. Record procedure on patient's chart.

CHARTING EXAMPLE:
2-16-XX
Bill's crutches were measured and adjusted for proper height. Hand pads and tips firmly attached. Demonstrated three-point gait, and had him return demonstration. Instructed not to bear weight on axillary area. Advised to select appropriate shoes to help prevent slipping or falling.

B. Cox, CMA (REW)

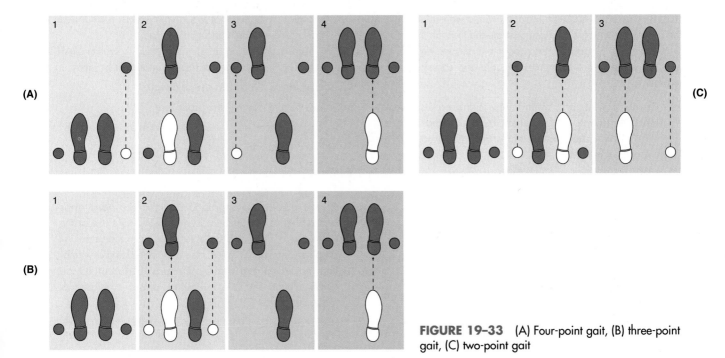

FIGURE 19–33 (A) Four-point gait, (B) three-point gait, (C) two-point gait

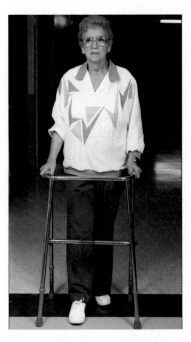

FIGURE 19–34 A walker provides stability and allows the patient to be mobile.

Some walkers come with wheels so that a patient can push it along as he walks and therefore can move a little quicker. This type of walker is less stable and may cause some patients to fall if it rolls away from them. Some more expensive wheeled walkers come with hand brakes that the patient can use to control the rolling, but this depends upon the response action and hand strength of the patient for control and safety. Some walkers even have a seating area so that the patient can stop and rest while walking. Many retirement and nursing home patients use walkers that they will bring to the physician's office. Become familiar with their use, and be able to instruct or correct a patient's usage.

Wheelchair

When a patient comes to your office in a wheelchair, you need to know how to help that patient from the wheelchair to the examination table and back to the wheelchair. This is not an easy task to do alone if the patient is unable to support his own weight. Always take care to enlist help from co-workers in order to prevent injury to a patient. Usually, examination rooms are limited in size, which

PROCEDURE

19-13 Use a Walker

PURPOSE: To adjust the walker's height and teach a patient the proper and safe use of a walker.

EQUIPMENT: Walker, handles, rubber tips.

PERFORMANCE OBJECTIVE: Provided with a walker, adjust it to the appropriate height and demonstrate the steps in the procedure to instruct a patient in the proper use of a walker. The patient will be able to demonstrate the safe and correct use of a walker.

1. Identify patient, and confirm physician's orders. **RATIONALE: Speaking to the patient by name and checking chart ensures that you are performing the procedure for the correct patient.**

2. Assemble equipment. Check walker for rubber tips, pads at handles, and stability.

3. Stabilize patient upright near wall or chair for support. **NOTE: Patient must be wearing non-skid shoes or foot coverings. RATIONALE: This helps prevent slipping or falling.**

4. The height of the walker should be adjusted so that the handles are at the patient's hip level, and the bend of the patient's elbows is at a comfortable 25° to 30° angle.

5. Position the walker around the patient (see Figure 19–34).

6. Instruct patient to pick up the walker, move it slightly forward, and walk into it.
   NOTE:
   - Instruct patient to keep all four feet of walker on the floor.
   - Explain to patient not to slide the walker. **RATIONALE: It may slip or catch and cause a fall.**
   - Instruct patient not to step too close to walker. **RATIONALE: This makes it difficult to maintain balance.**

7. Demonstrate the correct use of a walker.

8. Have patient practice the procedure.

9. Observe patient, and be ready to assist in case of possible fall.

10. Record and initial on patient's chart.

CHARTING EXAMPLE:
1-29-XX
Walker adjusted to appropriate height, and hand grips and rubber tips examined. Demonstrated safe use of the walker, and reminded Sally to wear non-skid shoes or slippers when walking. We also discussed being aware of floor coverings and possible hazards. She returned the demonstration and talked about the presence of hazards at her residence.

S. Moore, CMA, (RL)

PROCEDURE

19-14 Assist Patient from Wheelchair to Examination Table

PURPOSE: To safely move a patient from a wheelchair to an examination table.

EQUIPMENT: Examination table, wheelchair.

PERFORMANCE OBJECTIVE: Provided with necessary equipment, demonstate the steps in the procedure for assisting a patient from wheelchair to examination table in a safe manner.

1. Unlock wheels of chair, and wheel patient to examination room. **NOTE: Wheelchairs should always be locked in position when sitting still to prevent unexpected movement. This is accomplished by flipping brake on each wheel.**

2. Position chair as near as possible to place you want patient to sit on table.

3. Lower table to chair level. **NOTE: If this cannot be done, position footstool beside table, and determine if assistance will be needed.**

4. Lock wheels on chair.

5. Fold footrests back. If necessary, assist patient to move her feet.

6. Stand directly in front of patient with your feet slightly apart. To give a good base, place one foot forward.

7. Bend knees and have patient place hands on your shoulders while you place your hands under patient's armpits; assist patient to standing position. Pause in this position for a moment before next step.

8. Maintaining position of hands, pivot or side step to position in front of table (Figure 19–35).

9. Place one foot slightly behind you for support, and help patient to sitting position on table.

10. If it is necessary to use a stool, determine the assistance required, and enlist needed help *before* taking patient from wheelchair.

11. While supporting patient, stabilize stool by placing your feet on outside next to legs, and assist patient to step onto stool. **CAUTION: Be certain patient steps onto stool squarely to avoid tipping the stool.**

12. Assist patient to sit on table.

13. If patient still needs support, place one hand around patient's back. Help patient raise legs to table by placing free arm under legs and lifting them as patient turns. **NOTE: If patient needs to remove clothing, get someone to help you. One person balances patient while other removes necessary clothing.**

14. Place pillow under patient's head. Drape patient appropriately. **NOTE: Never leave a very ill or weak patient alone on a table. There is danger of a fall.**

15. Unlock chair wheels, and move chair out of way. **NOTE: If room is small, it may be necessary to place chair outside examination room.**

also adds to the difficulty of getting the patient to and from an examination table. Always remember to lock the wheels to prevent the chair from rolling away when assisting the patient to stand. It might be necessary to return her to the chair and adjust your position or hold. Refer to Procedures 19–14 and 19–15.

Patients who are residents of retirement or nursing facilities are often seen in the office. Many of them will arrive by wheelchair and may be accompanied by a nursing aide. To make it easier to assist these patients to stand or walk, a wide strap called a gait belt may be placed around their waist. The belt provides a way to hold and support the patient while she is trying to walk or being assisted in and out chairs or wheelchairs. The belt is grasped in front to assist the patient to rise and stand from a sitting position. It is held in the back to support the patient while walking. It would be advisable to practice using the gait belt so that when a patient does arrive, you will have some experience with the device. All of the procedures in

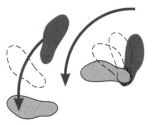

FIGURE 19–35 Position of feet when assisting patient from wheelchair onto examination table

this chapter need to be practiced many times so that you feel comfortable and confident when the need arises to use them.

Physical therapists, therapy aids, and medical supply representatives are trained to fit and instruct people in how to use various pieces of equipment. When it is known that a disability will occur, as with planned surgery, this is

PROCEDURE

19-15 Assist Patient from Examination Table to Wheelchair

PURPOSE: To safely move patient from examination table to wheelchair.

EQUIPMENT: Wheelchair, examination table.

PERFORMANCE OBJECTIVE: Provided with a wheelchair and an examination table, demonstrate the steps in the procedure to assist the patient from examination table to wheelchair in a safe manner.

1. Reposition chair and lock wheels.
2. Assist patient to sitting position on table. Support back if necessary. Lift patient's legs as patient is turned until feet dangle over side of the table.
3. Enlist help if needed and assist patient to dress.
4. Ask patient to put hands on your shoulders. Support patient on sides below armpits. Assist patient to step onto floor or have stepstool in place if table cannot be lowered to chair height. **CAUTION: Take special care to ensure that patient steps squarely on stool when getting down from examining table.** Place your feet against legs of footstool, on outside, to maintain its position.

5. Support patient into standing position on stool or floor.
6. Help patient step down from stool.
7. Side step or pivot patient to position in front of chair.
8. Have patient reach back to arms of chair as you help in lowering patient into chair.
9. Adjust footrests.
10. Unlock wheels, and return patient to reception room.

done prior to the procedure so that the patient is prepared to function as soon as possible after it is performed.

Being as careful as possible when assisting patients to walk or move about the office, you still may have one who becomes faint, slips, or suddenly becomes weak. Usually there is no way a single person can hold up someone who becomes "dead weight." The best option in this case is to ease the patient to the floor in such a way as to prevent injury. If you are supporting the patient from behind and he begins to fall backwards, grasp him under the arms, put one leg back with the foot at right angle, slide the other leg forward under the patient, and ease him to slide down your leg onto the floor (Figure 19–36A). If you are walking beside the patient, and she begins to fall forward, grasp her about the waist, extend your leg farthest from the patient forward, bend at the knees, and slowly lower the patient to the floor (Figure 19–36B). You must be careful to avoid injuring your own back by trying

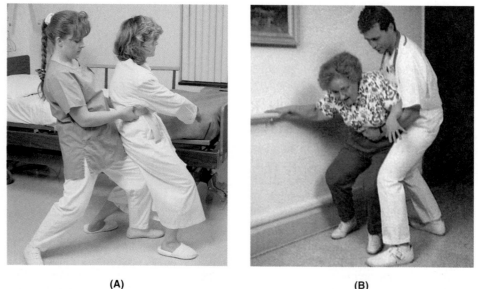

(A)   (B)

FIGURE 19–36 Easing the falling patient safely to the floor: (A) from behind, (B) from beside

to support too much weight. Keep your back as straight as possible, bend from the knees, and use your large thigh muscles to handle the weight. Whenever a patient falls, have the physician examine him as soon as possible, and be sure to carefully document the incident on the chart and on an accident/incident form if indicated by the office policy manual.

SAFETY AT HOME

Skills Menu:
- Safe Lifting
- Safe Falling

Patients and their families must be informed of the importance of maintaining a safe home environment for persons using ambulatory aids. Care must be taken to keep floors free of spills and clutter. It is especially important to remove all loose throw rugs or damaged floor covering which might cause the patient to fall. Any bare floor care product, such as floor wax, that might cause the floor to be slippery must be avoided. It is also important to ensure that appropriate footwear is worn. It should be well-fitting and have a non-slip walking surface.

RELATING TO ABHES

Chapter 19 discusses preparing for and responding to medical emergencies with acute illness, injuries, and accidents; recognizing diabetic coma and insulin shock symptoms; the signs of stroke; and providing immediate response to obstructed airway, respiratory, and cardiac arrest. The chapter also discusses the use of range of motion exercise and various mobility equipment to regain function. This content relates to the ABHES accreditation requirements of *Caring for patients with special and specific need,* and *Emotional crises/patients and/or family* within the content area of *Psychology of Human Relations,* and *Basic skills and procedures used in medical emergencies, Medical Equipment, First Aid,* and *CPR,* within the content area of the *Medical Office Clinical Procedures.*

ACHIEVE UNIT OBJECTIVES

Complete Chapter 19, Unit 4, in the workbook to help you obtain competency of this subject matter.

Medical-Legal-Ethical Scenario

Mary Santino was an 80-year-old Italian woman for whom English was a limited second language. She lived alone, but two of her children were only a few miles away. She was experiencing increased pain in her right hip, and it was becoming obvious that she was going to need a surgical procedure to correct her problem. Attempts to get her to take off her excess weight to reduce the stress on her hip had not been successful. Until an appointment could be arranged with an orthopedic surgeon and her surgery scheduled, Dr. Long suggested that she use a cane to take some of the weight-bearing load off her hip. Shelly, the medical assistant, retrieved an adjustable standard cane from the storage room for her to use temporarily. She had Mary stand up and shortened the cane for the proper height. Shelly explained to Mary to put the cane in her left hand and put weight on it at the same time she put weight on her right leg. She took Mary to the stairway to show her how to go up and down stairs because Mary lived in a two-story home. After watching Mary trying to use the cane, Shelly felt she was having a lot of difficulty. She didn't seem to have enough strength in her left arm to take much stress off her leg. She also seemed to have problems using the proper gait, often using the cane with the wrong leg. She was especially concerned about her not going up or down stairs correctly. But then she thought that maybe with a little more practice at home she would be more successful because Mary indicated she understood what to do.

CRITICAL THINKING CHALLENGE

1. What factors might be involved in Mary's problem with using a cane?
2. What options does Shelly have to help Mary with her mobility?
3. Does Shelly have an obligation to question the physician's order?
4. What risk factors may be involved in this situation?
5. Are there any options at home to be considered?
6. Review the Medical Assistant Role Delineation Chart, and identify at least four major areas that apply to this scenario.

RESOURCES

American Heart Association (2001). Advanced cardiovascular life support provider manual. Dallas: Author.

Beebe R. and Funk D. (2001). Fundamentals of emergency care. Clifton Park, NY: Delmar Learning.

American College of Emergency Physicians (1999). EMT-Basic field care: a care-based approach. St. Louis: Mosby.

Hegner, B.R., Caldwell E., and Needham J.F. (1999). Nursing assistant: a nursing process approach (8th ed.). Clifton Park, NY: Delmar Learning.

Lindh, W.Q., et al. (2002). Comprehensive medical assisting, administrative and clinical competencies (2nd ed.). Clifton Park, NY: Thompson Learning/Delmar Learning.

Simmers, L. (2001). Diversified health occupations (5th ed.). Clifton Park, NY: Delmar Learning.

WEB LINKS

www.aaem.org/home.html (American Academy of Emergency Medicine)

Provides current resources and news.

www.nceml.org (National Center for Emergency Medicine Informatics)

A collection of many items. Note clinical calculators and medical e-tools.

www.americanheart.org (American Heart Association)

Find symptoms of heart attack and stroke and information on association services, managing your weight, and cholesterol. Locate the CPR information, and find centers where you can train.

www.redcross.org (American Red Cross)

Learn about health and safety services and classes in first aid, CPR, and AED. Take the CPR quiz.

Behaviors and Health

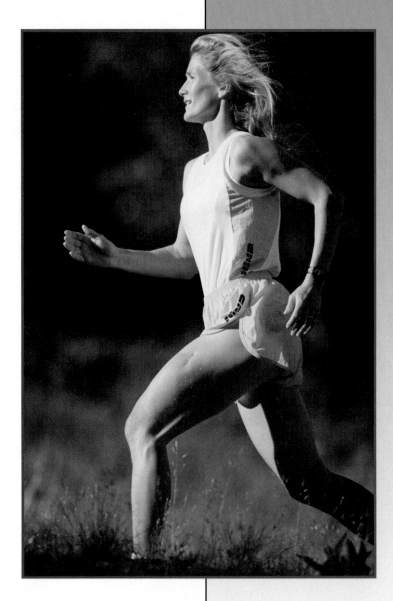

20

Behaviors Influencing Health

As you gain experience in the field, it will soon become apparent that patients have a tendency to depend on you for advice. The physician prescribes a treatment plan for the patient to follow and usually discusses it with the patient. Generally, the patient's next step is to ask you to explain the details. Therefore, you must have a complete understanding of the policies of the health care facility. Personal opinions should be restrained. This chapter concerns the significance of diet, exercise, weight control, sleep, and the way personal behaviors influence health. Habit-forming substances and treatment, the support groups for these patients, and a look at stress and how to use time well will be discussed. These areas are vitally important to you and to the patients you will serve.

UNIT 1

Nutrition, Exercise, and Weight Control

■ OBJECTIVES

Upon completion of the unit, meet the following performance objectives by verifying knowledge of the facts and principles presented through oral and written communication at a level deemed competent.

1. Spell and define, using the glossary at the back of the text, all of the **Words to Know** in this unit.
2. Explain the significance of diet and exercise to health.
3. Name and discuss the six food groups of the food pyramid.
4. Name the fat-soluble vitamins.
5. Name the water-soluble vitamins.
6. Name the essential minerals.
7. List ways to encourage patient compliance in weight control.
8. Explain how the body uses nutrients best.
9. Explain how to communicate dietary needs to someone who does not speak English.
10. Describe and discuss dietary and health concerns of adolescents.
11. Explain the importance of sleep and a positive outlook in regard to health.
12. Describe eating disorders in adolescence.
13. Describe nutrition labels on food products.
14. List guidelines for promoting good health.
15. Demonstrate stretching exercises.
16. Explain why sleep is essential to good health.

AREAS OF COMPETENCE (AAMA)

This unit addresses content within the specific competency areas of *Diagnostic orders, Patient care, Professionalism, Communication skills, Legal concepts,* and *Instruction,* as identified in the Medical Assistant Role Delineation Study. Refer to Appendix A for a detailed listing of the areas.

■ WORDS TO KNOW

amenorrhea	dietician
anorexia nervosa	emaciation
anorexic	health
beriberi	infirmity
binge	NREM (non-rapid eye
bulimia nervosa	movement)
calorie	nutrition
deprivation	obese

positive	scurvy
purge	sleep apnea
REM (rapid eye	tactile
movement)	therapeutic
rickets	

With today's attention to physical fitness, the medical assistant must be well informed to answer the countless inquiries patients make concerning diet and exercise programs. The physician will decide what is best for each patient after all data from the medical history, examination, laboratory findings, and other pertinent information have been evaluated. It is up to you to reinforce the physician's orders and help patients adapt those orders to their particular lifestyles.

As you begin to practice skills in communicating information to patients regarding treatment plans and their overall health, it is important for you to have a basic understanding of the meaning of health. **Health** is defined by the World Health Organization as a state of complete physical and mental or social well-being. Health is not merely the absence of disease or **infirmity**. All things

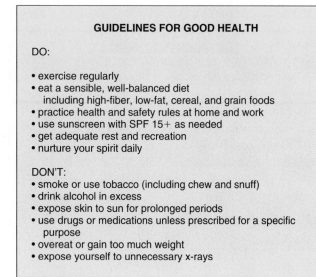

FIGURE 20–1   Guidelines for good health

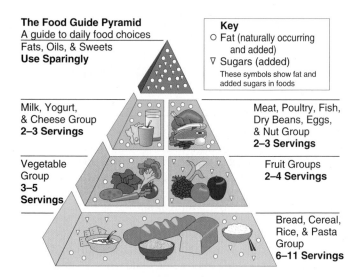

FIGURE 20–2   Food Guide Pyramid shows the recommended servings for daily nutritional needs (From How to Eat for Good Health, courtesy of National Dairy Council).

conducive to good health are referred to as healthful. Healthful living habits are essential for one to maintain good physical condition or to stay physically fit. Fitness, therefore, refers to being in good physical condition or being healthy. There are simple guidelines that can help to keep us in good health, increase vitality, and may even increase life expectancy. Figure 20–1 outlines the suggestions advised for the general population. Those who are in the health care professions are urged to set a good example to those patients we teach.

NUTRITION

Patient education in proper nutrition is one of your many responsibilities. **Nutrition** is defined as the sum of the processes involved in taking in, assimilating, and using nutrients. This includes the processes by which the body uses food for energy, maintenance, and growth.

The Food Guide Pyramid

The food guide pyramid was introduced in the spring of 1992 by the United States Department of Agriculture. This pyramid concept replaces the "food wheel" and the old basic four food groups that have been used since 1946. The pyramid is divided into six sections; the foods listed in the largest sections are those foods that should be consumed in the greatest quantities. Notice that at the top of the triangle, for example, are fats, oils, and sweets; this indicates that foods such as butter, salad oil, candy, and other sweets should be used sparingly. Explaining the food pyramid to patients will encourage healthful eating habits. Eating sensibly makes people feel better and more energetic. When people feel well, they have a more **positive** outlook on life.

It is a good idea to post the food guide pyramid shown in Figure 20–2 near the scale or on the wall of each examination room. Make it clear to patients that they are not expected to eat everything on the pyramid every day. En-

courage patients to select the bulk of their daily foods from the inner sections of the pyramid so they will likely eat sufficient amounts of fruits and vegetables. Some experts in nutrition think the non-starchy vegetables and fruits should take the bottom section of the pyramid and the refined grains the small triangle at the top, keeping the GI (glycemic index) low. Eating whole grain breads and fiber-containing foods can help you feel full longer. This food guide appears on many food products, such as cereals and breads, to remind people to eat sensibly. On television, there is a vast array of cooking shows. There are cooking magazines and cookbooks with recipes that can reinforce healthy eating habits. Helping patients in selecting materials that may benefit them is a way to keep them motivated in following a diet plan. Some of these patient education materials can be offered to patients in the reception area. Give patients support by letting them know that you are pleased that they are making progress in healthy choices in their diets. An attractive poster is an even better way to suggest good eating habits. Figure 20–3 illustrates an example of a colorful poster to catch the eye of patients to give them a visual reminder of healthy food choices. You may want to place a note regarding the "other" foods that have only slight nutritional value (fats, oils, and sweets) next to the poster. This reminder may help patients realize the importance of avoiding large amounts of the foods found at the top of the pyramid. Some patients have never been educated in this area of importance. Many pharmaceutical companies offer complimentary instructional materials to send home with patients to help reinforce your educational efforts.

Vitamins and Minerals

Vitamins are organic substances found in foods that are essential to good health and growth. Vitamins are called micronutrients. As the name implies, only a trace quantity

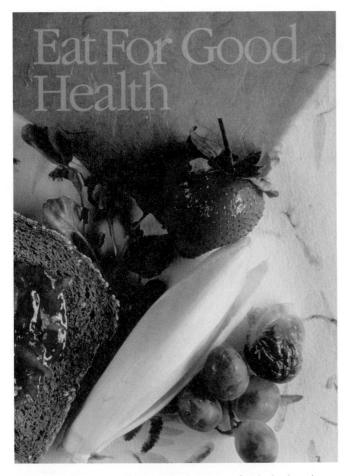

FIGURE 20–3 Colorful posters of nutritious foods displayed in your office, such as the one in this picture, can encourage dialogue between you and patients regarding healthy eating habits. (Courtesy of National Cancer Institute and Bill Branson, photographer.)

is required for enzymatic reaction in the body. If the body does not receive adequate vitamins or does not absorb them sufficiently, deficiency diseases may result. The major ones are **rickets**, **scurvy**, and **beriberi**. Rickets is the result of a deficiency of vitamin D; scurvy, of vitamin C or ascorbic acid; and beriberi, of vitamin B or thiamine. Vitamins A, D, E, and K are fat-soluble vitamins. Vitamin C and the B complex vitamins are water-soluble.

With a well-balanced diet, there is little likelihood of vitamin-deficiency diseases. Prepared foods display a list of their nutritional values on their labels for consumer information. Vitamins are added to many foods because of their loss in preparation. Patients will be advised by the physician if a vitamin or mineral supplement is necessary.

Minerals are naturally occurring nonorganic, homogeneous, solid substances. Thirteen are said to be essential to good health. They are supplied by a variety of meats and vegetables. Minerals found to be missing most often from the diet are calcium, iron, and iodine. Metabolic disturbances can be caused by insufficient amounts of zinc, copper, magnesium, and potassium.

The principal vitamins, minerals, and micronutrients are listed in Table 20–1 and 20–2 and a basic calorie chart in Table 20–3. Careful study of these charts will give you an understanding of the food sources, the function of each in the body's growth and repair, the effects of deficiency and toxicity, and the dosages recommended for daily intake.

Several servings of fiber-rich foods (fruits, vegetables, peas and beans, whole grain cereals) should be included in the daily diet to promote a healthy digestive tract and prevent constipation. Notice that the sections of the food pyramid that list these nutrients are more than half the size of the entire pyramid to show their importance. Encourage patients to modify cooking techniques by using less fats, oils, and sugars (smallest portion of pyramid) and by baking, broiling, boiling, roasting, grilling, poaching, or steaming meats and other foods instead of frying. These modified cooking practices can also help to reduce the amount of calories, cholesterol, sodium, sugar, and saturated and total fat from the diet. Review the information in Chapter 11 regarding the immune system and foods that aid the body in defense against disease.

Encourage patients to read food labels at the grocery store before they buy any food. As patients are planning their daily menu, advise them to again read food labels and note the percentage of each of the nutrients. They should also pay attention to the serving size, which is usually a half cup per item (likely not what is normally consumed). Explain to patients that if they plan a 2000 calorie per day diet, the percentage of total fat of the food products they eat is of that 2000 calorie per day total. The percentages refer to the total intake per day. Remind patients about attractive wording, such as no cholesterol and low fat. Some food labels claim to be low in fat or salt, or to contain no (zero) cholesterol, but they are generally high in sugar and calorie content. Table 20–3 lists single servings of some common foods with their total calorie content, carbohydrate and fat grams, and total calories from fats and carbohydrates. This may be used as a guide in meal planning. Prepared foods and many of the fast foods usually have more fat, sugar, and salt than those foods that we cook for ourselves. Advise patients that eating fast foods should be the exception and not a regular meal habit. Reduced-calorie food items also can often have a high salt or sodium content. The federal Nutritional Labeling and Education Act requires that labels list all ingredients in foods. An example of such labeling is shown in Figure 20–4. People who have food allergies will find the list very helpful in avoiding those foods that could cause them problems. It is important to understand how the ingredients are listed. The ingredient with the highest content in the product is listed first. The last ingredient listed is the one with the least amount contained in the product. A package of noodles, for example, may read: flour, eggs, niacin, iron, thiamin mononitrate, riboflavin. The main ingredient is flour with only a very small amount of riboflavin. All of the ingredients are listed in decreasing amounts, beginning with the most to the least.

Explaining to patients how to count calories, carbohydrates, fat grams, and so on will help them realize the importance of planning meals that are well balanced and sensible. For those who are interested in eating a healthier diet,

TABLE 20-1

FOOD AND NUTRITION BOARD, INSTITUTE OF MEDICINE—NATIONAL ACADEMY OF SCIENCES DIETARY REFERENCE INTAKES: RECOMMENDED INTAKES FOR INDIVIDUALS						
Life Stage Group	Calcium (mg/d)	Phosphorus (mg/d)	Magnesium (mg/d)	Vitamin D (μg/d)[a,b]	Fluoride (mg/d)	Thiamin (mg/d)
INFANTS						
0–6 mo	210*	100*	30*	5*	0.01*	0.2*
7–12 mo	270*	275*	75*	5*	0.5*	0.3*
CHILDREN						
1–3 y	500*	**460**	**80**	5*	0.7*	**0.5**
4–8 y	800*	**500**	**130**	5*	1*	**0.6**
MALES						
9–13 y	1,300*	**1,250**	**240**	5*	2*	**0.9**
14–18 y	1,300*	**1,250**	**410**	5*	3*	**1.2**
19–30 y	1,000*	**700**	**400**	5*	4*	**1.2**
31–50 y	1,000*	**700**	**420**	5*	4*	**1.2**
51–70 y	1,200*	**700**	**420**	10*	4*	**1.2**
>70 y	1,200*	**700**	**420**	15*	4*	**1.2**
FEMALES						
9–13 y	1,300*	**1,250**	**240**	5*	2*	**0.9**
14–18 y	1,300*	**1,250**	**360**	5*	3*	**1.0**
19–30 y	1,000*	**700**	**310**	5*	3*	**1.1**
31–50 y	1,000*	**700**	**320**	5*	3*	**1.1**
51–70 y	1,200*	**700**	**320**	10*	3*	**1.1**
>70 y	1,200*	**700**	**320**	15*	3*	**1.1**
PREGNANCY						
≤18 y	1,300*	**1,250**	**400**	5*	3*	**1.4**
19–30 y	1,000*	**700**	**350**	5*	3*	**1.4**
31–50 y	1,000*	**700**	**360**	5*	3*	**1.4**
LACTATION						
≤18 y	1,300*	**1,250**	**360**	5*	3*	**1.4**
19–30 y	1,000*	**700**	**310**	5*	3*	**1.4**
31–50 y	1,000*	**700**	**320**	5*	3*	**1.4**

Note: This table presents Recommended Dietary Allowances (RDAs) in **bold type** and Adequate Intakes (AIs) in ordinary type followed by an asterisk (*). RDAs and AIs may both be used as goals for individual intake. RDAs are set to meet the needs of almost all (97 to 98 percent) individuals in a group. For healthy breastfed infants, the AI is the mean intake. The AI for other life-stage and gender groups is believed to cover needs of all individuals in the group, but lack of data or uncertainty in the data prevent being able to specify with confidence the percentage of individuals covered by this intake.

[a]As cholecalciferol, 1 μg cholecalciferol = 40 IU vitamin D.

[b]In the absence of adequate exposure to sunlight.

TABLE 20-2

PRINCIPAL MICRONUTRIENTS				
Micro-Nutrient	Principal Sources	Functions	Effects Of Deficiency and Toxicity	Usual Therapeutic Dosage
Vitamin A	Fish liver oils, liver, egg yolk, butter, cream, vitamin A-fortified margarine, green leafy or yellow vegetables	Photoceptor mechanism of retina; integrity of epithelia; lysosome stability, glycoprotein synthesis	*Deficiency:* Night blindness, perifollicular hyperkeratosis, xerophthalmia; keratomalacia *Toxicity:* Headache; peeling of skin, hepatosplenomegaly, bone thickening	10,000–20,000 μg (30,000–60,000 IU/day)
Vitamin D	Fortified milk is main dietary source, fish liver oils, butter, egg yolk, liver, ultraviolet irradiation	Calcium and phosphorus absorption, resorption, mineralization, and collagen maturation of bone; tubular reabsorption of phosphorus (?)	*Deficiency:* Rickets (tetany sometimes associated); osteomalacia *Toxicity:* Anorexia; renal failure; metastatic calcification	*Primary Deficiency* 10–40 μg (1400–1600 IU)/day *Metabolic Deficiency* 1–2 μg/day 1.25–(OH)$_2$D$_3$ or 1α–(OH)D$_3$
Vitamin E group	Vegetable oil, wheat germ, leafy vegetables, egg yolk, margarine, legumes	Intracellular antioxidant; stability of biologic membranes	*Deficiency:* RBC hemolysis, creatinuria; ceroid deposition in muscle	30–100 mg/day
Vitamin K (activity) Vitamin K$_1$ (phytonadione) Vitamin K$_2$ (menaquinone)	Leafy vegetables, pork, liver, vegetable oils, intestinal flora after newborn period	Prothrombin formation; normal blood coagulation	*Deficiency:* Hemorrhage from deficient prothrombin *Toxicity:* Kernicterus	In situations conductive to neonatal hemorrhage, 2–5 mg during labor or daily for 1 wk prior; or 1–2 mg to newborn
Essential fatty acids (linoleic, arachidonic acids)	Vegetable seed oils (corn, sunflower, safflower); margarines blended with vegetable oils	Synthesis of prostaglandins, membrane structure	Growth cessation, dermatosis	Up to 10 g/day
Thiamine (vitamin B$_1$)	Dried yeast; whole grains; meat (especially pork, liver); enriched cereal products; nuts; legumes; potatoes	Carbohydrate metabolism, central and peripheral nerve cell function, myocardial function	Beriberi; infantile and adult (peripheral neuropathy, cardiac failure; Wernicke-Korsakoff syndrome)	30–100 mg/day
Riboflavin (vitamin B$_2$)	Milk, cheese, liver, meat, eggs, enriched cereal products	Many aspects of energy and protein metabolism integrity of mucous membranes	Cheilosis; angular stomatitis; corneal vascularization; amblyopia, sebaceous dermatosis	10–30 mg/day
Niacin (nicotinic acid, niacinamide)	Dried yeast, liver, meat, fish, legumes, whole-grain enriched cereal products	Oxidation-reduction reactions, carbohydrate metabolism	Pellagra (dermatosis, glossitis, GI and CNS dysfunction)	Niacinamide 100–1000 mg/day
Vitamin B$_6$ group (pyridoxine)	Dried yeast, liver, organ meats, whole-grain cereals, fish, legumes	Many aspects of nitrogen metabolism, e.g., transaminations, porphyrin and heme synthesis, tryptophan conversion to niacin. Linoleic acid metabolism	Convulsions in infancy, anemias; neuropathy; seborrhea-like skin lesions Dependency states	25–100 mg/day

(continues)

TABLE 20–2 *(continued)*

PRINCIPAL MICRONUTRIENTS—continued

Micro-Nutrient	Principal Sources	Functions	Effects Of Deficiency and Toxicity	Usual Therapeutic Dosage
Folic acid	Fresh green leafy vegetables, fruit, organ meats, liver, dried yeast	Maturation of RBCs; synthesis of purines and pyrimidines	Pancytoperia; megaloblastosis (especially pregnancy, infancy, malabsorption)	1 mg/day
Vitamin B$_{12}$ (cobalamins)	Liver, meats (especially beef, pork, organ meats); eggs; milk & milk products	Maturation of RBCs; neural function; DNA synthesis, related to folate coenzymes; methionine and acetate synthesis	Pernicious anemia; fish tapeworm & vegan anemias; some psychiatric syndromes, nutritional amblyopia Dependency states	In pernicious anemia 50 μg/day IM first 2 wk, 100 μg twice/wk next 2 mo, thereafter 100 μg/mo
Biotin	Liver, kidney, egg yolk, yeast, cauliflower, nuts, legumes	Carboxylation and decarboxylation of oxalocetic acid; amino acid and fatty acid metabolism	Dermatitis, glossitis Dependency states	150–300 μg/day
Vitamin C (ascorbic acid)	Citrus fruits, tomatoes, potatoes, cabbage, green peppers	Essential to osteoid tissue; collagen formation; vascular function; tissue respiration and wound healing	Scurvy (hemorrhages, loose teeth, gingivitis)	100–1000 mg/day
✷ Sodium	Wide distribution—beef, pork, sardines, cheese, green olives, corn bread, potato chips, sauerkraut	Acid-base balance; osmotic pressure; pH of blood; muscle contractility; nerve transmission; sodium pumps	*Deficiency:* Hyponatremia *Toxicity:* Hypernatremia; confusion, coma	
✷ Potassium	Wide distribution—whole and skim milk, bananas, prunes, raisins	Muscle activity, nerve transmission, intracellular acid-base balance and water retention	*Deficiency:* Hypokalemia; paralysis, cardiac disturbances *Toxicity:* Hyperkalemia; paralysis, cardiac disturbances	
✷ Calcium	Milk and milk products, meat, fish, eggs, cereal products, beans, fruits, vegetables	Bone and tooth formation; blood coagulation; neuromuscular irritability; muscle contractility; myocardial conduction	*Deficiency:* Hypocalcemia and tetany; neuromuscular hyperexcitability *Toxicity:* Hypercalcemia; GI atony, renal failure; psychosis	10–30 ml 10% calcium gluconate soln IV in 24 h
Phosphorus	Milk, cheese, meat, poultry, fish, cereals, nuts, legumes	Bone and tooth formation; acid-base balance, component of nucleic acids, energy production	*Deficiency:* Irritability; weakness; blood cell disorders; GI tract and renal dysfunction *Toxicity:* Hyperphosphatemia in renal failure	Potassium acid and di-basic phosphate parenteral 600 mg (18.8 mEq)/day

(continues)

TABLE 20-2 *(continued)*

PRINCIPAL MICRONUTRIENTS—continued

Micro-Nutrient	Principal Sources	Functions	Effects Of Deficiency and Toxicity	Usual Therapeutic Dosage
Magnesium	Green leaves, nuts, cereal grains, seafoods	Bone and tooth formation; nerve conduction; muscle contraction; enzyme activation	*Deficiency:* Hypomagnesemia; neuromuscular irritability *Toxicity:* Hypermagnesemia; hypotension, respiratory failure, cardiac disturbances	2–4 ml 50% magnesium sulfate soln/day IM
✶ Iron	Wide distribution (except dairy products)—soybean flour, beef, kidney, liver, beans, clams, peaches Much unavailable (<20% absorbed)	Hemoglobin, myoglobin formation, enzymes	*Deficiency:* Anemia; dysphagia; koilonychia; enteropathy *Toxicity:* Hemochromatosis; cirrhosis; diabetes mellitus; skin pigmentation	Ferrous sulfate or gluconate 300 mg orally t.i.d.
✶ Iodine	Seafoods, iodized salt, dairy products Water variable	Thyroxine (T_4) and triiodothyronine (T_3) formation and energy control mechanisms	*Deficiency:* Simple (colloid, endemic) goiter; cretinism; deaf-mutism *Toxicity:* Occasional myxedema	150 μg iodine/day as potassium iodide added to salt 1:10–40,000 ppm
Fluorine	Wide distribution—tea, coffee Fluoridation of water supplies with sodium fluoride 1.0–2.0 ppm	Bone and tooth formation	*Deficiency:* Predisposition to dental caries; osteoporosis (?) *Toxicity:* Fluorosis, mottling, pitting of permanent teeth; exostoses of spine	Sodium fluoride 1.1–2.2 mg/day orally
Zinc	Wide distribution—vegetable sources Much unavailable	Component of enzymes and insulin; wound healing; growth	*Deficiency:* Growth retardation; hypogonadism; hypogeusia; in cirrhosis; acrodermatitis enteropathica	30–150 mg zinc sulfate/day orally
Copper	Wide distribution—organ meat, oysters, nuts, dried legumes, whole-grain cereals	Enzyme component	*Deficiency:* Anemia in malnourished children; Menkes' kinky hair syndrome *Toxicity:* Hepatolenticular degeneration; some biliary cirrhosis (?)	0.3 mg/kg/day copper sulfate, orally
Cobalt	Green leafy vegetables	Part of vitamin B_{12} molecule	*Deficiency:* Anemia in children (?) *Toxicity:* Beer-drinker's cardiomyopathy	20-30 mg/day cobaltous chloride, orally
Chromium	Wide distribution—brewer's yeast	Part of glucose tolerance factor (GTF)	*Deficiency:* Impaired glucose tolerance in malnourished children; some diabetics (?)	

TABLE 20-3

NUTRITIONAL CONTENT IN A SINGLE SERVING OF COMMON FOODS

Food	Total Calories	Fat Grams	Calories from Fat	Carbohydrate Grams	Calories from C
BREADS/CEREALS					
Whole Wheat Bread 1 slice	56	.7	6.3	11	44
Biscuit (2-inch diameter)	103	4.8	43.2	12.8	51.2
Spaghetti (1 cup)	155	.6	5.4	32.2	128.8
Shredded Wheat (1 biscuit)	89	.5	4.5	20	80
Bran Flakes (1 cup)	106	.6	5.4	28.2	112.8
Granola (1 cup)	390	15	135	57	228
DAIRY PRODUCTS					
Milk (1 cup)					
Whole	159	8.2	73.8	11.4	45.6
2% low-fat	121	4.7	42.3	11.7	46.8
Skim (non-fat)	86	.44	4	11.8	47.2
Yogurt (1 cup) plain low-fat	144	3.5	31.5	16	64
Cottage Cheese (1 cup)					
Regular	217	9.4	84.6	5.6	22.4
Low-fat	203	4.4	39.6	8.2	32.8
Cheddar Cheese (1 oz)	112	9.4	84.6	.36	1.4
Swiss Cheese (1 oz)	107	7.8	70.2	.96	3.8
Egg (1 large, uncooked)	82	6.5	58.5	.5	2
FRUITS/VEGETABLES					
Apple (1 medium)	96	1	9	24	96
Avocado (1 medium)	334	32.8	295.2	12.6	50.4
Banana (1 medium)	127	.3	2.7	33	120
Broccoli (1 stalk, raw)	32	.3	2.7	5.9	24
Carrot (1 large, raw)	42	.2	1.8	9.7	38.8
Orange (1 medium)	64	.3	2.7	16	64
Potato, baked (1 large)	145	.2	1.8	32.8	131.2
Tomato (1 medium, raw)	33	.3	2.7	7	28
MEAT/POULTRY/FISH/LEGUMES					
Beef					
Ground, lean (1/4 lb)	203	11.3	101	0	0
Roast, chuck (1/4 lb)	226	18.7	168.3	0	0
Lamb, chop (1/4 lb)	286	24.2	217.8	0	0
Pork, chop (1/4 lb)	266	22.3	200.7	0	0
Chicken, breast (1/4 lb)	99	4.5	40.5	0	0

(continues)

TABLE 20-3 *(continued)*

NUTRITIONAL CONTENT IN A SINGLE SERVING OF COMMON FOODS—continued

Food	Total Calories	Fat Grams	Calories from Fat	Carbohydrate Grams	Calories from C
Turkey, light meat (1/4 lb)	199	4.4	39.6	0	0
Flounder (1/4 lb)	113	1.4	12.6	0	0
Shrimp, fresh (1/4 lb)	103	.9	8.1	6.8	27
Kidney beans, cooked (1 cup)	218	.9	8.1	39.6	158.4
Lentils, cooked (1 cup)	212	0	0	38.6	154.4
Split peas, cooked (1 cup)	230	.3	2.7	41.6	166.4
MISCELLANEOUS					
Butter (1 tablespoon)	102	11.3	102	0	0
Margarine (1 tablespoon)	102	11.3	102	0	0
Mayonnaise (1 tablespoon)	102	11.3	102	0	0

Nutrition Facts
Serving Size: 1/2 Cup
Servings Per Container: 4

Amount Per Serving

Calories 100   Calories from Fat 30

	% Daily Value*
Total Fat 3g	5%
Saturated Fat 0g	0%
Cholesterol 0mg	0%
Sodium 340mg	14%
Total Carbohydrate 15g	5%
Dietary Fiber 1g	4%
Sugars 0g	
Protein 2g	

Vitamin A 0% • Vitamin C 0%
Calcium 0% • Iron 2%

*Percent Daily Values are based on a 2,000 calorie diet. Your daily values may be higher or lower depending on your calorie needs:

	Calories	2,000	2,500
Total Fat	Less than	65g	80g
Sat Fat	Less than	20g	25g
Cholesterol	Less than	300mg	300mg
Sodium	Less than	2,400mg	2,400mg
Total Carbohydrate		300g	375g
Dietary Fiber		25g	30g

Calories per gram:
Fat 9 ∞ Carbohydrate 4 ∞ Protein 4

Ingredients: Flour, Water, Yeast Vegetable Oil, Salt, Artificial Flavor and Color.

FIGURE 20–4 Food companies are required to display nutritional facts about their products listing all ingredients, as this label shows.

guessing is eliminated. Having the contents listed on packages makes it easier for those who are on special diets and those watching their caloric intake, fat grams, cholesterol content, and so on. People find that reading the food labels is quite helpful because the guessing and estimating about what they are eating is eliminated. Food labels can also make menu planning a more pleasant and interesting project. Remind patients to read *all* labels carefully.

Supplements

When patients suffer from loss or lack of appetite or they cannot tolerate a normal diet, it may be necessary for the physician to prescribe a protein-vitamin-mineral food supplement. These food supplements come in the form of a powder or liquid for oral or tube feeding as required by the patient's condition. Patients who might need this type of treatment are the chronically ill, postoperative, underweight, anemic, and **anorexic**. This treatment should be conducted only under the supervision of a physician. Remind patients to take these supplements regularly as directed for their intended affect.

Health Concerns in Adolescents

Special focus should be directed to a predominantly adolescent condition called **anorexia nervosa**. Anorexia nervosa is a psychoneurotic disorder in which the patient—usually a female, but not exclusively—refuses to eat over a period of time. Often, vigorous exercise is a part of the daily routine to help burn calories. Many problems can stem from the ongoing weight loss, including **emaciation** and **amenorrhea**. This disorder may be the result of emo-

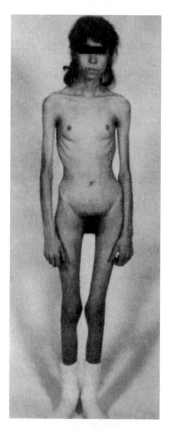

FIGURE 20–5 This photo shows an emaciated young woman, the long-term effects of anorexia. (From R.P. Rowlings, S.R. Williams, and C.K. Beck. *Mental health—psychiatric nursing,* 3rd ed., St. Louis: Mosby, 1992.)

tional stress or conflict. The patient has a poor self-image and is obsessed with a fear of becoming obese. Signs of this disorder are a change in personality, irritability, refusal to eat, and weight loss. Figure 20–5 shows the results of the disorder in an advanced case. A similar disorder, also seen mainly in adolescent females, is **bulimia nervosa.** Unlike the patient with anorexia, the patient with bulimia eats a very large quantity of food at one time (as much as 5,000 calories), but uses **purging** (vomiting, laxatives, and diuretics) to rid the body of the calories. Usually, the patient eats normal meals with others to keep the disorder secretive. This is one of the reasons that this disorder is sometimes difficult to diagnose. The bulemic's **binge** eating and purge behaviors also originate from poor self-image and feelings of inadequacy. Symptoms of bulimia are dark circles under the eyes, muscle wasting, dental cavities, and damage to tooth enamel caused by the acid from the stomach from frequent vomiting. Problems with gastrointestinal and cardiovascular systems are a potential danger in this disorder. Referral for psychiatric therapy and nutritional counseling as soon as possible are necessary to arrest these potentially fatal disorders. Make a sincere effort to give positive reinforcement to patients in an area of their personal interest (e.g., hobby, school project or activity). Your patience and understanding is extremely important in making these patients feel accepted and supported.

The adolescent in general needs a little extra attention in regards to the promotion of or in possibly the initial establishing of good health habits. Give this patient a chance to ask questions and discuss problems in private. Often there are fears about many timely issues, such as sexual behavior, STDs and HIV, pregnancy and birth control, substance abuse (drugs and alcohol), depression and suicide, domestic issues and abuse (emotional, physical, and sexual), peer pressure, and a wealth of other topics that she may feel she cannot talk to anyone else about because of being embarrassed or intimidated. You may be the only one who will treat her as an individual and listen objectively to her problems. Sometimes just getting a chance to let it out is helpful. Offer your listening ear, and support and refer the patient to the physician or to an appropriate service agency as necessary (i.e., mental health center, teen pregnancy free clinic). Some teenagers are reluctant to speak to the school nurse or other authoritative figure because of the possibility of having a parent called.

Being a teenager is a very stressful time. Many pressures begin to surface, creating many demands that pile up rapidly on an already-confused and mood-swinging young pre-adult. One very common problem that you may be influential in curbing is the cigarette habit. Giving adolescents and teenagers the facts about smoking and health may make all the difference in their decision to resist this temptation. Health care professionals have a responsibility to give this often neglected age group of patients their careful attention simply because they generally do not appear very often seeking health care services.

Weight Control

A good weight-control program should contain foods from the food guide pyramid to be nutritionally sound. Eating should be an enjoyable, relaxing experience. But in our fast-food society, people tend to eat more food with more calories more often. A **calorie** is a unit of heat, and all food substances have caloric value (Table 20–3). All of the body's processes burn calories to provide energy and sustain life. If you overeat regularly, the unused calories are stored as fat. If you reduce calorie intake, the fat will be used by the body for energy, and you will begin to shed the extra weight. You should make patients aware that they should eat their meals slowly because it takes approximately 20 minutes for the brain to realize that the stomach is full. Those who follow this practice in a relaxed atmosphere eat *less* and digest their food better. It is now recommended that eating several (five to six) small meals daily not only allows for better use of nutrients by the body for more energy, but it is much easier on the digestive tract. This practice also helps in weight control.

A variety of magazines, books, and businesses offer weight-control plans that promise success for each individual. Over-the-counter drugs promise miraculous weight loss in a matter of weeks. You can be influential in helping patients avoid possible health hazards by warning them of the danger in these quick-weight-loss programs. Many people do lose weight in a short time, but they gain it right back as soon as the program ends. Others do permanent damage to their health.

One respected and worthwhile weight-loss program is Weight Watchers. Most people who have reached their weight-loss goals through this program have maintained a satisfactory weight because they have learned how to change their eating habits. Many support groups offer similar programs. Positive reinforcement is one of the keys to their success. Many physicians realize the frustration of trying to reduce and suggest these support groups to patients. You may want to encourage patients who are trying to follow a diet by suggesting low-calorie recipes or cooking techniques. Showing genuine interest in patients' needs will help them reach their goals.

There is no "one list" that can be a low-calorie diet to follow for everyone who needs to lose weight. A list of foods with their calorie content or a basic diet as a guide can be helpful to those who wish to reduce their weight. The reason physicians want their patients to lose weight is because they are either on the threshold of obesity or have already been diagnosed as **obese**. Weighing more that 30% of your ideal body weight (obese) puts you at risk for developing serious health problems. A few that are considered serious are heart disease and stroke, diabetes, cancer, **sleep apnea**, osteoarthritis, and gallbladder disease. It is a service that patients appreciate because they realize that you are helping them toward a healthier life.

Diets

The number of special diets is far too numerous to list in this book. A few diets that may be helpful to you in providing education to patients are briefly discussed here. These are general guidelines to follow. You should follow the triage/patient education policy established by the physician(s) in your medical facility when advising patients either by phone or face-to-face. If you are uncertain or have any questions regarding what to tell patients about their treatment plan, you should ask the physician.

- **Clear liquid diet:** Pedialyte for infants and children, Gatorade for adults, clear gelatin, decaffeinated coffee and tea, clear broth, no-caffeine sodas, artificially-flavored drink mix, flavored frozen juice bars and treats, clear juice, and water as directed by physician—offered to patients at least every two hours the first 24 hours for patients with diarrhea.
- **Brat diet:** bananas, rice, applesauce, toast, and clear liquids/water (Pedialyte for infants) for 24 hours as tolerated by patients after diarrhea stops, as directed by the physician.
- **Soft diet:** creamed hot cereals, gelatin, pudding, ice cream, sherbet, mashed or baked potatoes, puréed vegetables, creamed soups, baked turkey/chicken/fish, meatloaf, milk, poached egg, macaroni and cheese, yogurt, applesauce, and graham crackers. These are suggestions for foods that may be more easily tolerated for patients who have gastrointestinal disorders, such as a duodenal ulcer or gastritis. These suggestions should be approved by the doctor for patients before telling them to follow this list of foods. This diet is also for those who are just getting over an intestinal virus.

- **Low-calorie diet:** Basically counting calories and fat grams every day and adding up the total will help those who wish to shed a few pounds, especially if there includes cardiovascular exercise at least three times a week for a minimum of 30 minutes. Eating no more than a total of 30% of calories from fat each day is recommended for a healthy heart, especially if there is a family history of heart disease.
- There are low-fat, no-sugar, high-fiber, low- or no-salt, and low-residue diets, and the list continues with specialized therapeutic diet plans for individual needs. Therapeutic diets are used in the treatment of patients with a specific disease or disorder. Standard printed diet sheets, pamphlets, booklets, and other patient education topics can be displayed on a wall-mounted rack for convenience to patients and you. Post information about nutrition, heart-healthy cooking classes, and other topics on the bulleting board for patients to get involved in their health care. Patients who have a medical condition with dietary needs beyond the printed materials in your facility, or who are ordered by the physician, should be referred to a registered dietitian (RD). Explain the need for this referral and how important it is that they give full cooperation. A patient's background and lifestyle will be considered and adjustments made as necessary. A dietician will work closely with other health care team members in individual **therapeutic** diet planning.

EXERCISE

In addition to a well-balanced diet, adequate exercise and sufficient rest are essential to good health. Special diets and exercise programs must be approved for individuals by the physician, who will determine the patient's needs and tolerance from careful examination and medical history. This is done to safeguard the patient from overexertion and stress.

Exercise is defined as physical exertion for improvement of health or correction of physical deformity. The safest form of exercise, and one almost everyone can participate in, is walking. Often patients are reluctant to walk if they have to walk alone because they fear for their safety. You may suggest that they seek a walking partner and try to go in daylight hours. The purchase of a treadmill is a good investment (for those who can afford it) because it is available at any time and in any weather. You may suggest that patients inquire at the local enclosed shopping mall about walking clubs that meet before the mall opens. This way the patients will have a safe and comfortable environment in the company of others with the same interest. This idea could be quite helpful in motivating them to stick to a routine for their better health. There are so many different exercise programs available that people can choose according to their individual needs and goals. A combination of proper diet and proper exercise brings satisfying results in overall good health.

Regular exercise improves circulation and muscle tone and relieves tension. People who have followed an exer-

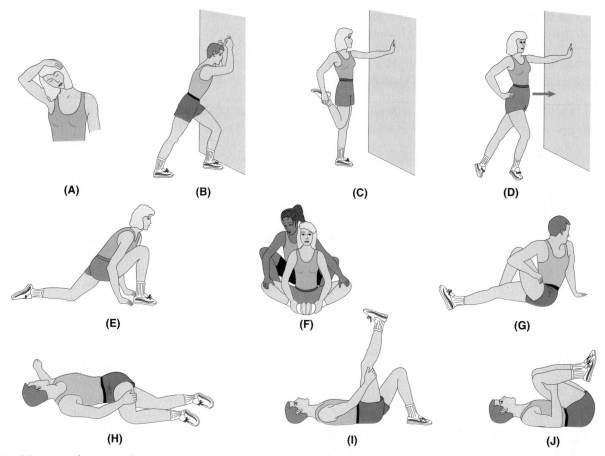

FIGURE 20–6 Ten basic stretching exercises: (A) To stretch the neck muscles, keep shoulders down while you tilt your head to the right. Then place your right hand on the left side of your head, and for approximately 15 to 25 seconds, pull gently toward your right shoulder. Repeat for the left side. (B) To stretch the calf muscles (gastrocnemius and soleus) place feet flat on the floor away from the wall (two to three feet). While leaning on your forearms flat against the wall, step toward the wall with the left foot, and bend the knee while keeping the heel of the right foot flat on the floor for approximately 15 to 25 seconds. Repeat for the right leg. (C) To stretch the thigh muscles (quadriceps), lean into the wall with your left hand to keep your balance, and pull your right ankle up gently with your right hand for 15 to 25 seconds. Repeat for the left ankle. (D) To stretch outer thigh muscle (iliotibial band), stand next to and press your left hand against the wall as you place your right hand on your right hip. Bend the right knee slightly, rest the left foot on its side, and hold for 15 to 25 seconds. Repeat for the left leg. (E) To stretch the hip muscles (hip flexor), get into a kneeling position with your foot flat on the floor, and bend the right knee up to touch your chest. Keep your left leg on the floor behind you (arms at your sides) and stretch and hold for 15 to 25 seconds. Repeat, bending the left knee with your right leg behind you. (F) To stretch the muscles in the groin (often called the butterfly stretch), while sitting on the floor, bring your heels together, and hold them with your hands. Gently push your legs down with your elbows (or ask someone to do it for you), and hold for 5 to 10 seconds; use resistance to feel stretching (avoid straining) and then relax. Repeat 5 to 10 times. (G) To stretch the back and side muscles, sit up straight on the floor with both legs straight out. Bring the left leg up with your knee bent, and place your foot on the floor to the right of the right knee. Then place your right elbow on the upper part of your left knee. Your left hand should be in back of you to help you look over your left shoulder. You should take in a deep breath before you begin to twist your upper body and exhale slowly while you hold this posture for 10 to 25 seconds. Repeat for the right leg. (H) To stretch muscles in the lower back, lie flat on your back and bring your left knee up. Cross it over to your right hip (keep your arms stretched out to your sides). Keep your shoulders against the floor, and turn your head to the left, then press your left thigh with your right hand to the floor, and hold for 10 to 25 seconds. Repeat for the right leg. (I) To stretch the hamstrings in the thigh, lie flat on your back and bend your knees, placing both feet flat on the floor. Raise your right leg up so that your heel is toward the ceiling. Hold your right leg behind the knee with both hands and pull into your chest. Relax your foot and keep straightening your leg until it becomes uncomfortable, and then hold the position for 10 to 20 seconds. Repeat for the left leg. (J) To stretch the lumbar muscles in the lower back, lie on your back with your knees bent up to your chest. Place your hands behind your knees, press into your chest, and hold for 10 to 25 seconds, then relax and repeat several times.

cise routine regularly report that they experience a better outlook on life, have more energy, and feel healthier. The degree of exertion in any exercise routine will vary with individuals, and the physician's advice should be taken. Even before walking, proper stretching is recommended as a warm-up to keep from straining muscles and to help prevent other possible injuries. Figure 20–6 illustrates the 10 basic stretching exercises to help prepare for exercise.

All of the behaviors which influence health are governed by one's mental (or social) health and vice versa. A positive outlook is most helpful in coping with life in general. (Refer back to Chapter 4.) Learning coping and problem-solving skills can help us deal with the everyday stress and the occasional crisis of routine living. Nurturing the spirit (the soul) has overall benefits as well. Practicing a chosen religious belief can help the feelings of completeness and belonging. Being a member of an organization where there are others who offer their support and caring is essential to one's sense of worth. It helps with fulfillment of our basic needs. Self-esteem needs can also be met with activities that reinforce our significance and our independence of one another. Many meaningful religious ceremonies give us a sense of direction and remind us of purpose. Meditation and other relaxation exercises including reflection have a calming effect. These are excellent ways to unwind and relieve stress and help one in getting a good night's rest.

SLEEP

Getting sufficient rest is also necessary for good health. Rest is usually thought of as another word for sleep and is defined as a time away from activity. Most people use the words rest and sleep interchangeably. Sleep is the natural way for the body to restore itself. Adequate rest/sleep equips us with strength to handle various daily activities. Winding down from strenuous or hectic activity is usually essential for a time for one to be able to rest and relax enough to go to sleep. Even though the number

of hours of sleep varies from person to person, quality sleep should not be interrupted. The average number of hours of sleep is between six and nine hours in a 24-hour period for most adults. Sleep patterns of the elderly become shorter and more like an infants, who sleep often for up to four or five hours at a time. Babies generally reduce the time of sleep during the day as they grow, gradually sleeping longer at night. Each of us has a pattern of sleep and sleep needs specific to us.

When a patient tells you he has not been getting any sleep at night, you must ask him how long he <u>does</u> sleep and <u>when</u> he sleeps. Often, there is sufficient sleep but not all at once at night when he thinks he should sleep. If the person is obviously not getting sufficient sleep, the physician needs to be alerted when the patient first mentions it. Often, the patient does not consider it a problem worth telling you because initially it is just annoying to him. Insomnia is a term used to describe not being able to sleep. There could be a serious physical or emotional (psychological) problem that is the reason for the insomnia. Generally, the physician will ask the patient to keep track of when and how long at a time the patient sleeps for a specific amount of time. Establishing a record of the sleep dysfunction helps the physician to make a decision about diagnostic and treatment plans. Being comfortable and ready to go to sleep should be stressed to those patients who have trouble sleeping. Patients who awaken once in a while, whether the reason is apparent or not, should not be alarmed. Those who wake up several times each night

Medical-Legal-Ethical Scenario

Mrs. Fletcher, an elderly patient, had an appointment for her blood pressure and weight to be checked. Darlene wanted to call her in, but they were running about a half hour behind schedule. Mrs. Fletcher waited for 25 minutes without a problem. Then she asked if Darlene could please bring her in because her back was getting stiff. Darlene brought her in and asked her to have a seat in the triage area. While she waited there, she became interested in the new pamphlet rack that Darlene had just put up the day before. Mrs. Fletcher had taken one of everything on the rack. When Darlene came to take her weight and blood pressure, she asked Darlene to explain each one to her. When Darlene told her she would during future visits, one at a time, Mrs. Fletcher replied, "Never mind, I will take them home and read them at night when I can't get to sleep."

CRITICAL THINKING CHALLENGE

1. Why was Mrs. Fletcher so interested in those pamphlets?
2. How did Darlene encourage the interest in the pamphlets without even knowing it?
3. What should Darlene have done about Mrs. Fletcher's complaint of a stiff back?
4. Why did Mrs. Fletcher's back complaint disappear?
5. Did Mrs. Fletcher disclose another problem? What is it?
6. What should Darlene have done in response to Mrs. Fletcher's request for her to explain each pamphlet?
7. What would you have done?

on a regular basis are at risk for health problems if sleep interruption continues. Sleep deprivation is a term that means lack of sleep. Many people experience times when sleep is not sufficient, but manage to function. Within a day or so of getting sufficient rest and sleep, they are back to a normal sleep pattern.

Those who suffer from sleep deprivation on a long-term basis exhibit irritability, fatigue, poor concentration and remembering ability, clumsiness, and sometimes visual or **tactile** hallucinations. Research studies have shown that a person needs both **REM (rapid eye movement)** and **NREM (non-rapid eye movement)** stages of sleep. The NREM stage begins approximately 90 minutes after a person goes to sleep. Those who can sleep for at least six hours uninterrupted feel better and more rested. That is because they have benefited from the effects of the proper sequence of sleep. Explain to patients that their sleep schedule may need to be altered. Patients often get stuck in a pattern because they think they have to sleep at a certain time. It is possible that some try to change their biological clock. Most people know that it is not easy to do. Sometimes all a patient needs to do is talk to someone about her concerns. Just listening and a little suggestion from you to read or play soft music or engage in a quiet activity can be helpful. One needs to realize that sleep is not a luxury, but it is necessary for the body to function well. Patients will appreciate your interest.

Each individual should find outlets to release tension and participate in activities that bring enjoyment and enrichment to his life. It is also important to practice the virtue of patience and maintain a sense of humor, for it has been said that laughter is the best medicine.

ACHIEVE UNIT OBJECTIVES

Complete Chapter 20, Unit, 1 in the workbook to help you obtain competency of this subject.

UNIT 2

Habit-Forming Substances

OBJECTIVES

Upon completion of the unit, meet the following performance objectives by verifying knowledge of the facts and principles presented through oral and written communication at a level deemed competent.

1. Spell and define, using the glossary at the back of the text, all of the **Words to Know** in this unit.
2. List the most commonly abused major groups of drugs and give an example of each.
3. Explain the effects of the most commonly abused substances.

4. Describe the difference between an alcohol-dependent drinker and alcoholic.
5. Describe research into the causes of alcoholism.
6. Describe ways you can be influential in assisting drug addicts and alcoholics toward rehabilitation.
7. Describe the action that tar, nicotine, and carbon monoxide have on the body.
8. List ways a person can stop smoking.
9. List diseases in which smokers have a higher probability rate.
10. Explain the effects of secondhand smoke.
11. List the stages of drug/alcohol abuse.
12. List signs of drug/alcohol abuse.
13. List organizations and facilities that assist in the rehabilitation of drug addicts and alcoholics.
14. Describe types of abusive behaviors and ways you can help those who are victims of abuse.
15. Describe the effects of the "date-rape drug" and the danger it presents.

AREAS OF COMPETENCE (AAMA)

This unit addresses content within the specific competency areas of *Diagnostic orders, Patient care, Professionalism, Communication skills, Legal concepts,* and *Instruction,* as identified in the Medical Assistant Role Delineation Study. Refer to Appendix A for a detailed listing of the areas.

WORDS TO KNOW

acetylcholine	euphoria
addiction	hallucinogen
advantageous	illicit
Al-Anon	intervention
Al-Ateen	malady
alcoholic	narcolepsy
Alcoholics Anonymous	nicotine
amphetamine	norepinephrine
barbiturate	proclivity
bizarre	pseudo
carbon monoxide	psychedelics
carboxyhemoglobin	stimulant
carcinogen	synergism
cholinergic	tar
depressant	traumatic
detrimental	veritable
enabler	

A habit is a pattern of behavior that is acquired over a time by repetition. Habits can be either **advantageous** or disadvantageous depending on the effects they have. Many of our habits are so much a part of us that we do not even realize they exist. Changing a behavior that has become a habit is difficult. It takes a great deal of patience and encouragement to repattern personal activities. Teach-

A CAAHEP CONNECTION

Patients of any age may disclose that they are involved in drugs, have been abused or raped, or know someone who needs help. Be careful not to categorize patients because of the way they wear their hair or dress or how they talk. Give your best effort in directing patients in need to the appropriate facility for treatment and support. *Communication* and *Patient education* is vitally important in serving patients and their families with these serious issues. Without making a fuss, make the physician aware of the request for help before the patient is examined. Encourage patients with problems to stay with their treatment and not give up.

ing good health habits to patients is an important duty of the medical assistant. The entire medical staff must strive to set a good example because example is the best teacher.

In times of stress, one may be temporarily inclined to relieve anxiety or depression by using chemical substances. Even individuals under the supervision of a physician may become dependent. Other persons turn to chemical substances to experiment with the feelings they produce. Often, this is a response to peer pressure, which can be strong indeed. Regardless of why persons turn to chemical substances, they need to know that dependency and abuse can follow and that the stakes can be very high.

Unfortunately, the influence of advertising has been to encourage chemical substance use by promoting fast relief, quick weight-loss, instant sleep and wakefulness, and a variety of other "feel-good" promises from the makers of chemical products. Although a substance may well relieve symptoms temporarily, the cause of the problem will still exist. If undetermined or undetected physical or emotional problems are not diagnosed and treated, they may balloon into more complex problems that are only worsened by the abuse of chemical substances. You can play an important part in recognizing potential chemical abusers and helping them take steps toward treatment.

ALCOHOL

Still the nation's number-one drug problem, alcohol is responsible for the destruction of many lives. Its use is commonly accepted by society and to a great degree encouraged. Most persons who drink alcoholic beverages do so moderately, probably because their effects have been learned from either first-hand observation or educational programs. The responsible social drinker can take alcohol or leave it alone.

On the other hand, a person who is dependent on alcohol has a difficult time doing without a drink. An alcohol-dependent drinker will say that cutting down is not a problem but is then unable to do so. Daily use of alcohol becomes a need and usually leads to increasingly compulsive drinking. Patients who indicate this during conversation or in giving a medical history may be indirectly asking for help with their problem. Privately disclosing this information to the physician may lead to a treatment or counseling program, which may prevent the patient from becoming an alcoholic. An **alcoholic** is a drinker who has become totally dependent on alcohol. All areas of the alcoholic's life are affected by it. It is the number-one priority, and control over drinking is nonexistent. More often than not, the occurrence of a tragedy is the reason the alcoholic seeks treatment, either by court order or sometimes voluntarily in an effort to put a productive life back together.

Alcoholism is now recognized as a disease, as serious as cancer or diabetes, which can be treated. It is a major health problem and recognized as such by the American Medical Association, American Osteopathic Association, and American Bar Association. Excessive long-term use of alcohol can reduce resistance to infections and eventually lead to cirrhosis of the liver. It can also add complications to other diseases and conditions. In effect, alcohol dissolves all tissues with which it comes in contact.

Research efforts continue in the search for the causes of the disease. Many theories have been offered but none are yet definitive. Current efforts are concentrating on brain chemistry, hereditary traits, and cultural influences. While certain ethnic groups show a **proclivity** toward alcoholism, others are virtually free of the disease. Studies in these areas suggest almost evolutionary relationships between habits, value systems, and brain chemistry. Many scientists feel that a combination of factors contributes to alcoholism.

Treatment

Alcoholics Anonymous (AA) is a well-known support group for the alcoholic, who must admit to being an alcoholic and be willing to start leading a productive life once again. AA was founded in the mid 1930s to help those who were looked on by society as hopeless degenerates. The program has become extremely successful over the years and has directly and indirectly helped millions to reorder their lives. Other support groups have branched from this initial organization. **Al-Anon** and **Al-Ateen** are for family members or close friends of the alcoholic to help them understand and cope with their loved ones' illness. Many companies maintain alcoholism assistance and rehabilitation programs for employees who are problem drinkers. It has been realized by employers that this practice is not only a service but is cost-effective as an alternative to training new personnel.

ABUSIVE BEHAVIORS

In addition to substance abuse behaviors prevalent in society, an equally serious **malady** also affects many people of all ages in this country. The combination of substance abuse and violence is common; however, it is not always the case. There may be an untreated mental disorder that can cause one to have a distorted view of reality and therefore can lead to a violent situation. These situations occur daily in various ways. Several forms of abuse, in all types of socioeconomic classes, cause multiple physical and emotional damage to victims—even death in some cases. Children who have been abused all of their lives are destined to repeat the cycle with their own children if there is no **intervention**. A learned hostile environment breeds more hostility. You may be instrumental in breaking this cycle. For assistance in reporting child abuse, call the national hotline: 800-4 A CHILD (800-422-4453).

Domestic violence is often reported to the authorities by the battered victim, but charges against the guilty ones are generally dropped because of threats to the victim if they pursue legal action. Victims range in age between newborns to the very elderly. Most domestic violence victims are female, although all children involved become victims in the end. There are safe and anonymous shelters for women and children in, or near, every community. You should become familiar with places of safety so that you can direct victims to a shelter in the event that a patient confides in you about a situation. Child, domestic, and elder abuse victims often reach out to physicians and other members of the health professions for help. Record all symptoms on the patient's chart and alert the physician of the situation. You have a responsibility to report any cases of physical or sexual abuse in children either disclosed to you during the course of a patient's visit or observed during the time they are in your facility. It is the law in many states for health care professionals, teachers, and other professional people to report all known cases of child abuse. It is further a criminal offense if a known case of child abuse is not reported. You may report any case of abuse anonymously. Even if you are not obligated by law to help victims of violent acts from another, your moral conscience will lead you to do the right thing. The importance of this matter is to get help for the victim as soon as possible. You may be saving a life by doing so.

DRUGS

(Refer to Table 20–4.) There was a time when we thought of drugs only in connection with a trip to the drugstore to have a prescription filled. Today the meaning has changed, and the term evokes the image of illicit chemical substances available on the street. Most of these are impure, diluted, extremely addictive, and expensive and dangerous.

Throughout civilized history people have had a desire to soothe the anxieties of life and obtain temporary relief from troubles. But our society, as a whole, is today more than ever before looking for instant gratification. Over-the-counter drugs are practically beyond number. It is a mind-boggling experience to look over a well-stocked drug shelf in a retail store and consider all the substances that can allegedly provide "fast and temporary" relief. In this age of fast food, instant car washes, one-hour dry cleaning, and express lanes, the art of patience has seemingly been lost. Our society has become accepting of drug use as a part of life, even a *way* of life, despite the physical and emotional damage, reflected in the high numbers of drug-related deaths from overdose and accident. In addition to the fear of the effects of the drugs themselves is the fear of the association with those who make these **illicit** drugs available. The increase in crime has been attributed to drug trafficking. Those unfortunate ones who become addicted to drugs must feed their habit in any way possible. That means that if there is no legal financial means for them, they turn to crime. Family and friends have no influence over the addict's habit. In fact, many loved ones become **enablers**, meaning that they help the person and thereby help promote the addiction without realizing it. Your help and support will be greatly appreciated because getting the addict to accept professional help is a very difficult and emotional ordeal.

The threat of nuclear war, unemployment, an uncertain economy, and a fast-paced lifestyle make it difficult for many to deal with the challenges of everyday living. For some people, the only way to cope with problems is by resorting to mood-altering drugs. But these drugs alter not only one's mood but also one's perception of reality, and they are dangerous not only to the user but to others as well. The **euphoric** state they produce exists only in the user's mind.

The reality of drugs in society and the seriousness of their abuse are not going to disappear. A **veritable** smorgasbord of legal and illegal drugs remains widely available and probably always will be. Educating the young children in schools, patients, and the general public to their dangers seems to be the only hope.

You could be most influential in helping someone, perhaps a patient or a family member of a patient (or someone in your personal life), recognize the signs of drug abuse so that intervention may be possible. You should always be supportive and understanding. Avoid being judgmental, sarcastic, or accusatory with patients or others seeking your help. The indications of drug abuse are outlined in Figure 20–7.

There are four basic stages of alcohol and drug abuse. In the first stage, one may show no visible signs in outward behavior. Unfortunately, society has taken somewhat an attitude of acceptance in the use of alcohol and drugs, especially in youth. Experimental use is considered normal, and abuse often goes unnoticed until the second stage has begun. In the second stage, use is more frequent, and the habit starts. Frequently signs may include a change in the type of friends one associates with and a decline in motivation and performance at school and work. Stage three shows a marked change in one's mood, and domestic problems are common. The abuser may exhibit signs of

---

INDICATIONS OF DRUG/ALCOHOL ABUSE

- Abrupt change in mood/attitudes
- Sharp decline in attendance/performance at school/work
- Resistance to discipline/rules at home/school
- Deterioration in relationships
- Sudden, unusual temper outbursts
- Increased frequency in borrowing money
- Stealing from others
- Increased intense secrecy about actions and belongings
- Associating with new friends

FIGURE 20–7 These are some of the common warning signs of possible drug or alcohol abuse. Be aware of these signs when dealing with patients and those in your personal life. Early intervention is critical.

depression and possibly talk of or attempt suicide. The person affected by abuse has an intense preoccupation to seek drugs for daily use. The fourth and last stage requires that the abuser take the drug in increasing amounts just to feel OK. Outward signs of stage four include coughing, frequent sore throats, weight loss, and fatigue. The person may also overdose and have blackouts. To maintain the habit, the person may have begun a life of crime. Deterioration of relationships and family is most evident. Obviously, the sooner help is initiated the better in dealing with this situation. Stay firm in your attitudes, explanations, and efforts in seeking help for one who requests it.

The most commonly misused major groups of drugs and medicines in the United States are **depressants**, **hallucinogens**, narcotics, and **stimulants**. The state of **addiction** stems from periodic or chronic intoxication (i.e., from repeated use). The abuser or addict has an overriding desire for the euphoric effect of the substance and will find a means of obtaining it to fulfill that desire. Because of increasing physiological tolerance of the drug, the user gradually must increase the dosage to maintain the desired effects. The user may also mix two or more drugs, including alcohol. This practice, referred to as **synergism**, greatly enhances the intoxicating qualities of each drug into a combined new effect, which can be quite erratic and unpredictable. Though the user may realize the damaging effects of the substance, dependence can become so great that it is quite impossible to stop using the drug without outside intervention and assistance.

Rarely does the drug abuser begin by taking medicine to relieve pain, but more typically it is to avoid a confrontation with emotional or psychological problems. Hence, the addiction is psychological and physical. These problems are only made more complex with the addition of mood-altering chemicals.

Depressants

Barbiturates, such as Butisol sodium, Donnatal, and Nembutal, are used in the treatment of patients who need sedation or for the relief of anxiety. They are also used to induce sleep and thus are frequently referred to as sleeping pills. They are also known as downers. They vary in strength and action but function by depressing the activity of the central nervous system. This affects the heart rate, respiration, blood pressure, and temperature. Tolerance to the drug is acquired after frequent use over a relatively short period. Psychological effects are similar to those of alcohol, and when used with alcohol, the danger to the user is great. A person under the influence of barbiturates appears to be intoxicated.

Immediate medical attention must be given in the case of overdose or death is imminent. For a victim who is still awake, the first step is to induce vomiting.

Hallucinogens

Hallucinogens are also referred to as **psychedelics** or sometimes as "mind-expanding" chemicals. Some of the most commonly used street drugs of this type are LSD (or acid), mescaline, and PCP (angel dust). These chemical substances give the user a distorted look at reality. "Taking a trip" refers to the visual hallucinations seen on those short chemical vacations. However, the images may be horrific, and "coming down" may be **traumatic**. Even though dependence does not seem to occur, the danger of hallucinogens is in the **bizarre** behavior that may result, which can cause accidental death to the user and others. In addition, some users experience undesirable "flashbacks" from some hallucinogens or effects long after the drug was taken.

Marijuana can have hallucinogenic effects on the user. The effects of marijuana are varied, and it can be classified in other drug categories as well. It is one of the oldest and probably most widely used drugs next to alcohol, and it has become more socially acceptable today than ever before. When mixed with other drugs, it becomes more powerful and dangerous. Marijuana stimulates the central nervous system and produces a euphoric effect. It also distorts the perception of time and reality and can give rise to feelings of paranoia.

Marijuana may have **detrimental** effects on the respiratory and reproductive systems, and these are being studied. Use in treating nausea in patients undergoing chemotherapy for cancer and use in treating glaucoma have prompted further investigation into potential medical applications.

There is ongoing debate regarding legalization of marijuana. Those who choose to use marijuana are likely to continue whether it is legal or not. There are reports of third-grade youngsters who have already smoked marijuana. Early usage frequently leads to later use of more dangerous drugs.

TABLE 20-4

COMMONLY ABUSED SUBSTANCES

Drug	Prescription (Brand Name)	Effect/Medical Use	How Administered	Street Name	Length of Effects (hrs)	Possible Symptoms of Use	Hazards of Long-Term Use/Overdose	Symptoms of Withdrawal
LSD D-lysergic acid, diethylamide	None	None	Orally, injected	Acid, cubes, purple haze microdots (tabs), tickets, blotters, wedge, window pane, Bevis & Butthead, Black Star, Cid, Dots, Microdot, paper acid, blue moons	Variable	Dilated pupils, illusions, mood swings, hallucinations, poor perception of time and distance	Breaks from reality, emotional breakdown, flashback	Not reported
Psilocybin, psilocin	None	None	Orally (ingested in natural form)	Magic mushrooms	Variable	Altered state of consciousness and mood	Not reported	Not reported
Inhalants: Gasoline, airplane glue, paint thinner, dry-cleaning solution	None	None	Sniffed, inhaled		Variable	Poor motor coordination, impaired vision, poor memory and thought processes, abusive and violent behavior	High risk of sudden death; weight loss; and damage to brain, liver, and bone marrow	
Nitrous oxide (N₂O)	Nitrous oxide	Anesthetic in dentistry	Inhaled	Laughing gas, whippets		Lightheaded feeling	Death by anoxia, muscle weakness, neuropathy	
Nitrites: Amyl, butyl	Amyl nitrite	Vasodilator	Inhaled, sniffed	Poppers, locker room, rush, snappers	Seconds to minutes	Slowed thought process, headache	Anemia, death by anoxia	
Marijuana, hashish	None	Limited use in CA and AZ in 1996	Orally, smoked	Pot, grass, reefer, jays, weed, Mary Jane, Columbian, hash, hash oil, joint, sinsemilla, shish, shishoil, oil, kif, charras, nup, Bale, blunt, Bo, Bo-Bo, Dube, Duby, bong, bone, Bud, Ganja, Hooch, Hydro, Cheeba, Spark it up	2–4	Euphoria, increase in appetite, short-term memory loss, disorientation, loss of interest and motivation, neglect of appearance	Lung damage, possible reproductive system damage, loss of motivation, damage to immune system and heart, interference with psychological maturation, impaired memory perception, psychological dependence	Insomnia, hyperactivity and decreased appetite reported in some individuals
Tranquilizers	(Librium, Valium, Tranxene)	Antianxiety, muscle relaxant, sedation	Orally		4–8	Drowsiness, confusion, slurred speech, impaired judgment, drunken behavior without odor of alcohol, constricted pupils	Nausea, addiction with severe withdrawal symptoms, loss of appetite, death from overdose, shallow respiration, cold and clammy skin, dilated pupils, weak and rapid pulse, coma	Anxiety, insomnia, tremors, delirium, convulsions, possible death
Narcotics	(Percodan)	Analgesic	Orally, injection	School boy	3–6	Nausea, drowsiness, respiratory depression, constricted pupils, lethargy, euphoria	Addiction, loss of appetite; in severe overdose, apnea, circulatory collapse, cardiac arrest, and death may occur.	Watery eyes, runny nose, loss of appetite, yawning, irritability, panic, chills, sweating, cramps, nausea
	Codeine	Analgesic	Orally, injection	Dreamer, junk, horse, smack, china white, crap, fix H, mother, pearl, stuff, boy, brown, bindle	3–6			
	Heroin	None	Injection, sniffed		3–6	Needle marks		
	Morphine	Analgesic	Injection, smoked		3–6			
Cocaine	Cocaine	local anesthetic for ENT surgery	Inhaling or snorting, Injection	Bernice, blow, chick, C, coke, Corine, dust, flake, nose candy (stuff), toot, snow, white (girl), uptown	Varies	Euphoria, hyperactivity, excitability	Rapid physical deterioration, paranoia, hallucinations, psychosis, convulsions, overdose illness, or death	(Same as narcotics in general)
Crack (a form of freebase cocaine)	None	None	Smoking	Crack, duff, rock, gravel, flake	Varies, usually 30 to 60 minutes	Euphoria, increase in pulse rate and blood pressure, elevated temperature, dilated pupils, hyperactivity, excitability	Rapid physical deterioration, paranoia, hallucinations, psychosis, convulsions, overdose illness, or death	(Same as narcotics in general)

Drug	Name/Examples	Medical use	How taken	Slang names	Duration (hrs)	Physical symptoms	Long-term/overdose effects	Withdrawal
Hallucinogens (drugs that alter one's perception of reality)	PCP, phencyclidine (Sernylan)	Veterinary anesthetic	Orally, smoked, inhaled, snorted, injection	Angel dust, killer weed, supergrass, pearly gates, hog, PeaCe Pill, acid, m&m's	Variable	Slurred speech, blurred vision, confusion, aggression, uncoordination, agitation, needle marks	Anxiety, depression, impaired memory and perception, death from accidents/overdose	Not reported
Mescaline	None	None	Orally, injection	Mesc, cactus, mescal, buttons		Illusions and hallucinations, poor perception of time and distance	Longer, more intense trip episodes, psychosis	
Alcohol	ethanol	None	Swallowed in liquid form	Booze, hooch, brew	Hours—depends on amount consumed	Impaired muscle coordination, and judgment	Heart and liver damage, death from overdose, death from auto accidents, addiction	Weakness, sweating, hyperreflexia, delirium tremens
Depressants (drugs that depress the CNS)								
Chloral hydrate	(Notec, Somnos)	Hypnotic	Orally	Downer	5–8	Drowsiness, confusion, slurred speech, impaired judgment, drunken behavior without odor of alcohol, constricted pupils	Nausea, addiction with severe withdrawal symptoms, loss of appetite, death from overdose, shallow respiration, cold and clammy skin, dilated pupils, weak and rapid pulse, coma	Anxiety, insomnia, tremors, delirium, convulsions, possible death
Barbiturates	(Butisol, Nembutal,) phenobarbital, (Seconal,) secobarbital	Anesthetic, anticonvulsant, sedation, sleep, epilepsy, heart disease	Orally, injection	Barbs, downers, yellow jackets, red devils, blue devils	1–16	Needle marks		
Glutehimide	(Doriden)	Sedation, sleep	Orally		4–8			
Methaqualone	(Parest, Quaalude, Somnafac)	Sedation, sleep	Orally		4–8			
Amphetamines	dextroamphetamine (Biphetamine) (Benzedrine)	Hyperkinesis, narcolepsy, weight control	Orally, injection	Speed, uppers, white crosses pep, pills, meth, whites, bennies, dexies, speed, black beauties, crank	2–4	Excess activity, mood swings, irritability, nervousness, needle marks, dilated pupils, increased pulse rate and blood pressure	Loss of appetite, hallucinations, paranoia, convulsions, coma, agitation, increase in body temperature, death from overdose	Apathy, long periods of sleep, irritability, depression, disorientation
Phenethylamines— MDMA (3,4- methylenedioxy-n- methylamphetamine) many variations	MDMA	(Schedule I) research	Ingested, snorted, or mixed with a liquid	XTC, Adam, Ecstasy MDA, MMDA	1 to 24 hrs (depends on drug & dose)	Euphoria, nausea, sweating, jaw tingling, fatigue, elevated blood pressure, relaxed feelings, enhanced mental clarity, euphoria, improved problem solving abilities, pseudo-hallucinations	Research continues, overdose illness or death	Not reported
Phenmatrazine	(Preludin)	Weight control	Orally	Lip poppers	2–4	Insomnia, loss of appetite		
Methylphenidate	(Ritalin, Cylert, Didrex)	Hyperkinesis	Orally	Meth crystals	2–4			
Nicotine	None	None	Smoked (snuff or chew)	Coffin nail, smoke, butt	Variable	Smell of tobacco, stained teeth and fingers, high carbon monoxide levels	Cancers of the lung, throat, mouth, esophagus, heart disease, emphysema, irritation/diseases of the GI and urinary tract; frequent URI, "smoker's cough"	Irritability, insomnia nervousness
Rohypnol	flunitrazepam	none	orally	date rape drug, forget pill, Rachas das, Roche, Roffies, Roples, Ruffies, Roaches (also name for butts of marijuana), Roapies, R2	Hours	Unconsciousness	rape/death	NA

Narcotics

A narcotic is a drug that produces insensibility or stupor. Legally, the term refers to habit-forming drugs, such as opiates: cocaine, heroin, meperidine, and morphine. The lesser narcotics are paregoric, which is used in the treatment of diarrhea and abdominal pain, and codeine, which is a pain reliever. These substances can be obtained legally by a physician's prescription. However, federal, state and local laws prohibit the sale of narcotics for other than medical purposes. These medications are extremely potent and highly addictive. The possibility of overdose is great. Because these medications may be stored in offices or clinics, great care must be taken to ensure their security. You have a tremendous responsibility in keeping accurate records of these drugs.

Stimulants

The medical uses for stimulants are few. They are used in the treatment of **narcolepsy**, some cases of mental depression and alcoholism, chronic rigidity following encephalitis, and in some cases of obesity. Ritalin and dexedrine have been prescribed in the treatment of Attention Deficit Disorder (ADD) and for Attention Deficit Hyperactive Disorder (ADHD). There has been a recent rise in the number of cases of abuse of these drugs. The central nervous system is stimulated by **amphetamines**, which are referred to as uppers or speed. Abusers take speed in pill form to stay awake, to feel more energetic, or to lose weight. Some abusers inject the drug directly into their veins for a faster, more intense reaction. Others "snort" or sniff it to obtain the effects.

Cocaine was used as a local anesthetic many years ago, but today it is rarely used for medical purposes. Its illegal use is nearly epidemic. Songs have been written about it, and some people use it in combination with other drugs for pleasure. Its effects are short-lived, usually about 12 minutes, and the user must constantly increase the dosage to reach the desired state. It is a stimulant that leaves the user depressed after it wears off. Most cocaine addicts must use other drugs to keep them going. The drug leads to frequent upper respiratory and gastrointestinal problems. A nasty side effect suffered by many heavy "snorters" is destruction of the nasal passages. It is an extremely dangerous and expensive addiction.

Heavy use of any stimulant results in physical and psychological dependence. Few deaths are reported from abuse of stimulants, but many result from mixing them with other drugs. Physical ailments and emotional problems are the most evident effects of abusing stimulants.

Over-the-counter diet aids are popular stimulants that are also abused. Their dangers arise when mixed with other drugs or alcohol. Pregnant women and patients with heart disease or hypertension must be particularly discouraged from using stimulants except under the direct supervision of a physician. This advice should be given to anyone who uses any stimulant.

Probably the most abused stimulant is caffeine, found in coffee, tea, chocolate, and many cola drinks. Caffeine stimulates the central nervous system and also acts as a diuretic. Moderation is advised in its use. Coffee "jitters," for instance, cause one to feel out of sorts and nervous. Abuse can result in many related physical and emotional problems.

Drug Abuse Treatment

Comprehensive rehabilitation programs to assist drug abusers are available in a variety of facilities, private and public.

Federal government facilities are located in Fort Worth, Texas, and Lexington, Kentucky. These are Public Health Service hospitals that offer treatment to addicts who volunteer for the program of rehabilitation.

Community hospitals and mental health centers provide these services as well. Staffed by psychiatrists, psychologists, counselors, and social workers, treatment centers give the addict the opportunity to receive therapy that can help in getting to the root of the problems leading to the addiction. Support from the health care team is necessary to assist in the return of the addict to a productive and meaningful life. Finally, Alcoholics Anonymous attracts many drug and alcohol abusers to its 12-step program for successful rehabilitation.

The Date-Rape Drugs

Three of the most dangerous drugs to enter the social scene and gain popularity in the past decade are the "date-rape drugs." Rohypnol (ro-hip-nal) flunitrazepam was the first to be used to commit date rape. This drug is dangerous because it is tasteless, and the victim cannot tell that it has been added to her drink. The effects of this drug are relaxation, confusion, and being spaced-out. The goal of the date is to take advantage of the victim while she is in this state. When she wakes up, she does not know what happened. If too much of the drug is consumed, the victim can become unconscious or even go into a coma. Another date-rape drug, GHB (gamma-hydroxybutyrate), is used in nightclubs for a euphoric effect and as a sedative. It is also used for body-building effects. Problems associated with GHB are seizures, coma, and if combined with other drugs (alcohol), nausea and dyspnea. Anxiety, tremors, sweating, and insomnia accompany withdrawal of this drug.

A drug that was developed for use in veterinary medicine is Ketamine. Veterinarians use it to tranquilize or anesthetize animals for procedures or surgery. Since it was approved for human and animal use in 1970, it is used in children in treating burns. These are the only uses that are legal. At raves and nightclubs, Ketamine is used in combination with other drugs. Its effects vary with who takes it and how his mental state is at the time. Common effects are hallucinations, feeling disconnected from reality, numbness of the extremities, and loss of muscle con-

A CAAHEP CONNECTION

It would be a great service to your young patients (and their parents) who may fall victim to this type of situation to be informed of the potential dangers. Remind them to keep watch over their drinks at parties and in other social gatherings. Contact drug crisis centers or check with web sites for informative materials you can use in patient education.

trol. An overdose of this drug puts the user in an anesthetized state like that of undergoing surgery.

Ecstasy is also a popular drug used in social gatherings, especially raves (all-night parties). This drug is extremely dangerous and deadly. The need to drink water constantly is essential to withstanding the accelerating activity that this drug produces. Physical activity (dancing) requires one to replace fluids lost in normal perspiration. Those who take this drug can become so dehydrated that their body temperature elevates to a dangerously high level very rapidly. There have been temperature readings reported as high as 108° F. Victims were unaware of the effect of this drug and unfortunately died.

SMOKING

According to recent government studies, the risk of premature death caused by smoking cigarettes is now the same for men and women. The saying, "You've come a long way, baby," is unfortunately true. Nicotine dependence, for those smokers who use 20 (or more) cigarettes per day, is responsible for decreasing life expectancy by one-half. There are over 2,000 substances that have been identified in tobacco smoke. Of these, the three poisons in tobacco smoke that do the most harm are **tar**, **nicotine**, and **carbon monoxide**.

Tar is the thick, sticky, dark brown or black substance that is carried in inhaling the smoke and deposited in the lungs. Tar is a **carcinogen**, which means that it is capable of producing cancer in tissues with which it comes in contact. Nicotine is believed to be the addictive drug that is absorbed in the lungs and first stimulates and then depresses the nervous system. The stimulation is caused by the release of **norepinephrine** and because nicotine acts similarly like **acetylcholine**. **Cholinergic** nerves are stimulated by nicotine; because nerve activity is blocked, depression results. Respiration rate is increased with stimulation of nerve receptors in the carotid arteries to supply more oxygen to the brain. The cardiovascular system is also stimulated with the release of norepinephrine, which causes an increase in blood flow to the heart and a rise in heart rate and blood pressure.

Nicotine seems to inhibit hunger, raises blood sugar levels slightly, and deadens taste buds in smokers.

Carbon monoxide produces still other dangerous effects. Red blood cells pick up carbon monoxide where it binds together to form **carboxyhemoglobin**. This could be the reason why smokers easily become short of breath with even moderate activity. Smokers have approximately 10% of their blood supply in the form of carboxyhemoglobin, which cannot carry oxygen. This is also a factor in the cause of heart attacks and lower birth weight and survival rate of babies of smoking mothers.

In addition, smokers are more at risk to have cancer of the lungs, larynx, lip, esophagus, and urinary bladder, chronic sinusitis and bronchitis, emphysema, URIs, cardiovascular diseases (CAD and ASHD), and peptic ulcers.

Even though these facts have been proven and efforts to discourage smoking in recent years have increased, men and women continue to smoke. The nicotine addiction is difficult for many to overcome. The key to success in the elimination of the smoking habit is first of all becoming thoroughly educated on the facts about smoking. Realizing the health hazards and the cost of this habit can be helpful to a smoker in making the decision to stop. Encourage patients, co-workers, family, and friends to consider attending a stop-smoking seminar. Post this information in the waiting room and on the employee's bulletin board. Reward those you know who have stopped smoking by giving them praise and recognition.

Some ways to help the smokers you know to get on the right track to stop their smoking habits are as follows:

1. Keep track of when and why you smoke for at least two weeks.
2. Compare a list of reasons why you should and should not stop.
3. Practice not smoking for a time (begin with an hour, a morning, a day, and so on).
4. Decide a target date when you are going to give up smoking.
5. Learn deep breathing relaxation exercises, and use at least twice a day when tension becomes apparent. Simply take a deep breath slowly and release slowly, thinking consciously of relaxing. Continue for five minutes unless you become dizzy.
6. Find a substitute to replace holding the cigarette.
7. Use sugar-free gums, mints, and mouth sprays to avoid overeating and to help curb the nicotine craving. (Transdermal nicotine patches available OTC may help patients break the habit successfully.) Note: Advise the patient to consider the amount of his nicotine habit per day before obtaining the transdermal nicotine patches because some dosage adjustment may be necessary. Many patients who are trying to quit smoking have already reduced their daily amount of nicotine. A large dose of a stimulant could cause heart dysfunction and elevated blood pressure, besides insomnia and other problems.

Tell patients that they may benefit also by using Nicotrol nasal spray (by prescription only). There is also Nicorette gum. Caution patients not to overuse these because they may cause them additional problems. Instruct patients to read the enclosed information about whatever product they purchase.

8. Drink plenty of water and eat sensibly. Pay special attention to caloric intake for the first four to eight weeks.

9. Include exercise to relieve tension and restlessness that comes with trying to overcome addiction.

10. Reward yourself with something special with the money saved from not buying cigarettes.

Involuntary smoking and *passive smoking* are terms describing secondhand smoke from active tobacco smokers. It is also called sidestream smoke. Both sidestream and mainstream smoke cause damage to the cells that line the heart and blood vessels. The buildup is a cause of atherosclerosis. Studies have shown that the platelets in the blood of smokers are more likely to clump together abnormally, which can lead to blood clots and the risk of a heart attack. Those exposed to secondhand smoke are not only at higher risk of heart disease and cancer, as are active smokers, they also are more likely to have respiratory illnesses often. Children who are exposed to passive smoke from parents may have poor development and reduced lung function, besides the diseases and disorders already mentioned. Those with chronic respiratory problems are obviously at greatest risk from passive smoke, and these individuals certainly should keep from contact to prevent further irritation and difficulty with breathing.

Remind those who smoke to at least think about stopping. Advise them to refrain from smoking around others, especially children and those with respiratory distress. Smoke-free areas should be encouraged, respected, and applauded by those especially in the health care fields. Figure 20–8 illustrates a commonly posted sign requesting "No Smoking."

In patient education pursuits, make sure that you make them aware that tobacco contains poisons that could be fatal to toddlers if swallowed. All smoking materials should be kept out of the reach of children.

Another type of tobacco that is used commonly, predominantly in young males, is chew or snuff, which is a smokeless tobacco. It is also known as chewing tobacco or as dipping. Often, young men think it is a cool thing to do. It is, however, a very addicting and harmful habit because the nicotine content must be increased continually to keep the "buzz" or "high" going. Blood pressure rises, and the heart beats faster the more the amount is increased. Other unpleasant and damaging effects include cancer of the mouth (cheeks, gums, and throat), exposure of roots of the teeth, staining of the teeth, bad breath, loss of ability to taste, and constant production of saliva. Irritability, shakiness, or dizziness results when trying to quit the habit. Remember, the United States Surgeon General's report applies to everyone. **Warning:** The Surgeon General has determined that cigarette smoking is dangerous to your health.

■ ACHIEVE UNIT OBJECTIVES

Complete Chapter 20, Unit 2, in the workbook to help you obtain competency of this subject.

UNIT 3
Stress and Time Management

■ OBJECTIVES

Upon completion of the unit, meet the following performance objectives by verifying knowledge of the facts and principles presented through oral and written communication at a level deemed competent.

1. Spell and define, using the glossary at the back of the text, all the **Words to Know** in this unit.
2. Describe the phenomenon of stress and differentiate between "good" stress and "bad" stress.
3. List and describe stress-related illnesses.
4. List positive methods for dealing with stress.
5. Describe type A and type B personalities.
6. List the four basic human physical needs.
7. List the four basic human developmental needs.
8. Describe steps you can take to eliminate unnecessary stress.
9. List mental health resources for referral of patients.
10. Explain the importance of time management.
11. Explain the purpose of a "to do" list and how it relates to successful time management.

FIGURE 20–8 This common symbol is displayed in most public places with the notation "Thank you for not smoking."

AREAS OF COMPETENCE (AAMA)

This unit addresses content within the specific competency areas of *Diagnostic orders, Patient care, Professionalism, Communication skills, Legal concepts,* and *Instruction,* as identified in the Medical Assistant Role Delineation Study. Refer to Appendix A for a detailed listing of the areas.

WORDS TO KNOW

absolute	nurture
absurdity	perspective
awry	prioritize
conflict	psychosis
discretion	psychosomatic
exemplify	receptors
impending	rejuvenate
implement	respite
leisure	

As you become familiar with patients' symptoms and their diagnoses, it will be evident that a great many illnesses may be ultimately stress-related. Some persons are more stress-prone than others, operating at such a hectic pace and with such compulsiveness or perfectionism that they create many stressful situations for themselves. In general, these persons are referred to as type A personalities. There is a type B personality as well, **exemplified** by a tendency to operate at a slower pace and not to worry as much. These typings are neither **absolute** nor evaluative; that is, one is not better than the other, and most people probably demonstrate characteristics of both types at different times and in different situations. For the most part, though, we lean toward one type or the other in our general actions. Although both type A and type B personalities inevitably face stressful situations, the type As probably face them more frequently than the type Bs. Hence, type A personalities should pay particular attention to recognizing stress and learning to deal with its effects.

Because there are so many different personalities and interests among people, we should consider what our stress stems from before discussing how to deal with it. Most people feel obligated to seek success because it is a self-expectation or they are expected to do so by one's family, peers, or spouse. Often, we can create our own stress, or at least much of it, without even realizing it. Much of the time, it seems that people tend to live too fast and pressure themselves into acquiring too many "things" in a short time. Sometimes, materialistic values override real needs to the point of **absurdity**. The quality of our health, personal relationships, and meaningful endeavors determines the quality of life more than material things. It is necessary, however, that our basic human survival needs are provided before advancing to another level.

All living beings require the physical needs of protection, food, water, and oxygen to maintain existence. As higher beings, we also have developmental needs that require **nurturing**, namely physical, emotional, intellectual, and spiritual. Each person whose physical needs are met on an ongoing basis can then begin to pursue other needs comfortably. Figure 20–9 shows Maslow's Hierarchy of Needs. Abraham Maslow, an American psychiatrist, realized the importance of all human needs beyond the physical ones. To fulfill these needs, we must first have the physical ones met before we can even think of

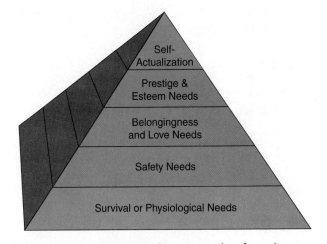

FIGURE 20–9 Maslow's Hierarchy of Needs

advancing to other levels. Motivating ourselves is achieved by our primary physical needs. Keeping a healthy perspective on our needs beyond the physical is necessary for happiness.

A certain amount of stress is necessary to provide motivation. This is "good" stress. The degree of stress that is necessary or helpful varies with the individual. Goals must be set realistically and kept in **perspective**. Reaching goals produces a sense of pride in accomplishment, and these positive feelings reinforce continued personal growth and development. Failure tends to produce feelings of worthlessness and even despair. These negative feelings, if not properly vented, can cause many **psychosomatic** problems. For example, they may lead to aggressive behavior, which is itself stress-producing to the one who displays it and to others. Feelings of hostility toward others may lead to difficulty in coping with pressures from change in employment or unemployment, family or personal **conflicts**, and many other problems, usually known only to the individual.

Difficulty in planning the use of time can produce stress. The feeling of being inefficient and unproductive can lead to a vicious cycle of defeat and despair. This negative attitude may encourage dependence on drugs or alcohol to find some pleasure in life and **respite** from feelings of worthlessness. Exaggeration? No. People vary in their coping skills for dealing with stress. Those who have no one to give them support and encouragement in stressful times may need to be given a little extra time from you. Showing empathy is a kindness that just may help someone over a particularly difficult period in his life.

OFFICE STRESS

The hectic pace of a medical office practice creates pressure. On some days, there may be little time to exchange even a complete sentence with a co-worker. Therefore, lunch and rest breaks are essential to your well-being

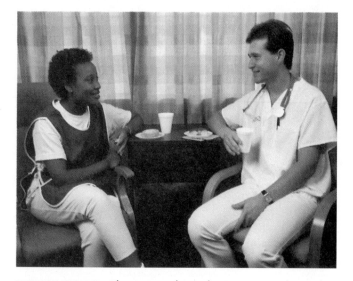

FIGURE 20–10 These co-workers take time out to relax and enjoy a pleasant conversation without interruption and then return to work with a renewed attitude.

(Figure 20–10). Time away from the responsibilities of patient care can give a whole new outlook on a problem. Some offices schedule time for the lunch period between morning and afternoon patients and block the time routinely in the appointment book. This is a good practice. You return to work refreshed and are more productive as a result. Most medical practices have a heavy schedule and working overtime is a frequent reality. Many find that trading evenings with another employee is a good practice. Because patients do not get sick by appointment, schedules will never run perfectly. Flexibility must be acquired early. A great number of problems stem from the high-pressure nature of the job itself. Realizing this will be of great help in learning to cope well with whatever situation presents itself. Coping skills will help to relieve stress. Each individual must find and use whatever works best for her. Prioritizing duties from the most important to the least is effective in reducing stress levels. Keeping a list of things to do and working at a comfortable pace is a sensible way to cope with stresses of daily living both in our personal lives and professionally. Learning how to say no to responsibilities that overload us is a smart coping skill, which is difficult for some to use. Many times, there is so much pressure that could be avoided if only an honest look at a situation were taken at the onset of the job. Realizing time schedules and personal abilities is a consideration that must be used.

Another stress reliever is venting of feelings. Office staff meetings and social gatherings are ways to discuss whatever may be a potential negative stressor affecting employees. It could be something as simple as a few employees disliking a particular color of uniform. Having time to get feelings out in the open may lead to a positive solution that would make everyone more comfortable and cooperative.

There may be times when you are tired, have a cold or a headache, or are worried about a personal problem that things will start to go **awry**, and it seems that everything follows suit. This is the time when it seems that every patient who calls has a major health problem or a mistake with their bill or insurance claim. Taking one thing at a time and completing it before starting something else can ease many tensions. There are times when it may become necessary to ask for assistance. It is wise to ask before things get too overwhelming. The right timing is not always apparent to inexperienced employees. Everyone must learn to help out on days when life itself seems to be a chore. Exchanging common courtesies and being considerate of each other's feelings can also help in stressful situations. Just knowing that someone cares is what patients need sometimes. You should give this consideration to colleagues as well.

Because you can be the target of patients', and sometimes coworkers', pent-up feelings from time to time, it is clear that your own feelings will need expression, too. Everyone needs to get rid of negative feelings. If this is not done, one may begin to feel over-burdened. The way that we communicate our feelings to others can determine the course of events. Delivering information in a non-threatening way is very important. Each one of us has personal feelings, and this also has to be remembered. Using tact and consideration is the key to getting along with others. We must also remember that there is a great difference between the things we can and cannot control.

STRESS AND RELATED ILLNESS

Stress in itself is a most useful reaction because it is a signal for one to respond to a stimulus. There is both good and bad stress. Good stress is known as *eustress,* such as special events we look forward to and plan for, or even deadlines to meet (when planned). Those things ultimately beneficial and rewarding to us are motivating and energizing. The stress is temporary and useful to us.

All of us are constantly processing various stimuli that aid us in our daily communications and activities. The difficulty in regard to stress occurs when the stressor is chronic (constant) and causes us to be troubled. Because no shortcut or fast relief can resolve the stressor or situation causing the stress, it becomes *distress* or bad stress. The effects of this chronic stress stay with the affected person so that a potentially dangerous physical and mental state ensues.

Stress manifests itself in individuals in many ways. The most commonly recognized stress-related illnesses are asthma, headaches (migraines), gastritis, heart disease, insomnia, mental (emotional) illness, and peptic ulcers.

The effects of stress are the nerve **receptors** send nerve impulses to the brain, where the sympathetic function of the autonomic nervous system reacts by sending a message of **impending** danger to the adrenal glands.

These glands pour adrenaline into the circulatory system, as do special nerve cells, to give the body extra strength to deal with the impending threat or danger. The heart beats faster, respirations are increased, and digestion slows down to allow the circulation of adrenaline. As the problem is resolved or removed, the body begins to reorganize impulses. The parasympathetic function sends impulses to slow the previously supercharged body functions back to normal levels. The sympathetic and parasympathetic functions work to create a balance of nerve impulses to regulate the activities of the body.

If one is living under constant stress, the heart and circulatory system, the lungs, and the intestinal tract are constantly being literally turned on and off, leaving insufficient time for normal body functioning. The human being, given too much to deal with too often, eventually breaks down and needs repair, as does an automobile run too hard and too long without proper maintenance.

The body reacts to stress by showing various symptoms. Constipation or diarrhea, frequent colds and flu, indigestion, and migraine headaches are a few of the common physical complaints of patients who overtax themselves. Those who seek medical attention for these types of complaints are usually referred to a counseling service, where the cause of the stress may be discovered and eliminated. Once this is accomplished, the symptoms usually disappear.

There are, of course, patients whose symptoms have developed over a long period and whose physical problems have progressed into a major illness. These patients need counseling, medical supervision, and treatment.

Referrals to a family counseling practice or a psychologist are generally the choice because time constraints are a factor in daily practice. Physicians have usually little or no time for counseling during a routine office visit. The general practitioner used to know the whole family and was often the counselor of all members. Some family and general practice physicians still do domestic counseling in a limited manner. You will notice if a patient who has always been pleasant and smiling during previous office visits suddenly demonstrates a change in mood. This patient may begin to complain of headaches or other aches and pains without apparent cause. After the physician's examination and lab reports have been reviewed, if no major cause has been found, the physician may suggest that the patient seek counseling.

In almost every community, large or small hospitals, health centers, and clinics offer mental health services. The county medical society will be helpful in referring patients to a physician, psychologist, or psychiatrist if listings are not available in the local phone directory.

Inquiries about mental health services should be treated with **discretion**. Mental illness can be a difficult and delicate problem to deal with, not only for the patient, but for family, close friends, and neighbors. As in all matters of medical records, confidentiality must be carefully maintained.

Depression

Depression is treated by physicians with both counseling and medication. Some patients may respond well with counseling only, however. Where medication is given, careful supervision of patients is a must. Alerting the physician to any changes that the patient reports by phone is vital in the direction of the patient's therapy.

Depression is a predictable reaction to the death of a relative, spouse, or close friend, for example. A person may take some time to overcome this grief, the amount of time varying with the individual. Usually, after a few months, the person should begin to adjust to the loss, however. When normal functioning does not return, assistance is necessary.

All ages can be affected by depression. The same symptoms can be recognized in varying degrees of any patient who is depressed: feelings of sadness, helplessness, lack of interest in everyday life, withdrawing from others, and a variety of other problems. Often, there are also feelings such as fear, anxiety, and hostility. When conducting telephone or face-to-face triage, the medical assistant should be alert to any signs of depression and report these findings to the physician. Many times patients or their family members simply do not recognize the signs of depression. Providing patient information in the reception area is a good way to offer passive assistance. Seeing this reading material may prompt those who are suffering from symptoms of depression to ask for help for themselves or for another person. **CAUTION:** A person who is severely depressed can be suicidal. Posting the suicide prevention hotline phone number and being kind and reassuring will show patients that you and your colleagues are caring individuals. You can be of great assistance in documenting these types of problems and be instrumental in the initiation of treatment for troubled patients.

There are many causes of depression, including a chemical imbalance. Initial treatment of depression may be medication in the form of an antidepressant drug. This medicine must be carefully monitored and documented. Any adverse reactions or side effects must be reported to the physician immediately. Getting to the root of the patient's depression must be determined along with the cooperation of the patient for a treatment plan to be effective. Management of depression cannot be rushed. Family and friends can be most helpful in showing understanding and support in the person's recovery. The medical assistant should remember that depression and mental illness are real problems that require empathy and consideration. Remaining non-judgmental and compassionate is required to help patients feel at ease.

There is still a certain amount of non-acceptance of mental illness in society even today. Patients sometimes feel that they are not treated with respect and that others make fun of them. This is certainly not a professional way to behave around patients no matter what their diagnosis is. The professional image that you project should show respect to all individuals. Many times patients and their family members or friends just need someone to listen to them so that they can vent their feelings. People expect members of the health care team to be compassionate and understanding, and they will look to you for support.

Psychosomatic Illness

Psychosomatic illness is not imagined. These patients have very real symptoms. However, the symptoms are usually emotional and not organic in nature. Patients with psychomatic illness may have deep-rooted guilt feelings, fears, frustrations, hostilities, anxieties, or phobias. The patient may not be conscious of these feelings. The stress-related illnesses described earlier are some of the common physical expressions of psychosomatic illness.

Anxiety

Anxiety is a stress-related condition in which the patient is in a constant state of worry. Those who are constantly feeling apprehension and fear have a variety of physical ailments as a result, which can lead to serious illness if not treated. Concerns over money or sexual dysfunction are common anxieties. Patients of this type usually need a combination of counseling and medication to regain a healthy outlook on life and function productively.

Psychoses

Psychosis is a more profound mental disorder characterized by impairment of normal intellectual and social functioning. These patients usually have either partially or completely withdrawn from reality. Their condition may become so severe that hospitalization is necessary. These patients have severe mood swings, sometimes experience hallucinations, and may not know who they are. Patients may be treated on an out-patient basis, but the most severe cases are hospitalized. Many persons in psychotic states can, with long-term treatment, return to normal functioning. Other psychotic states may be irreversible.

When dealing with patients who have, or appear to have, mental illness, it is best if you observe interactions between the patient and an experienced colleague and not attempt to take on such a responsibility if you do not know how to deal with it adequately. These patients need to be carefully assessed and their progress monitored closely and recorded accurately. In these matters, experience is often the best teacher.

Strategies for Coping with Stress

Many public service agencies, churches, colleges, businesses, and private organizations offer educational programs in stress management. Most programs deal with methods which can be practiced by individuals in coping with their personal lives. Significant life events, such as major changes in employment, geographic location, marital status, or health create varying levels of stress. Support groups can help; meetings are held to discuss problems or situations that are too complex or difficult to figure out alone. For that matter, a close friend can be a valuable resource. Simply identifying a source of stress may relieve some of it, but some action must usually be taken to relieve most stressful situations. Finding workable solutions to problems may take a considerable amount of time and patience. Counseling can help both in defining problems and in beginning to take definitive action to **implement** changes. Individuals must recognize the importance of **prioritizing** values and standing firm in beliefs, while at the same time remaining flexible enough to cope with new and challenging situations.

Activities that help you relax are a basic necessity. For some, it may be working a jigsaw puzzle, reading, or listening to music; for others, it may be taking a walk after supper, dancing, or gardening. Each person should find an enjoyable **leisure** activity. Something that refreshes the spirit and **rejuvenates** the soul is a must for sound mental and physical health. You also need to give yourself a pat on the back occasionally for doing a good job.

Following a dull pattern of work-eat-sleep-work is not enough. Boredom can also produce stress. Personal growth and development are rewarding and essential. A hobby or interest is vital to feeling good about yourself. Many find that physical activity is the answer (Figure 20–11). Regular exercise is not only a good way to relieve tension, it keeps you in shape and stimulates more energy. A daily

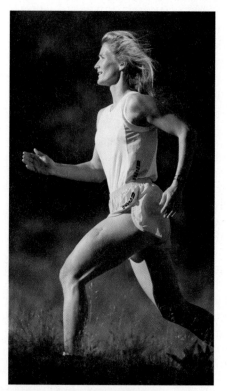

FIGURE 20–11
Exercise is good for the body and spirit, as shown by the trim body and pleasant expression.

program of physical activity is an excellent and refreshing outlet for stress relief.

Health conscious people today participate in exercise groups through community centers, schools, work, private health clubs, or public facilities, such as the YMCA/YWCA. Still others follow an individual exercise regimen. Whatever one does to stay physically fit, it will have a positive effect in reducing stress.

You may want to place exercise class announcements and other health-related tips on a bulletin board in the reception area or by the scale, or wherever patients have enough time to read and copy the information.

An excellent means of venting one's inner feelings is by associating with your peers. Talking "shop" for a while can be good therapy and can lead to friendships outside the workplace. Membership in a professional association will provide you with many growth opportunities. You can make strong friendships and participate in a variety of continuing education programs for personal and professional growth. Membership is encouraged because it adds a new perspective to your career.

Because stress is perceived by each of us differently, a personal evaluation to define the cause of our individual stress is necessary for relieving or eliminating it from our lives. Developing good habits of coping can include quiet "alone" time for reflecting, meditation (Figure 20–12), daydreaming (and visualization), imaging, or other techniques that help clear the mind and renew the spirit. The old saying, "a healthy mind—a healthy body" is becoming more evident. Maintaining a daily routine of physical and mental exercises to relieve anxiety and tension is a healthy way to cope with stress. A happier, healthier life results from successful stress management.

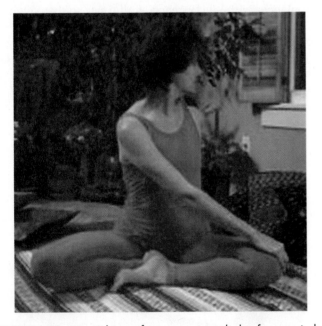

FIGURE 20–12 Taking a few moments each day for a period of quiet to meditate and organize your thoughts is a most healthy habit.

TIME MANAGEMENT

Effective time management involves careful assessment of one's personal routine and deciding how and when to accomplish priorities. Being in control of your time is both simple and complex. It is simple because *you* are ultimately the one who decides what you will do with your time. The complexity of time management is generated from relationships with others, responsibilities, interests, and goals. All of these factors influence us and how our time is spent. In addition, each of us has a personal body clock, physical and emotional strengths and weaknesses, and limits in what can be achieved in a 24-hour period.

Each of us has a unique biorhythm, or pattern of our biological body clock. We do not all function at peak performance all the time, at the same time, or in the same way; we function when our recurring biorhythm dictates it. Those who know themselves well can judge pretty accurately when the best time is for their maximum production, peak performance, and best coping abilities. Also, those who live a healthy lifestyle generally find that they have a greater capacity for dealing with the unpredictable events of life than those who do not. Thus, knowing when you function at your best can have a great influence on your success rate. Planning to present a topic at an inservice when you are at your peak, for example, will help you earn a successful outcome. As we all know, often there is nothing one can do to change a date to fit her own personal needs, but when there is a choice, it can make all the difference. On the days when we feel the best, our energy level is highest, a positive attitude is not easily shaken, and we can even push ourselves further if necessary to finish a task or project. Being flexible is far easier to do when you feel good. On the days when we are at our lowest, there is little reserve in our patience tank, energy source, and coping skills. Pushing to complete something takes everything out of us, if in fact we can even think about finishing it. The bad days should be few and far between if you take proper care of yourself.

We should pay attention to our own personal needs in order to function well. A regular routine of exercise and rest and a well-balanced diet are necessary for us to feel good physically. Just as the body needs adequate time to break down and assimilate the foods that are ingested for nourishment, so does one's mind and soul need time to process all that is taken in during the day. Everyone has a need for relaxation and recreation. Taking care of ourselves is necessary for productivity in both our personal and professional lives. We can motivate ourselves and give ourselves a boost in our outlook by setting realistic goals and working toward them by mapping out our own practical course to accomplish them. Taking advantage of opportunities to develop personally and professionally gives one's attitude a positive charge and keeps one's mind and spirit rejuvenated.

You must be realistic with goal setting and expectations. Allowing sufficient time, padded with some flexibility, built in for unexpected events and emergencies is a sensible way to schedule projects and other ventures. For example, when one is taking a class and has a number of assignments that are complex and time consuming, the due dates should be entered in your schedule book, calendar, or planner as soon as the dates are known. Among the necessary steps you will need to devote to this type of project are going to the library, taking notes, writing the first draft, making corrections, and typing your final copy, which all take varying amounts of time. Enter several time slots for doing each of the things listed above far in advance of the due dates. If each step is not taken into account with what is going on with the rest of your life, other classes, work schedule, personal affairs, rest, and all other responsibilities, pressures will mount, and you could get quite far behind in your work. This is the point where you can meet stress head-on.

This stress can be minimized by careful time management. The key is regular and faithful attention to keep a calendar of your life events. Whatever is important enough to accomplish is important enough to enter in your planner so that it will not be overlooked. Everything of significance to you should be considered: family activities and special events, private (meditation) time, parent-teacher conferences, work schedule (your late night or Saturday), staff meetings, seminars, professional development inservice dates, dental appointments, luncheon dates, exercise, concerts, vacation time, shopping, and deadlines. If you have never kept a planner before, and even before you begin, you should make a list of your short-term goals (it could be a week, a month, six months, or a year, depending on the goal and how short term it is). Then, list your long-term goals, usually thought of in years (five, ten, even lifetime goals) on a sheet of paper. After you have completed your goal sheets and made any new decisions about what you want to do, you need to prioritize what you want to accomplish first, and so on. The primary goal is to eliminate activities that are not worth the time they demand. Generally, a good rule to follow is to single out one issue at a time and deal with it thoroughly and appropriately.

Once you have made the choice or choices, you must make a list of all of the things that you need to do in a day, in a week, in a month, and in a year (or however long it may take to reach your goal), to succeed. Make out a "to do" list each day, and update your planner accordingly. Number them in the order of their importance, with one being the most important. Keep the list of what needs to be done in the planner for that particular day. As each of the items listed is accomplished, cross through it. This will help you visualize what you have done and gives you a feeling of accomplishment. The items that were not completed should be listed on the next day's list of things to do. If you find that an item is being put off until the next day's list too many times, you should evaluate the item and either eliminate it from your schedule or delegate it to someone to do it for you. Giving up a task that

may be worth doing, but does not rank high enough on your list to do it yourself, may be something as essential as hiring someone to do your housework or yard work. Avoid over-crowding and over-scheduling as much as possible. If, for instance, you have decided to take up a musical instrument, you must schedule time for lessons *and* practice. Your schedule must be updated on a regular basis (daily, and several times during the day if necessary). Your goal in using a planner may be simply to get yourself organized and make better use of your time. Keeping track of a personal schedule can be done easily and inexpensively by using a calendar that has large enough squares for writing in appointments and other important information. Scheduling appointments for patients to see the physician was discussed in Unit 2 of Chapter 6. The same basic principle of making the best use of time applies to us personally and professionally in a medical facility. Appointment schedule books are different from a personal planner in that they generally are scheduled for only the business day and week. Your personal planner should include all days in the week, and you should note all events in a 24-hour period, not just during the work day.

You can design your own planner for your particular needs, or you may purchase a more sophisticated schedule planner. There are many types and styles, sizes and colors made from a variety of materials. Figure 20–13 shows an example of a schedule planner. Office supply stores usually have a good selection of professional (one- or two-year) schedule planners from which to choose. There are also electronic pocket organizers available that can be used independently or in linking data with your personal computer. These can fit comfortably in your pocket, purse, tote bag, or briefcase. You must keep your schedule planner within your reach at all times so that you can refer to it when you are asked about a specific date or need to make an entry. As time passes and dates change, you must rearrange them in your schedule. There will be times when appointments or events are canceled and have

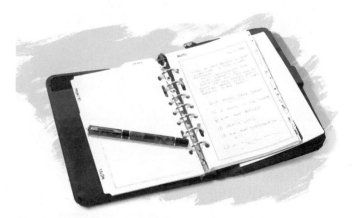

FIGURE 20–13 Example of a popularly used schedule planner

to be rescheduled. Often trying to find a date that is not already taken may place the rescheduled time too far ahead. It is a good idea, just as is done in the physician's appointment, to establish a matrix. That will block a day or so a week for just those kinds of situations. Adjustments may require that you schedule back-to-back appointments only for a day or two to catch up. Remember that this planner is your personal and your professional schedule. If you use it effectively and wisely, you will regularly write in time for yourself to have some "alone time," recreation, meditation, exercise, and spiritual and emotional nurturing. These are all most important for your well-being. The planner you select is a smart investment in yourself, if you use it, because it will help you use your time wisely and to the fullest.

ACHIEVE UNIT OBJECTIVES

Complete Chapter 20, Unit 3, in the workbook to help you obtain competency of this subject.

UNIT 4

Related Therapies

OBJECTIVES

Upon completion of the unit, meet the following performance objectives by verifying knowledge of the facts and principles presented through oral and written communication at a level deemed competent.

1. Spell and define, using the glossary at the back of the text, all the **Words to Know** in this unit.
2. Differentiate between complementary and alternative therapies
3. Explain the placebo effect.
4. List six guidelines to use when considering a related therapy.
5. List the four requirements for FDA (the Food and Drug Administration) approval.
6. Describe what is required for a therapy to be accepted as effective.
7. Briefly describe the related therapies discussed.

AREAS OF COMPETENCE (AAMA)

This unit addresses content within the specific competency areas of *Patient care, Professionalism, Communication skills, Legal concepts,* and *Instruction,* as identified in the Medical Assistant Role Delineation Study. Refer to Appendix A for a detailed listing of the areas.

WORDS TO KNOW

acupuncture	hypnosis
alternative	massage
aromatherapy	naturopathy
ayurvedic	placebo
biofeedback	reflexology
complementary	shiatsu
faith	therapeutic
herbal	visualization
homeopathy	yoga
humor	

A great deal of interest has arisen lately in methods of health care other than the traditional medical model with which we are familiar. Some of this interest comes from dissatisfaction with current, at times impersonal, care and the lack of "face time" with physicians. The impact of the HMO and the limiting coverage from insurance companies for certain procedures has also caused concern. Another factor may be expectations for "cures." When conventional medicine fails to improve or correct our problems, we are willing to resort to other possibilities, no matter how unconventional or expensive. We have heard about celebrities who are choosing **alternative** methods to treat their serious illnesses and people who travel to other countries to obtain treatment and medications that are not approved in the United States. Many of these people will testify to the effectiveness of their nonconventional treatment.

Interest in related therapies may also come from learning about health care methods from other cultures. The United States is a true "melting pot" of people from around the world. We live together and learn about the cultures of our neighbors and friends. We see and hear about the different approaches to disease and disorders used in their cultures. We see on television and read in our newspapers about the effectiveness of treatments not offered by conventional medicine. And of course, we are constantly bombarded with the documented "healed" testimonies from gravely ill people in sensational advertisements in magazines, "junk" mail, and gossip news.

Some authorities make a distinction between the various types of related therapies. One type is called **complementary** therapies. These are treatments that are considered to supplement or add to the conventional form of medicine. Some examples are the use of **massage**, acupressure, **acupuncture**, and **hypnosis**. Another type of therapy is called alternative. This is interpreted by some as meaning a method that is used instead of conventional medicine, such as the use of laetrile, shark cartilage, and other products made from various animal parts. Often alternative therapies are not validated by research, and no scientific evidence exists that they are or can be **therapeutic**. It is true that some people have claimed cures from these and other remedies, but without scientific study, the **placebo** effect or spontaneous healing can not be ruled out. (A placebo effect refers to the fact that some people respond favorably to a known ineffective treatment because they believe it is working. This occurs in about 30% to 40% of patients.) In this unit, the word "related" will also be used to mean any treatment, either complementary or alternative because the therapies may not be "labeled" by their practitioners, and to our knowledge, no authority has developed a classification standard.

The National Center for Complementary and Alternative Medicine defines these therapies as "medical practices that are not commonly used, accepted, or available in conventional medicine." In the booklet *Alternative Medicine* by Harvard Medical School, another definition states "those interventions not taught widely in U.S. medical schools nor generally available in U.S. hospitals." Currently, an effort is being made by medical science to become more knowledgeable of therapies from other cultures and those by previous generations in this country. They are trying to distinguish which ones are safe and effective, which are effective but may carry health risks, which are ineffective, and which ones are both ineffective and unsafe. Some medical schools are introducing courses on alternative therapies to provide physicians with a knowledge of non-conventional choices for their own evaluation and to be able to provide care and advice to patients who may select adjunct (added to) treatments.

INCREASED POPULARITY OF RELATED MEDICAL THERAPIES

There has been a dramatic increase in the use of alternatives to traditional medicine. Researchers from Harvard Medical School discovered that 42% of adults in the United States (82 million people) routinely use complementary medical therapies for treating common medical situations. It was estimated that Americans made 629 million office visits and spent an estimated $27 billion of their own dollars on complementary care. It was also documented that most of these therapies are used in addition to, not as a replacement for, their conventional medical care. In another study, it was determined that 60% of the related therapy users discuss their use with their medical doctor, which was a favorable and positive finding.

When selecting a related therapy, it is a good idea to use some guidelines. There are so many **herbal** therapies, healing techniques, and therapeutic approaches that it's difficult to know which ones might provide some benefit and which are a waste of money and time or even a risk to one's health. It is essential that the traditional medical provider be informed of a patient's related therapy treatments, especially when there are major health problems involved. Many herbal formulas contain compounds that react with prescription medications. In addition, products classified as "dietary supplements" are not under regulatory guidelines, so action or side effects have not been scientifically established. A good example is the interaction with the common herb St. John's Wort. It affects the action of drugs such as Coumadin (an anti-clotting drug) and Crixivan (an AIDS drug). It can reduce the level of cyclosporine (an immunosuppressant) in the blood, which has caused organ rejection in several transplant patients. It also reduces the effectiveness of birth control pills. Other drug interactions are known to be potentially dangerous. Remember, there is no regulatory agency governing the purity, stated strength, or method of production of herbal compounds.

There are two prime questions that need to be considered when choosing a related therapy approach: "Is it safe?" and "Does it work?" Some safety factors to think through before trying a therapy are:

- Are there any published studies on the effectiveness of this treatment in reputable medical journals or publications from known medical institutions or organizations?
- Is the treatment a "secret" that only certain providers can offer?
- Is it necessary to travel to another country to take advantage of the treatment?
- Does the provider oppose the person continuing to see their conventional medical doctor? (This is a reason to be skeptical because conventional medicine should not be abandoned while pursuing a complementary therapy.)

There are a growing number of studies on the effectiveness of related therapies. Information is available on the Internet, but reliable sources with evidence of careful analyses are difficult to find. The National Institute of Health and the National Library of Medicine have information available on their Web sites but may be difficult to evaluate (see resources at the end of this chapter).

If someone is thinking about trying unorthodox or related therapy treatments that are untested, they need to think twice and follow some specific guidelines.

- *Read up*—Read labels, look for research information, and talk to a doctor and a pharmacist about the ingredients before taking the medication or treatment. Also, consider the cost, especially if there is no medical evidence that the treatment works. Realize that insurance probably will NOT cover the therapy.
- *Be skeptical*—If it sounds too good to be true, it probably is. The more spectacular the claim and the more it costs, the more one needs to be skeptical.
- *Tell your doctor*—Physicians have become more aware of other therapies because of the increase in their popularity. The doctor needs to know if a patient is visiting a related therapist or taking any herbal remedy to watch for possible signs of drug interactions or adverse effects from the treatment.
- *Combine related and conventional therapies carefully*—Related therapies can be beneficial in some situations. For example, the American Cancer Society reports that options, such as aromatherapy, meditation, massage and biofeedback, appear to help patients deal with pain

and improve their quality of life. However, there are no proven related cures for cancer, and conventional treatment offers the best option and must be continued.

■ *Choose a professional who has appropriate training and credentials*—Some of the major related therapy providers are licensed or at least credentialed by their respective professions. This does not guarantee that the treatment will be effective, however; it just means that the person is trained in that specialty.

■ *Put safety first*—A label that reads "all natural" or "organic" does not necessarily mean it is safe because there is probably no regulation controlling the product. The same is true for some treatments. For example, body manipulations may be helpful for one person's condition but very harmful for an other. Read and understand the therapy. Discuss the option with the physician for medical insight before beginning treatment.

Foods

There are volumes written about the claims of certain foods. There is a strong body of evidence showing that *fruits and vegetables* promote good general health. Some foods may even protect against heart disease and certain cancers. Eating a diet with 9 servings of fruits and vegetables a day lowers the risk of ischemic stroke by 31%. The value of folates in the diet has shown that it reduces homocysteine in the blood—a substance that is linked to the risk of heart disease, stroke, and Alzheimer's. Fruits and vegetable also reduce obesity because they contain fewer calories and are filled with fiber to help people feel full. The most benefit comes from eating a variety of fruits and vegetables so that you consume a greater number of vitamins and minerals and benefit from the interaction between the nutrients. A general rule is: the brighter the color, the greater amount of protective phytochemicals (compounds that are known to be beneficial). Strawberries, blueberries, spinach, and kale are very colorful and have high antioxidant activity. Spinach, for example, not only has a lot of folate but also contains vitamin C, which helps the body to absorb the iron in the spinach. This natural combination of elements is much more beneficial than taking isolated nutrients in supplements.

The benefit from *whole grains* is well documented in its ability to lower the risk for heart disease, adult onset diabetes, hypertension, and some types of cancer. Whole grains contain complex carbohydrates, minerals, and antioxidants. There is also growing evidence that drinking *tea* may lower the rate of heart disease and cancer. This is based upon three areas of research. Tea has an antioxidant property that my help prevent the artery damage that can lead to heart attacks. Second, studies show tea drinkers have lower cholesterol levels, which also lowers heart disease risk. Third, when comparing sets of tea drinkers to non-drinkers, the drinkers have lower rates of heart attack. Tea has also been associated with lowering the risk of developing cancer. Green tea may help

protect against breast, colon, rectal, lung, and pancreatic cancer; however, there are contradicting studies showing increased rates in other cancers. Apparently, only regular tea is beneficial because herbal, instant ice tea mixes, or bottled teas contain undetectable levels of healthful substances.

Ginger is a food substance that can settle the stomach in certain instances. It has been studied for use in motion sickness, chemotherapy nausea, post-surgical nausea, and morning sickness with mixed results. The research did show taking a one-gram dose 30 minutes before travel could be recommended. *Garlic* is another food item that has been promoted as healthful. It does seem to have some ability to lower cholesterol and blood pressure, thereby preventing heart disease. It has been used for centuries to treat many conditions from tuberculosis to hemorrhoids and to ward off vampires. Laboratory studies have suggested that garlic might help fight cancer but *human studies* have not determined it lowers cancer risk. However, dietary histories of 564 Chinese people with stomach cancer were compared to 1,131 individuals without the disease. It was concluded the risk of developing stomach cancer was 60% lower among people who ate the most alliums (garlic, onions, leeks, and shallots), which seem to infer some protective benefit. Its cousin, the onion, was used for a poultice (a hot mashed mass inside a cloth) to treat chest congestion in years gone by.

Walnuts and other nuts in general have been identified as being able to reduce the risk of heart disease. Even though they are loaded with calories and fat, researchers believe that because they are rich in monounsaturated and polyunsaturated fats, they lower the LDL and raise the HDL cholesterol levels. However, this is possible only when these types of fat replace the saturated fats in meats and dairy products.

Our ancestors have used many other food type substances over the years. Native Americans used many wild berries, roots, and other things growing in their environment to make medicinal products. Early pioneers dug sassafras and ginseng root and used many herbs and compounds to treat their families. People still dig and use these roots today. A hundred years ago, women used a product called Lydia E. Pinkham's Vegetable Compound to ease "all those painful complaints and weaknesses so common to our best female population." One component of the product that did some of the "easing" was alcohol, which of course "ladies" did not consume in its other form. Its main ingredient was a woodland plant called black cohosh, which is still used today. Many of these former compounds have been studied and have been determined to contain beneficial properties.

Some other food items have been promoted as medicinal. Perhaps the most famous is Laetrile (the chemical compound anygdalin), a product of the kernels of fruit pits from peaches, almonds, and apricots. It is an alternative therapy for the treatment of cancer that was used in Russia in 1840s and in the U.S. in the 1920s. The theory behind its effectiveness is that the bacteria in the intestinal tract react to the compound and produce cyanide, which in turn increases the acid content of tumors, which then destroys lysosomes and kills the cancer cells. Scientific clinical trials were conducted that proved the treatment was not effective. Because of this finding and the fact that some patients even developed cyanide poisoning, the drug was banned from the U.S. It is still available in some foreign countries, including Mexico, where U.S. citizens who think it might provide them a cure most often obtain the drug.

Interesting information regarding many unusual treatments can be found on the Internet, but care must be taken to evaluate the content. You can read about the benefits of blue-green algae and vitamins you have never heard of like B$_{15}$. Two reliable sites operated by the National Cancer Institute of the National Institute of Health are in the resource information at the end of this chapter.

HERBAL PRODUCTS AND DIETARY SUPPLEMENTS

There has been a 380% increase in the use of herbal products since 1990, with an estimated 17% of people using herbal medicines regularly. In the past few years, dietary supplement business has skyrocketed into a $12-billion industry in the United States alone. In 1999, Congress appropriated funds for the Office of Dietary Supplements as part of the National Institutes of Health (NIH) to investigate the safety and effectiveness of herbal medicines. Scientific study is underway, and some results are beginning to be published. The most important thing to understand about dietary supplements is that there is a big difference in these products and conventional over-the-counter (OTC) drugs, even though they may be displayed on the same shelves in drug and grocery stores. The Food and Drug Administration (FDA) closely regulates OTC drugs but has virtually no responsibility over supplements. The FDA requires that OTC drugs be tested for stated effectiveness and that they meet standards for purity of their contents. With supplements you do not know for sure what you are buying. Substances passing OTC regulations require clinical trials, designated dosage establishment, documentation of side effects, and characteristics of people who had adverse reactions. Manufacturers are also required to show the product is at least as good as any previously-approved product for the same purpose. These reports are published in scientific journals for professional and public review. This whole process requires about 15 years from lab to consumer and costs about $500 million per item. It is no wonder that the manufacturers of supplements fight being brought under FDA control. At present, they have an exempt FDA status category of "dietary supplements" established by Congress in 1994. Untested products can be sold as supplements and direct claims as to the effectiveness or health benefit

cannot be made; however, indirect claims are allowed and have been stretched to the limit. Labels on dietary supplements should contain a list of ingredients and their strength, a suggested dosage, and any warning to its use. There should also be the standard statement, "These statements have not been evaluated by the Food and Drug Administration. This product is not intended to diagnose, treat, cure or prevent any disease." A few of the most common products that may have some benefit are:

St. John's Wort—Is widely used for herbal treatment for depression. A clinical trial in 1996 showed it worked as well as older antidepressant drugs for mid to moderate depression with few side effects. No standards for dosage, its preparation, or its long-term safety have been developed. Even though classified as a supplement, it has drug-like actions.

Black Cohosh—Is a large woodland plant found in eastern North America that is used for menopause relief as an alternative to traditional hormone therapy. It is effective in controlling hot flashes, night sweats, headaches, heart palpitations, and mood changes. Its effect seems to suggest that it contains a natural estrogen-like substance and the known salicylates found in aspirin. There are no recognized major studies on the compound and a lack of scientific trials common to all supplements. It appears the side effects are mild when taken in moderate amounts, but it can include vomiting, dizziness, and headaches in larger doses. Because it is not standardized, each manufacturer indicates the dosage. It is recommended that black cohosh should not be taken for more than six months because no long-term studies have be done on its safety.

Melatonin—Is a hormone produced naturally in the pineal gland within the brain. It plays a part in regulating sleep patterns. As a supplement, it is used to regulate sleep and prevent jet lag. It has also been promoted as an anti-aging agent. Evidence does seem to support its effect on sleep, and laboratory studies indicate it has antioxidant properties at much larger concentrations than in the body. No evidence exists that it slows the aging process or reduces the risk of developing cancer. A potential risk from melatonin is the resulting drowsiness that impairs function and may cause morning-after headaches. It has also been reported to interfere with conception.

Willow Bark—Has been used to relieve pain for more than 2,400 years. Hippocrates prescribed chewing on willow leaves to relieve childbirth pain. In the second century, it was used to reduce fever and inflammation. In 1897, a Bayer chemist determined that acetylsalicylic acid (aspirin) could be extracted from a willow-bark-related compound. Now, willow bark is being sold as a natural pain relief medication. Double-blind trials of 210 people with chronic low back pain determined willow bark extract to be a useful and safe treatment, at least for low back pain. Again, remember, it is not controlled or standardized. The recommended maximum daily dose is 240 mg, but it should not be used by people who have problems tolerating aspirin.

Echinacea—Is an herb reported to stimulate the immune system to help prevent developing a cold or the flu. It has been used for centuries by Native Americans to treat everything from coughs to burns and snakebites. Trials have reported milder symptoms and fewer sick days among echinacea users, but the studies were not totally scientific. It is difficult to recommend the product because it grows in three forms having different concentrations of ingredients. It also depends upon which part of the plant is used: the leaf, roots, or flowers. Analysis in 1999 of a dozen brands found great variety in concentrations and makes recommendations difficult. It is apparently more effective in liquid than tablet or capsule form. Potential side effects include severe allergic reactions, which indicates all people with asthma or allergic rhinitis should avoid usage. Echinacea can also be toxic to the liver if taken longer than eight weeks; therefore anyone using other drugs known to affect the liver are at potential risk.

Saw Palmetto—Is a plant that produces berries containing phytosterols compounds that scientists think might slow down the production of male testosterone that stimulates prostate growth. The compound is used to treat symptoms of benign prostate hypertrophy. Several traditional medications are available but are sometimes not effective and may cause a decline in sexual desire or impotency. Little research has been done in the U.S., but European investigation suggests it is safe and effective for the symptoms but can upset the gastrointestinal system and cause nausea in some. It is again noted that, without regulation, there's no guarantee of the purity or content of the product.

Glucosamine—Is a substance promoted as a product to relieve the pain of osteoarthritis. It reportedly promotes healthy cartilage formation to maintain or replace that which is worn away by age and use. European studies did confirm that it provides pain relief and increases mobility. It is widely used in the U.S. No side effects have been noted.

Ginseng—Is the root of a Chinese shrub and has been studied primarily in Asia. Varieties of ginseng come from other places, such as Siberia, Japan, and even the U.S. Scientific investigation has failed to support its claims as an aphrodisiac. There is evidence it improves circulation and elevates mood.

Gingko biloba—Is a product from the leaves of the ginkgo tree and is promoted as an agent to improve memory and mental function by increasing blood flow to the brain. European studies suggest that it may slow the progress of or even prevent Alzheimer's disease. It also appears to be an antioxidant and might help prevent atherosclerotic plaque. Side effects of nausea, vomiting, and diarrhea occur at extremely high doses.

This discussion of common herbs and supplements only scratches the surface of products that are available in grocery and health food stores. Remember, there is no industry control, so you are never sure of what you purchase. If the word "standardized" is used on the label, it is probably what it says it is. The use of supplements requires reading and careful consideration. Look for quality of evidence in reports, how many people are using the product, and their experiences. Discuss it with a physician; many are now familiar with supplements and can provide advice. Choose a brand tested in published studies if possible. For a database of medical literature, refer to the National Library of Medicine through a library, or find abstracts on their Web site listed at the end of this chapter. Learn as much as you can to make the wisest selection.

RELATED THERAPIES

The following is a brief look at several therapies that promote some form of medical intervention or treatment. If you find it interesting, there are many resources on alternative and complementary therapies for additional study.

Accupuncture

Accupuncture is a form of traditional Chinese medicine that is also practiced by the Japanese, Koreans, and the French. It consists of using extremely thin, sterilized needles, sometimes electrified with low-voltage, that are inserted on points along the network of 12 body meridians (channels) to connect the different levels from the organs to the skin. It is used as an anesthetic or to treat pain. Chinese medicine addresses the whole person when diagnosing or treating an illness. They have a fundamental philosophical idea of Qi (pronounced Chee) that believes the presence of this vital energy flows through the body and divides the living from the dead. Maintaining Qi is essential for good health. Illness results from disturbances in the flow of Qi, either too much or too little through the meridians. Qi is actually the balance of two opposing energies, yin and yang. Yin organs are those which are solid, such as the heart, spleen, lungs, kidney, and liver. There is an interacting corresponding hollow yang organ. These are the small intestine (heart), stomach (spleen), large intestine (lungs), bladder (kidney), and gallbladder (liver). (The organs do not necessarily correspond to Western anatomical organs. The spleen, for example, includes the entire digestive tract, while the heart is where one's conscious is, not the brain.) When yin and yang are in harmony, they work to achieve and maintain health. Acupuncture acts on Qi flowing through the meridians to help the body redirect the energy.

Acupuncture has a long history, but studies have not validated its effects. Western hypothesis is that acupuncture triggers the release of pain-killing molecules in the brain and central nervous system to provide relief from pain. Care needs to be taken in selecting a practitioner. Licensing requirements vary from state to state, and some have no requirements. A safe alternative is to find one who is certified from the National Certification Commission for Acupuncture and Oriental Medicine.

Aromatherapy

Aromatherapy is a treatment that uses essential oils extracted from plants for a therapeutic effect. Different oils are used for specific conditions, such as lavender for first aid of burns, neroli for anxiety, and tea tree for antibacterial and antifungal action. Use of oils goes back thousands of years. In 4500 BC, a Chinese emperor recorded therapeutic properties of plants that match those assigned properties today. Some of the oils have an estrogen-like effect; others are sedative or anti-infectious. There are a wide variety of chemical properties in the oils and their associated function. The issue of safety with using the oils has been discussed, but no definitive answers have been established. The quality and chemical content of the product changes because of conditions during growth, such as weather and altitude. Maintaining their composition is important. They must be stored in amber glass bottles to provide protection from light. Bottles must be sealed tightly and stored away from heat. They can be diffused through the air, inhaled, or absorbed through the skin with massage. Oils can also be used as a compress, in wound care, or as a mouth-rinse. There is therapeutic value in using oils for stress and anxiety; insomnia and restlessness; common colds and flu; muscular and neuralgic pain; arthritis; headaches and migraines; and digestive disorders and constipation. Many oils are sold in department, beauty, and drug stores that are supposed to affect your mood, but these are not the same as the medicinal therapeutic oils use by practitioners.

Ayurvedic Medicine

Ayurvedic Medicine is the traditional healing system of India and is perhaps the oldest formal medical system in the world. It addresses mental and spiritual well-being and physical health. Treatment is tailored to the individual's need with a strong emphasis on preventive self-care. Ayurveda identifies three types of energies that are present in all things: vata, pitta, and kapha. Vata energy is associated with movement. Pitta relates to metabolism and those types that tend to be intense, quick to anger, and have a medium build. Kapha is linked to structure and the types that are slow moving, calm, and have a larger body frame. Each person has a unique combination but is dominant in one. The practitioner tries to access the proportion of the energies and customize a health program to bring them into a health balance.

Sickness results from the energies being out of balance. The practitioner asks questions to determine the diet, sleep and elimination habits, emotional temperament, and personal and family history. He takes a pulse in both wrists and examines the tongue, eyes, and general appearance. He listens to the heart, lungs, and even the tone of the voice. Based on his opinion, he outlines a program of diet, herbal formulas, yoga postures, aerobic exercise, breathing techniques, meditation, and a variety of massages. In some cases, when cleansing is needed, he will order steam baths, laxatives, herbal enemas, and even induce vomiting. Practitioners are difficult to find in the U.S., but Indian communities, restaurants, and grocery stores might know of someone. There is an Ayurvedic Institute in Albuquerque, New Mexico that might know if there's a graduate in your area. They can be contacted at 505-291-9698. Herbal preparations from India are not recommended because of the lack of sanitary conditions in production.

Biofeedback

Biofeedback is a method that enables a person, usually with the help of electronic equipment, to learn to control otherwise involuntary bodily functions. It is also defined as any technique that increases the ability of a person to voluntarily control physiological activities by being provided with information about those activities. An example of this is learning to control heart rate by seeing or hearing its activity. The yogis of India have been reported to slow their heartbeat, increase their body temperature, and survive with little oxygen to influence bodily functions. Some methods of feedback involve skin response monitors to register autonomic tension or relaxation and skin temperature. Other monitors can indicate muscle activity or register brain waves. Therapeutic uses can be helpful with asthma, cardiovascular disorders, headaches, insomnia, controlling stress, and neuromuscular problems. Biofeedback has also been helpful in treating incontinence, migraines, and irritable bowel syndrome. Remarkable results have been attained with the electroencephalogram (EEG) application. Persons with learning difficulties, addiction, attention deficit, hyperactivity, and identity syndrome have reported benefits. The technique has been taught to persons with brainstem stroke or motor neuron disease who are totally paralyzed. By learning to control brain wave patterns, they can activate an alphabet board to communicate. It is believed this technique may some day be used to operate machines and vehicles.

Faith

One of the fastest-growing areas of study in medical schools is the healing power of prayer. Seventy-nine of the nation's 125 medical schools offer courses on prayer and spirituality; there were only three 10 years ago. There have been studies conducted that showed positive results with patients who have chest pains, heart attack, and AIDS. One study gave emergency room heart patients the opportunity to receive prayer. Those who agreed were divided into prayed-for and not-prayed-for groups. The names of the prayer group were sent to prayer gatherings around the world in every major religion. The prayed-for group experienced half as many and some times no side effects or complications from catheterization and angioplasty as did the other group. It was felt that prayer has a positive effect on recovery. Some skeptics felt it was a placebo effect, so the researcher repeated the study except this time they used mice and test tube microbes. It also showed the same type of outcome: the prayed-for mice made uneventful recovery, and the microbes flourished. A study of cardiac patients in 1995 reported those who lacked social support were much more likely to die within six months after cardiac surgery. Another group of older patients who had open heart surgery and who had no social support or received no comfort from religion were three times more likely to die within six months of surgery than those who received such support. Studies show that you don't have to believe in God or another higher being to benefit from intercessionary prayer. The empathy, love, and compassion of the prayer influence the effectiveness of prayer. If you think it is a sham, it won't work. Even though some physicians and health care providers do not accept the power of **faith** and prayer, many do recognize something or someone else was responsible for a patient's unexpected recovery.

Homeopathy

Homeopathy is a 200-year-old system of medicine based on the Law of Similars. This means that if a dose of a substance can cause a symptom, that same substance in minuscule amounts can cure the symptom. It is a highly controversial form of medicine and lacks any scientific explanation as to why it might work. Homeopathic medicines are produced from various natural sources, such as plants, metals, minerals, venoms and stings, and bacteria or human tissue. The materials are diluted many times in a base of water and alcohol. With each dilution, it is shaken vigorously, which practitioners believe gives the final product its power to heal. Sometimes, they are diluted to the point that no molecules of the ingredient remain. Practitioners contend that molecules leave a "memory" in the solution to which the body responds. Because the medicines are so dilute, it may take weeks before any therapeutic effect is seen. Critics believe any response is a placebo effect. Studies have shown insufficient evidence to arrive at any conclusion as to its effectiveness on any clinical condition. Homeopathic medicines are classified and regulated by the FDA as OTC drugs. Holistic healers, such as naturopaths, herbalists, chiropractors, acupuncturists, midwives, and even some medical doctors, also use the drugs. Because they are so dilute, they cause little

safety concerns. But patients should be cautioned to not rely on homeopathy or substitute it for conventional medicine, especially if they have a potentially life-threatening condition. Also, beware of the practitioner who says conventional medications will interfere with the homeopathic treatment and want them to be discontinued. Some also discourage immunization of children, which can be dangerous to the child and the community.

Humor

Humorous intervention by the health care professional or patient is used to produce a beneficial response. The physical response to **humor** and laughter affects most of the major systems of the body, increasing heart rate and blood pressure and improving muscle tone. In addition, following the viewing of a humorous video, IgA concentration and spontaneous lymphocyte multiplication increased while adrenalin and cortisol secretion decreased. Clinical significance of this reaction is unclear, but research has shown that humor can play a part in reducing anxiety. There is some evidence to indicate that humor can be used by patients to cope with cancer. One patient discovered that watching Candid Camera films would give him 10 minutes of "belly laughs" and resulted in two hours of painfree sleep. Dr. Hunter "Patch" Adams is one of this country's leading proponents of humor in medicine, as portrayed in the movie bearing his name. There are Laugh Mobiles and Humor Carts used in clinical settings to lift patient's spirits. They may contain Play Doh, finger paint, water guns, coloring books, Mr. Bubbles, humorous books, funny costumes, and video and audio tapes.

The patient must be assessed to determine if humor is appropriate. The criteria are:

- Timing—The patient might not think it is appropriate at present.
- Receptiveness—What might be funny one time may not be at another.
- Content—Be sure the content is not offensive in any way.
- Patient's beliefs—Determine whether the patient feels humor has a place in patient care.
- Relationship with patient—If a "joking relationship" has been established, it may be appropriate; if not, it may not be.

More research is needed to understand the role of humor in recovery or coping with illness. It is known that laughter increases NK cell activity, lymphocyte proliferation, monocyte migration, and the production of IL-2 and IgA, which are positive effects in the immune system.

Hypnosis and Self-Hypnosis

Hypnosis can be a very beneficial therapy to improve health and well-being. Most of us think of it as some theatrical trick that causes people to do funny things, but it can be a powerful therapeutic tool. It is effective against skin conditions, insomnia, stage fright, shyness, a habit such as smoking, weight gain, and pain, and it promotes rapid surgical recovery. It is something that a person can learn to do. The ability to achieve a " trance state" is inborn in about 90% of all people. Psychologist Dr. Fisher defines a trance as "a state of heightened attention in which your concentration is so focused that you are completely unaware of what's going on around you." In this state, both mind and body are very receptive to suggestions, and the right suggestions can change the way we act. He says it is possible to induce this state of trance yourself with self-hypnosis, so that you can give yourself specific instructions to make any changes you want. There are two essential steps to self-hypnosis:

1. Learn how to induce a trance whenever you want.
2. Use mental imagery to talk to your body and mind.

Dr. Fisher describes the steps to take to enter a trance and claims it should take less than a minute to achieve. A highly hypnotized person may feel totally detached, whereas a lesser state may only produce deep relaxation and alertness. The depth of the trance doesn't matter as much as the motivation to achieve the changes desired. He describes the steps to a trance as follows:

Step 1.   Sit or lie down with your head in a relaxed position. Focus your gaze upward as if you are trying to see your eyebrows. Close your eyes. Continue looking upward. Take a deep breath, and hold it for a count of three.

Step 2.   Exhale. Relax your eyes. Envision yourself gently floating downward, as if entering a safe and comfortable place.

Step 3.   When you're ready to come out of the trance, count backward slowly from three to one. Look upward. Open your eyes and slowly bring the world back into focus.

Dr. Fisher goes on to say that it is important to make your hypnotic suggestions concrete and very specific and express them to yourself in mental imagery. You need to see and feel yourself being the way you would like. The suggestions must be repeated 8 to 10 times each day for 90 seconds at a time. As an example, you want to loose weight, but you eat without really savoring the food or sensing when you are full. While in the trance, visualize yourself on a "TV screen" as you now appear. On an adjacent "screen," picture how you want to look after reaching your target weight. Twist the imaginary knob to turn the image on the first screen into the image on the second. (This will help keep you motivated.) Now, picture yourself eating slowly and consciously enjoying every bite. Picture pausing after each bite and asking yourself if you want more.

Obviously, this "treatment" will need to continue until you reach your goal. The format can be transferred to address other changes that are desired. Remember, hypnotherapy works only if the client wants it to.

Hypnotherapy provided by a therapist is actually supported by more scientific research than many other complementary therapies. Trance induction can be achieved by different techniques and may be adapted to the client. Often, the client is asked to focus on a point or concentrate on his breathing until his eyelids become heavy and he closes them and relaxes. The client controls the depth of his trance by his state of relaxation. In the trance, the therapist uses guided imagery to direct the client to address his concerns. The state is ended slowly by allowing the client to control the speed of return by counting from three to one or by the therapist slowly counting.

Clinically, hypnotherapy has been used in childbirth; to provide acute or chronic pain relief; for stress management; to control certain phobias; for post-amputation phantom limb pain, nausea, and hypertension; and in irritable bowel syndrome. It has even proved useful as a "numbing agent" in simple injuries that required suturing. Some physicians have incorporated hypnosis as a supplemental therapy in their practice. As with any therapy, it is important to choose a qualified professional practitioner. Hypnosis is not a substitute for treating a psychological condition, such as depression or a psychosis.

Magnet Therapy

Americans spend $500 million a year on magnetic devices to relieve headache, arthritis, tendonitis, foot pain, and other ailments. A neurologist, Dr. Michael Weintraub, recently completed a large study on the effectiveness of magnets. For 30 years, he had participated in many scientific studies using medications for treating headache and spinal pain. Relief was often inadequate, and side effects were common. He became interested in non-drug therapies like acupuncture and massage. He later was introduced to the use of magnets by one of his patients who had a cervical herniated disk. His recommendation of steroids helped until the patient returned to work, which worsened the pain. After consulting a neurosurgeon, the patient began using magnets instead of opting for surgery and had become pain-free. Dr. Weintraub's skepticism prompted him to investigate the use of magnets as a therapeutic device. He studied patients with unmanageable peripheral neuropathy common to patients with diabetes, with alcoholism, or receiving chemotherapy.

- His first small study used magnets in the shoes of 14 people and resulted in a 64% reduction in symptoms, a much higher rate than with conventional therapy.
- A second study used a real magnet in one shoe and a worthless device in the other. The results showed a 90% improvement in the magnetic-treated foot after four months of therapy.

- A recent study followed NIH protocol and involved 375 patients in 27 states with 95% having moderate to severe neuropathy pain. With 98% of the data in, results indicate a significant improvement in pain, numbness, and tingling.
- A small study was also conducted on 15 patients with carpal tunnel syndrome with a finding of 50% reduction in pain, numbness, and tingling. He also has had success in treating patients with arthritis and heel spurs.

It is theorized that magnets interrupt the action of small nerve fibers that cause pain and numbness and improve oxygen flow into the tissue. Further research is needed to explain why they work, but evidence shows they do in many instances.

Massage

Therapeutic massage is the second most popular related therapy in the U.S. It encompasses a wide range of approaches using hands to manipulate muscles and soft tissue. It is a powerful means to treat stress-related conditions, such as insomnia, headaches, and irritable bowel syndrome, and health conditions, such as sciatica and depression. There are different types of massage:

- *Swedish* is the most common type of Western massage using kneading and long strokes to reduce pain, relieve insomnia, reduce stress, and promote relaxation.
- *Sports* massage is a vigorous, deep-tissue manipulation to promote greater flexibility, loosen muscles, relieve muscle swelling, and treat injuries to tendons and ligaments.
- *Trigger-point* massage applies concentrated pressure to "trigger points," the areas of irritability in a muscle that are palpable as lumps or knots and may be painful or cause referred pain. This therapy attempts to apply enough pressure to release the chronic contraction of the muscle and stretch the surrounding muscles to prevent recurrence.
- *Shiatsu* massage comes from Japan and makes use of firm finger pressure applied to specific point on the body to balance the flow of chi (vital energy). The massage is done on the lightly clothed patient who lies on a pad on the floor. It has been used to treat low back pain, constipation, and nervous disorders.
- *Thai* massage is also performed through light clothing and on a floor pad. It combines stretches with hand pressure in a meditative, dance-like movement.

There are many other variations of massage. One that is strictly therapeutic is manual lymph drainage massage. This is particularly beneficial for correcting lymph fluid buildup in the arm following mastectomy and lymph node removal. This and some other forms are considered to be medically related and are being used with terminally ill and cancer patients. Insurance companies may cover them, especially if ordered by the physician.

It is recommended that care be taking in selecting a therapist. They are licensed in 25 states. Credentials from a training program accredited by the Commission on Massage Training Accreditation and a certificate from the National Certification Board of Therapeutic Massage and Bodywork are signs of the highest credential in the field.

Other Therapies

If this view into related therapies has been of interest to you, you may want to explore some others.

Hand Reflexology—This practice claims there is a map on the hands that matches a corresponding body part. Stimulating these points on the hand sends impulses to help the muscles in the corresponding body part relax, and blood vessels open to increase circulation, therefore allowing more oxygen and nutrients to enter and promote healing.

Naturopathy—This is a multidisciplinary approach to health care based on the belief that the body has power to heal itself. Treatment is based on assessment of the correct diet, rest, relaxation, exercise, fresh air, clean water, and sunlight the patient is receiving. Herbal products, detoxification procedures, massage, hydrotherapy, counseling, and advice on lifestyle may be used. They may also use homeopathy and acupuncture.

Tai Chi—This is a Chinese movement discipline that improves strength, flexibility, and sense of balance. It can help reduce frailty and falls in elderly patients. It involves a series of fluid movements performed while relaxed but maintaining focus on a pattern of movements. Proper breathing with the exercises helps to integrate the body and mind and enhance the flow of qi and overall health.

Visualization and Guided Imagery—Visualization refers to what you see in your mind's eye, whereas imagery involves all the senses. It can be effective in controlling heart rate, blood pressure, breathing, blood levels of stress hormones, and many other areas. It is a good adjunct therapy for cancer, heart disease, and chronic pain. There is good evidence that it reduces nausea with chemotherapy, reduces post-operative pain, shortens hospital stays, and reduces anxiety. The therapy works when patients visualize some activity affecting their problem. An example might be a patient with cancer visualizing immune cells attacking the malignant cells and destroying them. The more senses that are used, the more "real" it will seem to the brain. Scientists believe that the brain activity may influence the autonomic nervous system that controls important bodily processes.

Yoga—This is a discipline of breath control, meditation, and stretching and strengthening exercises that is thought to promote mental, physical, and spiritual well-being. It has been practiced for thousands of years. There are many types of yoga, such as bhaktri, jnana, karma, laya, raja, and hatha yoga. It places great emphasis on mental and physical fitness. It increases strength, balance, flexibility, and some claim energy and calmness. It consists of breathing exercises, assuming a number of positions, and meditation.

This introduction to the use of specific foods, herbs, supplements, and complementary and alternative therapies may give you a basic understanding of the vast amount of options that are available to patients who are searching for non-traditional methods of health care. Many have been proven to be beneficial when provided by a trained professional and are complementary to traditional medicine.

ACHIEVE UNIT OBJECTIVES

Complete Chapter 20, Unit 4, in the workbook to help you obtain competency of this subject matter.

Medical-Legal-Ethical Scenario

Renita, the office manager, opened the office early to make out the vacation schedules for office employees. Dr. Green was late for rounds and called the office to let Renita know that it would be at least an hour before he would get there. Renita began calling the first patients to delay or reschedule them at their choice. While she was on the phone, a patient without an appointment came in to see the physician. She did not know him. Renita held her hand over the phone receiver and greeted the man. She told him she would be right with him after she finished the call. Within seconds he started to yell and demanded to see the doctor! He pounded his fists on the door and repeated that he had to see the doctor! Renita was not sure, but she suspected that he had taken drugs to be in such a rage and so uncontrollable. She was alone in the office and did not expect the other assistant for another half-hour.

CRITICAL THINKING CHALLENGE

1. Discuss how you think Renita felt during this situation?
2. Who should she call? Why?
3. Should she call the doctor?
4. How should she speak to this patient? Why?
5. Should she continue the calls?
6. Is there any potential legal problem here?
7. What would you do in this situation?

RESOURCES

Alternative medicine: a selection of articles on complementary and integrative therapies (2001, March). Boston: Harvard Health Publications.

American Heart Association. An eating plan for healthy americans [brochure]. Dallas: Author.

Are you obese? (1999, October 27). *JAMA, 282*(16).

Can spirituality improve your health? (2001, July). *Bottom Line Health.*

Complementary medicine (1996, January). *Harvard Women's Health Watch,* p. 3.

Diet, glycemic index, and the food pyramid (2000, December). *Harvard Women's Health Watch.*

Hand reflexology. (2000, November). *Bottom Line Health.*

Magnet therapy does work. (2001, September). *Bottom Line Health.*

National Clearinghouse for Alcohol and Drug Information, P.O. Box 2345, Rockville, MD, 20847-2345.

NIDA National Institute on Drug Abuse, U.S. Department of Health and Human Services, National Institute of Health, P.O. Box 30652, Bethesda, MD, 20824-052.

Royal College of Nursing (2001). The nurses' handbook of complementary therapies (2nd ed.). London: Harcourt Publishers Limited.

Tai Chi: meditative movement for health (2000, December). *Harvard Women's Health Watch,* p. 6.

Weil, A. (2001, September). Ayurvedic medicine: living in balance. *Dr. Andrew Weil's Self Healing,* pp. 2-3.

Weil, A. (1999, August). The healing power of massage. *Dr. Andrew Weil's Self Healing,* pp. 2-3.

Weil, A. (2001, March). Visualization and guided imagery explained. *Dr. Andrew Weil's Self Healing,* p. 2.

WEB LINKS

http://www.eatright.org (**American Dietetic Association**)

Provides information on nutritional health.

http://www.niddk.nih.gov/index.htm (**United States National Institute of Diabetes & Digestive & Kidney Diseases**)

Provides information on weight control.

http://www.drugabuse.gov (**National Institute on Drug Abuse**)

Provides information on drug abuse.

http://www.health.org (**Department of Health & Human Services SAMHSA's National Clearinghouse for Alcohol and Drug Information**)

Provides alcohol and drug facts.

http://www.acupuncturealliance.org (**The Acupuncture and Oriental Medicine Alliance**)

http://www.aaom.org (**The American Association of Oriental Medicine**)

http://www.americanyogaassociation.org (**American Yoga Association**)

http://www.mindbody.harvard.edu (**Mind/Body Medical Institute**)

http://www.niam.com (**National Institute of Ayurvedic Medicine**)

http://www.nccam.nih.gov (**National Institutes of Health—Center for Complementary and Alternative Medicine**)

http://www.ncbi.nlm.nih.gov/pubmed (**National Library of Medicine—PubMed**)

http://www.medscape.com/prometheus/SRAM/publid/SRAM-journal.html (**The Scientific Review of Alternative Medicine on Medscape**)

SECTION 6

Employability Skills

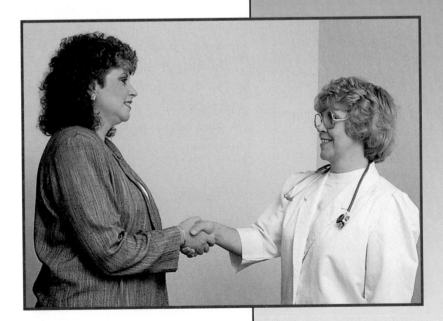

Achieving Satisfaction in Employment

A vast array of jobs require either administrative or clinical skills or a combination of both. Physicians in private practice usually have an average of three employees. In group practice, there may be from five to as many as forty or more, depending on the number of physicians and the size of the facility.

In seeking employment, you must be aware of the different opportunities and decide which area of medical assisting you would prefer. Many medical assistants prefer general or family practice because of its variety and challenge; others enjoy the specialty fields with their new developments and rapid change. There are still many health care facilities whose job descriptions specify particular duties, such as medical secretary, clinical office assistant, transcriptionist, insurance clerk, or receptionist. The generally-trained medical assistant should be able to perform the dual role of administrative and clinical assistant and will therefore be a valuable asset to any medical practice.

This chapter will discuss the steps involved in seeking employment in the health care field and present ideas for being a valuable employee. These job acquisition skills will be useful in other employment fields as well. Showing a genuine interest in others and the desire to work are the first steps in the job search.

UNIT 1

The Job Search

Upon the completion of the unit, meet the following performance objectives by verifying knowledge of the facts and principles presented through oral and written communication at a level deemed competent. Demonstrate the specific behaviors as identified in the performance objectives of the procedures.

1. Spell and define, using the glossary at the back of the text, all the **Words to Know** in this unit.
2. Prepare a neat, accurate, and well-organized resumé.
3. Describe information contained in a resumé and the purpose of each style of resumé.
4. Explain the purpose of and write a cover letter to accompany a resumé.
5. Explain how to reply to a classified ad in the newspaper.
6. Explain employment agency services.
7. List advantages and disadvantages of public and private employment agencies.
8. List three contacts to assist you in your job search.
9. Define the common abbreviations used in the newspaper "Help Wanted" section.

AREAS OF COMPETENCE (AAMA)

This unit addresses content within the specific competency areas of *Professionalism, Communication skills,* and *Legal concepts,* as identified in the Medical Assistant Role Delineation Study. Refer to Appendix A for a detailed listing of the areas.

■ WORDS TO KNOW

aspirations	functional
attribute	ingenuity
chronological	negotiable
classified	resumé
dual	targeted
elaborate	transcript

The job search begins with the desire to work. A medical assistant with skills in communication and medical office procedures should discover excellent opportunities for employment.

A personal review of your strengths and weaknesses will help you uncover some of your best qualities and remind you of what might need extra attention. Preparing yourself for your first employment in your chosen career is an exciting time. Ask for help from family and friends if you feel you need a few comments to help you sort out a few ideas. Often, good advice may come from those who know you well.

THE RESUMÉ

Ⓐ Employment Strategies:
Resume

One of the first steps in presenting yourself for employment is to develop a personal **resumé**. A resumé is an outlined summary of your abilities and experience. It should be complete, accurate, and neatly organized. The resumé will describe to prospective employers your educational background, previous work experience, professional affiliations, community service, personal interests, honors, employment objectives, and whatever else you feel is important for them to know. It need not contain personal information about your marital status, race, religion, age, or any other facts that may be used to discriminate against you illegally. The purpose of the resumé is to inform the prospective employer of how well you measure up to the position for which you are applying. Refer to Procedure 21–1.

There are several styles of resumés. You may arrange the information in a variety of ways. Some popular styles include: a traditional format in **chronological** order, a list of your career objectives, a **functional** plan, or a **targeted** layout. Figures 21–1A and B show examples of two types. Each of these designs is attractive and easy to read. The *traditional (chronological) approach* shows the reader your background information in an organized fashion. It is a good way to highlight your abilities when you are just beginning the job search. The *career objective* style shows your obvious career choice to the reader and is followed by your abilities and qualifications. It is also a frequently chosen style for the novice. A *chronologically arranged* resumé shows the prospective employer your employment history in dated order from present (or most recent) back to the beginning of your work experience. You should highlight the responsibilities of each position. Your present job duties should be emphasized. This will show the employer your strengths. The *functional type resumé* draws attention to the most important areas of your achievements and strengths. You may arrange the information to highlight your abilities but not necessarily in dated order of your employment experience. A *targeted resumé* is used for a precise field of employment. It shows the employer your expertise in a particular area. This type of resumé is directed to a specific job title. One that is basic but complete and properly arranged will attract an employer's attention. One that is flashy, too lengthy, or too wordy may well be discarded. A one-page resumé is a preferred length. It should be well-organized and grammatically correct. You should always have someone proofread your resumé because often our own mistakes go unnoticed. Spelling must be correct. There is no need for being **elaborate** in style. A simple typed or printed resumé on quality paper will make the information stand out, which is the sole purpose of it. The resumé that is printed on a soft pastel color of paper, such as light

PROCEDURE

21-1 Prepare a Resumé

PURPOSE: To document information concerning education, experience, and abilities for employment consideration.

Items needed: paper, pen, dictionary, thesaurus, telephone book, typewriter/word processor.

1. Write your complete legal name, address, and phone number. This information may be arranged flush left or centered at the top of the page.
   Refer to Figures 21–1A and B for the particular style of resumé that is appropriate for you and your needs. Use reference materials listed above for accuracy, expression, and correct spelling in composing your resumé.

2. Briefly state your qualifications and abilities, and list the position desired next to the heading of: Job Objective or Job Target.

3. List your educational background, beginning with the most recent or present date. You may note that you will furnish **transcripts**/certificates on request at the bottom of the resumé.

4. List all pertinent employment experience, beginning with the most recent or present date. Include the dates of employment, employer's name, address, and the position you held with a brief description of your responsibilities according to the style of resumé you have selected. **RATIONALE: Listing only the pertinent employment experience will allow you to provide necessary information and keep your resumé to the desired one page limit.**

5. List memberships/affiliations in professional organizations. These may be arranged alphabetically or ranked by order of importance.

6. List community service, including volunteer programs and activities as may be appropriate. This is optional.

7. List outside interests briefly as appropriate. This is optional.

8. List references on a separate sheet of paper. State on the bottom of the resumé that references will be furnished on request. You should have at least three references (persons *not* related to you) and no more than five. Permission should be obtained from these persons *before* they are listed.

9. Type the completed resumé on a sheet of bond paper, or use the word processor to enter your information. Underscore (underline) headings or use bold print for clarity and attractiveness. Check the finished copy for errors (use spellcheck program on word processor). Ask a reliable person to proofread your resumé. Have a number of copies printed on quality paper for distribution (off-white, beige, or ivory white are preferred colors).

10. Revise and update your resumé to document additional employment experience, educational achievements, certificates, awards, and personal development. Items of lesser importance should be deleted as more important accomplishments are added.

---

yellow or pale green, will stand out and is easily retrieved in a pile of others. Make sure that you refrain from dark colors that make print difficult to read. Describing your objectives clearly will direct the employer's attention to your qualifications for employment. Noting your **aspirations** will give the interviewer some insight into your long-term goals and your level of ambition. Although the main purpose of the resumé is to communicate your abilities to an employer, it also may spur interest in getting an interview for a specific position. Preparation of a resumé requires you to systematically list experiences that show your valuable **attributes**. Awards and special certificates should be listed along with the reasons for which they were given. These will interest an employer and may be the deciding factor when the final hiring decision is made.

In composing your resumé, you should be aware that some items are optional. Realizing that employers are people too will help you decide about including personal information. This section of your resumé can convey your genuine caring for others and good citizenship in your community. Interests and community service are not required, but they often communicate a human touch to the reader. Often, the employer can relate to the community service organization you have listed (or one similar). It is possible that you may be selected for an interview over others who are just as qualified because you have communicated to the reader that you are a well-rounded person. Employers are often interested in what you do with the other hours of your day besides work. A person who has a balance of life is usually happier, healthier, and more productive and full of life in general.

Sandy Lynn Beach, CMA **(A)**
4030 Newbank Road
Wheelersburg, Ohio 45794
(614) 555-1212
Qualifications: Certified Medical Assistant
Desired Position: Clinical Medical Assistant
Education:

XXXX to date:	Attending evening courses in Nursing, Southern Ohio Technical College, Lucasville, Ohio AAMA National Certification 19XX
XXXX–XX:	Certificate, Ohio Valley Training Academy, Wellston, Ohio. Major: Medical Assisting
XXXX:	Diploma, Portsmouth East High School, Portsmouth, Ohio. Major: General Business

EMPLOYMENT EXPERIENCE:

XXXX to date:	Administrative Medical Assistant to Wilber Roth, M.D., Rolling Hills, Ohio
XXXX–XX	Admissions Clerk, Green Meadows Community Hospital, Green Meadows, Ohio
XXXX–XX:	Cashier, Garden Inn Restaurant, Hilldale, Ohio

PROFESSIONAL ASSOCIATIONS:
American Association of Medical Assistants
Ohio State Society of Medical Assistants
Scioto County Chapter of Medical Assistants

COMMUNITY SERVICE:
Red Cross Volunteer
Big Sisters Association Volunteer
Interests: aerobics, camping, knitting, music, reading
References, transcripts and certificates, furnished upon request.

Sharon R. Beach **(B)**
4270 Hilldale Drive
Fernridge, CA 95061
(406) 555-1122
Job Target: Clinical Medical Assistant
Abilities:
• Communication skills—patient education
• CPR and first aid
• Phlebotomy
• Basic clinical laboratory skills
• Electrocardiography
Achievements:
• Certified Medical Assistant
• Bachelor's degree in Nutrition
• CPR certification
Employment Experience:

XXXX–Present	Fernridge Family Health Center Clinical Medical Assistant
XXXX–XXXX	Brownsville General Hospital Phlebotomist/ECG Technician
XXXX–XXXX	Ronald L. Botkin, D.O.—General Practice Administrative and Clinical Medical Assistant

Professional Affiliations:
• Member—American Association of Medical Assistants
Education:

XXXX	Baldwin Community College
XXXX	Brownsville University

FIGURE 21–1 Sample resumés: (A) traditional (chronological order format), (B) targeted resumé

THE COVER LETTER

A **Employment Strategies:**
Cover Letter

After you have perfected your resumé, you should do the same in composing a cover letter to send with it. It must state *why* you should be hired for the desired position. The cover letter should be addressed to the person who decides who is interviewed and hired. Finding out the name of the office manager or supervisor may be done by making a simple phone call and asking (be sure to get the correct spelling). Personalizing the letter will gain more attention than will the standard form letter. Let the employer know that your skills and qualifications will be an asset. Make the letter simple and direct to convey what makes you special for the job. Be sure to request an interview and make it clear when and how you can be reached for an appointment to be made. Figures 21–2A and B give sample cover letters. Remember that your resumé should provide a general overall description of your assets and qualifications. The cover letter should be specific and targeted toward a particular person or department. It should be sent in answer to an ad, in request for an interview, or at an individual's request.

Both cover letter and resumé must be error free. Employers eliminate numerous resumés by pitching those with spelling or grammatical errors and tears or smudges, or those that are too wordy or unorganized. Faxing a resumé may produce a "muddy" look and is only recommended when requested by an employer.

Date

Karla Baker, CMA-A
Office Manager
Hilldale Medical Center
Hilldale, Ohio 45102

Dear Ms. Baker:
My training in medical assisting at Ohio Valley Training Academy has provided me with skills in both administrative and clinical areas. I am very interested in securing a position in your health care facility as a dual Medical Assistant. I am nationally certified as my enclosed resumé states.

Please let me know if you wish an appointment for an interview. I can be reached at home on Tuesday and Thursday afternoons and every evening at 555-8131.

Thank you for your consideration.

Sincerely,

Sandy Lynn Beach, CMA

FIGURE 21–2A Cover letters for a resumé: sample A

4270 Hilldale Drive
Fernridge, CA 95061
(406) 555-1122
Date

Ms. Doreen Castle
Office Manager
Hopkin's Medical Clinic
739 Mountainview Way
Great Valley, CA 95068

Dear Ms. Castle:
I read your ad in the local paper about the opening for a full-time clinical medical assistant at Hopkin's Medical Clinic. I feel that my training and experience would make me a worthy candidate for this position. As you will see from my resumé, I am a Certified Medical Assistant and have a bachelor's degree in Nutrition.

In addition, my experience in patient education regarding therapeutic diets has helped me to sharpen my communication skills. I also have excellent clinical skills and am current in CPR certification.

I would like to meet with you for an interview to discuss the possibility of matching your needs with my qualifications at your earliest convenience. Please call me at the number listed above to schedule an appointment. I can be reached at home every evening and on Wednesday afternoons.

Yours truly,

(Miss) Sharon R. Beach, CMA

FIGURE 21–2B   Cover letter for a resumé: sample B

CLASSIFIED ADVERTISEMENTS

You may send your resumé to a prospective employer in response to a **classified** ad in the local newspaper. A classified ad is a request for qualified applicants to send information about themselves to a prospective employer. The employer may then request an interview with those who meet the requirements for the position instead of interviewing all persons who may wish to apply. This method of screening saves time for the employer and makes the resumé a most important means of communication. Figure 21–3 shows abbreviations commonly used in classified advertisements.

In responding to a classified ad, it is customary to write a cover letter to accompany your resumé. This cover letter expresses your desire to be interviewed for the position and describes briefly who you are and what you have to offer.

PUBLIC EMPLOYMENT SERVICES

All states offer assistance in locating jobs through the state employment service. Local offices of this agency will have job openings on file, possibly including the one you are looking for. You simply walk in, fill out the gen-

A CAAHEP CONNECTION

Applying for employment is a necessary part of establishing your career. Everyone has to start at the beginning. Dressing for success is an important part of the interview process. If you have the necessary qualifications for a position and your interview seems to go well, you may be called back for a second interview. If you are not called back, you can presume that someone with more experience or better qualifications was hired. If you have reason to believe that you were discriminated against because of your race, gender, age, beliefs, or any other reason, you should seek legal counsel. You must be sure of these accusations before taking these measures because this is a very serious matter. Falsely accusing someone of a discriminatory act is just as bad as doing it.

APPT—Appointment	MED—Medical
ASST—Assistant	MGR—Manager
BGN or BEG—Beginning	MOS—Months
COL—College	NEC—Necessary
DEPT—Department	NEG—**Negotiable**
EDUC—Education	OFC—Office
EOE—Equal Opportunity Employer	PD—Paid
	POS—Position(s)
EXP—Experience	PT—Part Time
F—Female	REF—References
FB—*Fringe Benefits*	REQ—Required
FT—Full Time	SAL—Salary
GRAD—Graduate	SEC—Secretary
H—Handicapped	T—Temporary
HS—High School	TRANSP—Transportation
HR—Hour	WPM—Words per minute
HRS—Hours	WK—Week
IMMED—Immediate	WKENDS—Weekends
INT—Interview	W/—With
LIC—License	Yrs—Years
M—Male	

FIGURE 21–3   Some abbreviations used in the "Help Wanted" section of the newspaper

eral forms, wait your turn, and then have a conference with an employment counselor. If there are listings that call for your kind of experience and training, you will have immediate leads to begin checking. If no appropriate listings are currently on file, the employment counselor will place your name on file and notify you when listings do materialize. Because this agency is supported by tax dollars, there is no fee for the service.

PRIVATE EMPLOYMENT AGENCIES

Private employment agencies offer similar services. A cover letter and resumé should be sent to the agency explaining your area of expertise and desired employment. Many agencies specialize in the medical field and can give efficient service in locating openings in medical assisting. Many potential jobs are "fee paid," meaning that the employer pays the agency's fees. In general, you should avoid positions that require you to pay the fee. This is too often a means of taking advantage of employees. The decision is obviously yours. You may be definitely interested in a particular position for which you have to pay the fee. Carefully weighing the advantages and disadvantages will help you decide if the cost is worth it to you in the long run. A substantial pay increase is an obvious advantage. If you have been waiting for a certain position to open for a relatively long time, it may well be a wise choice to secure it by paying a fee. Often, arrangements may be made for the fee to be paid in installments. Fees for finding employment positions are generally based on a percentage of the annual wages of an employee.

OTHER CONTACTS

A resumé with a cover letter requesting an interview may be sent to many medical offices or health care facilities even if there is no position available. If you ardently wish to be employed in a particular facility, making it known

may spark an interest in you as a prospective employee should there be an opening. Introducing yourself through correspondence and specifying your interest in employment should a position become available can be very productive. Employers may keep your letter and resumé on file for as long as a year and respond as the need arises.

Additional information about job opportunities may be obtained at the public library. There are many job opportunities you can check out by using the computer. Online information about jobs in every field is listed and updated regularly. Doing a job search is quick and easy. You can find opportunities without traveling miles and spending lots of time and money in the process. Taking advantage of one or all of the different ways to find employment should assure you of a position in an area of your liking. If you seek the services of an employment agency or register with the employment placement center on your campus, be sure to check back with a specific person often to reaffirm your interest in becoming employed. Many services, periodicals, and books deal with occupational information, and library personnel can be very helpful. Membership in professional associations is also quite helpful in the job search. Not only may an association's publications include classified ads, but personal contact with other members at meetings may provide invaluable information about job openings. Participation in community service groups can put you in touch with yet another network of persons who may have information about job openings. Finally, you should not overlook your friends and acquaintances; the job one of them happens to mention in conversation could turn out to be just the one you have been waiting for. If you have a sincere desire to be

Medical-Legal-Ethical Scenario

Anthony interviewed for a medical assistant position in a family practice office. He was well qualified, very interested in the position, and had left the interview feeling very positive about having the job. After all, the office manager asked him when would be the earliest he could start work. She had answered that next week sounded good to her. He waited to hear about his work schedule, and finally he called to ask

about it. He was told that the position had been filled. Anthony stopped in the office the next week and was surprised when he saw the new medical assistant at the reception desk. He recognized her but didn't know she was in medical assisting. He thought that he remembered her as a clothing store manager the last time he was at the mall. He just said hi and left feeling rather down.

CRITICAL THINKING CHALLENGE

1. How do you think Anthony got the idea he had the job?
2. What should he do about this situation?
3. Does Anthony have a reason to seek legal counsel?

4. Why do you suppose Anthony wasn't hired?
5. What do you think of having a new person at the reception desk who is not qualified?
6. What would you do in this situation?

employed, a job can be found. However, as most people have realized from time to time, it may take patience, persistence, and **ingenuity**.

ACHIEVE UNIT OBJECTIVES

Complete Chapter 21, Unit 1, in the workbook to help you obtain competency of this subject.

UNIT 2

Getting the Job and Keeping It

OBJECTIVES

Upon completion of the unit, meet the following performance objectives by verifying knowledge of the facts and principles presented through oral and written communication at a level deemed competent.

1. Spell and define, using the glossary at the back of the text, all of the **Words to Know** in this unit.
2. Complete a job application form.
3. Explain the importance of appearance when interviewing and/or applying for a job.
4. State the purpose of a job interview.
5. Explain the importance of promptness and courtesy in a job interview.
6. Explain the reasons for sending a follow-up letter after an interview.
7. Write a follow-up letter.
8. List the qualities employers regard as most important in employees.
9. List "dos and don'ts" in interviewing and applying for a job.
10. List the most important qualities necessary for job advancement.
11. Describe each of the 15 commonly asked questions on a job interview.
12. List questions that applicants may ask on a job interview.
13. Explain the purpose of a letter of resignation.
14. Describe reasons for employment termination.
15. Explain the purpose of a job description.
16. List and describe the contents of a job description.
17. Describe ways to advance in employment.

AREAS OF COMPETENCE (AAMA)

This unit addresses content within the specific competency areas of *Diagnostic orders, Patient care, Professionalism, Communication skills, Legal concepts,* and *Instruction,* as identified in the Medical Assistant Role Delineation Study. Refer to Appendix A for a detailed listing of the areas.

WORDS TO KNOW

apprise	demeanor
arbitrary	fringe
competent	negate
contemporary	reiterate

APPLICATION FORMS

Filling out an application for employment may be your next step. These forms may range from the simple to the complex. Figure 21–4 shows an example of an application form that asks for a minimal amount of information. Often, much of the information is the same as what is contained on your resumé. Remember to take a copy of your resumé with you to help you fill out the job application. Be sure to transcribe dates and all other information correctly, completely, and accurately. When you are nervous or if you are hurried, mistakes are often made, such as transposing numbers, leaving a space blank, or even placing the wrong information in a space. Take adequate time to complete whatever forms are necessary in a neat and attractive manner. Some applications are extremely lengthy (several pages). It may be best if this type is taken home to complete because it may take a considerable amount of time. It is not considered proper to ask for a phone directory or any other reference when applying for a job. You are supposed to show that you are prepared. In filling out an application for employment, you must be accurate and honest. Being prepared with dates, names, addresses, phone numbers, and other detailed information will expedite completion of the form. You should also be aware of the impression you may give when you apply for employment. Even if you are merely picking up an application to take home to complete or returning it after you have completed it, your appearance, including your attitude, will certainly be noticed. You should dress for success any time a prospective employer may see you. Other employees will surely notice you and relay the information to the employer, especially if there is a negative impression given.

Because of the professional setting (medical field) for which you are seeking employment, many employers require that the trust of prospective employees is checked. Among the areas of concern are the person's credit rating, police record, and chemical use/abuse. You may be asked to produce documents or give authorization for the employer to find out about your personal records before you may be considered for hiring.

Because the job application will probably reach the personnel manager's office before you do, it must speak well for you; it must make a good impression on the person who reads it. Applications must be complete, neat, and legible, or they will be discarded promptly. Reading and following the instructions on the form is of utmost importance. Take time to read the instructions and follow them precisely when completing an employment application

EMPLOYMENT APPLICATION FORM				
PERSONAL NAME				DATE _____
(LAST)		(FIRST)		(MI)
ADDRESS—STREET		CITY	STATE	ZIP
PHONE NUMBER		SOCIAL SECURITY NUMBER		
POSITION DESIRED:				
EXPECTED SALARY OR HOURLY WAGE:				
EDUCATION				
NAME OF SCHOOL		ADDRESS	DATE(S)	DEGREE/CERTIFICATE
HIGH SCHOOL				
VOCATIONAL/TECHNICAL				
COLLEGE				
OTHER				
WORK EXPERIENCE—Give present position (or last position held first).				
JOB TITLE:		EMPLOYER	ADDRESS	DATES
DUTIES PERFORMED:				
JOB TITLE:		EMPLOYER	ADDRESS	DATES
DUTIES PERFORMED:				
REFERENCES—LIST THREE PERSONS (OTHER THAN RELATIVES) WHO HAVE KNOWN YOU FOR AT LEAST 2 YEARS				
NAME/TITLE		ADDRESS		TELEPHONE NUMBER

FIGURE 21–4 An example of an employment application form. (Some applications can be completed online.)

form. If the printed instructions on the form say to print all information in black ink, you should do just that and not use cursive style in another color of ink. One of the functions served in having candidates complete the application form is to find out how well they follow directions. The applicant in Figure 21–5 is carefully thinking before writing on the form to avoid making any errors. Most forms begin with directions to print all information requested. Ignoring basic directions of this nature is not the work of a good candidate for employment. The application form will provide the employer not only with factual information about you but with many other insights as well.

If you take sufficient time and interest in completing the application, you will be more likely to be given a personal interview. Additionally, because of the Immigration Reform Act of 1986, employers are required by federal law to ask you for documents that show both your iden-

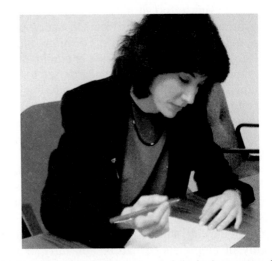

FIGURE 21–5 This applicant is carefully thinking over information before writing it on the application form to prevent making errors.

tity and eligibility to work in the United States. Employers will make copies of your documents and return them to you. Further, the Employment Eligibility Verification Form I-9 must be completed and filed in the employee's record along with other important documents. Employers must verify that you are legally entitled to work in the United States. All applicants and employers must comply with this law. Refer to Chapter 10, Medical Office Management, for more details.

THE INTERVIEW

An interview is a face-to-face meeting between you and your prospective employer. The day of the scheduled interview you should allow sufficient time to get ready. If you chew gum or smoke cigarettes, leave these at home for this trip. Neither has any place in a job interview.

When applying for a job, your appearance is extremely important. Appearance is an outward indication of who you are. Remember what you learned about nonverbal communication. If you are a sincere, **competent**, and dedicated person, then by all means attend to your appearance accordingly. Nonverbal messages, though silent, can speak loudly.

Most employers expect appropriate attire and some require adherence to a very specific policy concerning mode of dress and general appearance.

If you are interviewing for a clinical position, ask beforehand about what type of dress to wear. Your inquiry will most likely be taken as showing genuine interest. Often, employers will want to see you dressed in what you perceive as a "uniform" to see how you will look on the job.

Women who prefer to wear business attire should dress conservatively in a navy, gray, tan, or brown tailored suit. Bright colors, jewelry, miniskirts, pants, and frilly outfits are not considered professional attire. Men should also follow this advice and dress conservatively, avoiding outrageous ties, jewelry, and fad clothes. Remember that you should make every effort to make a positive impression with the interviewer concerning yourself and your qualifications, not your ability to show off fashions and accessories. It follows that those interested in employment at a facility should conform to the standards set forth. Following fads in fashion is usually not advisable. Trendy looks are for models for the most part. A medical assistant who is more interested in meeting the requirements of the job than in being the center of attention is more appealing to a personnel manager.

The same rules apply to job interviews that have already been mentioned in terms of the job. Because they are important, they will be **reiterated** once more. All matters concerning personal cleanliness are vital. The following attributes are sure to interfere with or **negate** the possibility of employment: bad breath, dirty or uneven fingernails, chipped nail polish, dirty or unkempt hair, overpowering aftershave or perfume, unclean teeth, unpleasant or offensive body odor, or untended complexion problems.

The point is this: no matter how well qualified or eager you are, you may not find anyone willing to pay for your services if you fail in certain matters of personal hygiene. Take nothing for granted. Make strict adherence to proper personal grooming a rigid daily rule.

Rushing usually detracts from your appearance and **demeanor**. If the address of the facility is not familiar to you, get directions and plan your time beforehand. (It is a good idea to go to the facility a day or two before the scheduled interview to scout out the area to determine the approximate travel time, exact location, parking, bus route, and so on to avoid getting lost or being delayed.) You should arrive about 10 to 15 minutes before the appointment. (You may be instructed to arrive up to an hour or more before the interview to complete an application form or to take required preemployment tests.) Arriving too early will make you appear insecure. Being late for almost any reason will make you appear irresponsible and a poor candidate for the position. If you happen to find yourself in this predicament, a telephone call explaining the delay and a sincere apology are in order. Being on time is a sign of reliability, dependability, and conscientiousness.

You will be able to give your undivided attention to the interviewer if all of your responsibilities are in order before you enter the facility. If you have children, it is best to leave them with a child care provider. Taking children to an interview is inappropriate and quite distracting. If you are preoccupied with worry about personal problems, illness, a parking meter, or anything else, you will not be able to interview well. As soon as you know the date of the interview, make plans to allocate your time so that you can be stress free to get ready, travel to the site, interview, and return without rushing. An interview can be an investment in yourself and your career. It is worth your giving sufficient time and effort toward a successful outcome.

Introducing yourself with a handshake should initiate a friendly and pleasant conversation. Your manner should tell the interviewer you are happy to be there.

The interview ought to allow sufficient time for each of you to inquire about the other and to discuss the requirements of the position. Often, the interviewer will have reviewed your resume.

You should be prepared to answer questions concerning your career goals and objectives, how you feel about changes, why you decided on this career, your further educational plans, and so on (Figure 21–6). Your answers should be brief, concise, and honest.

In terms of perspective and dimension, the section of the resume that lists community services is an appealing area to prospective employers. It is an indicator of your concern for others, your involvement, and your energy level and time management skills. Many employers will ask what prompted your interest in a particular service area.

1. What are your qualifications for employment in our facility?
2. Do you have plans for continuing education? If yes, what are your plans?
3. What were your favorite subjects in school and why?
4. Why are you seeking employment with us?
5. What made you decide to enter the medical assisting field?
6. What is your most rewarding experience in life thus far?
7. What are your long-range career goals?
8. What motivates you to do your best?
9. What is the most difficult problem you ever had to deal with? And how did you handle it?
10. What does success mean to you?
11. What relationship should exist between supervisors and those under their supervision?
12. How would you describe yourself?
13. Do you work well under pressure?
14. What are your strengths and weaknesses?
15. What two things are most important to you in a job?

FIGURE 21–6 A list of commonly asked questions during employment interviews

1. To see a job description
2. About hours—work day schedule
3. Rate of pay (if not discussed by the close of the interview)
4. Chances for advancement or promotion
5. About continuing education—in-service programs (are expenses paid?)
6. **Fringe** benefits:
    a. Health insurance plan
    b. Dental insurance plan
    c. Eye care
    d. Vacation/time off
    e. Membership dues in AAMA/ARMA
    f. Profit sharing
    g. Retirement plan
    h. Tuition reimbursement
    i. Other
7. Frequency of job performance evaluations

FIGURE 21–7 A list of questions *you*, the applicant, might ask during the interview

Contemporary federal laws are designed to deal with arbitrary discrimination in hiring practices. Toward this end, you should not be asked questions concerning your age, cultural or ethnic background, marital status, or parenthood. Nevertheless, these issues may come up in the course of your interview. You are not required to provide this information if you choose not to. The purpose of the interview is to ascertain the relevance of your experience and character to the job at hand. Should any of these unrelated issues come up, be careful to analyze the context in which they arose (it could be from something you said). In any case, if you are honestly convinced that you have been denied a job because of **arbitrary** discrimination, be advised that this is illegal, and you have legal recourse.

At some point during the interview, the interviewer may give you a written job description of the position for which you are applying. You will probably be given time to look it over and then asked if you would feel confident about performing the job described. An honest answer is the best. Avoid hedging or bluffing about issues because an experienced interviewer will pick up on your insecurities. Remember that body language tells the rest of the story. If there are one or two duties you have never performed before or one or two pieces of equipment that you know little about, say this but add that you are eager to learn. The employer will appreciate the initiative in your answer. If the job description sounds totally unfamiliar or if you feel it would be an impossible task, it is best to say so. The interviewer will appreciate your openness.

Some positions may have no job description, and the duties involved will be discussed during the interview.

Knowing that there are probably as many duties not mentioned as mentioned will give you an idea of the amount of work the job requires.

By the time all of these matters have been dealt with, the interview will be starting to wind down. The interviewer beginning to reach closure will **apprise** you of this by asking you if you have any further questions. If issues of salary, raises, and advancement have not been dealt with previously, this is an appropriate point to mention them. This is also the logical point for you to ask about any other matters you are uncertain about (Figure 21–7). See Figure 21–8 for the "dos and don'ts" of applying for a job. However, do not drag out this time. Let the interview end smoothly. When it is over, rise and thank the interviewer for his time. Firmly shake hands if the interviewer extends a hand (Figure 21–9). Remember to smile and be pleasant and polite as you exit with confidence.

WHEN INTERVIEWING OR APPLYING FOR A JOB:	
DO	*DON'T*
ARRIVE ON TIME (10–15 MINUTES EARLY)	BE LATE!
SHOW INTEREST—ENTHUSIASM!	ASK TOO MANY QUESTIONS
BE IMMACULATE IN APPEARANCE	MAKE EXCUSES
DISPLAY A POSITIVE ATTITUDE	TALK ABOUT PERSONAL PROBLEMS
USE COURTESY	ACT OVER-CONFIDENT
ACT COMPOSED & POISED	DRUM FINGERS, SWING LEG, TAP FOOT
DRESS APPROPRIATELY	OVERDRESS
KEEP GOOD POSTURE (SIT STILL AND STRAIGHT)	CHEW GUM OR SMOKE

FIGURE 21–8 Remember these tips when applying for a job or going for an employment interview.

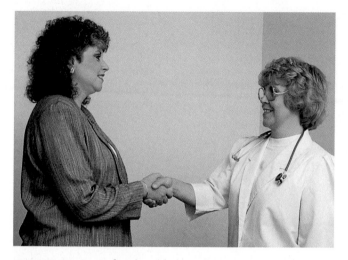

FIGURE 21-9 A firm handshake at the conclusion of the interview conveys courtesy and mutual respect.

The interviewer may talk to a number of people about a specific job opening in the office. To help the interviewer remember specific facts and traits about each individual, a form such as the one shown in Figure 21–10 may be filled out.

You may be one of many candidates interviewing for a particular job. Therefore, any decision may take some time. Out of courtesy and to enhance your image with the

INTERVIEW EVALUATION					
Subject	Excellent	Good	Satisfactory	Needs Improvement	Poor
Appearance					
Attitude					
Eye contact					
Self-control					
Voice					
Grammar					
Responses					
Manners					
Resumé					
Comments					
Date					
Employer		Title			
Address		Phone			
Applicant					

FIGURE 21-10 Employers may use a form such as this after an interview to record information about an applicant.

Date

Karla Baker, CMA-A
Office Manager
Hilldale Medical Center
Hilldale, Ohio 45102

Dear Ms. Baker:

Thank you very much for granting me an interview for the clinical medical assistant's position on your staff. The interview was both challenging and stimulating; I found it to be an enjoyable and rewarding experience.

You outlined the duties and responsibilities that come with the position very specifically. This is the type of position for which I have been trained; I feel confident that if I am offered the position, I can handle the responsibilities and become an asset to your staff.

Again, thank you for considering me for this position. I would be most appreciative if you would inform me of your final decision as soon as it is convenient for you (OR: I look forward to hearing from you soon).

Sincerely,

Sandy Lynn Beach, CMA

FIGURE 21-11 A sample follow-up letter

interviewer, take the time to compose a follow-up letter shortly after the interview has taken place. Figure 21–11 offers a sample letter. A typed thank you letter or a neat hand-written note is a polite gesture that shows your interest, persistence, and follow-through ability.

 Employment Strategies:
Thank You Letter

WHAT EMPLOYERS WANT MOST IN EMPLOYEES

The personal investment that you have made with regard to your education and skills training along with all of the effort you have put forth in producing a resumé and interviewing for employment does not stop with being hired. After securing a position, you must continually endeavor to look and do your best. An employer will expect you to perform with increasing expertise in your position as you continue to gain experience.

Desirable employee qualities that employers generally rank as most important are listed as follows:

1. Communication skills (oral and written)
2. Cooperation
3. Courteousness
4. Dependability
5. Enthusiasm
6. Initiative
7. Interest

8. Math skills
9. Punctuality
10. Reading skills
11. Reliability
12. Responsibility
13. Time management skills

These qualities are fast becoming increasingly more important and are a stark fact in holding a job. Becoming proficient in grammar, including both the written and spoken word, is a must. Speaking in a well-educated manner is necessary to portray a professional image of not only yourself but of the facility where you are employed. You become a member of a team of medical personnel who reflect each other to the public you serve. Good communication skills include refraining from the use of slang and phrases that are not familiar to patients and co-workers. Getting together with friends to relax and enjoy leisure time is the appropriate way to let down and have fun. Even though your work day should be pleasant and enjoyable, you must respect and remember the professional code of conduct and follow it. Effective communication in a professional setting requires that employees speak in an educated manner. The medical profession has long been respected for being knowledgeable and skilled. If one speaks as if there has been little formal schooling, it appears that there is also little knowledge and skill. To those who do not demonstrate the behavior of a well-educated person, respect from others may be lost quickly. The person who speaks politely using good communication skills in proper English imparts confidence to co-workers and patients. Many evening classes, such as a business English course, offer basic review in grammar. Taking the initiative to improve oneself is admirable. Employers recognize these efforts, and for those with ambition, rewards will surely follow.

Attendance is most important because schedules must be constantly changed and reassignments made when an employee is absent, especially when it is unexpected. An absent employee affects everyone because work must be divided among other team members. Scheduling personal appointments should be done on your day off or after working hours. If there is an important engagement for which you need time off from your job, you should ask for a meeting with your supervisor to discuss making arrangements for a day off well in advance of the date. Remember that *only when it is absolutely necessary* should you call in sick. If you are not sure about the office policy regarding this issue, you should ask your employer. Employees have a responsibility to report a personal or serious illness to their supervisor as soon as possible. When an emergency involves an accident or acute medical problem, notification of the circumstance will be received with sympathy and concern. Generally, employers are most understanding about illness when the reason is genuine. If child care is a problem, and the reason for absence is caused by needing someone to care for

children, the supervisor should be made aware of the situation. Often, supervisors may be helpful in assisting with information that could be a possible solution to the problem. However, repeated occurrences of calling in "sick" just to take a day off will become annoying and may lead to disciplinary action. Usually, offenders are more likely to take off on Mondays and Fridays for long weekends. These are days when schedules are full and all employees are most needed. If one is placed on probation and warned about poor attendance practices and the warnings go unheeded, it could ultimately result in the employee's dismissal.

It is equally important to be on time daily. If you are scheduled to be at work at 8:00 AM, you should be at the work site and ready to begin at 8:00 AM and not just coming in the door at that time. Arriving a few minutes early is a wise practice because it will allow time to put your personal belongings away and give you time to begin your day without being rushed. Being prompt is a valuable personal quality appreciated by both employers and patients. Leaving early is not advised unless absolutely necessary and with permission of the supervisor in advance. When one leaves before the scheduled time, it puts an added burden on other team members to finish your job. With each member of the health care team doing what is expected, the work will be shared, and the group's efficiency will be noticed by your employer. This makes for a harmonious working relationship among employees. You have studied throughout this text about various patient education materials and guidelines for better health. You must have realized by now that you should be practicing what you are expected to teach patients. This can only help you to feel better about yourself, which will be evident to others with whom you come in contact. In good health, you will be more productive, energetic, and display better coping skills. All of the qualities important to employers should also be important to you. The secret to success is simple. Strive toward fulfilling the goals you set, and do everything in your power to reach them, which simply means to always do the best you can. Your personal satisfaction is surely one goal that will be realized if you follow this plan.

In addition to these qualities, one in particular that the medical assistant must keep in mind is personal appearance. A medical assistant must continually strive to maintain an impeccable appearance; this is essential to ensure job security. Looking your best requires that you compliment your best assets and always keep neat, clean, and attractive to the public eye.

When you obtain employment, you must necessarily dedicate yourself first of all to the task of keeping the job. This is where your work history begins, and it will probably follow you throughout your working life. If the health care field remains your chosen career area and if medical assisting is your point of entry, then you must be determined to become the very best medical assistant you can. Ultimately, your eventual advancement into more responsible medical assisting duties and higher pay will depend largely upon your demonstrated capabilities in performing your administrative and clinical tasks. However, the aforementioned employee qualities will also become significant factors in paving the way for advancement.

Consider this scenario: A physician employs two medical assistants; both are the same age and possess relatively equal administrative and clinical skills. The only differences between the two come down to appearance and attitude. One maintains a considerably nicer appearance than the other, along with a more positive attitude. As the physician's volume of business expands and a promotion and salary increase for one of the positions becomes inevitable, guess which one will likely get the nod from the physician? You do not have to be a genius to figure this one out. In the end, it comes down to common sense.

THE JOB DESCRIPTION

The job description is an important document, especially in a health care facility. The health care team is made up of many team members who are delegated to perform specific functions to care for patient needs. Each member should have a detailed outline of the duties required of their employment position for expediency and efficiency in carrying out patient care. This detailed outline giving particular information regarding the performance of the duties and responsibilities of the position is called a job description. Because it can be helpful to both parties during the interview, this document may be referred to often during the interview process. The interviewer can show the applicant a detailed explanation of what would be expected of her on the job and observe her reaction to it. The applicant can be given a few minutes to read over the job description to get a better idea of what is involved in the job. Then, the applicant can formulate specific questions about the job and can see what steps are necessary to advance (if not already skilled in all procedures listed).

If there is no job description where you are applying for a job or you do not have one at your present job, it is wise to compose one. An example of a job description format is shown in Figure 21–12. This can be altered easily and used to document the duties and responsibilities of your job. The job description should contain the following information:

- title of the position
- person(s) responsible to
- summary of the position
- primary duties of the job
- expectations of the job (regarding job performance)
- requirements of the position (education, certification, and so on)
- qualifications of the job
- additional criteria per facility

As you may have realized, the job description is most helpful in setting guidelines, outlining educational re-

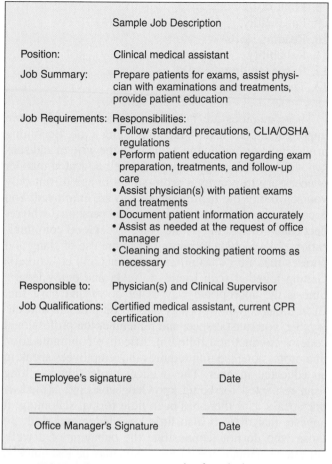

Sample Job Description	
Position:	Clinical medical assistant
Job Summary:	Prepare patients for exams, assist physician with examinations and treatments, provide patient education
Job Requirements:	Responsibilities: • Follow standard precautions, CLIA/OSHA regulations • Perform patient education regarding exam preparation, treatments, and follow-up care • Assist physician(s) with patient exams and treatments • Document patient information accurately • Assist as needed at the request of office manager • Cleaning and stocking patient rooms as necessary
Responsible to:	Physician(s) and Clinical Supervisor
Job Qualifications:	Certified medical assistant, current CPR certification

Employee's signature _____ Date _____

Office Manager's Signature _____ Date _____

FIGURE 21-12 An example of a job description

quirements and qualifications, and establishing standards and goals of the facility. This helps to keep employees on task and promotes consistency. Besides helping to motivate employees, the job description also serves as an evaluation guide. Knowing what is expected of you and having it in writing will safeguard misunderstandings and keep better communication links open. It also is important in protecting employees from being asked to perform duties and responsibilities for which they have little or no training and were not hired to perform.

THE EMPLOYEE EVALUATION/REVIEW

Most employers require that employees have regular, routine, or periodic reviews or evaluations regarding their work performance. The time schedule may vary from place to place, but usually the reviews are held initially every three months for the first year and then every six months thereafter. Some physicians/employers prefer to have annual reviews scheduled unless there is a problem or the employee requests it more often. Evaluations should be regarded in a positive light.

These are generally conducted by the supervisor, the office manager of the facility, and sometimes by the physician-employer. Whoever holds this meeting with

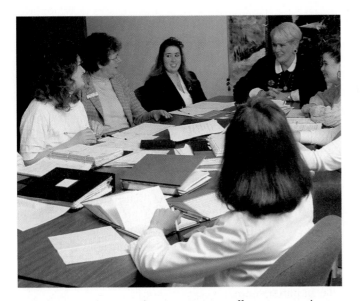

FIGURE 21-13 Attendance at routine staff meetings and in-service programs is a vital part of your job. Learning all you can about improving patient care and maintaining a good rapport with co-workers is essential to job success.

Employee's name	Job title/position	Date hired

Supervisor	Title	Date of evaluation

Scheduled evaluation/review: ___Initial ___3 month ___6 month ___annual ___*other

*Explain _____

Previous review date _____ Rating _____

Comments _____

Total days/times: absent_____ Tardy_____ Left early_____

Rate the following areas of the employee appropriately using the scale from 1 to 10:

                      1   2   3   4   5   6   7   8   9   10

Job knowledge: very little / limited / adequate / average / good / superior / outstanding ____

Quality of work: very poor / fair / good / acceptable / excellent / superior / outstanding ____

Quantity of work: inferior/ inadequate/ does just enough/ average/superior/outstanding ____

Speed: very slow / below average / average / above average / outstanding ____

Initiative: lacking / needs pushing / adequate / good / excellent / outstanding ____

Judgment: poor / unreliable / limited / reliable / superior / outstanding ____

Cooperation: very uncooperative / difficult / cooperative / excellent / outstanding ____

Adaptability: poor / slow / satisfactory / good / excellent / superior / outstanding ____

Appearance: poor/unprofessional/avg/reluctantly complies with dress code/outstanding____

Attendance: poor / average / good / excellent / superior / outstanding ____

                                                                  Total ____

Since last evaluation the employee has:

____improved ____made no noticeable change ____regressed

Recommendation for pay raise: ____Yes ____No

Overall impression:

____unsatisfactory ____fair ____satisfactory ____excellent ____outstanding

Comments of employee's strengths and weaknesses:_____

_____

Supervisor's signature_____

Employee's signature_____

FIGURE 21-14 An example of an employee evaluation (review) form, which employers may use in documenting employment progress

---

the employee offers insightful observations about the person. This is done to point out both positive and negative areas of which the employee may or may not be aware. Most facilities hold regular weekly staff meetings where suggestions, problems, and other important information is discussed. Figure 21–13 shows the health care team gathered to discuss important in-house matters, decisions regarding patient care, in-service scheduling, and other topics at a staff meeting. This is not the time or place to discuss personal problems or requests. It is vital, however, to have private meetings to discuss personal goals, promotion opportunities, pay increase possibilities, educational pursuits, etc. The review, or evaluation as it is also referred to, is meant for both employer and employee to have just this opportunity. You should use this meeting to your advantage. Let the employer/supervisor know your intentions regarding promotion goals. Ask questions tactfully about all concerns regarding policy, dress code, or whatever else you feel is important. You may ask about or schedule your vacation during this meeting. Your supervisor or evaluator may use a form similar to the one shown in Figure 21–14. Usually it will be completed and then offered to you to read. You should be asked to sign it at the bottom, indicating that you have read, discussed, and understood the rating on the form. You may request a copy if it is not offered. The original will remain in your employee record and filed with all of the other documents pertaining to your employment. It is a good idea to study the form and heed the rating scale. If you take the review seriously and with an open mind, you will most likely find out some good points and sometimes a couple of negative things about yourself that you may not have realized before. Try to improve on the negative things (e.g.,

poor attendance, poor grammar, appearance) before the next review. Showing improvement immediately and continuing on with the improvement will only make good points to remark about on the next review. If you show a poor attitude, it will only make matters worse. Remember that the supervisor's job responsibilities require that this evaluation be performed. You should not take the suggestions for improvement or reprimands about poor attendance, for instance, as personal insults.

The expression "constructive criticism" usually elicits a note of negativity that, even though spoken with good intentions, keeps us from listening to or taking the responsibility for whatever someone is trying to tell us. Usually, weaknesses are brought up and explained as objectively as possible, and suggestions are given for how one could go about changing the behavior or improving the lacking skill. The challenge to improve may be motivated by a reward appropriate to the success of the task. Those who have an excellent work performance may be surprised or even insulted that a supervisor would bring up a trivial weakness. Supervisors who see potential in others are obligated to encourage professional growth and development. All of us tend to ask more of those who are good at what they do and further expect the best from them. Employers are no different. This is actually a compliment but is often viewed as demanding and unfair. Try

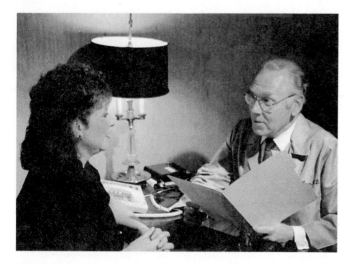

FIGURE 21-15 Employer discussing evaluation in an open communication manner

to remember the old saying "if the shoe fits, wear it," and consider the source of the remark. If you give the remark a chance to sink in and it does not, then possibly there is no just cause for it. Try to remain unaccusing and calm and discuss the problem. Chances are it may be a misunderstanding that can easily be talked out in a matter of seconds. Open dialogue and clear communication works wonders and leads to a better working relationship between you and your employer (Figure 21–15). Many positive results are achieved from reviews for both employee and employer.

ADVANCEMENT

Progressing in employment is up to you. The desire to advance in your field of choice is the first step to consider. Job satisfaction is also a major issue. If you enjoy your work and find your duties challenging and rewarding, you may want to stay in that position. If your salary meets your needs and you like what you do, staying with that job can be quite fulfilling. However, a motivating factor in moving up into a higher position or even changing jobs is most often for an increase in pay. Note: Cost-of-living raises (given to keep up with the economy) do not reflect one's job performance, but merit raises do. A merit raise is given to those employees who deserve recognition and praise for a job well done. Chances of advancement in your job will depend on several factors. Those employees who are offered better paying positions and positions with more responsibility are the ones who show the greatest interest. Interest can be displayed in several ways. Primarily, the person who shows initiative is the most dependable, seeks continuing education, acquires new skills, exhibits efficiency in a pleasant manner, and communicates well with others will be the first to be considered for a promotion. To move forward to a higher position in your place of employment means that you have

been recognized by your employer or supervisor for your efforts, and you are being rewarded with either a raise in pay, a promotion, or both.

Because the medical field in general is always changing and improving in health care technology, it is your responsibility to keep up with these changes. This is necessary if you want to reach peak performance at your job. To do this, you must acquire continuing education. This can be done in a variety of ways. Of course, the primary means of obtaining current information in the field of medicine is to read. Physicians usually subscribe to several medical news publications that you can read on breaks or at lunch time. Keeping up with the latest in managed health care, new medications, and other newsworthy items relating to patients is admirable and will be noticed by your employer. It will also help you perform your duties and give you a better appreciation for your role in patient care.

Other ways to better yourself and attain further education is to attend courses related to your area of interest in the medical field at a community college or university. Many night and weekend classes are offered for convenience to those who work during the day. You may want to take a refresher course in medical terminology or anatomy, for instance. Some find a favorite niche, such as medical records, transcription, or laboratory procedures, and realize that to advance in a particular area, additional education and credentialing is necessary. Discussing your goals with your supervisor is certainly advised so that reorganizing your work schedule to allow adequate time for classes can be arranged. The professional organizations AAMA and ARMA specifically address the needs of the medical assistant by offering continuing education programs at national, state, and local levels. Through these programs, there are continuing education units (CEUs) offered for keeping certification status current. There are also educational articles printed in the PMA (*The Professional Medical Assistant*) magazine that offer CEUs. AAMA will also consider CEU approval for educational programs offered by other professional organizations.

In addition, local hospitals offer educational seminars on a variety of topics for health care professionals. They welcome the attendance of those interested in learning more about patient care. You may ask to be put on the mailing list to keep you informed of future program offerings.

A perfect opportunity to inform your supervisor about your involvement in continuing education (if not already known) is during your scheduled evaluation. Employers are very receptive to and impressed by employees who take the initiative in self-improvement and involve themselves in professional organizations that offer continuing education to members. This conveys to the employer that you are interested in advancement and are willing to put forth the additional effort to move forward in your profession. Your involvement in leadership roles within the organization also gives the employer further insight into your appreciation of your career and its importance.

TERMINATING EMPLOYMENT

There are many reasons for terminating employment—relocation, advancement to a more responsible position, higher paying jobs, illness, educational pursuits, pregnancy, or a change in lifestyle. There is, however, a major responsibility that an employee has to an employer, that of giving at least two weeks' notice (Figure 21–16). This should be done to give the employer adequate time to fill the position that you will vacate. The notice that you give should be directed to your immediate supervisor, your physician-employer, or other appropriate member of the staff, with carbon copies to whoever else is appropriate for your place of employment. The letter should include the date that will be your last working day. Employers appreciate this considerate gesture because it allows for a smoother transition of personnel. There may be time for a new person to be hired to work with you so that you can help in the training and explain your job description in more detail. Often, however, this is not the case, and there is not sufficient time for the person who is leaving to train the new employee. If it is known that termination is evident because of a major move, or whatever the case may be, it is certainly a considerate gesture to inform your employer as far in advance as possible to assist in providing a smooth transition of your duties to another competent person. This is yet another reason to have a complete job description for every employee's position. Even without having a former employee to point out duties and responsibilities, the job description should have enough detail to help guide the new employee in the right direction with a minimum amount of difficulties.

Employment can also be terminated by the employer. This is an unpleasant experience for both employer and employee. The usual cause for termination initiated by the employer is failure of an employee to satisfactorily perform job responsibilities. Deficiencies can include being tardy, high absenteeism, failure to get along with co-workers and patients, poor work habits, undependability, dishonesty, poor attitude, and uncooperativeness. Another reason that the employer may terminate one's employment could be from irreconcilable issues caused by personality conflicts. After legitimate efforts to resolve differences have failed, there is often no other recourse but to terminate the employment of one who cannot, does not, or will not fit in with other staff members. On some occasions and in some situations, through employer–employee communication, one may be able to smooth over the conflict and ask if it is possible to change the situation from being fired to accepting a letter of resignation. This is mentioned because misunderstandings *do* happen from time to time. Having a poor work record is something that could follow a person and make it difficult to land another job in the future. After a new employee is hired, a file is established to keep all pertinent information regarding that person throughout his employment. It should be kept in strict confidence. The employee's

---

(A)   Date

Marlene Blackstone, CMA-A
Office Manager
Sports Medicine Center
7386 Canyon Road
Anywhere, U.S.A. 10000

Dear Ms. Blackstone:

It is with much regret that I submit this letter as my notice of resignation. My employment over the past five years in sports medicine has been a most interesting experience for me. I have learned so much in working with such a fine group of professionals. I am grateful for having had this opportunity.

From the date of this letter I am giving my two week notice; my last day will be (insert date).

Because my husband has taken a new position with his company, we are being transferred out of state. I will miss working with everyone at the center.

My thanks to all of you for making my years of employment at the center something that I can look back on with fond memories.

Sincerely,

Patsy J. Keene, CMA

(B)   Date

Maxwell S. Mitchell, M.D.
472 Circle Drive
Anywhere, U.S.A. 10000

Dear Dr. Mitchell:

Please accept this as my letter of resignation. During my employment in your practice I have learned a great deal, and I have greatly enjoyed working for you. However, (at this point the writer may choose to add a sentence or two elaborating on the specific reason for leaving).

My X years of employment with you have been a valuable experience for me; thank you for the opportunity to work and learn.

In accordance with your personnel regulations, this letter is also my two week notice; my last day in the office will be (at least two weeks hence).

Sincerely,

Your name and title or position with your signature

FIGURE 21–16 Sample letters of resignation A and B

---

record is kept just as a patient's record and all information should be entered in a timely and appropriate manner. The employment application form, resumé, reference letters, signed contract, tax forms, signed documents regarding compliance with OSHA/CLIA regulations and office policies, and any other relevant information must be placed in this file. There could be reason for the employer or the employee to refer to any of the filed information in the future. Dates of an employee's vacation, regularly scheduled day off, evaluations, incident/accident reports, reprimands/warnings, and all other relevant information must be recorded. Employees have the right to request a copy of any of the documents contained in their file. A formal written request signed by the employee is advised to obtain an expedient reply. Employees also have the right to request a conference with the employer or supervisor as needed to discuss concerns. Again, it is best to put all requests in writing to obtain a faster response.

Keeping on your toes can prevent this unwanted dilemma from happening. One should strive to do the best job possible for making a good reference if ever needed.

SUMMARY

Employers in medical practice have begun to realize the worth of trained medical assistants. Certified medical assistants (CMAs) or registered medical assistants (RMAs) are usually considered for employment over untrained applicants. In some managed care employment contracts, it may require that only CMAs or RMAs be hired. Currently, this is true in some states more than in others, but certification is becoming a nationwide requirement for employment in medical practice as regulations tighten. Keeping yourself up-to-date by attending continuing education programs, seminars, meetings, and other infor-

mative ways will make you a most valued employee. By opting to become certified or registered, you will demonstrate that you are knowledgeable in basic entry-level skills. Further, you will demonstrate to a prospective employer that you have pride in the profession and in your professional skills.

A FINAL NOTE

Throughout this chapter, much emphasis has been directed toward securing employment. Although it may seem to you that employers ask the impossible as you review their expectations, you must keep in mind that an employee is paid for work performed. Gainful employment is a mutually agreed to contract that is either written or implied. To assist you in gaining a better understanding of why employers have such expectations, you may find it interesting to know how and where they originated.

The concept of the "work ethic" originated from the 16th century's Protestant Ethic. During this period, work was considered a sacred task, and success in one's work was a sign of divine grace. One was looked down on by society in general if one was thought to have moral flaws, such as being lazy, having no ambition, or other undesirable characteristics. Essentially this ideal has not changed. The work ethics of today are basically the same as the original with some minor changes. The word *responsible* can be substituted for sacred. And being a success in one's work is a sign of *ambition, hard work, and perseverance.* These expectations are fair, realistic, and sensible. It sim-

Medical-Legal-Ethical Scenario

Juanita was in confused state when she got to work today. Her husband had just been offered a better job out of state, and he told her he wanted to take it. Juanita felt happy for her husband but felt awful that she couldn't continue in her job that she loved. She knew that her family had to move in a week so that the chil-

dren could enroll in school on time. She worried about it all the next week and decided to just leave a letter for the office manager to read after she was gone. She just knew she couldn't get through the conversation about having to resign without crying.

CRITICAL THINKING CHALLENGE

1. What is the first thing that Juanita should have done?
2. Do you think Juanita will get a good reference from her former employer when she applies for a job?
3. What do you think of Juanita? Do you understand what she did? Why?

4. What do you think was the reaction of the office manager? The physician(s)?
5. What should Juanita have done?
6. What would you tell Juanita?
7. What would you have done in her situation?

ply means that one should give an honest day's work for an honest day's wages. Taking the responsibility of providing for oneself financially usually makes most people aware of what is necessary to keep a job. Being a part of the health care team means that you have to be a team player!

Our best wishes for a successful and rewarding career in medical assisting!

ACHIEVE UNIT OBJECTIVES

Complete Chapter 21, Unit 2, in the workbook to help you obtain competency of this subject.

RELATING TO ABHES

Chapter 21 discusses the preparation, application, and interview process to obtain a job and the desirable behaviors to exhibit to maintain employment. This content relates to the ABHES accreditation requirements of *Job search, Professional development and success, Resume writing, Interviewing techniques and follow-up, Dress for success,* and *Professionalism* within the area of **Career Development**.

WEB LINKS

http://www.jobmedicalsupport.com (Job Science.com)

Provides information on searching for a medical assisting job through the Internet.

http://www.usawebpages.com (Mission of World Wide Webpages Corporation)

Maintains a world wide web directory that allows you to locate business webpages by geographic location and category.

Appendix A
Medical Assistant Role Delineation Chart

ADMINISTRATIVE

ADMINISTRATIVE PROCEDURES

- Perform basic clerical functions
- Schedule, coordinate, and monitor appointments
- Schedule inpatient/outpatient admissions and procedures
- Understand and apply third-party guidelines
- Obtain reimbursement through accurate claims submission
- Monitor third-party reimbursement
- Perform medical transcription
- Understand and adhere to managed care policies and procedures
- *Negotiate managed care contracts (adv)*

PRACTICE FINANCES

- Perform procedural and diagnostic coding
- Apply bookkeeping principles
- Document and maintain accounting and banking records
- Manage accounts receivable
- Manage accounts payable
- Process payroll
- *Develop and maintain fee schedules (adv)*
- *Manage renewals of business and professional insurance policies (adv)*
- *Manage personnel benefits and maintain records (adv)*

CLINICAL

FUNDAMENTAL PRINCIPLES

- Apply principles of aseptic technique and infection control
- Comply with quality assurance practices
- Screen and follow up patient test results

DIAGNOSTIC ORDERS

- Collect and process specimens
- Perform diagnostic tests

PATIENT CARE

- Adhere to established triage procedures
- Obtain patient history and vital signs
- Prepare and maintain examination and treatment areas
- Prepare patient for examinations, procedures, and treatments
- Assist with examinations, procedures, and treatments
- Prepare and administer medications and immunizations
- Maintain medication and immunization records
- Recognize and respond to emergencies
- Coordinate patient care information with other health care providers

GENERAL (TRANSDISCIPLINARY)

PROFESSIONALISM

- Project a professional manner and image
- Adhere to ethical principles
- Demonstrate initiative and responsibility
- Work as a team member
- Manage time effectively
- Prioritize and perform multiple tasks
- Adapt to change
- Promote the CMA credential
- Enhance skills through continuing education

COMMUNICATION SKILLS

- Treat all patients with compassion and empathy
- Recognize and respect cultural diversity
- Adapt communications to individual's ability to understand
- Use professional telephone technique
- Use effective and correct verbal and written communications
- Recognize and respond to verbal and nonverbal communications
- Use medical terminology appropriately
- Receive, organize, prioritize, and transmit information
- Serve as liaison
- Promote the practice through positive public relations

LEGAL CONCEPTS

- Maintain confidentiality
- Practice within the scope of education, training, and personal capabilities
- Prepare and maintain medical records
- Document accurately
- Use appropriate guidelines when releasing information
- Follow employer's established policies dealing with the health care contract
- Follow federal, state and local legal guidelines
- Maintain awareness of federal and state health care legislation and regulations
- Maintain and dispose of regulated substances in compliance with government guidelines
- Comply with established risk management and safety procedures
- Recognize professional credentialing criteria
- Participate in the development and maintenance of personnel, policy, and procedure manuals
- *Develop and maintain personnel, policy, and procedure manuals (adv)*

INSTRUCTION

- Instruct individuals according to their needs
- Explain office policies and procedures
- Teach methods of health promotion and disease prevention
- Locate community resources and disseminate information
- *Orient and train personnel (adv)*
- *Develop educational materials (adv)*
- *Conduct continuing education activities (adv)*

OPERATIONAL FUNCTIONS

- Maintain supply inventory
- Evaluate and recommend equipment and supplies
- Apply computer techniques to support office operations
- *Supervise personnel (adv)*
- *Interview and recommend job applicants (adv)*
- *Negotiate leases and prices for equipment and supply contracts (adv)*

*Denotes advanced skills.

Reprinted with permission of the American Association of Medical Assistants.

CORRELATION OF TEXT TO AAMA ROLE DELINEATION STUDY

CH	TEXT	Administrative		Clinical			General (Transdisciplinary)				
		Administrative Procedures	Practice Finances	Fundamental Principles	Diagnostic Orders	Patient Care	Professionalism	Communication Skills	Legal Concepts	Instruction	Operational Functions
1.	Health Care Providers					X	X	X	X	X	
2.	The Medical Assistant						X	X	X	X	
3.	Medical Ethics and Liability	X		X	X	X	X	X	X	X	
4.	Interpersonal Communications					X	X	X	X	X	
5.	The Office Environment	X	X	X		X	X	X	X	X	
6.	Oral and Written Communications	X	X	X	X	X	X	X	X	X	X
7.	Records Management	X	X			X	X	X	X	X	X
8.	Collecting Fees	X	X				X	X	X	X	X
9.	Health Care Coverage	X	X				X	X	X	X	X
10.	Medical Office Management	X	X				X	X	X	X	X
11.	Anatomy and Physiology of the Human Body	X	X		X	X		X		X	
12.	Preparing for Clinical Duties			X	X	X	X		X	X	
13.	Beginning the Patient's Record			X	X	X	X		X	X	
14.	Preparing Patients for Examination			X	X	X	X	X	X	X	X
15.	Specimen Collection & Laboratory Procedures			X	X	X	X	X	X	X	X
16.	Diagnostic Tests Procedures & X-rays			X	X	X	X	X	X	X	X
17.	Minor Surgical Procedures			X	X	X	X	X	X	X	
18.	Assisting with Medications			X		X	X	X	X	X	X
19.	Emergencies, Acute Illness, Accidents, and Recovery			X		X	X		X	X	X
20.	Behaviors Influencing Health			X	X	X	X	X	X	X	
21.	Achieving Satisfaction in Employment			X	X	X	X	X	X	X	
	Appendix	X		X	X	X	X	X	X	X	X
	Glossary	X						X		X	X
	Workbook	X	X	X	X	X	X	X	X	X	X
	Instructor's Guide	X	X	X	X	X	X	X	X	X	X

Appendix B
CAAHEP Standards

Content: To provide for student attainment of the Entry-Level Competencies for the Medical Assistant, the curriculum must include, but not necessarily be limited to:

a. Anatomy and Physiology
- (1) Anatomy and physiology of all the body systems
- (2) Common pathology/diseases
- (3) Diagnostic/treatment modalities

b. Medical Terminology
- (1) Basic structure of medical words
- (2) Word building and definitions
- (3) Applications of medical terminology

c. Medical Law and Ethics
- (1) Legal guidelines/requirements for health care
- (2) Medical ethics and related issues
- (3) Risk management

d. Psychology
- (1) Basic principles
- (2) Developmental stages of the life cycle
- (3) Hereditary, cultural, and environmental influences on behavior
- (4) Mental health and applied psychology

e. Communication
- (1) Principles of verbal and nonverbal communication
- (2) Recognition and response to verbal and nonverbal communication
- (3) Adaptations for individualized needs
- (4) Applications of electronic technology
- (5) Fundamental writing skills

f. Medical Assisting Administrative Procedures
- (1) Basic medical office functions
- (2) Bookkeeping and basic accounting
- (3) Insurance and coding
- (4) Facility management

g. Medical Assisting Clinical Procedures
- (1) Asepsis and infection control
- (2) Specimen collection and processing
- (3) Diagnostic testing
- (4) Patient care
- (5) Pharmacology
- (6) Medical emergencies
- (7) Principles of radiology

h. Professional Components
- (1) Personal attributes
- (2) Job readiness
- (3) Workplace dynamics
- (4) Allied health professions and credentialing

i. Externship
- (1) A minimum of 160 contact hours
- (2) Placement in an ambulatory health care setting

CORRELATION OF TEXT TO CAAHEP STANDARDS FOR CURRICULUM

CH	TEXT	Anatomy and Physiology	Medical Terminology	Medical Law and Ethics	Psychology	Communication (oral and written)	Medical Assisting Administrative Procedures	Medical Assisting Clinical Procedures	Professional Components	Externship
1.	Health Care Providers		X						X	
2.	The Medical Assistant		X						X	X
3.	Medical Ethics and Liability		X	X		X		X	X	
4.	Interpersonal Communications		X	X	X	X	X		X	
5.	The Office Environment		X	X	X	X	X		X	
6.	Oral and Written Communications		X			X	X		X	
7.	Records Management		X	X		X	X			
8.	Collecting Fees		X	X	X	X	X		X	
9.	Health Care Coverage		X	X		X	X			
10.	Medical Office Management		X	X		X	X		X	
11.	Anatomy and Physiology of the Human Body	X	X		X			X		
12.	Preparing for Clinical Duties		X	X		X		X	X	
13.	Beginning the Patient's Record		X	X	X	X		X		
14.	Preparing Patients for Examination	X	X	X	X	X		X	X	
15.	Specimen Collection & Laboratory Procedures	X	X	X	X	X		X		
16.	Diagnostic Tests Procedures & X-rays		X	X	X	X		X		
17.	Minor Surgical Procedures	X	X	X	X	X		X	X	
18.	Assisting with Medications	X	X	X	X	X		X	X	
19.	Emergencies, Acute Illness, Accidents, and Recovery	X	X	X	X	X		X		
20.	Behaviors Influencing Health	X	X	X	X	X		X	X	
21.	Achieving Satisfaction in Employment		X		X	X	X	X	X	
	Appendix		X			X		X		
	Glossary		X			X				
	Workbook	X	X	X	X	X	X	X	X	
	Instructor's Guide	X	X	X	X	X	X	X	X	X

Appendix C
ABHES Course Content Requirements for Medical Assistants

1. **Orientation**
   a. Introduction and review of program
   b. Employment outlook
   c. General responsibilities

2. **Anatomy and Physiology**
   a. Anatomy and physiology
   b. Diet and nutrition
   c. Study of diseases and etiology

3. **Medical Terminology**
   a. Basic structure of medical words (roots, prefixes, suffixes, spelling, and definitions)
   b. Combining word elements to form medical words
   c. Medical specialties and short forms
   d. Medical abbreviations

4. **Medical Law and Ethics**
   a. Ethical decisions, medical jurisprudence, and confidentiality
   b. Legal terminology pertaining to office practice
   c. Medical/ethical issues in today's society

5. **Psychology of Human Relations**
   a. Dealing with difficult patients with normal/abnormal behavior
   b. Caring for patients with special and specific needs
   c. Caring for cancer and terminally ill patients
   d. Emotional crises, patients, and/or family
   e. Various treatment protocols

6. **Pharmacology**
   a. Occupational math and metric conversions (drug calculations)
   b. Use of Physician's Desk References (PDRs) and medication books
   c. Common abbreviations used in prescription writing
   d. Legal aspects of writing prescriptions
   e. FDC and state laws
   f. Medications prescribed for the treatment of illness and disease based on a systems method

7. **Medical Office Business Procedures/Management**
   a. Manual and computerized records management
      1. Patient case histories (confidentiality)
      2. Filing
      3. Appointments and scheduling
      4. Inventory/control
   b. Financial management
      1. Basic bookkeeping
      2. Billing and collections
      3. Purchasing
      4. Banking and payroll
   c. Insurance (including Health Maintenance Organizations [HMOs], Preferred Provider Organizations [PPOs], co-pays, Current Procedural Terminology [CPT] coding, etc.)
   d. Equipment and supplies (including ordering, maintaining, storage, and inventory)
   e. Reception, public, and interpersonal relations
      1. Telephone techniques
      2. Professional conduct and appearance
      3. Professional office environment and safety
   f. Office safety and security

8. **Basic Keyboarding**
   a. Office machines, transcriptions, computerized systems, and medical data processing
   b. Transcribing medical correspondence and medical reports
   c. Medical terminology review

9. **Medical Office Clinical Procedures**
   a. Basic clinical skills (e.g., vital signs)
   b. Basic skills and procedures used in medical emergencies
   c. Patient examination
      1. Patient histories
      2. Patient preparation
      3. Physical exam
      4. Instruments
      5. Assisting the physician
      6. Housekeeping

d. Medical equipment
   1. Electrocardiogram, centrifuge, etc.
   2. Physical therapy
   3. Radiography
      a) Safety
      b) Patient preparation
      c) Radiography of chest and extremities
e. Medical asepsis/sterilization and minor office surgery
f. Specialties
g. First aid, cardiopulmonary resuscitation (CPR)
h. Injections (dosage calculations):
   1. IM (intramuscular)
   2. Sub q (subcutaneous)
   3. ID (intradermal)
i. Universal Precautions in the medical office

10. **Medical Laboratory Procedures**
    a. Orientation
       1. Laboratory equipment and maintenance
       2. Safety
       3. Storage of chemicals and supplies
       4. Fire safety
       5. Care of microscope (introduction)
    b. Urinalysis
       1. Specimen collection
       2. Physical exam
       3. Chemical analysis
       4. Microscopic exam
    c. Hematology
       1. Personal protective equipment
       2. Specimen collection
          a) Venipuncture
          b) Finger puncture
       3. Hemoglobin
       4. Hematocrit
       5. WBCs (white blood cells)
       6. RBCs (red blood cells)
       7. Slide preps
       8. Serology
          a) Blood typing
          b) Blood morphology
       9. Quality control
    d. Basic blood chemistries
    e. Human immunodeficiency virus (HIV)/acquired immunodeficiency syndrome (AIDS)
    f. OSHA (Occupational Safety and Health Administration) Compliance Rules and Regulations

11. **Career Development**
    a. Instruction regarding internship rules and regulations
    b. Job search, professional developmen, and success
    c. Goal setting, time management, and employment opportunities
    d. Resumé writing, interviewing techniques, and follow-up
    e. Dress for success
    f. Professionalism

12. **Guidelines for Acceptable Externship (160 Hours)**
    a. The externship should provide students practical experience in ambulatory health care facilities, including hospitals, physician's offices, or other health care facilities.
    b. Before assigning a student to an externship location, there must be a prior evaluation by the school that a viable externship site exists for an effective externship. In addition, the physician shall be provided with a written contract setting forth the conditions for the externship.
    c. Visitation by a qualified member of the school staff should be made during the externship of a trainee if the locale is within a reasonable distance from the school. In any event, telephone follow-up should be made to determine that the experience is a valid and satisfactory one for the trainee.
    d. The externship should include appropriately diversified learning experiences.
    e. A documented report on student performance must be submitted by the physician and/or the supervisory person involved. The report must be kept at the school in the student's file.

ABHES COURSE CONTENT REQUIREMENTS

	Chapter 1	Chapter 2	Chapter 3	Chapter 4	Chapter 5	Chapter 6	Chapter 7	Chapter 8	Chapter 9	Chapter 10	Chapter 11	Chapter 12	Chapter 13	Chapter 14	Chapter 15	Chapter 16	Chapter 17	Chapter 18	Chapter 19	Chapter 20	Chapter 21	Workbook	Instructor's Guide
Orientation	x	x	x		x			x	x		x									x		x	x
Anatomy & Physiology											x			x	x	x	x		x			x	x
Medical Terminology	x	x	x	x	x	x	x	x	x	x	x	x	x	x	x	x	x	x	x	x	x	x	x
Medical Law & Ethics		x			x	x	x	x	x		x					x	x	x				x	x
Psychology of Human Relations				x	x					x			x	x		x	x	x				x	x
Pharmacology											x						x		x			x	x
Medical Office Business Procedures/Management				x	x	x	x	x	x		x	x										x	x
Basic Keyboarding				x	x	x	x	x	x	x									x			x	x
Medical Office Clinical Procedures				x									x	x	x	x	x	x	x			x	x
Medical Laboratory Procedures										x				x	x							x	x
Career Development		x	x																x	x		x	x
Guidelines for Acceptable Externship																							x

Appendix D

Registered Medical Assistant (RMA [AMT]) Certification Competency Summary

I. GENERAL MEDICAL ASSISTING KNOWLEDGE
   A. Anatomy and Physiology
      1. Body systems
      2. Disorders of the body
   B. Medical Terminology
      1. Word parts
      2. Definitions
      3. Common abbreviations and symbols
      4. Spelling
   C. Medical Law
      1. Medical Law
      2. Licensure, certification, and registration
   D. Medical Ethics
      1. Principles of medical ethics
      2. Ethical conduct
   E. Human Relations
      1. Patient relations
      2. Other interpersonal relations
   F. Patient Education
      1. Patient instruction
      2. Patient resource materials

II. ADMINISTRATIVE MEDICAL ASSISTING
   A. Insurance
      1. Terminology
      2. Plans
      3. Claim forms
      4. Coding
      5. Financial aspects of medical insurance
   B. Financial Bookkeeping
      1. Terminology
      2. Patient billing
      3. Collections
      4. Fundamental medical office accounting procedures
      5. Banking
      6. Employee payroll
      7. Financial mathematics

   C. Medical Secretarial-Receptionist
      1. Terminology
      2. Reception
      3. Scheduling
      4. Oral and written communications
      5. Records management
      6. Charts
      7. Transcription and dictation
      8. Supplies and equipment management
      9. Computers for medical office applications
      10. Office safety

III. CLINICAL MEDICAL ASSISTING
   A. Asepsis
      1. Terminology
      2. Universal blood and body fluid precautions
      3. Medical asepsis
      4. Surgical asepsis
   B. Sterilization
      1. Terminology
      2. Sanitization
      3. Disinfection
      4. Sterilization
      5. Record keeping
   C. Instruments
      1. Identification
      2. Usage
      3. Care and handling
   D. Vital Signs
      1. Blood pressure
      2. Pulse
      3. Respiration
      4. Height and weight
      5. Temperature
   E. Physical Examinations
      1. Problem-oriented records
      2. Positions
      3. Methods of examination

4. Specialty examinations
5. Visual acuity
6. Allergy testing
F. Clinical Pharmacology
   1. Terminology
   2. Injections
   3. Prescriptions
   4. Drugs
G. Minor Surgery
   1. Surgical supplies
   2. Surgical procedures
H. Therapeutic Modalities
   1. Modalities
   2. Patient instruction
I. Laboratory Procedures
   1. Safety
   2. Quality control
   3. Laboratory equipment
   4. Urinalysis
   5. Blood
   6. Other specimens
   7. Specimen handling
   8. Records
   9. Microbiology
J. Electrocardiography
   1. Standard, 12-lead ECG (electrocardiogram)
   2. Mounting techniques
   3. Other ECG procedures
K. First Aid
   1. First aid procedures
   2. Legal responsibilities

COMPTENENCY INVENTORY NOTE

The tasks included in this inventory are considered by American Medical Technologists to be representative of the medical assisting job role. This document should be considered dynamic, to reflect the medical assistant's current role with respect to contemporary health care. Therefore, tasks may be added, removed, or modified on an ongoing basis.

(Reprinted with permission of American Medical Technologists.)

Appendix E

SITE VISIT GUIDELINES

Review Item	Y/N
Office sign is clearly identifiable with the name of the site and each doctor's name	
Reception room, exam rooms, lab, and all other waiting areas supply adequate lighting. Walls and doors are structured to assure confidentiality with regard to sound	
Stairwells, corridors, and exits are free from obstruction	
Exit signs are clearly visible	
Must supply log to show that fire extinguishers have been checked yearly and proof that staff members have been taught to use them	
Must have a written plan for medical/natural emergencies.	
Disaster/fire evacuation routes are posted throughout the facility	
Must show evidence of disaster/fire drills one to two times per year	
Reception counter is accessible to handicapped	
Reception room is clean and free from dust, dirt, and clutter. Reception room is well-ventilated	
Combustible items are not stored near furnace or water heater	

Review Item	Y/N
Educational items, such as pamphlets, are available, organized, and distributed to patients as indicated	
Must show proper labeling, logging, and storage of hazardous/infectious and flammable liquids	
Each patient care area provides proper hand washing stations with antibacterial soap and an adequate supply of paper towels	
Standard Precautions are practiced	
Gloves are located in each patient care area. Tables are disinfected and paper is changed between each patient	
Each physician has a minimum of two patient rooms	
Drape sheets/gowns are available to patients	
Work areas are designated as clean/dirty	
Site has a no-smoking policy that is posted and enforced	
Office policy that shows an assistant is always available (a female should always be available to male physicians during gynecological exams)	
Reception room had adequate seating for patient load (10 chairs for pediatric sites and 5 chairs for adult sites)	
Otoscope tips/thermometers are sterilized or disposable	

BUILDING/FACILITY

Review Item	Y/N
Facility has adequate parking	
Handicap parking is available	
Handicapped-accessible; if building was built prior to 1990, the site has a written plan for handling disabled patients; if building was built after 1990, the site has ramp accessibility; rooms and doors are handicapped accessible	
Restrooms have grab bars in place	
Building has a sprinkler system and smoke detectors in place according to building codes	

Review Item	Y/N
Bus service available to physician's office	
Entrance/exit doors are easy to open (automation preferable)	
Security system	
Buildings with multiple floors have elevators that are properly working, handicapped accessible, and currently licensed	
Adequate number of fire extinguishers are present, disbursed properly, and have had regular annual inspections	

SERVICE ACCESSIBILITY

Review Item	Y/N
Members requiring emergency care are seen the same day either in the office, hospital ER, or urgent care center, according to patient's condition and office availability. Should have an office protocol	
Members exhibiting minor symptoms are seen within two to three days	
Periodic health assessments are seen within four to six weeks	
There should be a written policy for telephone triage and walk-in triage procedures. A triage manual that has been approved by the physicians is preferred	
Callers should not be put on hold for more than two minutes	
After hours and weekend calls are maintained by a log	
Office hours should be posted both internally and externally for patient convenience along with after-hours phone number	
There should be consistency with scheduling regarding walk-in and scheduled patients. There must be a policy	
The office must accept new patients	
Preferred appointment intervals: Complete physical 30–45 minutes Routine exams 15–20 minutes Urgent/emergencies As necessary	

Review Item	Y/N
Members who are acutely ill, requiring urgent care, are seen with 24 hours	
Members wanting routine appointments, such as follow-ups for blood pressure, are seen in one to two weeks	
Emergency calls should be triaged immediately and treated within one hour (sooner if life-threatening)	
Telephone response time should be handled with 10 rings or less	
Callers should always be asked if it is permissible to be placed on hold	
Patients should have access to a physician 24 hours per day, including weekends, evenings, and holidays. Calls should be processed within 30 minutes for urgent calls and one to seven hours for non-urgent calls	
Patient wait times routinely should be less 15–30 minutes except in emergency situations	
There should be written policies that are given to patients on their first visit regarding broken appointments. There should be a written policy that is distributed to the staff regarding follow-up procedures for patients who break appointments	
Covering physicians must be located within 25 miles of PCP (primary care physician) office	

PHARMACEUTICALS

Review Item	Y/N
Medication logs are accessible and used for all immunizations and controlled substances	
Drug formularies are centrally located and accessible	
Light sensitive drugs are stored properly	
Controlled medications are locked and secured properly. Daily inventories are performed and logged	
Multiple use vials are dated upon opening and discarded according to manufacturer's instructions	
All drugs requiring refrigeration or freezing are stored properly. Medication refrigerators/freezers do not contain foods or lab specimens	

Review Item	Y/N
There should be no outdated medications anywhere, including emergency kit, sample room, refrigerator, drug cabinets, and patient rooms	
There should be clearly written policies regarding accessibility to, dispensing of, and disposal of medications, including samples, multi-dose vials, and expired medications	
Patient allergy immunotherapy medications are labeled	
There should be a clearly written plan concerning the drug sample area, including drug rep policy and procedures and proper inventory and disposal of expired samples	

LABORATORY

Review Item	Y/N
Should have lab policy and procedure manual that shows evidence of annual review and updating	
If Commission on Laboratory Accreditation (COLA) or Clinical Laboratory Improvement Amendments (CLIA) certified, must show current certificate and accreditation number	
Lab is following Standard Precautions for specimen handling	
There should be a written policy prohibiting eating, drinking, applying cosmetics or contact lenses, and smoking in the lab, x-ray room, and autoclave areas	
Controls and calibrations are performed on all instrumentation and test kits according to manufacturer's instructions. Logs should reflect this	

Review Item	Y/N
Quality control is maintained and documented	
Lab tests are performed and interpreted in a timely manner	
Personnel performing testing are qualitifed to perform testing. Training records should be in file	
There should be a written policy regarding reporting abnormal and normal lab findings after careful review by the physician	
Reagents and specimens are stored in labeled containers. Specimens should be stored appropriately (refrigerated, frozen, or at room temperature)	

EQUIPMENT

Review Item	Y/N
The following medications are available:	
Valium, 10 mg vial	
Dilantin 300 mg vial	
IV solutions	
Nitroglycerine 0.4 mg spray or sublingual	
Benadryl (Diphenhydramine) 50 mg IM	
Epinephrine 1:1000	
Procardia (Nifedipine) 10 mg PO	
Emergency equipment/medication is checked monthly or after each use	
Sites that perform IV sedation must have an emergency kit that is inspected on a regular basis and should contain: oxygen, ambu bag, face mask, atropine, adrenaline, suction equipment, and IV fluids and supplies	
Equipment should receive maintenance/calibration/service yearly; all records of maintenance should be readily available	
Sterilized and disinfected articles are current and are properly stored	
Housekeeping schedule shows proper cleaning and disinfecting of all counter tops, floors, tables, etc. Logs are accessible	
Freezer and refrigerator temperatures are checked and logged daily. Refrigerator temps are 36–45° F	

Review Item	Y/N
Ambu bags, airways, and pocket masks are readily accessible	
Oxgen should not be outdated and should be readily available, maintained, inspected, and secure	
Sites that perform cardiac stress testing must have a basic cardiac emergency kit, a cardiac monitor with a defibrillator (which is accessible and inspected regularly), and intubation equipment with an ambu bag	
Autoclaves should be maintained and in good working condition. Steri-gauges or equivalent should be run with each load, weekly spore checks should be performed. Autoclave should be cleaned on a regular basis. There should be evidence of a written procedure and log to show that all of these specifications are being followed.	
Prescription pads, drugs, and needles are secure (not accessible to patients) and disposed of properly	
Bacteriostatic solutions and cold sterilants are labeled, dated, and changed according to manufacturer's instructions	
Eyewash stations should be attached to plumbing. Hot water should be turned off. Log should show weekly/monthly inspections	

MEDICAL RECORDS GENERAL

Review Items	Y/N
Records are both safe and secure	
There is a written policy regarding patient confidentiality issues and proper release of medical information. These policies are consistently applied	
Each page of the record contains patient identification	
There is a policy for recording Advance Directives	
There is a protocol or policy on the proper technique for correcting errors in the patient chart	
The site has initials/signatures on files for all personnel who make chart entries	
There is a written policy or system for the storage and disposal of old records	

Review Items	Y/N
Records are maintained in a jacket marked with the patient's full name	
All applicable release and consent forms are signed	
Records are both readily available and easily retrievable; sections are divided and in chronological order; all pages are secure	
There is a written policy for documenting phone calls in the medical chart, both during and after office hours	
There is a written policy on patients who refuse treatment	
Records are retained according to state standards	
BP is recorded within 12 months prior to the last visit	

MEDICAL RECORDS CONTENT AND STRUCTURE

Review Items	Y/N
All entries are legible	
There is a complete history and physical documented for established patients (patients who have had three or more visits)	
Each chart has a summary list of current medications	
There is a complete medical and family history on each patient	
Heights and weights are documented. Growth charts are completed on pediatric patients	
Orders for all diagnostic testing documented	
All in-patient admissions are documented	
All entries are signed and dated	
Telephone advice is documented and signed	
Copies of advance directives or evidence of discussion is documented for appropriate members	
Drug allergies are listed or a prominent NKDA (no known drug allergies) is prominently displayed	

Review Items	Y/N
Each chart has a summary list for chronic illnesses	
Each chart contains current demographic information	
There is a complete and accurate social history on each patient, including tobacco, alcohol, and drug history	
There should be documentation of all medications dispensed, administered, and prescribed. Documentation should include dosage, route, frequency, and amount/number given	
Emergency care documented	
Broken appointments and follow-up procedures are documented	
All diagnostic testing and consultations are initiated by reviewing physician. Documentation shows that the patient was notified before filing and a follow-up plan is noted	
Referrals and results of referrals are documented	

STAFFING ISSUES

Review Item	Y/N
Staff records reflect current certifications and licensure	
Employee policy and procedure manual available to staff members	
All staff members must have proof of current OSHA training, disaster training, MSDS (material safety data sheets) training, and emergency preparedness training	
Must show current CPR certification for at least one staff member (the more staff members certified, the better)	
Employees should have access to the written exposure control plan and hazardous communication plan	
Policies, procedures, and protocols should be in place to ensure accountability and management of controlled substances, prescription pads and sample drugs.	
In-service programs should be provided as needed	

Review Item	Y/N
Written job descriptions are accessible	
Staff members must have a comprehensive, organized orientation program upon hiring	
Teaching activities are clearly delineated, and there is a defined scope of involvement in patient care	
Records should reflect the staff members availability for receiving the following immunizations: hepatitis B, flu vaccine, and purified protein derivative (PPD) skin testing. Staff refusal should be validated with declination forms	
Emergency numbers should be posted at all telephones	
All staff members should wear name tags which identify their title or position	
If the office has received OSHA/CLIA citations in the last year, a quality improvement plan must have been submited and accessible	

RADIOLOGY

Review Items	Y/N
Current certificate is available (registration number); state inspection certificate is current and visibly posted	
Must show a written order for all x-ray procedures	
Procedures are performed, interpreted, and reported in a timely manner	
Lead shields are available and used appropriately. The office has lead-lined walls or appropriate shielding	
Equipment is inspected on a regular basis and is re-calibrated every one to two years; equipment is appropriate for procedures. Routine maintenance is performed; x-ray chemicals are changed as recommended by the manufacturer and stored in a safe area not accessible to patients. A written policy exists on proper disposal	
There is a dedicated room to perform x-rays	
X-ray logs reflect each x-ray that is taken or sent out. Logs also reflect any repeat x-rays, equipment failure, and inadaquate visualization	

Review Items	Y/N
Dark room is clean and dust free	
Radiology and procedure manual is available outlining all procedures, including those related to safety	
All x-ray personnel should have current licensure or certification depending on the state's requirements	
All personnel wear x-ray exposure badges, which are monitored regularly	
Monthly records show x-ray badge exposure results	
Protective devices include warning signs and pregnant woman alert	
The table is either covered or cleaned after each use	
X-rays are stored in a central location	

PATIENT RIGHTS

Review Items	Y/N
Is there a written bill of rights that is either distributed or displayed where the patient can view it?	
Is there a written policy regarding the reporting of public health concerns to the appropriate authorities?	
Is there a written policy concerning the treatment of emancipated minors that are not accompanied by an adult?	

Review Items	Y/N
Is there a written description that is either distributed or displayed regarding the patient's right to file a grievance?	
Does the office have Advance Directive and Durable Power of Attorney material available and accessible for its patients?	
Does the office have a written "knock before entering" policy?	

MEDICAL RECORD PREVENTIVE MEDICINE ITEMS

Review Items	Y/N
Annual Physical: >50 years every 5 years	
Pap Smear: >18 years, 2 paps one year apart; then biennially, until age 70	
Sigmoidoscopy: at age 50, then every 5 years	
Immunizations: according to recommended schedules	
Diabetic Education: performed and documented A. **HgbA1C** done one to two times per year. Should be done more often if poorly controlled B. **Lipid profile** offered biennially C. **Annual eye exam** if on insulin, otherwise biennially D. **Annual foot exam, UA** (urinalysis) and **BP** (blood pressure) recorded	

Review Items	Y/N
Mammogram: offered every one to two years for ages 50–75	
Cholesterol Screening: men > 35 years every 5 years women > 45 years every 5 years	
Fecal Occult Blood: offered at age 50, then every year unless scoped	
Well Exam: done according to pediatric standards; adults biennially until age 70	

Appendix F

CONVERTING MEASUREMENTS

LENGTH	Centimeters	Inches	Feet
1 centimeter	1.000	0.394	0.0328
1 inch	2.54	1.000	0.0833
1 foot	30.48	12.000	1.000
1 yard	91.4	36.00	3.00
1 meter	100.00	39.40	3.28

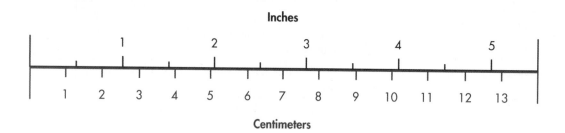

Comparison of Centimeters and Inches

VOLUMES	Cubic Centimeters	Fluid Drams	Fluid Ounces	Quarts	Liters
1 cubic centimeter	1.00	0.270	0.033	0.0010	0.0010
1 fluid dram	3.70	1.00	0.125	0.0039	0.0037
1 cubic inch	16.39	4.43	0.554	0.0173	0.0163
1 fluid ounce	29.6	8.00	1.000	0.0312	0.0296
1 quart	946.0	255.0	32.00	1.000	0.946
1 liter	1000.0	270.0	33.80	1.056	1.000

WEIGHTS	Grains	Grams	Apothecary Ounces	Pounds
1 grain (gr)	1.000	0.064	0.002	0.0001
1 gram (gm)	15.43	1.000	0.032	0.0022
1 apothecary ounce	480.00	31.1	1.000	0.0685
1 pound	7000.00	454.0	14.58	1.000
1 kilogram	15432.0	1000.00	32.15	2.205

RULES FOR CONVERING ONE SYSTEM TO ANOTHER

Volumes

Grains to grams—divide by 15
Drams to cubic centimeters—multiply by 4
Ounces to cubic centimeters—multiply by 30
Minims to cubic millimeters—multiply by 63
Minims to cubic centimeters—multiply by 0.06
Cubic millimeters to minims—divide by 63
Cubic centimeters to minims—multiply by 16
Cubic centimeters to fluid ounces—divide by 30
Liters to pints—divide by 2.1

Weights

Milligrams to grains—multiply by 0.0154
Grams to grains—multiply by 15
Grams to drams—multiply by 0.257
Grams to ounces—multiply by 0.0311

Temperature

Multiply centigrade (Celsius) degrees by $\frac{9}{5}$ and add 32 to convert Fahrenheit to Celsius
Subtract 32 from the Fahrenheit degrees and multiply by $\frac{5}{9}$ to convert Celsius to Fahrenheit

COMMON HOUSEHOLD MEASURES AND WEIGHTS

1 teaspoon	= 4-5 cc. or 1 dram
3 teaspoons	= 1 tablespoon
1 dessert spoon	= 8 cc. or 2 drams
1 tablespoon	= 15 cc. or 3 drams
4 tablespoons	= 1 wine glass or ½ gill
16 tablespoons (liq)	= 1 cup
12 tablespoons (dry)	= 1 cup
1 cup	= 8 fluid ounces or ½ pint
1 tumbler or glass	= 8 fluid ounces or 240 cc.
1 wine glass	= 2 fluid ounces, 60 cc.
16 fluid ounces	= 1 pound
4 gills	= 1 pound
1 pint	= 1 pound

Medical Symbols and Abbreviations

m̲	minim	s̄	without
℥	dram	c̄	with
℥	ounce	−	minus, negative, alkaline reaction
O	pint		
#	pound, number	+	plus, excess, acid reaction, positive
℞	recipe, prescription		
′	foot, minute	×	multiply
″	inch, second	÷	divide
a̅a̅	equal parts	=	equals
°	degree	>	greater than
%	percent	<	less than
♂	male	∞	infinity
♀	female	↑	increase
s̅s̅	one half	↓	decrease

Abbreviations

a, aa	of each
a.c.	before meals
ad lib	as desired
A & P	anterior and posterior
aq	aqueous, water
BE, ba.en.	barium enema
blf	black female
bib	drink
b.i.d., BID	twice a day
bm, BM	bowel movement
blm	black male
BP, B/P	blood pressure
BUN	blood urea nitrogen
c̄	with
C	centigrade
Ca	calcium
cap	capsule
CBC	complete blood count
cc	cubic centimeter
CCU	coronary care unit
CHF	congestive heart failure
cm	cubic centimeter
CNS	central nervous system
CO_2	carbon dioxide

Abbreviations (*continued*)

comp	compound
COPD	chronic obstructive pulmonary disease
CPR	cardiopulmonary resuscitation
CSF	cerebrospinal fluid
CVA	cerebrovascular accident
cysto	cystoscopy
D & C	dilatation and curettage
Dil, dil	dilute
DOA	dead on arrival
DPT	dephtheria, pertussis, tetanus
dr.	dram
dx, Dx	diagnosis
ECG	electrocardiogram
EEG	electroencephalogram
EENT	eye, ears, nose, throat
EKG	electrocardiogram
elix	elixir
ER	emergency room
et	and
expl lap	exploratory laparotomy
ext.	extract
F	fahrenheit
F	female
FBS	fasting blood sugar
fl	fluid
fl. dr.	fluid dram
fl. oz.	fluid ounce
Fx	fracture
GB	gallbladder
GI	gastrointestinal
Gm	gram
GP	general practitioner
gr	grain
gtt Gtt gtts	drop, drops
GU	genitourinary
GYN	gynecology
H, h	hour
HCL	hydrochloric acid
Hgb	hemoglobin
h.s.	hour of sleep, bedtime
Hx	history
hypo	hypodermic, under
ICU	intensive care unit
I & D	incision and drainage
IM	intramuscular
inj	injection
I & O	intake and output
IPPB	intermittent positive pressure breathing
IT	inhalation therapy
IUD	intrauterine device

IV	intravenous
IVP	intravenous pyelogram
k	potassium
KUB	kidney, ureter, and bladder
L, lb	pound
lat	lateral
liq	liquid
LLQ	left lower quadrant
LMP	last menstrual period
LUQ	left upper quadrant
m	minim
M	male
mm	millimeter
MS	multiple sclerosis
NB	newborn
no.	number
noxt.	at night
NPO	nothing by mouth
N & V	nausea and vomiting
O	pint
OB	obstetrics
OD	overdose
O.D.	right eye
OP	outpatient
OR	operating room
os	mouth
O.S.	left eye
O.U.	both eyes
oz	ounce
Path	pathology
PBI	protein bound iodine
p.c.	after meals
Peds	pediatrics
per	through, by
PID	pelvic inflammatory disease
PKU	phenylketonuria
PO, p.o.	by mouth
prn	as desired, needed
pro time	prothrombin time
Psych	psychiatry
pt	patient, pint
pulv	powder
Px	physical examination
q	every
qd	every day
q 4 h	every 4 hours
qh	every hour
q.i.d., QID	four times a day
qns	quantity not sufficient
qs	quantity sufficient

Abbreviations (*continued*)

qt	quart
R	right
Ra	radium
RBC	red blood cells
REM	rapid eye movement
rep	let it be repeated
R/O	rule out
ROM	range of motion
ROS	review of systems
Rx	prescription, take
s̄	without
sig	instructions, directions
SOB	short of breath
sol	solution
solv	dissolve
s.o.s.	distress signal
sp. gr.	specific gravity
ss	half
stat	immediately
subq	subcutaneous
syr.	syrup
T	temperature
T & A	tonsilectomy and adenoidectomy
tab	tablet
TIA	transient ischemic attack
t.i.d.	three times a day
tinct.	tincture
TPR	temperature, pulse, respiration
TUR	transurethral resection
UA	urinalysis
ung.	ointment
URI	upper respiratory infection
UTI	urinary tract infection
VD	venereal disease
vin	wine
VS	vital signs
WBC	white blood cells
WF	white female
WM	white male
WNL	within normal limits
wt. Wt.	weight

MEDICAL TERMINOLOGY DERIVATIVES

and—et
arm—brachium; brachion (Gr)
artery—arteria
attachment—adhaesio

back—dorsum

backbone—spina
backward—retro
belly—venter
bend—flexus
bile—billis; chole (Gr)
bladder—vesica
blind—obscurus
blister—pustulo
blood—sanguis; haima, aima (Gr)
blood vessel—vena
body—corpus; soma (Gr)
bone—os; osteon (Gr)
bony—osseus
bowels—intestina, viscera
brain—cerebrum
breach—ruptura
breast—mamma; mastos (Gr)
buttock—gloutos (Gr)

cartilage—cartilago; chondros (Gr)
chest—thorax
choke—strangulo
confinement—puerperium
corn—callus, clavus
cornea—cornu; keras (Gr)
cough—tussio
cramp—spasmus

dead—mortuus
deadly—lethalis
dental—dentalis
digestive—pepticus
disease—morbus
dose—potio

ear—auris
egg—ovum
entrails—viscera
erotic—amatorius
exhalation—exhalatio
expell—expello
expire—expiro
external—externus
extract—extractum
eye—oculus; ophthalmos (Gr)
eyeball—pupula
eyelid—palpebra

face—facies
fat—adeps; lipos (Gr)
feel—tactus
fever—febris
finger—digitus
flesh—carnis
foot—pedis; pous (Gr)
forearm—brachium
forehead—frons

Medical Terminology Derivatives (*continued*)

gall—bilis
gravel—calculus
gum—gingiva
gut—intestinum

hair—capillus
half—dimidius
hand—manus; cheir (Gr)
harelip—labrum fissum
head—caput; kephale (Gr)
healer—medicus
health—sanitas
hear—audio
heart—cor; kardia (Gr)
heat—calor
heel—calx, talus
hysterics—hysteria

illness—morbus
infant—infas, puerilis
infectious—contagiosus
infirm—debilis
injection—injectio
intellect—intellectus
internal—intestinus
intestine—intestinum; enteron (Gr)
itch—scabies
itching—pruritis

jaw—maxilla
joint—artus; anthron (Gr)

kidney—ren; nephros (Gr)
knee—genu
kneecap—patella

lacerate—lacero
larynx—guttur
lateral—lateralis
leg—tibis
limb—membrum
listen—ausculto
liver—jecur, hepar (Gr)
loin—lapara
looseness—laxitas
lukewarm—tepidus
lung—pulmo, pneumon (Gr)

mad—insanus
male—masculinus
malignant—malignus
maternity—conditio matris
milk—lac
moist—humidus
month—mensis
monthly—menstruus

mouth—os; stoma (Gr)

nail—unguis
navel—umbilicus; omphalos (Gr)
neck—cervis; trachelos (Gr)
nerve—nervus; neuron (Gr)
nipple—papilla
no, none—nullus
nose—nasus; rhis (Gr)
nostril—naris
nourishment—alimentus

ointment—unguentum
orifice—foramen

pain—dolor
patient—patiens
pectoral—pectoralis
pimple—pustula
poison—venenum
powder—pulvis
pregnant—gravida
pubic bone—os pubis
pupil—pupilla

quinsy—angina

rash—extanthema
recover—convalesco
redness—rubor
rib—costa
ringing—tinnitus
rupture—hernia

saliva—sputum
scab—scabies
scalp—pericranium
scaly—squamosus
sciatica—ischias
seed—semen
senile—senilis
sheath—vagina
shin—tibia
short—brevis
shoulder—humerus; omos (Gr)
shoulderblade—scapula
shudder—tremor
side—latus
skin—cutis; derma (Gr)
skull—cranium; kranion (Gr)
sleep—somnus
smell—odoratus
socket—cavum
solution—dilutum
sore—ulcus
spinal—dorsalis, spinalis
spine—spina

Medical Terminology Derivatives (*continued*)

spittle—sputum
sprain—luxatio
stomach—stomachus; gaster (Gr)
stone—calculus
sugar—saccharum
swallow—glutio

tail—cauda
taste—gustatus
tear—lacrima
teeth—dentes
testicle—testis; orchis (Gr)
thigh—femur
throat—fauces; pharygx (Gr)
throb—palpito
tongue—lingua; glossa (Gr)
twin—geminus

urine—urina

vagina—vagina; kolpos (Gr)
vein—vena; phleps (Gr)
vertebra—vertevra; spondylos (Gr)
vessel—vas

wash—lavo
water—aqua
wax—cera
weary—lassus
wet—humidus
windpipe—arteria aspera
woman—femina
womb—uterus; hystera (Gr)
worm—vermis
wrist—carpus; karpos (Gr)

yolk—luteum

PREFIXES AND SUFFIXES

a- an-	without, negative
ab- abs-	away from
ad-	toward
adeno-	gland
aero-	air
-aesthesia	sensation
-algia	pain
ambi-	both
angio-	blood vessel
ano-	anus
ante-	before
anti-	against
arterio-	artery
arthro-	joint
auto-	self
bi-	two, twice

brady-	slow
broncho-	bronchial
cardio-	heart
cata-	down
-cele	tumor, cysts
cent-	hundred
-centesis	puncture
cephal-	head
chole-	gall
chromo-	color
-cide	causing death
circum-	around
-cise	cut
co- com- con-	together
colo-	colon
colpo-	vagina
contra-	against
costo-	rib
cranio-	skull
cysto-	bag, bladder
-cyte -cyto	cell
dacry-	tears
de-	from, down
deca-	ten
deci-	tenth
demi-	half
dent-	teeth
derma-	skin
di-	double
dia	through, between
diplo-	double
dis-	negative, apart
dys-	difficult, painful
ecto-	out, on the outside
-ectomy	cutting out
-emesis	vomiting
-emia	blood
en-	in, into
encephalo-	brain
endo-	within
entero-	intestine
epi-	above, over
-esthesia	sensation
ex- exo-	out
extra-	on the outside
fibro-	connective tissue
fore-	before, in front of
-form	form
-fuge	to drive away
galact- galacto-	milk
gastro-	stomach
-gene -genic	origin, formation
glosso-	tongue
gluco- glyco-	sugar, sweet
-gram	a tracing, record
-graph	machine
-graphy	the process

Prefixes and Suffixes (*continued*)

gyne-	woman	necro-	dead
hema- hemato- hemo-	blood	neo-	new
hemi-	half	nephr- nephro-	kidney
hepa- hepato-	liver	neu- neuro-	nerve
herni-	rupture	niter- nitro-	nitrogen
histo-	tissue	non- not-	no
homo-	same, similar	nucleo-	a nucleus
hydra- hydro-	water	o-	ovum, an egg
hyper-	above, increased, over	ob-	against
hypo-	below, under, decreased	oculo-	eye
hyster-	uterus	-ode -oid	form, shape
-iasis	condition of	odont-	a tooth
ictero-	jaundice	oligo-	few
idio-	peculiar to the individual	-ology	study of
ileo-	ileum	-oma	a tumor
in-	in, into, not	oophor-	ovary
infra-	beneath	ophthalmo-	eye
inter-	between	-opia	vision
intra- intro-	within	orchid-	testicle
-ism	condition, theory	-orrhaphy	to repair a defect
-itis	inflammation of	ortho-	straight
-ize	to treat by special method	os-	mouth, bone
karyo-	nucleus, nut	-osis	disease, condition of
kata- kath-	down	oste- osteo-	bone
kera-	horn, indicates hardness	-ostomy	to make a mouth, opening
-kinesis	motion	oto-	ear
lact-	milk	-otomy	incision, surgical cutting
laparo-	abdomen	oxy-	sharp, acid
-lepsy	seizure, convulsion	pachy-	thick
leuco- leuko-	white	pan-	all, entire
lipo-	fat	para-	alongside of
lith-	a stone	path- -pathy	disease, suffering
-logia -logy	science of, study of	ped- (Greek)	child
-lysis	disintegration	ped- (Latin)	foot
macro-	large, long	-penia	too few, lack
mal-	bad, poor	per-	through, excessive
-mania	insanity	peri-	around
mast-	breast	pharyng-	throat
med- medi-	middle	phelebo-	vein
mega-	large, great	-phobia	fear
-megalia -megaly	large, great, extreme	-phylaxis	protection
melan-	black	-plasty	operate to revise
men-	month	-plegia	a stroke, paralysis
meso-	middle	-pnea	breathing
meta-	beyond, over, between, change, transportation	pneumo-	air, lungs
		poly-	many, much
-meter	measure	post-	after
metro- metra-	uterus	pre-	before
micro-	small	pro-	before, in behalf of
mio-	smaller, less	procto-	rectum
mono-	single, one	proto-	first
multi-	many	pseudo-	false
my- myo-	muscle	psych-	the mind
myel- myelo-	marrow	pyelo-	kidney, pelvis
narco-	sleep	pyo-	pus
naso-	nose	pyro-	heat
		re-	back, again

Prefixes and Suffixes (*continued*)

reni- reno-	kidney	super- supra-	above
retro-	backward, behind	syn-	with, together
-rhage -rhagia	hemorrhage, flow	tele-	distant, far
-rhaphy	a suturing, stitching	tetra-	four
-rhea	flow	-therapy	treatment
rhino-	nose	-thermy	heat
sacchar-	sugar	thio-	sulfur
sacro-	sacrum	thoraco-	chest
salpingo-	a tube, fallopian tube	thrombo-	clot
sarco-	flesh	thyro-	thyroid gland
sclero-	hard, sclera	trans-	across
-sclerosis	dryness, hardness	tri-	three
-scopy	to see	uni-	one
semi-	half	-uria	urine
septi-	poison, infection	urino- uro-	urine, urinary organs
stomato-	mouth	vaso-	vessel
-stomy	to furnish with a mouth	venter- ventro-	abdomen
sub-	under	xanth-	yellow

Glossary

abandonment—to desert, to give up entirely.

abbess—a mother superior; a woman who is the head of an abbey of nuns.

abbreviation—a shortened form.

abdomen—the cavity in the body between the diaphragm and the pelvis.

abdominal—pertaining to the abdomen.

abdominopelvic—pertaining to the anterior body cavity below the diaphragm.

abduct—to move away from the midline.

ablation—a surgical procedure using a resectoscope inserted into the uterus through the cervix.

abnormality—person, thing, or condition that is not normal.

abortion—the termination of pregnancy before the stage of viability; spontaneous or induced.

abrasion—an injury caused by rubbing or scraping off the skin.

abrupt—sudden; blunt, curt.

absolute—free as to condition, unlimited in power.

absorb—to suck or swallow up, to drink in.

abstract—a summary of the principal parts of a larger work.

absurd—contrary to sense or reason.

accelerator—increasing action or function.

accessible—capable of being reached.

accommodation—the process of the lens changing shape to permit close vision.

accountant—one who keeps, audits, and inspects the financial records of individuals or businesses.

account history—the past financial record.

accreditation—the assignment of credentials; approval given for meeting established standards.

accumulated—to pile up; collect; gather.

accuracy—correctness, exactness.

accurate—correct, exact, without error.

accurate and precise testing (APT)—refers to a standard for performing laboratory procedures to ensure reliability of results.

acetylcholine—a hormone released at the parasympathetic and skeletal nerve endings.

Achilles' tendon—a tendon attaching the gastrocnemius muscle of the leg to the heel.

acidosis—a disturbance of the acid–base balance of the body.

acne—a skin condition characterized by inflammation of sebaceous glands and producing pimples.

acquaintance—the state of knowing a person or subject.

acquire—to gain by one's own efforts or actions; to get.

acquisition—to acquire; to get by one's own efforts.

acromegaly—a chronic condition characterized by enlargement of bones of the extremities and some bones of the head; thickening of facial soft tissues.

acronym—a word formed from the initial letters of each major word in a term.

action potential—the temporary electrical charge within a cell.

activate—to make active or more active.

acupuncture—involves the insertion of needles at various points in the body to treat disease or relieve pain.

acute—sharp, severe; having a rapid onset, severe symptoms, and a short course; not chronic.

adaptability—the act of or the result of adjusting to a new circumstance or change.

addiction—the state of being governed or controlled by a habit, as with alcohol or drugs.

adduct—to draw together toward the midline.

adenitis—inflammation of lymph nodes or a gland.

adequate—equal to the requirement or occasion, sufficient.

adhere—to stick fast, become firmly attached; to be devoted to.

adjective—a word added to (modifying) a noun to quantify or limit it.

adjustments—changes to fit or bring into harmony.

administer—to manage; to conduct, as in business.

administrative—duties that manage or direct activities; in medical assisting, refers to tasks other than clinical in nature; front office duties.

admissions clerk—a person who processes information and forms for a patient who will be entering the health facility.

adrenal—pertaining to the adrenal glands which sit atop each kidney.

adrenaline—an internal secretion derived from the adrenal glands; can be commercially prepared from animal glands; acts as a stimulant.

adrenocorticotrophic hormone (ACTH)—a hormone secreted by the anterior lobe of the pituitary gland.

advantageous—beneficial, profitable.

adverb—a word added to (modifying) a verb, an adjective, or another adverb.

adverse—opposed to; unfavorable.

advocate—one who pleads for or defends a cause or a person.

aerobe—a microorganism that can live and grow only in the presence of oxygen.

aesthetic—relating to the principles of beauty and taste.

afebrile—without fever.

affiliate—to unite, to join or become connected.

agar—a dried mucilaginous substance, or gelatin, extracted from algae, used as a culture medium.

agent—one that acts or has the power or authority to act for another.

aggressive—pushy, assuming the offensive without cause; forceful.

Al-Anon—a support group for family members of alcoholics.

Al-Ateen—a support for teenagers with an alcoholic parent.

albino—a person who lacks pigment in the skin, hair, and eyes, either partial or total; a person with albinoism.

alcoholic—an individual who uses alcohol to excess.

Alcoholics Anonymous—an organization formed to assist alcoholics to refrain from the use of alcohol.

aldosterone—a mineralocorticoid hormone secreted by the adrenal cortex.

alignment—being in proper position.

alimentary canal—the intestinal tract, from the esophagus to the rectum, and accessory organs.

allege—to state positively but not under oath and without proof; to affirm.

allergic rhinitis—inflammation of the nose caused by an allergy.

allergist—a physician specializing in the care of patients with allergies.

allergy—an altered or acquired state of sensitivity; abnormal reaction of the body to substances normally harmless.

allosteric—a protein found in erythrocytes that transports oxygen in the blood; hemoglobin.

alopecia—the loss of hair; baldness.

alpha search—look by alphabetical order.

alveoli—microscopic air sacs in the lung.

amber—orange/yellowish color.

amblyopia—lazy eye; a condition characterized by the inward turning of the affected eye.

ambulate—to walk, not be confined to bed.

amenity—pleasantness, pleasant ways, civilities.

amenorrhea—absence of menses; without menstruation

American Society for Clinical Laboratory Science (ASCLS)

amniocentesis—the use of a needle to withdraw amniotic fluid from the amniotic sac.

amniotic—pertaining to the amniotic fluid within the amniotic membrane surrounding the fetus.

amphetamine—a central nervous system stimulant, often referred to as an upper.

amplifier—a device on an electrocardiograph that enlarges the EKG impulses.

ampule—a small glass container that can be sealed and its contents sterilized.

amputate—to cut off, remove a part.

anaerobe—a microorganism having the ability to live without oxygen.

anal—pertaining to the anus or outer rectal opening.

analysis—the examination of anything to determine its makeup; a description of the process or the examination, point by point.

analytical—characterized by a method of analysis, a statement of point-by-point examination.

anaphylaxis—a hypersensitive reaction of the body to a foreign protein or a drug; the term implies symptoms severe enough to produce serious shock, even death.

anatomic—pertaining to the anatomy or structure of an organism.

anatomy—the study of the physical structure of the body and its organs.

anchor—the attachment of a skeletal muscle; the wrapping at the start of a gauze or elastic bandage.

anemia—a deficiency of red blood cells, hemoglobin, or both.

aneroid—operating without a fluid; when used in reference to a sphygmomanometer, measuring by a dial instead of a mercury column.

anesthesia—without sensation, with or without loss of consciousness.

anesthesiology—the study of anesthesia.

anesthetic—an agent that produces insensibility to pain or touch, either generally or locally.

aneurysm—a widening, external dilation caused by the pressure of blood on weakened arterial walls.

angina—pain and oppression radiating from the heart to the shoulder and left arm; a feeling of suffocation.

angiography—a radiological study of an artery using a radiopaque medium.

angle—the inclination of two straight lines that meet in a point.

annotate—to provide with explanatory notes.

annotating—to provide critical or explanatory notes.

annuity—a sum of money to be received yearly, either in a lump sum or by installments.

anorexia—loss of appetite; with anorexia nervosa, loss of appetite for food not explainable by disease, which may be a part of psychosis.

antagonize—to annoy; to arouse opposition.

antecubital—the inner surface of the arm at the elbow.

anteflexed—abnormal bending forward.

anterior—before or in front of.

anteverted—a forward placement.

antibody—a protein substance carried by cells to counteract the effect of an antigen.

antibody-mediated—humoral immunity; when antibodies and complement work together to destroy antigens.

anticipation—expect, forsee.

anticoagulant—a substance that prohibits the coagulation of blood.

antigen—any immunizing agent that, when introduced into the body, may produce antibodies.

antihistamine—a class of drugs used to counteract allergic reactions or cold symptoms.

antiseptic—an agent that will prevent the growth or arrest the development of microorganisms.

antitoxin—a protein that defends the body against toxins.

anuria—the absence of urine.

anus—the external opening of the anal canal.

anxiety—a condition of mental uneasiness arising from fear or apprehension.

aorta—the main trunk of the arterial system of the body.

apex—the point, tip, or summit of anything; in reference to the heart, the point of maximum impulse of the heart against the chest wall.

apical—referring to the apex.

apnea—the absence of breathing.

aponeurosis—extension of connective tissue beyond a muscle in round or flattened tendons; a means of insertion or origin of a flat muscle.

apostrophe—a punctuation mark showing the absence of a letter or letters; possession.

apothocary—one who dispenses drugs and medicines.

appearance—outward show.

appendectomy—the excision of the appendix.

appendicitis—inflammation of the appendix.

appendicular—pertaining to the limbs or things that append (attach) to other parts.

applicable—capable of being applied, suitable.

appointment—an engagement; a meeting at a particular time.

apprehension—anticipation of something feared, dread; a mental conception.

apprenticeship—a training or learning period; study under the guidance of a skilled, experienced worker.

apprise—to inform.

appropriate—correct, suitable.

aqueous humor—a watery, transparent liquid that circulates between the anterior and posterior chambers of the eye.

arachnoid—a delicate, lacelike membrane covering the central nervous system.

arbitrary—depending on will or whim, self-willed; depending on choice or discretion.

ardently—eagerly, passionately, intensely.

areola—a ringlike coloration about the nipple of the breast.

arrhythmia—without rhythm; irregularity.

arteriography—a radiological study of an artery using a radiopaque medium.

arterioles—small blood vessels connecting arteries with capillaries.

arteriosclerosis—a degeneration and hardening of the walls of arteries.

artery—a blood vessel carrying blood away from the heart, usually filled with oxygenated blood.

arthritis—inflammation of a joint.

articulate—to join together, as in a joint.

artifact—something extraneous to what is being looked for. Activity that causes interference on EKGs.

ascending—referring to that portion of the colon that ascends from the lower right quadrant to the upper right quadrant of the abdomen.

ascertain—to make certain.

ASCLS—see American Society for Clinical Laboratory Science.

asepsis—a condition free of organisms.

aseptic technique—means of performing tasks without contamination by organisms.

asphyxiation—suffocation, loss of consciousness as the result of too little oxygen and too much carbon dioxide.

aspirate—to remove by suction.

assault—physical harm; a violent attack.

assess—to determine, to appraise the condition or state.

asset—anything owned that has exchange value, all the entries on a balance sheet that show the property or resources of a person or business.

associate—to connect in thought; to join in friendship or partnership; a degree granted by a junior college at the end of a two-year course.

asthma—an allergic reaction to a substance resulting in wheezing, shortness of breath, and difficulty in breathing.

astigmatism—blurring of the vision caused by an abnormal curvature of the cornea.

asymmetry—lack of same size, shape, and position of parts or organs on opposite sides.

atelectasis—lack of air in the lungs caused by the collapse of the alveoli of the lungs.

atherosclerosis—fatty degeneration of the walls of the arteries.

atmosphere—any surrounding influence.

atrial depolarization—the excitement and contraction caused by the SA node at the beginning of the cardiac cycle.

atrioventricular—see **AV node.**

atrium—cardiac auricle; the upper chamber of the heart.

atrophy—wasting away of a muscle.

attenuated—diluted; to reduce virulence of a pathogenic organism.

attitude—state of thought or feeling.

attribute—quality or characteristic; to give credit for.

atypical—deviated from normal.

audible—loud enough to be heard.

audiometry—testing of the hearing sense.

auditory—pertaining to the sense of hearing; the external canal of the ear.

aural—the ear; temperature measurement using tympanic infrared scanner.

augmented—refers to leads 4, 5, and 6 of the standard 12-lead EKG tracing; these leads are of different voltage.

auscultate—to listen for sounds produced by the body.

authorization—the giving of authority.

autoimmune—a condition wherein the person's antibodies react against their own normal tissues.

autologous—given by oneself.

automation—behavior in an automatic or mechanical fashion.

autonomic—spontaneous; the part of the nervous system concerned with reflex control of bodily functions.

autonomous—self-governing.

autotrophs—microorganisms that feed on inorganic matter.

AV node—atrioventricular node; the beginning of the Bundle of His in the right auricle/atrium; nerve fibers responsible for the contraction of the ventricles.

axial—pertaining to the spinal column, skull, and rib cage of the skeleton.

axilla—the underarm area, armpit.

axillary—referring to the underarm area.

axon—an extension from a nerve cell.

BSA—see **body surface area.**

bacteria—unicellular microorganism concerned with the fermentation and putrefaction of matter; disease-causing agent.

balance—to bring into or keep in equilibrium; to have equal weight and power.

bankruptcy—the state of being bankrupt, being legally declared unable to pay debts.

barbiturate—a sedative or hypnotic drug, also known as a downer.

barrier—to prevent access; bar passage.

barter—to give one thing in exchange for another.

Bartholin's glands—two small mucous glands, situated one on each side of the vaginal opening at the base of the labia minora.

baseline—the initial information on which additional data is based.

basophil—a granulated white blood cell.

battery—any illegal beating of another person.

benefits—anything that promotes or enhances well-being.

benign—non-malignant; not cancerous.

benign hypertrophy—nonmalignant enlargement.

bereavement—sadness as a result of death of a loved one.

beriberi—a disease resulting from lack of vitamin B, thiamine.

biceps—the muscle of the upper arm that flexes the forearm.

biconvex—the curving out on both sides.

bicuspid—heart valve between the left atrium and left ventricle, also known as the mitral valve.

biennially—happening once in two years.

bile—a secretion of the liver; a greenish-yellow fluid with a bitter taste.

bimanual—two-handed; with both hands.

bimonthly—occurring once in two months.

binge—a spree; to overindulge, such as with alcohol or food.

binocular—pertaining to the use of both eyes; possessing two eyepieces as with a microscope.

biochemistry—a science concerned with the chemistry of plants and animals.

biohazardous—any material that has been in contact with body fluid and is potentially capable of transmitting disease.

biopsy—excision of a small piece of tissue for microscopic examination.

birthday rule—a means to identify primary responsibility in insurance coverage.

bizarre—odd, unusual, strikingly out of the ordinary.

bladder—a membranous sac or receptacle for a secretion; the gallbladder, urinary bladder.

blood pressure—the amount of force exerted by the heart on the blood as it pumps the blood through the arteries.

body mechanics—the use of appropriate body positioning when moving and lifting objects to avoid injury.

body surface area (BSA)—refers to the total surface of the human body.

bolus—a mass of masticated food ready to be swallowed.

bookkeeper—one who records the accounts and transactions of a business.

booster—a subsequent injection of immunizing substance to increase or renew immunity.

bowel—refers to intestines.

Bowman's capsule—part of the renal corpuscle; surrounds the glomerulus of the nephron.

brachial—refers to the brachial artery in the arm; the artery used in measuring blood pressure.

bradycardia—slow heart rate.

braille—printing for the blind, using a system of raised dots.

brain scan—a diagnostic test using a scanner to measure radioisotopes within the brain.

breach—violation of a law, contract, or other agreement.

brochure—a small pamphlet or booklet of information.

bronchi—the primary divisions of the trachea.

bronchiole—small terminal branches of the bronchi that lack cartilage.

bronchitis—inflammation of the mucous membranes of the bronchial tree.

bruit—an adventitious sound of venous or arterial origin heard on auscultation; usually refers to the sound produced by the mixing of arterial and venous blood at dialysis shunts.

buccal—the mouth; oral cavity.

bulbourethral gland—two small glands, one on each side of the prostate gland, terminating in the urethra by way of a duct.

bulimia—a condition characterized by alternating periods of overeating followed by forced vomiting and the use of laxatives to remove food from the body.

bundle—a number of things bound together.

bunion—a bursa with a callus formation.

bursa—a sac or pouch in connective tissue chiefly around joints.

CAT scan—see **computerized axial tomography.**

CLIA—see **Clinical Laboratory Improvement Amendments (1988).**

COPD—see **chronic obstructive pulmonary disease.**

caduceus—the wand of Hermes or Mercury; used as a symbol of the medical profession.

calculate—to compute.

calculi—commonly called stones; usually composed of mineral salts.

calibrations—a set of graduated markings to indicate values.

callus—in fractures, refers to the formation of new osseous material around the fracture site.

calorie—a unit for measuring the heat value of food.

calyces—two or more calyx.

calyx—the cuplike division of the kidney pelvis.

cancellation—to strike out by crossing with lines; marking a postage stamp or check to delete an appointment or event.

cancellous—a latticework structure, as the spongy tissue of bone.

cancer—a malignant tumor or growth; specifically the hyperplasia of cells with infiltration and destruction of tissue.

cannula—a tube or sheath enclosing a trocar (triangular bore needle); after insertion, the trocar is removed.

capillary—a microscopic blood vessel connecting arterioles and venules.

capitation—a structure of payment based on the number served.

caption—heading, title, or subtitle.

carbohydrate—an organic combination of carbon, hydrogen, and oxygen as a sugar, a starch, or cellulose.

carbon dioxide—a gas found in the air, exhaled by all animals; the chemical formula is CO_2.

carbon monoxide—a colorless, odorless, poisonous gas caused by the incomplete combustion of carbon.

carboxyhemoglobin—combined carbon monoxide and hemoglobin in red blood cells.

carbuncle—a staphylococcal infection following furunculosis, characterized by a deep abscess of several follicles with multiple draining points.

carcinoembryonic antigen—a tumor marker that can be detected in the blood when tested.

carcinogenesis—the malignant transformation of a cell.

carcinogenic—cancer causing agents.

carcinoma—a malignant tumor from epithelial tissue.

cardiac—pertaining to the heart.

cardiac sphincter—the muscle that encircles the esophagus where it enters the stomach.

cardinal signs—principal signs: temperature, pulse, respiration, and blood pressure.

cardiologist—a physician specializing in the care of patients with diseases of the heart.

cardiology—the study of the heart and its diseases.

cardiovascular—pertaining to the heart and blood vessels.

carotid—pertaining to the carotid artery.

carpal tunnel syndrome—the symptoms associated with the entrapment of the median nerve within the carpal bones and the transverse ligament at the wrist.

carpals—bones of the wrist.

carrel—a small, partitioned space.

carrier—one who carries, transports; with insurance, it's the company who provides the policy.

cartilage—a strong, tough, elastic tissue forming part of the skeletal system; precalcified bone in infants and young children.

cataract—an opacity of the lens of the eye resulting in blindness.

catarrhal—pertaining to inflammation of mucous membranes; causing severe spells of coughing with little or no expectoration.

catastrophic—of great consequence; disastrous.

categorize—to arrange by class or kind; to place like things together.

catheterize—to insert a catheter into a cavity (for example, urinary bladder to remove urine) to remove body fluid.

caudal—pertaining to any taillike structure.

caustic—capable of burning; an agent that will destroy living tissue.

cauterize—to burn with an electrical cautery or chemical substance.

cautery—an iron or caustic used to burn tissue.

cavities—a hollow space, such as within the body or organs.

cecum—the beginning of the ascending portion of the large intestine that forms a blind pouch at the junction with the small intestine.

celiac disease—dilatation of the small and large intestines.

cell-mediated—direct cellular response to antigens.

cell membrane—the structure that surrounds and encloses a cell.

central—situated at or related to a center.

centrifuge—a machine for the separation of heavier materials from lighter ones through the use of centrifugal force.

centriole—an organelle within the cell.

cerebellum—lower or back brain below the posterior portion of the cerebrum.

cerebral—pertaining to the cerebrum of the brain.

cerebrospinal—referring to the brain and spinal cord.

cerebrospinal fluid—the liquid that circulates within the meninges of the spinal cord and ventricles and meninges of the brain.

cerebrovascular accident—a stroke; hemorrhage in the brain.

cerebrum—the largest part of the brain. It is divided into two hemispheres with four lobes in each hemisphere.

certificate—a written declaration of some fact.

certificate of waiver—refers to a list of basic laboratory tests that may be performed in the physician's office by non-laboratory personnel.

certification—written declaration.

certified—holding a certificate; being certificated; guaranteed in writing.

certified ophthalmic technician—a person trained and certified in diagnostic testing procedures and limited examination of the eye.

cerumen—waxlike brown secretion found in the external auditory canal.

cervical—pertaining to the neck portion of the spinal column; also to the entrance into the uterus.

cervix—the entrance into the uterus.

cesarean—surgical removal of an infant from the uterus.

cessation—ceasing or discontinuing.

chaos—a state of complete confusion; disorder.

charting—the recording of observations, subjective and objective findings, diagnostic procedures, treatments, and other pertinent data in the patient file.

chemical—a simple or compound substance used in chemical processes.

chemotherapy—the use of chemical agents in the treatment of disease, usually associated with cancer therapy.

Cheyne-Stokes—a breathing pattern characterized by alternating periods of apnea and hyperventilation.

chiropractic—a system of healing based upon the theory that disease results from a lack of normal nerve function; treatment by scientific manipulation and specific adjustment of body structures, such as the spinal column.

chiropractor—a health care provider who uses chiropractic methods to treat patients.

chlamydia—a sexually transmitted disease caused by a bacteria that lives as an intracellular parasite.

chloroform—a liquid compound that yields a gas that dulls pain and causes unconsciousness.

cholecystectomy—surgical removal of the gallbladder.

cholelithiasis—stones in the gallbladder.

cholenergic—nerve fibers capable of secreting acetylcholine.

cholera—an acute, specific, infectious disease characterized by diarrhea, painful cramps of muscles, and a tendency to collapse.

chorionic gonadotropin—a hormone detectable in the urine of a pregnant female soon after conception.

choroid—the vascular coat of the eye between the sclera and the retina.

chromosome—structures within the cell's nucleus that store hereditary information.

chronic—continuing a long time, returning; not acute.

chronic obstructive pulmonary disease (COPD)—a syndrome characterized by chronic bronchitis, asthma, and emphysema, or any combination of these conditions, resulting in dyspnea, frequent respiratory infections, and thoracic deformities from attempting to breathe.

chronological—the arrangement of events, dates, etc., in order of occurrence.

chyme—the mixture of partially digested food and digestive secretions found in the stomach and small intestines during digestion of a meal.

cilia—hairlike projections from epithelial cells as in the bronchi.

circulatory—refers to the circulatory system. The process of blood flowing through the vessels to all the cells of the body.

circumcision—surgical removal of the foreskin of the penis.

cirrhosis—an interstitial inflammation with hardening of the tissues of an organ, especially the liver.

civil—pertaining to the rights of private individuals; legal proceedings concerning rights that are not criminal.

clarity—clearness, absence of cloudiness.

classified—arranged in a group or classification according to some system.

clause—part of a sentence with a subject and a predicate.

claustrophobia—an abnormal fear of being in enclosed or confined places.

clavicle—the collar bone, articulating with the sternum and scapula.

clinical—based on observation; in medical assisting, pertains to duties considered "back office"; not administrative in nature.

Clinical Laboratory Improvement Amendments (CLIA)—legislation dealing with the operation of a clinical laboratory.

clitoris—an erectile organ located at the anterior junction of the labia minora.

clone—an exact copy.

coagulate—to lessen the fluidity of a liquid substance; to clot or curdle.

coccyx—the tailbone; the last four bones of the spine.

cochlea—the snail-shaped portion of the inner ear.

coercion—to force or compel; to restrain or constrain by force.

coitus—sexual intercourse between a man and a woman.

colitis—inflammation of the colon.

collaborate—to work together.

collateral—subordinate, secondary; property deposited as security for a loan.

colleague—an associate at work, usually one of similar status.

colon—the large intestine.

colorimeter—an instrument used for measuring the amount of pigments and determining the amount of hemoglobin in the blood.

colostomy—incision of the colon for the purpose of making a more or less permanent opening.

colposcopy—a diagnostic examination to visualize the cervix through a colposcope.

coma—an abnormal deep stupor from which a person cannot be aroused by external stimuli.

comminuted—a crushed bone fracture with many fragments.

commiserate—to feel or express sympathy or pity for.

commonality—people in general; a body corporate or its membership.

common bile duct—a duct carrying bile from the hepatic and cystic ducts to the duodenum.

communication—the act of communicating; information given; a means of giving information.

compatible—able to be mixed or taken together without destructive changes (as in blood typing and cross-matching); matching; not opposed to.

compensate—to make amends; be equivalent to.

compensation—anything given as an equivalent or to make amends; pay.

competent—fit, able, capable.

complement—a group of about 20 inactive enzyme proteins present in the blood.

complexity—the state of being complicated.

compliance—consent; conformity to formal or official requirements.

complicated—not simple, involved; having many parts; not easy to solve.

complimentary—express appreciation; given without charge.

compose—to form by putting together, creating.

compound—not simple, composed of two or more parts; with fractures, refers to bone fragments piercing the skin externally.

comprehensive—covering all areas; inclusive.

compression—to exert force against, press.

computer—a mechanical, electric or electronic device that stores numerical or other information and provides logical answers at high speed to questions bearing on that information.

computerized—to store in a computer; to put in a form a computer can use; to bring computers into use to control an operation.

computerized axial tomography (CAT)—a series of x-ray views of the body used to construct a three-dimensional picture.

conceal—to hide, to keep secret, to withhold, as information.

conceive—to become pregnant; the uniting of the sperm and ovum.

conception—the union of the sperm of a male and the egg of a female; fertilization.

concise—condensed, short.

condenser—part of a microscope substage that regulates the amount of light directed on a specimen.

confidential—revealed in confidence; secret information.

confidentiality—to be held in confidence; a secret.

confinement—restriction within certain limits.

confirm—to verify or ratify.

confirmation—making firm or sure; convincing proof.

conflict—a clash of opinions or interests; a fight or struggle; an inner moral struggle; to come into opposition.

confront—to stand face to face with.

congestive heart failure—a complex condition of inadequate heart action with retention of tissue fluids; may be either right or left side failure, or both.

congratulations—to express pleasure; a recognition of accomplishment.

conjunction—meeting; a word that connects.

conjunctiva—a mucous membrane that lines the eyelids and covers the anterior sclera of the eyeball.

connective—that which connects or binds together; one of the five main tissues of the body.

connotation—something implied or suggested.

consciousness—awareness, full knowledge of what is in one's own mind.

consecutive—following in order, successive.

consecutively—a series of things that follow each other.

conserve—to keep from damage or loss; to maintain.

constipation—a sluggish action of the bowel; usually refers to an excessively firm, hard stool that is difficult to expel or lack of a bowel movement over a time.

constrict—to narrow; to become smaller because of contraction of a sphincter muscle.

contact dermatitis—inflammation and irritation of the skin caused by contact with an irritating substance.

contagious—catching; able to be transmitted by contact.

contaminate—to place in contact with microorganisms.

contemporary—happening or existing at the same time; a person living at the same time as another.

content—the matter dealt with in a field of study; matter contained.

context—the part of a written or spoken statement that surrounds a particular word or passage and can clarify its meaning.

contraception—against conception.

contract—to draw together, reduce in size, or shorten.

contractions—the muscle action of the uterus during labor.

contracture—permanent shortening or contraction of a muscle.

contradiction—the act of contradicting; to deny; to assert to the contrary of.

contrast—to show difference; in radiology, refers to a radiopaque medium used to outline body organs.

contributory—giving a share; helping toward a result.

controversial—open to dispute; relating to discussion of opposing views.

conventional—growing out of custom; not spontaneous.

convey—to impart, as an idea; to transfer.

convulsion—attack of involuntary muscular contractions often accompanied with unconsciousness.

cooperate—to work together.

coordination—a state of harmonious adjustment or function.

cornea—the transparent extension of the sclera that lies in front of the pupil of the eye.

coronal plane—a line drawn through the side of the body from head to toe, making front and back section.

coronary—referring to the arteries surrounding the heart muscle; also refers to a "heart attack," which involves the coronary arteries.

corpus luteum—the yellow body that develops in the ruptured graafian follicle after the ovum has been discharged.

cortex—the outer portion of the kidney.

corticosteroids—hormones used to treat inflammation.

COT—see certified ophthalmic technician.

countershock—(in cardiology) a high intensity, short duration, electric shock applied to the area of the heart, resulting in total cardiac depolarization.

courteous—polite, considerate, and respectful in manner and action.

CPT—see current procedural terminology.

cramp—a spasmodic, painful contraction of a muscle or muscles.

cranial—pertaining to the cranium or skull.

cranium—the skull; the eight bones of the head enclosing the brain; generally applied to the 28 bones of the head and face.

crenated—notched or scalloped, as the crenated condition of blood corpuscles.

cretinism—a congenital condition caused by the lack of the hormone thyroxin.

criminal—of, involving, or having the nature of a crime.

crisis—the turning point of a disease; a very critical period; an emergency situation.

criterion—a standard of criticism or judgment (plural: criteria).

critique—a critical examination of a thing or situation, to determine its nature, worth, or conformity to standards.

Crohn's disease—an inflammation of the GI tract with debilitating symptoms.

cross-match—a blood test used to assure compatibility of the donor to the recipient when transfusing blood.

crutch—a staff with a cross-piece at the top to place under the arm of a lame person.

cryosurgery—the use of a substance at subfreezing temperature to destroy and/or remove tissue.

cryptorchidism—failure of the testicles to descend into the scrotum.

CTD—see cumulative trauma disorder.

CTS—see carpal tunnel syndrome.

cultivate—to form and refine; to improve.

cummulative trauma disorder (CTD)—an injury resulting from repetitive movement of a body part.

curette—an instrument to scrape material from a cavity.

currency—any form of money.

current—happening now; of the present time; the latest information.

current procedural terminology (CPT)—a numerical listing of procedures performed in medical practice; a standardized identification of procedures.

curriculum—a course of study at a school or university.

Cushing's syndrome—a disorder resulting from the hypersecretion of glucocorticoids from the adrenal cortex.

customarily—by custom, the usual course of action under similar circumstances.

cyanosis—a bluish discoloration of the caused by lack of oxygen.

cyst—a bladder; any sac containing fluid.

cystic—pertaining to a cyst; of disease, refers to a condition with multiple cysts.

cystic fibrosis—a disease condition of fibrous tumors that have undergone cystic degeneration, accumulating fluid in the interspaces; also known as fibrocystic disease.

cystitis—inflammation of the urinary bladder.

cystoscope—an instrument for examining the interior of the urinary bladder.

cytology—the study of cell life and cell formation.

cytoplasm—cellular matter, not including the nucleus of a cell.

cytotechnologist—a laboratory specialist who prepares and examines tissue cells to study cell formation.

cytotoxic—capable of destroying cells.

DACUM—an acronym for "design a curriculum."

D & C—see **dilatation and curettage.**

DEA—see **Drug Enforcement Administration.**

data—facts from which conclusions can be inferred.

debilitated—weaken; impaired the strength of.

debit—to deduct, to charge.

débridement—to clean up or remove, as is done with damaged tissue around a wound.

decline stage—becoming less intense, subsiding; a period of time when the symptoms of disease start to disappear.

dedicated—committed to; set apart for a special use.

deductible—an amount to be paid before insurance will pay.

deductions—to deduct or subtract; remove, take away.

defamation—to slander, or to attack the reputation of an individual or group.

defecate—to pass stool or move bowels.

defibrillation—to cause fibrillation to end; restore to normal action.

dehydration—withdrawal of water from the tissues naturally or artificially.

delegation—a person or group of persons officially elected or appointed to represent another or others.

delete—to remove, erase.

delirium tremens—a psychic disorder involving hallucinations, both visual and auditory, found in habitual users of alcohol.

deltoid—the muscle of the shoulder.

demeanor—behavior; bearing.

demography—the study of population statistics concerning births, marriage, death, disease, and many other indicators.

dendrite—an extension from a nerve cell.

denial—a refusal to believe or accept; disowning.

denomination—a category or classification of currency.

denote—to indicate, to mean.

dental assistant—a health care worker employed by a dentist to perform management and clinical functions and provide chairside assistance.

dental hygienist—a licensed health care provider who is trained to x-ray and perform prophylactic treatments on teeth.

dentist—a licensed health provider who cares for the teeth, repairing and replacing as needed.

deoxyribonucleic acid—DNA; material within the chromosome that carries the genetic information.

dependable—that which may be relied upon.

depict—to represent by a picture; portray.

depleted—consumed, emptied, exhausted.

deposit—to entrust money to a bank or other institution.

deposition—testimony given under oath.

depressant—a drug that causes a slowing down of bodily function or nerve activity.

depressed—a state of depression, a period of low spirits; referring to a fracture, usually a fracture of the skull where bone fragments are driven (depressed) inward.

deprivation—to be deprived; without; having to do without or unable to use.

dermatitis—an inflammation of the skin, often the result of an irritant.

dermatologist—a physician who specializes in the diseases and disorders of the skin.

dermatology—the study of the skin and its diseases.

dermis—true skin.

descending—refers to the portion of the large intestine from the splenic flexure to the sigmoid.

description—a word picture.

desensitization—the process of making an individual less susceptible to allergens.

design—working plan; layout; sketch.

designate—to point out; indicate; appoint.

detection—find out or discover.

detrimental—harmful, injurious.

devastate—to lay waste, plunder, destroy.

dextrose—a simple sugar, also known as glucose.

diabetes mellitus—a metabolic disease caused by the body's inability to use carbohydrates.

diabetic—one afflicted with the condition diabetes.

diagnostic—referring to measures that assist in the recognition of diseases and disorders of the body.

dialysis—removal of the products of urine from the blood by passage of the solutes through a membrane.

diaphanography—a type of transillumination used to examine the breast, using selected wavelengths of light and special imaging equipment.

diaphoresis—profuse sweating.

diaphragm—the muscle of breathing that separates the thorax from the abdomen.

diarrhea—frequent bowel movements, usually liquid or semisolid.

diarthroses—a movable joint; another word for synovial.

diastole—the relaxation phase of the heartbeat; the period of least pressure.

dictation—spoken words; recorded voice communication.

dietician—one who is trained in dietetics, which includes nutrition, and in charge of the diet of an institution.

differential—refers to determining the number of each type of leukocyte in a cubic millimeter of blood.

diffuse—to scatter or spread.

diffusion—a process whereby gas, liquid, or solid molecules distribute themselves evenly through a medium.

digestion—the process by which food is broken down, mechanically and chemically, in the gastrointestinal tract and converted into absorbable forms.

digestive—pertaining to digestion.

digital—pertaining to or resembling a finger or toe, as an examination using a finger or fingers.

dilatation and curettage (D & C)—dilation of the cervix and scraping of the interior lining of the uterus.

dilate—to enlarge, expand in size; to increase the size of an opening.

dimpling—a condition characterized by indentations in the skin.

diphtheria—an acute infectious disease characterized by the formation of a false membrane on any mucous surface, usually in the air passages, interfering with breathing.

diplomate—an advanced status of medical practice.

disability—a legal incapacity.

disaster—an occurrence inflicting widespread destruction and distress.

disciplinary—designed to correct or punish breaches of conduct.

discipline—self-control, conduct, system of rules.

disclose—to uncover, reveal.

discoid—a type of Lupus that is confined to the skin; also called cutaneous.

discreet—wisely cautious, prudent.

discrepancy—inconsistencies; variances.

discretion—the use of judgment, prudence.

disease—sickness, illness, ailment.

dislocate—the displacement of a part; usually refers to a bone temporarily out of its normal position in a joint.

dispense—to distribute; to deal out in portions.

displacement—the transfer of emotions about one person or situation to another person or situation.

disposition—the act or manner of putting in a particular order; arrange.

dissect—to cut into parts for examination; to separate.

distal—farthest from the center, from the medial line, or from the trunk.

distend—to become inflated, to stretch out.

distinctive—unmistakable, different from anything else.

distort—to misrepresent; to twist out of usual shape.

diversion—the act of diverting or turning aside.

diverticulitis—inflammation of the diverticula.

diverticulum—a sac or pouch in the walls of a canal or organ, particularly the colon.

divulge—to make public; to make known; reveal.

DNA—see deoxyribonucleic acid.

doctorate—a postgraduate degree conferred following extensive course work, an individual research project, and the writing of a dissertation; a PhD.

doctrine—the principles of any branch of knowledge; a belief held or taught.

documentary—presenting facts without inserting fictional matter.

domestic—not foreign; private.

dominant—strongest; prevailing, the prime or main.

dorsal—pertaining to the back.

dorsalis pedis—a pulse point palpable on the instep of the foot.

douche—an irrigation of the vagina.

downtime—refers to being off-line; computer failure; time when nothing is scheduled.

dribbling—uncontrolled leakage of urine from the bladder.

drill—disciplined repetitious exercises as a means of perfecting a skill or procedure.

droplet—a very small drop.

Drug Enforcement Administration (DEA)—a division of the federal government responsible for the enforcement of laws regulating the distribution and sale of drugs.

duodenum—the first segment of the small intestine.

dura mater—the outer membrane covering the brain and spinal cord.

duration—the amount of time a thing continues.

dwarfism—a condition caused by inadequate growth hormone during childhood.

dysmenorrhea—painful menstruation.

dyspnea—difficult or labored breathing.

dystrophy—progressive atrophy or weakening of a part, such as the muscles.

dysuria—painful urination; difficulty in urination.

ECG/EKG—see **electrocardiogram.**

echocardiography—ultrahigh-frequency sound waves directed toward the heart to evaluate function and structure of the organ.

echoes—reflections of sound.

ectopic—in an abnormal position; in pregnancy refers to the embryo or fetus being outside the uterus.

eczema—a non-contagious skin disease characterized by dry, red, itchy and scaly skin.

edema—a condition of body tissues containing abnormal amounts of fluid, usually intercellular; may be local or general.

effacement—the thinning out of the cervix during labor.

efficiency—the ratio of energy expended to results produced.

ejaculation—the expulsion of seminal fluid from the male urethra.

ejaculatory duct—the duct from the seminal vesicle to the urethra.

elasticity—ability to return to shape after being stretched.

electrical—charged with electricity; run by electricity.

electrocardiogram (EKG, ECG)—a graphic record of the electric currents generated by the heart; a tracing of the heart action.

electrocardiograph—a machine for obtaining a graphic recording of the electrical activity of the heart.

electrocautery—an apparatus used to cauterize tissue with heat from a current of electricity.

electrocoagulation—coagulation of tissue by means of a high-frequency electric current.

electrode—an instrument with a point or a surface that transmits current to the patient's body.

electroencephalogram—a graphic record of the electric currents generated by the brain; a tracing of brain waves.

electrolyte—a substance that, in solution, conducts an electric current.

electromagnet—a soft iron core that temporarily becomes a magnet when an electric current flows through a coil surrounding it.

electromagnetic radiation—rays produced by the collision of a beam of electrons with a metal target in an x-ray tube.

electromyography—the insertion of needles into selected skeletal muscles for the purpose of recording nerve conduction time in relation to muscle contraction.

electron—a minute particle of matter charged with the smallest known amount of negative electricity; opposite of proton.

electronic—operated by the use of electrons.

elements—substances in their simplest form; the basic building blocks of all matter.

elicit—to draw out, to derive by logical process.

eliminate—to remove, get rid of, exclude; also to pass urine from the bladder or stool from the bowel.

elite—choice, superior, select.

ellipses—a mark or series of marks used in writing or printing to indicate an omission, especially of letters or words.

emaciated—to become abnormally thin; the loss of too much weight.

emancipated minor—no longer under the care, custody, or supervision of a parent or guardian.

embolus—a circulating mass in a blood vessel; foreign material that obstructs a blood vessel.

embryo—the first 8 weeks of development after fertilization.

emergency—an unexpected occurrence or situation demanding immediate action.

emergency medical technician (EMT)—an individual trained to respond in emergency situations and provide appropriate initial medical treatment.

emesis—to vomit.

emetic—medication that induces vomiting.

empathy—sympathetically trying to identify one's feelings with those of another.

emphysema—a chronic lung disease characterized by overdistention of the alveolar sacs and inability to exchange oxygen and carbon dioxide.

empyema—exudate (pus) within the pleural space of the chest cavity.

enact—to make into law.

encompass—to surround, enclose.

encounter—to meet, unexpectedly or by chance.

endocardium—the serous membrane lining of the heart.

endocervical—the lining of the canal of the cervix.

endocrine—a gland that secretes directly into the blood stream.

endocrinologist—a physician specializing in the diseases and disorders of the endocrine system.

endocrinology—the study of the endocrine or ductless glands of internal secretion.

endocytosis—a cellular process to bring large molecules of material into the cytoplasm of the cell.

endometrium—the mucous membrane lining of the uterus.

endoplasmic reticulum—an organelle within the cytoplasm of a cell.

endorse—to approve, recommend, or sponsor.

endorsement—the act of endorsing; approving.

endoscope—an instrument consisting of a tube and optical system for observing the inside of an organ or cavity.

enema—the instillation of fluid into the rectum and colon.

engorge—to fill with blood to the point of congestion; to devour or engulf.

enhance—to intensify, improve.

enthusiasm—intense interest; zeal; passion.

entity—a thing having reality.

enucleation—surgical excision of the eyeball.

enumerate—to count separately, name one by one.

enunciate—to speak or pronounce clearly.

envelope—to enclose completely with a cover; a paper container for a letter.

environment—surroundings.

enzyme—a complex chemical substance produced by the body, found primarily in the digestive juices, that acts upon food substances to break them down for absorption.

eosinophil—a white blood cell or cellular structure that stains readily with the acid stain eosin; specifically an eosinophilic leukocyte.

epidemic—affecting many persons at one time.

epidermis—the outer layer of the skin; literally *over the true skin*.

epididymis—a convoluted tube resting on the surface of the testicle that carries sperm from the testicle to the vas deferens.

epigastric—pertaining to the area of the abdomen over the stomach.

epiglottis—a cartilagenous lid that closes over the larynx when swallowing.

epilepsy—a chronic disease of the nervous system characterized by convulsions and often unconsciousness.

epinephrine—a hormone produced by the adrenal medulla.

epiphysis—a portion of bone not yet ossified; the cartilagenous ends of the long bones that allow for growth.

episiotomy—an incision in the perineum to avoid tearing during childbirth.

epistaxis—nosebleed; hemorrhage from the nose.

epithelial—pertaining to a type of cell or tissue that forms the skin and mucous membranes of the body.

equity—the value of property beyond the total amount owed on it.

equivalent—equal to in value, size, or effect.

erectile—refers to tissue that is capable of erection, usually caused by vasocongestion.

ergonomics—the applied science of being concerned with the nature and characteristics of people as they relate to design and activities with the intention of producing more effective results and greater safety.

erythema—diffuse redness over the skin because of capillary congestion and dilation of the superficial capillaries.

erythrocyte—a red blood cell (RBC).

erythropoiesis—the formation of red blood corpuscles.

eschar—slough, especially after following a cauterization.

esophagus—a collapsible tube from the pharynx to the stomach through that passes the food and water the body ingests.

essential—necessary; when referring to blood pressure, indicates an elevation without apparent cause.

estrogen—a female hormone produced by the ovaries.

ether—a colorless liquid used to produce unconsciousness and insensibility to pain.

ethical—right, according to the principles of ethics.

ethics—standards of conduct and moral judgement.

etiology—the study of the cause of disease.

etiquette—conventional rules for correct behavior.

euphoria—a feeling of well-being, elation.

eustachian tube—refers to the tube of the middle ear that connects to the pharynx.

evacuate—to empty, especially the bowels.

evacuation—withdrawal, to remove, to make empty.

evaluation—assessment; judgment concerning the worth, quality, significance, or value of a situation, person, or product.

evoke—to call forth or up; summon; elicit.

excretion—the process of expelling material from the body.

exemplify—to show by example.

exempt—excluded; not liable; freedom from duty or service; privileged.

exemption—freed from or not liable for something to which others are subject.

exfoliate—to scale off dead tissue.

exhale—to breathe out.

exocrine—a gland that secretes substances through a duct into the body.

exocytosis—a cellular process that moves materials within the cell to the outside.

exogenous—originating outside an organ or part.

exophthalmia—abnormal protrusion of the eyeball.

exorcism—the act of expelling an evil spirit.

expectorate—to spit, to expel mucus or phlegm from the throat or lungs.

expedient—suitable means for achieving or attaining a purpose or end; of immediate advantage, convenient.

expedite—to hasten.

expend—to spend or use, as with money or energy.

expertise—special knowledge or skill.

expiration—the expulsion of air from the lungs in breathing.

explicit—clearly and definitely expressed; unambiguous; leaving no room for questions.

express—to utter; to make known in words or by action.

expressed—said in words or by action.

extensive—having a wide range.

extensor—the muscle of a muscle team that extends a part, allowing the joint to straighten.

externship—a supervised employment experience in a qualified health care facility as part of the educational curriculum.

extinguish—to put out; put an end to.

extinguisher—a device for putting out fire.

extracellular—outside the cell.

extract—a substance distilled or drawn out of another substance.

extremity—refers to the terminal parts of the body—the arms, legs.

exudate—pus; the collection of purulent material in a cavity.

eyewash—a device using water to remove foreign material from the eyes, usually in emergency situations.

facility—a building; in medical situations, a building for the care and treatment of patients.

facsimile—an exact copy.

facultative—able to live under conditions of temperature or oxygen supply that vary; having the capability to adapt to more than one condition, as a facultative anerobe.

fallopian tube—the ovaduct; the passageway for the ova from the ovary to the uterus.

family practice—one which cares for patients of all ages and all conditions not requiring specialization.

fascia—a fibrous membrane covering, supporting, and separating muscles; may also unite the skin with underlying tissue.

fasting—to abstain from food; without food or water.

fatal—causing death.

feasible—possible; practicable.

febrile—pertaining to a fever.

fecal—pertaining to feces.

feces—stool, bowel movement.

fee schedule—listing of allowable charge.

femoral—pertaining to the artery that lies adjacent to the femur.

femur—the thigh bone of the leg.

fenestrated—having a window or opening.

fertilization—impregnation of the ovum by the sperm; conception.

fetal—pertaining to a fetus, pregnancy beyond the third month.

fetal monitor—a device to access fetal heart beat.

fetus—an embryo after eight weeks of gestation.

fibrillation—the quivering of muscle fibers; ineffective, rapid but weak heart action.

fibroid—a tumor made up of fibrous and muscular tissue.

fibrosis—abnormal formation of fibrous tissue.

fibula—a long bone in the leg from the knee to the ankle.

filtration—the movement of solutes and water across a semipermeable membrane as a result of a force, such as gravity or blood pressure.

fiscal—of or pertaining to finances in general.

fissure—an ulcer, split, crack, or tear in the tissue.

fistula—an abnormal tubelike passage from a normal cavity or an abscess to a free surface.

flatulence—the existence of flatus or intestinal gas.

flatus—intestinal gas.

flexed—bent, as at a joint.

flexibility—easily bent, compliant, yielding to persuasion.

flexor—the muscle of a muscle team that bends a part.

flextime—refers to the practice of permitting work hours within a range of time.

flora—plant life as distinguished from animal life; plant life occurring or adapted for living in a specific environment, as flora in the intestines.

flu—an abbreviation for the word influenza; a respiratory or intestinal infection.

fluoroscope—a device consisting of a fluorescent screen in conjunction with an x-ray tube to make visible shadows of objects interposed between the screen and the tube.

flush—sudden reddish coloration of the skin.

follicle—a small excretory duct or sac or tubular gland; a hair follicle.

folliculitis—a staphylococcal infection of a hair follicle.

foreign—anything that is not normally found in the location; usually refers to dirt, splinters, etc.

foreskin—loose skin covering the end of the penis.

forge—to imitate, especially to counterfeit, as a signature.

formaldehyde—a colorless, pungent gas used in its liquid form to harden tissue for pathological study, or as a germicide, disinfectant, or preservative, according to the strength of the solution.

formalin—wood alcohol containing 40% formaldehyde.

fortitude—courageous endurance.

fovea centralis—a depression in the posterior surface of the retina that is the place of sharpest vision.

fracture—the sudden breaking of a bone.

fraudulent—characterized by cheating and deceit; obtained by dishonest means.

frequency—the need to void urine often, though usually only a small amount at one time.

friction—resistance of one surface to the motion of another surface rubbing over it.

fringe benefits—benefits included in or added to the salary paid, such as health insurance, retirement fund, etc.

frontal—anterior; the forehead bone; refers to the plane drawn through the side of the body from the head to the foot.

functional—practical, working, useful.

fungus—a vegetable, cellular organism that subsists on organic matter, such as bacteria or mold; a disease condition that causes growth of fungal lesions on the surface of the skin.

furuncle—the medical term for a boil.

GYN—see **gynecology.**

gait—manner of walking.

gallbladder—a small sac suspended beneath the liver that concentrates and stores bile.

galley proof—printed matter in preliminary form, to be corrected.

galvanometer—an instrument that measures current by electromagnetic action.

gamete—a germ cell; any reproductive body.

ganglion—a mass of nerve tissue that receives and sends out nerve impulses.

gangrene—a form of necrosis; the putrefaction of soft tissue.

gastric—pertaining to the stomach.

gastrocnemius—the large muscle in the calf of the leg.

gastroenterologist—a physician specializing in the care of patients with diseases and disorders of the gastrointestinal tract.

gastroenterology—the study of the stomach and intestines and their diseases.

gastrointestinal (GI)—pertaining to the stomach and intestines.

gastroscopy—examination of the stomach with a gastroscope.

gauge—the size of a needle bore; the smaller the number the larger the needle bore.

gene—a substance within the chromosome that dictates heredity.

generate—to produce, as heat, ideas, power.

generic—general; characteristic of a genus or group.

genetic—pertaining to the genes.

genital herpes—fluid-filled lesions on the external genitalia, which are contagious upon direct contact.

genitalia—the external sexual organs.

genucubital—pertaining to the elbows and knees; the knee-elbow position.

genupectoral—pertaining to the knees and chest; the knee-chest position.

geriatrics—the study and treatment of the diseases of old age.

gerontologist—a physician specializing in the care of the aged.

gestation—period of intrauterine fetal development.

gigantism—a condition resulting from the overproduction of growth hormone during childhood.

glance—a quick look or view.

glaucoma—a disease of the eye characterized by increased intraocular pressure.

glomerulonephritis—inflammation of the glomerulus of the nephron of the kidney.

glomerulus—the microscopic cluster of capillaries within the Bowman's capsule of the nephron.

glucohemoglobin—sugar in the blood.

glucose—a colorless or yellow, thick, syrupy liquid obtained by the incomplete hydrolysis of starch; a simple sugar.

gluteus maximus—the large muscle of the buttocks.

glycosuria—sugar in the urine.

goiter—an enlargement of the thyroid gland.

golgi apparatus—an organelle within the cytoplasm of a cell.

gonadotrophic—related to stimulation of the gonads.

gonads—the sex glands, the ovaries in the female and the testicles in the male.

gonorrhea—a venereal disease of the reproductive organs, which is highly contagious upon direct contact.

graafian follicle—the vesicle in which ova are matured and which releases them when ripened.

graft—a constructed part.

gram-negative—bacteria that take on a pink color with Gram staining process.

gram-positive—bacteria that take on a purple color with Gram staining process.

greenstick—an incomplete fracture, occurring in children.

grillwork—a bar-like device, usually constructed of heavy metal; an open grating for a door or window.

groin—the depression between the thigh and the trunk of the body; the inguinal region.

gross—exclusive of deductions; total; entire.

gross anatomy—refers to the study of those features that can be observed with the naked eye by inspection and dissection.

guaiac—a solution used to test for the presence of occult blood in the stool.

guarantee—assurance that something will be done as specified; a pledge.

guarantor—a person who makes or gives a guarantee or pledge, often to pay another's debt or obligation in the event of default.

guilds—associations of persons engaged in the same trade or calling for mutual protection.

gynecologist—a physician specializing in the care of diseases and disorders of women, particularly the genital organs.

gynecology (GYN)—the study of diseases of the female, particularly of the organs of reproduction.

HCFA—Health Care Financing Administration.

HHS—Health and Human Services.

HIB/hib—hemophilus influenzae type B.

haemophilus—bacterial strains that grow best in hemoglobin.

hallucinogen—a substance that causes hallucinations.

hamstring—a group of muscles of the posterior thigh.

handicap—to hinder; with (people) those who are physically disabled or mentally retarded.

harassment—continual annoyance; persecution.

hard copy—information printed on a solid surface, such as paper, instead of displayed on a CRT screen or stored on a disk.

harmonious—having parts combined in a proportionate, orderly, or pleasing arrangement; being peaceable or friendly.

hazardous—dangerous; risky.

health—a state of complete physical and mental or social well-being.

heart block—a condition in which impulses from the SA node fail to carry over to the AV node, resulting in a slow heart rate and a different rate of contraction between the upper and lower heart chambers.

heartburn—a burning sensation beneath the breastbone, usually associated with indigestion.

hematocrit—an expression of the volume of red blood cells per unit of circulating blood.

hematologist—a physician specializing in the care of patients with disorders and diseases of the blood and blood-forming organs.

hematology—the study of the blood and its diseases.

hematoma—a tumor or swelling that contains blood.

hematuria—blood in the urine.

hemodialysis—a process whereby blood is passed through a thin membrane and exposed to a dialysate solution to remove waste products.

hemoglobin—the combination of a protein and iron pigment in the red blood cells that attracts and carries oxygen in the body.

hemolysis—dissolution; the breaking down of red blood cells.

hemophilia—hereditary condition, transmitted through sex-linked chromosomes of female carriers; affects males only, causing inability to clot blood.

hemorrhage—abnormal discharge of blood either internally or externally from venous, arterial, or capillary vessels.

hemorrhoidectomy—surgical excision of hemorrhoidal tissue.

hemorrhoids—varicose veins of the anal canal.

hemothorax—blood within the pleural space of the chest cavity.

heparin—a substance formed in the liver that inhibits the coagulation of blood.

hepatic—pertaining to the liver.

hepatitis—inflammation of the liver.

hernia—a projection of a part from its normal location.

herniorrhaphy—the surgical repair of a hernia.

herpes simplex—the medical term for fever blister, an acute viral infection of the face, mouth or nose.

herpes zoster—the medical term for shingles, an acute viral infection of the dorsal root ganglia.

hesitancy—difficulty in starting a urine stream.

heterosexual—sexual attraction toward the opposite sex.

heterotrophs—microorganisms that feed on organic matter.

hiatus—pertains to a herniation of the stomach through an opening or hiatus.

hiccough—(also hiccup) a result of the spasmodic closing of the epiglottis and spasm of the diaphragm.

hilum—the recessed area of the kidney where the ureter and blood vessels enter.

hinge—a type of joint.

Hippocratic—refers to the oath taken by a doctor bonding him to observe the code of medical ethics contained in the oath by Hippocrates in the 4th century.

histamine—a substance normally present in the body.

histologist—(histotechnologist) a person engaged in the study of the microscopic structure of tissue.

histoplasmosis—a fungal infection caused by an organism found in bird and bat droppings.

holistic—considering the whole or entire scope of a situation.

Holter monitor—a device that attaches electrodes to a patient's chest for the purpose of obtaining a 24-hour EKG tracing in an accessory tape recorder.

homeostasis—maintenance of a constant or static condition of internal environment.

homosexual—sexual attraction toward the same sex as oneself.

honesty—the state of being truthful, trustworthy; genuine.

horizontal—not vertical; flat and even; level; parallel to the plane of the horizon.

hormone—a chemical substance secreted by an organ or gland.

hostility—unfriendliness, enmity.

hpf—high-power field; refers to microscope lens.

humble—modest, unassuming.

humerus—the long bone of the upper arm.

humoral—antibody-mediated immunity.

hyaline membrane disease—a condition resulting from incomplete development of the respiratory system in premature infants.

hydrocele—the accumulation of fluid in the scrotum.

hydrochloric acid—a digestive juice found in the stomach.

hygiene—the study of health and observance of health rules.

hygienist—one who provides health related services, such as dental procedures.

hymen—a membranous fold partially or completely covering the vaginal opening.

hyperglycemia—increase of blood sugar, as in diabetes.

hyperopia—a defect of vision so that objects can only be seen when they are far away; farsightedness.

hypersensitive—over sensitive; abnormally sensitive to a stimulus of any kind.

hypertension—elevated blood pressure.

hyperthermia—higher than normal temperature.

hyperthyroidism—a condition caused by excessive secretion of the thyroid glands.

hypertonic—having a higher concentration of salt than found in a red blood cell.

hyperventilation—excessive deep and frequent breathing.

hypoallergenic—unlikely to cause an allergic reaction.

hypochondriac—pertaining to the upper outer regions of the abdomen below the thorax; also someone with a morbid fear of disease, resulting in abnormal concern about one's health.

hypogastric—referring to an abdominal area in the middle lower third of the abdomen.

hypoglycemia—deficiency of sugar in the blood.

hypotension—abnormally low blood pressure.

hypothalamus—a structure of the brain between the cerebrum and the midbrain; lies below the thalamus.

hypothermia—below normal body temperature.

hypothyroidism—a condition caused by a marked deficiency of thyroid secretion.

hypotonic—having a lower concentration of salt than found in a red blood cell.

hypoxia—a lack of oxygen.

hysterectomy—surgical removal of the uterus.

hysteroscopy—a procedure using the hysteroscope to view the endometrium of the uterus.

ICD—see International Classification of Diseases.

I & D—see **incision and drainage.**

IVP—see **intravenous pyelography.**

identification—anything by which a person or thing can be identified.

idiopathic—disease without recognizable cause.

ileocecal—the valve between the end of the small intestine and the cecum.

ileostomy—a surgical opening from the ileum onto the abdominal wall.

ileum—the last section of the small intestine.

iliac—the edge or crest of the pelvic bone.

ilium—the hip bone.

illegible—impossible to read.

illicit—improper; unlawful; not sanctioned by custom or law; illegal.

illuminate—to enlighten, throw light on.

imaging—a representation or visual impression produced by a lens, mirror, etc.

immobilize—to keep out of action or circulation; stationary.

immune—protected or exempt from a disease.

immunization—becoming immune or the process of rendering a patient immune.

immunodeficiency—lacking the components necessary to mount an immune response.

immunoglobulin—a large protein molecule which assists in the immune response.

immunological—pertaining to immunology.

immunosuppressed—a condition wherein the immune system has been overpowered and cannot function adequately.

impacted—refers to a fracture where the broken ends are jammed together.

impaction—a collection of hardened feces in the rectum that cannot be expelled.

impending—to be at hand or about to happen.

implant—something implanted into tissue; a graft; artificial part.

implement—a tool or instrument for doing something; to put into effect.

implementation—put into effect.

implication—involvement, bringing into connection.

implied—hinted, suggested.

impotence—inability of a male to obtain or maintain an erection.

impulse—a charge transmitted through certain tissues, especially nerve fibers and muscles, resulting in physiological activity.

inappropriate—not appropriate, out of place.

incinerate—to burn, set afire.

incision—cut.

incision and drainage (I & D)—cutting into for the purpose of providing an exit for material, usually a collection of pus.

inclined—leaning or tending toward.

incompetent—not capable; not legally qualified; deficient.

incomprehensible—beyond belief, not to be grasped by the mind.

incongruous—lacking harmony or agreement.

incontinent—unable to control the bladder or bowel.

increments—becoming greater; amount of increase; gain.

incubation—the interval between exposure to infection and the appearance of the first symptom.

incus—the anvil, the middle bone of the three in the middle ear.

indemnity—to compensate for damage done or loss caused.

indigent—needy, poor, destitute.

indigestion—difficulty in digesting food.

inevitable—unavoidable, destined to occur.

infarct—infiltration of foreign particles; material in a vessel causing coagulation and interference with circulation.

infectious—capable of producing infection; denoting a disease in the body caused by the presence of germs; tending to spread to others.

inferior—below, under.

infertility—inability to achieve conception.

infirmity—illness, disease.

inflict—to strike, to cause punishment.

influenza—an acute illness characterized by fever, pain, coughing, and general upper respiratory symptoms.

infrared—pertaining to those invisible rays just beyond the red end of the visible spectrum that have a penetrating heating effect.

infusion—to instill; introduction of a substance into a vein.

ingest—to eat.

inguinal—referring to the region where the thigh joins the trunk of the body; the groin.

inguinal canal—a passageway in the groin for the spermatic cord in the male.

inguinal hernia—the presence of small intestine in the inguinal canal.

inhale—to breathe in.

initial—the first; beginning; the first letter of each of a person's names.

initiate—to get something started, begin.

initiative—the action of taking the first step; ability to originate new ideas.

innate—inborn; inherent.

inoculating loop—a laboratory instrument used to transfer organisms from one source to another.

inorganic—not living; occurring in nature independently of living things.

inseminate—to impregnate with semen.

insertion—the place where a muscle is attached to the bone that it moves.

insidious—hidden, not apparent.

insignificant—unimportant; petty; of little or no value.

insomnia—abnormal inability to sleep.

inspect—to examine closely.

inspection—the first part of a physical examination; close observation.

inspiration—to breathe in, inhale.

institute—to originate as a custom.

insufficient—not as much as needed.

insulin—a hormone secreted by the Islets of Langerhans in the pancreas.

insurance—a contract to guarantee compensation for a specified situation.

intact—unbroken, undamaged.

intangible—that which cannot be touched, easily defined or grasped.

integrity—soundness of character; honesty in particular.

integumentary—the skin; a covering.

intellectualization—to employ reasoning to avoid confrontations or stressful situations.

intelligence—the ability to learn or understand.

interaction—to act upon one another.

intercede—to mediate, plead on behalf of another.

intercostal—between the ribs.

interference—confusion of desired signals caused by undesired signals, as in artifacts on an EKG.

interferon—a lymphokine that helps regulate the activities of macrophages and NK cells.

interjection—a part of speech; an exclamation.

interleukin—a substance that is a messenger between leukocytes.

intermediate—in the middle.

intermittent—stopping and starting again at intervals.

intermuscular—within the muscle.

Internal Revenue—the division of federal government charged with implementing tax laws and collecting taxes.

International Classification of Diseases—ICD; a comprehensive listing of diseases and disorders of the human body.

interneurons—neurons connecting sensory to motor neurons.

internist—a physician specializing in the care of patients with internal diseases.

internship—a time following graduation wherein practice of the profession is performed.

interpersonal—between persons.

interpret—to explain, translate; to determine the meaning.

interval—time between events; space.

intervention—taking action to modify, hinder, or change an effect.

intervertebral—between the vertebrae.

intestine—the alimentary canal extending from the pylorus of the stomach to the anus.

intimidate—to make afraid, to frighten.

intimidation—to make afraid; to deter with threats.

intracellular—within the cell.

intradermal—within the skin.

intraocular—within the eyeball.

intrauterine device (IUD)—an object inserted into the uterus to prevent pregnancy.

intravenous—to insert into the vein.

intravenous pyelography (IVP)—the insertion of a radiopaque material into the vein for the purpose of x-raying the kidneys and ureters.

intricate—complicated, complex, elaborately interwoven.

intubation—insertion of a tube into the larynx for entrance of air.

intuition—the immediate knowing or learning of something without the conscious use of reasoning.

inunction—the process of administering drugs through the skin.

invasive—diagnostic methods involving entry into living tissue.

inventory—an itemized list of goods in stock.

involuntary—independent of or even contrary to will or choice.

iodine—a nonmetallic element belonging to the halogen group.

iris—the colored, contractible tissue surrounding the pupil of the eye.

irrational—lacking the power to reason; senseless.

irreparable—damaged beyond possibility of repair.

ischemia—temporary and localized anemia caused by obstruction of the circulation to a part.

ischium—posterior and inferior portion of the hip bone.

Ishahara—refers to an eye test to determine color vision.

Islets of Langerhans—clusters of cells in the pancreas.

isotonic—having the same concentration of salt as found in a red blood cell.

issue—to send forth; to put into circulation.

Jaeger—a system for measuring near vision acuity.

jaundice—a yellowish discoloration of the sclera and skin due to the presence of bile pigments in the blood.

jejunum—the middle segment of the small intestine, which measures approximately 8 feet in length.

journal—a record of happenings; a diary.

journalizing—entries on the daily log.

judgment—a decision; ability to make the right decisions.

keloid—an overgrowth of new skin tissue; a scar.

keying—pressing a lever or button, as on a typewriter, that is pressed with the finger to operate the machine.

kidney—a bean-shaped organ that excretes urine and is located retroperitoneally, high in the back of the abdominal cavity.

KUB—kidneys, ureters, and bladder; refers to a radiological study.

kyphosis—a convex curvature of the spine; humpback.

L & A—light and accommodation.

labia majora—the two large folds of adipose tissue lying on each side of the vulva of the female; external genitalia.

labia minora—the two mucocutaneous folds of membrane within the labia majora.

laboratory—a room or building in which scientific tests or experiments are conducted.

laboratory technician—a health care worker who performs specialized chemical, microscopic, and bacteriologic tests of blood, tissue, and body fluids.

laceration—a cut or tear.

lacrimal—pertaining to tears; the glands and ducts that secrete and convey tears.

lamaze—a program or method of managing labor during birth.

laminectomy—the removal of a portion of the vertebral posterior arch.

lancet—a sharp, pointed instrument used to pierce the skin to obtain a capillary blood sample.

laryngeal—pertaining to the larynx.

laryngectomy—surgical removal of the larynx or voice box.

larynx—the voice box.

lateral—pertaining to the side.

latissimus dorsi—the large muscle of the back.

laxative—a substance which induces the bowels to empty.

ledger—the principal account book of a business establishment, containing the credits and debits.

legible—easy to read, readable.

Legionnaires disease—an acute bronchopneumonia.

leisure—spare or free time, away from the pressure and responsibilities of work.

lens—a part of the eye that bends or refracts images onto the retina.

lesion—an injury or wound; a circumscribed area of pathologically altered tissue.

lethal—deadly; capable of causing death.

leukemia—a disease characterized by a great excess of white blood cells; it exists in a lymphatic and myelogenous form; it is often fatal, especially in adults.

leukocyte—a white blood cell.

liability—anything to which a person is liable, responsible, legally bound.

liaison—intercommunication between two entities.

license—a legal permit to engage in an activity.

licensed practical nurse (LPN)—an individual trained in basic nursing techniques, to provide direct patient care under the supervision of an RN or physician.

ligament—fibrous tissue that connects bone to bone.

ligation—to tie off; the process of binding or tying.

limbs—refers to the arms and legs.

limited—to restrict; to hold within fixed bounds.

liter—a unit of measure; 1,000 ml or approximately 1 quart.

liver—the largest gland in the body, located in the upper right quadrant of the abdomen beneath the diaphragm.

lithotomy—an examination position wherein the patient lies upon the back with thighs flexed upon the abdomen and legs flexed upon the thighs.

lithotripsy—destruction of stone; stonecrusher.

LMP—last menstrual period.

longevity—a long duration of life; lasting a long time.

longitudinal fissure—the deep cleft between the two hemispheres of the cerebrum.

lordosis—abnormal anterior curvature of the lumbar spine.

lpf—low-power field; refers to microscope lens.

lubb dupp—sounds made by the heart.

lumbar—pertaining to the back, specifically to the five vertebrae above the sacrum.

lumbar puncture—the insertion of a needle between the vertebrae in the lumbar area for the purpose of withdrawing spinal fluid.

lumen—the space within an artery, vein, or capillary; the space within a tube.

lung—the organ of respiration, located within the thoracic cavity.

lupus erythematosus—a chronic autoimmune disease which causes changes in the immune system.

luteinizing—a hormone effect which causes ovulation and progesterone in the female and sperm production and testosterone in the male.

Lyme disease—a disease caused by a spirochete that is carried by the deer tick.

lymph—a body fluid formed within the tissue spaces and circulated throughout the body.

lymphatic system—a network of transparent vessels carrying lymph fluid throughout the body.

lymphocyte—a type of white blood cell.

lysosomes—an organelle within the cytoplasm of the cell.

MI—see **myocardial infarction.**

MRI—see **magnetic resonance imaging.**

MUGA—see **multiple-gated acquisition scan.**

macrophage—a phagocytic cell that destroys antigens.

macule—a discolored spot or patch on the skin neither elevated nor depressed.

magnetic—having the properties of a magnet, able to attract.

magnetic resonance imaging (MRI)—a diagnostic test using magnetic waves to visualize internal body structures.

magnify—to make something look larger than it really is.

mailable—a standard for judging written correspondence as satisfactory for sending.

maintenance—to preserve; the act or work of keeping something in proper condition.

malaise—a feeling of discomfort or uneasiness.

malignant—a cancerous growth; tumor.

malinger—to pretend illness to escape dealing with a situation or obligation.

malleus—the largest of the three bones of the middle ear, also called the hammer.

mammary glands—the breasts.

mammograph—an x-ray of the breast.

management—the act, manner, or practice of managing, handling, or controlling something.

mandate—an order of authorative command; instruction.

manifestation—act of disclosing; revelation; display.

manipulation therapy—any treatment or procedure involving the use of the hands; movement of a joint to determine its range of extension and flexion; additional manual skills used by osteopathic physicians.

marginal—close to the lower limit of acceptability.

marrow—the soft tissue in the hollow of long bones.

masses—a multitude; a large number of people.

mastectomy—surgical removal of a breast.

matrix—a format for establishing a time schedule for appointments.

maturation—refers to a stage of cellular development.

maturation index (MI)—a measurement of cellular maturity.

maturity—a state of full development.

measles—a highly contagious disease characterized by the presence of maculopustular eruptions.

mechanical—pertaining to machinery.

medial—pertaining to the middle or midline.

Medicaid—a government health care program.

Medicare—a federal health program for paying certain medical expenses of the aged.

Medigap—refers to situations not covered by Medicare insurance.

medulla—the inner section of the kidney.

medulla oblongata—enlarged portion of the spinal cord; the lower portion of the brainstem.

melanin—a pigment which gives color to the skin, hair, and eyes.

melanocyte—cells which produce the pigment of the skin, melanin.

membrane—a thin, soft, pliable layer of tissue that lines a tube or cavity or covers an organ or structure.

menarche—the first menstrual period.

Meniere's disease—a disorder of the ear characterized by nausea, vomiting, tinnitus, and hearing loss.

meninges—the membranes covering the brain and spinal cord.

meningitis—inflammation of the meninges of the brain and/or spinal cord.

meniscus—a concave level of fluid in a tube or cylinder.

menopause—the permanent cessation of menstruation.

menorrhagia—excessive menstrual flow, hemorrhage.

menstruate—to periodically discharge bloody fluid from the uterus.

mensuration—the process of measuring.

mercury—a liquid metal used in measurement devices such as thermometers and sphygmomanometers; chemical symbol, Hg.

merit—to deserve reward or praise; excellence.

mesentery—a peritoneal fold connecting the intestine to the posterior abdominal wall.

metabolism—the successive transformations to which a substance is subjected from the time it enters the body to the time it or its decomposition products are excreted, and by which nutrition is accomplished and energy and living substance are provided.

metacarpals—pertaining to the five bones of the hand between the wrist and the phalanges.

metastasis—movement of cancer cells from one part of the body to another.

metatarsals—the five bones of the feet between the instep and the phalanges.

methodical—systematic, following a plan or method.

microbial—related to microbes.

microfiche—a sheet of microfilm capable of accommodating and preserving a considerable number of book pages in reduced form.

microorganism—a microscopic living body not perceivable by the naked eye.

microscopic—visible only with a microscope.

microscopic anatomy—an area of study that deals with features that can be seen only with a microscope.

micturation—the passing of urine.

midbrain—that portion of the brain connecting the pons and the cerebellum.

midline—the middle.

migraine—a severe headache with characteristic symptoms.

minute—a measurement of time equal to 60 seconds; very small, tiny.

misalignment—out of alignment; not straight.

misspelled—to spell incorrectly.

mitochondria—an organelle within the cytoplasm of the cell.

mitosis—the division of a cell.

mitral—the valve in the heart between the chambers of the left side, also known as the bicuspid.

mobility—quality of being mobile; easy to move.

modifier—changes; limits the meaning.

modifies—changes the form or quality of; alters slightly.

molten—melted.

monilia—a family of parasitic fungi or molds.

monitor—to oversee or observe.

monoclonal—a laboratory-produced hybrid cell that produces antibodies.

monocular—possessing a single eyepiece as with a microscope.

monocyte—single nucleated cells that leave the blood and enter into tissues to become macrophages.

monotone—a single, unvaried tone; having the same pitch; a tiresome sameness.

mons pubis—a pad of fatty tissue and coarse skin overlying the symphysis pubis in the female.

morality—right living; virtue.

mores—folkways that, through general observance, develop the force of a law.

morphology—a branch of biology dealing with the form and structure of organisms.

motor—refers to the nerves that permit the body to respond to stimuli.

mouth—the oral cavity; can also refer to the opening to organs.

mucosa—pertaining to mucous membrane.

multi-channel—refers to the capability of ECG equipment of processing impulses from multiple leads.

multi-skilled—having more than one skill area for employment.

multiple-gated acquisition scan (MUGA)—a diagnostic test to evaluate the condition of the myocardium of the heart.

mumps—an acute contagious disease characterized by inflammation of the parotid gland and other salivary glands.

murmur—a soft blowing or rasping sound heard on auscultation of the heart.

muscle—a type of tissue composed of contractile cells or fibers that effect movement of the body.

muscle team—a pair of skeletal muscles, one that flexes and one that extends the joint.

muscle tone—a state of muscle contraction in which a portion of the fibers are contracted while others are at rest.

muscular—pertaining to muscles.

musculoskeletal—pertaining to the muscular and skeletal systems.

mutation—a change in an inheritable characteristic; cellular change caused by an influence.

myelin—a fatlike substance forming the principal component of the myelin sheath of nerve fibers.

myelography—an x-ray examination of the spinal cord following an injection of a radiopaque material.

myocardial infarction (MI)—blockage of a coronary artery that interrupts the flow of blood to the heart muscle.

myocardium—the muscle layer of the heart.

myometrium—the muscular structure of the uterus.

myopia—a defect in vision so that objects can only be seen when very near; nearsightedness.

myxedema—a condition resulting from the hypofunction of the thyroid gland.

narcolepsy—overwhelming attacks of sleep that the victim cannot inhibit; sleeping sickness.

narcotic—a drug capable of producing sleep and relieving pain or inducing unconsciousness and even death, depending upon the dosage.

nasal—pertaining to the nose.

nausea—an inclination to vomit.

negate—to deny the existence or truth of.

negligent—guilty of neglect; lacking in due care or concern; act of carelessness.

negotiable—capable of being discussed and terms arranged.

neoadjuvant—new attachment process; giving chemotherapy prior to surgery to shrink the tumor before removal.

neonate—a newborn infant.

neoplastic—new abnormal tissue formation; cancer related.

nephrologist—a physician specializing in the diseases and disorders of the kidney.

nephrology—the study of the kidney and its diseases.

nephron—the structural and functional unit of the kidney.

nephrotic syndrome—term applied to renal disease of whatever cause characterized by massive edema, proteinuria, and usually elevation of serum cholesterol and lipids.

nerve—a group of nervous tissues bound together for the purpose of conducting nervous impulses.

nervosa—loss of appetite for food not connected with a disease; part of a psychosis.

net—remaining after all deductions have been made; to clear as profit.

neurilemma—a thin membranous sheath enveloping a nerve fiber.

neurologist—a physician specializing in the diseases and disorders of the nervous system.

neurology—the study of the nervous system and its diseases.

neuron—a nerve cell.

neurosurgery—surgical procedures performed on the nervous system.

neutrophil—a granulated white blood cell.

nicotine—a poisonous alkaloid extracted from tobacco leaves.

nit—the egg of a louse or other parasitic insect.

nocturia—having to void at night.

node—a knot, knob, protuberance, or swelling.

nomenclature—a system of technical or scientific names.

nominal—too small to be considered, or a very small amount.

nomogram—representation by graphs, diagrams, or charts of the relationship between numerical variables.

nonchalant—unconcerned, indifferent.

non compos mentis—general legal term for all forms of mental illness.

non-invasive—a diagnostic method not requiring entry into body tissue.

nonpathogen—an organism that does not produce a disease.

nonspecific urethritis—inflammation of the urethra in males and vaginitis or cervicitis in females caused by bacteria or an allergy to substances used by a sexual partner.

norepinephrine—a hormone secreted by adrenal medulla in response to sympathetic stimulation.

normal saline—a solution with the same salt content as that found within a red blood cell.

nuclear—pertaining to the nucleus of an atom.

nuclear medicine—the branch of medicine that uses radionuclides in the diagnosis and treatment of disease.

nucleolus—a structure found within the nucleus of the cell.

nucleus—the vital body in the protoplasm of a cell.

numeric—denoting a number or system of numbers.

nurse practitioner—an RN with advanced clinical experience and education in a special branch of practice.

nurture—to care for, train, or educate.

nutrition—refers to edible material, food, things that nourish.

nutritionist—a member of the health care team who studies and applies the principles and science of nutrition.

OSHA—Occupational Safety and Health Administration.

OTC—see **over the counter.**

objective—the end toward which action is directed; of a disease symptom, perceptible to persons other than the one affected; on a microscope, a lens or series of lenses.

obligate—to bind legally or morally.

obliterate—to blot out; leave no trace; destroy.

observant—quick to notice, watchful.

obsolete—out of use, discarded, no longer useful.

obstetrician—a physician who specializes in the care and treatment of women during pregnancy and childbirth.

obstetrics—the branch of medicine dealing with women during pregnancy, childbirth, and postpartum.

obturator—anything that obstructs or closes a cavity or opening; refers to that internal portion of an examining instrument that facilitates the introduction of the instrument into the body and is then withdrawn, permitting visualization of the internal area.

occipital—pertaining to the back part of the head, the posterior lobe of the cerebrum.

occlude—to close up, obstruct.

occult—obscure; hidden.

occulta—obscure; hidden.

occupational medicine—diagnosing and treating disease or conditions arising from occupational circumstances.

occupational therapist—a health care worker involved in the use of purposeful activity with individuals who are limited by physical injury or illness, psychosocial dysfunction, developmental or learning diabilities, poverty and cultural differences, or the aging process to maximize independence, prevent disability, and maintain health.

occupational therapy assistant—OTA; a person trained to assist an occupational therapist.

O.D.—oculus dexter, or right eye.

office manager—(business office manager) an individual responsible for the overall operation of the medical office.

ointment—a salve; a fatty, soft substance having antiseptic or healing properties.

olfactory—pertaining to the sense of smell.

oliguria—scanty production of urine.

oncogenes—a gene in a tumor cell.

oncology—the branch of medicine dealing with tumors, usually malignant.

ophthalmologist—a physician specializing in the diseases and disorders of the eye.

ophthalmology—the study of the eye and its diseases.

opportunistic—seizing the opportunity; taking advantage of the situation.

opposition—action against, resistance.

optic—pertaining to the eye or sight.

optic disc—the blind spot where the optic nerve exits from the retina of the eye.

optometrist—a person who measures the eye's refractive power and prescribes correction of visual defects when needed.

oral—pertaining to the mouth.

orbital—refers to the cavity within the skull where the eye is located.

organ—a part of the body constructed of many types of tissue to perform a function.

organ of Corti—terminal acoustic apparatus in the cochlea of the inner ear.

organelles—functional structures within the cytoplasm of a cell.

organic—pertaining to or derived from animal or vegetable forms of life.

origin—the beginning or source of anything; of muscles, the anchor.

orthopedics—the branch of medicine dealing with the structure and function of bones and muscles.

orthopedist—a physician who corrects deformities and treats diseases and disorders of the bones, joints, and spine.

orthopnea—respiratory condition in which breathing is possible only in an erect sitting or standing position.

orthostatic—standing; concerning an erect position.

O.S.—oculus sinister, or left eye; also a mouth or opening.

oscilloscope—an instrument that displays a visual representation of electric variations on the fluorescent screen of a cathode ray tube.

osmosis—the process of diffusion of water or another solvent through a selected permeable membrane.

osseous—bonelike, concerning bones.

osteopathy—any bone disease; also refers to a school of medicine based on the belief that the bony fragment of the body largely determines the structural relations of its tissues.

osteoporosis—a condition resulting from a decrease in the amount of calcium stored in the bone.

OTA—see occupational therapy assistant.

otitis—inflammation of the ear; can be referenced to the external, middle, or internal ear.

otorhinolaryngologist—a physician specializing in diseases and disorders of the ear, nose, and throat.

otorhinolaryngology—the study of the ear, nose, and larynx and their diseases.

otosclerosis—condition characterized by progressive deafness caused by the fixation of the stapes of the middle ear.

O.U.—oculus uterque, or each eye.

ovary—the female gonad, which produces hormones causing the secondary sex characteristics to develop and be maintained.

over the counter (OTC)—referring to accessible, nonprescription drugs.

overdraft—an amount beyond what is currently in the account.

ovulation—the periodic ripening and rupture of a mature graafian follicle and the discharge of the ovum.

ovum—an egg, the female gamete or reproductive cell.

oxalate—a salt of oxalic acid.

oxygen—a colorless, odorless, tasteless gas found in the air; chemical symbol, O_2.

oxygenate—combine or supply with oxygen.

PDR—*Physician's Desk Reference.*

PKU—see **phenylketonuria.**

POL—physician's office laboratory.

PS—see **postscript.**

pacemaker—the SA node of the heart; also refers to an artificial device which initiates heartbeat.

pallor—lack of color, paleness.

palpate—to feel; to examine by touch.

pancreas—an organ which secretes insulin and pancreatic digestive juice.

pancreatitis—inflammation of the pancreas.

pandemic—epidemic over a large region; epidemic in many regions.

pantomime—motions or gestures used for expressive communication.

Papanicolaou (Pap) smear—a test to detect cancer cells in the mucus of an organ.

papillae—small protuberances or elevations, such as the taste buds of the tongue.

papillary muscles—muscular attachments to the undersides of the heart valves from the walls of the ventricles, which open the valves during the relaxation phase of the heartbeat.

papule—red, elevated area on the skin.

parabasal—beside, near, an accessory to the base or lower part.

paralytic ileus—paralysis of the intestinal wall with symptoms of acute obstruction.

paramedic—health care providers who provide emergency and supportive medical care. Have additional training beyond EMT status.

parameter—quantity to which an arbitrary value may be given as a convenience in expressing performance or for use in calculations.

parasite—an organism that lives in or on another organism without rendering it any service in return.

parasympathetic—a division of the autonomic nervous system.

parathyroid—small endocrine glands located close to the thyroid gland.

parenteral—other than by mouth.

parietal—a central portion of the cerebrum located on each side of the brain.

paroxysmal—a sudden attack of a disease; fit of acute pain, passion, coughing, or laughter.

patella—the kneecap.

pathogen—any microorganism or substance capable of producing a disease.

pathological—a condition caused by a disease.

pathologist—a physician specializing in the interpretation and diagnosis of changes caused by disease in tissues and body fluids.

pathology—the study of the nature and cause of disease.

pathophysiology—the study of mechanisms by which disease occurs, the responses of the body to the disease process, and the effects of both on normal function.

patience—calm in waiting, endurance without complaint.

patient care technician—PCT; a health care worker who uses both nursing and medical assisting skills to provide patient care in a hospital setting.

payee—a person to whom money is paid.

PCT—see **patient care technician**.

pectoralis major—the principal muscle of the chest wall.

pediatrician—a physician specializing in the diseases and disorders of children.

pediatrics—the branch of medicine dealing with the care of children and their diseases.

pediculosis—the scientific name for lice.

peer—equal; usually refers to someone of similar standing or status.

pelvic—pertaining to the pelvis.

penis—the male external sex organ.

peptic—pertaining to digestion; can also refer to an ulcer of the upper digestive tract.

per capita—for each person.

perceive—to become aware of through the senses; to understand.

percentage—rate or proportion of each hundred.

percentile—any value in a series dividing the distribution of its members into 100 groups of equal frequency.

perception—awareness through the senses; the receipt of impressions; consciousness.

percussion—tapping the body lightly but sharply to determine the position, size, and consistency of an underlying structure.

perfusion—passing of a fluid through spaces; the act of pouring over or through.

pericarditis—inflammation of the pericardium, the covering of the heart.

pericardium—the membranous sac that covers the heart.

perineum—the region between the vagina and anus of the female and the scrotum and anus of the male.

periodic—occurring, appearing, or done again and again, at regular intervals.

periodical—appearing at regular intervals of time.

periosteum—the fibrous membrane covering the bone except at the articulating surfaces.

peripheral—pertaining to a portion of the nervous system; an item attached to a computer system.

peristalsis—a progressive, wavelike muscular movement that occurs involuntarily in the urinary and digestive system.

peritoneal—pertaining to the peritoneum.

peritoneum—the membrane that lines the abdominal cavity and covers the abdominal organs.

permeable—capable of being penetrated; allowing entrance.

pernicious anemia—a severe anemia characterized by progressive decrease in the production of red blood cells.

perplexing—troubling with doubt, puzzling.

persecute—treat badly; do harm to again and again; pursue to injure.

perserverance—the act of continuing steadfastly, especially in the face of discouragement.

personality—the personal or individual qualities that make one person different from another.

perspective—a view of things, or facts, in which they are in the right relations.

pertinent—having to do with what is being considered; relevant or to the point.

pertussis—an acute infectious disease characterized by a paroxysmal cough, ending in a whooping inspiration.

petechiae—small, purplish, hemorrhagic spots on the skin.

petition—a written plea in which specific court action is sought.

petty—small, having little value, mean, narrow-minded.

pH—a measure of acidity or alkalinity.

phagocyte—a white blood cell that engulfs and destroys antigens.

phagocytosis—ingestion and digestion of bacteria and particles by phagocytes.

phalanges—bones of the fingers and toes.

phalanx—any one of the bones of the fingers or toes.

phantom limb—an illusion following amputation of a limb that the limb still exists.

pharmaceutical—concerning drugs or pharmacy.

pharmacist—a licensed health care provider who prepares and dispenses drugs.

pharmacology—the study and practice of compounding and dispensing medical preparations.

pharmacy technician—PT; an assistant to a pharmacist who prepares and in some situations administers medication.

pharynx—the throat; that portion of the alimentary canal between the mouth and the esophagus.

phenylalanine—an amino acid of a protein.

phenylketonuria (PKU)—a genetic disorder resulting from the body's failure to oxidize an amino acid, perhaps because of a defective enzyme.

phimosis—a narrowing of the opening of the foreskin of the penis.

phlebitis—inflammation of a vein.

phlebotomist—a health care worker who specializes in obtaining blood samples.

photocopy—a photographic reproduction of written matter made by a special device.

photophobia—sensitive to light; avoiding light.

physical—pertaining to the body; also used for the examination of the body.

physical medicine—the branch of medicine dealing with the treatment of disorders and diseases with mechanical devices, as in physical therapy.

physical therapist—one who is licensed to assist in the examination, testing, and treatment of physically disabled or handicapped people through the use of special exercise, application of heat or cold, use of sonar, and other techniques.

physician—a medical doctor; one skilled in the practice of medicine.

physician's assistant—a person trained in certain aspects of the practice of medicine to provide assistance to the physician.

physician's office laboratory—a designated room in the physician's office where laboratory procedures and tests are performed by qualified persons.

physiology—the study of the function of the cells, tissues, and organs of the body.

pia mater—innermost of the three meninges of the brain and spinal cord.

pigment—any coloring matter.

pineal body—a small endocrine gland attached to the posterior part of the third ventricle of the brain.

pinocytosis—the process whereby a cell engulfs large amounts of liquid.

pitch—the frequency of vibrations of sound that enable one to classify sound on a scale from high to low.

pitfall—trap or hidden danger.

pituitary—a small endocrine gland attached to the base of the brain; the "master" gland.

PKU (phenylketonuria)—a genetic disorder resulting from the body's failure to oxidize an amino acid, perhaps because of a defective enzyme.

placenta—the structure through which the fetus obtains nourishment during pregnancy; the afterbirth.

plague—a deadly epidemic or pestilence.

planes—a flat or relatively smooth surface; points of reference by which positions or parts of the body are indicated.

plasma—the liquid part of the lymph and blood.

platelet—a type of cell found in the blood that is required for clotting.

pleura—a serous membrane that covers the lungs and lines the thoracic cavity.

pleurisy—inflammation of the pleura.

plexuses—a network of nerves.

plight—unfavorable situation or distressed condition.

pneumoconiosis—a respiratory condition caused by inhalation of dust particles from mining or stone cutting.

pneumoencephalography—an x-ray examination of ventricles and subarachnoid spaces of brain following withdrawal of cerebrospinal fluid and injection of air or gas via a lumbar puncture.

pneumonia—inflammation of the lung caused primarily by microbes, chemical irritants, vegetable dust, or allergy.

pneumothorax—a collection of air or gas in the pleural cavity which displaces lung tissue.

podiatrist—(chiropodist) a person trained to diagnose and treat diseases and disorders of the feet.

podiatry—the branch of medicine dealing with disorders of the feet.

POL—see **physician's office laboratory**.

polio—(poliomyelitis) an acute, infectious, systemic disease which causes inflammation of the grey matter of the spinal cord.

polling—pertains to obtaining an unauthorized FAX transmission.

polycystic disease—a condition of multiple cysts.

polycythemia—an excess of red blood cells.

polyp—a tumor with a pedicle, especially on mucous membranes, such as in the nose, rectum, or intestines.

polyuria—excessive secretion and discharge of urine.

pons—a portion of the brainstem connecting the medulla oblongata and cerebellum with upper portions of the brain.

popliteal—pertains to the area back of the knee.

portal—pertaining to the portal circulation of blood from impaired internal organs to the liver for processing before entering the inferior vena cava.

positive—strongly affirmative.

post—to transfer charges from the day sheet to patient account records.

posterior—toward the rear or back or toward the caudal end.

postmark—a dated cancellation of a stamp by the post office which also identifies the place of posting.

postoperative (post-op)—after or following a surgical procedure.

postpartum—the period following delivery of a baby.

postscript (PS)—an addition to a letter written after the writer's name has been signed.

posture—the position and carriage of the body as a whole.

potential—possible; ability to develop into actuality.

Power of Attorney—a legal document authorizing a person to act as another's attorney, legal representative, or agent.

PPMP—see provider-performed microscopy procedures.

practitioner—one who practices the profession of medicine.

preauthorization—prior approval of insurance coverage and necessity of procedure.

precancerous—a state just prior to the development of cancer.

precautions—care beforehand; a preventive measure.

precise—exact; definite; very accurate.

precision—exactness, accuracy.

precordial—pertaining to that area of the chest wall over the heart for the placement of EKG chest leads.

pregnancy—the condition of being with child.

preliminary—coming before, leading up to.

premium—the amount paid or payable (for example, an insurance policy premium).

prenatal—the period before birth.

preoperative (pre-op)—the preparatory period preceding surgery.

presbycusis—impairment of acute hearing in old age.

presbyopia—a defect of vision in advancing age involving loss of accommodation.

prescribe—to lay down as a rule or direction; to order or advise the use of.

prescription—a written direction for the preparation of a medicine.

prevention—the act of keeping something from coming to pass; to hinder.

preventive—tending to prevent or hinder. Something used to prevent disease.

primary—occurring first in time, development, or sequence; earliest.

prioritize—to arrange in order of importance.

priority—preference; state of being first in time, place or mark.

process—to treat or prepare by some method.

processor—performing a whole sequence of actions or operations.

proclivity—an inclination or predisposition toward something.

procrastination—intentionally delaying action of something that should be done; to postpone.

proctology—the study of the rectum and anus and their diseases.

proctoscope—an instrument for the inspection of the rectum.

proctoscopy—instrumental inspection of the rectum.

procure—to get or obtain.

procurement—to obtain; acquire.

productivity—the amount of work accomplished in a period of time.

professional—conforming to the technical or ethical standards of a profession.

professionalism—professional status, methods, character, or standards.

proficiency testing—PT; the measurement of acquired knowledge and skills; a means of assessing the competency of someone or of something.

proficient—well advanced in an art, occupation, skill, or branch of knowledge; unusually knowledgeable.

profit sharing—a system by which employees receive a share of the profits of a business enterprise.

progesterone—a hormone secreted by the graafian follicle following the expulsion of the ovum.

programmed—arranged; planned; a sequence of actions performed by a computer.

progress notes—record of the continuing progress and treatment of a patient.

project—to produce and send forth with clarity and distinctness.

prolapse—dropping of an internal part of the body; usually refers to uterus or rectum.

prominent—conspicuous, outstanding.

promissory—containing a pledge to pay.

prompt—to urge to action, to inspire.

prone—a position, lying horizontal with the face down.

pronoun—a word used instead of a noun, to indicate without naming.

proofread—reading of printed proofs to discover and correct errors.

proprietary—privately owned and managed and run as a profit-making organization.

proprietorship—the amount by which assets exceed liabilities.

prostaglandins—a group of chemical substances secreted by mast cells or basophils that constricts smooth muscles in some organs.

prostate—a gland of the male reproductive system that surrounds the proximal portion of the urethra.

prostatectomy—excision of part or all of the prostate gland.

prosthesis—an artificial replacement of a missing body part.

pro tem—acting as (a temporary position); for the time being.

prothrombin—chemical substance existing in circulating blood which aids in the clotting process.

protocol—a plan of treatment, usually experimental, used to determine effectiveness of new treatments or medications.

protozoan—a single-cell animal.

provider-performed microscopy procedures (PPMP)—refers to microscopic procedures done in the POL.

provisions—the act of providing; something provided for the future; a stipulation.

proximal—nearest the point of attachment.

proxy—one who has authority to vote or act for another; a certificate of authorization to vote.

prudent—careful; wise in practical affairs.

pruritus—severe itching.

pruritus ani—itching about the anus.

psoriasis—a chronic inflammatory disease characterized by scaly patches.

psychedelics—hallucinogenic drugs.

psychiatrist—a physician specializing in the diseases and disorders of the mind, including neuroses and psychoses.

psychiatry—the branch of medicine dealing with the diagnosis, treatment, and prevention of mental illness.

psychological—of the mind; mental.

psychologist—a person specializing in the study of the structure and function of the brain and related mental processes.

psychology—the study of mental processes, both normal and abnormal, and their effects upon behavior.

psychoneuroimmunology—a science studying the connection between the brain, behavior, and immunity.

psychopathic—concerning or characterized by a mental disorder.

psychosis—mental disturbance of such magnitude that there is personality disintegration and loss of contact with reality.

psychosomatic—pertaining to interrelationships between the mind or emotions and body.

psychotherapy—the treatment of disease by hypnosis, psychoanalysis, and similar means.

PT—see **pharmacy technician** or **proficiency testing**.

ptosis—a drooping or dropping of an organ or part, for example the eyelid or the kidney.

puberty—the period of life at which one becomes functionally capable of reproduction.

pubic—pertaining to the middle section of the lower third of the abdomen, also referred to as the hypogastric.

pulmonary—concerning or involving the lungs.

pulmonary edema—the presence of interstitial fluid in the lung tissue.

pulmonary embolism—a blockage in the pulmonary artery or one of its branches.

pulse—throbbing caused by the regular alternating contraction and expansion of an artery.

pulse deficit—the difference between the pulse rate measured radially and apically.

pulse pressure—difference between the systolic and diastolic measurements.

punctual—prompt; being on time.

punctuation—standardized marks in written matter to clarify meaning.

puncture—a hole made by something pointed.

pupil—the contractible opening in the center of the iris for the transmission of light.

purge—to empty; to cleanse of impurities; clear.

purkinje—network of fibers found in the cardiac muscle that carries the electrical impulses resulting in the contraction of the ventricles.

pustule—small elevation of the skin filled with lymph or pus.

pyelonephritis—inflammation of the kidney, pelvis, and nephrons.

pyloric—pertaining to the opening between the stomach and the duodenum.

pyrogen—capable of producing fever.

QNS—quantity not sufficient.

quackery—the pretense to knowledge or skill in medicine.

quad-based—refers to a cane with four "feet."

quadrant—one of four regions, as of the abdomen, divided for identification purposes.

quadriceps femoris—a large muscle on the anterior surface of the thigh which is composed of four separate muscles.

quality assurance (QA)—inclusive policies, procedures, and practices as standards for reliable laboratory results that includes documentation, calibration, and maintenance of all equipment, quality control, proficiency testing, and training.

quality control (QC)—inclusive laboratory procedures as standards to provide reliable performance of equipment, including test control samples, documentation, and analyzing statistics for diagnostic tests.

R/O—rule out.

ROM—see **range of motion.**

radial—referring to the radial artery or pulse taken in the radial artery.

radiation—the emission and diffusion of rays; a product of x-ray and radium.

radioactive—capable of emitting radiant energy.

radiograph—a record produced on a photographic plate, film, or paper by the action of x-ray or radium.

radiologic technologist—(x-ray technician) a person with specialized training in the techniques to prepare x-ray films to visualize the tissues and organs of the body.

radiologist—one who diagnoses and treats disease by the use of radiant energy.

radiology—the study of radiation and its uses.

radionuclides—a type of atom used in nuclear medicine for the diagnosis and treatment of disease.

radiopaque—impenetrable to the x-ray or other forms of radiation.

radius—a long bone of the forearm.

râles—an unusual sound heard in the bronchi on examination of respirations.

ramification—a subdivision or consequence.

random—by chance; without plan.

range of motion (ROM)—refers to the degree of movement of the body's joints and extremities.

rapport—relationship characterized by harmony and cooperation.

rational—based on reasoning, sensible.

rationalization—to explain on rational grounds, to devise plausible explanations for one's acts.

Raynaud's phenomenon—a symptom of lupus characterized by fingers that turn white or blue in the cold.

reactivity—rate of nuclear disintegration in a reactor.

reagent—a substance involved in a chemical reaction.

realm—kingdom or empire, as used in text.

reason rule—refers to the purpose or reason for doing a test or procedure, an insurance company criteria for reimbursement.

receipt—a written acknowledgement that something has been received.

reception—the fact or manner of being received; a social gathering.

receptionist—one employed to greet telephone callers, visitors, patients, or clients.

receptor—peripheral nerve ending of a sensory nerve that responds to stimuli.

recessive—tending to recede; apparently suppressed in crossbred offspring in preference for a characteristic from the other parent; an organism having one or more recessive characteristics.

recipient—one who receives.

reciprocity—mutual exchange, especially the exchange of special privilege.

reconcile—process to bring checkbook and bank statement into agreement.

rectal—referring to the rectum.

rectocele—the protrusion of the posterior vaginal wall with anterior wall of rectum through the vagina.

rectum—the lower part of the large intestine between the sigmoid and the anal canal.

recumbent—lying down.

recurrent—returning at intervals.

reduce—to restore the ends of a fractured bone to their usual relationship.

redundant—extra, not needed, repetitive.

reference—a source of information or authority.

reflex—an involuntary response to a stimulus.

reflux—a return or backward flow.

refractive—the degree to which a transparent body deflects a ray of light from a straight path.

regimen—regulation of diet, sleep, exercise, and manner of living to improve or maintain health.

register—a formal or official recording of items, names, or actions.

registered—legally certified or authenticated.

registry—a list of persons qualified in a particular area of expertise.

regulate—control or direction.

Regulations in the POL—standards set for QA and QC in the physician's office laboratory to ensure reliable diagnostic tests.

regulatory—to control according to a rule; to adjust so as to make work accurately.

rehabilitate—to put back in good condition; to restore.

reimburse—to pay back or compensate for money spent, or losses or damages incurred.

reiterate—to say or do again.

rejuvenate—to make young again; to give youthful qualities to.

reliable—dependable, can be relied upon.

reluctant—marked by unwillingness.

rely—to depend on, to trust.

remedy—anything that relieves or cures a disease.

remission—a period that is disease- and symptom-free.

remote—from a distance; far removed in time and place; indirect.

renal—pertaining to the kidney.

renal failure—loss of function of the kidneys' nephrons.

renal threshold—the concentration at which a substance in the blood normally not excreted by the kidney begins to appear in the urine.

render—to present or to deliver, as a service or statement.

renovate—restore; to make new again.

repolarization—reestablishment of a polarized state in a muscle or nerve fiber following contraction or conduction of a nerve impulse.

repression—to force painful ideas or impulses into the subconscious.

reproductive—concerning reproduction.

reputable—having a good reputation; well thought of.

res ipsa loquitur—the thing speaks for itself.

residency—physician training period in a specialty field of medicine.

residual—pertaining to that which is left as a residue.

residual barium—barium remaining in the intestinal tract following evacuation at the completion of x-ray studies.

resistance—opposition, ability to oppose.

resonance—(1) quality of the sound heard on percussion of the chest; (2) the intensification and prolongation of a sound by reflection or by vibration of a nearby object.

resource—a source of support or supply.

respectful—showing respect; honoring; treat with consideration.

respiration—the taking in of oxygen and its use in the tissues and the giving off of carbon dioxide.

respiratory—pertaining to respiration.

respiratory therapy technician—a person trained to perform procedures of treatment that maintain or improve the ventilatory function of the respiratory tract.

respite—a temporary cessation of something that is painful or tiring; to delay, postpone.

respondeat superior—let the master answer.

restricted—limited; only for a certain group.

retardation—slowing, delay, lag; slow in development, mental or physical.

retention—inability to void urine that is present in the bladder.

reticuloendothelial—pertaining to that group of cells that appear to aid in the making of new blood cells and the disintegration of old ones.

retina—the innermost layer of the eye that receives the image formed by the lens.

retinopathy—a degeneration of the retina caused by a decrease in blood supply.

retraction—a shortening; the act of drawing backward or state of being drawn back.

retroflexed—refers to the body of the uterus being bent backward.

retrograde—refers to an x-ray procedure in which a radiopaque material is instilled by catheter into the bladder, ureters, and kidneys.

retroperitoneal—behind the peritoneum; posterior to the peritoneal lining of the abdominal cavity.

retroverted—refers to the entire uterus being tilted backward.

retrovirus—one with RNA genetic material.

revalidation—the renewing or reconfirmation of credentials.

revoke—to cancel, withdraw, take back.

Rh factor—an antigenic substance in human blood similar to the A and B factors which determine blood groups; apparently present only in red blood cells.

rhinitis—inflammation of the nasal mucosa.

rhinoplasty—plastic surgery of the nose.

rhythm—a measured time or movement; regularity of occurrence.

ribosome—an organelle within the cytoplasm of the cell.

rickets—a disease of the bones primarily due to the deficiency of vitamin D.

risk—chance; hazard; chance of loss or injury; degree of probability of loss.

roentgen—refers to x-rays.

Role Delineation Study—occupational analysis study conducted by AAMA and the National Board of Medical Examination in 1997, which identifies the most up-to-date entry-level areas of competence of the medical assisting profession.

rotate—to move around; to turn on an axis.

rubella—(German measles) a mild contagious viral disease which may cause severe damage to an unborn child.

rubeola—(measles) an acute, highly contagious disease marked by a typical cutaneous eruption.

SA node—see **sinoatrial node.**

sacrilege—the crime of misappropriating what is consecrated to God or religion.

sacrum—five fused vertebrae that lie between the coccyx and the lumbar vertebrae of the spinal column.

safety—freedom from danger or loss.

sagittal—refers to a plane that is made by dividing the body down the center creating a right and left side.

saliva—a digestive secretion of the salivary glands that empties into the stomach.

salivary glands—three pairs of glands that secrete the saliva that begins the digestion of food, primarily the breakdown of starch or complex carbohydrates.

salpingectomy—surgical removal of the fallopian tube or tubes.

salpingo-oophorectomy—surgical excision of the ovary and fallopian tube.

salve—an ointment.

sarcoma—malignant tumors of the connective, muscle, or bone tissue.

sartorius—a long narrow muscle of the thigh; the longest muscle of the body.

scan—to look over quickly but thoroughly.

scapula—the shoulder blade.

schedule—to arrange a timetable; to place in a list of things to be done.

sciatica—inflammation and pain along the sciatic nerve felt at back of thigh running down the inside of the leg.

scientific—based upon or using the principles and methods of science; systematic; exact.

sclera—the white or sclerotic outer coat of the eye.

scoliosis—lateral curvature of the spine.

screening—a preliminary or indicating procedure.

script—manuscript; type designed to look like handwriting.

scrotum—the double pouch containing the testes and part of the spermatic cord.

scurvy—a disease caused by lack of fresh fruits, vegetables, and vitamin C in the diet.

sebaceous—an oily, fatty matter; glands secreting such matter.

sebum—oily secretion of the sebaceous glands of the skin.

secondary—one step removed from the first; not primary.

secretary—one employed to conduct correspondence; a person responsible for records and correspondence.

secretion—separation of certain materials from the blood by the activity of a gland.

sector—a section or division.

security—freedom from fear or anxiety.

sedentary—pertaining to sitting; inactivity.

sedimentation—formation or depositing of sediment; of blood, refers to the speed at which erythrocytes settle when an anticoagulant is added to blood.

segment—a part or section of an organ or a body.

seizures—a sudden attack of pain, disease, or certain symptoms.

self-control—control of ones emotions, desires.

semen—the mixture of secretions from the various glands and organs of the reproductive system of the male, which is expelled at orgasm.

semicircular canals—structures located in the inner ear.

semilunar—the valves of the heart located between the ventricles and the pulmonary artery and aorta.

senility—feebleness of body or mind caused by old age.

sensitivity—abnormal susceptibility to a substance.

sensorineural deafness—a loss of hearing caused by transmission failure of the nerves within the inner ear or the auditory nerve.

sensory—refers to the nerves that receive and transmit stimuli from the sense organs.

septum—a membranous wall dividing two cavities, as within the heart or the nose.

sequence—order of succession.

sequentially—arranged in sequence; in an order.

series—a group; a set of things in the same class coming one after another.

serrated—notched, toothed.

sharps—any object that can cut, prick, stab, or scrape the skin.

sheath—a covering structure of connective tissue, such as the membrane covering a muscle.

shock—a condition in which the pulse becomes rapid and weak, the blood pressure drops, and the patient is pale and clammy.

sickle cell anemia—a blood disorder in which the red blood cells are shaped like sickles.

sigmoid—an S-shaped section of the large intestine between the descending colon and the rectum.

sigmoidoscopy—an inspection of the sigmoid with an instrument.

signature—a signing of one's own name.

simple—referring to a bone fracture, one without involvement of the skin surface.

simultaneous—occurring at the same time.

sinoatrial (SA) node—the source of the nerve impulse that initiates the heartbeat; the pacemaker.

sinusitis—inflammation of the sinuses.

skeletal—pertaining to the skeleton or bony structure; also to the muscles attached to the skeleton to permit movement.

skip—a person who owes money but cannot be located.

sling—a hanging support for an injured arm.

slough—to cast off, as dead tissue.

smooth—a type of involuntary muscle tissue found in internal organs.

snap locks—metal locking devices.

Snellen chart—the chart of alphabetic letters used to evaluate distant vision.

solace—an easing of grief, to comfort.

sole—only.

solicit—to ask for.

somatic—pertaining to the body as distinguished from the mind; physical.

sonar—a device that transmits high-frequency sound waves in water and registers the vibrations reflected back from an object.

sonogram—record obtained by ultrasound.

sophisticated—not simple or natural; very refined; highly complex or developed in form, technique, etc.

sound—that which is or can be heard; free from damage, safe, secure.

spasm—an involuntary sudden movement or convulsive muscular contraction.

spastic colon—spasmodic contractions of the large intestine.

specificity—something specially suited for a given use or purpose; a remedy regarded as a certain cure for a particular disease.

specified—named particularly; mentioned in detail.

specimen—a sample; a representative piece of the whole.

sperm—the male gamete or sex cell.

spermatozoon—a sperm cell.

sphincter—a circular muscle constricting an opening.

sphygmomanometer—a device that measures blood pressure; also called manometer.

spina bifida—a disorder characterized by a defect in the spinal vertebrae with or without protrusion of the spinal cord and meninges.

spinal—pertaining to the spinal column, canal, or cord.

spinal fusion—the surgical implanting of a bone fragment between the processes of two or more spinal vertebrae to render them immobile.

spiral—having a circular fashion.

spirometer—an apparatus that measures the volume of inhaled and exhaled air.

spleen—an oval, vascular, ductless gland below the diaphragm in the upper left quadrant of the abdomen.

splinter—a thin sharp piece of wood.

spontaneous—involuntary; produced by itself; unforced.

spores—hard capsules formed by certain bacteria that allow them to resist prolonged exposure to heat.

sports medicine—the branch of medicine dealing with the care of athletes to prevent and treat sports-related injuries.

sprain—the forcible twisting of a joint with partial rupture or other injury of its attachments.

sputum—substance ejected from the mouth containing saliva and mucus; usually refers to material coughed up from the bronchi.

stabilize—to make steady; firmly fixed; constant.

standardization—process of bringing into conformity with a standard; pertaining to EKG, a mark made at the beginning of each lead to establish a standard of reference.

stapes—one of the three bones of the middle ear.

stasis ulcer—an open lesion caused by stagnant or inadequate blood supply to an area.

STAT (statim)—immediately.

stationery—writing materials, especially paper and envelopes.

stature—height.

statutory—legally enacted; deriving authority from law.

stenosis—narrowing or constriction of a passage or opening.

sterile—without any organisms.

sternocleidomastoid—a muscle of the chest arising from the sternum and inner part of clavicle.

sternum—the breastbone.

stethoscope—an instrument used in auscultation to convey to the ear the sounds produced by the body.

stimulant—a substance that temporarily increases activity.

stipulations—terms of an agreement.

stomach—a dilated, saclike, distensible portion of the alimentary canal below the esophagus and before the small intestine.

stool—bowel movement, feces.

strabismus—an eye disorder caused by imbalance of the ocular muscles.

strain—injury to muscles from tension caused by overuse or misuse.

stratagem—a trick or deception.

stress—to put pressure on; emphasize; urgency; tension, strained exertion. Topical; causing strain or injury to the skin.

striated—a type of muscle tissue marked with stripes or striae.

stricture—the narrowing of an opening, tube, or canal, such as the urethra or esophagus.

stylus—a pen; the EKG writer.

subarachnoid—the space between the pia mater and the arachnoid containing cerebrospinal fluid.

subcutaneous—beneath the skin.

subdural—beneath the dural mater; the space between the arachnoid and the dura mater.

subjective—relating to the person who is thinking, saying, or doing something; personal; of a disease symptom, felt by the individual but not perceptible to others.

sublimation—to express certain impulses, especially sexual, in constructive, socially acceptable forms.

sublingual—under the tongue.

subpoena duces tecum—court process initiated by party in litigation, compelling production of specific documents and other items, and material in relevance to facts in issue in appending judicial proceedings.

subsequent—coming after, following.

substantial—considerable, large.

suction—withdrawal by pressure; a sucking action.

sudden infant death syndrome (SIDS)—the sudden, unexplainable death of an infant.

superficial—on the surface.

superior—above or higher than.

supernatant—floating on the surface.

supine—lying horizontally on the back.

supplement—something added; an additional or extra section.

support—to hold up; to bear part of the weight of.

suppository—a medicated conical- or cylindrical-shaped material that is inserted into the rectum or vagina.

suppression—the shutdown of kidney function; the absence of urine excretion.

suppression—in psychology, it is the deliberate exclusion of an idea, desire, or feeling from consciousness.

suppressor—one that holds back or stops an action.

suprapubic—above the pubic arch.

surfactant—a fatty molecule on the respiratory membranes.

surgeon—a physician with advanced training in operative procedures.

surgery—the branch of medicine dealing with manual and operative procedures for correction of deformities and defects and repair of injuries.

surrogate—a substitute; in place of another.

susceptible—having little resistance to a disease or foreign protein.

suture—to unite parts by stitching them together.

symmetry—the state in which one part exactly corresponds to another in size, shape, and position.

sympathetic—a portion of the autonomic nervous system.

symphysis pubis—the junction of the pubic bones on the midline in front.

symptom—any perceptible change in the body or its functions that indicates disease or the phase of a disease.

synapse—the minute space between the axon of one neuron and the dendrite of another.

syncope—fainting; a transient form of unconsciousness.

syndrome—the combination of symptoms with a disease or disorder.

synergism—something stimulating the action of another so that the effect of both is greater than the sum of the individual effects.

synovial—a movable joint; also called diarthroses.

syphilis—a communicable venereal disease spread by sexual contact.

system—a group of organs working together to perform a function of the body.

systematic—by a system or plan.

systole—the contraction phase of the heart; the greatest amount of blood pressure.

tachycardia—abnormal rapidity of heart action.

tact—delicate perception of the right things to say and do without offending.

tar—a sticky, brown or black carcinogenic substance.

tarry—a stool that has the appearance of tar.

tarsals—pertaining to the seven bones of the instep of the foot.

taut—tightly drawn; tense.

technical—relating to some particular art, science, or trade; also, requiring special skill or technique.

technologist—one skilled in technology; able to apply the technical methods in a particular field of industry or art.

technology—the practice of any or all of the applied sciences that have practical value and/or industrial use.

teleconference—a meeting held over phone lines incorporating video equipment.

temperature—degree of heat of a living body; degree of hotness or coldness of a substance; usually refers to an elevation of body heat.

temporal—relating to the temporal bone on the skull.

tendon—fibrous connective tissue serving to attach muscles to bones.

tendonitis—inflammation of the tendon.

tentative—experimental, provisional, temporary.

terminal—final, end; a terminal illness, refers to a condition that cannot be reversed.

termination—ending.

testes—the male gonads of the scrotum that produce sperm.

testosterone—a male hormone secreted by the testes that causes and maintains male secondary sex characteristics.

tetanus—an acute infectious disease caused by the toxins of the bacillus tetani.

tetany—intermittent tonic spasms resulting from inadequate parathyroid hormone.

thalamus—a portion of the brain lying between the cerebrum and the midbrain.

theories—beliefs not yet tested in practice; the general principles on which a science is based.

therapeutic—having medicinal or healing properties; pertaining to results obtained from treatment.

therapist—one who practices the curative and preventive treatment of disease or an abnormal condition.

thermal—characterized by heat; heat activated.

thermography—a technique for sensing and recording on film hot and cold areas of the body by means of an infrared detector that reacts to blood flow.

thermometer—an instrument used to measure temperature.

thesaurus—a treasury of words, quotations, knowledge; a collection of words with their synonyms and antonyms.

third party—(insurance) someone other than the patient, spouse, or parent who is responsible for paying all or part of the patient's medical costs.

thoracic—pertaining to the thorax or chest.

thorax—the chest; the body cavity enclosed by the ribs and containing the heart and lungs.

thready—term used to describe a weak pulse that may feel like a thread under the skin surface.

thrombophlebitis—inflammation of a vein associated with the formation of a blood clot.

thrombosis—the formation of a blood clot or thrombus.

thymus—an unpaired organ located in the mediastinal cavity anterior to and above the heart.

thyroid—an endocrine gland located anteriorly at the base of the neck.

thyroidectomy—the surgical removal of the thyroid gland.

tibia—a long bone in the leg from the knee to the ankle.

tibialis anterior—a muscle of the leg.

tinnitus—a ringing or tinkling sound in the ear that is heard only by the person affected.

tissue—a collection of similar cells and fibers forming a structure in the body.

tolerance—the difference between the maximum and minimum; the amount of variation allowed from a standard.

tongue—the muscular organ of the mouth that assists in the production of speech, contains the taste buds, and provides the ability to swallow.

tonometer—instrument for measuring intraocular tension or pressure.

topical—pertaining to a specific area; local.

tort—any wrongful act, damage, or injury done willfully, negligently.

torticollis—stiff neck caused by spasmotic contraction of neck muscles drawing the head to one side with the chin pointing to the other; can be congenital or acquired.

total quality management (TQM)—refers to a management style that uses QA and QC to maintain quality of performance throughout the total process, not just to assure the end result is satisfactory or corrected.

tourniquet—any constrictor used on an extremity to produce pressure on an artery and control bleeding; also used to distend veins for the withdrawal of blood or the insertion of a needle to instill intravenous injections.

toxin—poisonous substance or compound of vegetable, animal, or bacterial origin.

toxoid—a toxin treated so as to destroy its toxicity, but it is still capable of inducing formation of antibodies on injection.

TQM—see total quality management.

trace—the production of a sketch by means of a stylus passing over the paper, as in electrocardiography.

trachea—a cartilaginous tube between the larynx and the main bronchus of the respiratory tree.

tracheostomy—a surgically-made opening in the trachea through which a person will breathe.

traction—the process of pulling; with fractures, traction is applied in a straight line to stretch the contracted muscles and permit realignment of the bone fragments.

trait—a feature; a distinguishing feature of character or mind.

transactions—dealings accomplished.

transcript—a copy made directly from an original record, especially an official copy of a student's educational record.

transcription—writing over from one book or medium into another; typing in full in ordinary letters.

transdermal—through the skin.

transducer—a device that transforms power from one system to another in the same or different form.

transfusion—injection of the blood of one person into the blood vessels of another.

transient ischemic attack (TIA)—temporary interruption of blood flow in the brain caused by small clots closing off blood vessels.

transillumination—inspection of a cavity or organ by passing a light through its walls.

transition—passing from one condition, place, or activity to another.

transmitted—sent from one person, thing, or place to another.

transpose—putting one in place of another, the accidental misplacing of words or letters.

transurethral—literally means through the urethra; refers to the removal of the prostate by going through the urethral wall.

transverse—lying across; the segment of large intestine that lies across the abdomen; a line drawn horizontally across the body or a structure.

trapezius—the large muscle of the back and neck.

traumatic—caused by or relating to an injury.

traumatize—to cause trauma or injury.

treadmill—an apparatus with a movable platform that permits walking or running in place.

Trendelenburg—a position with the head lower than the feet.

trephining—cutting out a circular section.

trial balance—bookkeeping strategy to confirm accuracy in debits and credits in ledger.

triangular—having three angles and three sides.

triceps—the posterior muscles of the arm that work as a team with the biceps; the triceps straighten the elbow.

trichomoniasis—infestation with parasitic protozoa; usually refers to vaginal involvement.

tricuspid—a valve in the right side of the heart, between the chambers; literally means three cusps or leaflets.

trimester—divided into three sections; the third segment or period.

trivial—of little value, insignificant.

truncated—to cut the top or end off; to lop; with insurance.

tuberculosis—an infectious disease caused by the tubercle bacillus; pulmonary tuberculosis is a specific inflammatory disease of the lungs that destroys lung tissue.

tumor—a swelling or enlargement; a neoplasm; often used to indicate a malignant growth.

turbidity—flaky or granular particles suspended in a clear liquid giving it a cloudy appearance; usually refers to cloudy urine.

tympanic membrane—the eardrum.

typhoid—an acute infectious disease acquired by ingesting contaminated food or water.

Tzanck smear—examination of tissue from the lower surface of a lesion in vesicular disease to determine the cell type.

URI—see **upper respiratory infection.**

UTI—see **urinary tract infection.**

ulcer—an open lesion on the skin or mucous membrane of the body characterized by loss of tissue and the formation of a secretion.

ulceration—suppuration of the skin or mucous membrane; an open lesion.

ulna—a long bone in the forearm from the elbow to the wrist.

ultimately—in the end, finally.

ultrasonic scanning—a process of scanning the body with sound waves to produce a picture on a screen of underlying internal structures.

umbilical—pertaining to the umbilicus or navel of the abdomen.

unemployed—the state of being without work.

unique—one of a kind, unmatched.

unit clerk—a secretarial position on the health care team of a patient care facility.

universal—relating to the universe; general or common to all.

unobtrusive—not forced upon others; not thrusted forward or pushed out.

unproductive—not productive; no accomplishment.

unstructured—without specific arrangement.

unwittingly—not knowing, unaware; unintentional.

upper respiratory infection (URI)—inflammatory process involving the nose and throat, may include the sinuses; refers to symptoms associated with the common cold.

uremia—a condition in which products normally found in the urine are found in the blood.

ureter—a tube carrying urine from the kidney to the urinary bladder.

urethra—a membranous canal for the external discharge of urine from the bladder.

urgency—the sudden need to expel urine or stool.

urinalysis—an analysis of the urine; a test performed on urine to determine its characteristics.

urinary meatus—the opening through which urine passes from the body.

urinary tract infection (UTI)—infection occurring within the kidneys, ureters, and/or urinary bladder.

urination—the act of urinating or voiding of urine.

urine—fluid secreted from the blood by the kidneys, stored in the bladder, and discharged from the body by voiding.

urology—the study of the urine and diseases of the urinogenital organs.

urticaria—an inflammatory condition characterized by the eruption of wheals that are associated with severe itching; commonly called hives.

uterus—a muscular, hollow, pear-shaped organ of the female reproductive tract in which a fertilized ovum develops into a baby.

utilization—to put to profitable use.

utilize—to use or make use of.

vaccination—inoculation with modified harmless viruses or other microorganisms to produce immunity, a preventative against diseases.

vaccine—any substance for prevention of a disease.

vagina—a musculomembranous tube that forms the passageway from the uterus to the exterior.

vaginitis—inflammation of the vagina.

vagus—the tenth cranial nerve that has both motor and sensory function, affecting the heart, stomach, and other organs.

valve—any one of various structures for temporarily closing an opening or passageway or for allowing movement of fluid in one direction only.

varices—enlarged, twisted veins.

varicose—pertaining to varices; distended, swollen veins, most commonly found in the legs.

vas deferens—the excretory duct of the testes.

vasectomy—the cutting out of a portion of the vas deferens.

vein—a blood vessel carrying blood toward the heart after receiving it from a venule.

vena cava—one of two large veins that empty into the right atrium of the heart.

venipuncture—the puncture of a vein; the insertion of a needle into a vein for the purpose of obtaining a blood sample or instilling a substance.

venous—pertaining to a vein.

ventilatory—that which ventilates, lets in fresh air.

ventral—pertaining to the anterior or front side of the body.

ventricle—one of the two lower chambers of the heart; also used in reference to cavities within the brain.

venule—a minute vein; a blood vessel that connects a capillary with a vein.

verb—the part of speech that expresses an action.

verify—to prove to be true; to support by facts.

veritable—actual, genuine.

vermiform appendix—the appendix; a small tube attached to the cecum.

verrucae—warts; small, circumscribed elevations of the skin formed by hypertrophy of the papillae.

vertebrae—the bones in the spinal column.

vertex—the top of the head, the crown.

vesicle—a small sac or bladder containing fluid; a small, blisterlike elevation on the skin containing serous fluid.

vested—settled; complete; absolute; continuous.

viable—capable of living.

vial—a small glass tube or bottle containing medication or a chemical.

video display terminal—the computer monitor.

villi—tiny projections from a surface; the villi of the small intestine that absorb nutrients during the process of digestion.

villous adenoma—a type of polyp that is invasive and malignant.

viral shedding—that time when a virus is the most active and most contagious.

virulent—full of poison; deadly; malignant.

virus—a very simple, frequently pathogenic, microorganism capable of replicating within living cells.

visceral—pertaining to viscera, the internal organs, especially the abdomen.

vital—essential; pertaining to the preservation of life (the vital signs).

vital capacity—the total volume of air exchanged from forced inspiration and forced expiration.

vitreous humor—the substance that fills the vitreous body of the eye behind the lens.

void—to pass urine from the urinary bladder; to make ineffective or invalid.

volatile—easily changed into a gas or tending to change into a vapor; usually considered potentially dangerous.

voltage—a measure of electromotive force.

volume—the amount of space occupied by an object as measured in cubic units.

voluntary—under one's control; done by one's own choice.

vomit—to expel the contents of the stomach through the mouth.

voucher—a document that serves as proof that terms of a transaction have been met.

vulnerable—liable to injury or hurt; capable of being wounded.

vulva—the female external genitalia, including the clitoris, the labia minora, and the labia majora.

waiver—to give up; forgo; waiving of a right or claim.

warrant—to justify, to give definite assurance as to the value of; to authorize.

warranted—justification for some act, belief.

wart—see **verrucae.**

watermark—a mark imprinted on paper that is visible when it is held to the light, usually a sign of quality.

wheals—more or less round and evanescent elevations of the skin, white in center with a pale red edge, accompanied by itching.

wheelchair—a chair fitted with wheels by which a person can propel oneself.

whorl—a type of fingerprint in which the central papillary ridges turn through at least one complete circle.

withdrawal—a removal of something that has been deposited.

womb—nonmedical name for the uterus.

work-in—to make time or space for.

writer—the person who writes; the author.

xiphoid—a process that forms the tip of the sternum.

x-linked—connected to the cell's sex chromosome; a characteristic of the sex chromosome.

Z-tract—a method of injecting medication intramuscularly.

zygote—a cell produced by the union of an ovum and a sperm.

Index

Page references followed by "*f*" indicate figures, "*t*" indicate tables, and "*b*" indicate boxes

Delmar's Medical Assisting Administrative Skills CD-ROM
and
Delmar's Medical Assisting Clinical Skills CD-ROM

Set-Up Instructions for both CD-ROMs

1. Insert disk into CD-ROM player.
2. From the Start Menu, choose *RUN*.
3. In the *Open* text box, enter **d:setup.exe** then click the *OK* button. (Substitute the letter of your CD-ROM drive for **d:**)
4. Follow the installation prompts from there.

System Requirements
Administrative Skills CD-ROM

166 MHz Intel Pentium processor or greater
Microsoft® Windows® 95, 98, NT4, 2000
32 MB of installed RAM
100 MB of available disk space
256-color monitor capable of 800 X 600 resolution
CD-ROM drive
Microsoft® Windows® compatible sound card

System Requirements
Clinical Skills CD-ROM

100 MHz Intel Pentium
Microsoft® Windows® 95 or later
32 MB or more of RAM
Approx. 8 MB free disk space
SVGA monitor with 24-bit (16 million colors) display
4x or faster CD-ROM drive
Sound card and speakers

License Agreement for Delmar Learning, a division of Thomson Learning